Archives *of* Internal Medicine

VOLUME 128

July through December, 1971

American Medical Association Publication

Archives of Internal Medicine

Internal medicine at large

Experiment in space

Much thought and a number of microorganisms are going into a container which will fly on the next-to-last Apollo moon mission.

The container, smaller (4½ x 4½ x 9¾ inches) than a cigar box, is to be placed aboard Apollo XVI, scheduled for next March.

According to National Aeronautics and Space Administration microbiologist Gerald R. Taylor, PhD, this is essentially "a study to see what the difference is between ultraviolet-mediated changes on the ground and ultraviolet-mediated changes in space."

As a hypothetical example of what some previous space studies have shown, he told an interviewer: "You do a lot of base line work, and you say, 'If we irradiate these organisms under these conditions, 83% of them will die.' Then you fly them, bring them back, and–lo and behold–50% of the organisms still are alive."

Insofar as possible in one experiment, this 1972 study will try to follow leads provided by previous studies to determine what is happening.

"In a nutshell," Dr. Taylor said, "we're using the solar ultraviolet light as a mutagenic force." Then, the rate of ultraviolet-mediated change in flight will be compared with the known rate of ultraviolet-mediated change on the ground. Enough variables will be built into the experiment to try to determine which components of the space flight environment produced the change.

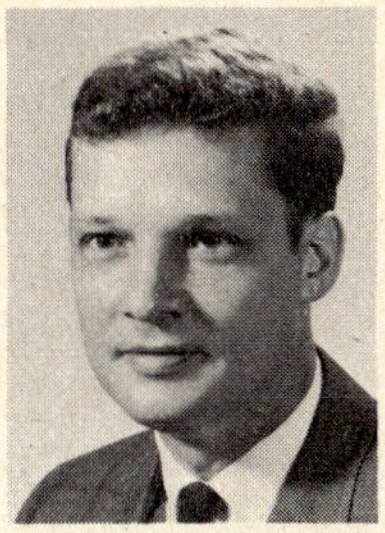

Dr. Taylor

"What we're not doing," Dr. Taylor emphasized, "is sending a bunch of bugs up there, bringing them back, and seeing if the space flight environment caused them to do something they wouldn't otherwise do.

"We're not expecting the green ones to turn brown and the big ones to become little and that sort of thing. What we are doing is sending up organisms that, say, are green, generally with about 5% brown. If we look at them post-flight and 25% are brown, that's something they ordinarily do, but they are doing it differently. There's a big difference in biology between generating a brand new substance and changing the rate at which that substance is formed."

Although this will not primarily be a survival study, Dr. Taylor said, "you can't really do an experiment like this without doing survival studies because you have to count the organisms when they get back. You know how many you sent up, so you automatically have a survival study."

Generally, however, he noted, the scientific community already has tested everything from tobacco mosaic virus to fecal bacteria, and scientists have a pretty good idea which organisms will survive in the space environment.

For the upcoming experiment, NASA scientists are selecting vari-

continued

Highlights This Month

Vaccines for two strains of meningitis have undergone preliminary trials in children . . . page 8

Virus theory of breast cancer is further supported by recent findings . . . page 7

Work continues on eradication of and treatment for tuberculosis . . . page 9

Internists in the news . . . pages 13, 16

Experiment continued

ous wave lengths of ultraviolet light—such as wave lengths known to interfere with nucleic acids or proteins and amino acids, for example—in which they are interested. The experiment will also include "a wave length which really doesn't do anything, a control as it were."

In addition to this type of ultraviolet energy, the experiment will allow control of the amount of energy to which the organisms are exposed. Cultures can be sent up in either fluid or dry condition, with some of the "dry" cultures in a portion of the container vented to the outside to see what happens in vacuum.

Some lunar soil also will be sent back to the moon—as a covering for some organisms. This, Dr. Taylor said, is "so we can get some idea how well lunar material protects the organism from ultraviolet light."

The experiment requires extra-vehicular activity, and will be performed as Apollo XVI returns from the moon. The container will be attached to the end of a television boom which in turn is fastened to the hatch handle on the craft.

Apollo XVI crewmen then will turn their craft toward the sun. (Dr. Taylor considers this extremely important, because shadows across the container could "throw the data all off.") An astronaut will reach up and open the box, exposing the organisms to ultraviolet light for exactly 10 minutes. There are three compartments in the container; one compartment in the back will receive no light as a control.

"After 10 minutes," Dr. Taylor said, "this (container) is closed up, carried back inside the command module, and stored. Nobody looks at it again until they take it out on recovery and send it here (to the Manned Spacecraft Center, Houston)."

Dr. Taylor is assigned to the Preventive Medicine Division of NASA's Houston center.

Space Medicine

As National Aeronautics and Space Administration specialists prepare the Apollo XV mission, and the Mariner races toward Mars, IMBLMS is taking shape at the Manned Spacecraft Center, Houston.

IMBLMS, in the acronym-infested world of space research, stands for Integrated Medical and Behavioral Laboratory Measurement System.

Expected to be ready for flight by

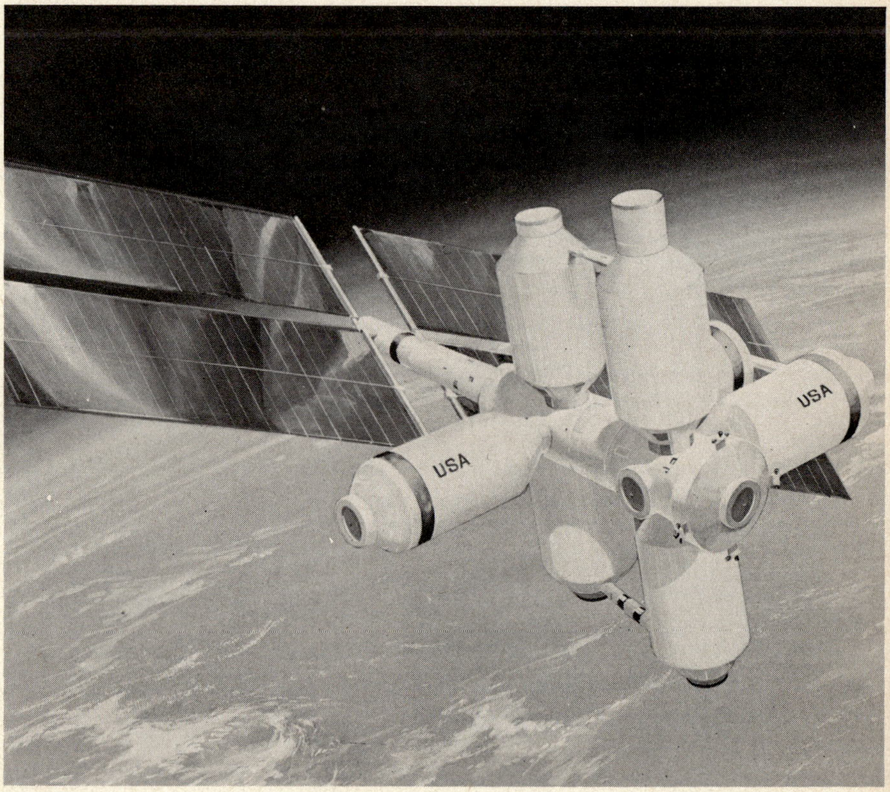

A six-man space station, shown here in an artist's concept, might be transported to orbit by a space shuttle, then assembled in space. Such a station could contain the Integrated Medical and Behavioral Laboratory Measurement System.

early 1973, IMBLMS is being designed for medical research in the first space stations. It will also see use in later earth-orbiting, lunar, and interplanetary missions.

However, long before it flies, the spacegoing laboratory is expected to have implications for earthbound medicine. According to Charles A. Berry, MD, NASA's director of medical research and operations, "IMBLMS is one of our very exciting programs, with great potential for medicine on the ground."

Potential applications of IMBLMS equipment in "earth medicine" which have been suggested by NASA scientists and others include mobile health clinics, diagnostic data banks, extended measurement parameters, and even predictive medicine.

Thus, the United States' space program remains a combination of missions in progress (the unmanned Mariner's flight toward a November orbit around Mars), missions in preparation (the three-man Apollo XV moon flight, scheduled to launch July 26), and missions well in the future (the vehicles for IMBLMS, which will perhaps fly later in the 1970s and 1980s).

Several of these efforts, however, have obvious "spin-off" potential for earth-bound medicine, Dr. Berry emphasized. One reason for the development of IMBLMS is because bioinstrumentation for recording vital functions and medical studies (dependent in part on pre-flight and post-flight tests) cannot answer questions about man's physiological and behavioral status during prolonged space missions.

The system is being designed to evaluate crew responses, perform research, and help in diagnosis and treatment of illness during lengthy space missions.

The measurements' list for the functional "breadboards" includes: Clinical evaluation (history, physical examination), neurological (EEG, electronystagmogram, electromyogram), cardiovascular (ECG, vectorcardiogram, cardiac output, arterial blood pressure, venous pressure, phonocardiogram, vibrocardiogram, heart rate, pulse wave velocity, arterial pulse contour), respiratory (lung volume, timed vital capacity, airway resistance, total airway compliance, distribution of blood flow and gas in lungs, diffusion capacity), metabolism (energy metabolism, balance studies, body mass, total body water, muscle size and strength, core and skin temperature).

Clinical laboratory measurements called for include: Blood count, urinalysis, plasma volume, blood and urine electrolytes, total protein, blood glucose, blood pH-pO_2-pCO_2, reticulocyte count, red blood cell fragility-mass-survival, bleeding and coagulation times, and the Rumpel-Leede test for capillary fragility.

Body and environmental microflora—bacterial, viral, and fungal—can be checked, and other proposed environmental measurements include temperature, pressure, humidity, motion, and atmospheric composition.

Proposed behavioral measurements include time and motion studies, level of consciousness, learned activity, sensory and perceptual evaluation, higher thought processes, memory, vigilance, vision, and audiometry.

After the ground-bound "breadboards" are evaluated, versions of the equipment suitable for flight are to be developed. Computer-based data management is a vital aspect. NASA sums up IMBLMS as "a biomedical support system that integrates medical measurement, clinical support, and data-management capabilities for space application."

Breast cancer virus?

The theory that breast cancer is caused by a virus has received new support with the discovery of two groups of women whose milk contains particles that look identical to a virus that causes breast cancer in mice. The "B-type" particles were found in the milk of American women with a familial history of breast cancer and Parsi women from Bombay, India.

Both these groups have a higher than normal incidence of breast cancer. Among the Parsi, a sect whose members have intermarried for 1,300 years, breast cancer accounts for half of all the cancers in women.

Dan H. Moore, PhD, and co-workers reported recently that the particles were found in the milk of 18 of 46 Parsi women and 12 of 20 American women with familial histories of breast cancer. In contrast, only 5% of

continued

Breast cancer continued

American women without such a family history had such particles in their milk.

The virus-like particles in human milk closely resemble the mouse mammary tumor virus, formerly called the Bittner virus or "milk factor." Both are RNA viruses. Dr. Moore said there was some evidence that incubating the mouse virus with the serum of women with breast cancer makes mice less susceptible to developing cancer from the virus.

A monkey mammary tumor virus has also been isolated; this is also an RNA virus and its developmental stages resembles a B-type particle. Its mature form is that of a C-type particle, however. Both B-type and C-type particles have been found in milk from former breast cancer patients; some of the milk samples in Dr. Moore's series contain C-type particles.

These findings and similar ones by other researchers lead to the question of which animal model—mouse or monkey—furnishes a better system for the study of human breast cancer. Mouse mammary tumor virus injected into a normal mouse will produce tumors, but so far the virus has failed to infect normal cells in tissue culture. On the other hand, according to Harish C. Chopra, PhD, of the National Cancer Institute, monkey mammary tumor virus readily propagates itself in tissue culture and infects normal cells, but so far it has not caused any breast tumors. The incubation period of the virus is not known, however, and tumors may appear eventually.

All the particles and viruses involved contain an enzyme called RNA-dependent DNA polymerase ("reverse transcriptase"). The enzyme is believed to allow an RNA virus to use its single-strand RNA as a template to make a complementary DNA molecule, which can integrate with a cell's own DNA and change it into a cancer cell. The same enzyme has been found in all other tumor-producing RNA viruses, but it has been demonstrated in other viruses which are not known to be oncogenic.

The significance of these findings is not yet clear, but researchers seem to agree that the particles found in the milk of women who are considered susceptible to breast cancer may indeed be a virus, similar to those that cause such tumors in the laboratory.

Electromicrophotographs below show a B-type particle in which the outer membrane has stretched into a tail (left). Right: A fixed particle from a thin preparation.

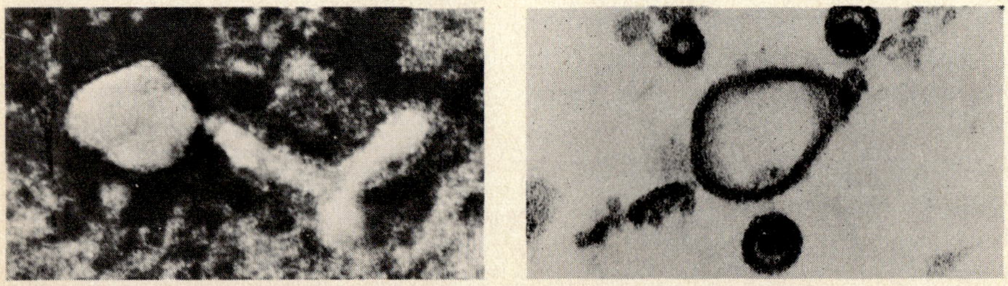

Meningitis vaccine

Vaccines for two strains of meningococcal meningitis have produced no adverse effects in 50 children inoculated in March 1970, and antibody responses have been generally satisfactory in the tested children who are over two years of age.

Martha Lepow, MD, reported on results of the preliminary field trials at the Society for Pediatric Research-American Pediatric Society meeting in Atlantic City, NJ. She said that in 10 of the 50 children there has been little decline in antibody titers, and even though more time is needed to see whether the vaccines will protect the children, previous experience with adults indicates that "there is every reason to believe that a polysaccharide vaccine will be protective."

Dr. Lepow is associate professor of pediatrics, University of Connecticut Medical School.

The C strain vaccine proved to be 95% effective in earlier tests with military recruits. Both the A and C strain vaccines have been found safe to use in adults.

The group of 50 Connecticut children consisted of 26 who had chronic orthopedic or neurologic problems, but were otherwise healthy, and 24 healthy children. Six children in each group received 50μg of vaccine subcutaneously (equal to an adult dose), while the others were given 25μg.

Antibody response was determined on the basis of four serologic tests:

- Indirect immunofluorescence testing showed that all the children produced specific IgG, IgM, and IgA antibodies.
- Bactericidal antibodies were produced in serum from 48 of the 50 children when the serum was tested against either the A or C-strain pathogen. Children under three years of age produced less antibody.
- Hemagglutination tests in which red cells were coated with specific polysaccharide C or A antigens provoked an antibody response in 49 of the 50 children.
- Quantitative immunoprecipitation assays in which the A or C polysaccharide was labelled with tritium showed that 47 of the 50 children produced at least 5μg/ml specific antibody concentrations. The mean response was 25μg/ml.

Although types B and C meningococci are responsible for nearly all the 4,000 cases occurring here yearly, attempts to produce vaccine have been successful only against types A and C. The antigenic potential of polysaccharides is dependent upon their molecular weight. Type A and C vaccines were developed from large, high-molecular weight polymers of sialic acid. Type B meningococcal polysaccharides have been isolated, but these have thus far been too small to be consistently antigenic in humans.

"The emergence of sulfonamide-resistant pathogenic meningococci during the past decade has significantly reduced the usefulness of these drugs in preventing outbreaks of meningococcal disease," Dr. Lepow said. "There is genuine need for other means of prophylaxis.

Dr. Lepow's co-authors were Irving Goldschneider, MD, assistant professor of pathology, University of Connecticut medical and dental school, and Emil C. Gotschlich, MD, associate professor at Rockefeller University, New York. Drs. Goldschneider and Gotschlich worked with Malcolm S. Artenstein, MD, director of the bacteriology department, Walter Reed Army Institute of Research, Washington, DC, in developing the vaccine.

Tuberculosis

"Tuberculosis eradication programs have a way of getting wiped out before the disease," was the wry comment from Vernon N. Houk, MD, deputy chief of the Tuberculosis Branch at the Center for Disease Control in Atlanta.

In an interview, Dr. Houk pointed to epidemiologic studies that showed 37,187 "new active" cases in the United States during 1970. Although this figure represents an all-time low of 18.3 cases per 100,000 people, 5,340 persons died from tuberculosis as recently as 1969. In that same year, the total number of known active cases in this country was 114,620.

To help identify more of these patients, Dr. Houk and Phyllis Q. Edwards, MD, chief of the Tuberculosis Branch would like to enlist the help of community leaders and neighborhood health aides in house-to-house screening. Also needed are conveniently located and efficiently run tuberculosis care facilities and a one-shot tuberculosis test that would eliminate the need for return visits to interpret the results.

Officials at the Federal Tuberculosis Branch also hope to find an agent that will awaken dormant tubercle bacilli and destroy them during this vulnerable stage. This "wake 'em and whack 'em" approach is important, he explained, because the infection may remain dormant for two or even three years. Perhaps eight out of ten "new active" cases reported each year represent breakdowns to overt disease of tuberculosis infection acquired years ago when the disease was more common.

There is also need for a technique that can pick out the vulnerable 10% of infected persons who will experience breakdown into active disease.

Research directed toward development of a vaccine continues. The *Bacillus Calmette-Guerin* vaccine protects only persons who have never been infected, and causes a positive reaction to tuberculin testing in those who have been vaccinated.

Therapy, another important aspect of the tuberculosis eradication program, was the subject under discussion by an ad hoc committee to the Public Health Service.

The committee was specifically

continued

An intestinal autobiography of rage, contentment and horror

"Feeling unfairly taxed by the government (Internal Revenue Service) and not given enough attention by A.U.O. [an experimenter to whom the subject became very attached], he became overtly critical and accusatory. He shouted, raged, and threatened to quit."*

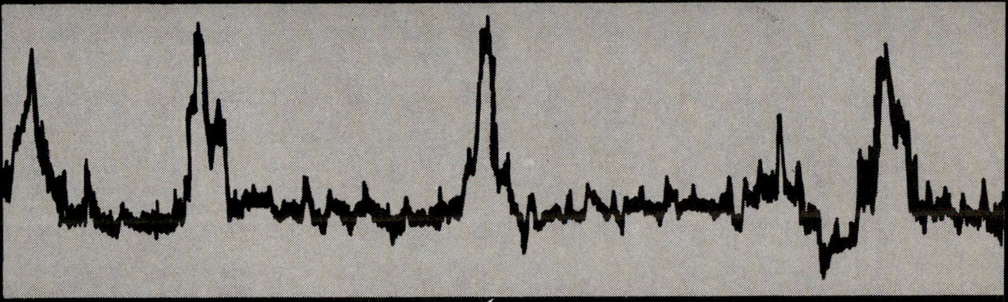

"The motility that day was quiet. This type of recording is seen regularly when he is relaxed and contented and the laboratory seems peaceful."*

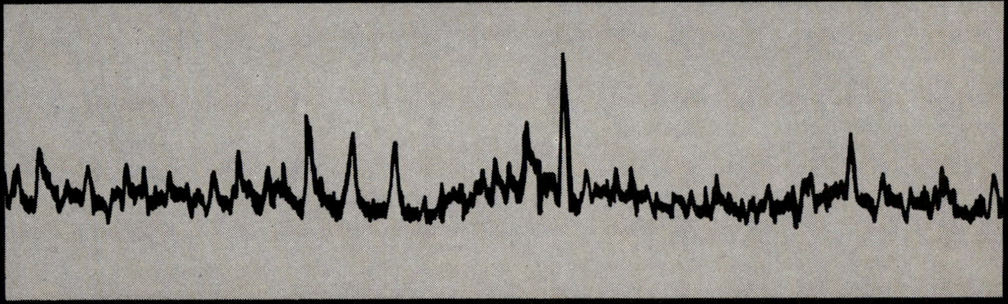

He was overwhelmed by "paralyzing horror" when told he would need a partial laryngectomy for removal of an early carcinoma; "...the activity of the ileum virtually ceased for over a five-minute period...."*

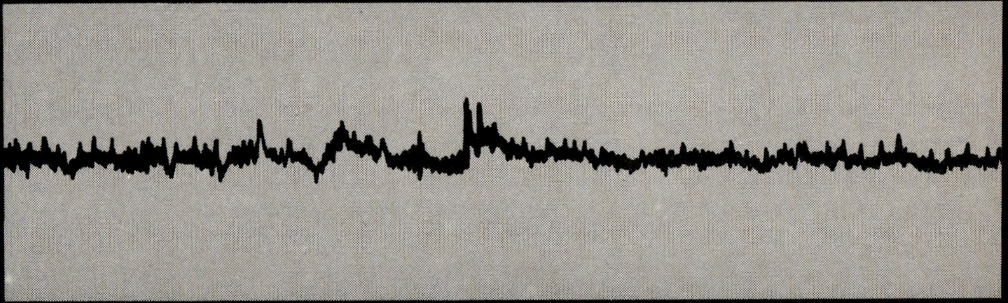

Background

*Data presented here derive from a 13-year ongoing study by Henry Harrison Sadler, M.D., and Aline Underhill Orten, Ph.D., at Wayne State University. Their findings, which demonstrate a correlation between the emotional state of a human subject and the motility of an isolated segment of his ileum, were published in the April, 1968, *American Journal of Psychiatry*, volume 124, page 1375.

The subject is a 56-year-old man with a 40 Thiry loop of ileum created as a result of emergency surgery. A person of modest attainment and simple tastes, the subject depends on the investigators as he might h own family. His full-time job is as a "huma laboratory," and throughout the 13-year pe of the study, he has taken great personal p in his own participation.

A story charged with emotion

The graphs on the facing page are intestinal motility readings on a human subject experiencing the emotions of rage, contentment and horror (see "Background" below left). This "intestinal autobiography" dramatizes the point that certain emotions correlate with specific patterns of G.I. motility.

The visceral clutch and functional G.I. disorders

The gut response to stress has been amply demonstrated in many functional G.I. disorders. Nervous diarrhea and irritable colon syndrome, for example, are disorders associated with abnormal G.I. motility. And these disorders are commonest among patients sensitive to life-stress situations productive of conflict and excessive anxiety.

Librax® calms anxiety, calms the gut

In these areas of G.I. pathology, Librax has become a mainstay of adjunctive therapy. Reason? Effective two-way calming action. Librax, by relieving excessive anxiety, not only helps calm emotional overreaction to stress, it controls intestinal hypermotility, too. Depend on Librax—the only drug that combines the well-known antianxiety action of Librium® (chlordiazepoxide HCl) and the potent, dependable antisecretory/antispasmodic action of Quarzan® (clidinium Br).

1 or 2 capsules, 3 or 4 times daily in the treatment of nervous diarrhea and irritable colon syndrome

Before prescribing, please consult complete product information, a summary of which follows:

Indications: Indicated as adjunctive therapy to control emotional and somatic factors in gastrointestinal disorders.

Contraindications: Patients with glaucoma; prostatic hypertrophy and benign bladder neck obstruction; known hypersensitivity to chlordiazepoxide hydrochloride and/or clidinium bromide.

Warnings: Caution patients about possible combined effects with alcohol and other CNS depressants. As with all CNS-acting drugs, caution patients against hazardous occupations requiring complete mental alertness (*e.g.*, operating machinery, driving). Though physical and psychological dependence have rarely been reported on recommended doses, use caution in administering Librium (chlordiazepoxide hydrochloride) to known addiction-prone individuals or those who might increase dosage; withdrawal symptoms (including convulsions), following discontinuation of the drug and similar to those seen with barbiturates, have been reported. Use of any drug in pregnancy, lactation, or in women of childbearing age requires that its potential benefits be weighed against its possible hazards. As with all anticholinergic drugs, an inhibiting effect on lactation may occur.

Precautions: In elderly and debilitated, limit dosage to smallest effective amount to preclude development of ataxia, oversedation or confusion (not more than two capsules per day initially; increase gradually as needed and tolerated). Though generally not recommended, if combination therapy with other psychotropics seems indicated, carefully consider individual pharmacologic effects, particularly in use of potentiating drugs such as MAO inhibitors and phenothiazines. Observe usual precautions in presence of impaired renal or hepatic function. Paradoxical reactions (*e.g.*, excitement, stimulation and acute rage) have been reported in psychiatric patients. Employ usual precautions in treatment of anxiety states with evidence of impending depression; suicidal tendencies may be present and protective measures necessary. Variable effects on blood coagulation have been reported very rarely in patients receiving the drug and oral anticoagulants; causal relationship has not been established clinically.

Adverse Reactions: No side effects or manifestations not seen with either compound alone have been reported with Librax. When chlordiazepoxide hydrochloride is used alone, drowsiness, ataxia and confusion may occur, especially in the elderly and debilitated. These are reversible in most instances by proper dosage adjustment, but are also occasionally observed at the lower dosage ranges. In a few instances, syncope has been reported. Also encountered are isolated instances of skin eruptions, edema, minor menstrual irregularities, nausea and constipation, extrapyramidal symptoms, increased and decreased libido—all infrequent and generally controlled with dosage reduction; changes in EEG patterns (low-voltage fast activity) may appear during and after treatment; blood dyscrasias (including agranulocytosis), jaundice and hepatic dysfunction have been reported occasionally with chlordiazepoxide hydrochloride, making periodic blood counts and liver function tests advisable during protracted therapy. Adverse effects reported with Librax are typical of anticholinergic agents, *i.e.*, dryness of mouth, blurring of vision, urinary hesitancy and constipation. Constipation has occurred most often when Librax therapy is combined with other spasmolytics and/or low residue diets.

In functional G.I. disorders, adjunctive Librax®

Each capsule contains 5 mg chlordiazepoxide HCl and 2.5 mg clidinium Br.

calms anxiety, calms the G.I. tract

ROCHE

Roche Laboratories
Division of Hoffmann-La Roche Inc.
Nutley, N.J. 07110

Internal medicine at large

TB continued

concerned with reports of liver disease associated with administration of isoniazid, one of the major drugs used to treat tuberculosis.

However, members of the committee concluded that there should be no changes in the present program of preventive treatment with isoniazid, or in the guidelines for selection of patients for therapy. They said screening should emphasize exclusion of patients who have had an adequate course of isoniazid and those who have reacted adversely. Patients who have had other long-term medication or a history of current liver disease should be considered individually.

Angiography

What is the significance of angiography in operative evaluation of chest disease, diagnosing pelvic masses, or managing esophageal varices?

Three investigators offered their views on these applications of the procedure at the American College of Angiology meeting in New Orleans:

Operative evaluation in chest disease—Neopito Robles, MD, former chief of vascular surgery at Veterans Administration Hospital in Tucson, said that newer, safer dyes, and more thorough instruction in angiographic techniques in medical schools mean there is no reason to avoid the procedure.

Intravenous angiography, he said, can prevent needless surgery by revealing tumors that are too extensive for resection. The procedure also helps to identify patients whose symptoms could be relieved by surgery, snd it allows study of changes in hemodynamic function as reflected in uptake of contrast medium.

Pelvic mass diagnosis—Reed Altemus, MD, University of Pittsburgh clinical assistant professor of radiology, listed several indications for pelvic angiography: obesity that prevents palpation of a mass, palpable asymptomatic uterine tumors in young women, all trophoblastic tumors, suspected nonacute ectopic pregnancy or missed abortion, amenorrhea lasting for over three months without uterine enlargement, and questionable diagnosis of salpingitis.

Managing esophageal varices—Andrew B. Crummy, MD, University of Wisconsin Medical School professor of radiology, said that angiography makes it possible to locate the source of gastroesophageal bleeding, infuse the patient with vasopressin, then evaluate the effect of the procedure. This type of management should be most valuable for patients with arterial bleeding, he said, because they do not necessarily follow the "inexorable course" seen in most variceal bleeders.

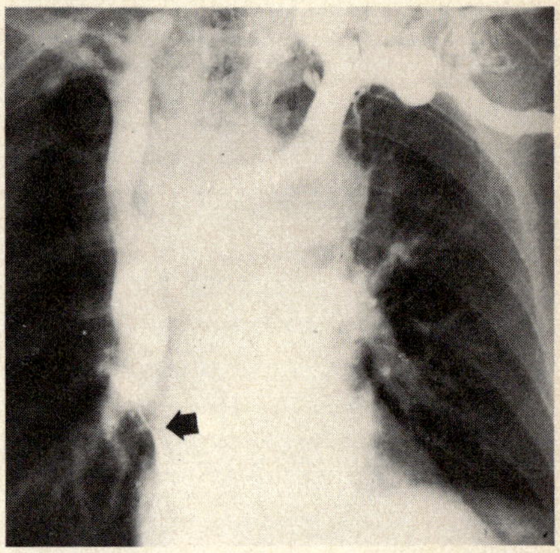

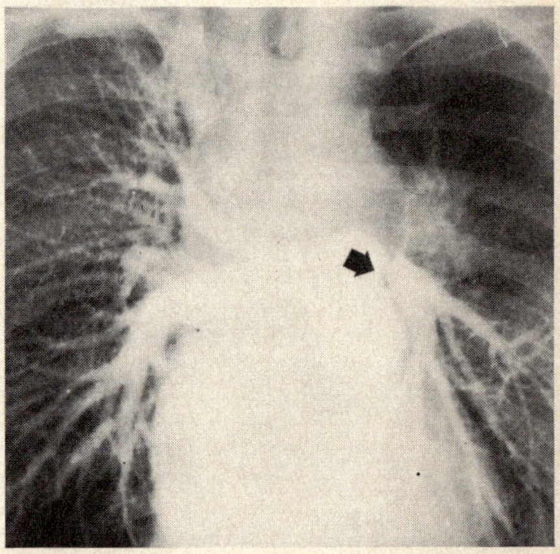

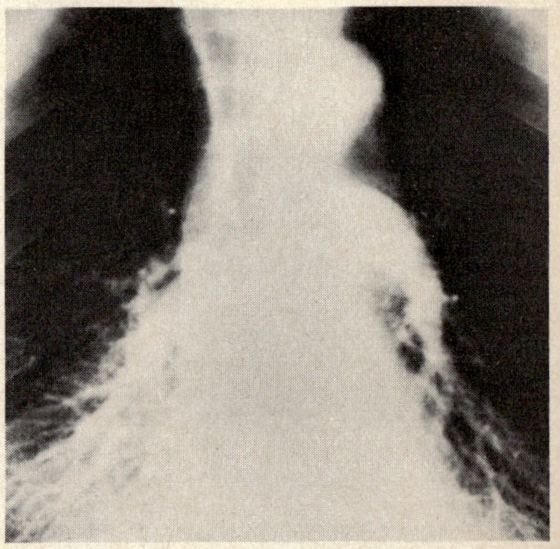

Top photograph shows pulmonary angiogram of unresectable solid tumor in patient's mediastinum. Angiogram of another patient in center photograph shows obstruction of left pulmonary artery—an indication that the tumor had invaded the artery, thus blocking circulation to the lung. The bottom photograph is an angiogram showing absence of perfusion in the upper portion of the lungs. A cyst, crowding the vasculature into the lower lobes, prevented exchange of gas.

Myron P. Walzak MD, has been appointed to head the newly created Department of Urology at Creighton University School of Medicine, Omaha. Previously he was assistant and associate professor in the Department of Urology at the University of Virginia Hospital.

The new president-elect of the American Thoracic Society is **Alan K. Pierce,** MD, professor of medicine at the University of Texas Southwestern Medical School at Dallas.

Morris E. Chafetz, MD, acting director of the Division of Alcohol Abuse and Alcoholism in the National Institute of Mental Health, will retain that position in its successor agency, the National Institute of Alcohol Abuse and Alcoholism.

George F. Stevenson, MD, has been appointed executive vice-president and the first full-time Commissioner of Continuing Education of the American Society of Clinical Pathologists. Dr. Stevenson is professor of clinical pathology and dean of the School of Allied Health Sciences at the Medical University of South Carolina and has served as commissioner on a part-time since 1967.

George F. Wilkins, MD, has received this year's **Knudsen Award** of the Industrial Medical Association. Dr. Wilkins is medical director of New England Telephone Co, Boston, and associate clinical professor of occupational medicine at Harvard Medical School.

The first president of the recently-formed Society of Critical Care Medicine is **Max Harry Weil,** MD, PhD, associate professor of medicine at University of Southern California School of Medicine and director of the Center for the Critically Ill of Hollywood Presbyterian Hospital. **David Allan,** MD, professor of anesthesia at Northwestern University Medical School, was elected secretary-treasurer of the group which accepts as members physicians, scientists, engineers, nurses and other allied health professionals who spend much of their time caring for patients with acute life-threatening illnesses and injuries.

Joseph Kirsner, MD, the Louis Block Professor of Medicine, has been appointed deputy dean of Medical Affairs and chief of staff of the division at the University of Chicago Pritzker School of Medicine and Division of the Biological Sciences. **Irwin H. Rosenberg,** MD, associate professor or medicine, succeeds Dr. Kirsner as chief of the gastroenterology section at the university.

The American Urological Association has presented its annual **Hugh Hampton Young Award** for contributions to treatment of urinary infections to **Grayson Carroll,** MD, clinical professor emeritus of medicine at St. Louis University. Dr. Carroll is a member of the editorial board of the *International Journal or Urology and Nephrology* and formerly served on the editorial board of the *Journal of Urology.*

Ronald G. Evens, MD, will become professor and head of the Department of Radiology at Washington University School of Medicine August 1. He will also become director of the Edward Mallinckrodt Institute of Radiology.

Samuel Hellman, MD, has been named to the Alvan T. and Viola D. Fuller-American Cancer Society Professorship at Harvard. He is also director of the Harvard Joint Center for Radiation Therapy and serves on the editorial board of the journal, *Blood.*

Stephen H. Richardson, PhD, has been promoted to professor of microbiology at the Bowman Gray School of Medicine of Wake Forest University.

McGill University has awarded the degree of professor emeritus of investigative medicine to **J.S.L. Browne,** MD, PhD, former chairman of the Department of Investigative Medicine. Dr. Browne joined the McGill faculty in 1933, and is a former president of the Endocrine Society and the American Society of Clinical Investigation.

Edward C. Lynch, MD, formerly associate professor of medicine at Baylor College of Medicine, has been appointed associate dean of the medical school. His duties include recruiting applicants, counseling students regarding health career opportunities, and implementing Baylor's new curriculum.

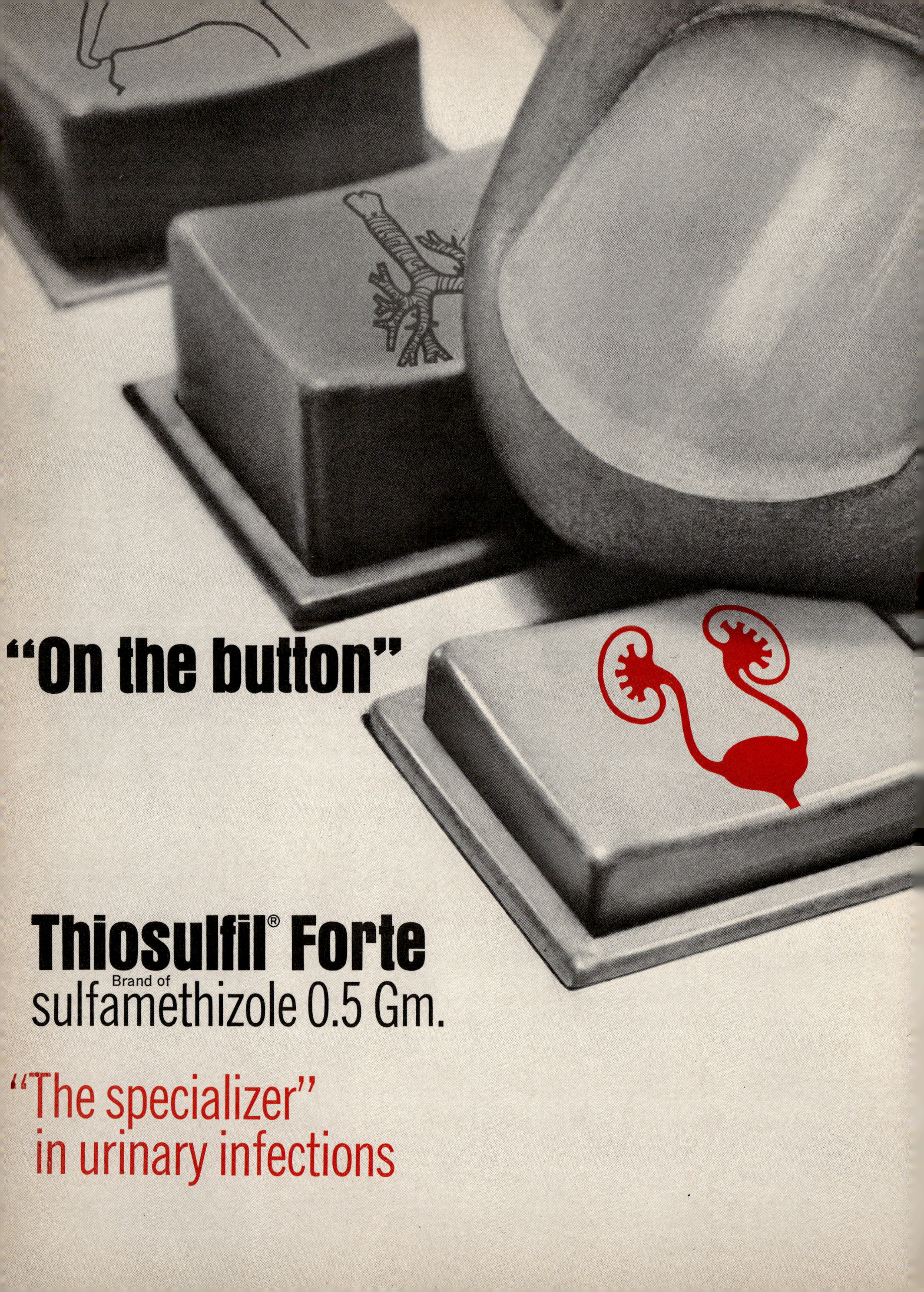
"On the button"
Thiosulfil® Forte
Brand of
sulfamethizole 0.5 Gm.
"The specializer"
in urinary infections

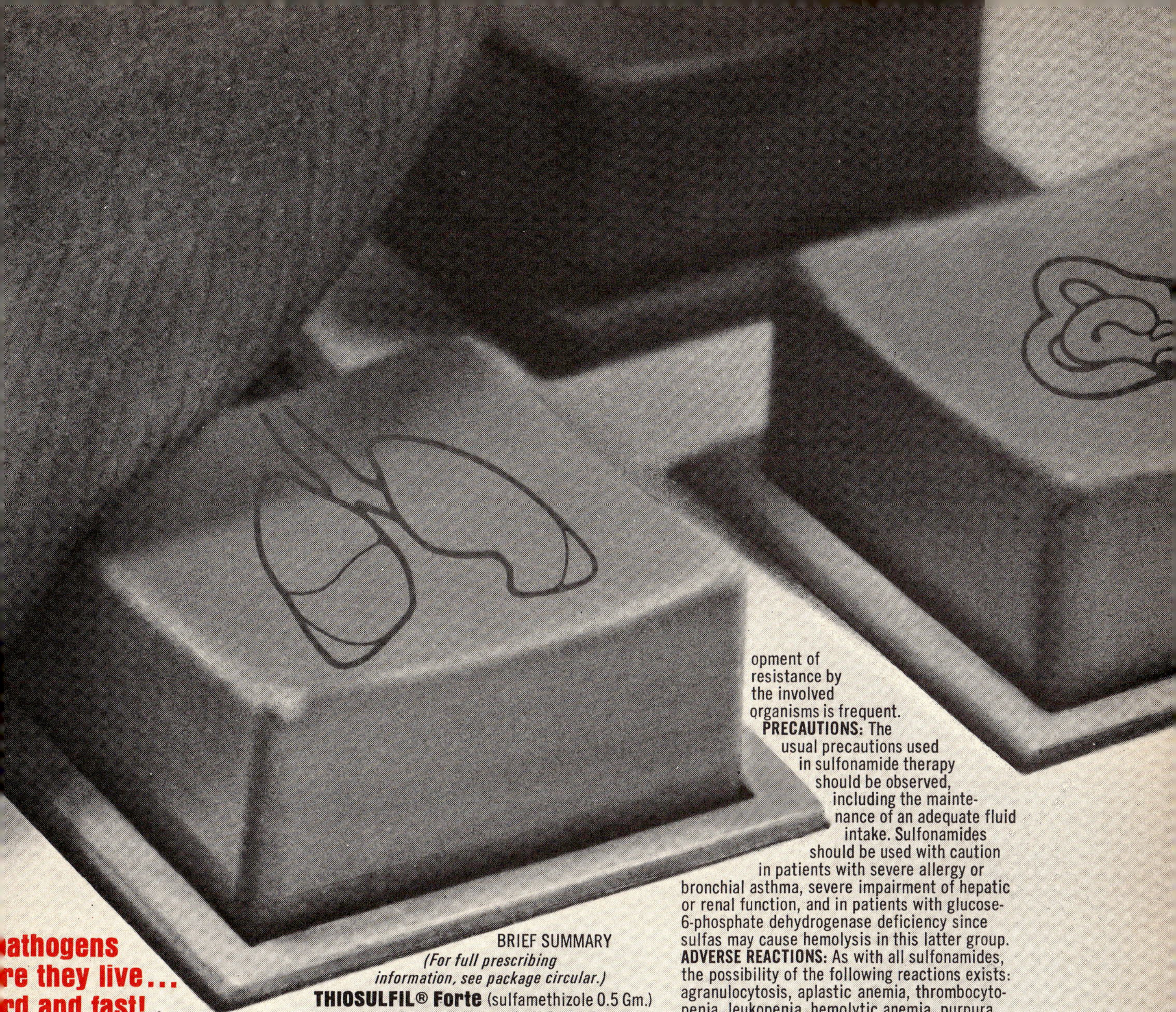

Internal Medicine at large

Paul A. Marks, MD, dean of the Faculty of Medicine and vice president in charge of medical affairs at Columbia University, has been elected president of the American Society for Clinical Investigation. Dr. Marks has been editor-in-chief of the *Journal of Clinical Investigation* since 1967.

David G. Nathan, MD, has been promoted to associate professor of pediatrics at the Harvard Medical School.

Eli M. Nadel, MD, professor of pathology and associate dean at St. Louis University School of Medicine, now holds a secondary appointment as professor of community medicine.

Postgraduate Course on Chronic Inflammatory Disease of the Gut. A postgraduate course on chronic inflammatory disease of the gut, sponsored by the American Gastroenterological Association, will be given July 29 through 31, 1971, at Aspen, Colo. The course chairman is Marvin H. Sleisenger, MD, University of California School of Medicine. Associate chairmen are Fred Kern, Jr., MD, University of Colorado School of Medicine, and Jerry S. Trier, MD, Boston University School of Medicine.

For information write Mrs. Bernie C. Kern, 740 Krameria St, Denver 80220.

Col **Robert W. Morrissey,** USAF, MC, has been appointed director of the Armed Forces Institute of Pathology in Washington, DC, and will assume command on August 1. He has been deputy director since August 1969.

Thomas D. Kinney, MD, has succeeded **Peter C. Nowell,** MD, as president of the American Society for Experimental Pathology. Dr. Kinney is chairman of the Department of Pathology and director of medical and allied health education at Duke University Medical Center as well as editor of the *American Journal of Pathology.* He is a past editor of *Laboratory Investigation.*

Richard D. Amelar, MD, director of the male infertility clinic at Bellevue Hospital Center, has been promoted to clinical professor of urology at the New York University School of Medicine.

John A. Shively, MD, professor of pathology at the University of Missouri School of Medicine, has been appointed professor and chairman of the Department of Pathology at the University of Tennessee Medical Units. The Tennessee position has been vacant since **Douglas Sprunt,** MD, retired in 1968. **Cyrus C. Erickson,** MD, who held the position on an interim basis, will return to full-time teaching and research as professor of pathology. Dr. Shively is immediate past president of the American Association of Blood Banks.

J. Thomas Grayston, MD, is succeeding **John R. Hogness,** MD, as head of the University of Washington Health Sciences Center, Seattle, and the university's vice president for health affairs. Dr. Grayston had been dean of the School of Public Health and Community Medicine at the university since the school's formation a year ago. **Donovan J. Thompson,** PhD, professor of biostatistics, was named acting dean of the school.

Neal S. Bricker, MD, has been named president-elect of the American Society of Clinical Investigation. Dr. Bricker is professor of medicine and director of the Division of Nephrology at Washington University School of Medicine, St. Louis.

The recipient of the 1971 **Hofheimer Prize for Research** of the American Psychiatric Association is **Joseph J. Schildkraut,** MD, associate professor of psychiatry at the Massachusetts Mental Health Center and Harvard Medical School. Dr. Schildkraut received the award for his studies of the biochemical changes that accompany manic and depressive disorders.

Paul Wozencraft, MD, professor of pathology at the University of Cincinnati College of Medicine, was named acting director of the Department of Pathology. He succeeded **Edward A. Gall,** MD, who has been named vice president of the university and director of the University of Cincinnati Medical Center.

Volume 128, Number 1, July 1971

Archives of Internal Medicine

Original Articles

Ophthalmologic Manifestations of Sickle Cell Thalassemia

Morton F. Goldberg, MD, Chicago;
Samuel Charache, MD, Baltimore; and
Ireneo Acacio, MD, Chicago

Vascular abnormalities were studied in the eyes of 14 patients with sickle cell thalassemia (S-thal). Angioid streaks were observed for the first time in a patient with S-thal. "Black sunbursts," which are seen more often in the fundi of patients with sickle cell anemia (SS disease) than in those with sickle cell hemoglobin C disease (Hb SC) were generally few in number in the fundi of patients with S-thal. Proliferative sickle retinopathy, which is much more characteristic of Hb SC than of SS disease, was seen in nine patients with S-thal. The retinas of S-thal thus resemble those of Hb SC more than SS. The hemoglobin composition of a patient's red blood cells can be predicted, to a degree, from the presence and type of certain retinal anomalies in sickling disorders. Overall clinical status is not usually as good as indicator of hemoglobin composition.

A variety of ocular abnormalities has been reported in sickling disorders. The "conjunctival sign" of sickle cell disease, for example (vascular segmentation which can be observed with the +40 diopter lens of a hand ophthalmoscope or with a slit lamp), was shown to occur in patients with several types of sickling.[1-5] It was suggested that this sign was more evident in those individuals with sickle cell hemoglobin C disease (Hb SC) and sickle thalassemia (S-thal) who had the most se-

Received for publication Dec 1, 1970; accepted Feb 2, 1971.

From the Department of Ophthalmology, University of Illinois Eye and Ear Infirmary, Chicago (Drs. Goldberg and Acacio), and the Department of Medicine, Johns Hopkins University and Hospital, Baltimore (Dr. Charache).

Reprint requests to 1855 W Taylor St, Chicago 60612 (Dr. Goldberg).

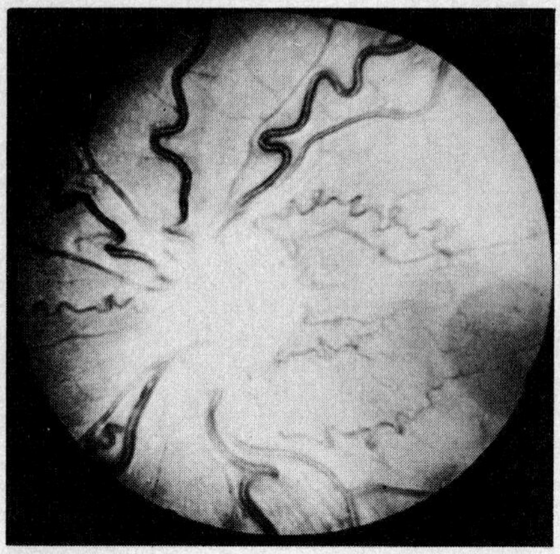

Fig 1.—Tortuosity of the retinal arterioles and venules is demonstrated in Negro woman with sickle-thalassemia (patient 5). Vision is not affected.

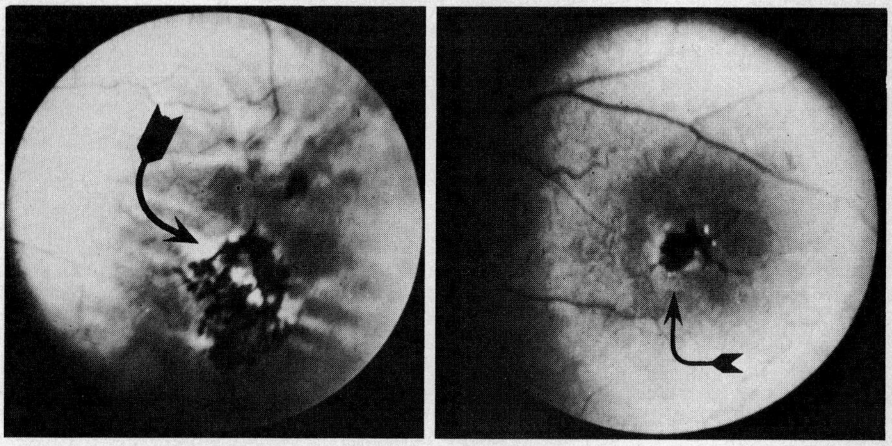

*Fig 2.—*Left and Right, *Black sunbursts[6] (black chorioretinal lesions) are seen (arrow) in the fundi of a male patient with sickle thalassemia (patient 9). They are also characteristic of sickle cell anemia.*

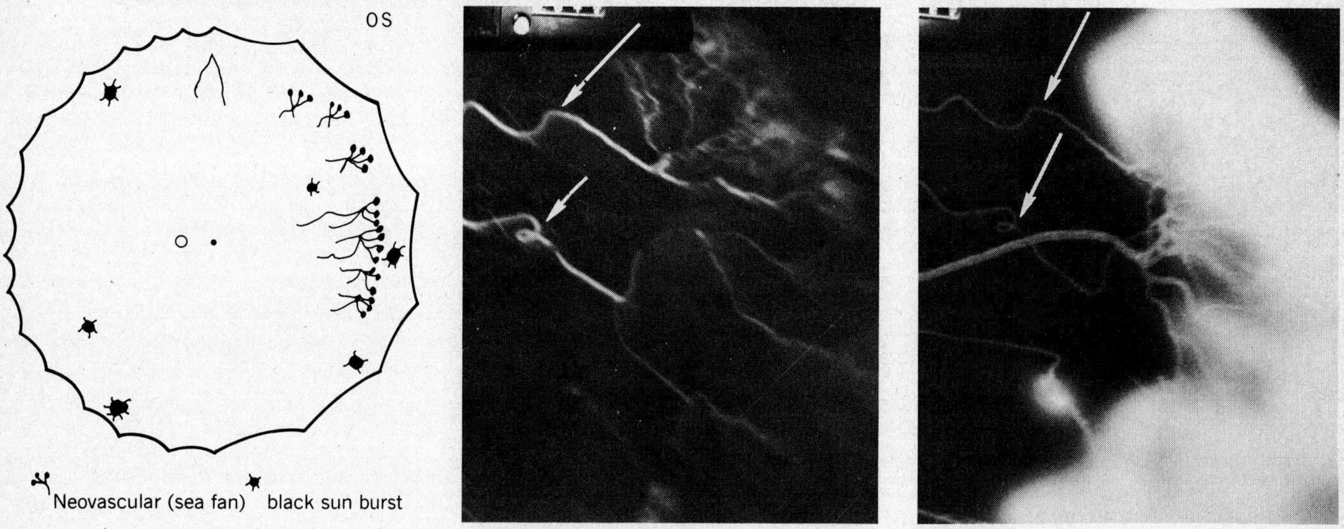

*Fig 3.—*Left, *Left fundus (patient 11). Optic disk and macula are in the center. Scalloped border represents ora serrata. Multiple neovascular proliferations (sea fans)[6] are seen in temporal periphery, photographs of which are seen in center and at right.* Center, *Arterial phase of fluorescein angiogram. Early perfusion of sea fans (patient 11). Venous return of fluorescein has not yet occurred.* Arrows *indicate vessels seen in arteriovenous phase (compare right).* Right, *Later arteriovenous phase of fluorescein angiogram. Large white areas represent fluorescein leaking from neovascular tissue into vitreous.* Arrows *are placed similarly in Fig 3, center.*

vere systemic manifestations.[1]

Tortuosity of the retinal vessels was also noted in early descriptions of the sickling disorders[6] (Fig 1) but is nonspecific, and is of little diagnostic or clinical significance. More impressive and significant abnormalities can be visualized through dilated pupils by direct and indirect ophthalmoscopy, but these have been infrequently noted by internists. Characteristic of sickle cell anemia (SS) are circular, black chorioretinal scars, so-called "black sunbursts"[6] (Fig 2). These lesions, which may represent the sequelae of small infarctions or hemorrhages, were found in 43% of patients with SS, but in only 18% of patients with Hb SC. Their presence does not ordinarily affect visual acuity.

Most significant is proliferative retinopathy (Fig 3), which may be responsible for vitreous hemorrhage,[7] retinal detachment,[8] and loss of vision. These neovascular lesions can be prophylactically obliterated by photocoagulation[9] (Fig 4). Recent evidence[10,11] suggests that the initial event in the development of proliferative sickle retinopathy is a peripheral arteriolar (and probably capillary) occlusion (Fig 5). Rather than producing a scar, this ultimately develops into a tuft of proliferating vessels, the "sea fan"[6] (Fig 3). These neovascular abnormalities are commonly observed in the superotemporal quadrant of the retina, approximately midway between the optic nerve and the anterior pole of the eye. They were found in 60% to 70% of patients with Hb SC disease, but in less than 10% of patients with sickle cell anemia.[6] By use of fluorescein angiography, it is usually possible to visualize leakage of dye from these lesions into the vitreous[6,9-12] (Fig 3 and 4). None of these retinal lesions has been observed with an appreciable incidence in patients with sickle cell trait (AS).[6] In patients with S-thal, previous reports indicated similarly that there were either no abnormal retinal findings or retinal vascular tortuosity only.[13,14]

The hemoglobin components of patients with S-thal do not differ qualitatively from those of patients with sickle cell trait. Because of the inherited defect in synthesis of normal hemoglobin A, however, S-thal red blood cells contain 60% to 95% hemoglobin S, rather than the 35% found in individuals with AS.[14-16] Although systemic manifestations of S-thal are extremely variable, severity of these manifestations can some-

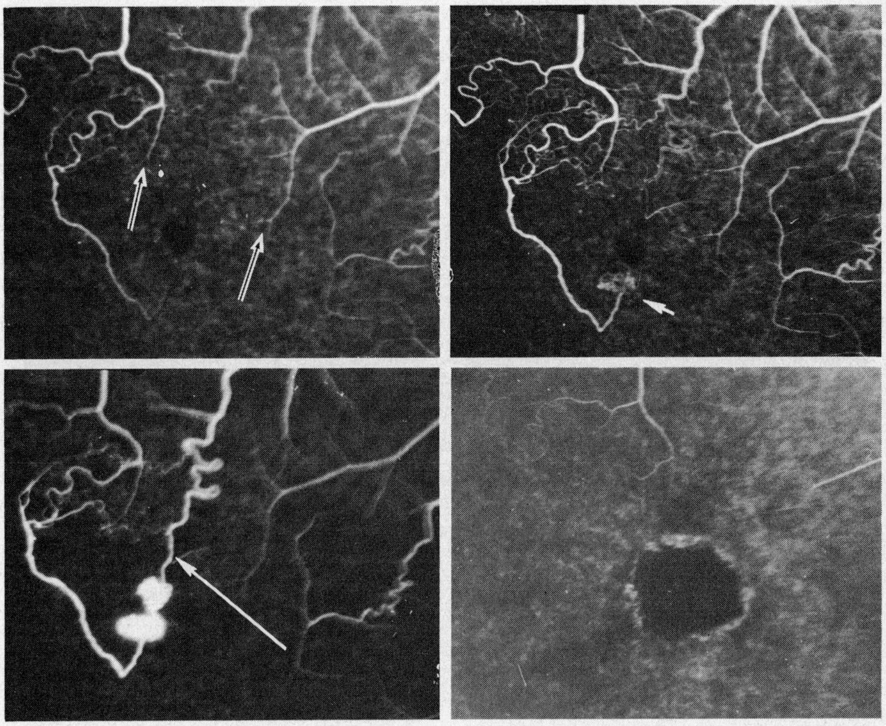

Fig 4.—Top left, *Arterial phase of fluorescein angiogram of (patient 7) a Negro man with sickle thalassemia. Peripheral retina (lower left corner) is not perfused, due to capillary and arteriolar obstruction* (arrows). Top right, *Two seconds later, angiogram reveals small neovascular patch* (arrow). Bottom left, *Five seconds after photograph was taken in Fig 4, top right, angiogram reveals extent of neovascular tissue. Fluorescein is beginning to leak into the vitreous. Venous drainage of sea fan is now seen* (arrow). Bottom right, *Several weeks following prophylactic photocoagulation of sea fan seen in Fig 4, bottom left, only an atrophic chorioretinal scar is observed in fluorescein angiogram. Neovascular tissue has been obliterated, and there is no leakage of fluorescein.*

Table 1.—Systemic and Hematologic Findings in Patients With S-thal

Patient	Age-Sex (At First Exam)	Systemic Status	Hct (%)	Hgb A_2 (%)	Hgb A (%)	Hgb F (%)	Hgb S (%)	Reticulocytes (%)
1	8 M	Very mild	44	31.1	...	2.4	66.5	4.7
2	10 F	Moderate	28	16	3.73	3.7	76.6	3.1
3	18 M	Mild	20-33	0	...	5-14	83-92	5
4	20 M	Mild	34	19.5	...	3.1	77.4	3.7
5	22 F	Very mild	33	15.3	...	9.1	75.6	3.3
6	24 F	Very mild	41	39.1	...	0.8	60.1	2.3
7	27 M	Moderate	30-35	S>A	...	3	S>A	8
8	29 F	Moderate	38	35.1	...	3.3	61.6	2.4
9	36 M	Mild	33-40	S>A	...	...	S>A	1
10	37 M	Moderate	...	10	5	5	80	...
11	41 F	Mild	43.9	27.7	...	2.3	66.4	3.1
12	42 M	Moderate	...	22.4	1.2	...	74.6	...
13	52 M	Moderate	25-40	20-25	...	2.5	66	4
14	64 M	Moderate	37-43	22	3.2	5.2	69	2.1

Table 2.—Ophthalmologic Findings in Patients With S-thal

Eye	Vision (at First Exam) R	Vision (at First Exam) L	Conjunctiva* R	Conjunctiva* L	Refractile Retinal Deposits R	Refractile Retinal Deposits L	Black Sunbursts R	Black Sunbursts L	Retinal Vascular Tortuosity R	Retinal Vascular Tortuosity L	Angioid Streaks R	Angioid Streaks L	PSR† Stage I (Peripheral Arteriolar Occlusions) R	PSR† Stage I (Peripheral Arteriolar Occlusions) L	PSR Stage II (Peripheral Arteriolar-Venular Anastomoses) R	PSR Stage II (Peripheral Arteriolar-Venular Anastomoses) L	PSR Stage III (Neovascularization) R	PSR Stage III (Neovascularization) L	PSR Stage IV (Vitreous Hemorrhage) R	PSR Stage IV (Vitreous Hemorrhage) L	PSR Stage V (Retinal Detachment) R	PSR Stage V (Retinal Detachment) L	Negative Fundi R	Negative Fundi L
1	20/25	20/25	+	+	+	0	0	1	0	0	0	0	0	0	0	0	0	0	0	0	0	0	0	0
2	20/20	20/20	+	+	+	+	1	2	0	0	0	0	0	1	0	1	0	1	0	0	0	0	0	0
3	20/30	20/20	+	+	+	+	4	10	+	+	0	0	2	3	1	0	0	0	0	0	0	0	0	0
4	20/20	20/20	2+	2+	+	0	0	0	0	0	0	0	0	0	0	0	0	0	0	0	0	0	0	+
5	20/30	20/30	+	+	0	0	1	0	+	+	0	0	0	0	0	0	0	0	0	0	0	0	0	0
6	20/20	20/20	—	—	0	0	2	0	0	0	0	0	0	0	0	0	0	0	0	0	0	0	0	+
7	20/20	20/30	?	?	0	0	2	1	0	0	0	0	3	2	3	2	1	1	0	2	0	0	0	0
8	20/20	20/25	0	0	0	+	0	3	0	0	0	0	1	2	0	0	0	0	0	0	0	0	0	0
9	20/20	20/20	0	0	+	+	multiple OU§		0	0	0	0	0	0	0	0	0	0	0	0	0	0	0	0
10	20/20	20/20	+	+	0	0	5	6	0	0	0	0	1	1	1	1	1	1	0	0	0	0	0	0
11	20/50	20/50	4+	4+	+	0	4	6	0	0	0	0	1	3	1	3	1	3	0	0	0	0	0	0
12	NLP‡	20/20	+	+	—	+	—	2	—	0	—	+	—	2	—	2	—	2	4	0	—	0	0	0
13	20/20	20/20	0	0	0	0	1	2	0	0	0	0	2	0‖	2	0‖	2	0‖	1	0	0	0	0	0
14	20/20	20/20	0	0	0	0	2	0	0	0	0	0	1	0	0	0	0	0	0	0	0	0	0	+

* Vascular segmentation in bulbar conjunctiva.

† PSR = proliferative sickle retinopathy. Roman numerals refer to stages in classification; Arabic numerals refer to substages in classification: 0 = none: 1 = ≤30° of circumferential fundus involvement and ≤ three occluded arterioles (or ≤ three anastomoses or neovascularizations); 2 = 31° to 60° of circumferential fundus involvement or four to six occluded arterioles (or four to six anastomoses or neovascularizations); 3 = 61° to 90° of circumferential fundus involvement or seven to nine occluded arterioles (or seven to nine anastomoses or neovascularizations); 4 = ≥ 91° of circumferential funds involvement or ≥ ten occluded arterioles (or ≥ ten anastomoses or neovasculariations).

‡ NLP = No light perception. Massive vitreous hemorrhage obscured details of the right fundus of this patient.

§ OU = each or both eyes.

‖ Nine months later: I = 1 II = 1, III = 1, IV = 0, V = 0.

Fig 5.—Fluorescein angiogram in retinal periphery of Negro man with sickle thalassemia (patient 13). Multiple spontaneous arteriolar obstructions are present (arrows). *Extreme retinal periphery (at left) is completely nonperfused.*

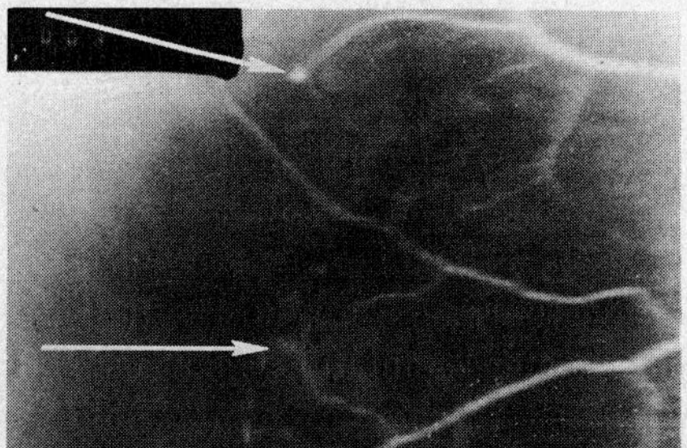

times be related to the proportion of hemoglobin S in patients' red blood cells. It was, therefore, of interest to examine the eyes of 14 patients with S-thal, and attempt to relate their ophthalmologic findings to both clinical status and to hematologic findings.

Materials and Methods

All 14 patients were Negroes who were referred from the hematology clinics of the Johns Hopkins Hospital, Baltimore, the West Side Veteran's Administration Hospital, Chicago, and the University of Illinois Hospital, Chicago.

The diagnosis of sickle thalassemia was established by quantification of the proportions of hemoglobin S in patients' hemolysates by elution after starch block or cellulose acetate electrophoresis (S. Charache, M. Bartalos, and V. Schneider, unpublished data). If it can be determined that the patient has not had a transfusion, a hemolysate containing 60% to 95% hemoglobin S, a small amount of hemoglobin F, and the remainder hemoglobin A is diagnostic of S-thal. Family studies are required to establish a diagnosis in patients with higher proportions of hemoglobin S. One parent must have sickle cell trait, and the other beta-thalassemia trait. The latter diagnosis is established by demonstration of an increased proportion of hemoglobin A_2 (> 3.5%). Such family studies were carried out in patients 1, 3, 5, 6, 8, and 13 (Tables 1 and 2).

All patients' conjunctivas were examined with a slit lamp in order to determine the presence or absence of the characteristic vascular segmentation of sickling disease.[1-5] Each retina was evaluated through dilated pupils by indirect ophthalmoscopy and scleral indentation. Large (8 × 12 in) fundus drawings were made. Fluorescein angiography was performed according to techniques published elsewhere.[6,12,17] Black sunbursts were counted. Each retina was graded according to a recently described classification[10,11] of proliferative sickle retinopathy (PSR) (Table 2).

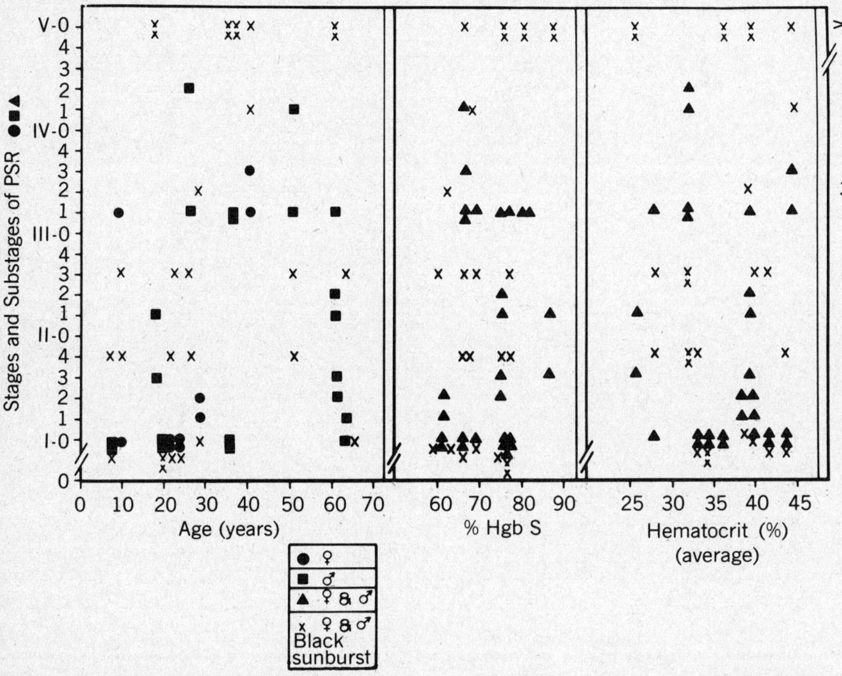

Fig 6.—Stages and substages of proliferative sickle retinopathy and number of black sunbursts are plotted on vertical axes. A precise relationship between these factors and patient age, percent of hemoglobin S, and hematocrit value is not apparent.

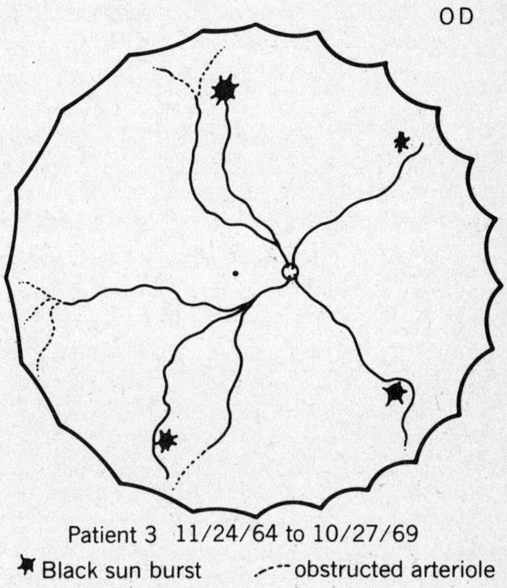

Fig 7.—Right fundus of a Negro man with sickle thalassemia (patient 3). Multiple black sunbursts and occluded arterioles. There was no change in the fundus appearance from Nov 24, 1964, to Oct 27, 1969.

Results

A summary of findings is presented in Table 1 and Fig 6. Vascular segmentation in the conjunctiva was seen in eight of the 14 patients. These lesions were qualitatively similar to those described by Paton and others[1-5] in homozygous sickle cell anemia and in Hb SC disease, in that they were isolated comma and curlicue-shaped segments of small-caliber vessels. Granular flow, sludging, and erythrocytic clumping are *not* diagnostic of sickling disorders, and were *not* observed. In S-thal, the isolated vascular segments were much fewer and far less noticeable than in SS disease.

Fundus abnormalities similar to those described in SC and in SS diseases were observed in all but three of the 28 eyes studied. Refractile deposits in the retina,[6,18] which may or may not be true lipid, were noted in 11 eyes. Black sunbursts were present in 20 eyes (Fig 7), and were numerous in eight of the eyes. Retinal vascular tortuosity was present in only two patients and was pronounced in only one. Angioid streaks were observed in one patient (Fig 8).

Proliferative retinopathy was graded according to the classification in Table 2. Fourteen of the eyes had at least the earliest signs of proliferative retinopathy (peripheral arteriolar obstruction, stage I). Many of the remaining retinas showed evidence of arteriolar-venular anastomoses (stage II) and neovascular and fibrous proliferations (stage III). The sea fan neovascularization was present in nine of the retinas (Fig 9). Spontaneous vitreous hemorrhage (from the neovascular proliferations) had occurred unilaterally in three patients (stage IV) (Fig 10). In one of these, the hemorrhage was massive. Retinal detachment (stage V) was not observed in this series.

There appeared to be no precise relationship between either extent of PSR or number of black sunbursts and patient age, percent of hemoglobin S, and hematocrit value (Fig 6). However, black sunbursts were especially numerous in patient 3, whose red blood cells contained the highest percentage of hemoglobin S in this series (Table 1).

Comment

Significant ocular abnormalities in thalassemia were first reported by Rudd et al in 1953.[19] They observed areas of hemorrhage and retinal detachment in a 22-year-old Negro man, who was initially considered an example of thalassemia minor. Subsequent evaluation, however, revealed latent sickling, and the cor-

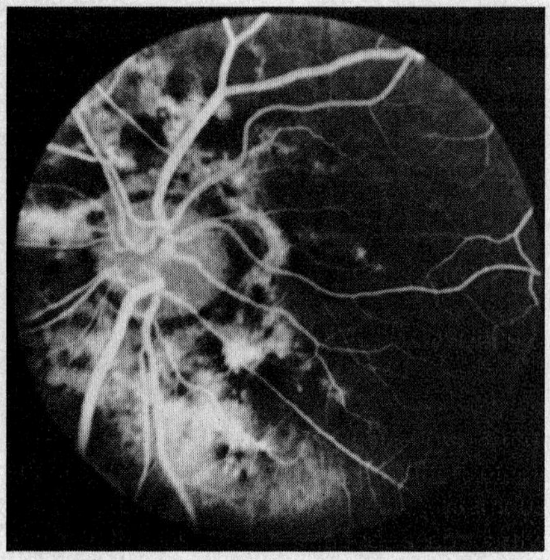

Fig 8.—Fluorescein angiogram of a Negro man with S-thal (patient 12). Irregular white areas represent angioid streaks. Optic disk and retinal vessels appear normal.

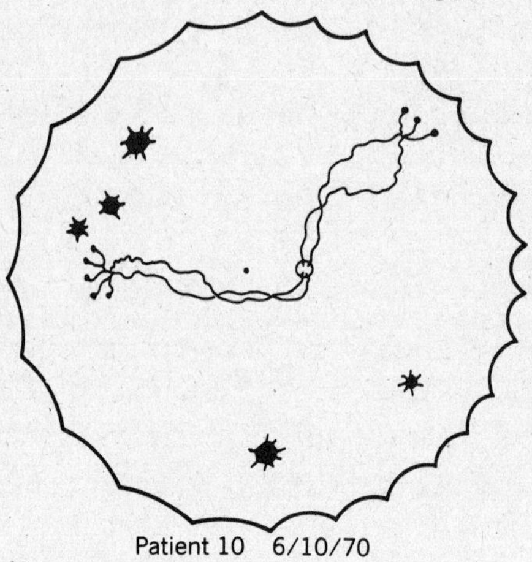

Fig 9.—Right fundus of a Negro man with sickle thalassemia (patient 10). Two sea fans and five black sunbursts are seen.

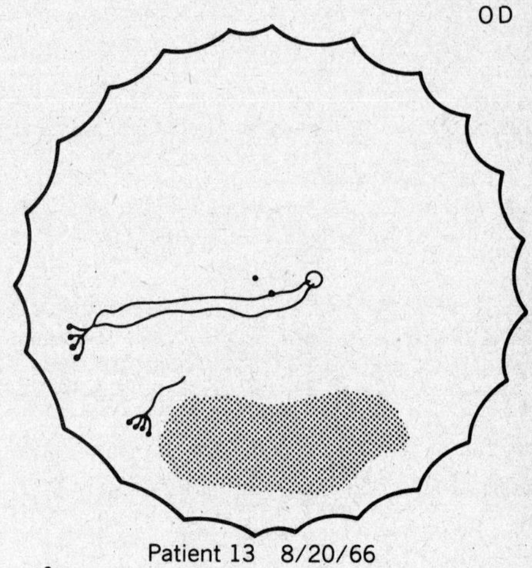

Fig 10.—Right fundus of a Negro man with sickle thalassemia (patient 13). Two sea fans are seen. One of them had bled spontaneously, and the blood had gravitated to inferior vitreous, where it obscures a black sunburst.

rect diagnosis may well have been S-thal. Kahan et al[20] then called attention to vitreous hemorrhage in a case of thalassemia minor, and vascular veils in the vitreous of a patient with thalassemia minima. In 1969, Toselli et al[21] studied 13 individuals with unexplained intraocular hemorrhages. Six of them were found to have thalassemia minor or minima, but not S-thal. Conjunctival signs similar to those described here have never been described in thalassemia.

Conjunctival lesions are much more numerous and obvious in patients with SS than in patients with SC.[1] In our series, the conjunctival vasculopathy observed in eight patients with S-thal was qualitatively similar to that seen in patients with SC and SS, but was less pronounced. Its presence could not be related to severity of disease, age, percent of hemoglobin S, or to hematocrit value.

Angioid streaks have been reported previously in SS and in Hb SC diseases.[22-24] One patient with Hb AS was reported to have angioid streaks,[25] but also apparently had pseudo-xanthoma elasticum. To our knowledge, patient 12 is the first S-thal case to be reported with angioid streaks. The pathogenesis of these cracks in the elastic lamina (Bruch's membrane) separating the retina from the choroid remains obscure.[22] However, it is possible that chronic hemolytic anemia may result in chronic iron deposition in Bruch's membrane, and cause brittleness and crack formation.

Vitreous hemorrhages arising from patches of neovascular, proliferative retinopathy have also been reported in various sickle cell diseases. Although proliferative retinopathy (with or without vitreous hemorrhage) may occur in SS disease, and even in sickle cell trait, it is decidedly uncommon in any of these disorders when compared with its prevalence in SC diseases. For example, neovascular and fibrous proliferations (stage III) have been reported in a majority of patients with SC hemoglobin and in a small minority of patients with SS hemoglobin. Conversely, the black sunbrust lesions (circular, black, chorioretinal scars) are more characteristic of SS than of SC disease, having been observed more than twice as commonly in the former than in the latter condition.

The retinas of our patients appear more similar to those of patients with Hb SC disease than to those of patients with sickle cell anemia, in that proliferative lesions were frequently observed. In vitro studies can be interpreted to predict such findings.[26] When blood from a patient with a sickling disorder passes through a deoxygenated vascular bed, its viscosity increases. The magnitude of the increase depends upon the rate at which the cells sickle and the hematocrit value of the blood. In the extreme case, vascular occlusion results. Rates of sickling in S-thal and SC diseases are very similar, as are hematocrit values, and one might expect retinal manifestations to follow suit.

Susceptible cells will not sickle until a critical *concentration* of deoxygenated hemoglobin is exceeded.[26] That concentration depends on the degree of interaction between hemoglobin S and any other hemoglobins present within the cell. The SC cells contain about 70% hemoglobin S (ie, less than that of S-thal cells), but Hb C interacts with Hb S to a greater degree than does the Hb A of S-thal. The two factors (percent of S and degree of interaction) more or less cancel out, and, during controlled deoxygenation, the two types of cells sickle at much the same rate. Hematocrit values for patients with Hb SC disease and for those with S-thal are approximately the same: average hematocrit value for 50 patients with SC is 33.5%; average value for 7 patients with S-thal is 33.4% (S. Charache, MD, unpublished data).

One might also expect systemic manifestations to parallel in vitro factors. They do, in general terms, but degree of incapacitation in an individual patient may be impossible to predict from the blood alone. Patient 5, for instance, considers herself to be in good health, whereas patient 13, whose red blood cells contain less hemoglobin S, has recurrent, painful crises. It was, therefore, of interest to find the most black sunbursts (which are characteristic of SS disease) in the patient with the highest concentration of Hb S, although his general clinical status was no more severe than that of other patients. Certain retinal abnormalities, such as the black sunburst and the sea fan, thus, may be more directly related to the in vitro behavior of red blood cells than is overall clinical status, which appears to be a resultant of additional factors.

This investigation was supported in part by Public Health Service training grant EY-24-13, research grant 5-R01-HE-02799-14, the Illinois Eye Bank, and a research fellowship from the Illinois Society for the Prevention of Blindness.

References

1. Paton D: The conjunctival sign of sickle cell disease. *Arch Ophthal* **68**:627-632, 1962.

2. Comer PB, Fred HL: Diagnosis of sickle cell disease by ophthalmoscopic inspection of the conjunctiva. *New Eng J Med* **271**:544-546, 1964.

3. Fink AI, Funahashi T, Robinson M, et al: Conjunctival blood flow in sickle cell disease. *Arch Ophthal* **66**:824-829, 1961.

4. Fink AI, Funahashi T, Robinson M, et al: Conjunctival blood flow in sickle cell disease: Responses to local stimuli. *Trans Amer Acad Ophthal Otolaryng* **68**:301-315, 1969.

5. Fink AI: Vascular fine structure changes in the bulbar conjunctiva associated with sickle cell disease. *Amer J Ophthal* **69**:563-572, 1970.

6. Welch RB, Goldberg MF: Sickle cell hemoglobin and its relation to fundus abnormality. *Arch Ophthal* **75**:253-262, 1966.

7. Hannon JF: Vitreous hemorrhages associated with sickle cell hemoglobin C disease. *Amer J Ophthal* **42**:707-712, 1956.

8. Ryan SJ, Goldberg MF: Anterior segment ischemia following scleral buckling in sickle cell hemoglobinopathy. *Amer J Ophthal*, to be published.

9. Goldberg MF: Treatment of proliferative sickle retinopathy. *Trans Amer Acad Ophthal Otolaryng*, to be published.

10. Goldberg MF: Proliferative sickle retinopathy: Classification and pathogenesis. *Amer J Ophthal* **71**:649-665, 1971.

11. Goldberg MF: Natural history of untreated proliferative sickle retinopathy. *Arch Ophthal*, to be published.

12. Newcomb N, Goldberg MF, Welch RG: Intravenous fluorescein photography of the ocular fundus in sickle cell anemia. *Med Biol Illus* **17**:95-98, 1967.

13. Smith EW, Conley CL: Clinical features of the genetic variants of sickle cell disease. *Bull Johns Hopkins Hosp* **94**:289-318, 1954.

14. Weatherall DJ: *The Thalassemia Syndromes*. Oxford, England, Blackwell Scientific Publications, 1965.

15. Necheles TF, Allen DM, Finkel HE: *Clinical Disorders of Hemoglobin Structure and Synthesis*. New York, Appleton-Century-Crofts, Inc, 1969, p 60.

16. Pearson HA: Hemoglobin S-thalassemia syndrome in Negro children. *Ann NY Acad Sci* **165**:83-92, 1969.

17. Hyvarinen L, Maumenee AE: Fluorescein angiography of the choriocapillaris. *Amer J Ophthal* **67**:653-666, 1969.

18. Levine RA, Kaplan AM: The ophthalmoscopic findings in C&S disease. *Amer J Ophthal* **59**:37-42, 1965.

19. Rudd C, Evans PJ, Peeney ALP: Ocular complications in thalassemia minor. *Brit J Ophthal* **37**:353-358, 1953.

20. Kahan A, Kahan IL, Benko A: Erythrocyte anomalies in hereditary vitreo-retinal degeneration (degeneratio hyaloideoretinalis). *Brit J Ophthal* **47**:620-631, 1963.

21. Toselli C, Bertoni G, Alessio L, et al: High incidence of thalassemia in patients with intraocular hemorrhages. *Ophthalmologica* **157**:343-348, 1969.

22. Paton D: The significance of angioid streaks. *Mid East Med J* **1**:301-336, 1962.

23. Paton D: Angioid streaks and sickle cell anemia. *Arch Ophthal* **62**:852-858, 1959.

24. Geeraets WJ, Guerry D III: Angioid streaks and sickle cell disease. *Amer J Ophthal* **49**:450-470, 1960.

25. Collomb H, Graneline J, Diop M, et al: Elastorrhexie systematisee chez une sicklemique. *Bull Soc Med Afr Noire Lang Franc* **10**:597-602, 1965.

26. Charache C, Conley, CL: Rate of sickling of red cells during deoxygenation of blood from persons with various sickling disorders. *Blood* **24**:25-46, 1964.

Pathologic Findings In the Pancreas of Mice Infected With Coxsackievirus B4

George E. Burch, MD;
Ching-Ya Tsui, MD;
Joseph M. Harb, PhD; and
Harry L. Colcolough, MD,
New Orleans

Pathologic changes in the exocrine and endocrine portions of the pancreas were observed in suckling and young adult mice infected with coxsackievirus B4. Thirty-two of 56 infected mice studied histologically showed significant cellular alterations. Generally, the changes ranged from focal and mild degeneration to widespread necrosis and inflammation. Electron micrographs of other infected mice showed derangement of the endoplasmic reticulum in acinar cells and various degrees of degranulation and cellular disruption in the islets. It seems likely that viruses may produce similar damage to the pancreas in man, and it is postulated that viral pancreatitis may cause subclinical diabetes as well as overt diabetes mellitus of varying degrees.

For some time we have been interested in the pathologic changes in a variety of organs of animals infected with the coxsackievirus B4. Our attention has been primarily directed toward the myocardium and associated structures, ie, endocardium and valves,[1-6] and to the kidneys.[7,8] From our first experience with this virus we have been impressed with the widespread vasculitis which frequently accompanies infection.[9] A less well recognized but equally frequent series of pathologic changes, however, has been consistently present in the pancreas of mice infected with the virus by the intraperitoneal route. It is the purpose of this paper to describe some of these changes as they affect the acinar and islet portions of the pancreas.

Received for publication June 10, 1970; accepted Aug 25.

From the Department of Medicine of the Tulane University School of Medicine, and Charity Hospital of Louisiana, New Orleans.

Reprint requests to the Department of Medicine, Tulane University, 1430 Tulane Ave, New Orleans 70112 (Dr. Burch).

Materials and Methods

The coxsackievirus B4 used in these experiments was originally recovered by Kibrick and Benirschke[10] from a 10-day-old infant who died of encephalo-hepatomyocarditis. The virus was obtained as monkey kidney culture passage strain and was prepared for these studies in rhesus monkey kidney cell culture according to techniques previously described.[11] Control fluid which was free of virus was also obtained. Both the virus and control fluid were stored at −65 C.

A random breed of HaM/ICR mice was used in these experiments. Nine adult mice approximately 2 months old were inoculated intraperitoneally with 0.2 ml of monkey kidney culture fluid containing coxsackievirus B4 10^3 50% tissue culture infective dose ($TCID_{50}$). Also, sixty-one 2-

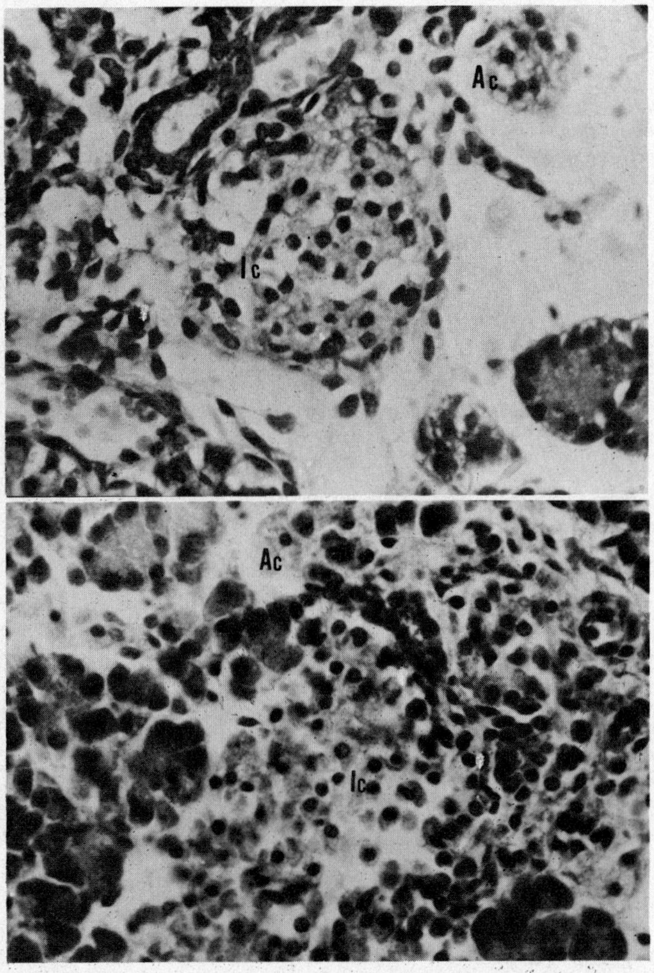

Fig 1.—Pancreas of suckling mice infected with coxsackievirus B4. Top, *Section from a 6-day-old mouse killed three days after infection which shows degenerating islet (Ic) and acinar (Ac) cells with cytoplasmic vacuolation and deeply basophilic nuclei (hematoxylin-eosin stain, ×450).* Bottom, *Section from a four-day-old mouse killed two days after infection which shows necrosis of individual islet (Ic) and acinar (Ac) cells (hematoxylin-eosin stain, ×450).*

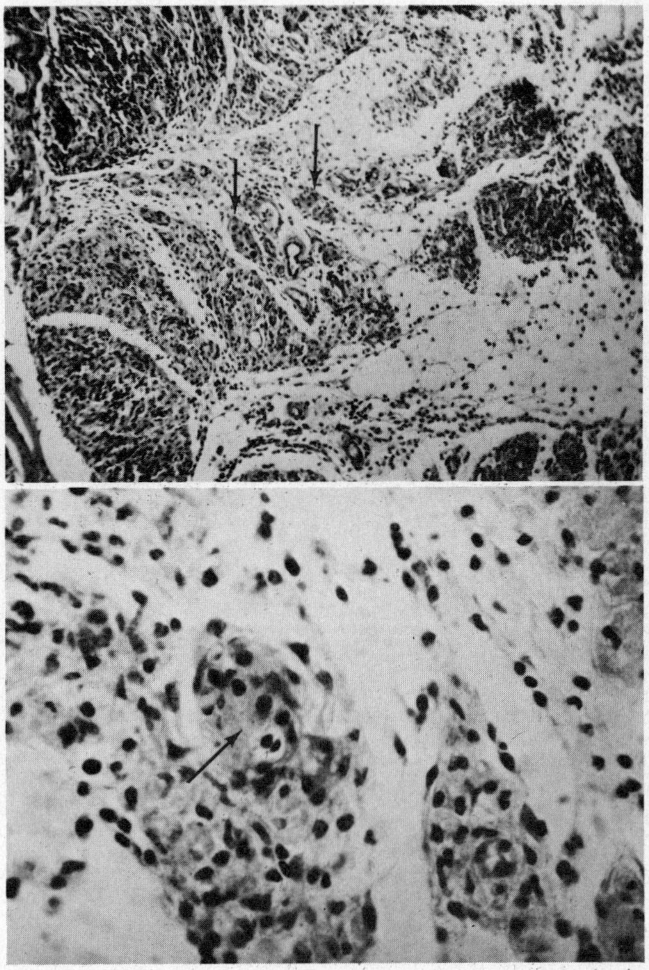

Fig 2.—Pancreas of adult mice infected with coxsackievirus B4. Top, *Section from a mouse seven days after inoculation. Note extensive lobular necrosis with widespread inflammatory cell infiltration. Two degenerative islets* (arrows) *are shown (hematoxylin-eosin stain, ×120).* Bottom, *Section from a mouse eight days after infection. Note islet cell degeneration and cell necrosis* (arrow) *in the extensively damaged pancreas (hematoxylin-eosin stain, ×450).*

to 11-day-old suckling mice were inoculated in the same manner with 0.05 to 0.1 ml of monkey kidney culture fluid containing coxsackievirus B4 10^5 $TCID_{50}$. Forty-four animals, including the nine adults, were killed from the first day through the 21st day after inoculation, and 26 were killed after 26 days of infection. For control studies, eight adult mice about two months of age and twenty-two 2- to 11-day-old suckling mice were inoculated intraperitoneally with 0.2 ml and 0.05 to 0.1 ml virus-free culture fluid, respectively, and killed at various intervals with the infected animals.

For light microscopy, the pancreatic tissues of 26 control and 56 infected mice were fixed in neutral formaldehyde solution, embedded in paraffin, and cut in serial sections of 6μ thickness. Sections were stained by routine hematoxylin-eosin methods.

The pancreas of 5 control and 15 infected suckling mice were studied with an electron microscope. For electron microscopy, 1 cu mm pieces of tissue were fixed in cold (4 C) phosphate-buffered 3% glutaraldehyde[12] for two hours and then rinsed six to eight times at 30-minute intervals in cold (4 C) phosphate buffer to remove excess glutaraldehyde. Tissues were postfixed in cold (4 C) 1% osmium tetroxide in phosphate buffer for 1½ hours. Dehydration was initiated with a ten-minute rinse in cold 50% ethyl alcohol and continued through a graded series of cold 70%, 80%, 95%, and anhydrous alcohol. Dehydration was completed with three 30-minute changes of anhydrous alcohol at

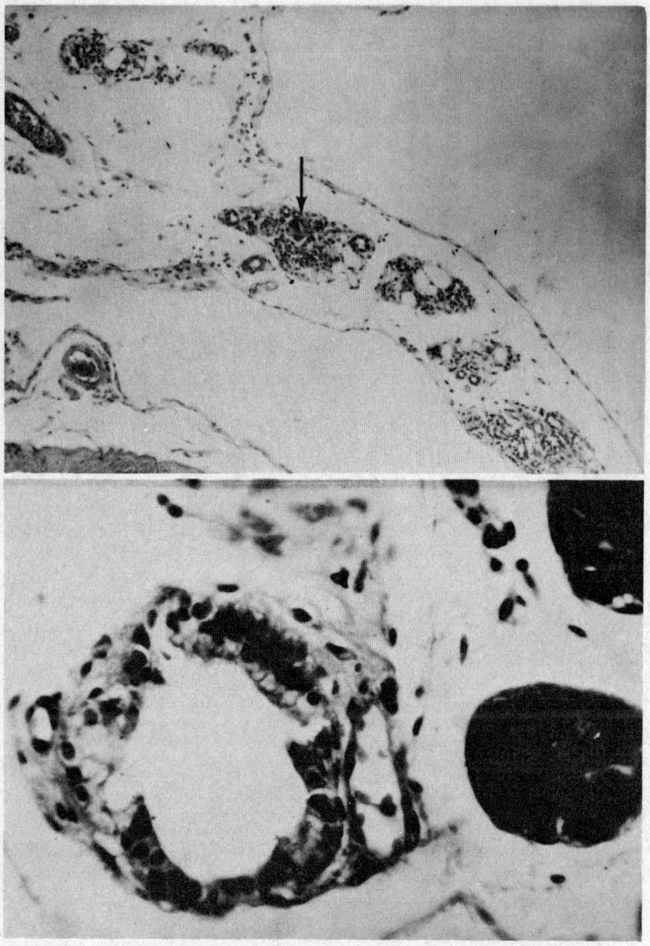

Fig 3.—Pancreas of adult mice killed 15 days after infection with coxsackievirus B4. Top, *Note the necrotic lobules replaced with fatty infiltration and inflammatory cells. An atrophic islet can be seen* (arrow) *(hematoxylin-eosin stain, ×120).* Bottom, *A metaplastic duct is shown (hematoxylin-eosin stain, ×450).*

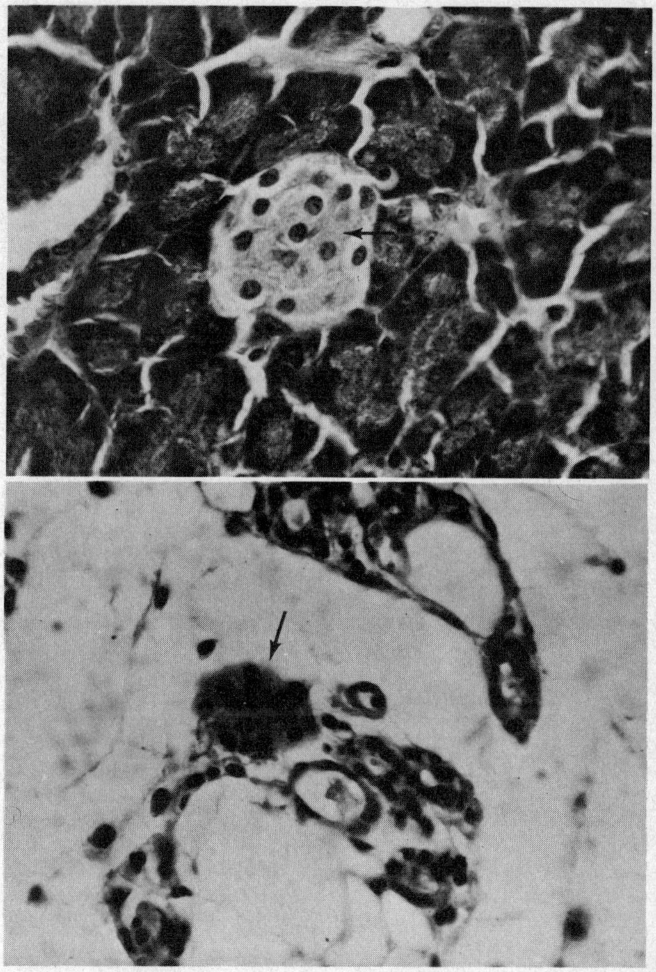

Fig 4.—Pancreas of (top) *control (normal) adult mouse and* (bottom) *adult mouse 14 days after infection with coxsackievirus B4. Note the slightly basophilic and granular islet cells with nuclei showing a distinct chromatin pattern* (arrow) *in the normal animal* (top) *as compared with the atrophic islet showing smaller cells with homogeneous eosinophilic cytoplasm and dense basophilic nuclei* (arrow) *in the infected animal* (bottom) *(hematoxylin-eosin stain, ×450).*

room temperature. After two 15-minute changes in propylene oxide, the tissues were embedded in epoxy (Maraglas)[13] or in epoxy resin (Epon 812).[14] Thin sections were cut with an ultramicrotome, stained with the lead stain of Sato,[15] and examined with an electron microscope.

Results

Gross Pathology.—Of 56 inoculated animals examined grossly, 7 adult (2 months old) and 25 suckling (2 to 11 days old) mice showed gross pancreatic lesions which were later substantiated in histologic sections. The gross appearance of the pancreas 2 to 15 days after infection was gray and edematous, whereas after 26 days the gross appearance was not remarkable. The 2-month-old adult animals generally tended to have more widespread damage to the pancreas than the suckling animals. The pancreatic tissues of all control animals appeared normal.

Microscopic Pathology.—The microscopic changes in the suckling and 2-month-old groups were essentially the same. Pathologic alterations were seen in the acinar and islet portions of the pancreas as early as two days after infection. Islets and acini showed eosinophilic vacuolated cytoplasm with deeply basophilic nuclei

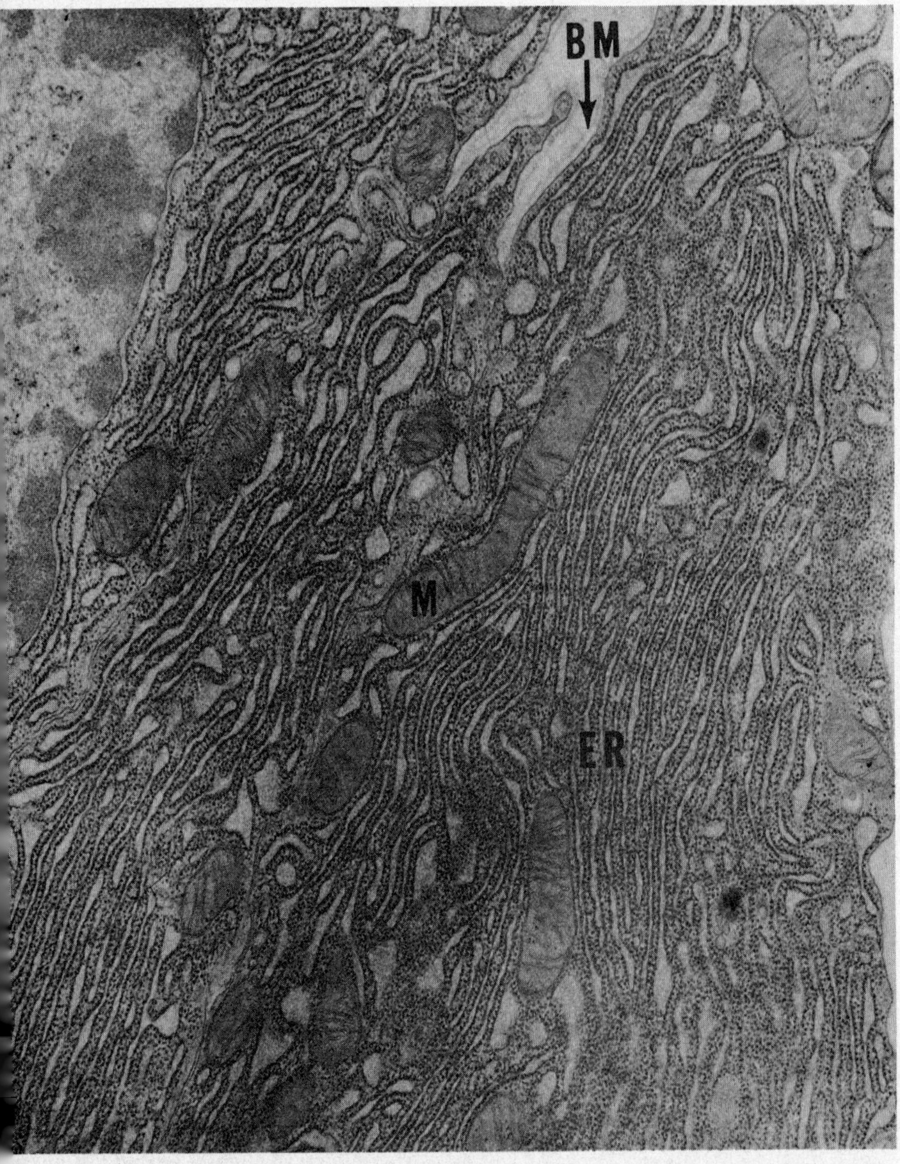

Fig 5.—Electron micrograph of three adjacent acinar cells of the pancreas of a control (normal) adult mouse. N indicates nucleus; ER, endoplasmic reticulum; M, mitochondria; BM, basement membrane (× 25,000).

(Fig 1, *top*). Individual cells of both islet and acinus frequently showed necrosis with dissolving cytoplasm and pyknotic nuclei (Fig 1, *bottom*). Acinar changes were most marked after the seventh day after infection. Extensive lobular destruction and marked inflammatory cell infiltration were widespread (Fig 2). The inflammatory cells were predominantly mononuclear leukocytes, but some were neutrophils. Islet cell degeneration persisted, and occasional cell necrosis was seen (Fig 2, *bottom*). By the 14th day after infection the necrotic areas of the pancreas were frequently replaced with fatty infiltration and inflammatory cells (Fig 3, *top*). Metaplastic ducts were sometimes seen (Fig 3, *bottom*). The damaged islets usually showed changes in their size and tinctorial properties. The normal slightly basophilic islets (Fig 4, *top*) became atrophic, deeply eosinophilic, and the nuclei took on a dense homogeneous basophilia (Fig 4, *bottom*). Of the animals killed 26 days after inoculation, one showed marked fatty tissue replacement. Islets scattered between the fatty tissue were less in number, and some of them were still atrophic. Slight acinar cell degeneration and inflammatory cell infiltration were also encountered.

The electron micrographs of the acinar cells of the control animals were normal. For example, Fig 5 shows portions of three adjacent normal acinar cells from a control mouse. The cisternae of the rough endoplasmic reticulum (ER) are flattened sacs which are in a parallel arrangement. Ribosomes are attached to the membranes of the ER along their length. Nuclei with peripheral chromatin are seen, and ribosomes are attached to the outer nuclear membrane. The mitochondria are located among the cisternae of the ER. Zymogen granules are numerous in the acinus of control mice.

The granules of the alpha cells from the pancreatic islet of the control mouse are more dense and smaller than those of the beta cells (Fig 6, *top*). The membrane sac is separated from the dense portion of the granule by a clear space which is wider in the beta granule than in the alpha granule. The delta granules are less dense than the alpha and beta granules and are about the same size as the beta cell granules (Fig 6, *bottom*). The matrix of the delta cell granule is homogeneous and completely fills the sac. The granules of the delta cell are more tightly clustered than those of the alpha and beta cells. All cells contain profiles of rough ER scattered among the pancreatic granules (Fig 6).

Figure 7 shows cells of adjacent acini from the pancreas of an infected mouse. One cell (lower portion of figure) appeared well organized, with the cisternae of the rough ER lamellar and evenly parallel. Ribosomes were attached to the membranes of the endoplasmic reticulum. In the second cell (upper part of figure) the chisternae of the ER were no longer flat, parallel-arrayed sacs, but, instead, were distended vesiculated structures distributed randomly throughout the cytoplasm. Vesicles of this type were probably formed from the breakdown of the tubular elements of the ER. The vesicular profiles of the ER still had the ribosomes attached. Other ribosomes were free in the cytoplasm. The cisternae of the ER contained a material of similar electron density as the cytoplasm. The mitochondria resembled those of the control pancreas.

In some acinar cells, the damage was more extensive. The intracellular architecture became greatly disorganized (Fig 8, *top*) and highly vesiculated (Fig 8, *bottom*). Several vesicles had ribosomes attached, indicating that they might be remnants of the rough surfaced endoplasmic reticulum. It is difficult to state with certainty whether or not other vesicles were remnants of the rough ER with the ribosomes detached. The nucleus remained intact, with an intact nucleolus, but there was often clumping of the chromatin (Fig 8, *bottom*). The nuclear envelope was scalloped and dilated and occasionally broken, and the outer and inner membranes lost their close parallel apposition (Fig 8, *bottom*). The mitochondria remained intact. Dense bodies probably of lysosomal

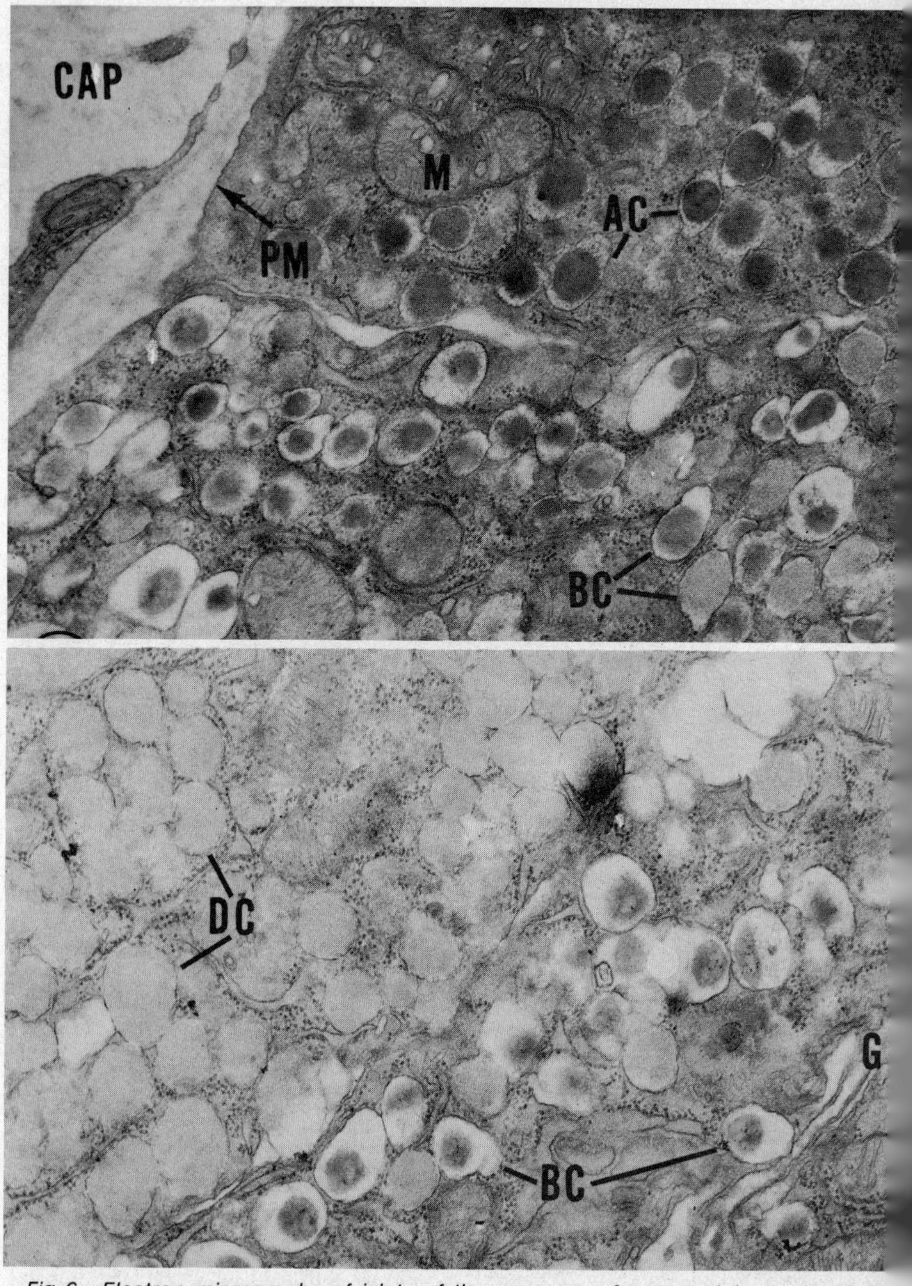

Fig 6.—Electron micrographs of islets of the pancreas of a control (normal) adult mouse. Top, *Note small dense alpha cell granules (AC) and larger, lighter beta cell granules (BC). M indicates mitochondrion; PM, plasma membrane; CAP, capillary.* Bottom, *Delta cell granules (DC) are larger than beta cell granules (BC) and their membrane sacs are fully packed. G signifies Golgi element (× 28,800).*

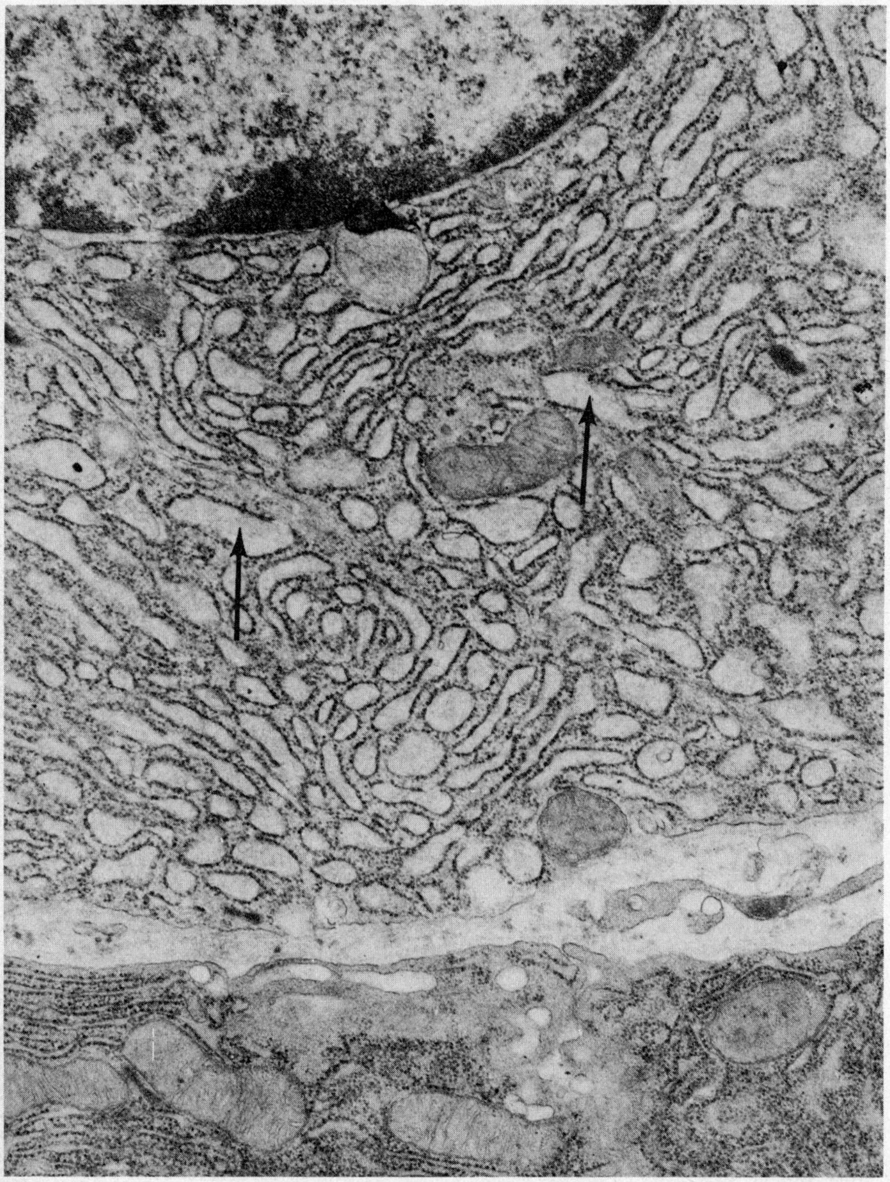

Fig 7.—Electron micrograph of two adjacent acinar cells of the pancreas of a 14-day-old mouse killed three days after infection with coxsackievirus B4. One cell (bottom) *appears well organized, whereas the ER in the other cell* (arrows) *is disorganized and distended (×21,600).*

nature were visible within the cytoplasm. In one such body (Fig 8, *top*) remnants of a mitochondrion and other cytoplasmic materials were seen. In one instance, beta granules were seen in an acinar cell (Fig 9).

In the infected animals, islet cells frequently showed extensive changes. In some areas beta cells were found in which the cellular architecture was markedly distorted (Fig 10, *top*). The ER became fragmented, dilated, and lost its lamellar arrangement. Large vesicles formed, the granules became dispersed, and the ground substance lost its usual electron density (Fig 10, *bottom*). Some of the remaining intact granules lost their contents. The mitochondria were intact but the cristae became slightly dilated (Fig 10, *top*).

Comment

The pancreatic damage caused by coxsackievirus B4 infection in experimental animals has received relatively little attention. A diabetes-like syndrome in coxsackievirus infected mice has been described by Robertson[16] and Minkowitz and Berkovich.[17] Since pancreatic damage is so wide-spread and involves both the exocrine and endocrine portions of the pancreas, it is not surprising that diabetes is a frequent concomitant of sublethal infection in experimental animals. The results of infection in experimental animals reported here have suggested to us that an analogous situation may occur in clinical medicine. The frequency of viral infections in childhood and early adulthood is well known. In general, these infections are self-limited, and recovery is uneventful. Nevertheless, we wonder if infections with viruses that may have a tropism for the pancreas could be one of the initiating or contributing causes of the subsequent development of overt clinical diabetes mellitus. It would seem that if islet cell damage is extensive and irreversible, diabetes mellitus may be expected in childhood or early adulthood; whereas if the damage is milder or relatively less irreversible, diabetes would not develop at all or only in later life. Thus, one may postulate that viral pancreatitis may produce subclinical diabetes as well as overt diabetes mellitus of varying degrees. Whether or not a slightly damaged islet can function adequately for a time and deteriorate

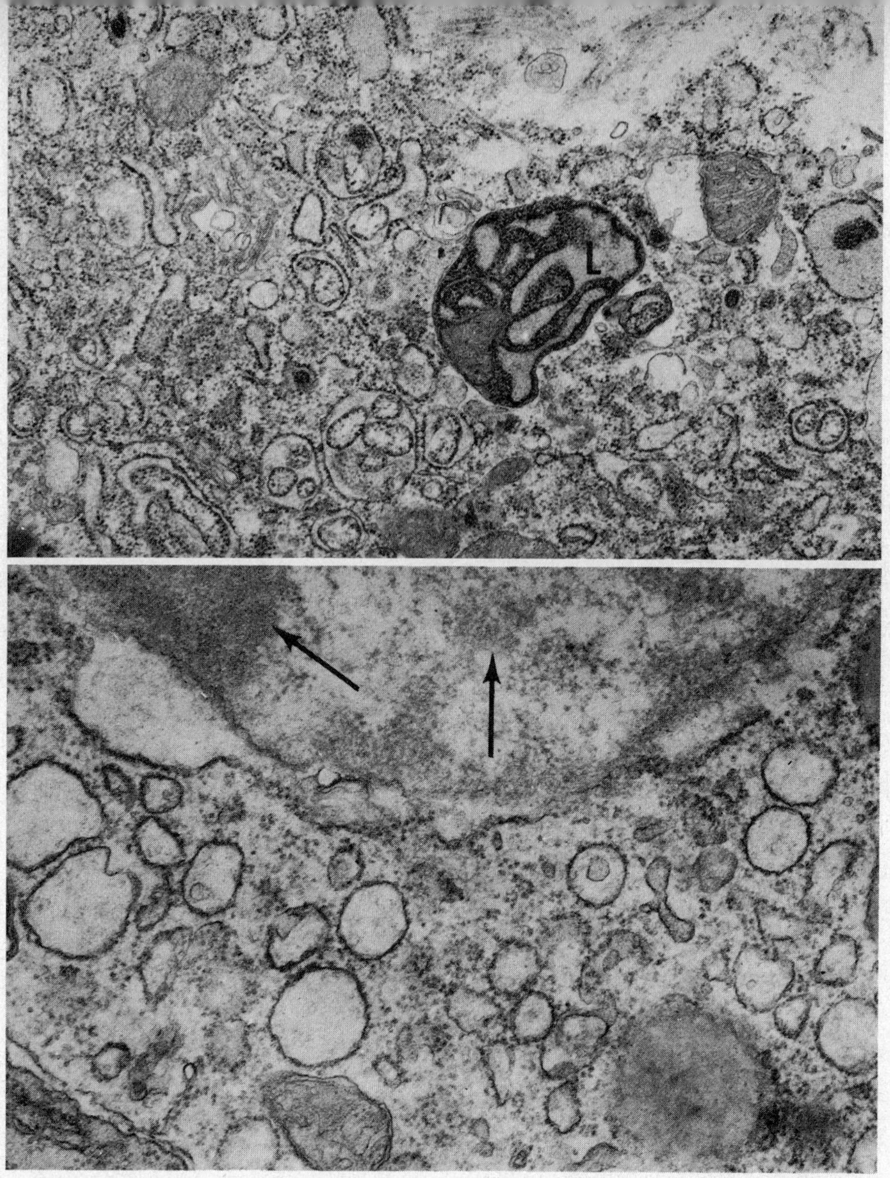

Fig 8.—Electron micrographs of acinar cells of the pancreas of a 12-day-old mouse killed one day following infection with coxsackievirus B4. Note intracellular disorganization, vacuole formation, and loss of ground substance. Top, *Dense bodies (L), which are probably lysosomes are seen throughout the cytoplasm.* Bottom, *Clumping of nuclear chromatin was also seen* (arrows). Top, *×18,400;* bottom, *×32,400.*

Fig 9.—Electron micrograph of acinar cell of pancreas from a 28-day-old mouse killed 17 days after infection with coxsackievirus B4. Note presence of beta granules (arrows) *within acinar cell. Cisternae of the rough ER contain an electron dense material of unknown nature (×24,800).*

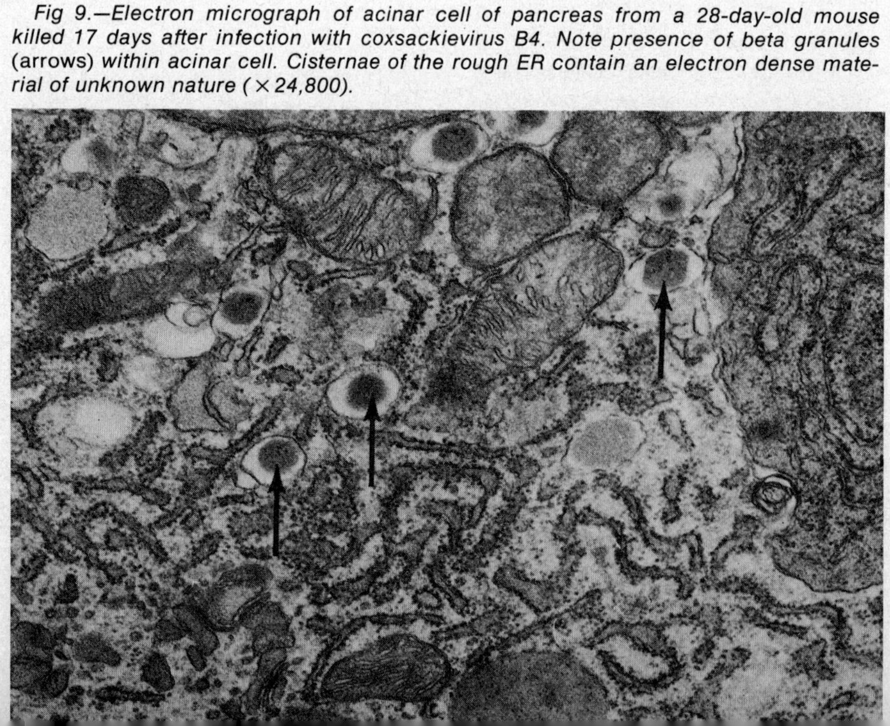

at some later date under the influence of a number of conditioning factors or subsequent viral infections is unknown at this time. The possible role of viral diseases in the production of pancreatitis and pancreatic dysfunction needs investigation. It is rather interesting that this has received essentially no attention.

A delineation of the types of viruses that can infect the pancreas in the experimental animal is needed in order to stimulate further research into the mechanisms of pancreatic infections as a possible cause of diabetes mellitus. We believe that essentially the same events described here in infected mice could occur in man and that some cases of diabetes in man may be caused by viral infection.

It is worth noting that recent studies of Gamble et al[18,19] suggest that diabetes mellitus can be produced in man by the coxsackieviruses. The finding of high titers of neutralizing antibodies in patients with diabetes is also worthy of note.[18] The great frequency of viral diseases in man and the wide spectrum of abdominal pain and discomfort in association with these infections are well known. Rarely, if ever, does the physician attempt to explain or investigate the epigastric pain which is such a frequent complaint of children, and even of adults, with respiratory and other viral infections. That coxsackievirus B4 can produce pancreatitis in mice is evident from our studies. Knowledge concerning the initiation and perpetuation of the clinical syndrome of chronic relapsing pancreatitis is quite meager. The relationship of Coxsackie B4 viral pancreatitis to disturbances in endocrine and exocrine function is under in-

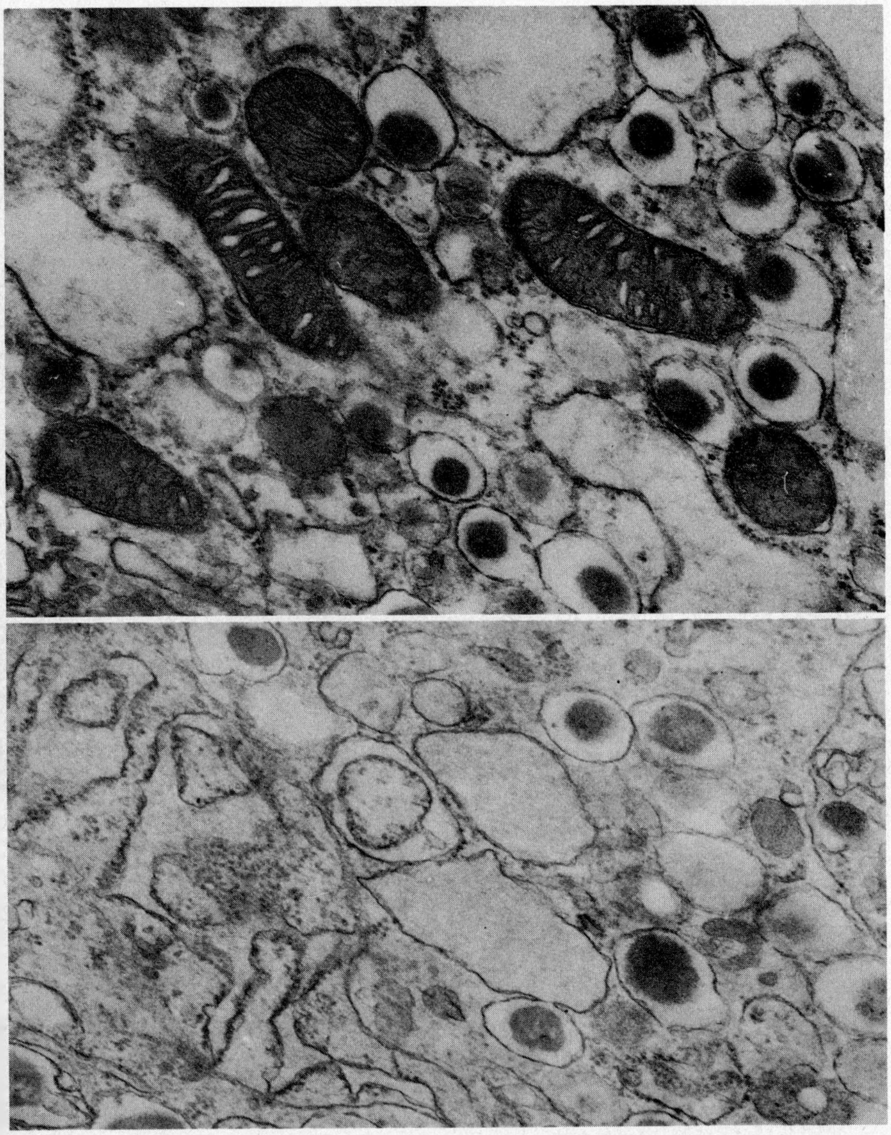

Fig 10.—Electron micrographs of islet cells of pancreas from 12-day-old mouse killed one day after infection with coxsackievirus B4. Note cellular disorganization, vacuolation and dispersion, and dissolution of granules (× 30,000).

vestigation in our laboratory.

The subtle-ultrastructural changes in the acinar and islet cells of the pancreas in our infected mice attest to the wide spectrum of damage that coxsackievirus B4 can produce in the pancreas. The effect of repeated infections with the same as well as other viruses is being studied. The role of adjuvants, conditioning factors, and multiple infections (bacterial and viral; viral and viral) also remains unknown but should be studied.

This investigation was supported by Public Health Service research grant HE-06769 from the National Heart Institute, by the Rudolph Matas Memorial Fund for the Kate Prewitt Hess Laboratory, and by the Rowell A. Billups Fund for Research in Heart Disease. W. J. Mogabgab, MD, provided and prepared the coxsackievirus B4 fluid used in this study.

References

1. Burch GE, DePasquale NP, Sun SC, et al: Experimental coxsackievirus endocarditis. *JAMA* **196**:349-352, 1966.

2. DePasquale NP, Burch GE, Sun SC, et al: Experimental coxsackie virus B_4 valvulitis in cynomolgus monkeys. *Amer Heart J* **71**:678-683, 1966.

3. Sun SC, Colcolough HL, Burch GE, et al: Immunofluorescent study of B_4 coxsackievirus valvulitis in mice. *Proc Soc Exp Biol Med* **125**:157-162, 1967.

4. Burch GE, Sun SC, Colcolough HL, et al: Coxsackie B viral myocarditis and valvulitis identified in routine autopsy specimens by immunofluorescent techniques. *Amer Heart J* **74**:13-23, 1967.

5. Burch GE, Sun SC, Chu KC, et al: Interstitial and coxsackie B myocarditis in infants and children. *JAMA* **203**:1-8, 1968.

6. Burch GE, Colcolough HL: Viral valvulitis. *Amer Heart J* **78**:119-123, 1969.

7. Sun SC, Burch GE, Sohal RS, et al: Coxsackie B_4 viral nephritis in mice and its autoimmune-like phenomena. *Proc Soc Exp Biol Med* **126**:882-885, 1967.

8. Burch GE, Chu KC, Colcolough HL, et al: Immunofluorescent localization of coxsackievirus B antigen in the kidney observed at routine autopsy. *Amer J Med* **47**:36-42, 1969.

9. Sohal RS, Burch GE, Chu KC, et al: Ultrastructural changes in cardiac capillaries of coxsackie virus B_4 infected mice. *Lab Invest* **19**:399-405, 1968.

10. Kibrick S, Benirschke K: Severe generalized disease (encephalohepato myocarditis) occurring in the newborn period and due to infection with coxsackie virus, group B. *Pediatrics* **22**:857-875, 1958.

11. Mogabgab WJ: Viruses associated with upper respiratory illnesses in adults. *Ann Intern Med* **59**:306-322, 1963.

12. Millonig G: Advantages of a phosphate buffer for OsO_4 solution in fixation. *J Applied Physics* **32**:1637, 1961.

13. Freeman J, Spurlock B: A new epoxy embeddment for electron microscopy. *J Cell Biol* **13**:437, 1962.

14. Luft J: Improvements in epoxy resin embedding methods. *J Biophys Biochem Cytol* **9**:409-414, 1961.

15. Sato T: A modified method for lead staining of thin sections. *J Electron Micr* **17**:158-159, 1968.

16. Robertson JS: The pancreatic lesion in adult mice infected with a strain of pleurodynia virus: I. Electron microscopical observations. *Aust J Exp Biol* **32**:393-410, 1954.

17. Minkowitz S, Berkovich S: Hepatitis produced by Coxsackievirus B_1 in adult mice. *Arch Path* **89**:427-433, 1970.

18. Gamble DR, Kinsley ML, Fitzgerald MG, et al: Viral antibodies in diabetes mellitus. *Brit Med J* **3**:627-630, 1969.

19. Gamble DR, Taylor KW: Seasonal incidence of diabetes mellitus. *Brit Med J* **3**:631-633, 1969.

Oxidants and Lung Biochemistry

A Brief Review

F. Gordon Hueter, PhD, and Martin Fritzhand, MD, Research Triangle Park, NC

A brief review of the literature relative to the biochemical effects of oxidant air pollutants of mammalian systems is presented. Specific oxidants discussed are ozone, nitrogen dioxide, and the photochemical oxidant mixture. Enzyme alterations precede many of the structural indications of tissue degradation and offer a sensitive method for detection prior to actual irreversible damage. The initiation of additional biochemical research concerning normal lung metabolic processes is necessary in order to interpret the effects of air pollution more intelligently. A total research approach for determining the health effects of air pollution must include laboratory animal toxicological studies, laboratory clinical investigation of humans, and epidemiological studies under naturally occurring conditions.

Oxidants such as ozone, nitrogen dioxide, and peroxyacyl nitrates, when inhaled at sublethal concentrations, may alter, impair, or otherwise interfere with normal physiological systems. Because all living systems depend upon complex biochemical processes, an understanding of these processes is essential for assessing normal or altered body mechanisms.

The physiological and pathological effects of the oxidant gases have only recently been studied, while the biochemical and biophysical effects resulting from short-term and prolonged exposure to these gases have not yet been defined. Part of this difficulty results from the paucity of basic knowledge concerning biochemical and biophysical indices of the normal pulmonary system. Assessment of abnormality must be founded on a factual description of normality. A serious effort to bridge this gap would allow a more meaningful interpretation of the results of oxidant effects research and a more systematic research approach.

The following is a brief, limited review of biochemical research relative to the potential health effects of oxidant air pollution.

Biochemical Effects and Implications of NO_2 Toxicity

Experimental studies in man and animal indicate that continuous exposure to low concentrations of nitrogen dioxide results in pathological alterations in the lung consistent with the histological and physiological diagnosis of emphysema.[1,2] There is an enlargement of the alveoli,[3] loss of exfoliative activity (ie, an apparent inactivity of cells exposed to nitrogen dioxide), decreased blebbing of the cytoplasm into airways, a decrease in or loss of cilia, and the appearance of rod-shaped intracytoplasmic crystalloid inclusions.[4-6] The significance of the inclusions is unknown, but they apparently represent a paracrystalline accumulation of protein, which suggests a metabolic disturbance due to the low concentration of nitrogen dioxide.[5] These pathological findings and metabolic disturbances could result from the action of nitrogen dioxide on enzymes present in the lung. The gas may act via enzyme systems or directly on the structural proteins of the lung. The structural conformation of collagen and elastin may undergo irreversible changes during prolonged exposure to nitrogen dioxide with a resultant lung disease of striking similarity to emphysema.[7] Alterations in serum or tissue enzyme activity levels or both resulting from short- or long-term inhalation of nitrogen dioxide should

Received for publication Oct 21, 1970; accepted Feb 2, 1971.
From the Division of Effects Research, National Air Pollution Control Administration, Environmental Health Service, Public Health Service, Research Triangle Park, NC.
Read in part before the Tenth Annual Hanford Biology Symposium on Pollution and Lung Biochemistry, Richland, Wash, June 4, 1970, jointly sponsored by the Battelle Memorial Institute-Pacific Northwest Laboratories, National Air Pollution Control Administration, National Institute of Environmental Health Sciences, and the US Atomic Energy Commission.
Reprint requests to Division of Effects Research, Bureau of Air Pollution Sciences, Environmental Protection Agency, Technical Center, Research Triangle Park, NC (Dr. Hueter).

be a sensitive indicator of toxicity or of possible tissue damage (with subsequent structural changes). In fact, previous studies of alterations in enzyme activity levels following exposure to irritants have revealed that these changes may occur early, even before clinical signs of tissue damage.[8-10]

The literature concerning the biochemical effects of nitrogen dioxide deals largely with the enzymatic alterations following exposure to that gas. Buckley and Balchum have related nitrogen dioxide exposure to changes in enzyme activity.[8] They felt that lactic dehydrogenase (LDH) was one of the important regulating steps in the metabolic scheme, mediating the pyruvate-lactate interconversion. Lactic dehydrogenase is found throughout the body and functions under widely varying physiological and biochemical conditions.[9] Its enzyme activity level was determined in a series of experiments to add information about alterations in tissue metabolism resulting from nitrogen dioxide exposure. In 1965, these authors first noted that the activity levels of LDH and aldolase are altered by exposure to nitrogen dioxide.[8] However, they were unable to locate the site of release of these enzymes.

After Buckley and Balchum discovered that enzyme alterations occur in the course of nitrogen dioxide inhalation, they determined the manner in which the LDH and aldolase activity levels changed during the course of long-term exposure to nitrogen dioxide.[11] Because enzymes are responsible for biological regulation, the change of activity should appear early, precede many of the structural indications of tissue degradation, and offer a sensitive method for detection prior to actual irreversible damage. Also, knowledge of the time relationship between metabolic changes in tissues and time of exposure to nitrogen dioxide might point to a possible mechanism by which these enzyme alterations are brought about.

In a study designed to determine whether regular inhalation of nitrogen dioxide resulted in changes in the LDH isoenzyme distribution patterns, in addition to the previously reported alterations in total enzyme activity, Buckley and Balchum found that LDH enzyme activity was grossly elevated in lung, liver, and kidney tissue homogenates, while the isoenzyme pattern was significantly altered (from that of controls) only in lung tissue.[9] The changes suggest that nitrogen dioxide favors conditions which inhibit aerobic and stimulate anerobic oxidation in lung tissue. However, the possibility of an alteration in isoenzyme activity due to endogenous factors cannot be ruled out.

It is well known that the body's response to a noxious substance can result in elevated tissue enzyme activity. However, the alteration in the lung LDH isoenzyme pattern following nitrogen dioxide inhalation appears to result from a direct effect on the lung tissue itself rather than to a generalized stress response, since lung tissue, which was in direct contact with the inhaled oxidant, showed a significant alteration in its isoenzyme pattern, whereas kidney and liver homogenates showed no such changes.[9] On the other hand, studies demonstrating nitrogen dioxide transport across the alveolar wall through the blood stream to other organs have not been performed. The extreme chemical reactivity of nitrogen dioxide would make it unlikely, however, that the substance would exist long enough to be transported to tissue sites and result in isoenzyme alteration.

The lack of difference in kidney and liver tissue patterns suggests that the factors responsible for the elevation of total LDH activity may very well not be the same as those causing the alterations in the isoenzyme distribution.[9,11] The nonspecific elevation of enzyme activity in organs other than the lung could be explained as a physiological stress response. Circulating substances resulting from either the interaction of nitrogen dioxide, lung tissue, and blood, or the physiological stress response might well result in nonspecific alteration of enzyme activity in other tissues of the body.[11]

The real meaning of these enzyme alterations is difficult to interpret without knowledge of possible alterations in the activity levels of other glycolytic enzymes. Histochemical techniques have been used to determine whether the detected enzyme changes represent general changes in all the cells of a tissue or are localized effects due to direct contact and interaction between nitrogen dioxide and various cells of the respiratory system.[11] Sherwin et al[12] noted large numbers of macrophages in the lungs of guinea pigs that had been exposed to nitrogen dioxide. Later, they found that LDH activity was primarily localized in the alveolar cells with slight activity in the endothelial and epithelial cells of the alveolar wall.[12] Only minimal abnormalities were found in any of the lung sections. The presence of increased numbers of alveolar cells in the absence of overt lesions indicates that the index should be useful in detection of low levels of air pollutants.[12]

These findings were confirmed by

exposing germ-free mice to 37 ppm nitrogen dioxide for 37 days.[13] The lungs of the exposed mice showed intense LDH activity. Staining for LDH was heavy in the hyperplastic epithelium lining the bronchial tree, particularly along the terminal bronchioles. The alveolar septal cells stained heavily in the lungs of both the exposed control groups, but the number of LDH-positive cells in the bronchiolar epithelium and alveoli near the terminal bronchioles was greatly increased in the mice exposed to nitrogen dioxide. The normal cytoplasmic distribution of LDH was not altered.

The effect of nitrogen dioxide inhalation on other enzymes has also been studied. Mice exposed to 37 ppm nitrogen dioxide for periods up to 37 days were examined both for acid and alkaline phosphatase activity.[13] The enzymes were found distributed nonspecifically throughout the lung fields, and neither histochemical nor biochemical data indicated that the enzymatic activities were increased following nitrogen dioxide inhalation.

There is a possibility that enzyme systems of various tissues studied may respond differently to nitrogen dioxide exposure since liver oxygen consumption (Q_{O_2}) in animals exposed over a long period increased.[8] However, it was previously shown that exposure to nitrogen dioxide favors the appearance of the anerobic form of lung LDH while depressing the level of activity of the aerobic form; one would therefore expect oxygen consumption to decrease likewise. Rounds and Bils[14] measured the oxygen consumption of rabbit endothelial cells in vitro before, during, and after exposure to 20 ppm sodium nitrite. The addition of sodium nitrite did indeed depress respiratory activity, though this was reversible in all cases.

It appears that the primary effect of nitrogen dioxide is on lung tissue itself, with only those cells in contact with nitrogen dioxide undergoing definitive structural and metabolic changes. The solubility and chemical activity of nitrogen dioxide probably results in its removal from inspired air prior to its reaching the distal alveoli where transfer to the bloodstream takes place. The metabolic effects noted in other organ systems may represent the body's physiologic response to a noxious irritant, though a direct effect through a chemical intermediary cannot yet be ruled out.

The possibility that nitrogen dioxide alters lung protein leads to another area of discussion. Nitrogen dioxide may induce these protein changes by various mechanisms: through enzymatic changes previously discussed, direct alteration of collagen and elastin conformation through chemical interaction, or modification of cell membranes which would, in turn, be reflected by changes in the conformation of the attached protein.

Phospholipids are compounds basic to cell membrane structure. Insoluble monomolecular films of phospholipids have been widely used as cell membrane models to simulate the interaction of materials with living membranes at the molecular level. Felmeister et al[15] exposed monomolecular films composed of the phospholipids dipalmitoyl lecithin (DPL) and egg lecithin (EL) to various nitrogen dioxide-olefin gas atmospheres. Films of DPL (the saturated phospholipid) showed no interaction with any of the test atmospheres used. On the other hand, the unsaturated phospholipid, EL, showed a significant change in the surface pressure and surface area curves in the presence of all atmospheres containing nitrogen dioxide. The resultant increase in area per molecule of the EL film in the presence of nitrogen-dioxide appears to be the result of a chemical reaction between nitrogen dioxide and the double bonds of EL rather than a simple physical penetration of the film. This step will be discussed later in this review.

A similar experiment performed by Weiner et al[16] using membrane phospholipid extracted from *Escherichia coli* verified the oxidative activity of nitrogen dioxide on materials present in cell membranes.

The in vivo work of Thomas[17] confirms the previously described in vitro studies. Rats were killed 24 to 48 hours after a 4-hour exposure to 1 ppm nitrogen dioxide, and lung lipid was extracted at autopsy. The absorption spectra characteristic of diene conjugation (oxidation of double bonds) typical of peroxidized polyenic fatty acids was found only in those rats exposed to nitrogen dioxide. The intense spectroscopic peak at 230 to 235 mμ is characteristic of the peroxidation of linoleate, arachidonate, and other methyl-interrupted unsaturated fatty acids. Oxidation could be partially prevented by large doses of an antioxidant (vitamin E) but only when it is added prior to exposure with nitrogen dioxide.

Cell membrane lipoprotein contains a large proportion of unsaturated phospholipids that support the structural and functional proteins. Changes in the supporting phospholipid would in turn be reflected by changes in the conformation of the attached protein (ie, elastin and collagen). In the case of a functional protein, these changes in conformation would most likely be accompanied by a modification of enzyme activity. It is conceivable that some of the observed effects of nitrogen dioxide described are the direct result of its interaction with lipids responsible for cell membrane integrity, causing cell membrane expansion and subsequent changes in cell membrane permeability or enzymatic activity or both.[15,16]

The effect of nitrogen dioxide on the pulmonary tree does not appear to be limited to enzyme activity or cell membrane alteration alone. A direct effect on the structural proteins (collagen and elastin) found in lung tissue has been reported by Buell.[18] Collagen and elastin were isolated from the lungs of rabbits killed after a one-hour exposure to 1 ppm nitrogen dioxide. Using differential ultraviolet spectrophotometry, they found a change in the conformation of both proteins that was reversible within 24 hours. The observed denaturation is consistent with the hypothesis that the acidic products of nitrogen dioxide hydrolysis result in the rupture of H-bonds that normally maintain the configuration of the proteins. The extreme chemical activity of nitrogen dioxide (or its acidic breakdown products) as an oxidant could result in protein denaturation on direct contact with these tissues.[11] Lowering the pH of the lung environment through the acidic products of nitrogen dioxide should result in the denaturation of lung proteins, though intimate contact between the irritant and lung tissue itself may be required.[19]

The reversibility of these changes may indicate that the natural buffering system in the rabbit is able to restore a normal pH within 24 hours. It is also likely that the normal metabolic activity in lung tissue, particularly those activities mediated by enzymes, is reduced in the acidic environment that occurs with nitrogen dioxide exposure.

Familial emphysema is characterized by early onset of severe and fatal obstructive lung disease. Absence of α_1-antitrypsin, an enzyme normally present in the α_1-globulin portion of blood, leads to excessive breakdown of the structural lung proteins. At the present time, it is not known that this enzyme is depressed in those animals with emphysema secondary to nitrogen dioxide inhalation.

There is still the possibility that low concentrations of nitrogen dioxide profoundly affect at least one of the many enzymes concerned with collagen and elastin metabolism. For example, the enzyme aldolase, whose activity is affected by nitrogen dioxide inhalation, has been implicated in various cross-linking reactions with collagen. Milch[20] has identified certain monoaldehyde compounds that are remarkably similar to the type produced by aldolase. These compounds cause changes in collagen that are similar to those found in degenerative connective tissue diseases or aging.

Though the concentration of nitrogen dioxide in ambient air is quite low, carbon particles inhaled with the gas could act as a carrier mechanism and exaggerate the effects of nitrogen dioxide[5,6,21] by permitting high local concentrations of the gas to occur within the lung.

In short, research indicates that nitrogen dioxide exposure causes enzymatic modifications, cell membrane alteration, and changes in the conformation of collagen and elastin. The exact mechanism of its effect on lung properties has not yet been elucidated, but it is probably a combination of the aforementioned systems.

Biochemical Effects and Implications of Ozone Toxicity

Ozone has been shown to lower resistance to respiratory bacterial infection, weaken lung structure, reduce pulmonary function, and disrupt cellular biochemistry. It has also been implicated as an accelerator for the aging process, as well as a radiomimetic agent.

Biochemical studies have indicated that ozone may affect both fixed tissue elements and pulmonary surfactant. Buell et al[22,23] exposed rabbits to 1,960μg/cu m (1 ppm) and 9,800μg/cu m (5 ppm) ozone for one hour and then analyzed hydrolyzed lung protein for the presence of carbonyl compounds. Positive identification of carbonyl compounds indicated the possible occurrence of structural changes in lung tissue. Similar effects were still noted 24 hours after exposure indicating nonreversibility of the process within that period of time. The authors postulated that this effect may occur with collagen and elastin and result in decreased flexibility of lung tissue.

Ozone has been demonstrated to interfere with biochemical entities associated with the normal protective mechanisms of the lung. Holzman et al[24] found a reduction in active lysozyme obtained by bronchopulmonary lavage from animals exposed to ozone and theorized that the loss of lysozyme activity was due to the in vivo oxidation of lysozyme. Coffin et al[25] have demonstrated a decrease in the phagocytic activity of pulmonary cells following ozone inhalation by rabbits which may be associated with metabolic disturbances in the macrophage.

Using a unilateral lung preparation, Frank et al[26] exposed rabbits to 4,300μg/cu m to 23,500μg/cu m (2.2 to 12.1 ppm) ozone for three hours and observed that an edematous change in the exposed right lung resulted in altered surfactant properties in the unexposed left lung. This experiment suggests that products of ozone exposure may prove deleterious to unexposed tissue or cause a compensatory response by the exposed subject—a pertinent suggestion relative to ozone's effect at the cellular level as evidenced by effects similar to radiation damage.[27-29] The studies of Goldstein et al[30-32] suggest that ozone affects red blood cells (RBC) via ozonolysis or lipid peroxidation resulting from the products of ozonolysis.

Brinkman et al[27] found that inhalation of 390μg/cu m to 490μg/cu m (0.20 to 0.25 ppm) ozone for 30 to 60 minutes may accelerate the aging of RBC. Studies utilizing techniques relative to the biochemistry of aging should prove useful when applied to the study of ozone and oxidant toxicology.

Ozone has also affected other nonpulmonary tissues such as the cell membranes and nuclei of myocardial muscle fibers,[27] brain serotonin levels,[33] liver DNA:RNA ratios,[34] and alkaline phosphatase.[35] The mechanisms producing such alterations are yet to be elucidated.

More definitive biochemistry is also required to validate, explain, and quantitate the reported effects of ozone relative to lung tumor acceleration,[36] aging,[27,37-39] and the tolerance phenomena.[39-43]

Biochemical Effects and Implications of Oxidants

The study of oxidants has usually involved photochemical smog either naturally occurring or synthetically produced in the laboratory. In all cases, the primary oxidizing compounds are ozone and NO_2. Biochemical studies have been limited but will be necessary to determine whether the factors demonstrated to be affected by ozone and NO_2 as single entities are similarly affected by the combination. Indirect biochemical effects on fertility and neonatal mortality have been demonstrated by Hueter et al[44] and Lewis et al,[45] while stress effects have been reported by Harvey and Maxfield,[46] and Hueter et al.[44]

It is interesting to note that Sapse et al[47] reported a decrease in human tear lysozyme in subjects experiencing eye irritation from photochemical smog. This effect may be similar to the inactivation of lung lysozyme reported by Holzman et al.[24]

Air Pollution Health Effects Research

A number of studies have provided clues about biochemical alterations resulting from animal exposures to oxidant type air pollutants. There is a need for expanded research concerning normal biochemistry of the mammalian lung in order to interpret and interrelate air pollution health effects studies more intelligently.

Any research on air pollution health effects, biochemical or otherwise, should consider the following total approach.

Initial health effects research for any pollutant requires the qualitative and quantitative identification of the prime effect. This effect is usually identified via an extreme exposure and must be subsequently verified as the result of long-term low level exposures, ie, dose:time effects research. A pollutant rarely exists as a single discrete entity. Consequently, the identified effects must be studied in relation to the interaction of other components of the total milieu. Such information provides a firm basis for initiating meaningful air quality standards. Subsequent modification of such standards will then be based upon additional research that identifies other environmental factors, eg, temperature and humidity, as potentiators or attenuators of known effects. Research related to identifying susceptible populations determined by age, existing disease, stress, etc, may also dictate the need for modifying established standards.

Identification and interpretation of health effects requires input from the integration of three scientific approaches: (1) laboratory animal toxicological studies, (2) laboratory clinical investigations of human subjects, and (3) epidemiological studies under naturally occurring conditions. Animal toxicology research is needed to identify prime effects via controlled experimental designs that minimize confounding environmental variables normally existing under field conditions. Such studies also allow for the use of exposure concentrations unsuitable for human studies due to ethical and medicolegal limitations. Animal toxicology allows for in vitro and manipulative approaches, which produce techniques for subsequent application to clinical and epidemiological investigations. Laboratory clinical investigations on human subjects are used to test techniques developed by animal toxicology and to verify, in a cause and effect manner under controlled conditions, correlative epidemiological results. The final test of any indicated effect is its expression in human populations exposed to ambient pollution as measured by sensitive epidemiological techniques. Such field studies are the proving grounds for all laboratory research. In addition, epidemiological results provide an important input toward designating the direction of laboratory animal and human clinical experimentation. Thus, this triphasic, integrated research effort is deemed essential for the most expeditious obtainment of meaningful health effects information.

References

1. Gray ELeB: Oxides of nitrogen: Their occurrence, toxicity, hazard. *Arch Industr Health* **19**:479-486, 1959.

2. McAdams A Jr: Bronchiolitis obliterans. *Amer J Med* **19**:314-322, 1955.

3. Blair WH, Henry MC, Ehrlich R: Chronic toxicity of NO_2: II. Effect on histopathology of lung tissue. *Arch Environ Health* **18**:186-192, 1969.

4. Freeman G, Crane SC, Stephens RJ, et al: Environmental factors in emphysema and a model system with NO_2. *Yale J Biol Med* **40**:566-575, 1968.

5. Freeman G, Stephens RJ, Crane SC, et al: Lesions of the lung in rats exposed to 2 ppm of NO_2. *Arch Environ Health* **17**:181-192, 1968.

6. Freeman G, Crane SC, Stephens RJ, et al: Pathogenesis of the NO_2-induced lesion in the rat lung: A review and presentation of new observations. *Amer Rev Resp Dis* **98**:429-443, 1968.

7. Gray ELeB, Palton FM, Goldberg SB, et al: Toxicity of the oxides of nitrogen: II. Acute inhalation toxicity of NO_2, red fuming nitric acid, and white fuming nitric acid. *Arch Industr Hyg* **10**:418-425, 1954.

8. Buckley RD, Balchum OJ: Acute and chronic exposures to NO_2. *Arch Environ Health* **10**:220-223, 1965.

9. Buckley RD, Balchum OJ: Effects of NO_2 on LDH isoenzymes. *Arch Environ Health* **14**:424-428, 1967.

10. Scheel LD, Dobragorski OJ, Mountain JT, et al: Physiologic, biochemical, immunologic, and pathologic changes following ozone exposure. *J Appl Physiol* **14**:67-72, 1959.

11. Buckley RD, Balchum OJ: Enzyme alterations following NO_2 exposure. *Arch Environ Health* **14**:687-692, 1967.

12. Sherwin RP, Winnick S, Buckley RD: Response of LDH-positive alveolar cells in the lungs of guinea pigs exposed to nitrogen dioxide. *Amer Rev Resp Dis* **96**:319-323, 1967.

13. Buckley RD, Loosli CG: Effects of NO_2 inhalation on germfree mouse lung. *Arch Environ Health* **18**:588-595, 1969.

14. Rounds DE, Bils RF: Effects of air pollutants on cells in culture. *Arch Environ Health* **10**:251-259, 1965.

15. Felmeister A, Amanat M, Weiner ND: Interaction of NO_2-olefin gas mixtures with lecithin monomolecular films. *Environ Sci Techn* **2**:40-43, 1968.

16. Weiner ND, Amanat M, Felmeister A: Monomolecular films as a model to study air pollutant-membrane interactions. *Arch Environ Health* **18**:636-640, 1969.

17. Thomas H: Lipoperoxidation of lung lipids in rats exposed to NO_2. *Science* **159**:532-536, 1968.

18. Buell G: Lung collagen and elastin denaturation in vivo following inhalation of NO_2, abstracted. *Program of the Section on Biological Effects at the 59th annual meeting of the Air Pollution Control Association*, San Francisco, 1966.

19. Patty FA, Sterner JH: *Industrial Hygiene and Toxicology*. New York, Interscience Publishers Inc, 1967, vol 2, p 921.

20. Milch RA: Possible role of aldehyde metabolites in the aging processes of connective tissue. *South Med J* **58**:153-156, 1965.

21. Boren HG: Carbon as a carrier mechanism for irritant gases. *Arch Environ Health* **8**:119-124, 1963.

22. Buell GC, Tokiwa Y, Mueller PK: Potential crosslinking agents in lung tissue: Formation and isolation after in vivo exposure to ozone. *Arch Environ Health* **10**:213-219, 1969.

23. Buell GC, Jeung E, Fenninger W: Chemical changes in respiratory tissue following ozone exposure. Read before West Coast Section Air Pollution Control Association, Monterey, Calif, 1963.

24. Holzman RS, Gardner DE, Coffin DL: In vivo inactivation of lysozyme by ozone. *J Bacteriol* **96**:1562-1566, 1968.

25. Coffin DL, Gardner DE, Holzman RS, et al: Influence of ozone on pulmonary cells. *Arch Environ Health* **16**:633-636, 1968.

26. Frank NR, Brain JD, Sherry DE: Unilateral lung exposure to ozone. *Fed Proc* **27**:279, 1968.

27. Brinkman R, Lamberts HB, Venings TS: Radiomimetic toxicity of ozonized air. *Lancet* **1**:133-136, 1964.

28. Fetner RH: Ozone-induced chromosome breakage in human cell cultures. *Nature* **194**:793-794, 1962.

29. Brinkman R, Lamberts HB: Ozone as a possible radiomimetic gas. *Nature* **181**:1202-1203, 1958.

30. Goldstein BD, Balchum OJ: Effect of ozone on lipid peroxidation in the red blood cell. *Proc Soc Exp Biol Med* **126**:356-358, 1967.

31. Goldstein BD, Pearson B, Lodi C, et al: The effect of ozone and mouse blood in vivo. *Arch Environ Health* **16**:648-650, 1968.

32. Goldstein BD, Lodi C, Collinson C, et al: Ozone and lipid peroxidation. *Arch Environ Health* **18**:631-635, 1969.

33. Skillen RG: Brain 5-hydroxytryptamine in ozone-exposed rats. *Proc Soc Exp Biol Med* **108**:121-122, 1961.

34. Scheel LD: Physiologic, biochemical, immunologic and pathologic changes following ozone exposure. *J Appl Physiol* **14**:67-80, 1959.

35. Murphy SD, Davis HV, Zaratzian VL: Biochemical effects in rats from irritating air contaminants. *Toxic Appl Pharmacol* **6**(5):520-528, 1964.

36. Stokinger HG: Effects of air pollution on animals, in Stern AC (ed): *Air Pollution*. New York, Academic Press Inc, 1962, vol 1, pp 282-334.

37. Bjorksten J: Aging: Primary mechanism. *Gerontologia* **8**:179-192, 1963.

38. Bjorksten J, Andrews F: Chemical mechanisms underlying the biological mechanisms of the aging process. *J Amer Geriat Soc* **12**:627-631, 1964.

39. Stokinger HE: Ozone toxicology: A review of research and industrial experience: 1954-1964. *Arch Environ Health* **10**:719-741, 1965.

40. Coffin DL: Effect of air pollution on alteration to susceptibility to pulmonary infection. Read before the Third Annual Conference on Atmospheric Contamination in Confined Spaces, Dayton, Ohio, 1967.

41. Pace DM, Landolt PA, Aftonomos BT: Effects of ozone on cells in vitro. *Arch Environ Health* **18**:165-170, 1969.

42. Henschler D: Reactions of the lung to repeated and long-term exposures to respiratory irritants. Read before the Gordon Research Conference on Toxicology, Meriden, NH, 1962.

43. Henschler D: Mechanism of tolerance increase during repeated inhalation of lung-node-producing gases. *Arch Exp Pathol Pharmakol* **249**:343-356, 1964.

44. Hueter FG, Contner GL, Busch KA, et al: Biological effects of atmospheres contaminated by auto exhaust. *Arch Environ Health* **12**:553-560, 1966.

45. Lewis TR, Hueter FG, Busch KA: Irradiated automobile exhaust: Its effects on the reproduction of mice. *Arch Environ Health* **15**(1):26-35, 1967.

46. Harvey H, Maxfield M: *Biologic Response of Animals Exposed to Urban Atmospheres Characterized by Automotive Emissions in the Los Angeles Area.* Berkeley, California State Dept of Public Health, 1961.

47. Sapse AT, Bonavida B, Stone W Jr, et al: Human tear lysozyme: III. Preliminary study on lysozyme levels in subjects with smog eye irritation. *Amer J Ophthal* **66**:76-80, 1968.

Oxygen Effect on Lung Cells

Ewald R. Weibel, MD, Bern, Switzerland

Breathing pure oxygen at one atmosphere leads to primary destruction of alveolar capillary endothelial cells; squamous epithelial cells are damaged secondarily, whereas granular pneumocytes are found to regenerate a cuboidal epithelium lining and air spaces. Interstitial and alveolar edema ensue as a consequence of permeability changes in the cell layers. The role of hematological changes in the development of pulmonary oxygen toxicity is discussed.

It has long been known that breathing higher partial pressures of oxygen results in lung abnormality which is ascribed to a toxic effect of oxygen on lung tissue.[1] Best known are the development of interstitial and alveolar edema when breathing pure oxygen at atmospheric pressure. On the other hand, as it is well known that high oxygen pressures can damage cells by either inhibiting enzyme functions or by peroxidation of lipids,[2] it appears likely that the lung abnormality observed is a result of cell damage in alveolar epithelium and capillary endothelium, those cells which are directly exposed to the oxygen-rich atmosphere. We have been engaged during the past years in a series of studies with the aim to elucidate what oxygen does to lung cells. The following shall be a summary of our present state of knowledge.

Received for publication Jan 29, 1971; accepted Feb 1.

From the Department of Anatomy, University of Berne, Switzerland.

Read in part before the Tenth Annual Hanford Biology Symposium on Pollution and Lung Biochemistry, Richland, Wash, June 4, 1970, jointly sponsored by the Battelle Memorial Institute-Pacific Northwest Laboratories, National Air Pollution Control Administration, National Institute of Environmental Health Sciences, and the US Atomic Energy Commission.

Reprint requests to Anatomisches Institut, Bühlstrasse 26, 3000 Bern, Switzerland (Dr. Weibel).

Destruction of Capillary Endothelium.—If rats are brought into pure oxygen at 1 atmosphere they will do rather well for two days, but their health will deteriorate during the third day: they may gradually turn cyanotic, develop dyspnea, and become lethargic. Most strains will not survive for much more than 72 hours: they die of suffocation.

A study of these lungs by electron microscopy[3] has shown that these rats had developed interstitial edema already at 48 hours, which was further aggravated after 72 hours. Fixation of such lungs by vascular perfusion[4] revealed also the development of alveolar edema. By morphometric analysis it was found that the air-blood barrier became significantly thickened (Fig 1), and that the capillary volume was greatly reduced. From this it was estimated that diffusion capacity must have dropped to 10% to 20% of the control value.[3]

The cytological changes observed were peculiar: the damage seemed to be much more pronounced in the endothelial than in the epithelial cells. Figure 1 reveals that, at 72 hours, the mean thickness of the endothelium was reduced to about 60% of its control value. This could be explained by massive destruction of endothelial cells which underwent cytoplasmic condensation or vacuolation as well as fragmentation, cellular changes which were quite evident in electron micrographs.[3] This also explained the reduction of capillary volume and gave a clue for the formation of interstitial edema: the destroyed endothelium would allow plasma to leak out into the tissue.

Epithelial Destruction and Proliferation.—It was surprising to find that the epithelial layer showed little signs of cellular damage; morphometry even indicated that its mean thickness had increased to 160% of its control value after 72 hours of oxygen breathing (Fig 1). Nevertheless, this epithelium could be expected to be leaky because of the occurrence of alveolar edema.[3]

This apparently paradoxical finding found its explanation when the effect of pure O_2 breathing on the monkey lung was studied.[5] The monkey survives oxygen toxic changes for almost two weeks.[6] Initially, it is again the capillary endothelium which undergoes destruction.[5] But secondarily, between the second and fourth day, the epithelial lining also disappears over vast areas of the alveolar surface. Indeed, after seven days the entire alveolar surface is pathologically altered. At this time we note a peculiar change: the occurrence of a large number of cuboidal cells; and after 12 days of pure oxygen breathing the entire alveolar surface is lined by a cuboidal epithelium,[5,6] a finding which has also been described for the human lung in oxygen poisoning.[7] What has happened?

The alveolar epithelium consists of two cell types: the squamous pneumocytes (type I) resemble endothelial cells and normally line the major part of the alveolar surface with thin cytoplasmic extensions; the cuboidal granular pneumocytes (type II) are

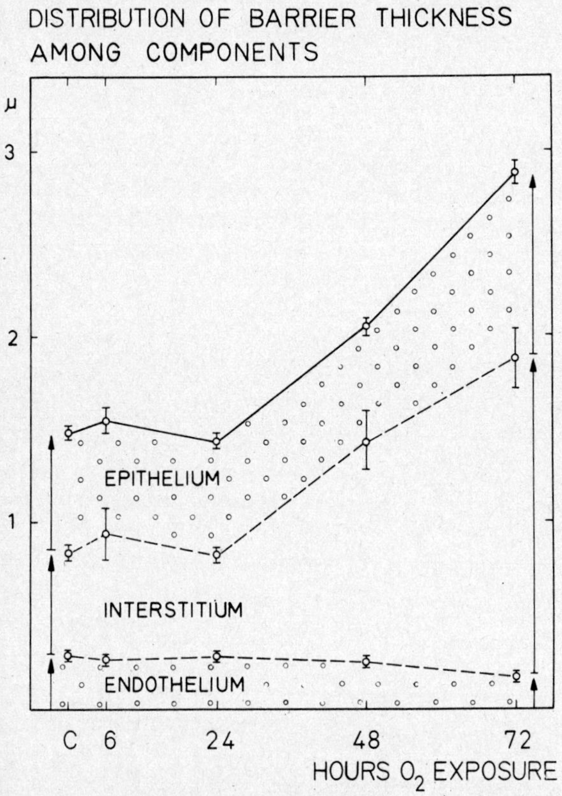

Fig 1.—Change in average thickness τ of air-blood barrier in rats breathing pure oxygen for up to 72 hours. Subdivision of barrier into epithelium, interstitium, and endothelium.

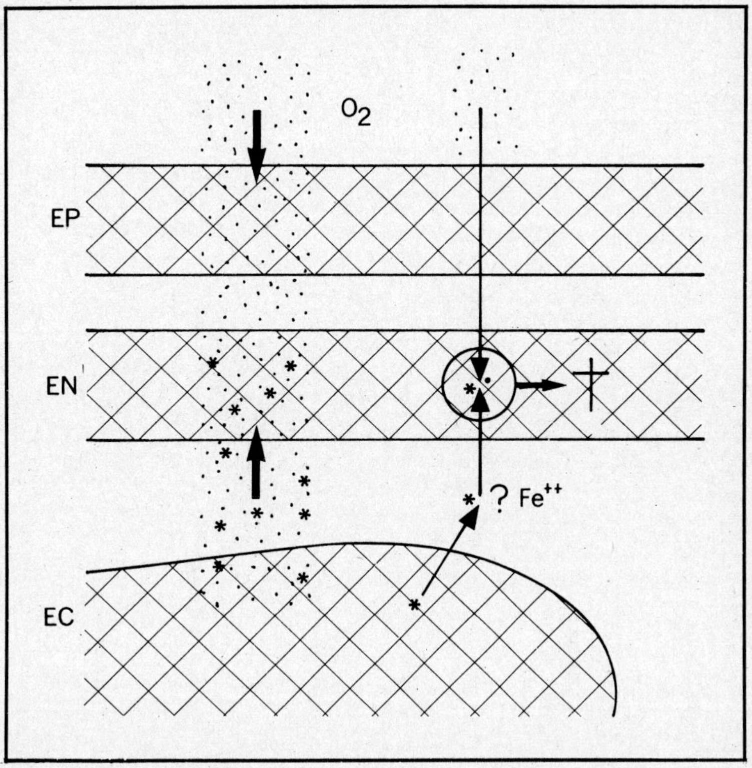

Fig 2.—Possible way of interaction of O_2 and additional factors originating from hemolysed erythrocytes (EC) in endothelial cells (EN).

interspersed in the epithelium and are thought to be responsible for secreting surfactant.[4] Oxygen has apparently destroyed the squamous cells, whereas the granular pneumocytes survive and can regenerate an epithelial lining by mitotic division and multiplication.[5,6] Practically all cells of the cuboidal epithelium in monkeys that survived oxygen breathing for 12 days contained some lamellated bodies, the characteristic granules of the granular pneumocyte.[5]

The reason for this different effect of oxygen on the two epithelial cell types may reside in their different cytological differentiation. The granular pneumocyte is rich in organelles, particularly in mitochondria, and has a well developed endoplasmic reticulum. If high oxygen partial pressures cause damage to some cell constituents, especially to membranes, these are likely to be rapidly repaired. Indeed, protracted application of high levels of oxygen leads to alterations in the organelles of the type II cell[8] which appear compatible with increased anabolic function. In contrast, the squamous cell is rather

Fig 3.—Effect of oxygen breathing on osmotic fragility of erythrocytes in vitamin E-deficient rats (TD). Shaded area indicates range of hemolysis curves in normal rats exposed to oxygen for 24 to 48 hours.

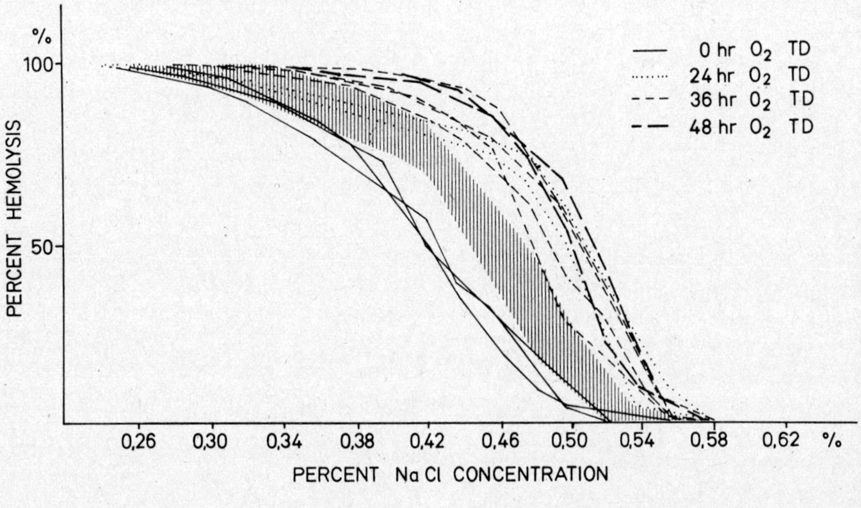

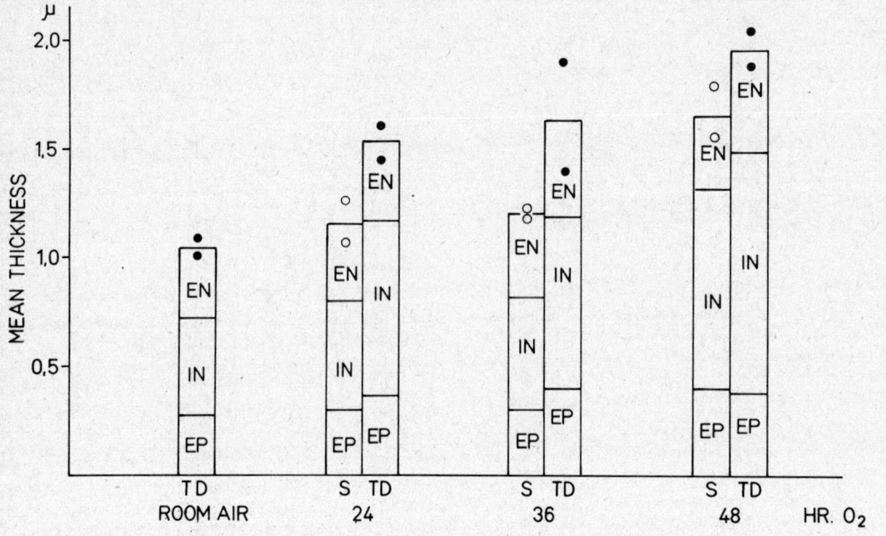

Fig 4.—Change in thickness of air-blood barrier and its composition in terms of epithelium (EP), interstitium (IN), and endothelium (EN) in tocopherol-deficient rats (TD) as compared to normal rats (S) exposed to pure oxygen for 24 to 48 hours. Compare with Fig 1.

poor in organelles. Its vast cytoplasmic extensions consist only of cell membranes and a little cytoplasmic matrix; endoplasmic reticulum elements are exceedingly rare. Membrane deterioration due, eg, to peroxidation of lipids, therefore, cannot be repaired easily and rapidly; destruction of the thin cytoplasmic laminae may ensue.

Possible Mechanism of Cellular Damage.—It was most puzzling to find that endothelial cells were first to be damaged by high oxygen tensions in the air, and not the epithelial cells although the latter were directly exposed to the toxic environment. This led to the hypothesis that "additional factors" were necessary for oxygen to become toxic and that these were supplied by the blood as shown in Fig 2.[3] It had been shown that enzyme inhibition and lipid peroxidation by oxygen depends on the presence of heavy metal compounds.[2] On the other hand, red blood cells were known to be hemolysed by increased oxygen tensions.[9] This led us to suspect a close correlation between hematological and pulmonary changes in oxygen poisoning.

As a first step towards elucidation of this problem we have studied the correlation between blood and lung changes in vitamin E (α-tocopherol)-deficient rats.[11] Vitamin E deficiency was known to greatly increase sensitivity of erythrocytes to oxygen.[10] As shown in Fig 3 osmotic fragility of red blood cells of tocopherol-deficient rats increases drastically after only 12 hours of pure oxygen breathing. Thickening of the air-blood barrier due to interstitial edema formation occurred already after 24 hours (Fig 4), whereas it takes at least 48 hours for the first signs of pulmonary changes to occur in normal rats (Fig 1 and 4).

These preliminary studies merely show that there is a close correlation between erythrocytic and pulmonary oxygen toxicity, but it will need further studies to elucidate the role played by the blood in the development of a primary cellular damage in the alveolar capillary endothelium, a damage which eventually leads to vast destruction of the gas exchange function to an extent incompatible with life.

These studies have been supported by contracts with the 6,570th Aerospace Medical Research Laboratories, Air Force Systems Command, Wright-Patterson Air Force Base, Ohio, through the European Office of Aerospace Research and by grant 3-5-68 from the Swiss National Foundation. Dr. Carmen Conradi aided in this investigation.

References

1. Bean JW: Effects of oxygen at increased pressures. *Physiol Rev* **25**:1, 1945.

2. Davies HC, Davies RE: Biochemical aspects of oxygen poisoning, in Fenn WO, Rahn H (eds): *Handbook of Physiology.* Washington, DC, American Physiological Society, 1965, vol 2, p 1047.

3. Kistler GS, Caldwell PRB, Weibel ER: Development of fine structural damage to alveolar and capillary lining cells in oxygen-poisoned rat lungs. *J Cell Biol* **32**:605, 1967.

4. Gil J, Weibel ER: Improvements in demonstration of lining layer of lung alveoli by electron microscopy. *Resp Physiol* **8**:13, 1969.

5. Kapanci Y, Weibel ER, Kaplan HP, et al: Pathogenesis and reversibility of the pulmonary lesions of oxygen toxicity in monkeys: II. Ultrastructural and morphometric studies. *Lab Invest* **20**:101, 1969.

6. Kaplan HP, Robinson FR, Kapanci Y, et al: Pathogenesis and reversibility of pulmonary lesions of oxygen toxicity in monkeys: I. Clinical and light microscopic studies. *Lab Invest* **20**:94, 1969.

7. Nash G, Blennerhasset JB, Pontoppidan H: Pulmonary lesions associated with oxygen therapy and artificial ventilation. *New Eng J Med* **276**:368, 1967.

8. Rosenbaum RM, Wittner M, Lenger M: Mitochondrial and other ultrastructural changes in great alveolar cells of oxygen-adapted and poisoned rats. *Lab Invest* **20**:516, 1969.

9. Kann HE, Mengel ChE, Clancy WT, et al: Effects of in vivo hyperoxia on erythrocytes: VI. Hemolysis occurring after exposure to oxygen under high pressure. *J Lab Clin Med* **70**:150, 1967.

10. Jacob HS, Lux SE: Degradation of membrane phospholipids and thiols in peroxide hemolysis: Studies in vitamin E deficiency. *Blood* **32**:4, 1968.

11. Weibel ER, Conradi C: Pulmonary pathology of oxygen toxicity, in *Proceedings of the Fifth Annual Conference on Atmospheric Contaminations in Confined Spaces.* Wright-Patterson AFB, Ohio, Aerospace Medical Research Laboratories, 1969, p 227.

Effects of Nitrogen Dioxide on Cell Renewal in the Rat Lung

Michael J. Evans, PhD; Robert J. Stephens, PhD; and Gustave Freeman, MD, Menlo Park, Calif

In order to determine the effects of continuous exposure to 17 ± 2 ppm NO_2 in air on cell renewal in bronchiolar and alveolar cells, young rats were exposed continuously for as long as seven days, removed at intervals, and killed. One hour before the killings, dividing cells were labeled with tritiated thymidine. In terminal bronchioles, labeling index increased fourfold, the mathe first 24 hours. The index decreased slowly and by seven days had returned to the original level. In the alveolar walls, the labeling index increased fourfold, the majority being labeled type II cells. Here, too, the labeling indexes had returned to control levels by the seventh day. Cell renewal, thus, is initially stimulated by NO_2 and then returns to control levels.

Effects of subacute concentrations of atmospheric nitrogen dioxide on mammalian tissues, particularly on the lungs, have been studied for several years.[1] Studies have shown that such levels of NO_2 can significantly alter the morphology, physiology, and biochemistry of cells and tissues. Of particular importance are changes in the lungs which may be associated with pulmonary emphysema.[2]

The purpose of this study was to determine the effects of NO_2 on cell renewal (as measured by changes in the labeling index) in the terminal bronchioles and alveoli of rats. To accomplish this we exposed rats to NO_2 and then labeled cells which were preparing to divide with tritiated thymidine. Such labeled cells were visualized and counted in the light microscope by the use of autoradiography and the results expressed as a labeling index. The preliminary results are reported here.

Received for publication Oct 21, 1970; accepted March 5, 1971.

From the Life Sciences Division, Stanford Research Institute, Menlo Park, Calif.

Read in part before the Tenth Annual Hanford Biology Symposium on Pollution and Lung Biochemistry, Richland, Wash, June 5, 1970, jointly sponsored by the Battelle Memorial Institute-Pacific Northwest Laboratories, National Air Pollution Control Administration, National Institute of Environmental Health Sciences, and the US Atomic Energy Commission.

Reprint requests to Stanford Research Institute, 333 Ravenswood Ave, Menlo Park, Calif 94025 (Dr. Evans).

Materials and Methods

Young male rats (Wistar), weighing about 100 gm, were exposed continuously to NO_2 (17 ± 2 parts per million [ppm]) in exposure chambers described in a previous report.[3] A group of equivalent rats maintained at ambient conditions served as controls.

At intervals, after 6, 24, 48, 72, and 168 hours of exposure, rats were removed from the chambers, injected intraperitoneally with 300 microcuries of tritiated thymidine (specific activity 6.7 curies/millimol) and killed 1 hour later with pentobarbital (Nembutal) sodium. The intact lungs and trachea were then removed together from the thoracic cavity and the left main bronchus was ligated at the bifurcation near the trachea. Fixative (1% osmium tetroxide buffered with veronal acetate and containing 7.8% sucrose) was gently perfused into the airways of the left lung through a 22-gauge needle inserted into the main bronchus distal to the ligature. After the lung was filled with fixative, a ligature was placed near the hilus and the main bronchus severed between the ligatures. The lung was then placed in a vial of the same fixative for one hour.

Following fixation in OsO_4, the lung was sliced longitudinally into thin (1 mm) leaf-like pieces, dehydrated in alcohol, and infiltrated with resin (Araldite). The infiltrated slices of tissue were examined with a dissecting microscope and small squares of tissue, each containing a longitudinal section of a terminal bronchiole with its alveolar ducts and adjacent alveoli, were removed. The small squares were then embedded in resin. This preparation of terminal bronchioles was previously described by Freeman et al.[4]

The remaining lung was fixed by perfusing Zenker's solution through the trachea. Following fixation it was embedded in paraffin, and 6μ sections were stained with hematoxylin-eosin. Mitotic figures were counted in the areas used for determining labeling indexes as described below.

For autoradiography, 1μ sections were cut from the resin-embedded specimens with a glass knife on an ultramicrotome (Porter-Blum MT-II) and then mounted on glass slides dubbed with a solution of 0.1% gelatin containing 0.01% chromic potassium sulfate. The mounted slides were then coated with a 1:1 dilution of nuclear emulsion (Ilford L-4) and stored in light-tight boxes at 0 to 4 C. After three weeks they were developed in a 13.5% developing agent (Microdol X) for five minutes, rinsed in distilled water, fixed in 15% sodium thiosulfate for five minutes, and washed for ten minutes. The tissues were stained with toluidine blue, rinsed in alcohol, and dried and a cover slip was mounted on them.

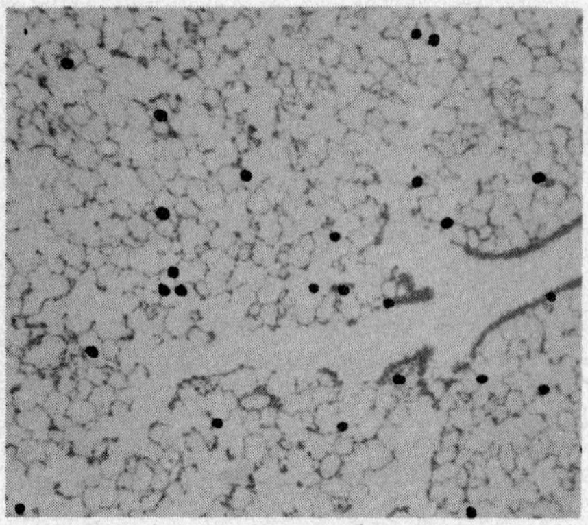

Fig 1.—Distribution of labeled cells in a control animal. Each black dot represents where a labeled cell was observed (×55).

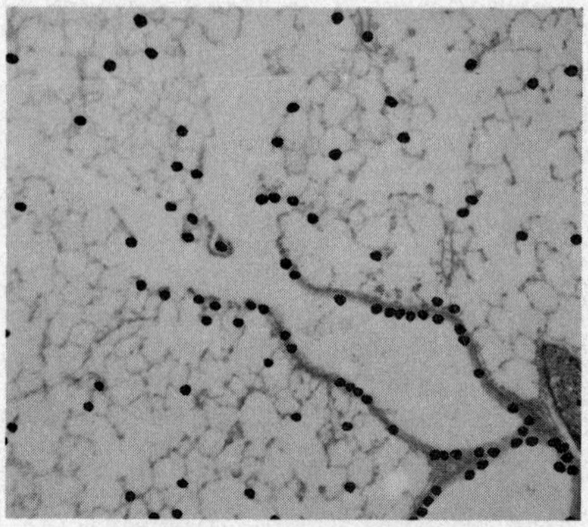

Fig 2.—Distribution of labeled cells in an animal exposed to 17 ppm NO_2 for 24 hours. Each black dot represents where a labeled cell was observed. Note the increased labeling of the terminal bronchiole (×55).

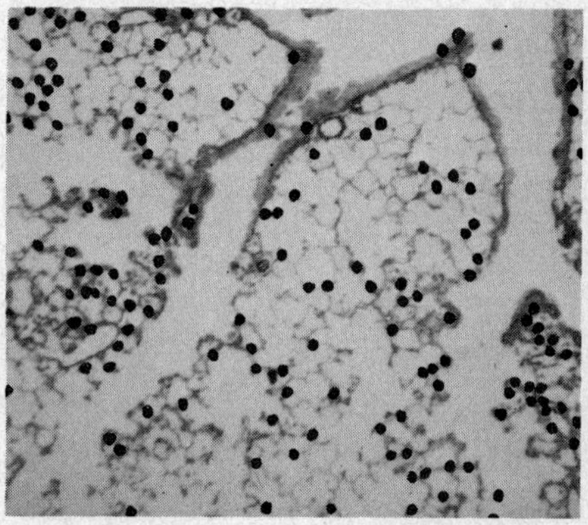

Fig 3.—Distribution of labeled cells in an animal exposed to 17 ppm NO_2 for 72 hours. Each black dot represents where a labeled cell was observed. Note the lack of labeling in the terminal bronchioles and the increased labeling in the alveoli (×55).

Cells that had incorporated tritiated thymidine into their nuclei (labeled cells) were counted and expressed as a percentage of the total cell population (labeling index). Two areas of tissue were studied, terminal bronchioles and alveoli. In the former, the percentage of labeled, ciliated, and nonciliated cells together was determined from the total of all cells from ten different terminal bronchioles. In the alveoli, the percentages of labeled type II cells, alveolar macrophages, and other labeled cells of the alveolar walls were determined from all the cells counted in ten different specimens. Approximately 200 cells were counted in each specimen. Cells of the adventia around the bronchioles and large vessels were excluded.

Results

General Observations.—Several publications have previously appeared describing the morphological changes in rats chronically exposed to subacute concentrations of NO_2 (Freeman et al[1]). More recently, the early lesion has been reported by Freeman[5] and R.J. Stephens, PhD, et al (unpublished data) and the data agrees with the current observations made on young rats exposed to 17 ± 2 ppm NO_2 for up to seven days. The epithelium in the normal terminal bronchiole is irregular, the nonciliated cell protruding into the lumen above the ciliated cells. By 24 hours after exposure this irregularity had substantially disappeared, presenting a smooth profile and in addition there was a marked loss of cilia. Some piling up of cells in isolated areas along the terminal bronchioles was noted after 48 to 72 hours of exposure; mitotic figures were numerous and an increase in the nonciliated cells was evident. More peripheral regions are less noticeably affected, however. Animals receiving tritiated thymidine one hour after being killed showed a marked increase in the number of cells labeled even after as little as 24 hours exposure to NO_2. The data shows that the greatest increase was observed in the nonciliated cells of the terminal bronchiole and the type II alveolar epithelial cells although a more modest increase was also evident in other cell types.

Fig 4.—Labeling index of cells in the terminal bronchioles during exposure to 17 ppm NO_2.

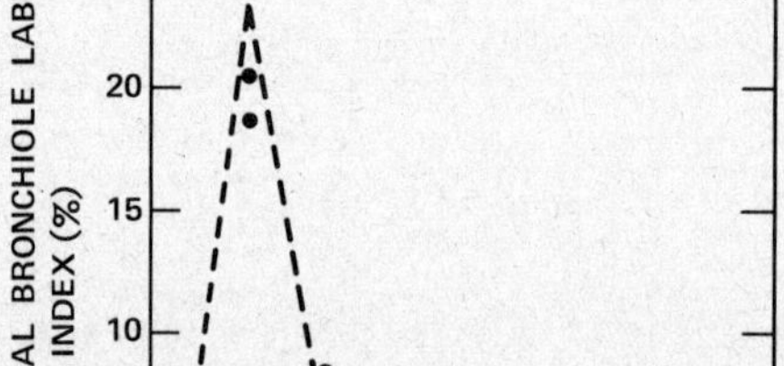

Terminal Bronchiolar Labeling Index.—The distribution of labeled cells in the terminal bronchioles and alveoli are shown after 0, 24, and 72 hours of exposure in Fig 1, 2, and 3, respectively. These animals received a single injection of tritiated thymidine one hour before being killed. Data accumulated from numerous sections of this type was used to establish the labeling index graph for the terminal bronchioles (Fig 4). In the terminal bronchiole the values represent both ciliated and nonciliated cells.

Control groups had a mean labeling index of 1.1% ± 0.7%. After 24 hours of exposure, the index had increased to 23.5%, the increase being due almost entirely to labeling of noncilliated cells (Fig 5). Ciliated-

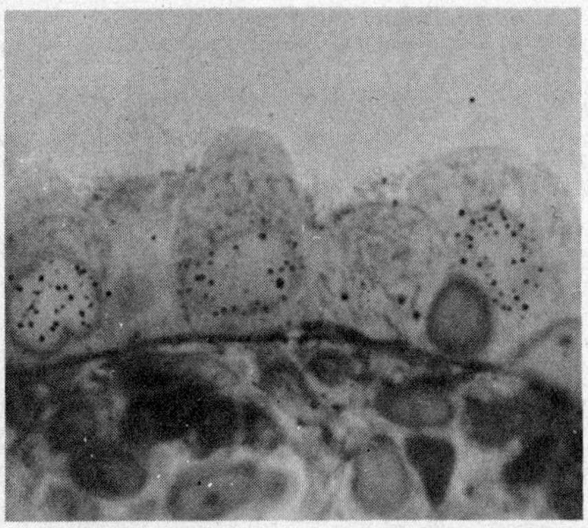

Fig 5.—Labeled nonciliated cells in the terminal bronchiole after 24 hours exposure to 17 ppm NO_2 (×1,250).

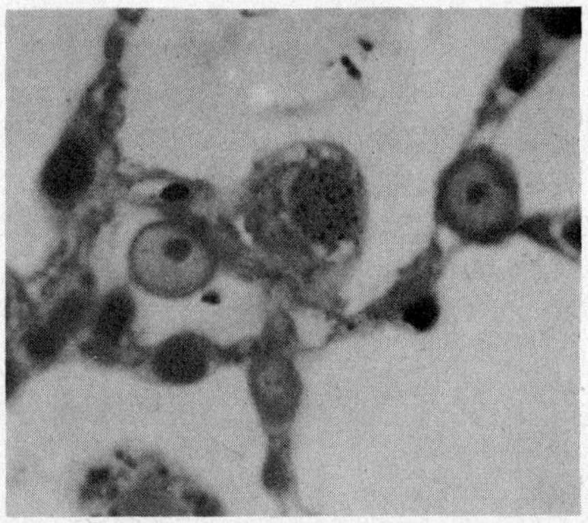

Fig 6.—Labeled type II alevolar cell after 48 hours exposure to 17 ppm NO_2 (×1,250).

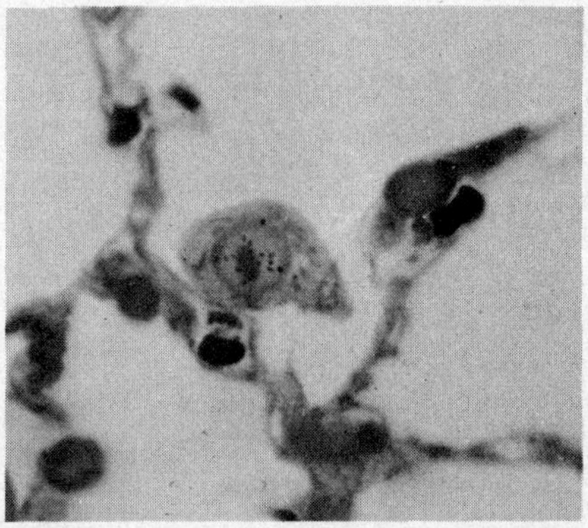

Fig 7.—Labeled alveolar macrophage after 48 hours exposure to 17 ppm NO_2 (×1,250).

type cells that had lost cilia could be recognized by the persistence of the ciliary basal bodies but it is conceivable that an occasional deciliated cell may have changed enough morphologically to have been classified as a nonciliated cell. After 48 and 72 hours of exposure, the mean labeling indexes fell to 6.4% and 5.0%, respectively, levels still considerably higher than control values. After 168 hours of continuous exposure, however, the labeling index had returned to the preexposure values (1.2%). Corresponding in time to the rise in cell labeling, there was a considerable increase in mitosis by 24 hours which gradually returned to the approximate initial level during the 168 hours of continuous exposure.

Alveolar Labeling Index.—Control animals had a random distribution of labeled alveolar cells. Animals exposed to NO_2 generally showed more labeled alveolar cells in the region of the terminal bronchiole and alveolar duct than in the more distal alveolar areas. Therefore, proximal alveolar areas were avoided in the determination of the alveolar labeling index. Figures 1, 2, and 3 illustrate the distribution of labeled cells in alveoli.

The total number of alveolar cells labeled with tritiated thymidine during exposure increased from a control mean of 2.1% ± 0.7% to 4.7% after 24 hours, to 6.3% after 48 hours, and to 4.8% after 72 hours, and then decreased to 1.8% after 168 hours of exposure. Labeled cells were classified into three groups, type II cells (Fig 6), alveolar macrophages (Fig 7), and cells of the alveolar walls (Fig 8). The major increase in labeling took place in type II cells (Fig 9), although increased labeling in macrophages contributed. The increase in cell labeling was accompanied by an increased number of mitosis in type II alveolar cells.

The labeling indexes of cells in the alveolar walls remained about the same as control values (Fig 10), although there was a slight increase due to more labeled type I cells.

Comment

It is generally considered that cells of the pulmonary alveoli constitute a renewing cell population.[6,7] In a renewing cell population cell division takes place but because some cells are sloughed off, there is no net increase in the total number of cells. The purpose of a renewing cell population is to maintain the integrity of a tissue by acting as a source of new cells, eg, bone marrow and intestine.[8]

Fig 8.—Labeled cell in the alveolar wall after 24 hours exposure to 17 ppm NO_2 (×1,250).

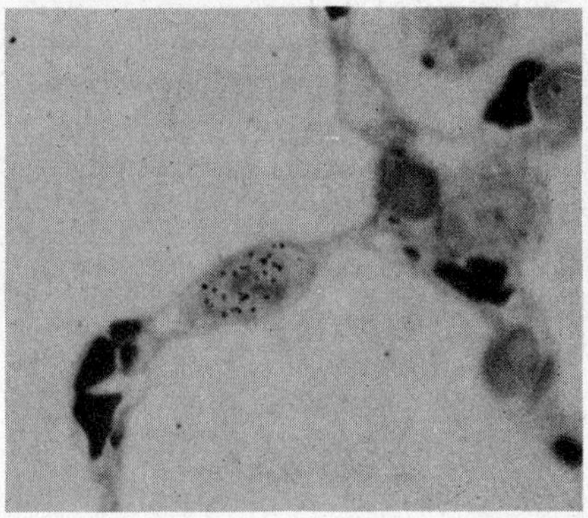

In the lung, the role of each cell type involved in the renewal process has not been determined. Traditionally, lung cell renewal has been looked upon primarily as a source of alveolar macrophages, but recent information suggests the process may also be involved in maintaining the integrity of the tissue.[6,9]

In previous studies we have shown that oxygen and ozone can inhibit cell renewal in the pulmonary alveoli (unpublished data).[10] This was thought to result from an alteration of some aspect of cell division, such as depressing DNA synthesis. The pathology that results from such a condition may be reflected as either

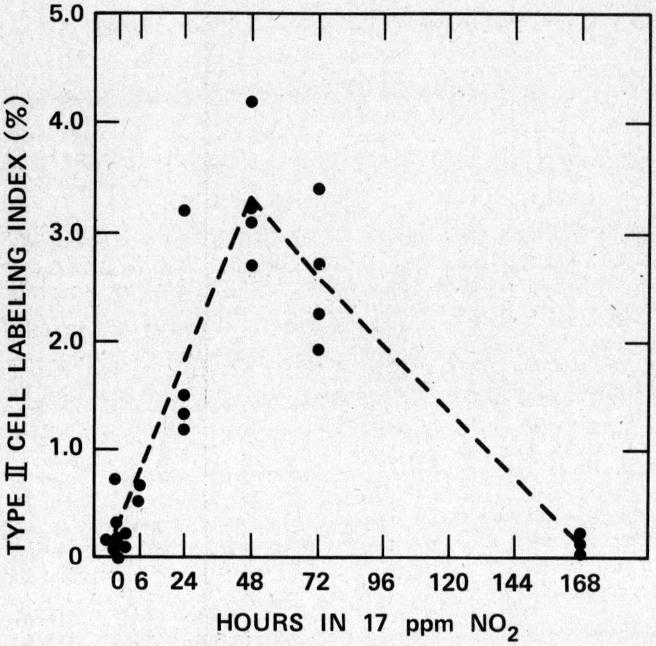

Fig 9.—Labeling index of type II alveolar cells during exposure to 17 ppm NO_2.

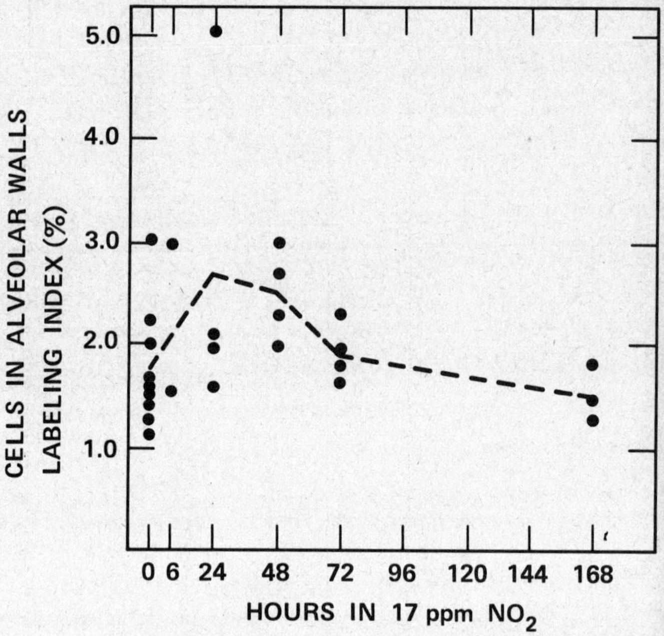

Fig 10.—Labeling index of cells in the alveolar walls during exposure to 17 ppm NO_2.

fewer cells of a specific type or a breakdown in the integrity of the tissue.

The present experiments show that subacute concentrations of NO_2 cause an increase in the number of cells incorporating tritiated thymidine. The cell types most stimulated were nonciliated cells of the terminal bronchioles and type II cells of the alveolar walls. Other cells within the alveolar walls (leukocytes, and endothelial and interstitial cells) were not similarly affected. This is an important point because it illustrates that cells of the epithelium are the principal type affected by NO_2. Mitotic events were confirmatory of the suspected rise in cell division. In the terminal bronchioles and adjacent alveoli there was a slight piling up of cells, which suggests that the rate of cell renewal was faster than that of cell loss. After 168 hours exposure to NO_2 the labeling indexes had returned to control levels.

Enhanced cell renewal may reflect direct stimulation by NO_2 of some process associated with cell division or, on the other hand, may be an indirect secondary response to a demand for either additional cells or replacement of cells injured by NO_2. At present the answers to these questions are not known. They are currently being investigated in this laboratory.

This investigation was supported by Public Health Service grants HE-13373-01, AI-0835-4-01A1, and AI-08723-09 and Department of Health, Education, and Welfare contract PH 86-65-27 from the Health Effects Research Program.

Dr. S. C. Crane and N. J. Furiosi assisted in maintaining the equipment used to expose the animals. Linda Cabral and Marlene Sloan provided technical assistance.

References

1. Freeman G, Crane SC, Stephens RJ, et al: Environmental factors in emphysema and a model system with NO_2. *Yale J Biol Med* **40**:566-590, 1968.

2. Freeman G, Haydon GB: Emphysema after low-level exposure to NO_2. *Arch Environ Health* **8**:125-128, 1964.

3. Freeman G, Crane SC, Stephens RJ, et al: Pathogenesis of the nitrogen dioxide-induced lesion in the rat lung: A review and presentation of new observations. *Amer Rev Resp Dis* **98**:429-443, 1968.

4. Freeman G, Crane SC, Stephens RJ, et al: The subacute nitrogen dioxide-induced lesion of the rat lung. *Arch Environ Health* **18**:609-612, 1969.

5. Freeman G: *Discussion of Alteration Mechanisms of Air Pollutants*, publication 18, Atomic Energy Symposium Series, Oak Ridge, Tenn, US Atomic Energy Commission, Technical Information Branch, 1970, pp 267-268.

6. Evans MJ, Bils RF: Identification of tritiated thymidine labeled cells in the pulmonary alveolar walls of the mouse. *Amer Rev Resp Dis* **100**:372-378, 1969.

7. Simnett JD, Heppleston AG: Factors controlling renewal of alveolar wall cells in adult mouse lung: An organ culture study in relation to sex, strain and age. *Exp Cell Res* **46**:488-494, 1967.

8. Bullough WS: Mitotic and functional homeostasis: A speculative review. *Cancer Res* **25**:1683-1727, 1965.

9. Evans MJ, Hackney JD, Bils RF: Effects of a high concentration of oxygen on cell renewal in the pulmonary alveoli. *Aerospace Med* **40**:1365-1369, 1969.

Lung Capillary Permeability

Nitrogen Dioxide Exposure and Leakage of Tritiated Serum

Russell P. Sherwin, MD, and Valda Richters, Los Angeles

A method has been developed for detection of altered lung capillary permeability and epithelial cell damage by low levels of nitrogen dioxide. Leakage of tritiated serum, injected intravenously before or at intervals after NO_2 exposure, was detected by scintillation counting of dialyzed pulmonary lavage fluid. In experiments with mice, elevated readings were obtained for those exposed to continuous low levels of NO_2. Determinations were also made of plasma levels and lung tissue content. Although good reproducibility and significant differences were not achieved in respect to the accumulation of reabsorbed serum and its large degradation products in lung tissue, evidence (including data from ultrastructural autoradiography) was found that serves to encourage further exploration. The results of the lavage fluid study by itself warrant strong consideration of the methodology as a highly sensitive and biologically meaningful indicator of adverse air pollutant levels.

A major consideration in the development of standards for tolerable levels of nitrogen dioxide and other air pollutants is the demonstration of physiopathologic effects of ambient levels. Although histopathologic findings[1-3] have been equivocal in experiments dealing with NO_2 at "near maximal" ambient levels (< 10 parts per million [ppm]), recent ultrastructural[4-6] and pathobiologic studies[7-10] indicate that cellular abnormalities do occur at such levels and may ultimately be found at high ambient concentrations. A potentially important consequence of structurally subtle but nonetheless functionally significant damage is a correspondingly slight increase in capillary permeability and congestion. Pertinently, the latter two factors are well known as flagrant common denominators in the response of the lung to essentially all *overt* airborne insults. Since blood protein transudation accompanies increased capillary permeability and the associated congestion, it would thus seem that the measurement of increased intraalveolar protein would be a sensitive, early, and physiologically meaningful indicator of lung damage secondary to the inhalation of an air pollutant. Further, the use of a radioactively labeled blood protein, such as albumin, would appear to be particularly advantageous since it would permit the dectection of very small amounts of protein leaking through damaged epithelium.

With the foregoing factors in mind, several pilot studies have been carried out in an attempt to develop a feasible methodology. A tritium-labeled serum was selected as a tracer substance since the β-emitter nature of the label not only affords extraordinary sensitivity in respect to scintillation counting but also allows concomitant histologic, ultrastructural, and autoradiographic investigations. The specific aim of the study has been to demonstrate not only intraalveolar but intracellular accumulation of protein which follows continuous exposure of mice to low levels (2 to 8 ppm) of NO_2.

Received for publication Oct 21, 1970; accepted April 5, 1971.

From the Department of Pathology, University of Southern California School of Medicine, Los Angeles.

Read in part before the Tenth Annual Hanford Biology Symposium on Pollution and Lung Biochemistry, Richland, Wash, June 5, 1970, jointly sponsored by the Battelle Memorial Institute-Pacific Northwest Laboratories, National Air Pollution Control Administration, National Institute of Environmental Health Sciences, and the US Atomic Energy Commission.

Reprint requests to 2025 Zonal Ave, Los Angeles 90033 (Dr. Sherwin).

Materials and Methods

The tritiated blood proteins were obtained by subjecting lyophilized rabbit serum to a Wilzbach procedure. The lyophilized tritiated serum had a specific activity of 91.5 microcuries/gm of dry weight. The serum was reconstituted in small lots as needed, generally 15 mg/5 ml of sterile distilled water, and was dialized for 24 hours prior to use. The working solution was found to have a specific activity of generally 7.5×10^6 counts per minute (cpm)/0.1 ml (corrected to 100% efficiency), or approximately 3 microcuries/0.1 ml. In a few of the early experiments, the specific activity was very high, as much as 200 microcuries/0.2 ml being given to a single animal. The serum was injected into the tail veins of mice with the use of a 1-ml tuberculin-type syringe and a No. 27 needle. To facilitate injection, the mice were exposed to a heat lamp placed 50 cm above them to produce a temperature of 32 C for approximately 20 minutes prior to injection. The total dose for each injection was 0.2 ml for most of the experiments. In any instance where a question of incomplete administration was raised (eg, suspected partial subcutaneous extravasation), the animal was killed and discarded.

The bronchial washing procedure for the recovery of tritiated serum in the lung was accomplished by anesthetizing the animal with 0.3 ml of pentobarbital sodium (18 mg/1 ml) intraperitoneally. At a point shortly before the animal succumbed to this lethal dose, both jugular veins were incised and the extravasating blood collected for analysis. An average of 0.6 ml of blood was collected from each animal in a 1.0-ml tuberculin syringe con-

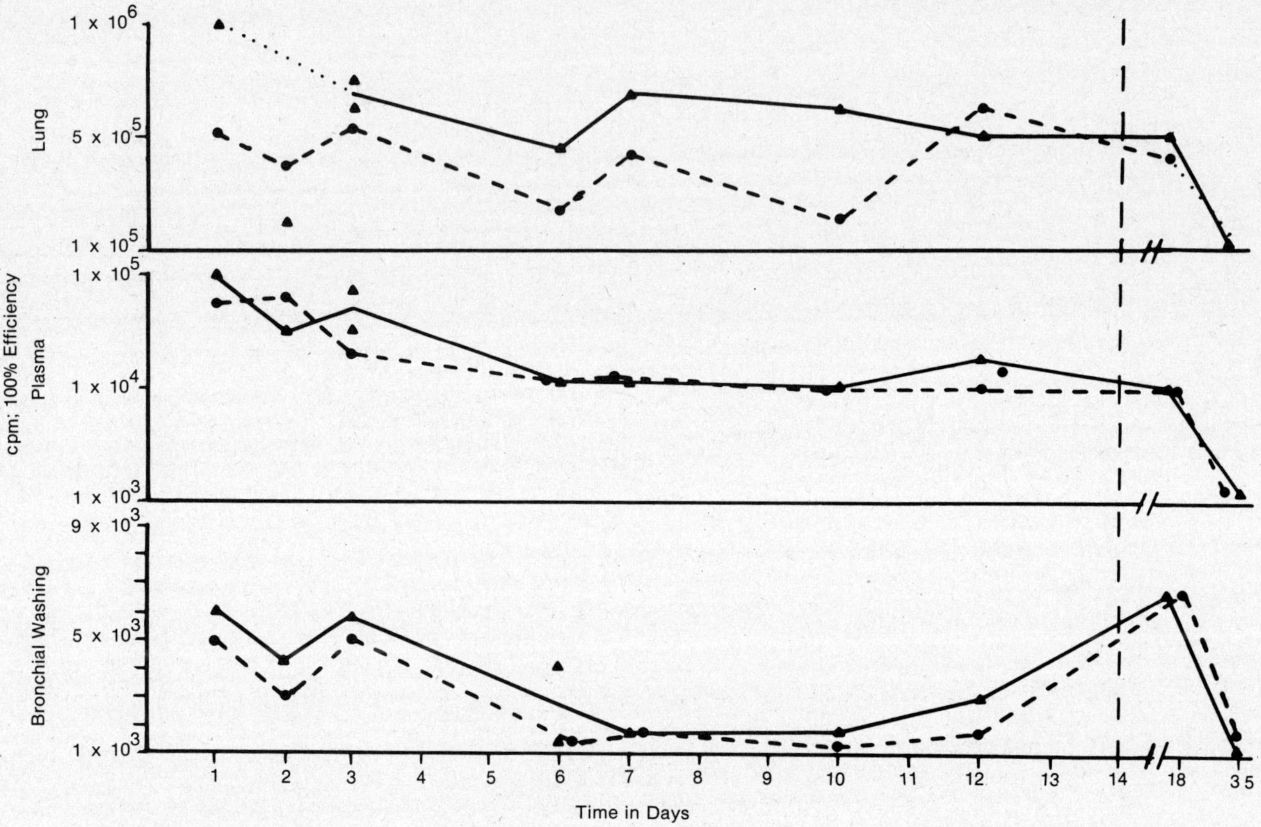

Fig 1.—Tritiated rabbit serum injected prior to 7 to 4 ppm NO_2 exposure. The exposed animals tended to have higher radioactive counts for undialyzed lavage fluid, plasma, and lung tissue. The findings here are not considered reliable in view of a number of inconsistent readings. Notable sources of error were the use of slightly hemolyzed serum and pipetting procedures not applicable to solubilized tissue. ● = control animals ▲ = exposed animals. Note: lung tissue analysis per 100 mg of lung tissue. On day 3, two exposed animals were killed.

taining 0.05 ml of 3.8% sodium citrate and centrifuged at 1,500 × g for 10 minutes at 4 C. The plasma was collected to provide two 100μl aliquots for analysis. The trachea was then carefully stripped of surrounding tissues and a large portion of the anterior rib cage removed widely to expose both lungs. The exterior of the trachea was washed with saline and carefully sponged free of blood. Cannulation was achieved by inserting a No. 22 cannula with its attached, saline-filled 1-ml syringe. The cannula was anchored in place by two sutures and lavage was accomplished by filling the lungs with 0.6 ml of saline under direct observation and then withdrawing the fluid. The number of excursions varied in the different experiments, from 12 initially to 5 in the final set of experiments. It was possible to recover, as a rule, all but 0.1 ml of the lavage fluid; maximal retention in the lung was no more than 0.2 ml. With each excursion of the lavage cycle, a portion of the air within the lung could be seen to undergo fluid replacement. Generally five excursions filled all of the air spaces with fluid insofar as gross examination was concerned. On removal of the cannula and syringe, the first two drops expelled were discarded. In the first of the experiments, the lavage fluid was allowed to stand at room temperature overnight to effect breakdown of cellular components. Following this, three 100μl aliquots were digested by means of a tissue solubilizer. Subsequently, the lavage fluid was placed in a dialysis bag and dialyzed overnight in a refrigerator.

The lung tissue was analyzed for tritium content by removing both lungs after bronchial lavage, mincing each lobe (2 to 4 lobes) finely, weighing the minced tissue of each lobe, washing in normal saline, centrifuging, and weighing out respective aliquots of wet tissue. Since the washings contained a negligible amount of radioactive material, the washing procedure was discontinued for the last two experiments. The minced tissue was digested by a solubilizer, and 100μl ali-

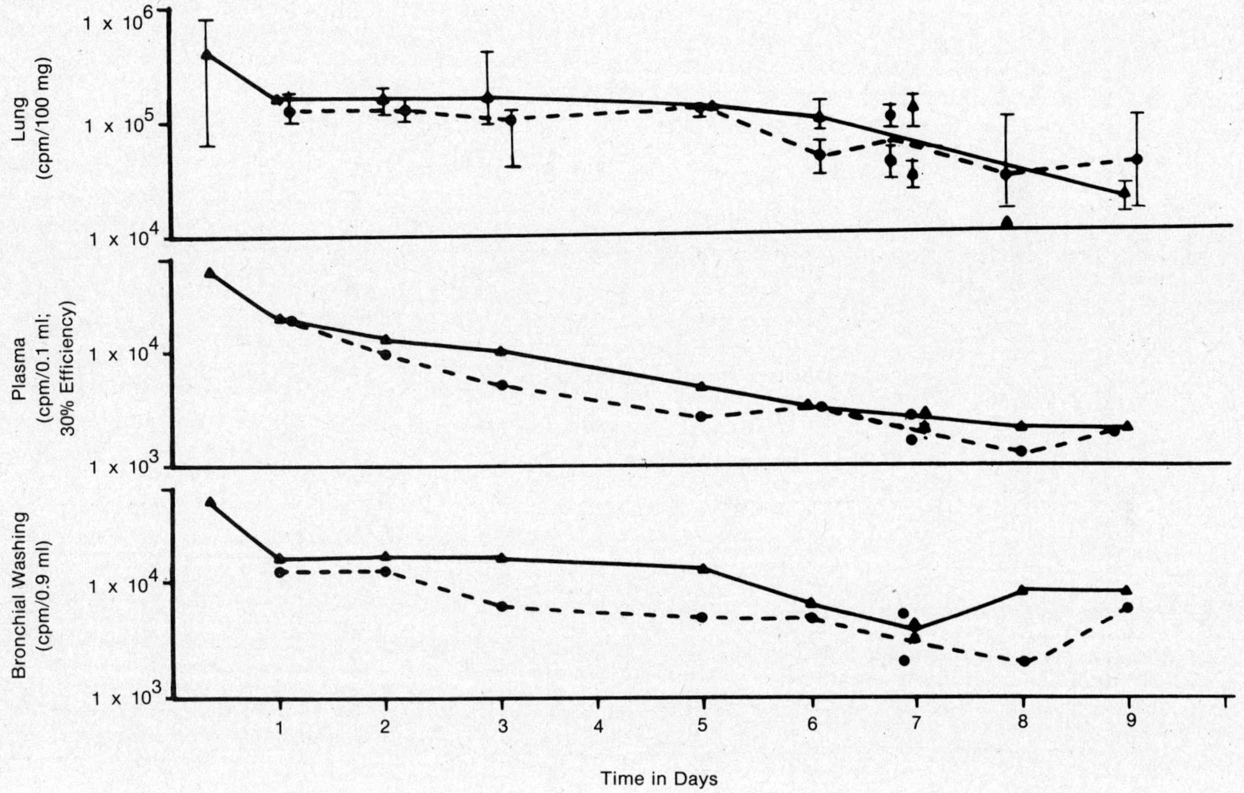

Fig 2.—In this experiment, entire lobes of the lung were digested in scintillation vials, bypassing the pipetting procedure used in experiment 2A. The undialyzed lavage fluids show consistently higher counts for the exposed animals. Reproducibility of lung tissue analyses was poor, apparently due to severe quenching. ● = control animals ▲ = exposed animals. Note: On day 7 two pairs of animals were killed.

quots were used for scintillation counting. In one experiment, a similar procedure was carried out for the analysis of liver and kidney tissues. A procedure carried out in one experiment consisted of pressure blotting of each lobe of the lung in several saline-moistened sponges to remove intravascular blood. In one other experiment, four lobes of the lung were processed individually and in their entirety by placing the minced fragments from each lobe directly into scintillation vials where digestion was carried out.

The scintillation counting involved the use of a commercial solubilizer (NCS). Glacial acetic acid was used to neutralize the solubilizer and 10-ml standard scintillation counting fluid added. A limited study was carried out to evaluate the usefulness of benzoyl peroxide as a decolorizer for the plasma and tissues.

Five of 13 experiments (involving 103 mice of the Swiss-Webster [S-W] strain and 45 of the A/Jax strain) are reported here. The experiments were designed to obtain data in the following major areas: (1) Experiment 1: pilot studies were done with 26 A/Jax mice to develop the methodology of injection and tissue analysis. (2) Experiment 2A: a study was done of 19 A/Jax mice divided into control and NO_2-exposed groups injected with tritiated serum (1.6×10^7 cpm/0.2 ml). The NO_2 exposure was continuous and varied from 4 to 7 ppm over a period of 14 days. (3) Experiment 3: this was essentially a repeat of experiment 2A except for the use of S-W mice (total 19) and digestion of entire lobes directly in vials, rather than pipetting small aliquots of solubilized lung tissue. (4) Experiment 4: 12 S-W mice were equally divided into control and exposed (5 ppm NO_2) groups. At periodic intervals after NO_2 exposure was started; one control and one exposed mouse were injected with tritiated serum (7.4×10^6 to 1.0×10^7 cpm/0.2 ml) and each killed 18 minutes after injection. In this experiment, the bronchial fluid recovered from lavage was dialyzed for 24 hours prior to analysis. Aliquots of both the dialyzed bronchial fluid and the dialysate were processed for scintillation counts. (5) Experiment 5: this experiment was limited to two pairs of S-W mice, one pair being exposed for 24 hours to 30 ppm of NO_2. At the end of the exposure period, the mice

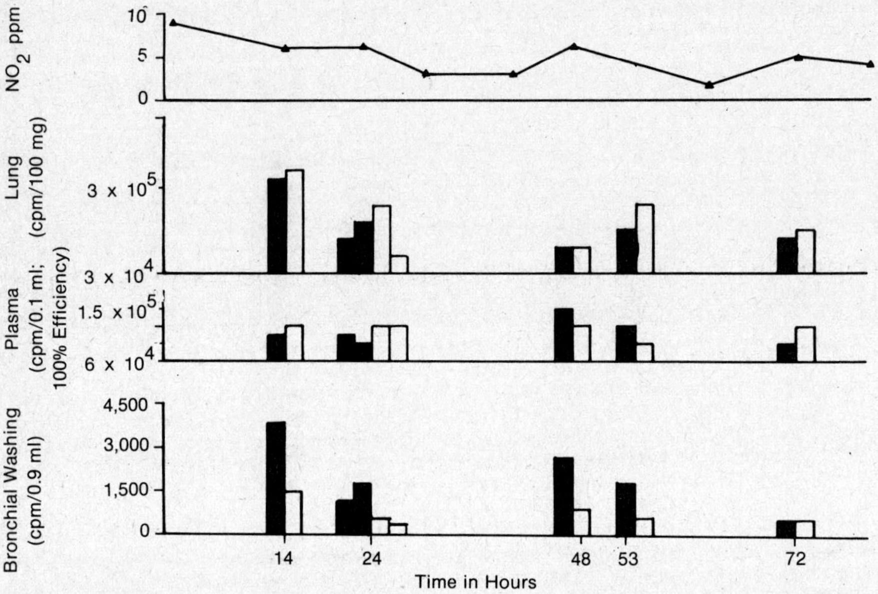

*Fig 3.—Tritiated serum was injected at intervals varying from 14 to 72 hours after 5 ppm NO_2 exposure of the animals. The dialyzed lavage fluids of exposed animals showed levels which were consistently higher and also more variable than those of the control animals. Plasma levels for the control animals were remarkably uniform in contrast to those of the exposed animals. The lung tissue findings were inconclusive. (*Solid bar *indicates exposed animals).*

were injected with tritiated serum (1.2 x 10^7 cpm/0.3 ml) and were killed three hours after injection for analysis of dialyzed bronchial lavage fluid only.

For electronmicroscopy, the middle lobe of the right lung from all mice was sectioned into small cubes and fixed in 2% glutaraldehyde in cacodylate buffer. The tissues were postfixed in 1% osmium and processed routinely thereafter. Plastic-embedded (Araldite) sections were obtained for routine electronmicroscopy and autoradiographic studies (including 1μ-thick sections). For electronmicroscopy, emulsion (Gilford L-4) was employed and NTB (Eastman Kodak) for the thick sections. Coated (Formvar) copper and stainless steel grids were used. The sections were examined after one to three weeks of exposure and following uranyl acetate and lead citrate staining.

Results

The weights of the paired animals when killed showed relatively little variation, there generally being no more than 1 to 2 gm difference, with a range of animal weight from 18 to 26 gm. However, the control animals were generally the heavier ones since the exposed animals apparently failed to gain weight as readily. All of the lung lobes were weighed after mincing and, in one experiment, after saline washing. The weights varied from 20 to 30 mg for the right lower lobe, 35 to 50 mg for the left lower lobe, 15 to 25 mg for the right upper lobe, and 8 to 15 mg for the left upper lobe. The variation in weight was due to the size of the animal, occasional lung abnormalities, and minor technical complications.

In respect to the overall behavior of the animals during the various experiments, no overt abnormalities could be attributed to the NO_2 exposure, although a few suggestive relationships to NO_2 exposure were encountered, ie, a slight decrease of overall activity, a questionably longer bleeding time, and less collapse of the lungs on opening the chest. There were occasional instances of attritional deaths in both control and exposed groups.

Of the experiments the following are reported: In experiment 2A (4 to 7 ppm NO_2 exposure), the *plasma levels* of tritiated serum protein of both control and exposed groups were roughly parallel, but in four of six instances the exposed animals showed higher levels than the controls with also slight domination by exposed animals at 18 and 35 days (Fig 1). The radioactivity measurements of the *undialyzed lavage fluid* of control and exposed animals again showed a slight to moderate dominance for the exposed group, with unusually high readings at 18 days for both animals. At 35 days, radioactivity in the lavage fluid was still high for both animals, 1,000 cpm/0.1 ml of lavage fluid. In respect to the radioactivity of *lung tissue* following lavage, there was a dominance by the exposed group, with high levels for both groups towards the end of the experiment. At 35 days the findings were 100,000 cpm/100 mg lung tissue for the exposed animal and an almost tenfold higher level for the control.

Duplicate samples of lavage fiuid varied less than 4% when three or more counts of each sample were averaged. Fair reproducibility with plasma counts was achieved, but there were several instances of wide disparity in association with low efficiency readings and hemolysis of the plasma. Up to 100% variation in duplicate samples of lung tissue was

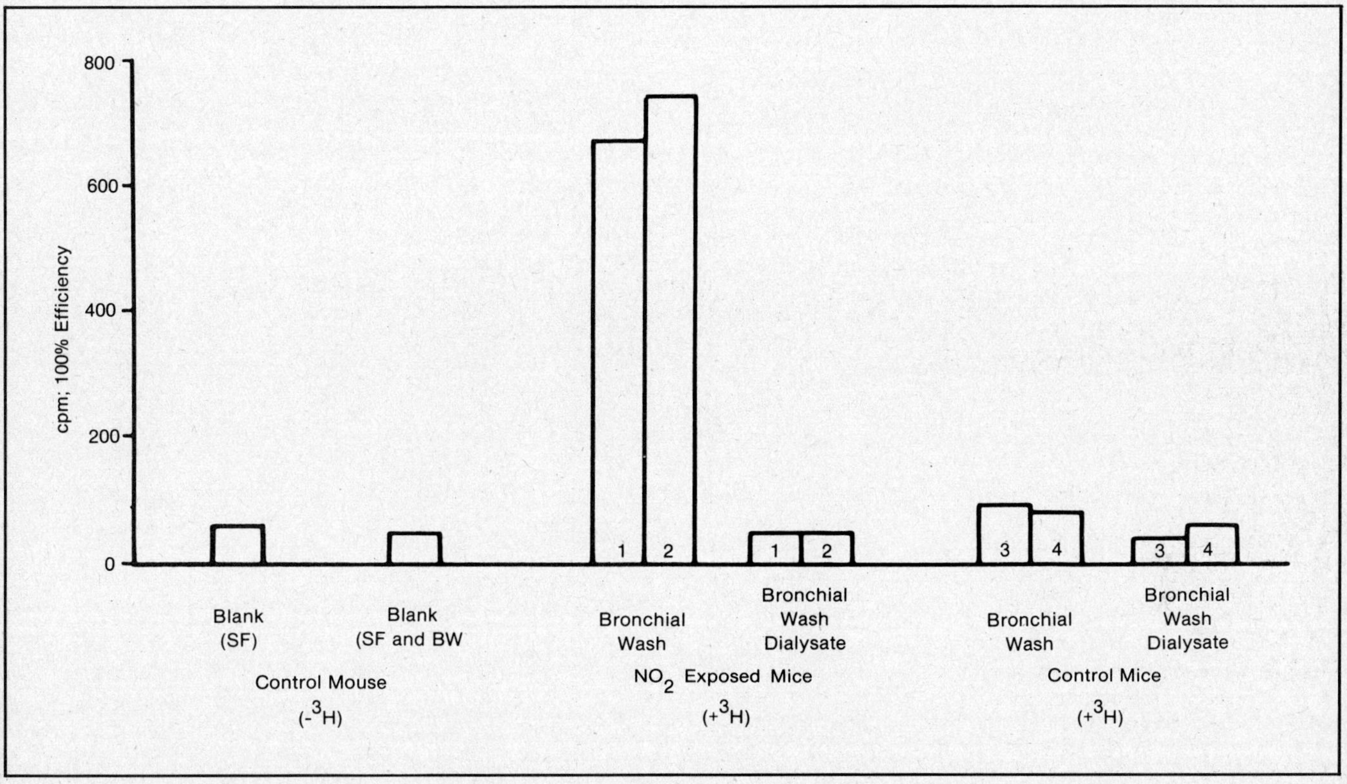

Fig 4.—Experiment 5: Exposure of mice to 30 ppm NO_2. The dialyzed lavage fluids of the exposed mice are overtly higher than those of the controls. The dialysates of both the control and experimental lavage fluids are at background levels. Note: The 100% efficiency for the cpm was derived from a tritium channel ratio quench curve. SF = scintillation fluid; BW = bronchial washing.

recorded, presumably due in large part to pipetting difficulties with solubilized lung tissue.

Experiment 3 was similar to experiment 2 except that the NO_2 exposure level was 8 ppm ± 1 ppm and entire lobes were digested directly in scintillation vials as opposed to the use of pipetted aliquots of digested lung in all other experiments. Again the plasma and undialyzed lavage fluid levels of the exposed animals dominated those of the control group (Fig 2). In respect to *lung tissue* content, the averages of the three lobes of matched animal pairs were roughly parallel, but great variation in the individual readings was often noted. Also, the counting efficiency was very low, only 1% to 8% efficiency as compared to the 40% generally obtained for the aliquot preparations of the other experiments.

In experiment 4, six pairs of animals, half of which were exposed to 5 ppm NO_2, were injected intravenously with serum at five selected intervals after beginning the NO_2 exposure (Fig 3). For four pairs of animals the amount of labeled albumin injected was identical, 8.4 × 10 cpm/0.2 ml. For the other two pairs, the figures were 5.4×10^6 and 7.8×10^6. The *plasma levels* of the control animals sacrificed 18 minutes after injection averaged 1.05×10^5 cpm and those of the exposed animals 1.04×10^5 cpm. However, there was a moderate variation in the levels for the exposed animals as compared to the relatively constant control levels. No differences were attributable to animal weights, the range being 23.1 to 27.4 gm.

All 12 *lavage fluids* were dialyzed and 24 hours later the analyses showed that five of the six exposed animals had levels substantially higher than those of the control animals, and the level of the sixth animal, three days after the beginning of NO_2 exposure and at a time following a substantial fall in the NO_2 level, was the same as that of the control.

The *lung tissue radioactivity* 18 minutes after intravenous injection of tritiated albumin showed considerable variation; some consistency

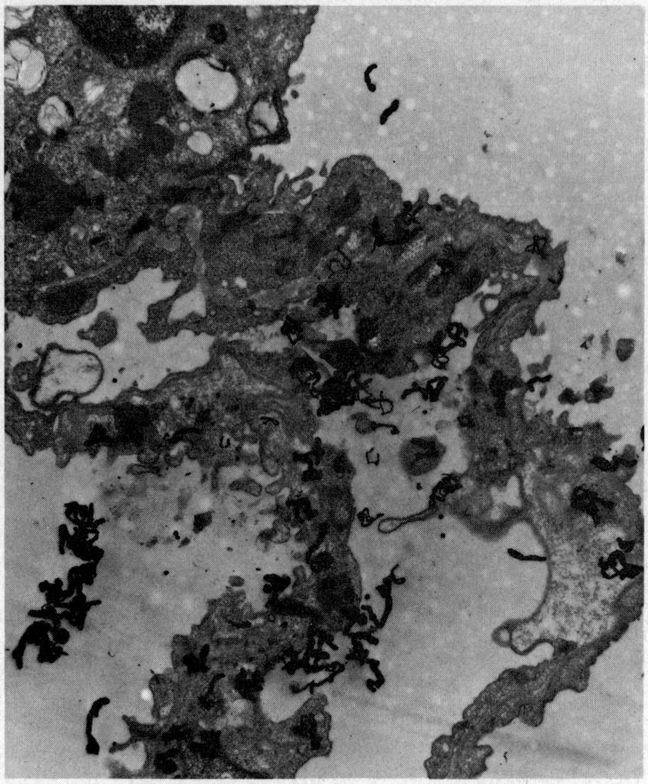

Fig 5.—Electron micrograph of lung of mouse injected with 3_H-labelled serum and killed 24 hours after exposure to 8 ppm NO_2 (experiment 3). A type II pneumocyte is seen (top left margin) *and the central alveolar walls show a pronounced localization of labeled substances. Damage to the wall cannot be demonstrated with certainty. This large amount may reflect local obstruction or some other trapping mechanism, as well as residue after lavage.*

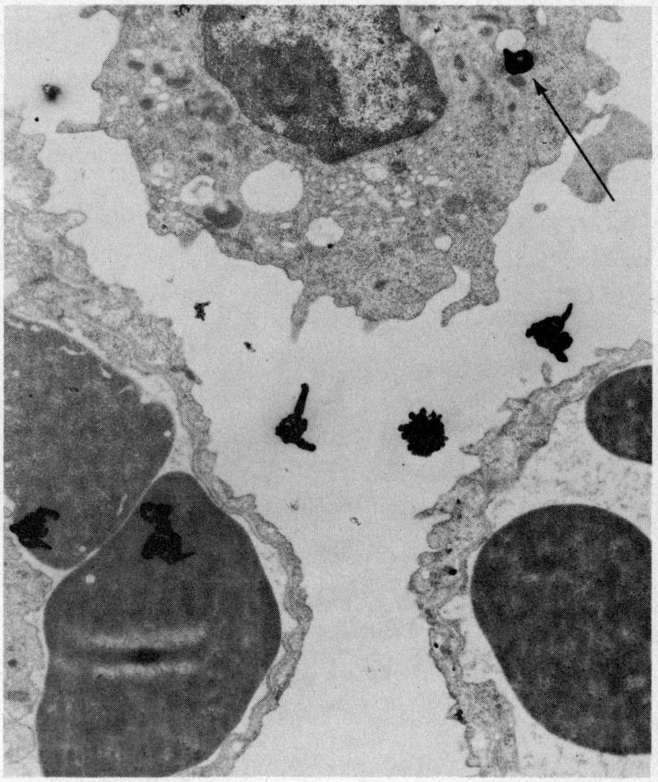

Fig 6.—Electron micrograph of lung of control animal which shows intraalveolar and intracapillary aggregates of silver filaments 11 days after injection of 3_H-labelled serum (experiment 2A). An aggregate is also present over the cytoplasm of a macrophage, near an introcytoplasmic vacuole of similar size (arrow).

was noted in that four of the six control lungs had slightly higher values than the corresponding exposed group levels.

In experiment 5, two mice were exposed to 30 ppm of NO_2 for 24 hours and two others were maintained as controls. Three hours following tail-vein injection of tritiated serum, each mouse was killed and the bronchial tree and air sacs were lavaged with normal saline. As shown in Fig 4, the levels for the dialyzed lavage fluid of the exposed animals were very high, whereas those for the control animals were near background counts. All dialysate counts were also at background levels.

The electron microscopic study confirmed the presence of labeled substances within capillaries and alveolar lumina (Fig 5 and 6). Apparent intracytoplasmic labeling occurred with endothelial cells, macrophages, type II pneumocytes, and bronchial mucosal lining cells (Fig 7 to 9).

Comment

The primary purpose of the multiple experiments was the development of a methodology for the detection of blood protein leakage into airsacs and airways in response to NO_2 exposure at less than 10 ppm. Throughout the investigation many constructive modifications were made and errors in procedure corrected. The methodology in respect to lung lavage is now considered to be readily reproducible, although questions remain as to the level of NO_2 exposure that will produce leakage and the percentage of intra-alveolar and intrabronchial protein that can be recovered. The findings of experiments 3 and 4 in particular, with injections before and after NO_2 exposure, respectively, show clear and consistent elevations of labeled substances in lavage fluids for the exposed animals as opposed to the control groups. Dialysis of the lavage fluid apparently greatly accentuated the differences. The use of a protein precipitating agent for the lavage fluid, eg, trichloroacetic acid, may be equally effective, with the advantages of faster processing and possibly a higher yield. Insofar as *lung tissue* analysis is concerned, experiment 2A is most suggestive that resorption of leaked protein leads to intracellular accumulation but the wide variation in some samples and the fact that cell synthesis will incorporate free tritium indicates that gel electrophoresis or some other means of separating serum protein

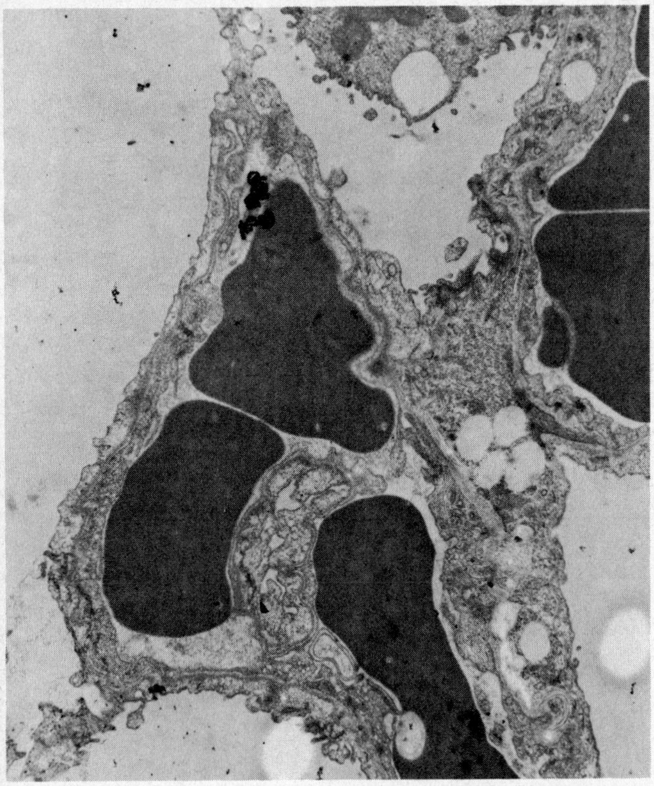

Fig 7.—Electron micrograph of lung of control animal (same as in Fig 6) which shows two silver filament aggregates over the cytoplasm of an endothelial cell. It is not certain whether this is within endothelial cell cytoplasm or a displacement from the capillary lumen.

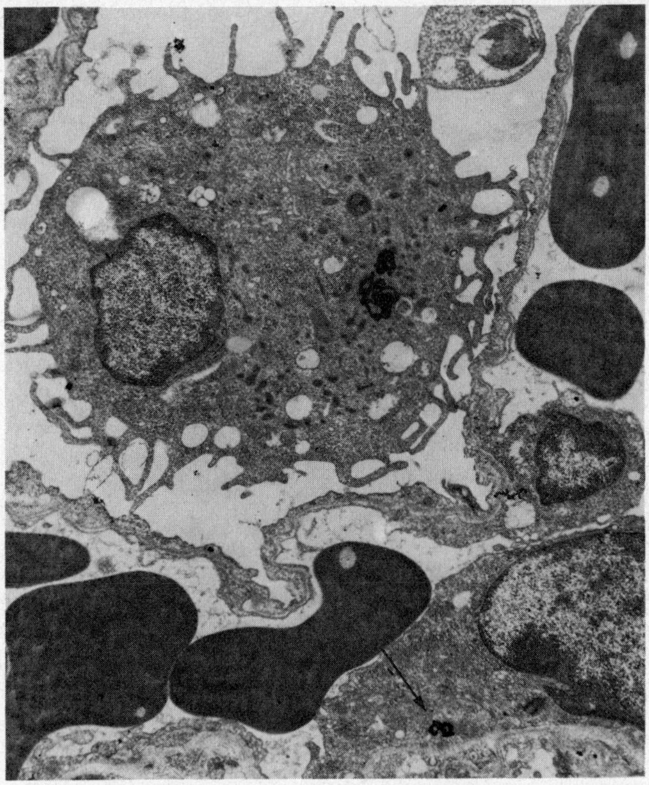

Fig 8.—Electron micrograph of lung of animal (same as Fig 6) which shows two silver filament aggregates over cytoplasm of macrophages and one over the cytoplasm of an endothelial cell near the basement membrane (arrow).

from other proteins must be incorporated in the methodology. Further, the unsatisfactory experience in experiment 3 was clearly due to excessive quenching, no doubt related to the 15 to 50 mg of tissue content, despite the addition of an oxidizer. The sampling of lobes and improved weighing,[11] as well as improved pipetting of solubilized tissue solutions (a spring bellows has been constructed for this purpose), should help to resolve the problems. In respect to the plasma levels, fair to good reproducibility was obtained. The differences found did not appear to be critical factors in influencing the lavage fluid content and, in retrospect, it was realized that the blood-collecting procedure had an error in dilution that could account for the differences.

Tritiated albumin (or serum) as a tracer substance has several outstanding attributes: (1) albumin is a normal constituent of the blood; (2) it has a moderately high molecular weight (69,000 vs 400,000 for fibrinogen) and abnormal extravasation into the pulmonary alveoli is unquestionably an early and significant indicator of altered capillary permeability; (3) tritium labeling is an excellent means of detecting very small quantities of specifically labeled substances, with the use of scintillation counting procedures; (4) lung lavage permits the recovery of free and macrophage-bound labeled albumin in the airsacs and airways; (5) a correlative study, using histologic and ultrastructural autoradiography, adds an extremely fine dimension to detection and at the same time affords insight into the nature and location of the abnormality; and (6) albumin is known to be reabsorbed from the alveolar lumina and temporarily accumulates in lining cells. Thus, an additional mea-

Fig 9.—Electron micrograph of lung of exposed animal (cf Fig 5) which shows lamellar bodies and other organelles of a type II pneumocyte. Note the intracytoplasmic inclusion with an overlying silver filament aggregate (bottom center) and a second filament (center).

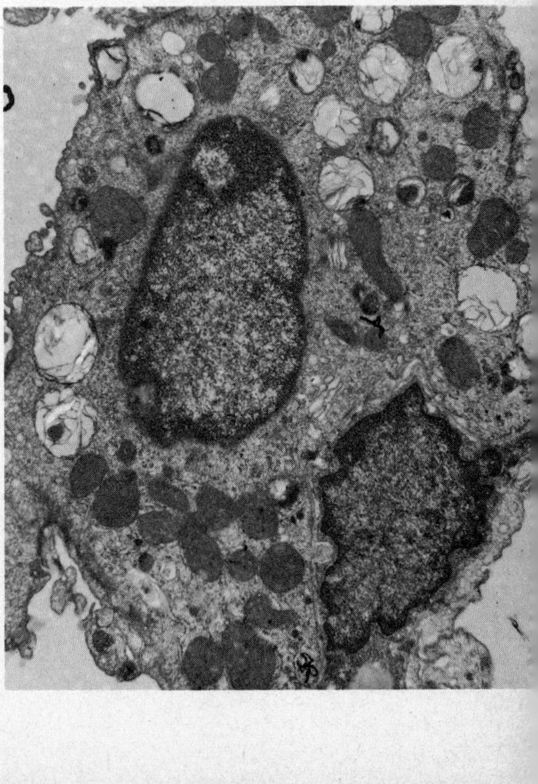

surement of protein leakage is potentially available through analysis of the lung tissue itself.

Certain questions arise with the use of albumin or serum, such as obtaining a uniformly high level of labeling without serious alteration of the molecular structure, either during storage or following injection into the blood stream. As judged by the preliminary studies, many of the potential difficulties mentioned do not seem to be serious obstacles inasmuch as gel electrophoresis of the dialyzed serum indicated the presence of intact albumin and reconstitution of the lyophilyzed serum over the period of several experiments yielded relatively constant values for the working solutions. To minimize breakdown of albumin, it would, of course, be highly desirable to use isologous albumin; in this experiment rabbit serum was used in view of the difficulty and expense of starting a pilot study with mouse albumin. Although radioactive iodine (^{131}I) labeled albumin (other than mouse) has been employed as a protein tracer,[12,13] it has the limitations of being a γ-emitter and is therefore unsuitable for autoradiography. Also, it would seem advisable not to use the macroaggregate form,[14,15] in view of properties which may influence capillary permeability.

The injection of labeled protein at various intervals after the start of air pollutant exposure and killing of the animal 18 minutes after injection has the advantage of producing a relatively constant quantity of labeled serum into the circulation. Conversely, degradation and variable clearance of labeled serum in each animal over a period of days or weeks apparently leads to less reliable findings. A presently unsolved problem with the 18-minute after-injection time is a level of lung tissue labeling higher than expected (Fig 3). Possibly this reflects foreign protein (rabbit serum) clearance by the lung but may be explained simply on the basis of failure to remove capillary blood or labeled small molecules absorbed to the tissues. The report by Hapke and Pederson[14] is support for a rapid protein absorption in that they found a remarkable degree of albumin phagocytosis by *type 1* alveolar wall cells 40 minutes after the intravenous injection of ^{131}I macroaggregated albumin. Also Dominguez et al[16] state that over 50% of albumin introduced into alveoli is resorbed by six hours afterwards. Although the initial findings have fallen short of establishing the *tissue* analysis methodology, there are nevertheless good indications that further exploration will lead to a feasible technique.

This investigation was supported in part by Public Health Service grants AP 00607 and AP 00774 from the National Air Pollution Control Administration and by the Hastings Foundation.

References

1. Kleinerman J, Cowdrey CR: The effects of continuous high level nitrogen dioxide on hamsters. *Yale J Biol Med* **40**:579-590, 1968.

2. Buckley RD, Loosli CG: Effects of nitrogen dioxide inhalation on germfree mouse lung. *Arch Environ Health* **18**:588-595, 1969.

3. Blair WH, Henry MC, Ehrlich R: Chronic toxicity of nitrogen dioxide: II. Effect on histopathology of lung tissue. *Arch Environ Health* **18**:186-192, 1969.

4. Yuen TGH: Ultrastructural abnormalities in the lungs of guinea pigs. *Fed Proc* **28**:804, 1969.

5. Bils RF, Romanovsky JC: Ultrastructural alterations of alveolar tissue of mice: II. Synthetic photochemical smog. *Arch Environ Health* **14**:844-858, 1967.

6. Freeman G, Stephens RJ, Furiosi NJ: The subacute nitrogen dioxide induced lesion of the rat lung. *Arch Environ Health* **18**:609-612, 1969.

7. Sherwin RP, Winnick S, Buckley RD: Response of lactic acid dehydrogenase-positive alveolar cells in the lungs of guinea pigs exposed to nitric oxide. *Amer Rev Resp Dis* **96**:319-323, 1966.

8. Sherwin RP, Richters V, Brooks M, et al: The phenomenon of macrophage congregation in vitro and its relationship to in vivo NO_2 exposure of guinea pigs. *Lab Invest* **18**:269-277, 1968.

9. Valand SB, Acton JD, Myrvik QN: Nitrogen dioxide inhibition of viral-induced resistance in alveolar monocytes. *Arch Environ Health* **20**:303-309, 1970.

10. Freeman G, Furiosi NJ, Haydon GB: Effects of continuous exposure of 0.8 ppm NO_2 on respiration in rats. *Arch Environ Health* **13**:454-456, 1966.

11. Atherton JC, Green R, Hai MA: Evaluation of a method for weighing small tissue samples: Investigations into freezing and evaporation. *Pflugers Arch* **309**:203-211, 1969.

12. Meyer EC, Dominguez EAM, Bensch KG: Pulmonary lymphatic and blood absorption of albumin from alveoli: A quantitative comparison. *Lab Invest* **20**:1-8, 1969.

13. Liebow AA: Aspects of transcapillary fluid and protein exchange in the lung, in Fishman AP, Hecht HH (eds): *The Pulmonary Circulation and Interstitial Space.* Chicago, University of Chicago Press, 1969, pp 99-112.

14. Hapke EJ, Pederson HJ: Ultrastructural changes in rat lungs induced by radioactive macroaggregated albumin. *Amer Rev Resp Dis* **100**:194-205, 1969.

15. Haddad RG, Luchsinger PC: Disappearance rate of ^{131}I-tagged macroaggregated albumin from the lung. *J Nucl Med* **10**:560-561, 1969.

16. Dominguez EAM, Liebow AA, Bensch KG: Studies on the pulmonary air-tissue barrier: I. Absorption of albumin by the alveolar wall. *Lab Invest* **16**:905-911, 1967.

Alveolar Protein Accumulation

A Sensitive Indicator of Low Level Oxidant Toxicity

Stephen M. Alpert, MD; Barry B. Schwartz, MD;
Si Duk Lee, PhD; and Trent R. Lewis, PhD, Cincinnati

Studies of response to low doses of edematogenic gases have been hampered by the insensitivity and the nonquantitative nature of the major indicators of response. A new and more sensitive indicator, the recovery of ^{131}I-albumin from the alveolar spaces six hours after its intravenous injection in rats, has been applied. Significantly increased albumin recovery was found for all concentrations of ozone at and above 0.5 ppm. No wet weight changes were noted below 2.5 ppm ozone, and there was no consistent histologic finding except for slight sloughing of bronchial epithelium at 2.5 ppm. Application of these methods to studies of steroid effects revealed increased sensitivity to ozone following administration of methylprednisolone sodium succinate. In addition, animals treated with steroids prior to exposure to 0.25 ppm ozone became tolerant to subsequent ozone challenge, whereas animals given preexposure but no steroids did not.

Received for publication Oct 20, 1970; accepted Feb 25, 1971.

From the National Air Pollution Control Administration, Environmental Health Service, Public Health Service, Cincinnati. Drs. Alpert and Schwartz are now with the Department of Medicine, Kings County Hospital, Brooklyn, NY.

Read in part before the Tenth Annual Hanford Biology Symposium on Pollution and Lung Biochemistry, Richland, Wash, June 5, 1970, jointly sponsored by the Battelle Memorial Institute-Pacific Northwest Laboratories, National Air Pollution Control Administration, National Institute of Environmental Health Sciences, and the US Atomic Energy Commission.

Reprint requests to 1055 Laidlaw Ave, Cincinnati 45237 (Dr. Lewis).

Short-term studies of edematogenic oxidizing air pollutants have previously involved concentrations greater than those found in the environment. At present, ways to assess edema produced by air pollutants, including histologic study, increase in percent wet weight, and mortality, are largely ineffective at ambient levels of pollutants, especially with short exposure periods. Histology has traditionally been the most sensitive indicator of pollutant toxicity; however, rats exposed to ambient concentrations for short periods show no consistent pathologic changes. Moreover, histology does not easily lend itself to quantitation and statistical analysis short of the very cumbersome methods of pulmonary morphometry. Increase in percent wet weight, while easily quantitated, is considerably less sensitive than histology, and pollutant concentrations necessary to cause death over a short period of exposure are orders of magnitude higher than those in the environment.[1] With no sound methods to measure ambient pollutant damage, subtle changes caused by modifications in the exposure conditions or in the experimental animal are not detectable.

The need for a new approach to these problems is obvious. We present a technique of sufficient sensitivity to measure pulmonary effects of ozone in rats after a six-hour exposure to 1 ppm (1 ppm ozone = 2 mg/cu m) or less. This method has been employed in a study of the effect of corticosteroid administration on response to ozone exposure and of the tolerance phenomenon at ambient ozone levels.

Methods

Experimental Animals.—Female, CD strain, random bred rats weighing 150-200 gm were maintained on rat chow ad libitum except during exposure periods.

Exposures.—Groups of rats were exposed in chambers with a 25 cu ft volume, provided with 30 air changes per hour. Ozone was generated from a stream of oxygen flowing through a standard neon arc generator before entering the chamber. Ozone concentrations within the chamber were monitored continuously with a meter (Mast) calibrated by the neutral-buffered potassium iodide method.[2] The desired ozone concentration was maintained within limits of ± 5%. All exposure periods were six hours.

Albumin.—Iodinated I 131 serum albumin (RISA-131) was injected via the lateral tail vein immediately prior to exposure. The lots used varied from 109 microcuries to 119 microcuries/10 mg albumin per milliliter. In all lots at least 95% of the ^{131}I was precipitated by 10% trichloroacetic acid. Additionally, six hours after injection at least 95% of ^{131}I in the plasma could still be precipitated in this way. Injections of approximately 80 microcuries/kg of body weight were made. Exact amounts were computed by weight of the syringe before and after injection. All results were then corrected to a dose of 80 microcuries/kg of body weight.

Lavage.—After six hours of exposure, animals were anesthetized with pentobarbital sodium administered intraperitoneally. A tracheostomy was performed and a polyethylene catheter tied in place. Lavage was gently performed with five successive 5 ml aliquots of normal saline. Twenty-three ± 0.5 ml of lavage fluid was recovered. As an indication

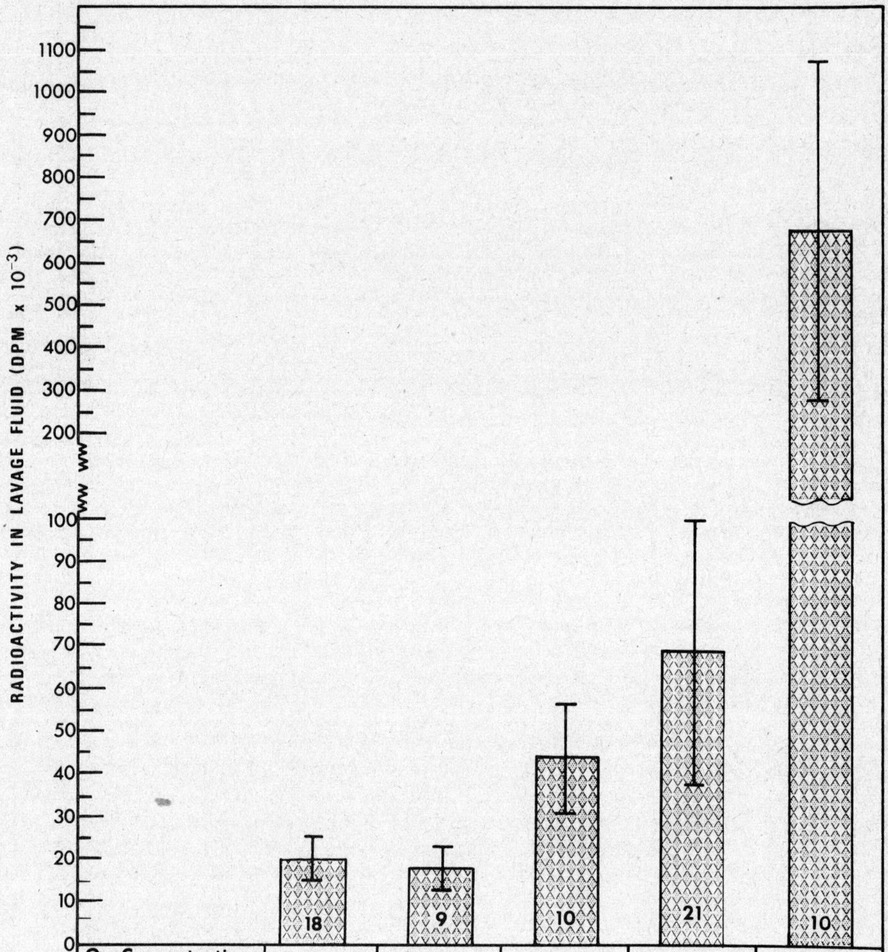

O3 Concentration (ppm) 6 hr Exposure	0	0.25	0.50	1.00	2.50
p (vs Animals Exposed at 0 ppm)	——	>0.20	<0.001	<0.001	<0.001

Fig 1.—Pulmonary alveolar protein accumulation in response to ozone exposure (values ± 1 SD—No. of animals per group on columns).

of the efficiency of the lavages, washing with an additional 25 ml of fluid produced less than 20% of ^{131}I recovered in the initial 25 ml. At least 90% of ^{131}I in the lavage fluid was precipitated with 10% trichloroacetic acid.

Histolic Findings and Percent Wet Weight.—Groups of ten animals were exposed as previously described. No lavage was performed. Immediately after exposure the lungs were removed, trimmed, gently blotted, and weighed. They were then heated at 110 C until constant weight was obtained, and again weighed. Results were expressed in wet weight as a percent of total weight. (The equation is given at the bottom.)

Additional groups of five animals were exposed for histologic study. Their lungs were removed immediately and fixed in formaldehyde solution. Sections through the hilar regions were stained with hematoxylin-eosin. These sections were studied under double blind conditions and were studied again after treatment groups were identified. Knowledge of the treat-

$$\% \text{ wet weight} = \frac{\text{total weight} - \text{dry weight}}{\text{total weight}} \times 100$$

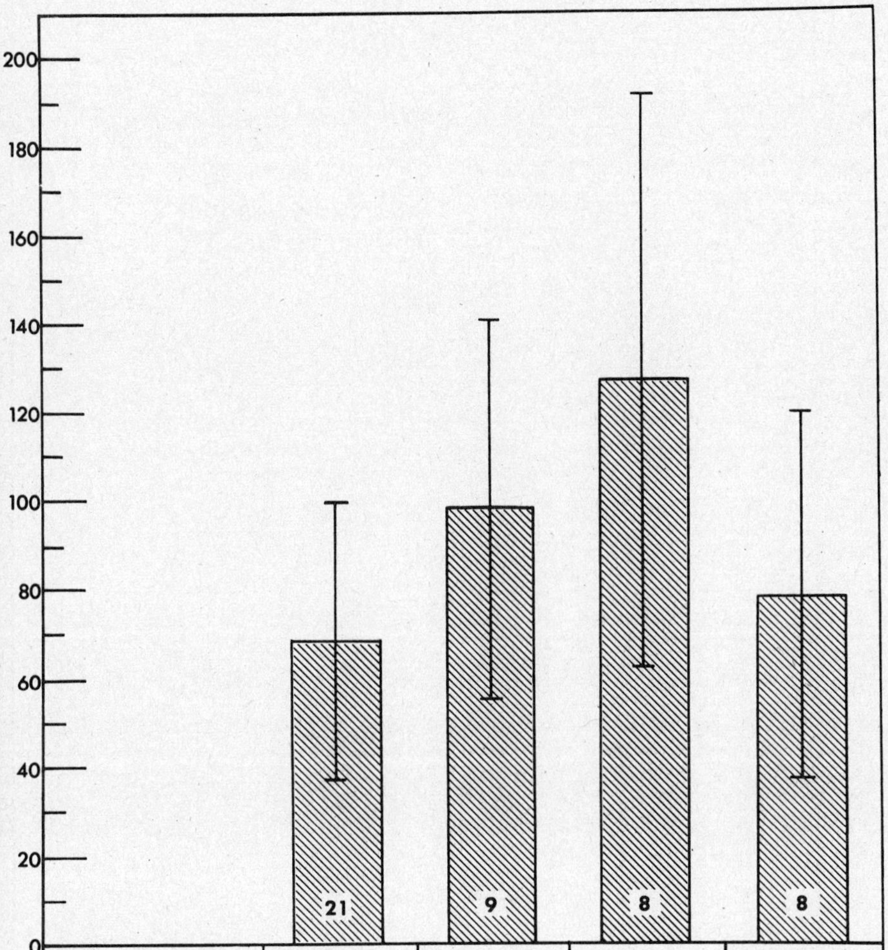

Methylprednisolone Given Day 1 & Day 2	NO	YES	YES	YES
Day of Exposure	—	2	4	6
p (vs Group Given No Steroids)	—	<0.05	<0.01	>0.40

Fig 2.—Effect of corticosteroid administration on response to ozone exposure (values ± 1 SD—No. of animals per group on columns).

ment of the animals produced no new histologic findings.

Steroids.—All animals receiving corticosteroids were given 5 mg of methylprednisolone sodium succinate (Solu-Medrol) intraperitoneally on each of two successive days.

Estimation of Radioactivity.—All gamma counting was done in a shielded well-type scintillation spectrometer with an efficiency of approximately 4×10^5 counts per minute (cpm)/microcurie of ^{131}I over a background of 38 cpm. Two-milliliter aliquots of lavage fluid were counted until the standard error of the net counts was less than 2%. All results were expressed as discharges per minute per 25 ml of lavage fluid. Corrections for decay were made as necessary.

Statistical Analysis.—Student's *t*-test was used to test the equality of treatment means.

Results

The Table shows the effects of ozone at 0 ppm to 2.5 ppm on histologic appearance and on percent wet weight. The histologic techniques used failed to detect a consistent effect below 2.5 ppm. At this level, three of the five animals showed sloughing of bronchial epithelium, a finding previously described.[3] Only one animal at this level (indeed, the only animal at any ozone concentration) exhibited intra-alveolar fluid, the classical effect of short-term ozone exposure. The percent wet weight of the lungs of animals exposed to 1.0 ppm ozone or less was not statistically different from animals breathing no ozone. Animals exposed to 2.5 ppm showed an increase in percent wet weight ($P <$ 0.01).

Figure 1 shows alveolar protein accumulation under the same exposure conditions as above, ie, 0 ppm to 2.5 ppm ozone. Exposure to 0.25 ppm produced no increase in recoverable ^{131}I-albumin. However, at 0.5 ppm and above, recovery was at least twice that seen in animals exposed to no ozone. These differences were statistically significant ($P < 0.001$).

The influence of methylprednisolone on alveolar protein accumulation in response to ozone challenge is shown in Fig 2. Methylprednisolone was administered to three groups of animals on days 1 and 2. Challenge with 1.0 ppm ozone for six hours on days 2 and 4 showed a statistically significant increase in ^{131}I-albumin recovery ($P < 0.05$, and $P < 0.01$, respectively), while challenge on day 6 showed no difference from animals not receiving steroids. Therefore, the presence of a steroid effect was confirmed up to two days after administration; by the fourth day, the steroid was no longer detectable. Recovery of ^{131}I-albumin from animals receiving the same steroid regimen, but not exposed to ozone was not different at any time from control animals receiving no steroids and no ozone ($P < 0.40$ for all groups).

In order to assess the role of steroids in the etiology of tolerance, it was necessary to study four treatment groups. The sequential regimen underlying the formation of these groups was as follows (appropriate groups referenced in parentheses): a 5 mg intraperitoneal injection of methylprednisolone sodium succinate on day 1 and 2 (groups 2 and 4), tolerance inducing ozone exposure of 0.25 ppm ozone for six hours on day 4 (group 3 and 4), and an ozone challenge of 1.0 ppm for six hours on day 6 (groups 1 to 4). Three types of control groups were employed, ie, animals which received neither steroid injection nor tolerance inducing ozone exposure (group 1), animals which received steroid injection but no tolerance inducing exposure (group 2), and animals which received the tolerance inducing ozone exposure but no steroid injection (group 3). A fourth group, the experimental, received both steroid injection and a tolerance inducing ozone exposure (group 4). All four groups received the ozone challenge exposure to assess the edematogenic response relative to the prior experimental regimen.

A comparison of groups 1 and 3 demonstrated that there was no significant difference ($P < 0.40$) in the amount of recoverable ^{131}I-albumin attributable to a six-hour pre-exposure to 0.25 ppm ozone (Fig 3). Likewise, the other pairwise comparisons of the three control groups showed no significant difference ($P < 0.40$) in recoverable ^{131}I-albumin. Group 4, however, demonstrated a significant decrease in the amount of recoverable ^{131}I-albumin when compared to each control group. As witnessed in the last line of Fig 3, the levels of significance were no pretreatment ($P < 0.05$), prior injection of steroid alone ($P < 0.02$), or prior exposure to 0.25 ppm ozone alone ($P < 0.01$).

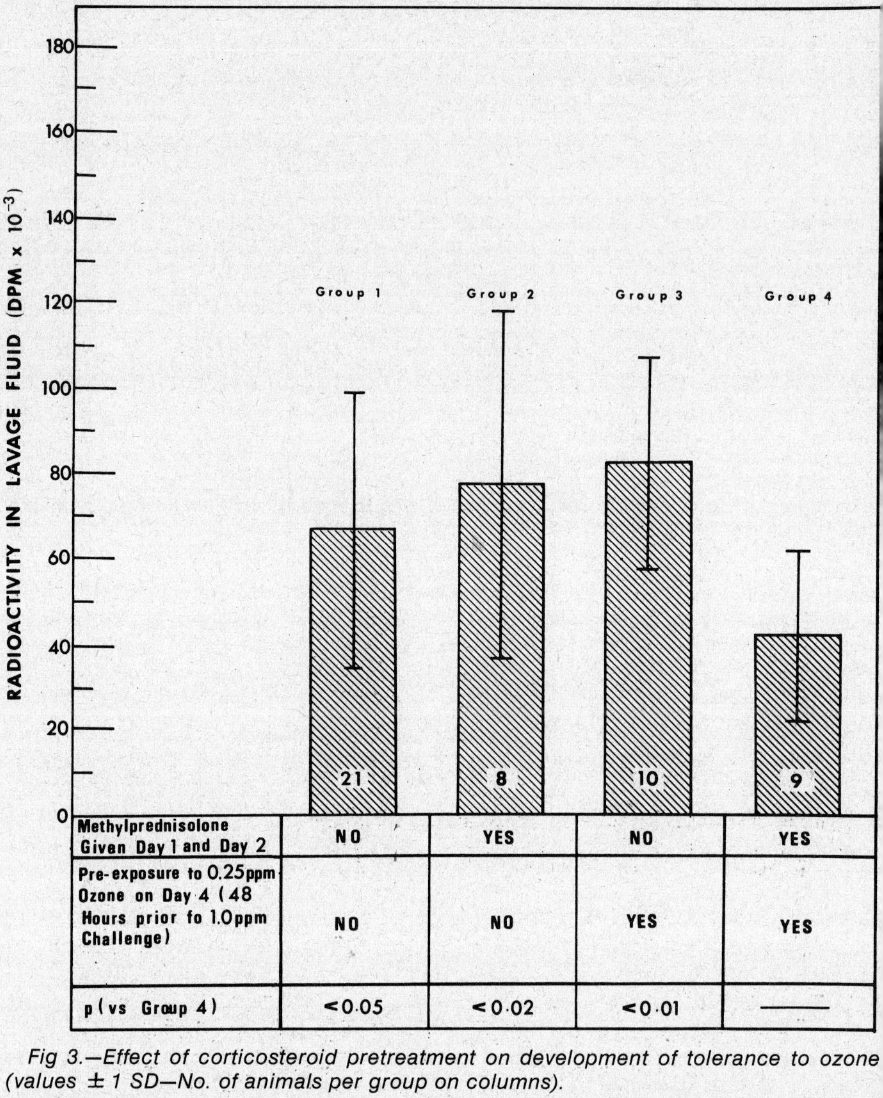

Methylprednisolone Given Day 1 and Day 2	NO	YES	NO	YES
Pre-exposure to 0.25ppm Ozone on Day 4 (48 Hours prior to 1.0ppm Challenge)	NO	NO	YES	YES
p (vs Group 4)	<0.05	<0.02	<0.01	——

Fig 3.—Effect of corticosteroid pretreatment on development of tolerance to ozone (values ± 1 SD—No. of animals per group on columns).

Comment

There is extensive evidence that iodinated I 131 serum albumin injected intravenously undergoes a rapid phase of disappearance from the vascular space, lasting from one to several days, followed by a more gradual disappearance lasting many weeks.[4-6] The rapid phase is attributed mainly to distribution of the albumin to extravascular fluid, while the second phase is attributed to elimination and degradation. There is also evidence that, at least over the short term, heterologous albumin in a nonimmune recipient is handled in a manner indistinguishable from native albumin with respect both to disappearance from the intravascular space and to appearance in various tissues and lymph.[7] The fact that over 90% of ^{131}I in the lavage fluid was precipitated with 10% trichloroacetic acid indicates that ^{131}I

Studies of Pulmonary Percent Wet Weight and Histology in Response to Ozone

Ozone Concentration (6-hr Exposure)	% Wet Weight ±1 SD (10 Animals per Group)	*P* (vs 0 ppm)	Histologic Findings (5 Animals per Group)
0 ppm	79.71 ± 0.23	. . .	3 animals normal; 1 with interstitial swelling, and 1 with focal perivascular hemorrrage
0.25 ppm	79.94 ± 0.43	>0.20	4 animals normal; 1 with focal intra-alveolar hemorrhage
0.50 ppm	79.95 ± 0.44	>0.10	4 animals normal; 1 with interstitial swelling
1.00 ppm	79.69 ± 1.72	>0.40	All animals normal
2.50 ppm	80.32 ± 0.58	<0.01	No normal animals; 1 with intra-alveolar edema and one with interstitial swelling; 2 with sloughing of bronchial epithelium; 1 with both sloughing of bronchial epithelium and focal intra-alveolar hemorrhage

reflects true protein accumulation in the alveoli. Thus, over the six-hour time course of this experiment, the ^{131}I-albumin recovered from rats not exposed to ozone reflects normal passage of albumin into the alveoli of the lung. The demonstrated excess of ^{131}I-albumin in response to ozone indicates increased accumulation caused by the edematogenic toxicity of this pollutant. Furthermore, this increased accumulation can be detected in the alveolar spaces long before the fluid which accompanies the protein can be demonstrated by increase in percent wet weight or by histology.

These three methods of analysis were simultaneously compared here because no previous studies used exactly comparable conditions, and sensitivity to ozone is dependent upon many variables, eg, species, breed, age, and sex of the experimental animals.[8] The methodology developed here, therefore, offers unique advantages in the study of low concentrations of edematogenic gases.

Alveolar protein accumulation was used to study the effect of steroid administration on the toxicity of ozone exposure at levels below the sensitivity of the other methods tested. This is a confused subject in the existing literature. Exogenous steroids may protect against acute ozone lethality while having no detectable effect on the percent wet weight of the lungs.[9] Adrenalectomy, on the other hand, has also been observed to protect against ozone mortality. Administration of steroids to adrenalectomized animals exerts a further protective effect.[10]

Our experiment demonstrated that administration of methylprednisolone, a corticosteroid known for its potent antiinflammatory effect, increased sensitivity to low concentrations of ozone on the same day and two days following administration. This increased sensitivity was demonstrated both by direct means—the increased recovery of ^{131}I-albumin in response to 1.0 ppm of ozone—and by indirect means—the development of a decreased edematogenic response only after the combination of steroid administration and preexposure to 0.25 ppm ozone. Presumably, the mechanism of the latter is an increased response to the preexposure ozone dose of 0.25 ppm caused by prior administration of methylprednisolone.

The histologic sections were interpreted by Ralph Powell, MD, of the National Cancer Institute.

•

References

1. Werthamer S, Schwarz LH, Carr JJ, et al: Ozone-induced pulmonary lesions. *Arch Environ Health* **20:**16-21, 1970.

2. Byers DH, Saltzman BE: Determination of ozone in air by neutral and alkaline iodide procedures. *J Amer Industr Hyg Assoc* **19:**251-257, 1958.

3. Scheel LD, Dobrogorski OJ, Mountain JT, et al: Physiological, biochemical, immunologic and pathologic changes following ozone exposure. *J Appl Physiol* **14:**67-80, 1959.

4. Sterling K: The turnover rate of serum albumin in man as measured by I^{131} tagged albumin. *J Clin Invest* **30:**1228-1237, 1951.

5. Margen S, Tarver H: Comparative studies on the turnover of serum albumin in normal human subjects. *J Clin Invest* **35:**1161-1172, 1956.

6. Tyor MP: Human serum albumin tagged with I^{131} in patients with ascites caused by abdominal carcinomatosis and portal cirrhosis: The rates of interchange between the vascular compartment and peritoneal cavity. *J Lab Clin Med* **44:**110-117, 1954.

7. Wasserman K, Mayerson HS: Exchange of albumin between plasma and lymph. *Amer J Physiol* **165:**15-26, 1951.

8. Stokinger HE: Ozone toxicity: A review of research and industrial experience: 1954-1964. *Arch Environ Health* **10:**719-741, 1965.

9. Matzen RN: Effect of vitamin C and hydrocortisone on the pulmonary edema produced by ozone in mice. *J Appl Physiol* **11:**105-109, 1957.

10. Fairchild EJ: Neurohumoral factors in injury from inhaled irritants. *Arch Environ Health* **6:**79-86, 1963.

Short-Term Exposure to Nitrogen Dioxide

Effects on Pulmonary Ultrastructure, Compliance, and the Surfactant System

Anthony R. Dowell, MD; Kaye H. Kilburn, MD; and Philip C. Pratt, MD, Durham, NC

Eleven beagles were exposed to nitrogen dioxide in concentrations ranging from 3 to 16 ppm for one hour. Two control dogs were air-ventilated for one hour. Widespread bleb formation, loss of pinocytotic vesicles, and mitochondrial swelling of endothelial cells ensued. Intraalveolar edema occurred in most dogs exposed to 7 ppm NO_2 or higher and membrane damage without edema occurred in the others. Intraalveolar edema by light microscopy was associated with impaired surfactant activity and lung compliance. Exposure to NO_2 of 5 ppm or greater resulted in decrease of recovered lung lavage saturated lecithin. Exposure to 3 ppm NO_2 resulted in bleb formation in alveolar endothelium without biochemical or physiological changes.

Inhalation of nitrogen dioxide produces acute pulmonary edema if the concentration is sufficiently high. Human subjects exposed to silo gas containing up to several hundred parts per million of NO_2 have developed acute pulmonary edema. If they survive, a diffuse alveolitis and bronchiolitis obliterans follows.[1-3] Lowry and Schuman coined the term "silo filler's disease" to categorize such patients.[4] Similar clinical patterns of lung damage have been induced by accidental exposure to NO_2 during electric arc welding, combustion of organic compounds, and etching and acid-dipping of metals.[5] The present threshold limit of 5 ppm of NO_2 has been set for human industrial exposure.[5,6] Some urban communities report as high as 1.3 ppm NO_2 in the ambient air due chiefly to the internal combustion automobile engine.[7]

The present study was designed to evaluate the acute effects of low-level NO_2 inhalation on lung structure and function with the use of the anesthetized dog as a model. Changes in lung morphology and ultrastructure were related to alterations in static lung compliance, surface tension lowering capacity, and lipid composition of the lung wash material. Concentrations of NO_2 from 16 down to 3 ppm were used to define the sensitivity of the various sensors used to detect lung damage.

Received for publication Oct 21, 1970; accepted March 11, 1971.

From the departments of medicine and pathology, Duke University Medical Center, Durham, NC.

Read in part before the Tenth Annual Hanford Biology Symposium on Pollution and Lung Biochemistry, Richland, Wash, June 5, 1970, jointly sponsored by the Battelle Memorial Institute-Pacific Northwest Laboratories, National Air Pollution Control Administration, National Institute of Environmental Health Sciences, and the US Atomic Energy Commission.

Reprint requests to Muncie Clinic, 420 Washington St, Muncie, Ind 47302.

Methods and Materials

Thirteen beagle dogs weighing between 8 and 13 kg were studied. Anesthesia was produced by either pentobarbital sodium (30 mg/kg) administered intravenously or a combination of morphine sulfate (1 mg/kg) parenterally and chlorolose (80 mg/kg) intravenously. The latter anesthesia was better because it avoided low cardiac output and shock at NO_2 levels of 16 ppm. Direct, percutaneous tracheal cannulation was performed with the use of a cuffed, Teflon endotracheal tube. Aortic blood pressure and central venous pressure or pulmonary artery pressure were continually monitored in all studies using strain gauges (Statham, P_{23} AA) connected to a dual channel recorder (Sanborn). Cardiac outputs were measured in four dogs with the use of the green dye dilution technique.[8] Arterial P_{CO_2}, P_{O_2}, and pH were measured during each study, before and during NO_2 exposure.

The thoraxes of dogs 12, 13, and 14 were opened following the connection of the endotracheal tubes to a volume respirator (Harvard). In these dogs, sections of preexposed lung were removed surgically for electron microscopic examination and dry weight/wet weight determination. Postexposure lung samples were removed prior to killing the dogs. In the remaining dogs, the thorax was not opened until NO_2 exposure had been completed. The NO_2 was administered via the inspiratory port of the respirator and the expired air vented into a hood. The de-

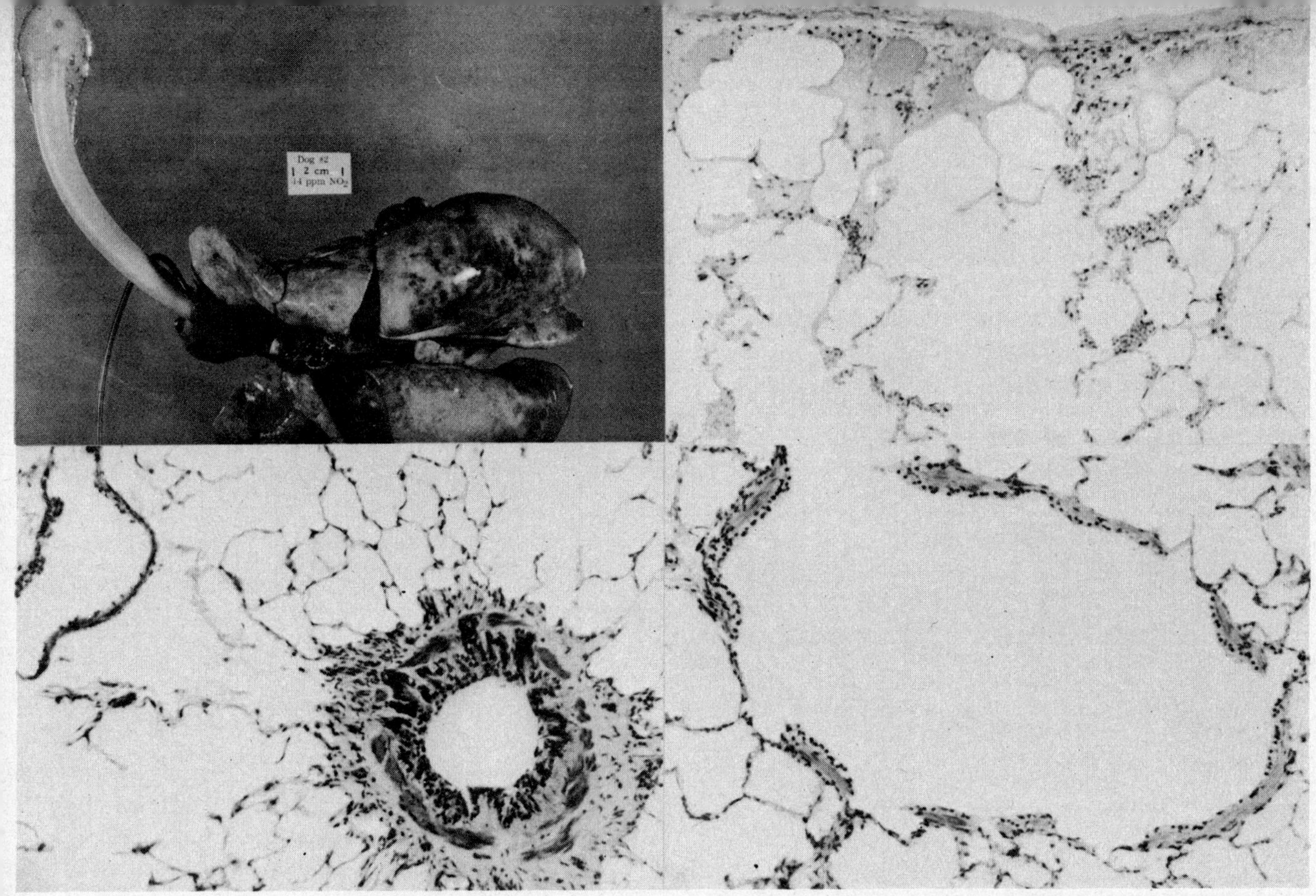

Fig 1.—Top left, *Lung from dog exposed to 16 ppm NO_2 for one hour. Airway edema is shown issuing from the endotracheal tube.* Top right, *intraalveolar edema and hemorrhage are shown in lung exposed to 13 ppn NO_2 for one hour (hematoxylin-eosin stain, ×100).* Bottom left, *Section of lung (×100) from animal exposed to 5 ppm NO_2 for one hour. Perivascular lymphatic dilatation and bronchiolar construction with inflammatory cell infiltration are shown.* Bottom right, *Lung section (×100) from animal exposed to 3 ppm NO_2 for one hour. No abnormalities are noted.*

sired NO_2 concentration was mixed in a 300-liter bag (Mylar) by diluting given volumes of 1% NO_2 with compressed air. Duplicate analyses for NO_2 content were performed using the Saltzman colorimetric technique.[9] Eleven dogs were exposed, each to a selected NO_2 concentration ranging from 3 to 16 ppm for one hour. Two dogs were ventilated for one hour with air alone. The dogs were killed by bleeding (shock lung) and the lungs excised. Static pressure-volume curves were obtained on ten lungs. One lung was lavaged with 150 ml of normal saline and the lavage material centrifuged at 1,000 × g for ten minutes at 4 C. Thirty milliters of supernatant was used to measure surface tension lowering capacity on a surface tension balance equipped with a Teflon barrier which completed one cycle in two minutes.[10] The rest of the supernatant was lyophilized and lipids extracted under nitrogen with the use of the technique of Folch et al.[11]

Individual phospholipids and neutral lipids were separated on silica gel thin-layer ascending chromatograms.[12] Spots were identified with appropriate standards using I_2 vapor except when fatty acid analysis was performed and then 2,4-

Table 1.—Effect of Intense NO_2 Exposure Upon Cardiopulmonary Performance in Dog 4 (16 ppm NO_2 × One Hour)*

Time	Cardiac Output (Liters/min)	Heart Rate (Beats per Minute)	Systemic Arterial Pressure (mm Hg)	Pulmonary Arterial Pressure (mm Hg)	Minute Ventilation (Liters/min)	Pa_{O_2} (mm Hg)	Pa_{CO_2} (mm Hg)	pH
11:00 AM	1.29	162	142/109	18/13	3.5	81	37	7.290
12:00 noon	1.05	160	140/100	10/7	3.5	84	35	7.305
1:30 PM	1.02	160	160/124	15/9	3.5	94	29	7.325
1:45 PM				NO_2 started				
2:00 PM	0.43	90	86/64	13/7	3.5	69	33	7.260
2:15 PM	0.42	90	86/64	9/5	3.5	41	40	7.180
2:30 PM	0.26	120	102/80	10/5	3.5	31	51	7.060
2:45 PM				NO_2 stopped				
3:00 PM	0.23	80	62/42	11/7	3.5	30	47	6.950

* Pentobarbital sodium (30 mg/kg) anesthesia with respirator (Harvard).

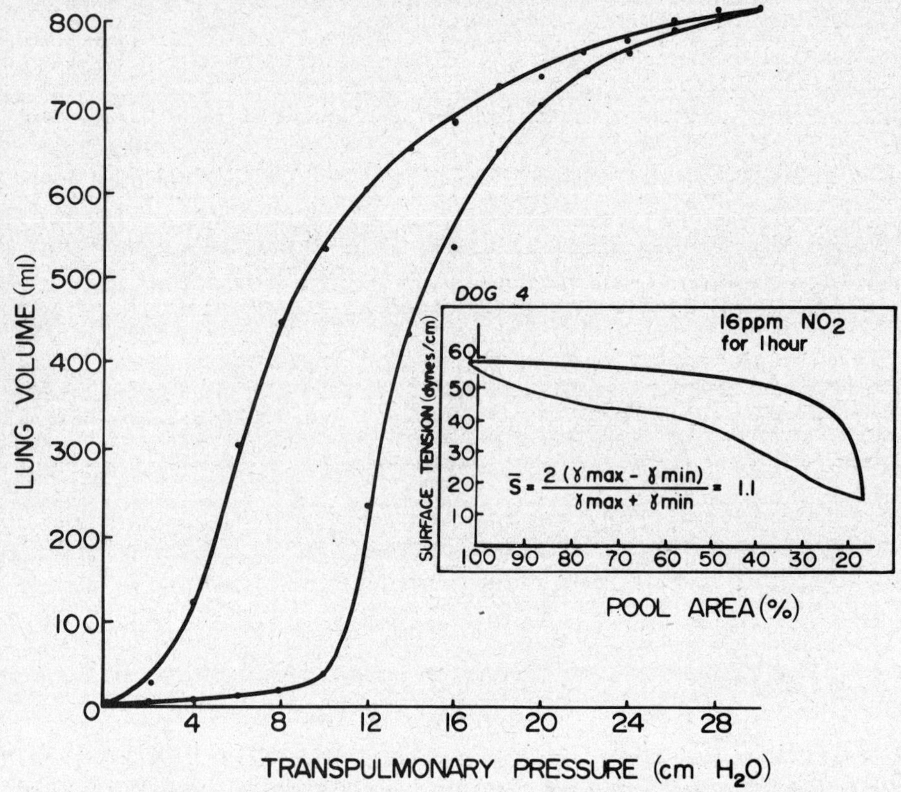

Fig 2.—Static pressure-volume curve on excised lung and surfactant activity of lung wash material from dog exposed to 16 ppm NO_2 for one hour. Lung required high transpulmonary pressure for inflation and deflation limb was shifted to the right which indicates premature alveolar closure. Surfactant minimum surface tension was 16 dynes/cm V_{max} (volume in milliliters at P_{TP} of 30 cm) = 3.4 ml/gm. LSI (lung stability index, computed from deflation limb) = $\frac{2V_5 + V_{10}}{2V_{max}}$ = 0.88. % V_{15} (percent total lung volume [milliliters] at a deflation P_{TP} of 15 cm H_2O) = 0.83.

Table 2.—Effect of Intense N

Study	LSI*	% V_{15}†	V_{max}‡ (ml/gm)
2	...	...	...
3	0.57	76	3.1
4	0.88	83	3.4
5	1.20	96	8.8
6	...	...	...
14	0.68	79	3.2
7	1.02	90	10.0
8	...	...	...
10	1.53	96	10.7
12	0.96	95	13.1
13	0.91	92	12.8
9	...	...	...
11	1.12	90	9.1

* Lung stability index (LSI) =

† % V_{15} = percent of total lung volume
‡ V_{max} = volume (milliliters) per gram of
§ S = (2 maximum surface tension [dynes/

dichlorofluorescein spray was used. Lipid phosphorus was determined and the micrograms of phospholipid calculated as micrograms of lipid phosphorus ×25.[13] Cholesterol,[14] glycerides,[15] and free fatty acids[16] were also quantified. Hydrolysis of lecithin fatty acids was done by heating in 0.5M methanolic NaOH and methyl esterification was performed with the use of boron trifluoride-methanol.[17] The composition of fatty acids was determined by gas-liquid chromatography with the use of an EGSS-X column at 180 C.

Sections for electron microscopy were cut into 1-mm cubes and fixed in 2% glutaraldehyde in cacodylate buffer. They were postfixed in 1% osmium tetroxide, dehydrated in alcohol followed by propylene oxide and embedded in epoxy resin (Epon). Sections were cut with a diamond knife and grids were stained with uranyl acetate followed by lead citrate. Lungs were pressure-fixed for three days with a solution of Jores' solution. Parafin-embedded sections were stained with hematoxylin-eosin for light microscopy.

Results

Exposure to 7 to 16 ppm NO_2 was frequently associated with acute pulmonary edema within 60 minutes. Hypotension was accompanied by a decrease in cardiac output and stroke volume (Table 1). The heart rate tended to become slower and pulmonary artery pressure either was unchanged or decreased. Systemic acidosis was out of proportion to the rise in arterial carbon dioxide pressure (Pa_{CO_2}) and paralleled the decrease in cardiac output and arterial oxygen pressure (Pa_{O_2}). The excised lungs frequently showed gross pulmonary edema with froth emanating from the endotracheal tube (Fig 1, top left). The mean lung dry weight/wet weight ratio was 12.9 in these animals as compared to 18.2 in the animals without intraalveolar edema. Static lung compliance (C_L) was abnormal in three of four studies with obvious intraalveolar edema (Table 2). Increased pressures were needed to open airways during inflation and a low volume of air per gram of wet lung at 30 cm H_2O transpulmonary pressure (P_{TP}) with poor stability of the deflation limb was noted (Fig 2). Light microscopy always revealed the presence of perivascular lymphatic dilation when intraalveolar edema was present (Fig 1, top right).

The lung wash material showed an impaired tendency to lower surface tension when intraalveolar edema was present irrespective of the NO_2 concentration used (Table 2). That the surfactant itself was not directly destroyed by the NO_2 was indicated by the fact that in vitro exposure of normal dog surfactant to NO_2 did not impair its ability to lower surface tension despite marked lowering of its pH (Table 3). The mean lipid composition of lung wash material taken from lungs with intraalveolar edema showed a low concentration of total phospholipid (36%) as opposed to neutral lipid (64%).

posure on Dog Lung Compliance, Surface, Activity, and Lipid Composition of Lung Wash Material

γ-min ynes/cm)	S̄§	Total Lipid (mg)	Lyso-lecithin (%)	Sphingo-myelin (%)	Lecithin (%)	Phos-Serine, Phos-Inositol (%)	Phos-Ethanol-amine (%)	Total Cholesterol (%)	Total Glycerides (%)	Free Fatty Acids (%)
	Intraalveolar Edema (7 to 16 ppm NO_2)									
20	0.7	...	...	...	...	...	...	...	...	...
15	1.3	...	...	...	...	...	...	...	...	...
17	0.9	...	...	...	...	...	...	...	...	...
12	1.2	1.6	4.4	6.5	9.1	0.0	8.0	40.0	24.6	0.0
22	0.8	1.2	0.0	2.0	7.8	0.9	8.7	16.3	60.3	2.1
12	1.2	13.4	2.3	9.7	29.9	0.7	17.7	23.0	6.9	9.9
Membrane Damage Without Intraalveolar Edema (3 to 12 ppm NO_2)										
3	1.6	2.6	0.0	2.5	25.6	0.8	5.5	24.4	30.1	11.0
3	1.5	3.6	0.0	1.2	25.2	1.6	3.5	15.3	39.7	10.8
1	1.9	7.0	1.2	3.6	53.9	2.9	15.3	17.1	4.5	0.0
5	1.6	3.2	0.0	0.9	53.9	0.0	13.0	1.8	9.6	20.6
4	1.6	7.7	0.0	5.9	51.6	2.7	9.6	1.8	16.7	11.5
		Unexposed								
3	1.8	6.3	0.0	0.0	39.1	0.0	3.2	27.5	29.8	0.0
4	1.7	9.2	0.6	2.1	44.6	1.8	13.4	19.1	14.1	4.4

$$\frac{\text{2 volume (milliliters) at } P_{TP} = 5 \text{ cm } H_2O + \text{volume (milliliters) at } P_{TP} = 10 \text{ cm } H_2O}{\text{2 volume (milliliters) at } P_{TP} = 30 \text{ cm } H_2O} = \frac{2V_5 + V_{10}}{2\,V_{max}}$$

(milliliters) at deflation $P_{TP} = 15$ cm H_2O.

vet lung at $P_{TP} = 30$ cm H_2O.

cm]) − minimum surface tension (dynes/cm)/maximum surface tension + minimum surface tension = (2 γ-max − γ-min)/γ-max + γ-min.

Whereas normal dog lung lavage lipid contained a preponderance of phospholipid (52%) the reverse was true in the edematous lungs. Phosphatidyl choline (lecithin) accounted for 42% of the total lavage lipid from normal lungs but was less than 30% in the lungs with intraalveolar edema. The fatty acid profile of lung lavage lecithin was examined in three animals and showed an increase in the content of unsaturated fatty acids, chiefly the C-18 unsaturates, and a decrease in the content of saturated fatty acids, chiefly C-16 palmitic acid. The lecithin fatty acid composition in these dogs resembled that of normal lung homogenate lecithin (Table 4).

Cell membrane damage without intraalveolar edema was noted histologically in five animals exposed to concentrations of NO_2 ranging from 3 to 12 ppm. In none of these dogs were there appreciable hemodynamic alterations although blood oxygen tensions tended to decrease late during the hour exposure (Table 5). The inflation and deflation limbs of the C_L curves were normal and the minimum surface tension of the lavage supernatants was 5 dynes/cm or less in each (Table 2). The mean total phospholipid percentage of total recovered lavage lipid was 55% for this group of animals. In two dogs (7 and 8) the percentages of total phospholipid were 26% and 25%, respectively, but the surface tension lowering capacity of the lavage supernatants was normal. The lung lavage lecithin fatty acid profile from one animal (7) showed an increase in the C-18 unsaturated fatty acids and a decrease in the palmitic acid content similar to those dogs with intraalveolar edema (Table 4). This animal was exposed to 5 ppm NO_2 for one hour with no effect on hemodynamics, arterial blood gas tensions, or pH. Histology showed no intraalveolar edema but perivascular lymphatic dilation and bronchocon-striction were noted (Fig 1, bottom left and right). Although the lipid composition of the lung wash material showed phospholipid and lecithin concentrations below normal and increases in neutral lipid concentrations, the C_L and surfactant activity were normal.

Three parts per million of NO_2 did not result in hemodynamic, blood gas tension, C_L, or surfactant changes. No evidence of lymphatic enlargement or intraalveolar edema was seen and the lung wash lipid composition was normal.

Ultrastructural Effects.—One-hour exposure to 3 to 12 ppm of NO_2 in air damaged cell membranes and mitochondria to produce swelling, (Fig 3 and 4). The swelling of mitochondria in all alveolar cells with loss of pinocytotic vesicles and swelling of endothelial cells was evident but scattered in 3 ppm exposure and became more general with higher exposure. The cristae and inner membranes of mitochondria disappeared. Blisters or blebs in endothelial cells reduced capillary lumina and appeared to trap erythrocytes and leukocytes or obliterate lumina. Intercellular junctions were not altered. Alveolar epithelial cells (type I cells) showed absence of pinocytotic vesicles, blebbing with clear cytoplasm, and loss of outer membranes. The alveolar spaces contained cell debris, especially small vesicles. Widening or swelling of the basement membranes between alveolar epithelial cells and capillary endothelial cells was in-

Table 3.—Exposure of Normal Dog Surfactant to 10^3 ppm NO_2 in Vitro

Exposure Time (Minutes)	pH of Hypophase	γ-min* (Dynes/cm)	$\bar{S}$†
0	6.80	4	1.6
5	2.80	4	1.6
10	2.20	3	1.7
15	1.70	4	1.6
30	1.20	3	1.7

*Minimum surface tension.

† Stability index $= 2 \frac{(\gamma\text{-max} - \gamma\text{-min})}{\gamma\text{-max} + \gamma\text{-min}}$.

Table 4.—Fatty Acid Composition of Dog Lung Wash Lecithin and Lung Homogenate Lecithin

NO_2 (ppm)	Intraalveolar Edema	14:0*	15:0	16:0	16:1	18:0	18:1 18:2 18:3	20.4
Dogs Exposed to NO_2 (n = 7)								
10	+	0	tr†	7	tr	9	82	tr
13	0	tr	2	53	tr	12	32	0
5	0	0	tr	11	0	15	73	0
10	+	0	tr	25	0	13	62	0
7	+	tr	tr	35	5	30	30	0
3	0	0	tr	49	10	20	21	0
3	0	0	tr	56	7	16	21	0
Unexposed (n = 2)								
	0	tr	tr	58	2	19	20	0
Normal Lung Homogenate (n = 5)								
	0	tr	tr	23	2	11	59	tr

* Number of carbons in fatty acid: number of unsaturated bonds.
† tr = trace.

Table 5.—Effect of Intense NO_2 Exposure Upon Cardiopulmonary Performance in the Dog (D_7 5 ppm of NO_2 × One Hour)

Time	Cardiac Output (Liters/min)	Heart Rate (Beats per Minute)	Systemic Arterial Pressure (mm Hg)	Central Venous Pressure (mm Hg)	Minute Ventilation (Liters/min)	Pa_{O_2} (mm Hg)	Pa_{CO_2} (mm Hg)	pH
12:30	1.10	150	140/100	1	2.75	79	47	7.290
12:45	1.03	150	140/100	1	3.00	105	31	7.340
1:00 PM	1.12	150	130/100	1	3.00	...	...	...
1:10				NO_2 started				
1:20	1.11	140	140/100	1	3.00	90	38	7.300
1:30	0.95	150	140/110	1	3.00	86	36	7.260
1:35	0.83	150	140/115	1	3.00	80	35	7.280
1:50	1.16	140	140/120	1	3.00	79	37	7.290
2:00	1.18	160	135/120	1	3.00	...	...	...
2:10	1.34	180	145/120	1	3.00	85	40	7.320
2:11				NO_2 stopped				
2:25	1.50	180	150/130	1	3.00	82	41	7.330

Morphine (1.0 mg/kg) and chloralose (80 mg/kg) anesthesia; with the use of a respirator (Harvard).

frequent and was not related to damage to the surrounding cells. Large numbers of polymorphonuclear leukocytes and platelets were observed against the membranes of the narrowed lumina of capillaries. Although mitochondria in the leukocytes were swollen, the cell membranes were intact. The presence of granular and vesicular debris, erythrocytes in alveolar spaces, and edema was observed after exposure to 7 ppm NO_2 and higher concentrations. In summary, the ultrastructural changes were characterized by swelling of organelles and cells and were most evident on the membranes of mitochondria and pinocytotic vesicles and in endothelial cells and epithelial cells (type I). Sticking of leukocytes in capillaries and leakage of plasma and erythrocytes were secondary effects. The acute effects were not proportional to concentration of NO_2 but membranes appeared to have a threshold of 3 ppm of NO_2.

Comment

The swelling of mitochondria in alveolar cells, including macrophages, and of endothelial cells is a sensitive manifestation of damage to membrane function. Membrane damage permits water to move into organelles and cells. The distribution of acute effects of low levels of NO_2 (3 to 5 ppm) in these dogs may be more uniform because anesthesia and positive pressure breathing from a volume respirator overcome normal regulation of distribution of inspired gas. Higher exposures cause further membrane leakiness and damage to alveolar epithelial cells which produces intraalveolar edema. This sequence appears to operate in alveolar damage from a wide variety of agents including shock, hypoxia, antilung antibodies, oxidants, paraquat, and 2,4-dinitrophenol.

As little as 7.5 ppm NO_2 for one hour produced acute intraalveolar edema in the model. In general, concentrations above this level resulted in acute pulmonary edema but not invariably. Because pulmonary artery and central venous pressure was unchanged or decreased during exposure, the intraalveolar edema was related to the toxic action of NO_2 on lung cells. One animal exposed to 12 ppm NO_2 for one hour showed only irregular ultrastructural lung damage. Subtle differences in exposure technique, as well as host factors from dog to dog, may be responsible for varying degrees of tissue damage. The critical concentration of one hour of NO_2 in this dog model appears to be about 5 ppm since exposures to lower concentrations produce only subtle ultrastructural changes in cell membranes and mitochondria. Although extrapolation from this anesthetized dog model to man is questionable, the data support the present industrial threshold

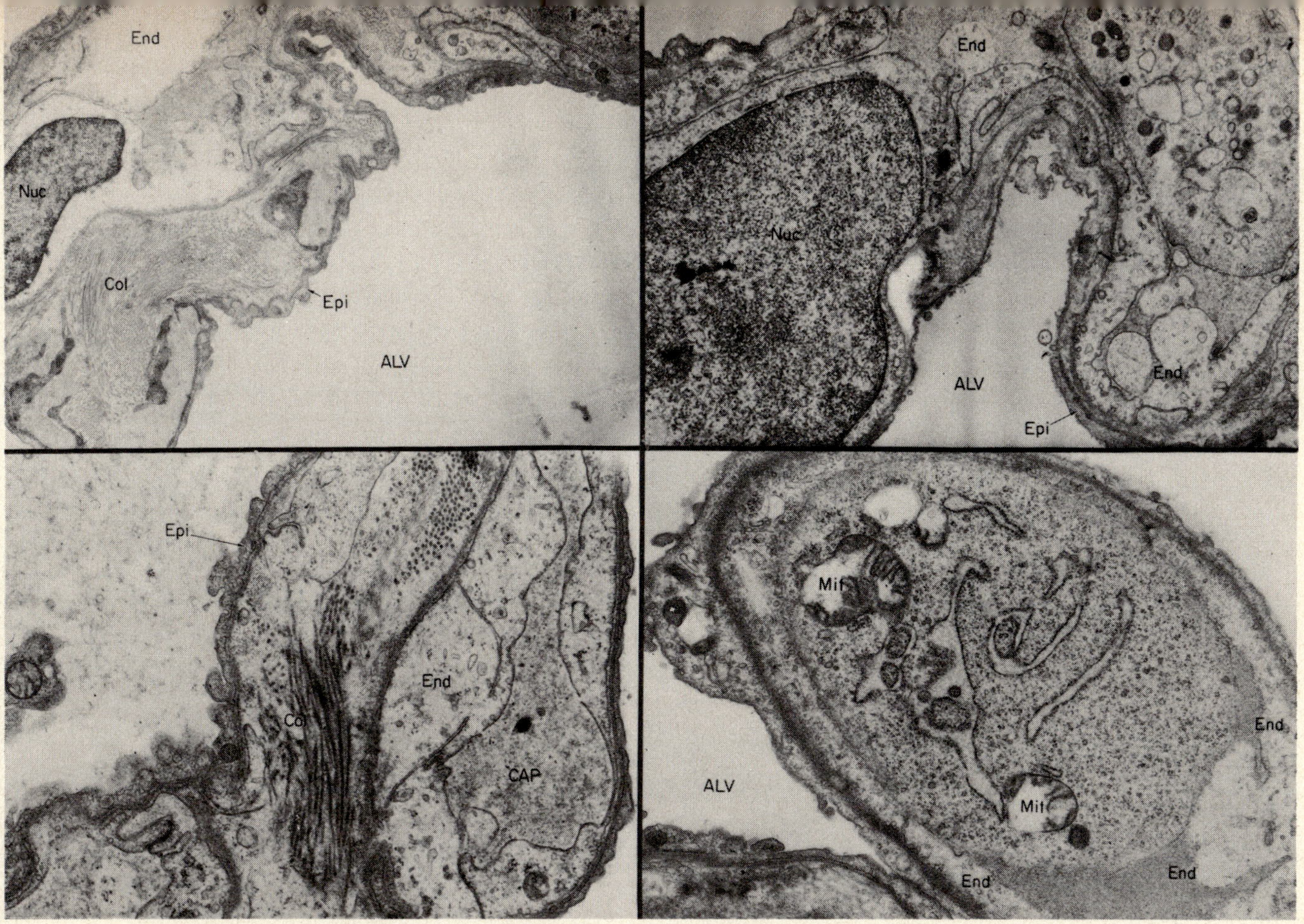

Fig 3.—Electron micrographs of alveoli from dogs exposed to NO_2 for one hour. Fixation was with glutaraldehyde 2%, postfixed with osmium tetroxide. It was embedded in epoxy resin and thin-sectioned with diamond knives, and the grids were stained with uranyl acetate and lead citrate. Top left, *5 ppm NO_2 ($\times$17,500);* top right, *5 ppm NO_2 ($\times$26,250);* bottom left, *5 ppm NO_2 ($\times$30,000);* bottom right, *12 ppm NO_2 ($\times$26,250).*

Fig 4.—Electron micrograph of normal alveoli (left, $\times$*10,500;* right, $\times$*35,000).*

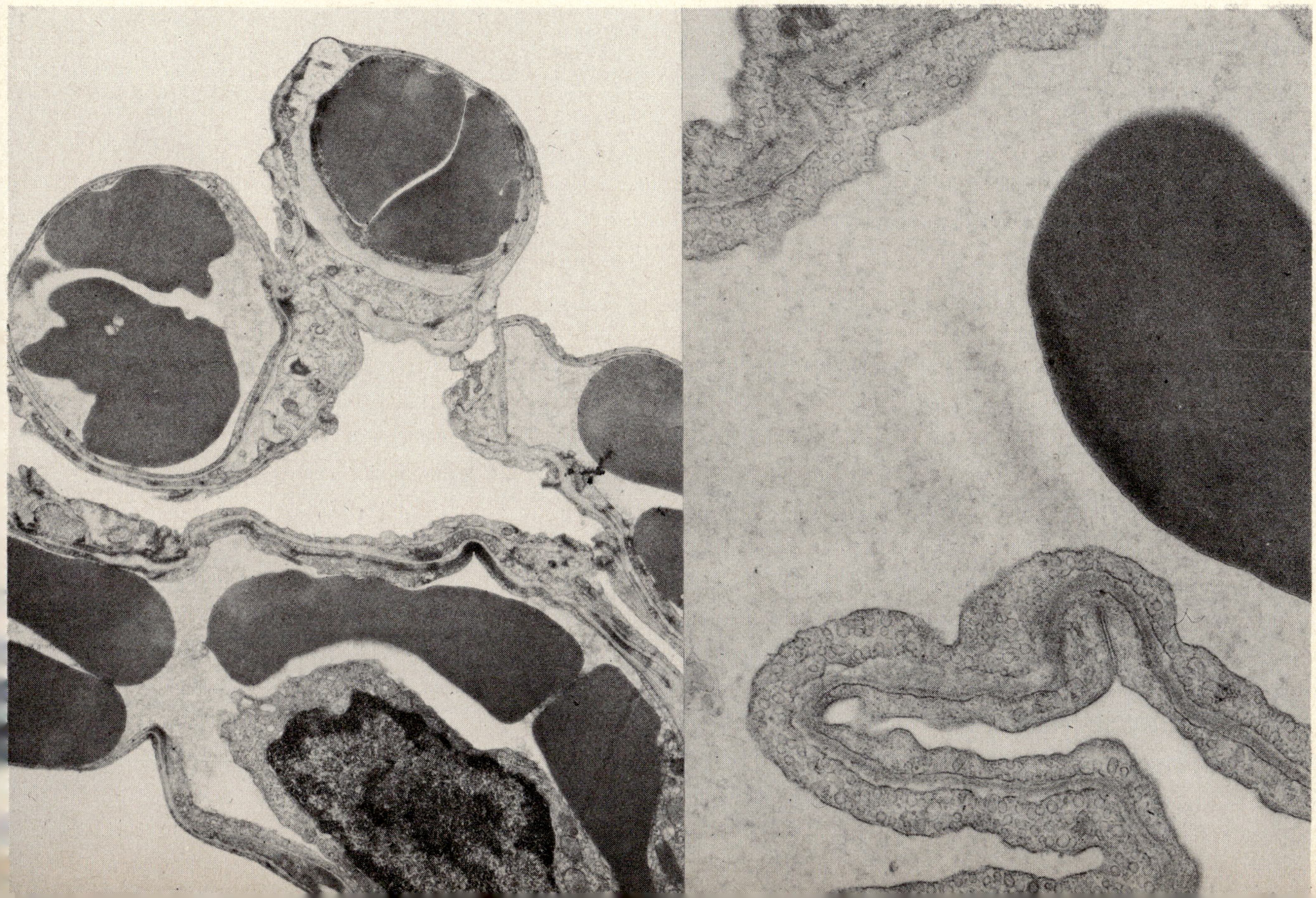

limit of 5 ppm[5,6] at least for short-term exposure.

Only when atelectasis or intraalveolar edema occurred did the C_L or surfactant become abnormal. Similar findings have been published for oxygen-induced lung damage.[18] Fibrinogen from serum impairs the surfactant activity and may partly explain the loss of surface tension lowering capacity in the presence of intraalveolar edema.[19] In addition, neutral lipids such as cholesterol impair the surface tension lowering effect of phospholipid.[20] The present finding of impaired surface active material from the NO_2 exposed lungs with intraalveolar edema lends support to those observations. In addition, the lecithin recovered, which is the chief surface active phospholipid in normal lung, was abnormal in that it contained a preponderance of unsaturated fatty acids. The optimal lecithin for normal surface activity is one which contains an abundance of saturated fatty acids (palmitic) which allows a greater concentration of surface active molecules per unit area of interface.[21] It is likely that several factors are operative in impairing surfactant activity in the presence of intraalveolar edema: binding of active phospholipid sites, alteration of phospholipid structure, and dilution by nonsurface active lipids derived from damaged tissue and plasma.

The poor recovery of lung wash lipid from some NO_2 damaged lungs may represent an inability to recover alveolar surfactant lipid. The high surface tension within edematous alveoli may interfere with the ingress and subsequent egress of the saline lavage fluid. The result would be recovery of nonsurfactant lipid from upper airways. However, the poor recovery of such nonsurfactant lipid from dogs without intraalveolar edema would not be in accord with this hypothesis. Nitrogen dioxide causes marked bronchoconstriction in such concentrations[5] and this may impair the recovery of alveolar surfactant lipid. Further studies are needed to elucidate this point.

Endothelial damage seems to be an early stage of lung destruction produced by NO_2. Such damage permits transudation of fluid into the lung interstitial spaces and finally into the alveoli, depending on the severity. After intraalveolar edema occurs, surfactant activity is impaired, C_L is diminished, and airway closure results. The increased P_{TP} needed to initially inflate the lung probably represents recruitment of such closed airways, while the unstable deflation limb reflects early alveolar closure due to high surface tensions.[22]

Impairment of surfactant synthesis would not explain the changes which follow acute NO_2 exposure, because the surfactant lecithin pool has a half-time of about 14 hours.[23] However, more prolonged exposures to low NO_2 levels may impair sufactant lecithin synthesis.

This investigation was supported in part by Public Health Service contract 22-69-105 from the National Air Pollution Control Administration.

References

1. Delaney LT Jr, Schmidt HW, Stroebel CF: Silo-filler's disease. *Proc Staff Meet Mayo Clin* **31**:189-198, 1956.
2. Grayson RR: Silage gas poisoning: Nitrogen dioxide pneumonia, a new disease in agricultural workers. *Ann Intern Med* **45**:393-408, 1956.
3. Moran TJ, Hellstrom L: Bronchiolitis obliterans. *Arch Path* **66**:691-707, 1958.
4. Lowry T, Schuman LM: Silo-filler's disease: A syndrome caused by nitrogen dioxide. *JAMA* **162**:153-160, 1956.
5. Wagner WD, Duncan BR, Wright PG, et al: Experimental study of threshold limit of NO_2. *Arch Environ Health* **10**:455-466, 1965.
6. Tabershaw IR, Ottoboni F, Cooper WC: Oxidants: Air quality criteria based on health effects. *J Occup Med* **10**:464-480, 1968.
7. Biological effects of air pollutants, in Stern AC (ed): *Air Pollution*. New York, Academic Press, 1968, pp 446-533.
8. Fox IJ, Brooker LGS, Haseltine DW, et al: A new dye for continuous recording of dilution curves in whole blood independent of variations in blood oxygen saturation. *Circulation* **14**:937-938, 1956.
9. Saltzman BE: Colorimetric microdetermination of nitrogen dioxide in the atmosphere. *Anal Chem* **26**:1949-1955, 1954.
10. Greenfield LJ, Ebert PA, Benson DW: Effect of positive pressure ventilation on surface tension properties of lung extracts. *Anesthesiology* **25**:312-316, 1964.
11. Folch J, Lees M, Sloane-Stanley GH: A simple method for the isolation and purification of total lipid from animal tissues. *J Biol Chem* **226**:497-509, 1957.
12. Skipski VP, Peterson RF, Barclay M: Separation of phosphatidyl ethanol amine, phosphatidyl serine, and phospholipids by thin-layer chromatography. *J Lipid Res* **3**:467-470, 1962.
13. Bartlett GR: Phosphorus assay in column chromatography. *J Biol Chem* **234**:466-468, 1959.
14. Mann GV: A method for measurement of cholesterol in blood serum. *Clin Chem* **7**:275-284, 1961.
15. Walsh D: Thin-layer chromatographic separation and colorimetric analysis of barley or malt lipid classes and their fatty acids. *J Chromatogr* **17**:278-287, 1965.
16. Dole VP: A relation between non-esterified fatty acids in plasma and the metabolism of glucose. *J Clin Invest* **35**:150-154, 1956.
17. Metcalfe LD, Schmitz AA, Pelka JR: Rapid preparation of fatty acid esters from lipids for gas chromatographic analysis. *Anal Chem* **38**:514-515, 1966.
18. Morgan TE, Finley TN, Huber GL, et al: Alterations in pulmonary surface active lipids during exposure to increased oxygen tension. *J Clin Invest* **44**:1737-1744, 1965.
19. Taylor FB Jr, Abrams ME: Effect of surface active lipoprotein on clotting and fibrinolysis, and of fibrinogen on surface tension of surface active lipoprotein. *Amer J Med* **40**:346-350, 1966.
20. Tierney DF, Johnson RP: Altered surface tension of lung extracts and lung mechanics. *J Appl Physiol* **20**:1253-1260, 1965.
21. Scarpelli EM: *The Surfactant System of the Lung*. Philadelphia, Lea & Febiger, 1968, p 269.
22. Gruenwald P: A numerical index of the stability of lung expansion. *J Appl Physiol* **18**:665-667, 1963.
23. Tierney DF, Clements JA, Trahan HJ: Rates of replacement of lecithins and alveolar instability in rat lungs. *Amer J Physiol* **213**:671-676, 1967.

Alterations in the Lung Following the Administration of Ozone

Gary L. Huber, MD, Boston; Robert J. Mason, MD, Bethesda, Md; Marc LaForce, MD, and Nancy J. Spencer, MS, Boston; and Donald E. Gardner, MS; and David L. Coffin, DVM, Cincinnati

Inhalation of ozone (5 ppm for three hours) by rabbits resulted in morphologic alterations in the pulmonary alveolar macrophages recovered from the lungs of exposed animals. These structural alterations were characteristic of cellular injury or cell death and included intracellular vacuolization, dilatation of the endoplasmic reticulum and perinuclear envelope, swelling of mitochondria, cell lysis, and formation of myelin figures and autophagic vacuoles. Exposure to ozone had no significant effect on pulmonary surface activity, phosphatide composition, or fatty acid composition of phospholipids recovered from extracts of whole lung or by bronchioalveolar lavage from exposed animals. A dose-related functional impairment in alveolar macrophage intrapulmonary antibacterial defense mechanisms resulted from exposure to lower levels of ozone. Similar dose-related impairments in macrophage function were induced with prolonged oxygen administration.

The fundamental host defense mechanism against inhaled bacteria is the pulmonary alveolar macrophage system.[1,2] A wide variety of environmental and endogenous influences have been shown to depress this macrophage defense network and to alter the rate at which inhaled bacteria are inactivated by the lungs.[3,4] Since experimental exposure to high levels of ozone increased the mortality of animals subsequently challenged with aerosolized pathogenic bacteria,[5,6] an alteration in alveolar macrophage function or structure was suspected. Further studies supported this hypothesis by demonstrating a dose-related functional impairment of phagocytosis of bacteria by alveolar macrophages following experimental exposure to ozone in vivo.[7] Because of this critical importance of the alveolar macrophage system, structural alterations in alveolar macrophages recovered from animals experimentally exposed to ozone were investigated. In addition, since inhalation of ozone has been reported to cause peroxidation of lipids in the lung,[8] the effect of ozone on pulmonary phospholipids was evaluated.

Received for publication Oct 21, 1970; accepted April 27, 1971.

From the Channing Laboratory and Thorndike Memorial Laboratory, Harvard Medical Unit, Boston City Hospital; the Department of Medicine, Harvard Medical School; and the Department of Physiology, Harvard School of Public Health, Boston; the Molecular Disease Branch of the National Heart and Lung Institute, Bethesda, Md; and the Consumer Protection and Environmental Health Service, Division of Health Effects Research, National Air Pollution Control Administration, Cincinnati and Durham, NC.

Read in part before the Tenth Annual Hanford Biology Symposium on Pollution and Lung Biochemistry, Richland, Wash, June 5, 1970, jointly sponsored by the Battelle Memorial Institute-Pacific Northwest Laboratories, National Air Pollution Control Administration, National Institute of Environmental Health Sciences, and the US Atomic Energy Commission.

Reprint requests to Channing Laboratory, Harvard Medical Unit, Boston City Hospital, Boston 02118 (Dr. Huber).

Methods

Ozone was generated by passing commercial oxygen through a neon-tube silent arc generator and delivered to an exposure chamber, as previously described.[6,7] Ozone concentrations were evaluated every 45 to 60 minutes by the neutral buffered potassium iodide method.[9] The period of exposure was in all cases three hours. White, male, New Zealand rabbits (1.5 to 2.0 kg in weight), maintained on commercial rabbit chow, were placed in the exposure chamber. Ten experimental animals were exposed to 5 ppm of ozone for three hours. Ten control animals were exposed to room air. Immediately after exposure all rabbits were killed by intravenous administration of pentobarbital sodium (50 mg/kg). In five ozone-exposed rabbits and in five control animals, alveolar macrophages were obtained by washing the lung in situ with three 30-ml aliquots of isotonic saline at room temperature and harvested according to a modification of the method of Myrvik.[7,10] Recovered cells were separated from lavaging fluid by centrifugation at 100 g for ten minutes. The supernatant was decanted and immediately frozen at −70 C. The pellet of recovered cells was fixed for three hours by gentle resuspension in 3% glutaraldehyde in 0.1M sodium cacodylate buffer at pH 7.4, with 0.01% calcium chloride.[11] The cells were kept in suspension by periodic, gentle shaking. After aldehyde fixation, the cells were washed twice in cacodylate buffer and kept in the same medium for two to seven days at 8 C. The cells were then postfixed at 4 C for one hour in 1.3% osmium tetroxide in pH 7.4 s-collidine buffer,[12] with 0.01% calcium chloride. They were dehydrated in increasing concentrations of alcohol, infiltrated with propylene oxide-Epon 812 and embedded in Epon 812 at the bottom of plastic capsules.[11,13] When the cell pellets were over 1 mil in thickness, aliquots were distributed to additional capsules. Thick sections (0.5μ to 1.0μ) were stained with toluidine blue and prepared for light microscopy.[14] Ultrathin sections were cut with a diamond knife on an ultramicrotome (LKB III Ultratome) and stained with a combination of uranyl acetate and lead citrate.[15,16] A minimum of 100 cells from each animal was examined with an electron microscope (Philips EM 200), and representative cells photographed. Differential cell counts were performed on several samples by serial sectioning whole blocks to assure random sampling.

An additional five ozone-exposed (5 ppm) and five control animals were studied for alterations in pulmonary phospholipids, light and electron microscopic structural changes, and pulmonary surface activity. After death, each hemithorax and the heart were exposed through a midline sternotomy and median pericardectomy. The left main-stem bronchus

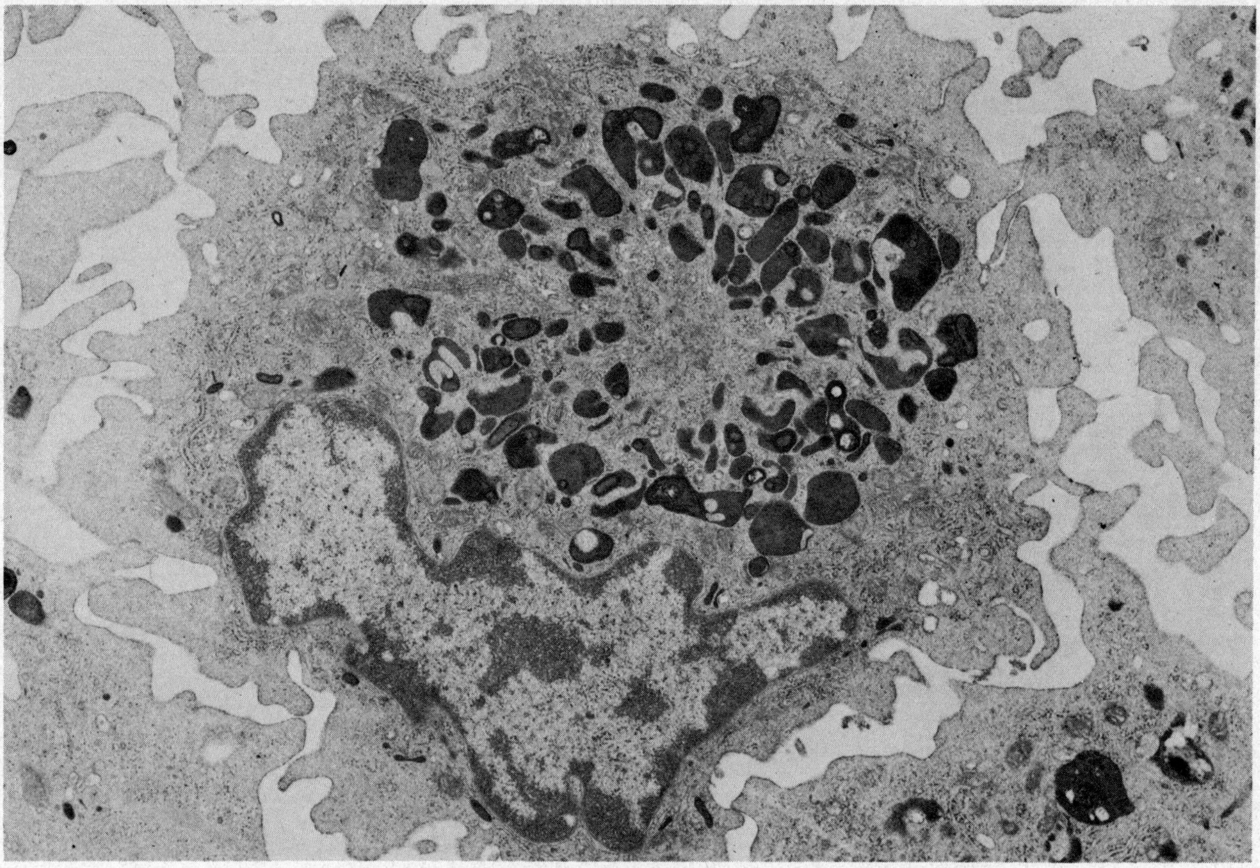

Fig 1.—Electron micrograph of a pulmonary alveolar macrophage recovered from the lungs of a control rabbit by bronchioalveolar lavage (× 18,000).

was intubated with a rubber catheter and the left lung lavaged in situ with isotonic saline. The recovered lavage fluid was centrifuged (500 g for ten minutes), separated from cells, and stored at −70 C. Multiple lung biopsy specimens (10 to 30) were taken from the right upper lobe for light and electron microscopy.[17] The pulmonary arteries to the right middle and lower lobes were gently perfused (less than 10 to 15 mm Hg pressure) with saline until the effluent from the pulmonary veins was grossly free of blood. These lobes were then excised and immediately frozen at −70 C.

Minimal surface tension of extracts of the right middle lobes of these five ozone-exposed and of five control rabbits was measured on a modified Wilhelmy balance at room temperature.[18] Extracts were prepared from approximately 1.5-gm specimens of lung, minced, and mixed with 30 ml of isotonic saline for 30 minutes. The solution was then filtered through gauze and placed in the Teflon trough of the balance. The surface film of the trough was alternately compressed to 20% of its maximum surface area and then expanded to maximum area in 20-minute to 30-minute cycles. The lowest surface tension found after prolonged cycling (up to 12 hours) was considered the minimal surface tension. Minimal surface tension of the recovered lavage fluid from the additional five ozone-exposed and control animals was evaluated in a similar manner.[18]

The right lower lobe and the lyopholized fluid of the lavaged left lung from control and ozone-exposed animals were extracted by the method of Folch et al.[19] All solvents were of analytical grade and subsequently glass distilled. Lipids thus extracted were stored in benzene-acetone (8:1, volume/volume) at −70 C until analyzed. An aliquot of total lipids was examined for ultraviolet absorbency at 225 to 300 mμ in hexane-ethanol (1:1, v/v) to estimate conjugated dienes formed by lipid peroxidation.[8] 4-Methyl-2,6-di-*tert*-butylphenol (BHT) was added to all samples except those subject to direct fatty acid analysis or chromatography with diethylaminoethyl cellulose (DEAE). Phospholipid composition was determined in triplicate by one-dimensional thin-layer chromatography.[20] Phospholipid phosphorus was quantified, as described by Bartlett.[21] Lecithins to be analyzed for fatty acid composition were partially purified by DEAE column chromatography[22] and were then further isolated by thin-layer chromatography.[20] These isolated lecithins were saponified and the fatty acids con-

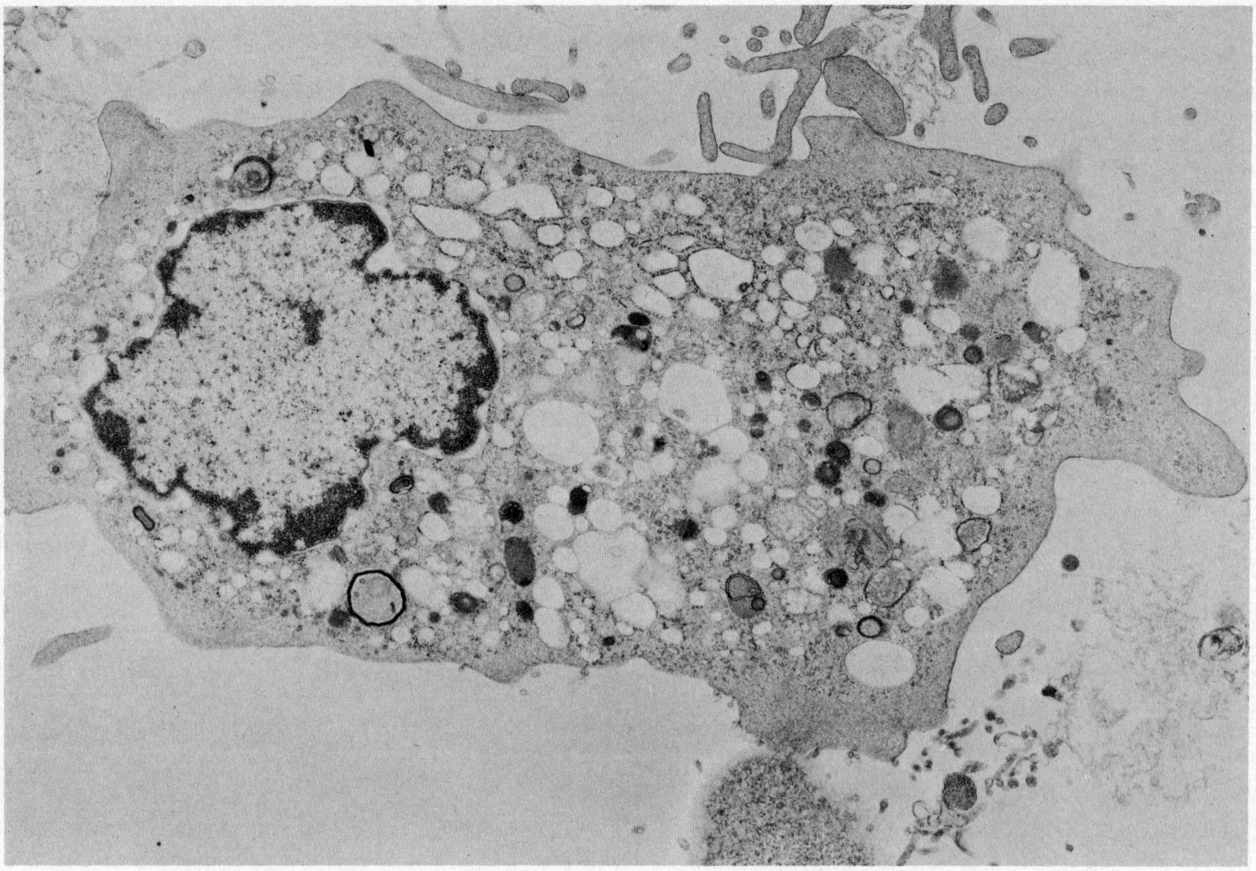

Fig 2.—Electron micrograph of an alveolar macrophage recovered from the lungs of a rabbit exposed to ozone (5 ppm for three hours), which demonstrates intracellular vacuolization, swollen mitochondria, and dilatation of the endoplasmic reticulum and perinuclear envelope (×20,000).

verted to the methyl esters,[23] which were determined by gas-liquid chromatography on an ethylene glycol succinate. Quantitative results with National Heart Institute fatty acid standards (KD,KF) agreed with the stated composition data, with a relative error of less than 5% for major components (greater than 10% of total mixture) and of less than 15% for minor components (less than 10% of total mixture). After formation of mercuric acid adducts[24] and removal of excess mercuric acetate by repeated Folch washings, disaturated lecithins were separated from unsaturated lecithins by thin-layer chromatography on silica-H plates in chloroform-methanol-8M ammonium hydroxide (75/25/3.5). Lipid analyses on the cell pellet recovered by bronchioalveolar lavage of control and exposed animals were not performed because of the variable change in differential cell profile following ozone inhalation, as previously noted.[7]

Results

The majority (84% to 94%) of cells recovered by bronchioalveolar lavage from control rabbits had the morphologic characteristics of pulmonary alveolar macrophages.[25] These cells, as seen in Fig 1, have a single, eccentric nucleus, an abundance of mitochondria and endoplasmic reticulum, and were devoid of desmosomes. They contained, in variable number, a variety of pleomorphic inclusions, the phagosomes or secondary lysosomes, that are considered to represent the end products of phagocytosis.[25] Only an occasional (2% to 3%) heterophil was noted in cells recovered from control animals. Granular pneumocytes (alveolar type II cells, greater alveolar cells) comprised less than 0.5% of recovered cells, as identified by electron microscopy. The remainder of cells harvested from control animals included lymphocytes (2% to 3%), ciliated epithelial cells (1% to 2%), and an occasional Clara cell. The remainder of cells could not be definitively identified by ultrastructural criteria.

Differential cell counts on cells

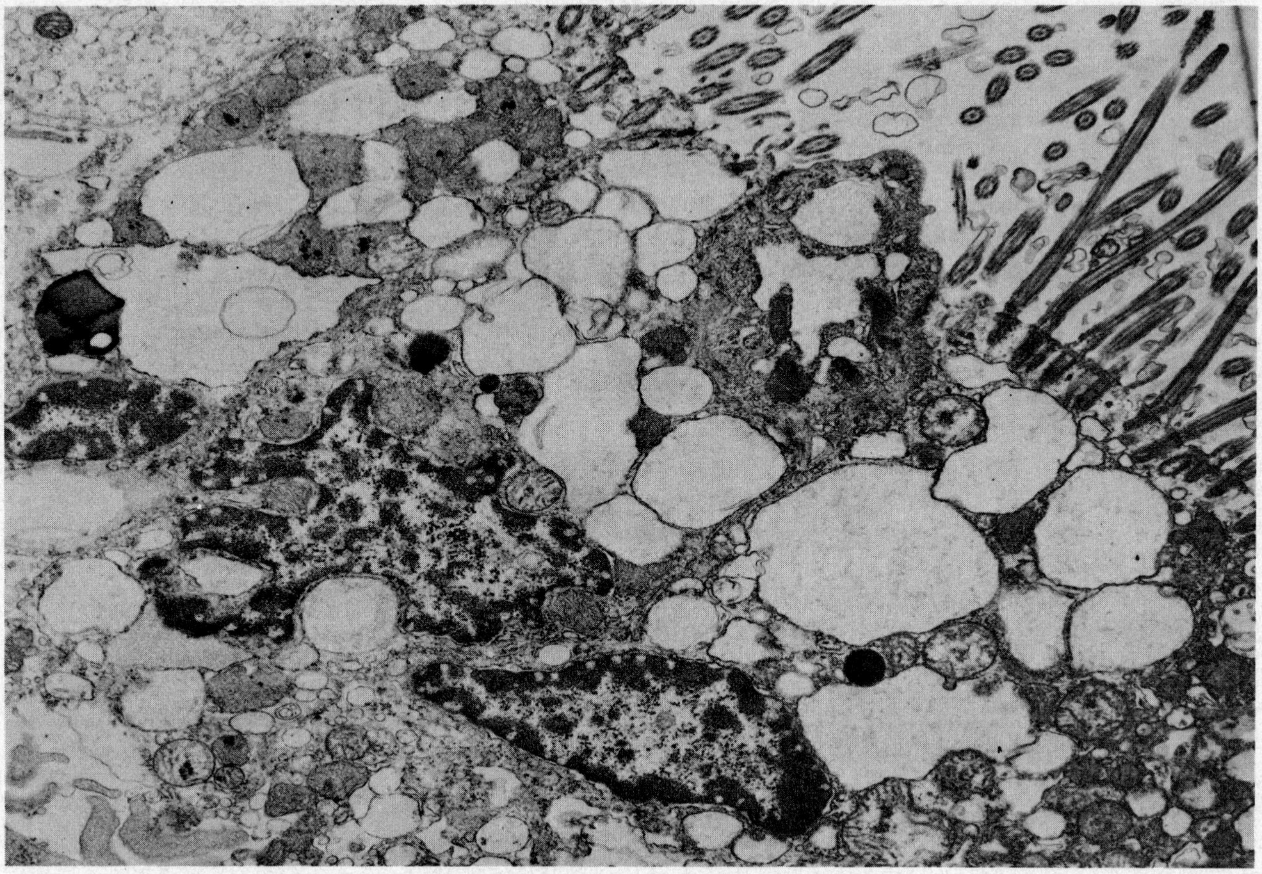

Fig 3.—Electron micrograph of a ciliated epithelial cell recovered from the lungs of a rabbit exposed to ozone, with profound intracellular vacuolization, dilatation of the endoplasmic reticulum, and swollen mitochondria (×25,000).

harvested from ozone-exposed animals demonstrated an increase predominantly in the percentage of heterophils (34% to 50%) and ciliated epithelial cells (8% to 16%) which were often recovered as sheets of cells often apparently adherent to a layer of mucus. There was no demonstrable increase in the number of granular pneumocytes or lymphocytes recovered. An abundance of red blood cells was present in the lavage fluid of ozone-treated animals; red blood cells were only infrequently noted in control animals.

Essentially all alveolar macrophages and ciliated epithelial cells recovered from ozone-exposed animals had morphologic alterations characteristic of cellular injury or cell death (Fig 2,3). These ultrastructural alterations included intracellular vacuolization, dilatation of the endoplasmic reticulum and perinuclear envelope, swelling of mitochondria, cell lysis, and, to a lesser degree, formation of myelin figures and autophagic vacuoles. These morphologic changes were also seen, to a lesser degree, in heterophils recovered from ozone-exposed rabbits. Similar alterations were noted in a much smaller fraction (8% to 16%) of alveolar macrophages recovered from control animals.

The results of surface tension measurements on extracts of whole lung and in recovered lavage fluid from control and ozone-exposed animals are presented in Table 1. Surface activity was measured on the lung extracts and endobronchial washings at varying intervals after freezing. Normal surface activity (less than 15 dynes/cm) was present in both control and ozone-exposed animals. Moderate increases in surface tension on samples from the ozone-exposed group did not appear to be significant.

Light and electron microscopy of lung parenchyma revealed minimal interstitial edema and an apparent increase in cellular elements (red

Table 1.—Effect of Ozone on Pulmonary Surface Tension*

	(Dynes/cm) Control	Ozone
Pulmonary lavage	8.0 ± 1.4	9.8 ± 2.5
Whole lung extract	10.6 ± 2.7	12.8 ± 1.3

* (Mean ± SE, n = 5). This table presents the minimum pulmonary surface tensions (dynes/cm) obtained after prolonged cycling on pulmonary lavage fluid and extracts of whole lung obtained from control and ozone-exposed animals.

Table 2.—Effect of Ozone on Lung Lipids and Lung Weight

Right Lower Lobe	Control	Ozone
Weight (gm)	2.49 ± 0.16	2.73 ± 0.08
Lipid P (mg)	3.03 ± 0.19	3.44 ± 0.24
Weight/lipid P (gm/mg)	0.837 ± 0.021	0.804 ± 0.042
Disaturated lecithin (mg/gm lung)	5.21 ± 0.21	5.53 ± 0.36

* (Mean ± SE, n = 5). Presented in this table are the lungs weights (gm), total lipid phosphorus (mg) the lung weight-lipid phosphorus ratio (gm/mg) and the amount of disaturated lecithin (mg/gm lung) for the right lower lobe of control and ozone-exposed animals.

Table 3.—Phosphatide Composition of Pulmonary Lavage Fluid and of Whole Lung*

	% Total Lipid Phosphorus			
	Pulmonary Lavage Fluid		Whole Lung	
Phosphatide	Control	Ozone	Control	Ozone
Lecithin	81.9 ± 0.8	82.8 ± 0.9	47.1 ± 1.2	48.3 ± 0.5
Phosphatidyl ethanolamine	11.8 ± 0.7	11.3 ± 0.6	26.4 ± 0.4	25.7 ± 0.2
"X"†	4.8 ± 0.2	3.7 ±0.6	12.8 ± 0.4	12.2 ± 0.2
Sphingomyelin	0.7 ± 0.1	1.3 ± 0.1	12.4 ± 0.2	12.3 ± 0.2
Lysolecithin	0.4 ± 0.1	0.3 ± 0.1	0.9 ± 0.2	0.8 ± 0.1
Base and top	0.1 ± 0.1	0.5 ± 0.2	0.7 ± 0.4	0.7 ± 0.4

* (Mean ± SE, n = 5). This presents the phosphatide composition, expressed as a percent of the total lipid phosphorus, of pulmonary lavage fluid and whole lung for control and ozone-exposed animals.

† "X" group = pooled values for phosphatidyl serine, phosphatidyl inositol, and phosphatidyl dimethyl ethanolamine.

Table 4.—Fatty Acid Composition of Total Lecithin*

		(mol %)								
		14:0	16:0	16:1	18:0	18:1	18:2	18:3	20:4	Percent Disaturated Lecithin†
Pulmonary lavage fluid	Control	3.6	69.8	6.5	1.4	12.9	5.5	0.2	0	49.7 ± 2.1
	Ozone	3.9	68.4	6.3	1.7	12.2	7.3	0.2	0	52.3 ± 1.4
Whole lung	Control	2.2	61.0	4.8	6.1	14.4	10.7	0.1	0.8	37.4 ± 1.0
	Ozone	2.1	61.4	5.7	5.6	12.7	11.2	0.4	0.9	37.1 ± 0.5

* (Mean ± SE, n = 5)
† Percent of total lecithin

blood cells, heterophils) in the alveoli of animals treated with ozone. Intra-alveolar edema was not demonstrable. Except for the presence of heterophils and red blood cells in the alveoli of the ozone-treated group, tissues from control and experimental animals could not be readily distinguished morphologically either by light or electron microscopy.

Lung weights (right lower lobe) and analyses of whole lung lipids are shown in Table 2. Phospholipid composition of whole lung and of pulmonary lavage fluids are summarized in Table 3. The fatty acid composition of the isolated lecithins and the percent of disaturated lecithin, as determined by mercuric acid adduction, are shown in Table 4. Lecithin was the predominant phosphatide component recovered from both sources. There were no demonstrable differences in lung weights, total lipid phosphorus, phosphatide composition or lecithin fatty acid saturation in the control and ozone-exposed animals. There was also no difference in the ultraviolet absorbency of whole lung lipids and, as such, there was no indication of conjugated diene formation following exposure to ozone.

Comment

The relatively pure yield of pulmonary alveolar macrophages from control animals, with the use of electron microscopic criteria of identification, correlates with light microscopic observations of previous investigators.[7] The absence of desmosomes in the alveolar macrophages and the paucity of granular pneumocytes in both groups of animals suggest that the harvest of cells by this technique recovers cells that were free in the alveolar spaces and airways and not washed off the parenchymal walls. The significant increase in the number of heterophils, red blood cells, and ciliated epithelial cells recovered from the ozone-exposed animals reflects the inflammatory response of exposure to this level of oxidant.

The ultrastructural alterations demonstrable in the macrophages recovered from the ozone-exposed animals are characteristic of a nonspecific, toxic cellular reaction.[26] Preliminary results of studies with exposure to lower concentrations of ozone suggest that the degree of cellular injury, characterized by the above morphologic criteria, may be closely related to the concentration of ozone exposure. Fewer cells recovered from animals exposed to lower levels of ozone (3 and 1 ppm for three hours) have these demonstrable ultrastructural changes and the magnitude of the cellular alterations appears to be less. Other investigators have noted significant ultrastructural alterations in the lung parenchyma of mice exposed to oxidants.[27] The absence of these changes in our animals may be due to species-specific differences in response to a given level of ozone,[28] a different duration or level of oxidant exposure,[29] the relative concentration of cells exposed,[30] or differences in methods of fixation.[27]

The severity of morphologic alterations in alveolar macrophages in our studies parallels the degree of functional impairment and the alterations in alveolar macrophage hydrolases reported in earlier observations.[7,31] In additional studies, we have demonstrated that the intrapulmonary inactivation of an aerosolized bacterial challenge is progressively impaired by prior exposure to increasing concentrations of ozone[32] or to increasing duration of exposure to high oxygen tensions.[33] These functional alterations in alveolar macrophage antibacterial host defenses were accompanied by morphologic alterations in macrophage structure.[32,33]

Acute exposure to ozone did not appear to have a significant effect on pulmonary surface activity in either the alveolar lining material, as harvested by saline lavage, or in saline extracts of whole lung (Table 1). It must be emphasized, however, that surface tension studies of this type are purely qualitative in nature,[18] that a minimum surface tension of 15 dynes/cm reflects simply an arbitrary evaluation for the "presence" or "absence" of the so-called pulmonary surfactant,[18] and that quantitative conclusions cannot be drawn from these data.[18] These results are in accord with the oxidant exposure studies of Morgan et al,[34] who found no alteration in pulmonary surface activity in the absence of pulmonary edema. The data also support the work of Frank and co-workers, who demonstrated that exposure to ozone, in levels as high as 12 ppm for three hours, had little effect on pulmonary surface activity or volume-pressure behavior of the lung in the absence of pulmonary edema.[35]

Earlier work had demonstrated the induction of pulmonary edema following in vivo exposure of ozone levels of 5 ppm and higher.[36] It has been well demonstrated that there are not only significant variations in species response to oxidant exposure but also considerable variability in response of individual animals within the same species.[36,37] In the current experiments, however, pulmonary edema did not appear to be significant and the effect of exposure to ozone on pulmonary lipids and lung weight appears to be negligible.

There were no changes in the composition of the major phosphatides, the fatty acid composition of the isolated lecithins, or the percentage saturation of the lecithins following exposure to ozone. The precise reason for the low percent polyunsaturated fatty acids (18:3, 20:4) in the lecithins isolated from whole lung is unclear. (Levels of arachidonate in plasma lecithins from these animals were also low [2% to 5%]). The lungs were perfused with saline, to remove red blood cells, and plasma prior to analyses, and this process may have removed the primary source of arachidonate in whole lung from these animals. The correlation of normal pulmonary surface tension forces with a high percentage of lecithin disaturation is inherently consistent and in accord with previous studies.[34]

The mechanism by which ozone-exposure induces functional and structural alterations in the pulmonary alveolar macrophage system is unclear. At a level of exposure which produces extensive morphologic changes in alveolar macrophages, there was no alteration in the phospholipid composition or pulmonary surface activity of the whole lung or of the lavaged material recovered. Therefore, it would appear that these alterations in structure are not mediated directly through an alteration in a protective function that can be provided by dipalmitoyl lecithin alone,[38] as there was no demonstrable biochemical alteration in this phosphatide following ozone exposure. In fact, pulmonary surfactant has been shown by DuBois and co-workers to increase cell fragility and lysis of cell membranes, which would be in keeping with the lytic action and detergent function of surface active agents in general.[39] Ultrastructural changes in alveolar macrophages, which can synthesize disaturated lecithins,[40] without a change in phosphatide composition or fatty acid saturation of lipids harvested from lungs of ozone-exposed rabbits, may suggest that the majority of lipids analyzed were not synthesized during the period of exposure or that structural alterations cannot be correlated with lipid synthesis. Since there were no demonstrable significant alterations in lipids recovered from whole lung or in recovered lavage material from animals exposed to a relatively high level of ozone (5 ppm), further biochemical evaluations at lower, more environmentally physiologic levels were not pursued. Significant functional impairment of intrapulmonary bacterial inactivation, however, was demonstrable at lower levels of exposure to ozone. Further studies will be needed to evaluate this impairment in alveolar macrophage function, the structural alterations noted above, and the mechanisms of cellular injury following exposure to ozone.

This investigation was supported in part by Public Health Service research grants 72-080-7028, HD-03693, and AI-08558-03 and by the National Air Pollution Control Administration.

John Clements, MD, and Richard King, MD, assisted with the development of the methods for isolating disaturated lecithins. Stephanie Burley, Iris Hagmann, Abbie Huber, Robert Kass, and Hunter Nicholas provided technical assistance.

References

1. Laurenzi G, Berman L, First M, et al: A quantitative study of the deposition and clearance of bacteria in the murine lung. *J Clin Invest* **43**:759-768, 1964.

2. Green GM, Kass EH: The role of the alveolar macrophage in the clearance of bacteria from the lung. *J Exp Med* **119**:167-176, 1964.

3. Green GM, Kass EH: Factors influencing clearance of bacteria by the lung. *J Clin Invest* **43**:769-776, 1964.

4. Kass EH, Green GM, Goldstein E: Mechanisms of antibacterial action in the respiratory system. *Bact Rev* **30**:488-496, 1966.

5. Miller S, Ehrlich R: Susceptibility of respiratory infections of animals exposed to ozone: I. Susceptibility to *Klebsiella pneumoniae*. *J Infect Dis* **103**:103-145, 1958.

6. Coffin DL, Blommer EJ, Gardner DE, et al: Effect of air pollution on alteration of susceptibility to pulmonary infection, in *Proceedings of the Third Annual Conference on Atomic Contamination in Confined Spaces.* Wright-Patterson Air Force Base, Ohio, Aerospace Medical Research Laboratories, 1958, pp 71-80.

7. Coffin DL, Garner DE, Holzman RS, et al: Influence of ozone of pulmonary cells. *Arch Environ Health* **16**:633-636, 1968.

8. Goldstein BD, Lodi C, Collinson C, et al: Ozone and lipid peroxidation. *Arch Environ Health* **18**:631-635, 1969.

9. Saltzman B: *Selected Methods for Measurement of Air Pollutants,* publication 99-AP-11. Department of Health, Education and Welfare, Public Health Service, 1965.

10. Myrvik ON, Leake ES, Fariss B: Studies on pulmonary alveolar macrophages from the normal rabbit: A technique to produce them in a high state of purity. *J Immun* **86**:128-132, 1961.

11. Cotran RS, Litt M: The entry of granule-associated peroxidase into the phagocytic vacuoles of eosinophils. *J Exp Med* **129**:1291-1306, 1969.

12. Bennett HS, Luft JH: s-Collidine as a basis for buffering fixatives. *J Biophys Biochem Cytol* **6**:113-118, 1959.

13. Luft JH: Improvement in epoxy resin embedding methods. *J Biophys Biochem Cytol* **9**:409-414, 1961.

14. Trump BF, Smuckler EA, Benditt EP: A method for staining epoxy sections for light microscopy. *J Ultrastruct Res* **5**:343-348, 1961.

15. Huxley HE, Zubay G: Preferential staining of nucleic acid-containing structures for electron microscopy. *J Biophys Biochem Cytol* **11**:273-296, 1961.

16. Karnovsky MJ: Simple methods for staining with lead at high pH in electron microscopy. *J Biophys Biochem Cytol* **11**:729-732, 1961.

17. Huber GL, Edmunds LH Jr: Pulmonary artery occlusion: II. Morphologic studies. *J Appl Physiol* **22**:1002-1011, 1967.

18. Clements JA: Surface tension of lung extracts. *Proc Soc Exp Biol* **95**:170-172, 1957.

19. Folch J, Lees M, Sloanestanley GH: A simple method for the isolation and purification of total lipids from animal tissues. *J Biol Chem* **226**:497-509, 1957.

20. Parker F, Peterson RF: Quantitative analysis of phospholipid and phospholipid fatty acids from silica gel thin layer chromograms. *J Lipid Res* **6**:455-460, 1965.

21. Bartlett GR: Phosphorus assay in column chromatography. *J Biol Chem* **234**:466-468, 1959.

22. Rouser G, Bauman A: Kritchevsky G, et al: Quantitative chromatographic fractionation of complex lipid mixtures: Brain lipids. *J Amer Oil Chem Soc* **38**:544-555, 1961.

23. Radin NS, Hajro AK, Akahori Y: Preparation of methyl esters. *J Lipid Res* **1**:250-251, 1960.

24. Blank ML, Nutter LJ, Privett OS: Determination of the structure of lecithins. *Lipids* **1**:132-135, 1966.

25. Cohn ZA, Hirsch JG, Fedorko ME: The in vitro differentiation of mononuclear phagocytes: IV. The ultrastructure of macrophage differentiation in the peritoneal cavity and in cultures. *J Exp Med* **123**:747-756, 1966.

26. Trump BF, Goldblatt PJ, Stowell RE: An electron microscopic study of early cytoplasmic alterations in hepatic parenchymal cells of mouse liver during necrosis in vitro (autolysis). *Lab Invest* **11**:986-1015, 1962.

27. Bils RF, Romanovsky JC: Ultrastructural alterations of alveolar tissue of mice: II. Synthetic photochemical smog. *Arch Environ Health* **14**:844-858, 1967.

28. Stokinger HE, Wagner WD, Dobrogorski OJ: Ozone toxicity studies: III. Chronic injury to lungs of animals following exposure to a low level. *Arch Environ Health* **16**:514-522, 1957.

29. Rounds DE, Bils RF: Effects of air pollutants on cells in culture. *Arch Environ Health* **10**:251-259, 1965.

30. Pace EM, Landolt PA, Aftonomos BT: Effects of ozone on cells in vitro. *Arch Environ Health* **18**:165-170, 1969.

31. Hurst DJ, Gardner DE, Coffin DL: Effect of ozone on acid hydrolases of the pulmonary alveolar macrophage. *J Reticuloendothel Soc,* to be published.

32. Huber GL, Spencer NJ: Alterations in pulmonary antibacterial defense mechanisms following exposure to ozone. *Amer Rev Resp Dis* **101**:1016, 1970.

33. Huber GL, LaForce FM, Mason RJ: Impairment and recovery of pulmonary antibacterial defense mechanisms following oxygen administration. *J Clin Invest* **49**:47a, 1970.

34. Morgan TE, Finley TN, Huber GL, et al: Alterations in pulmonary surface active lipids during exposure to increased oxygen tension. *J Clin Invest* **44**:1737-1744, 1965.

35. Frank NR, Brain JD, Sherry DE: Unilateral lung exposure to ozone. *Fed Proc* **27**:279, 1968.

36. Stokinger HE: Evaluation of the hazards of ozone and oxides of nitrogen. *Arch Indust Health* **15**:181-190, 1957.

37. Stokinger HE: Ozone toxicology. *Arch Environ Health* **10**:719-731, 1965.

38. Gardner DE, Pfitzer EA, Christian RT et al: Loss of protective factor for alveolar macrophages when exposed to ozone. *Arch Intern Med* **127**:1078-1084, 1971.

39. Swada H, Valasquez BJ, DuBois AB: Effect of pulmonary surfactant on cell fragility. *Fed Proc* **27**:279, 1968.

40. Mason RJ, Huber GL, Vaughan M: Synthesis of dipalmityl lecithin by lung and alveolar macrophages. *J Clin Invest* **49**:62a, 1970.

Antioxidants vs Lung Disease

Jeffery N. Roehm, PhD; John G. Hadley;
and Daniel B. Menzel, PhD, Richland, Wash

Oxidation of fatty acid methyl esters was markedly increased by trace quantities (1.5 ppm) of nitrogen dioxide or ozone. Nitrogen dioxide-catalyzed oxidation occurred through conventional peroxidation mechanisms. Ozone reacted in thin films by directly attacking the double bond. Phenolic antioxidants retarded NO_2—but not O_3—oxidation. In aqueous media, O_3-oxidation occurred by direct attack and peroxidation; NO_2-oxidation by conventional peroxidation. Both were retarded by phenolic antioxidants. Exposure of rats to 10 ppm NO_2 for four weeks resulted in reduction of polyunsaturated fatty acids in the vitamin E-depleted group. Exposure to 1.0 ppm ozone resulted in death from pulmonary edema of all animals within 22 days. Lethal time for 50% of the population (LT_{50}) was 8.2 days for vitamin E-depleted animals, and 18.5 days for those receiving vitamin E. Vitamin E appears to protect against the biological effects of photochemical air pollutants.

The photochemical air pollutants, nitrogen dioxide and ozone, are similar in that they are both strong oxidizing agents. This common property has been proposed as a mechanism for their toxicity.[1-3] Unsaturated lipids, major constituents of all biological membranes, are liable to oxidation and are therefore logical cellular sites for NO_2 or ozone-induced damage. Ultraviolet (uv) absorbance at 235 nm, indicative of peroxidation,[4] has been observed in lipid extracts from mice exposed to ozone[1] and NO_2.[2]

We report a study undertaken to determine the effect of low levels of NO_2 or ozone on the oxidation of purified lipids. The usefulness of phenolic antioxidants in preventing oxidation under these conditions was also studied. Animal exposures were carried out to study the influence of dietary vitamin E, a biologically active antioxidant, on the effects of ozone and NO_2.

Experiment

In Vitro Oxidation of Fatty Acids.—Multiple samples of purified fatty acid methyl esters were exposed as thin films (2 mg per sq cm) to atmospheres containing 1.5 ppm of either O_3 or NO_2. The oxidizing atmospheres were regulated by gas mixing in methyl methacrylate (Plexiglas) glove boxes of 340 liter capacity with a gas flow of 28.3 liters/min. Temperature was maintained at 24 C with a relative humidity of 55%. Animal exposures were also carried out in these boxes. Ozone was generated by passing filtered air through a silent arc generator similar to that described by Bonner.[5] Nitrogen dioxide was obtained as a 1% mixture in nitrogen. Methods described by Saltzman and Gilbert were used periodically to determine the concentration of ozone[6] and NO_2.[7]

At various time intervals, samples were removed from the exposure chamber, dissolved in methanol, and extent of oxidation determined by uv analysis at 235 nm or by the 2-thiobarbituric acid (TBA)

Received for publication Oct 21, 1970; accepted March 3, 1971.

From the Biology Department, Pacific Northwest Laboratories, Battelle Memorial Institute, Richland, Wash. Dr. Menzel is now with Ross Laboratories, Columbus, Ohio.

Read in part before the Tenth Annual Hanford Biology Symposium on Pollution and Lung Biochemistry, Richland, Wash, June 5, 1970, jointly sponsored by the Battelle Memorial Institute-Pacific Northwest Laboratories, National Air Pollution Control Administration, National Institute of Environmental Health Sciences, and the US Atomic Energy Commission.

Reprint requests to Ross Laboratories, Columbus, Ohio 43216 (Dr. Menzel).

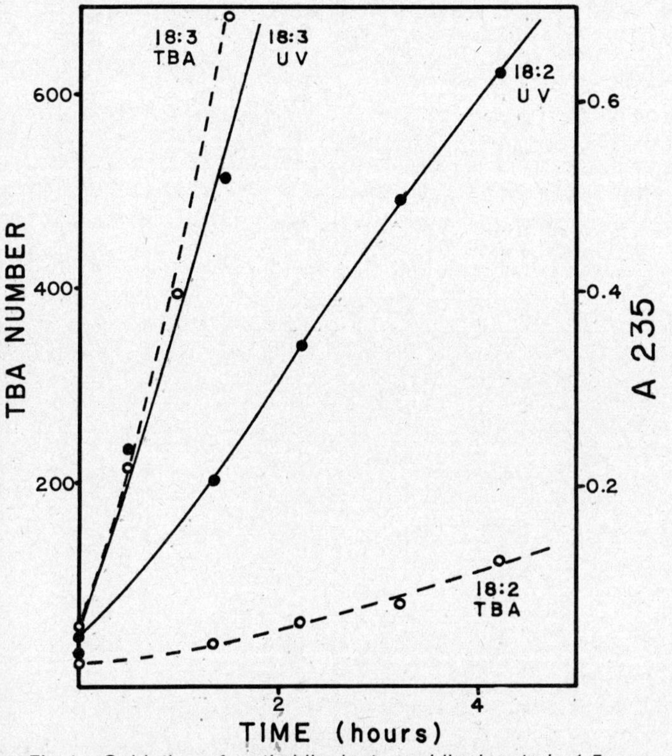

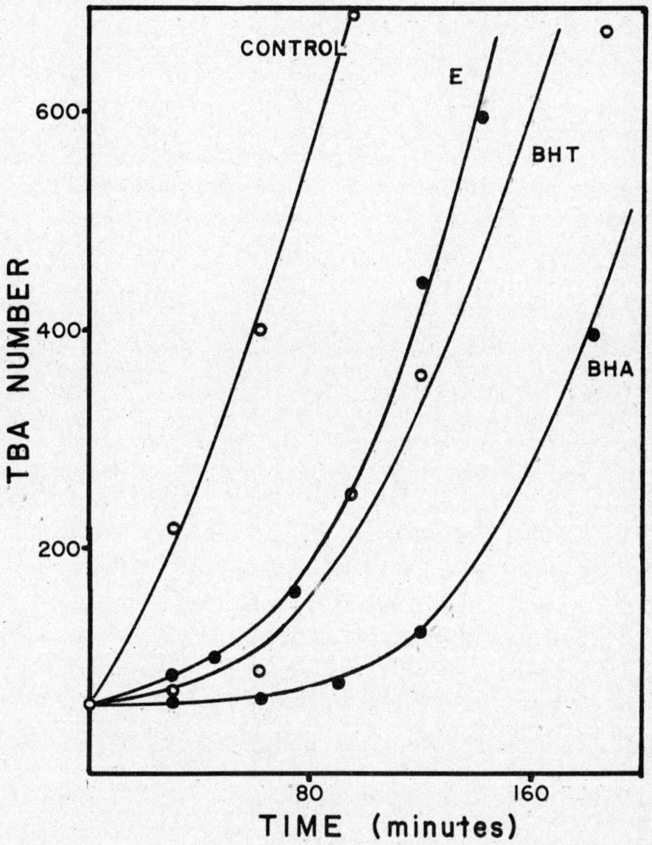

Fig 1.—Oxidation of methyl linoleate and linolenate in 1.5 ppm NO_2. A_{235} signifies absorbence at 235 nanometers.

Fig 2.—Influence of antioxidants on the oxidation of methyl-linolenate films in 1.5 ppm NO_2.

reaction. Diene conjugation (A_{235}) was determined via difference spectra of methanol solutions containing 0.1 mg of oil per milliliter. For the TBA reaction, which determines malonaldehyde, the ester sample was dissolved in 1 ml methanol and placed in a Teflon-sealed test tube. To this was added 1 ml water, 2 ml TBA reagent (0.1M TBA in 0.01N hydrogen chloride), and 2 drops of 5% butylated hydroxytoluene (BHT) in methanol. The solution was sealed under nitrogen and heated at 100 C for 30 minutes. The sample was then cooled, shaken with 1 ml chloroform, and centrifuged. The upper phase was then analyzed colorimetrically at 532 nm. This method showed typical standard curves, and was suitable for analysis of purified lipids in both thin films and aqueous emulsions. In the latter case the oxidized emulsion was added in place of the distilled water. Results of these analyses were reported as TBA number[8] which is simply parts per million malonaldehyde.

Aqueous emulsions of the purified esters were prepared in 0.1N sodium phosphate buffer (pH 7.0) containing 0.02% octylphenoxy polyethoxyethanol. (Triton X-100). The emulsions contained 2 mg ester per ml and were stirred continuously during exposure.

Antioxidants were added to the oils at a concentration of 0.01μmol/mg of ester. Antioxidants used were butylated hydroxyanisole (BHA), BHT, and vitamin E (d1-α-tocopherol).

Animal Exposures.—Male rats of the Sprague-Dawley strain weaned 10 days previously were placed on a synthetic diet which was either vitamin E-free or supplemented with 100 mg/kg vitamin E acetate (*dl*-α-tocopherol acetate). The dietary lipid consisted of a randomized synthetic triglyceride containing 50% linolenic acid (18:3). (Numbers in parentheses denote number of carbon atoms: number of double bonds.) This highly peroxidizable lipid would, according to Witting and Horwitt,[9] increase the peroxidizable of tissue lipids and therefore increase the vitamin E requirement of the rat. After four weeks of dietary equilibration, groups of ten rats each from the vitamin E-depleted and supplemented groups were exposed simultaneously to either 10 ppm NO_2 or 1.0 ppm ozone.

At various time intervals, rats were removed from the chamber and anesthetized with 50 mg/kg pentobarbital sodium. The lungs were removed and endobronchial saline lavage performed. The lungs were then homogenized in chloroform:methanol (2:1) and the lipids extracted according to the method of Folch et al.[10] Each saline lavage was evaporated to approximately 1 ml volume under vacuum and extracted in an identical manner. These lipids were esterfied in 2% sulfuric acid in methanol and the resultant methyl esters were analyzed using a gas chromatograph equipped with dual flame ionization detectors.

Results

Exposure of methyl linoleate (18:2) and methyl linolenate (18:3) to 1.5 ppm NO_2 resulted in extremely rapid oxidation (Fig 1). Methyl linolenate generated over 400 ppm malonaldehyde in 1 hour, while the same compound exposed to room air (not shown) required 30 hours to reach a

TBA number above 200 ppm. Ultraviolet absorbance at 235 nm, which in this system is a measure of conjugated dienoic hydroperoxides, increased in a similar manner.

Methyl linoleate formed conjugated dienes rapidly at a predictable rate somewhat greater than one third that observed with linolenate. Corresponding concentrations of malonaldehyde, however, were not observed. The normal mechanism for lipid peroxidation requires three or more double bonds in order for malonaldehyde to be formed through primary peroxide decomposition.[11,12] In fatty acids of three or more double bonds, malonaldehyde has a linear relationship with oxygen uptake and hydroperoxide formation.[8,13] Nitrogen dioxide-catalyzed lipid oxidation appears to occur via the normal mechanism of lipid autoxidation. This autoxidation should be retarded by phenolic antioxidants which terminate the autocatalytic chain reaction by interacting with peroxy-free radicals.[14]

Figure 2 shows the oxidation of 18:3 films in 1.5 ppm NO_2 with the addition of phenolic antioxidants. Oxidation curves typical of antioxidant activity were observed with BHA (by far the most effective), BHT, and vitamin E. Similar results were also observed using aqueous emulsions.

The oxidation of 18:3 and 18:2 films in 1.5 ppm ozone is shown in Fig 3. Although 18:3 formed TBA-reactive compounds at a rate approximately 1.5 times that found with NO_2, no significant diene conjugation (A_{235}) was detected. In this case, 18:2 also formed TBA-positive compounds at a rate of approximately one half that of 18:3. Again, no significant diene conjugation was detected. These observations suggest that oxidation is occurring by direct attack of the double bond by ozone, possibly via the Criegee mechanism[15] (Fig 4).

Since naturally occurring fatty acids contain unsaturation that is methylene interrupted, ie, separated by three carbons, formation of an aldehydic function (Fig 4, [2]) at the double bond could give rise to malonaldehyde. This is supported by the observation that 18:3, which contains two such 3-carbon moieties, formed TBA-positive compounds twice as fast as 18:2 which contains only one.

Infrared analysis of 18:2 which had been exposed to 1.5 ppm ozone for 16 hours showed an intense absorption band at 9.0μ which is typical of the ozonide ring structure (Fig 4, [3]). This ester was completely destroyed, as shown by analysis on thin layer chromatography, and had an extremely high TBA number of 31,000. A similarly exposed film or methyl oleate (18:1) also formed ozonides, but had no TBA reaction or uv absorbance.

Ozone oxidation would not be expected to be influenced by antioxidants. This was, in fact, the case with 18:3 films exposed with antioxidants in a manner identical to that described for NO_2. Ozone exposure of 18:3 in aqueous emulsion (Fig 5) resulted in some retardation of oxidation as measured by the TBA reaction, suggesting that peroxy free radicals were forming. The atypical nature of these oxidation curves suggests mixed kinetics—perhaps a combination of direct attack by ozone and normal lipid autoxidation. Ozone exposure of 18:2 in aqueous emulsions produced both TBA-positive compounds and conjugated dienes. Since direct attack by ozone did not produce conjugated dienes, and autoxidation did not produce a TBA color

Table 1.—Total Fatty Acid Composition of Lung Lavage Lipids From Rats Exposed to 10 ppm NO_2 for Four Weeks*

Fatty Acid	Supplemented Control	Deficient Control	Supplemented Exposed	Deficient Exposed
12.0	1.00 ± 0.15	0.96 ± 0.22	0.09 ± 0.10	1.04 ± 0.29
14:0	4.30 ± 0.17	4.30 ± 0.30	3.34 ± 0.18	4.19 ± 0.77
16:0	52.15 ± 1.15	55.78 ± 0.77	47.33 ± 3.67	50.90 ± 6.27
16:1	8.43 ± 0.55	8.84 ± 0.58	8.10 ± 0.80	8.81 ± 0.61
17:1	0.92 ± 0.16	0.92 ± 0.24	1.17 ± 0.20	1.25 ± 0.46
18.0	8.79 ± 0.41	8.63 ± 0.49	7.83 ± 1.08	9.87 ± 2.58
18:1	14.44 ± 0.96	13.76 ± 0.26	16.58 ± 2.33	16.69 ± 2.64
18:2	4.96 ± 0.30	3.59 ± 0.31	5.38 ± 0.57	3.79 ± 0.36
18:3	4.33 ± 0.73	2.83 ± 0.19	8.72 ± 2.23	2.49 ± 0.70

* Minor components omitted for clarity.

Table 2.—Total Fatty Acid Composition of Lung Lipids From Rats Exposed to 10 ppm NO_2 for Four Weeks*

Fatty Acid	Supplemented Control	Deficient Control	Supplemented Exposed	Deficient Exposed
16:0	25.60 ± 0.13	25.94 ± 0.64	28.27 ± 0.95	28.59 ± 0.25
16:1	4.55 ± 0.32	4.66 ± 0.16	5.43 ± 0.07	5.80 ± 0.30
18:0	10.29 ± 0.50	10.74 ± 0.36	10.03 ± 0.13	9.57 ± 0.54
18:1	24.56 ± 0.66	24.25 ± 1.43	25.10 ± 0.05	28.62 ± 1.36
18:2	7.86 ± 0.27	7.85 ± 0.16	6.61 ± 0.36	6.43 ± 0.13
18:3	6.02 ± 1.02	6.67 ± 0.45	4.81 ± 0.55	4.89 ± 0.53
20:4	5.57 ± 0.16	4.90 ± 0.43	5.14 ± 0.17	4.58 ± 0.88
20:5	3.07 ± 0.34	3.28 ± 0.24	3.06 ± 0.08	2.15 ± 0.24
22:5	4.61 ± 0.57	4.69 ± 0.43	3.79 ± 0.09	2.78 ± 0.42
22:6	1.17 ± 0.20	1.47 ± 0.00	1.16 ± 0.13	1.04 ± 0.12

* Minor components omitted for clarity.

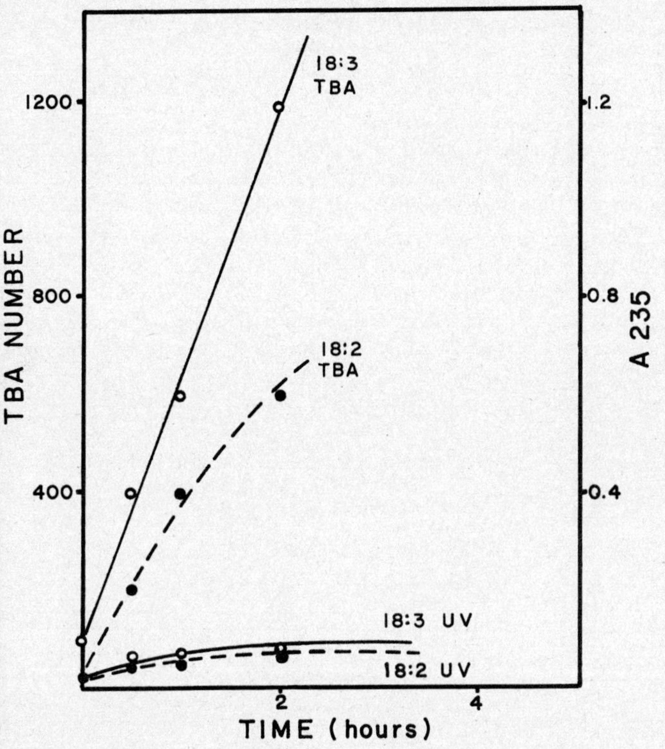

Fig 3.—Oxidation of methyl linoleate and linolenate films in 1.5 ppm ozone.

Fig 4.—Oxidation via the Criegee mechanism.

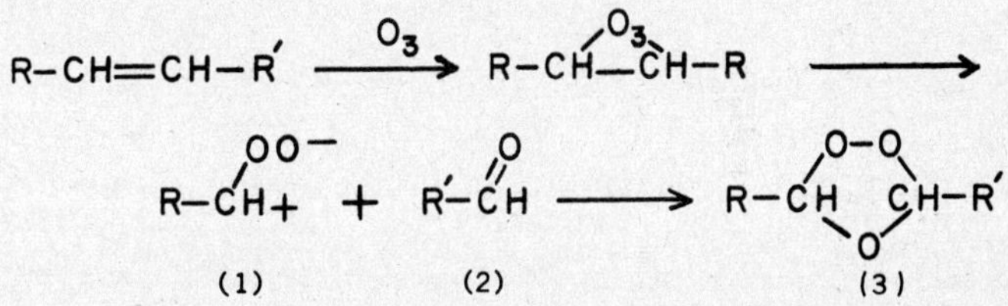

reaction, both mechanisms must be occurring in aqueous media.

Simultaneous exposure of both vitamin E-depleted and vitamin E-supplemented rats in 10 ppm NO_2 resulted in changes in the polyunsaturated fatty acid content of lung tissue lipids. Table 1 shows the total lung tissue fatty acids after four weeks continuous exposure. Rats fed the vitamin E-free diet showed significant reductions ($P <$ 0.05) in 18:2, 18:3, 20:5, 22:5, and 22:6, with corresponding increases in 18:0, 16:1, and 18:1. No changes in 20:4 were observed. Rats fed vitamin E, 100 mg/kg, also had reduced levels of 18:2, 18:3, and 22:5, but these differences were not significant at the 5% level of probability. A comparison of the two exposed groups, which is possible because the controls are identical, shows 20:5 and 22:5 significantly reduced in the depleted group. It appears, therefore, that vitamin E has a protective influence on the maintenance of normal lung fatty acid composition during exposure to NO_2. These findings follow closely those of Witting[16] with vitamin E deficient rats. Their observations were characterized by a decrease in the most highly unsaturated fatty acids with a concomitant increase in archidonic acid (20:4). These authors theorize that these changes in composition reflect the preferential peroxidative destruction of polyunsaturated fatty acids and an increased synthesis of arachidonate in a homeostatic attempt to maintain normal membrane lipid fatty acid composition. It appears that NO_2 exposure accelerates these changes.

The fatty acids from lipids recovered from endobronchial saline lavage are shown in Table 2. A comparison of the two control groups revealed fatty acid changes attributable to vitamin E deficiency. The concentrations of both 18:2 and 18:3 were significantly reduced ($P < 0.05$) with a corresponding increase in 16:0, in contrast to findings with lung tissue lipids at the same sampling period (Table 1) which showed no differences. The lipids lining the air-tissue interface may be more susceptible to the effects of vitamin E deficiency because they are in more direct contact with the atmosphere.

A comparison of the NO_2-exposed, vitamin E-supplemented group with its air-exposed control revealed a marked increase ($P < 0.05$) in the concentration of 18:3. This increased level of 18:3 may be due to an alteration in some transport function by NO_2. This action would not be influenced by vitamin E and should, therefore, occur in both exposed groups. A similar comparison of the vitamin E-depleted, NO_2-exposed rats with their controls, however, revealed no significant changes.

A consideration of the lavage lipids of the two exposed groups revealed several interesting features. The standard deviation calculated for 16:0, 18:0, 18:1, and 18:3 were very

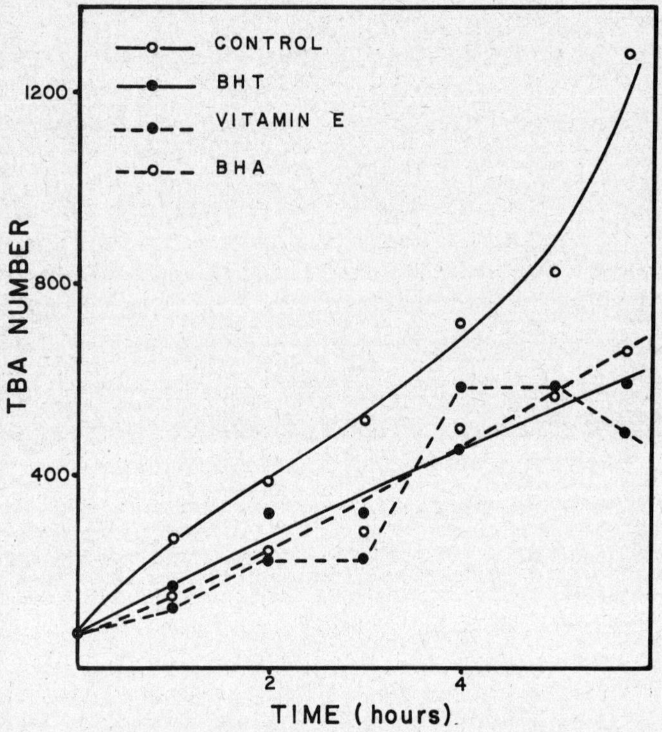

Fig 5.—Influence of antioxidants on the oxidation of methyl-linolenate emulsions in 1.5 ppm ozone.

Fig 6.—Mortality curves of vitamin E depleted (solid line) *and vitamin E supplemented* (broken line) *rats exposed in 1.0 ppm ozone.*

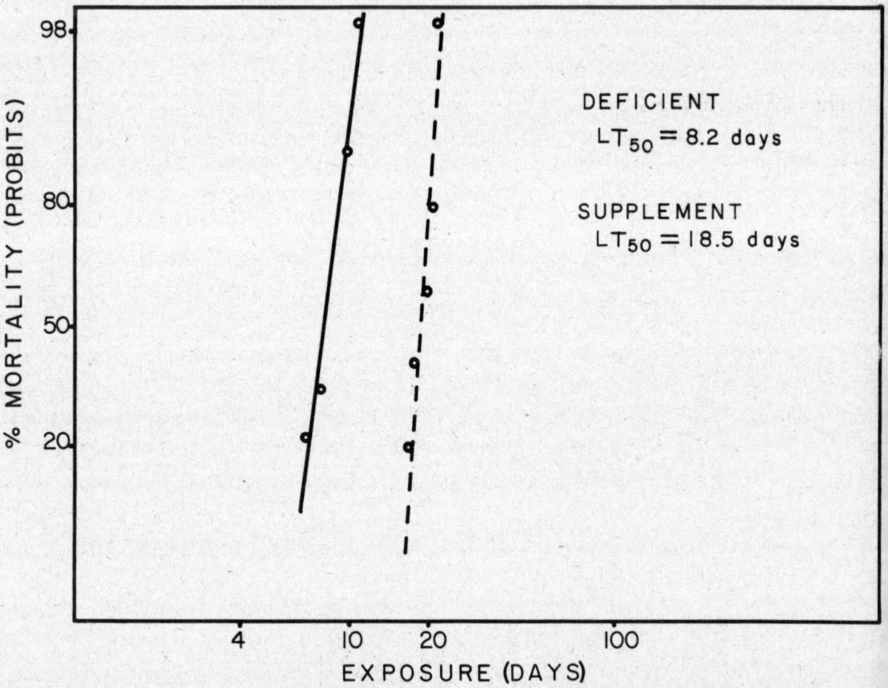

high in comparison to the controls. An increased variation within treatments could possibly be due to the stress conditions of NO_2. The vitamin E-depleted group contained significantly reduced levels of 18:2 and 18:3 ($P < 0.05$). If, indeed, any effect of NO_2 on lipid transport was identical in both groups, then the data show that oxidation of unsaturated fatty acids was occurring at an increased rate in the vitamin E-depleted group.

Rats fed the vitamin E-free diet and exposed to 1.0 ppm ozone began to show symptoms of respiratory stress within two days of exposure, characterized by increased respiratory rate and abdominal respiration. The vitamin E-supplemented group, however, did not exhibit these symptoms until the 11th day of exposure, although their feed consumption was reduced almost immediately. Prior to the first planned sampling, the vitamin E-deficient rats began to die. Autopsy of these rats revealed massive pulmonary edema and lung hemorrhaging. All of the vitamin E-deficient rats were dead after 11 days of exposure, during which time the supplemented rats showed normal respiration. Figure 6 shows the mortality curves for both vitamin E-supplemented and deficient rats simultaneously exposed to 1.0 ppm ozone. Lethal time for 50% of the population (LT_{50}) calculations of 8.2 days for the deficient group and 18.5 days for the supplemented group indicate a clearly defined protective effect of vitamin E. It is important to consider that these rats had been fed a vitamin E-free ration for only four weeks prior to exposure, and did not display any vitamin E deficiency symptoms. The supplemented group, on the other hand, had not been fed massive doses of vitamin E, but were given a normal dietary level of 100 mg *dl-α*-tocopherol acetate per kilogram added directly to the dietary triglyceride.

Comment

The apparent mechanistic difference observed between lipid oxidations in ozone-containing vs NO_2-containing atmospheres is pertinent to any consideration of their biological effects. The data reported here show that NO_2 catalyzes lipid autoxidation by the well-known mechanism originally proposed by Farmer et al, as reported by Witting.[16] This mechanism involved the initiation of a free radical at the methylene carbon of the 1,4-pentadiene system common to fatty acids, followed by addition of molecular oxygen and hydrogen abstraction to form a hydroperoxide. A second free radical is generated by the hydrogen abstraction, and if this specie is of high enough energy the reaction is autocatalytic. The addition of NO_2 to the double bond of lipids to form a nitroso-free radical is well documented[17] and probably initiates this chain reaction. Thin-layer chromatography of 18:1 exposed overnight to 1.5 ppm NO_2 showed only a slight formation of polar degradation products, indicating that direct attack of the double bond was not a major reaction.

With ozone-containing atmospheres direct attack of the double bond is the predominant reaction in thin films. In aqueous systems normal autoxidation can be detected, but direct attack is still a major consideration.

The importance of these differences in a biological system is obvious. Autocatalytic reactions are characterized by a slow buildup of the products of initiation followed by a rapid reaction after a critical concentration is reached. Normal methods of repair which exist within the cell (including antioxidant activity) may extend this "induction" period indefinitely. Direct attack of lipid double bonds would not be autocatalytic and biological repair would be much less effective. In this case of ozonolysis of lipids, this consideration is even more important because phenolic antioxidants, the principal natural biological antioxidants, will not retard this reaction.

If lipid oxidation is related to the toxicity of nitrogen dioxide and ozone, then ozone would be expected to be much more toxic and less sensitive to protection by antioxidants. The edematogenic effect observed for ozone at concentrations of only 1 ppm supports this contention. The extension of LT_{50} observed also suggests that lipid autoxidation is also occurring in vivo.

This study was supported by Public Health Service contract PH 22-68-61 from the National Air Pollution Control Administration.

References

1. Goldstein BD, Lodi C, Collison C, et al: Ozone and lipid peroxidation. *Arch Environ Health* **18**:631-635, 1969.
2. Thomas HV, Mueller PK, Lyman RL: Lipoperoxidation of lung lipids of rats exposed to nitrogen dioxide. *Science* **159**:532-534, 1968.
3. Menzel DB: Toxicity of ozone, oxygen and radiation. *Ann Rev Pharmacol* **10**:379-394, 1970.
4. Privett OS, Lundbert WO, Khan NA, et al: Structure of hydroperoxides obtained from autoxidized methyl linoleate. *J Amer Oil Chem Soc* **30**:61-66, 1953.
5. Bonner WA: A portable semimicro ozonizer. *J Chem Educ* **30**:452-453, 1953.
6. Saltzman BE: Colorimetric microdetermination of nitrogen dioxide in the atmosphere. *Anal Chem* **26**:1949-1955, 1954.
7. Saltzman BE, Gilbert N: Iodometric microdetermination of organic oxidants and ozone: Resolution of mixtures by kinetic colorimetry. *Anal Chem* **31**:1914-1920, 1959.
8. Yu TC, Sinnhuber RO: Improved 2-thiobarbituric acid procedure for the measurement of autoxidation in fish oils. *J Amer Oil Chem Soc* **44**:256-258, 1967.
9. Witting LA, Horwitt MK: Effect of degree of fatty acid unsaturation in tocopherol deficiency-induced creatinuria. *J Nutr* **82**:19-33, 1964.
10. Folch J, Lees M, Stanley GHS: A simple method for the isolation and purification of total lipids from animal tissue. *J Biol Chem* **226**:497-509, 1957.
11. Tarladgis BG, Watts BM: Malonaldehyde production during the controlled oxidation of pure, unsaturated fatty acids. *J Amer Oil Chem Soc* **37**:403-406, 1960.
12. Dahle LK, Hill EG, Holman RT: The thiobarbituric acid reaction and the autoxidation of polyunsaturated fatty acid methyl esters. *Arch Biochem* **98**:253-261, 1962.
13. Kenaston CB, Wilbur KM, Ottolenghi A, et al: Comparison of methods for determining fatty acid oxidation produced by ultraviolet irradiation. *J Amer Oil Chem Soc* **32**:33-35, 1955.
14. Bolland JL, Ten Haven P: Kinetic studies in the chemistry of rubber and related materials: IV. Inhibitory effect of hydroquinone on the thermal oxidation of ethyl linoleate. *Trans Faraday Soc* **43**:201-210, 1947.
15. Criegee R: Course of ozonization of unsaturated compounds. *Rec Chem Prog* **18**:111-120, 1957.
16. Witting LA: The effect of antioxidant deficiency on tissue lipid composition in the rat: IV. Peroxidation and interconversion of polyunsaturated fatty acids in muscle phospholipids. *Lipids* **2**:109-113, 1967.
17. Estefan RM, Gause EM, Rowlands JR: Electron spin resonance and optical studies of the interaction between NO_2 and unsaturated lipid components. *Environ Res* **3**:62-78, 1970.

Reaction of Nitrogen Dioxide With Blood and Lung Components

Electron Spin Resonance Studies

John R. Rowlands, PhD, and Emily M. Gause, MS, San Antonio, Tex

Electron spin resonance studies of the effects of nitrogen dioxide and cigarette smoke upon blood and lung tissue components were performed. In vivo exposure of small animals to NO_2 and cigarette smoke has been interpreted in terms of pollutant reaction with the heme moiety of hemoglobin. Results imply that the pollutants have migrated through the erythrocyte membrane. So as to understand the effects of these pollutants upon the membranes themselves, various model systems have been studied, particularly the interaction of nitrogen dioxide with unsaturated lipids. Three stable free radicals have been characterized as products of these reactions; and a short-lived initial free radical was observed, the structure of which provides evidence as to the initial reaction site and mechanism.

Specific physiological damage has been attributed to the oxidants present in the atmosphere—especially nitrogen oxides and ozone. Arioka[1] demonstrated that pulmonary damage was experimentally induced in rats by inhalation of nitrogen dioxide. He successfully demonstrated a relationship between the mortality rate and the NO_2 concentration, and he also showed that the blood of the exposed rats contained an elevated concentration of both metmyoglobin (4% to 6%) and potassium ions. Symon[2] has reported that elevated levels of metmyoglobin (3% to 5%) have been observed in children living in an environment containing high concentrations of oxides of nitrogen.

Studies by Thomas et al[3] concerned with the effects of NO_2 on young rats have demonstrated that the inhalation of 1 ppm for one hour or 0.5 ppm for four hours leads to significant morphological changes in their lung-mast cells. The morphological changes are thought to occur both as a result of the chemical interaction of NO_2 with the cell membrane and as a result of the interaction of NO_2 with certain specific but undefined cellular elements which lead to a loss in cell integrity.

Thomas et al[4] have reported absorption spectroscopic evidence of lipid peroxidation from extracts of the lungs of rats which have been exposed to 1 ppm atmospheres of NO_2 for both single periods of four hours and repeated four-hour exposures over a period of six days. Their results suggested that the extent of peroxidation was cumulative. These authors also report that structural changes are induced in the lung lipids upon exposure to NO_2.

In vitro studies aimed at elucidating products and mechanisms associated with observed in vivo effects have included work by Felmeister et al[5] on surface pressure measurements of films of both saturated and unsaturated phospholipids. They find that, whereas no observable interactions were observed in the case of the saturated phospholipids, films of egg lecithin, an unsaturated phospholipid, showed significant changes in the surface pressure-surface area curves in the presence of all atmospheres studied which contain NO_2. They attribute their observed effects to a chemical interaction of NO_2 with the double bonds of the lecithin.

Our studies, described herein, support this observation. Evidence is presented to indicate that this is, indeed, a general mode of attack upon biological molecules, and a reaction pathway is suggested. In addition, another type of biological reaction of nitrogen oxides—the interaction with hemoglobin—is also described.

Nitric oxide and NO_2 are both free radical molecules, as are some of their reaction intermediates and products. A brief discussion of the nature and characteristics of certain types of free radicals therefore appears appropriate at this time.

Received for publication Oct 21, 1970; accepted Feb 10, 1971.

From the Department of Physical and Biological Sciences, Southwest Research Institute, San Antonio, Tex.

Read in part before the Tenth Annual Hanford Biology Symposium on Pollution and Lung Biochemistry, Richland, Wash, June 5, 1970, jointly sponsored by the Battelle Memorial Institute-Pacific Northwest Laboratories, National Air Pollution Control Administration, National Institute of Environmental Health Sciences, and the US Atomic Energy Commission.

Reprint requests to Southwest Research Institute, 8500 Culebra Rd, San Antonio, Tex 78228 (Dr. Rowlands).

Electron Spin Resonance as a Technique for the Study of Lung/Pollutant Interactions

Electron spin resonance (ESR) studies have had considerable success in the study of systems containing unpaired electrons such as free radicals and paramagnetic complexes. The technique is widely used for in vitro studies of biological systems which exhibit paramagnetism (heme proteins, certain enzyme-substrate reactions, tissue homogenates, etc). It therefore lends itself well to the study of the effects of exogenous substances such as air pollutants (several of which are themselves free radical in nature) upon biological systems. For study of effects of air pollutants, the technique can be used for direct observation of in vitro reactions and these results compared and correlated with measurements made before and after in vivo exposures. The nature of the information obtained is unique to the ESR technique and is providing a depth of knowledge of several important biochemical pathways—for example, respiratory electron transport and photosynthesis, which would not be possible without the ESR technique.

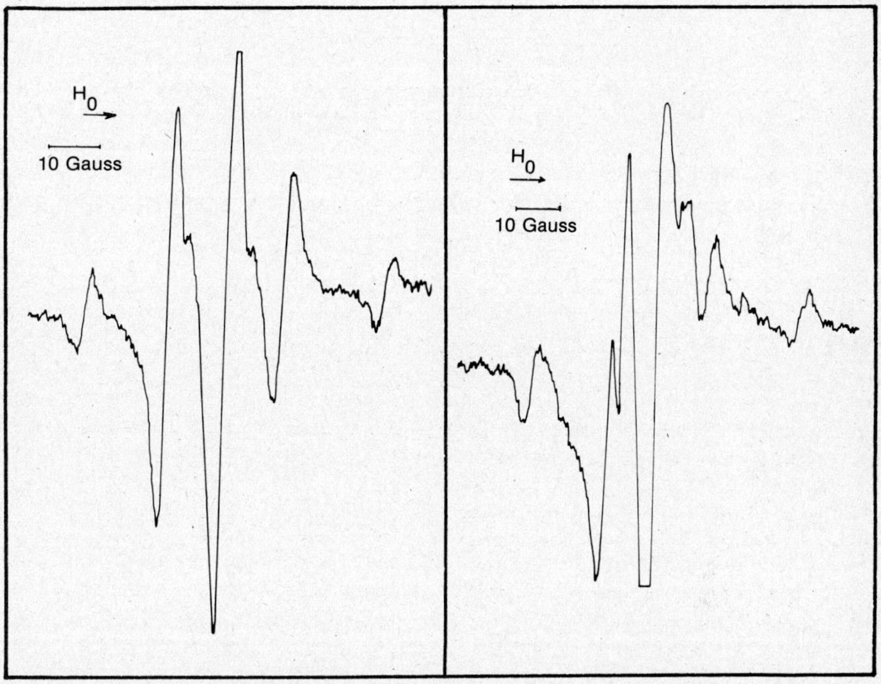

Fig 1.—Left, *The ESR spectrum of 0.1M L-a-lecithin in chloroform mixed with 0.15 ml of NO_2-saturated chloroform.* Right, *The ESR spectrum of 0.1M phosphatidyl enthanolamine in chloroform mixed 0.15 ml of NO_2-saturated chloroform.*

The technique relies upon the fact that the unpaired electron has two possible spin states which differ in energy when allowed to interact with a magnetic field. It is then possible to excite the electron from its lower state into its upper state. Experimentally, the samples containing the paramagnetic materials are contained in a microwave resonance cavity. Transitions between the two levels are effected by applying the electromagnetic radiation at a fixed frequency and varying the applied field until an absorption of energy corresponding to the excitation of the electrons is observed. The radiation is supplied by a klystron and is led through a wave guide to the resonant cavity which contains the specimen. Most commercial spectrometers operate at a frequency of about 9,000 megacycles/sec. At this frequency, free radicals are observed at magnetic field strengths of approximately 3,000 gauss. Paramagnetic metals, on the other hand, give rise to resonance signals at field strengths of as little as 1,000 gauss up to fields of greater than 3,500 gauss. The field strength at which a particular resonance is observed is referred to by means of a dimensionless quantity called the g factor.

The g factor of a free electron takes the value $g = 2.0023$. The g factors of most organic free radicals are within 1% of the free spin value and are significantly larger for sulphur, oxygen, and nitrogen radicals than for carbon radicals where the deviation is seldom more than 0.1%. For the case of paramagnetic metal complexes, their g-factor variations are much more significant and provide considerable structural information. For free radicals in particular, the appearance of structure on the ESR signal is of great importance. The analysis of this hyperfine structure leads to identification of the type of free radical that is being observed.

There are three types of free radicals that are of importance in studies of the reactions between oxidizing air pollutants with lipid materials. The general characteristics of these types of free radicals, and also a brief outline of the ESR characteristics of paramagnetic heme protein complexes, will be given prior to a discussion of some of the results that have been obtained in our air pollution studies.

Aliphatic Hydrocarbon Radicals.—

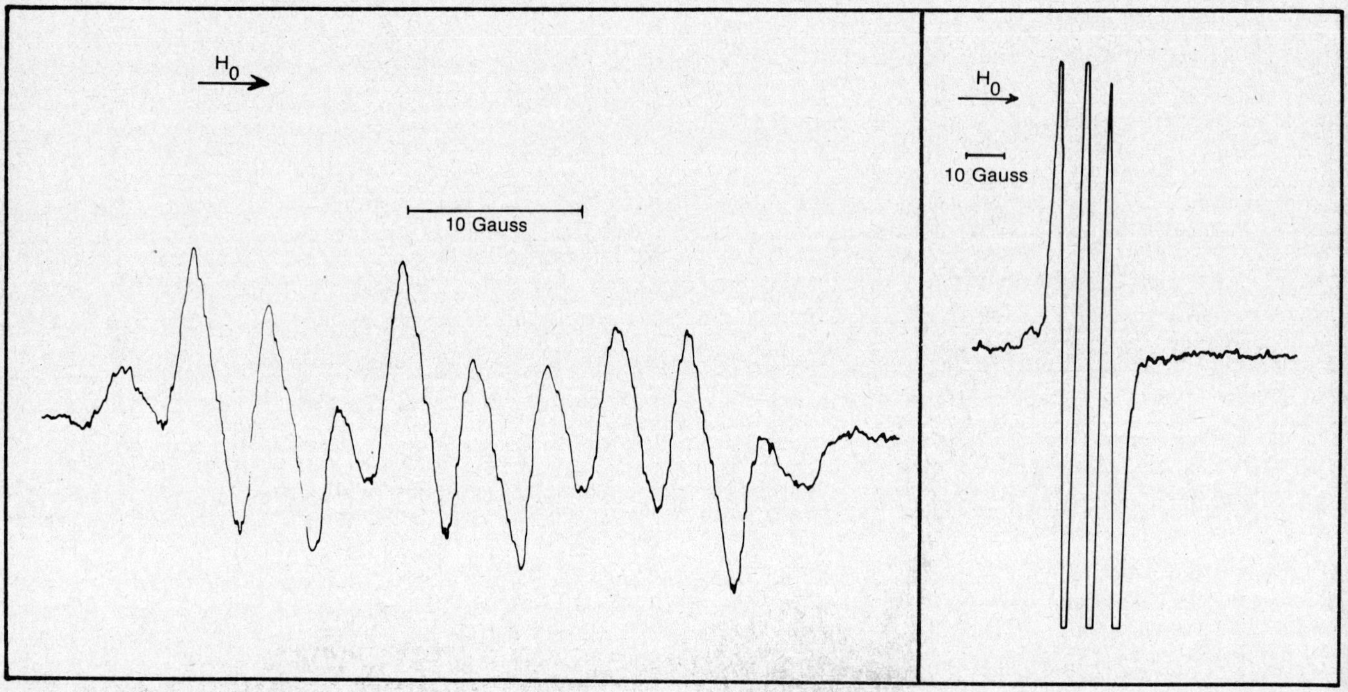

Fig 2.—Left, The ESR spectrum of radical produced under continuous flow conditions in reaction of 20% (volume) oleic acid in dioxane with NO_2 in dimethoxyethane. Right. *The ESR spectrum of type 1 radical formed upon stopping flow in oleic acid-NO_2 reaction.*

Aliphatic hydrocarbon radicals are very reactive and are usually too short-lived to be studied in the liquid state except by special techniques such as continuous irradiation of the sample within the ESR cavity by ionizing radiation or by rapid flow techniques. Considerable information has been obtained on this type of free radical, however, by studies of γ-irradiation of frozen samples and by γ- and x-irradiation both at room temperature and at 77 K of aliphatic acids and amino acids.

The values of the g factors of aliphatic hydrocarbon radicals, as we previously mentioned, depart from the g factor of the free electron by less than 1%. The principal means of identification of such radicals has been the analysis of the observed hyperfine structure.

Radicals Containing Nitrogen.—Another very common magnetic nucleus in free radicals is the nitrogen atom, which has a spin $I = 1$, so that a single nitrogen nucleus splits the electron resonance line into three equally intense lines from $mI = 0$ and ± 1.

There are two main types of nitrogen-containing free radicals which are important from the point of view of air pollution research. These are the nitroxide and iminoxy free radicals. In each case, a spectrum of three lines of equal intensity is observed, the principal difference being in the magnitude of the coupling, or splitting, which is approximately 15 gauss for the case of the nitroxide radical and 30 gauss for the iminoxy. The g factors of nitroxide and iminoxy radicals are found to be in the range $g = 2.0060$ to 2.0066 and $g = 2.0050$ and 2.0060, respectively. A third nitrogen-containing free radical has also been observed in NO_2-unsaturated fatty-acid reactions.[6] The nature of this species will be discussed later in the text.

Oxy and Peroxy Radicals.—Both alkoxy ($R\dot{O}$) and alkyl peroxy ($RO\dot{O}$) radicals have the unpaired electron mainly concentrated on oxygen atoms, the abundant isotope of which contains no nuclear spin, and hence gives rise to no hyperfine structure. The g factors of several oxy radicals and peroxy radicals that have been reported are found to be in the range $g = 2.0137$ to $g = 2.0155$.[7] The lack of hyperfine structure makes the distinction between oxy and peroxy radicals difficult to make.

Paramagnetic Complexes.—Electron spin resonance has been observed in the hemoglobin (Fe III) complexes, both for low ($S = \frac{1}{2}$) and high ($S = 5/2$) spin derivatives. In the low spin hemoglobin derivatives such as the azide, there are three distinct g values; while the high spin derivatives like the fluoride are characterized by two g values, $g \parallel = 2$ and $g \pm = 6$, where parallel and perpendicular refer to the fourfold symmetry axis perpendicular to the porphyrin plane.

In the hemoglobin (Fe II) complexes, low spin compounds like oxyhemoglobin and carboxyhemoglobin have $S = 0$ and, hence, are diamagnetic; while high spin ($S = 2$) ferrous compounds, although paramagnetic, have not been observed.

Experimental Studies

Reaction of NO_2 With Lipids.—We found that NO_2 reacts in vitro with lecithin and phosphatidyl ethanolamine to produce three different nitrogen-containing free radical species (Fig 1). These three radicals were quite stable in that they persisted in solution for periods of several hours to several days. In addition, a fourth free radical (single line, $g = 2.0069$) was observed in the reaction of phosphatidyl ethanolamine with NO_2. These reactions assume particular biological significance due to the function of these two phospholipids as surfactants of the alveolar lining; therefore, a study of the reaction mechanisms leading to the formation of these free radicals was undertaken.

We soon confirmed that the same three free radicals were produced upon exposure to NO_2 of any lipid compound containing a double bond. The reaction of NO_2 with olefins at the unsaturated linkage has been recognized and has been the subject of many previous investigations by organic chemists over a period of many years. However, the results of these studies have been conflicting and confusing, and a multitude of reaction products have been reported,

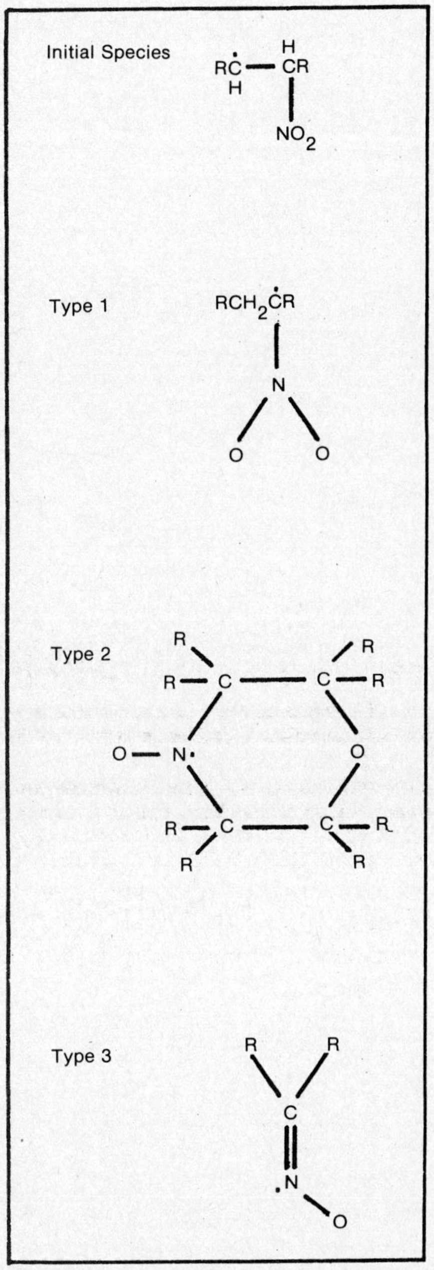

Fig 3.—Free radicals observed by the reaction of NO_2 with unsaturated lipids.

including dinitro compounds, nitronitrites, nitronitrates, nitronitroso derivatives, nitrosonitrites, nitronsonitrates, dinitrites, and nitronitrates. Surprisingly enough, until our results were published, no one had reported the production of free radical species from this reaction, although Bielski and Gebicki[8] had recently reported observing similar free radicals which they attributed to the formation of NO_2-olefin π-complexes when NO_2 was dissolved in unsaturated solvents.

We have provided fairly conclusive evidence that π-complexes are not involved in the reaction. (This has subsequently been confirmed by the work of Jonkman et al.[9]). The three types of stable nitrogen-containing free radicals were observed consistently in the reactions between NO_2 and a series of olefinic hydrocarbons and fatty acids.

In addition to these long-lived free radicals, we observed a fourth, very short-lived free radical when the reaction was carried out in a flow system through the sample cavity of the ESR spectrometer. The nature of this initial transient free radical (Fig 2, *left*) was such that it was obvious we were observing the initial step in the reaction of NO_2 with a double bond, in which NO_2 breaks the double bond and adds to one side of the bond, leaving an unpaired electron on the carbon atom on the other side (Fig 3).

Immediately after stopping the flow of the reactants through the cavity, the ESR spectrum of this initial radical was shown to have disappeared and to have been replaced by a type 1 free radical (Fig 2, *right*). The principal features of the ESR spectrum of this species consist of a triplet of equal intensity lines of 7 gauss splitting consistent with the interaction of the unpaired electron with a nitrogen nucleus. The formation of this type 1 species from the initial radical most probably occurs as a result of a hydrogen atom transfer reaction.

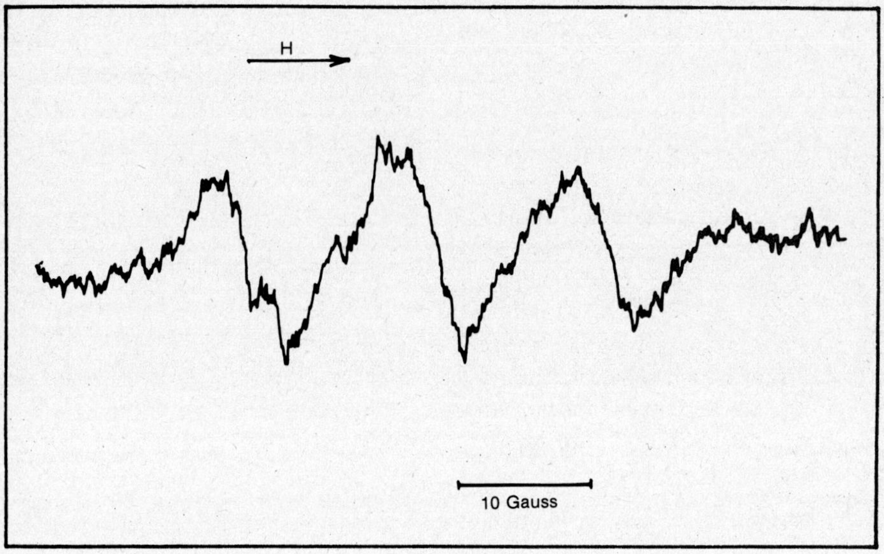

Fig 4.—The ESR spectrum of tryptophan (0.5N NaOH) exposed to less than 5 ppm NO_2 for 20 hours.

Type 2 free radicals, which were shown to be produced in all systems studied, were produced in greatest concentration relative to the type 1 radicals both at higher nitrogen dioxide concentrations studied and in the presence of ultraviolet radiation. Free radicals with hyperfine coupling constants comparable to type 2 radicals have been previously reported to be produced in the reaction of NO_2 with methylmethacrylate.[10]

Type 3 free radicals have been shown to be present in systems which contained appreciable concentrations of the type 2 free radicals. These type 2 radicals exhibit nitrogen hyperfine coupling constants and g factors characteristic of iminoxy radicals.

In view of the findings that the formation of both type 2 and type 3 radicals, ie, nitroxide and iminoxy radicals, are enhanced by ultraviolet radiation, it appears likely that the photochemical dissociation of NO_2 into nitric oxide and oxygen atoms plays an important role in their formation. Whether or not this dissociation reaction is a necessary precursor to the formation of these species will require detailed study.

Reaction of NO_2 With Protein Constituents.—The reactions of NO_2 with unsaturated linkages in lipids to produce the four different free radical species described took place in essentially nonaqueous systems; however, we have also observed a stable free radical species with a 13.4 gauss ^{14}N hyperfine coupling to be produced in aqueous solutions of tryptophan by exposure to less than 5 ppm levels of NO_2 (Fig 4), an atmospheric concentration of NO_2 encountered in pollution episodes.

We have also observed that NO_2 reacts with serum albumin in aqueous solutions to quench the fluorescence of the typtophan residues of the protein.

Interaction of NO_2 with a protein constituent such as tryptophan to produce a stable free radical has many implications. Not only are the tryptophan residues affected directly, but the stable free radical species produced might enter into secondary reactions with other sites on the protein or with neighboring molecules.

Effects of NO_2 Upon Hemoglobin and Related Molecules.—We found that both NO and NO_2 react with hemoglobin solutions to give rise to paramagnetic solutions characterized by a well-defined triplet ESR spectrum.[11] Kon[12] has recently published a detailed study of the NO-hemoglobin reaction. He was able to show that the appearance of the triplet ESR spectrum with a ^{14}N hyperfine coupling of 17 gauss coincided with a detergent-induced organic change in protein structure. Prior to the addition of the detergent, he showed from the observed g factors that the complex was consistent with rhombic symmetry, with no evidence of ^{14}N hyperfine coupling. Further changes in the spectrum were observed at very high detergent concentration when the spectrum indicated an axial symmetry with hyperfine structure to its ^{14}N nucleus still observable on the high field component ($g_{\parallel}$), but reduced in magnitude from 17 to 15 gauss. The same author reports similar spectral changes occurring in a study of sodium salicylate-NO-hemoglobin interactions. At high salicylate concentrations, he also observed further peaks appear with apparent g factors of 2.28, 2.19, 1.93, and 1.83. From the point of view of air pollution research, these observations are extremely interesting, as they parallel very closely some of the observations that we have made on the effects of tobacco smoke on whole blood. Tobacco smoke is known to contain NO in appreciable quantities. With respect to the biological significance of such complexes, it is of interest to note that Woolum and Commoner[13] have recently reported the isolation

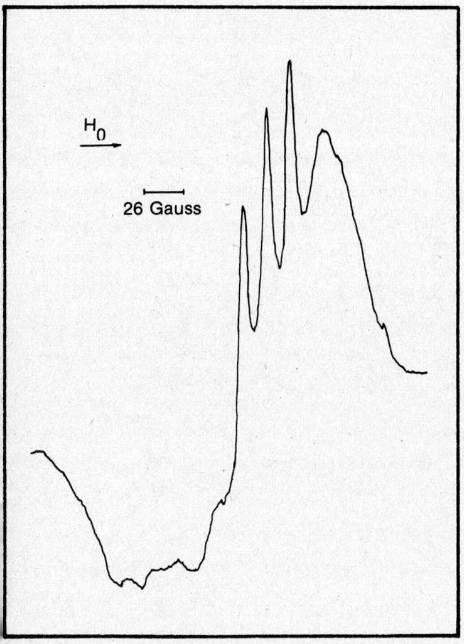

Fig 5.—The ESR spectrum of hemoglobin/cigarette smoke (narrow scan; 77 K).

of similar complexes from livers of carcinogen-fed rats.

We found that blood samples taken from mice and rabbits that have been exposed to tobacco smoke give ESR spectra with a broad resonance in the region of $g = 2$, with a well defined triplet high field component of ^{14}N hyperfine coupling of 16 gauss. Similar spectra can also be produced by exposing hemoglobin solutions in vitro to smoke and smoke fractions. The precise details of the observed spectrum were found to vary with different boiling point smoke fractions, but in all cases the triplet hyperfine structure was plainly visible. Based upon Kon's interpretation, this would indicate that considerable protein denaturation occurs in the reaction, along with formation of the NO-hemoglobin complex. A spectrum of the $g = 2$ region obtained from the reaction of hemoglobin with total tobacco smoke is illustrated in Fig 5.

We have also found that the reaction of NO_2 with hemoglobin solutions in vitro and in the blood of rats exposed in vivo to 1 to 3 ppm NO_2 gives rise to a broad resonance at ca $g = 2$, with a nitrogen hyperfine coupling of 16 gauss plainly observable on the high field side of the signal (Fig 6). In view of the close correspondence between both the observed hyperfine coupling and g factor of this feature and the similar spectrum obtained in the NO reaction, it is difficult to definitively assign the nature of the species giving rise to the observed spectrum. Nitrogen dioxide is known to react with water to give rise to nitric acid and NO according to the following equations:

$$2NO_2 + H_2O \rightarrow HNO_2 + H^+ + NO_{3^-}$$
$$3HNO_2 \rightarrow H^+ + NO_{3^-} + 2NO + H_2O$$

It is therefore possible that the observed triplet arises from an NO-hemoglobin complex formed subsequent to this reaction. Another although similar possibility is that NO_2 is reduced to the nitrite anion which subsequently reacts with hemoglobin. Ferrous ions are known to reduce nitrite ions to NO. The reaction of sodium nitrite with hemoglobin rapidly gives rise to a paramagnetic solution with an ESR spectrum identical to that obtained from the NO_2 reaction.

However, the reaction of NO_2 with hemoglobin is more complex than just that of disproportionation to NO to produce a NO-hemoglobin complex.

We have shown, in studies of the reaction of NO_2 with hematoporphyrin, the basic porphyrin ring system of the heme group without the metal ion, that two free radicals are produced, characterized by ^{14}N coupling constants of 7 and 12 gauss. Both radicals must be formed by the reaction of NO_2 with double bonds of the porphyrin structure. The precise nature of these radicals is not known; however, a possible structure for the 7 gauss species can be predicted by analogy to the reactions of NO_2 with oleic acid and a knowledge of the chemistry of porphyrin molecules. Cleavage of a double bond at one of the methine groups followed by a hydrogen transfer would give a radical of structure (Fig 7), which would be magnetically similar to the type 1 radical observed in oleic acid. The radical with the 12 gauss hyperfine

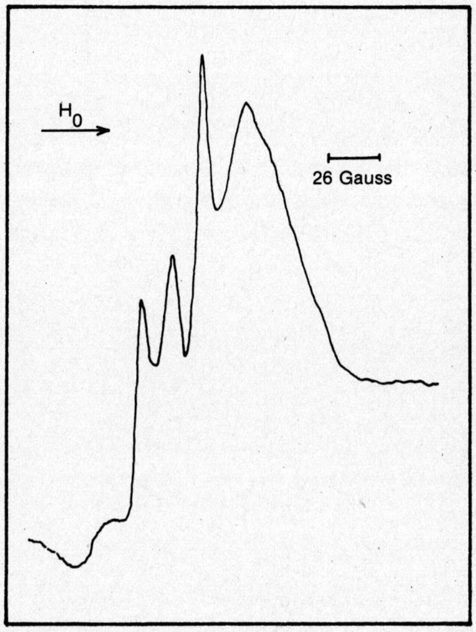

Fig 6.—The ESR spectrum of hemoglobin plus NO_2 (narrow scan, 77K).

Fig 7.—Diagram of a possible structure for the 7 gauss species of radical.

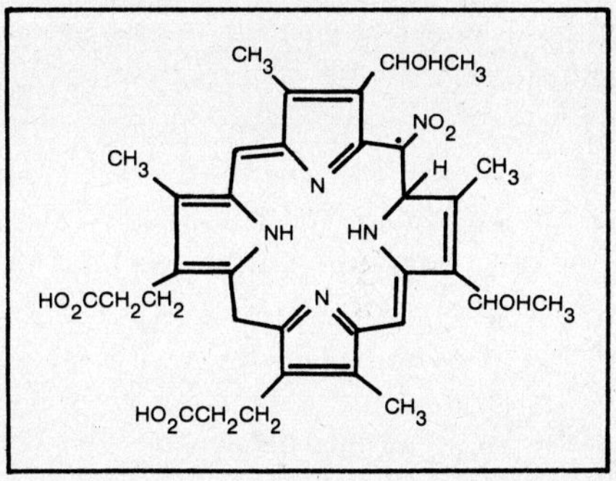

coupling could be a nitroxide type; however, its mode of formation is not immediately obvious. These reactions are accompanied by significant changes in the optical spectrum of the hematoporphyrin solution. Furthermore, since we have shown that NO_2 is capable of reacting with an aqueous solution of tryptophan to produce free radicals, then the possible reaction of NO_2 with the globin moieties of hemoglobin need also be considered.

Conclusions

The foregoing has been a summary of some of the ESR studies that have been conducted to date relevant to air pollution research. Most of the reactions that have been discussed on lipid components have been conducted on model systems under nonrealistic environmental conditions. This is perfectly reasonable for preliminary work designed merely to characterize some of the possible free radical reactions. Nitrogen dioxide has been known for some time to react with unsaturated compounds at the double bond; however, the mechanism of reaction has not been known. Our work has established the pathways of reaction by proving the existence of the short-lived initial radical species and the three subsequent stable free radicals. This evidence that at least two of the free radical products of this reaction are quite long-lived (several hours) must be considered in the light of their potential interactions with either distant sites on the same biological molecule or with neighboring molecules. Furthermore, the formation of the nitroxide radicals necessitates the crosslinking of two lipid molecules, a factor which may have significance in understanding the changes induced by NO_2 in membrane structure. There are some clues as to the fate of nitroxide radicals (type 2) in biological systems from spin labeling experiments. It is known that, in the presence of living cells, the nitroxide radical is sometimes destroyed either by reduction or by interaction with natural free radical biochemical intermediates. As an example, nitroxides are reduced by ascorbic acid and by cysteine in the presence of traces of ferric ions. Nitroxides are also known to rea with light-induced radicals essenti to photosynthesis.[15]

Much remains to be determined a to the effects of nitroxide radica upon biological systems, and th question of the effects of iminox radicals (type 3) upon biological sys tems has not even been considere yet.

Further work, however, needs t be directed towards both in vitro an ain vivo studies conducted under co trolled exposure conditions.

Some aspects of the reaction o NO_2 with hemoglobin have been dis cussed. Evidence has been presente that indicates that the NO_2-hemo globin reaction may involve direc reaction with both the heme and th globin moieties of the hemoglobi molecule, as well as binding to th iron atoms. Studies of this reactio which utilize an interplay of severa spectroscopic techniques would ac vance our knowledge significantly.

This investigation was supported in part b the US Council for Tobacco Research grant 085-80492.

References

1. Arioka I: Experimental pulmonary damage by the inhalation of NO_2. *Hakkaido Igaku Zasshi* **40**:457, 1967; cf *Chem Abst* 58251c, vol 68, 1968.

2. Symon K: Air pollution research in Czechoslovakia. *Proc Roy Soc Med* **57**:988-990, 1965.

3. Thomas HV, Mueller PK, Wright R: Response of rat lung mast cells to nitrogen dioxide inhalation. *J Air Pollution Control Assoc* **17**:33, 1967.

4. Thomas HV, Mueller PK, Lyman RL: Lipoperoxidation of lung lipids in rats exposed to nitrogen dioxide, *Science* **159**:532, 1968.

5. Felmeister A, Amanat M, Weiner ND: Interaction of nitrogen dioxide-olefin gas mixtures with lecithin monomolecular films. *Environ Sci Technol* **2**:1, 1968.

6. Estefan RM, Gause EM, Rowlands JR: Electron spin resonance and optical studies of the interaction between NO_2 and unsaturated lipid components. *Environ Res* **3**:62-78, 1970.

7. Ayscough PB: *Electron Spin Resonance in Chemistry.* London, Methuen & Co Ltd, 1967, p 349.

8. Bielski BHJ, Gebicki JM: Electron spin resonnance studies of the mechanism of interaction between nitrogen dioxide and olefinic solvents. *J Phys Chem* **73**:1402, 1969.

9. Jonkman L, Muller H, Kiers C, et al: Electron spin resonance of radicals formed in the reaction of nitrogen dioxide with olefins. *J Phys Chem* **74**:1650, 1970.

10. McRae JA, Symons MCR: Nitroxide radicals from methylmethacrylate interacting with oxides of nitrogen. *Nature* **206**:1259, 1966.

11. Rowlands JR, Estefan RM, Gause EM, et al: An electron spin resonance study of tobacco smoke condensates and their effects upon blood constitutents. *Environ Res* **2**:47-71, 1968.

12. Kon H: Paramagnetic resonance study of nitric oxide hemoglobin. *J Biol Chem* **243**:4350, 1968.

13. Woolum JC, Commoner B: Isolation and identification of a paramagnetic complex from the livers of carcinogen-treated rats. *Biochem Biophys Acta* **201**:131-140, 1970.

14. McConnell HM, McFarland BG: Physics and chemistry of spin labels. *Quart Rev Biophys* **3**:91, 1970.

15. Corker GA, Klein MP, Calvin MC: Chemical trapping of a primary quantum conversion product in photosynthesis. *Proc Nat Acad Sci USA* **56**:1365, 1966.

The Response of Lung Tissue and Surfactant to Nitrogen Dioxide Exposure

Ronald A. Williams, PhD; Rodney A. Rhoades, PhD;
and William S. Adams, PhD, University Park, Pa

A control group of rats was exposed to filtered air and an experimental group to nitrogen dioxide levels of 15 ppm. Surface tension-area curves were recorded from fresh lung washings of excised lungs. Total phospholipid and lecithin concentrations were determined as an index of surfactant quantity, and an analysis of the surface tension-area curves was made by computer techniques. Total phospholipid and lecithin concentrations from the experimental animals were significantly higher, but the percentage contributed by lecithin was nearly identical for both groups. Nitrogen dioxide exposure at this level appears to alter the properties of surfactant demonstrated on surface tension balance, since higher trough concentrations of the experimental wash produced nearly normal surface tension-area loops. Changing surface tension properties of surfactant may be important in nitrogen dioxide-induced pulmonary injury.

The mechanical properties of the lungs are primarily governed by two forces—tissue forces and surface tension forces.[1] The surface forces are considered the most important and are the result of the air-liquid interface formed by the surfactant lining of the alveoli.[2] Hence, the surfactant lining layer is doubly important since it acts as both an interface between the gaseous environment and the lung tissue and significantly contributes to the mechanical properties of the lungs.

Pulmonary damage is the major toxic effect from exposure to nitrogen dioxide.[3] Because of its molecular weight and solubility, nitrogen dioxide has the capacity to cause damage at the alveolar level.[4] This

Received for publication Oct 22, 1970; accepted March 3, 1971.

From the Center for Air Environment Studies, Human Performance Research Laboratory, and Electrical Engineering Department, Pennsylvania State University, University Park, Pa. Dr. Williams is now with the Battelle Memorial Institute, Columbus, Ohio.

Read in part before the Tenth Annual Hanford Biology Symposium on Pollution and Lung Biochemistry, Richland, Wash, June 5, 1970, jointly sponsored by the Battelle Memorial Institute-Pacific Northwest Laboratories, National Air Pollution Control Administration, National Institute of Environmental Health Sciences, and the US Atomic Energy Commission.

Reprint requests to Battelle Memorial Institute, Columbus Laboratories, 505 King Ave, Columbus, Ohio 43201 (Dr. Williams).

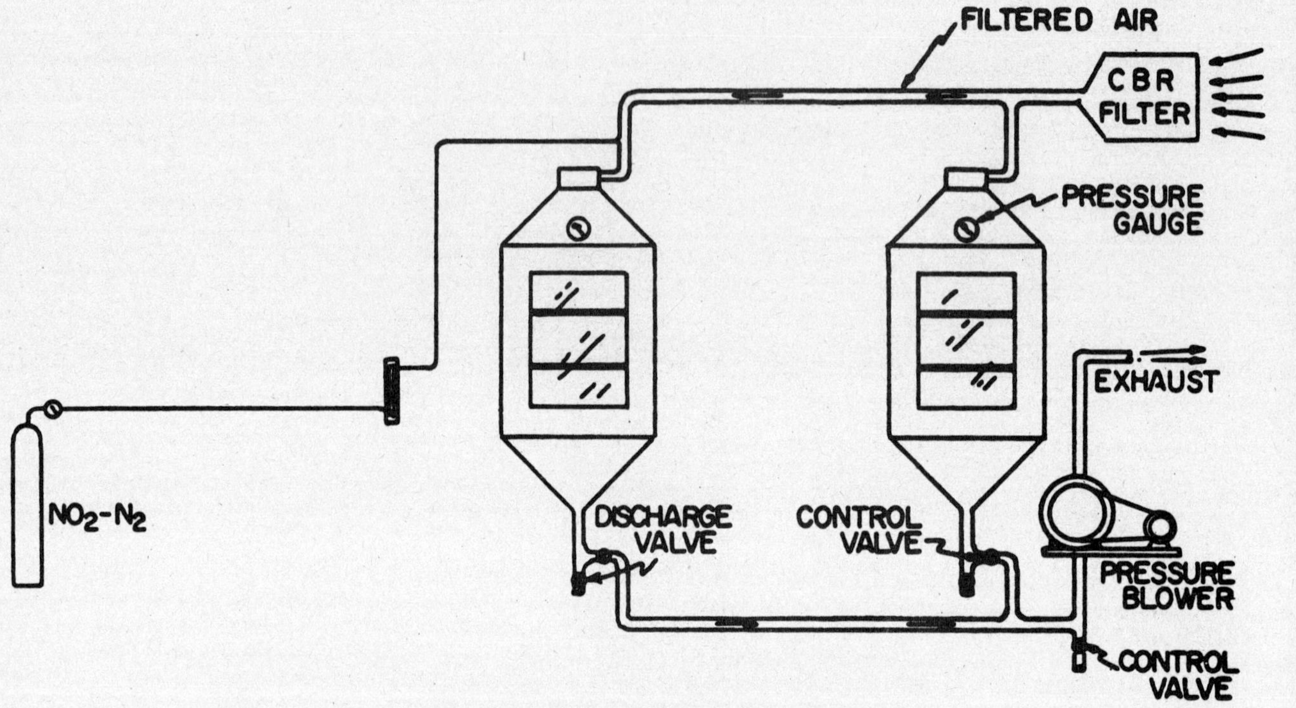

Fig 1.—Nitrogen dioxide exposure system.

manifests itself as atelectasis, edema, and alveolar thickening. Increased surface tension forces via the loss of surface active material (surfactant) have been postulated as a possible injury mechanism,[4] but little data exists to support such a mechanism. It was felt that further information on the nature of the action of the nitrogen dioxide on the lung could be obtained by a study in which measurements on the lipid content and surface properties of the lung washings from exposed lungs were obtained. Such information would be pertinent to describing any alteration of the surfactant system or the lung tissue which is the site of the surfactant manufacture.[5]

Methods

Male Long Evans Hooded rats of average weight 265.8 gm (15.7 SD, 12 rats), were continuously exposed to 15 ppm (1.0 SD) nitrogen dioxide for 28 days in a stainless steel exposure chamber similar in design to those described by Hinners.[6] The animals received filtered air through a chemical biological radiological filter, and nitrogen dioxide was metered in from a gas cylinder which contained 2% nitrogen dioxide in nitrogen. Control rats of average weight 266.8 gm (22.9 SD, 12 rats) were placed in an identical chamber which received only filtered air. Air flow rate was sufficient to produce an air change in the chamber once every four minutes, thereby preventing a build-up of waste material. Temperature and relative humidity were controlled between 72 to 75 F and 40% to 65%, respectively. The nitrogen dioxide concentration was monitored three times daily on a nitrogen dioxide meter. Food and water were supplied ad libitum. A block diagram of the complete exposure system is shown in Fig 1.

Following the 28-day exposure, the animals were killed by intraperitoneal pentobarbital injection and exsanguination via a carotid artery. The lungs were quickly removed and alveolar surfactant was collected. The method of Godish and Rhoades[7] was used to collect the alveolar wash. This method is shown schematically in Fig 2. This procedure consisted of cannulating the pulmonary artery, and pumping 0.9% saline into the vasculature while alternately compressing and expanding the lungs. The lipid material was dispersed in the saline and collected from the trachea. One hundred milliliters of alveolar wash was collected from each animal. The wash gave normal surface active properties, and the 100-ml volume provided optimal phospholipid recovery from the lungs. A particulate count done on the alveolar wash was very low, indicating that little tissue debris was being collected.

Surface tension-area loops were obtained on a modified surfactometer (Kimray).[8] The procedure for obtaining these curves was as follows: First, the Teflon trough and platinum flag (Wilhelmy plate) were thoroughly cleaned. The platinum flag was cleaned with chromic acid cleaning solution, rinsed thoroughly with double distilled water, and dried using a purified nitrogen jet. The Teflon trough and barrier were cleaned with benzene and rinsed with acetone, followed by thorough rinses with double distilled water. The balance was calibrated, and the surface tension of double distilled water was recorded over a complete compression and expansion cycle to check both the calibration and cleanliness of the trough and flag. No saline-surfactant material was tested until a constant surface tension of 72 dynes/cm was achieved during this cyclic compression and expansion. Twenty milliliters of test material was then placed into the trough and aged for ten minutes. Subsequently, it was cyclically compressed and expanded three times between the 100% and 15% area; the third cycle was recorded for analysis. Duration of a full cycle was nine minutes. Surface tension-area curves of the material were recorded directly on an X-Y plotter with surface tension on the abscissa and trough area on the ordinate. A typical surface tension-area curve is shown in Fig 3. All measurements were made at room temperatures (25 to 27 C).

After completion of the surface tension analysis, the contents of the surfactometer trough were salvaged and stored under purified nitrogen for subsequent chemical analysis. Lipids were extracted from this salvaged material by using the basic method of Godish and Rhoades.[7] Phospholipids were separated from other lipids by thin layer chromatography on silica gel (H.R. extra pure, Brinkman Inc.); the solvent system was $CHCl_3$:-MeOH;H_2O:29% NH_4OH, 130:70:6.5:0.6 (volume:volume).[9] To determine total phospholipid and phosphatidyl choline concentrations, replicate spots were aspirated into test tubes and their phosphorus content determined as described by Morrison.[10]

Computer techniques were used to analyze the surface tension-area curves. An application program (IBM System 350, 360A-CX-16X, the Continuous System Modeling Program [CSMP]) was used to maintain the analog nature of the curves. This program was used to compute the hysteresis area, coefficient of compressibility, average limbs, and average hysteresis area for each group. The analysis process is shown more clearly in Fig 4 which is the analog schematic of the program for the calculation of hysteresis areas and average limbs. The various function generators contain the data ob-

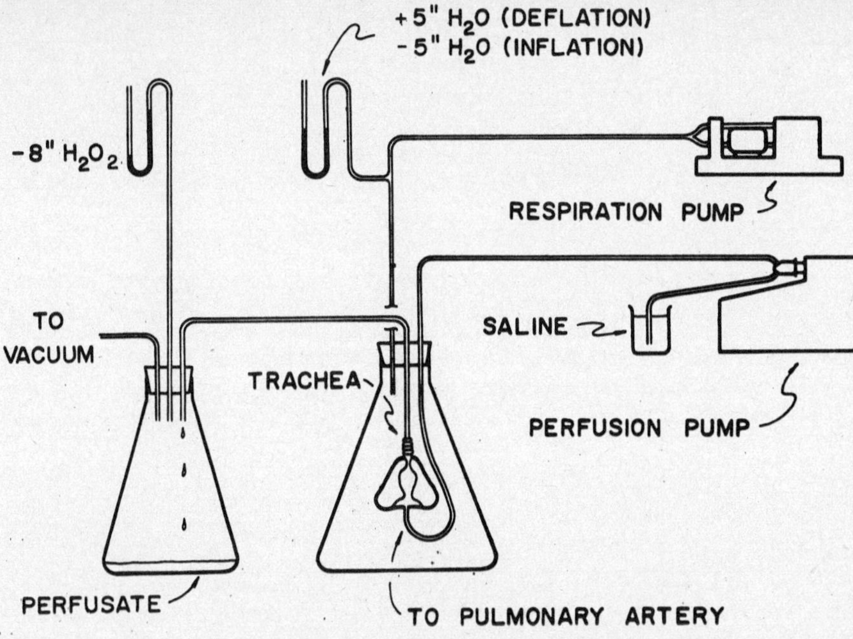

Fig 2.—Alveolar surfactant removal method.

Fig 3.—Typical surface tension-area curve from alveolar wash.

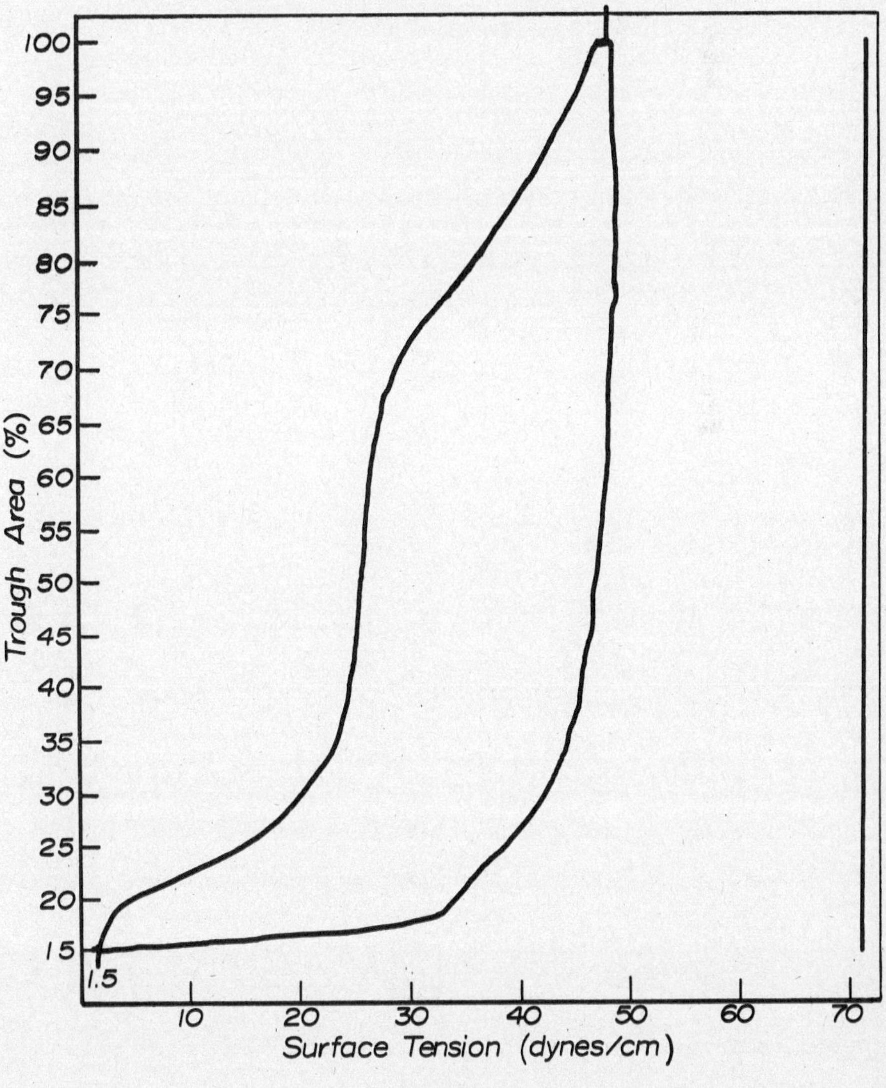

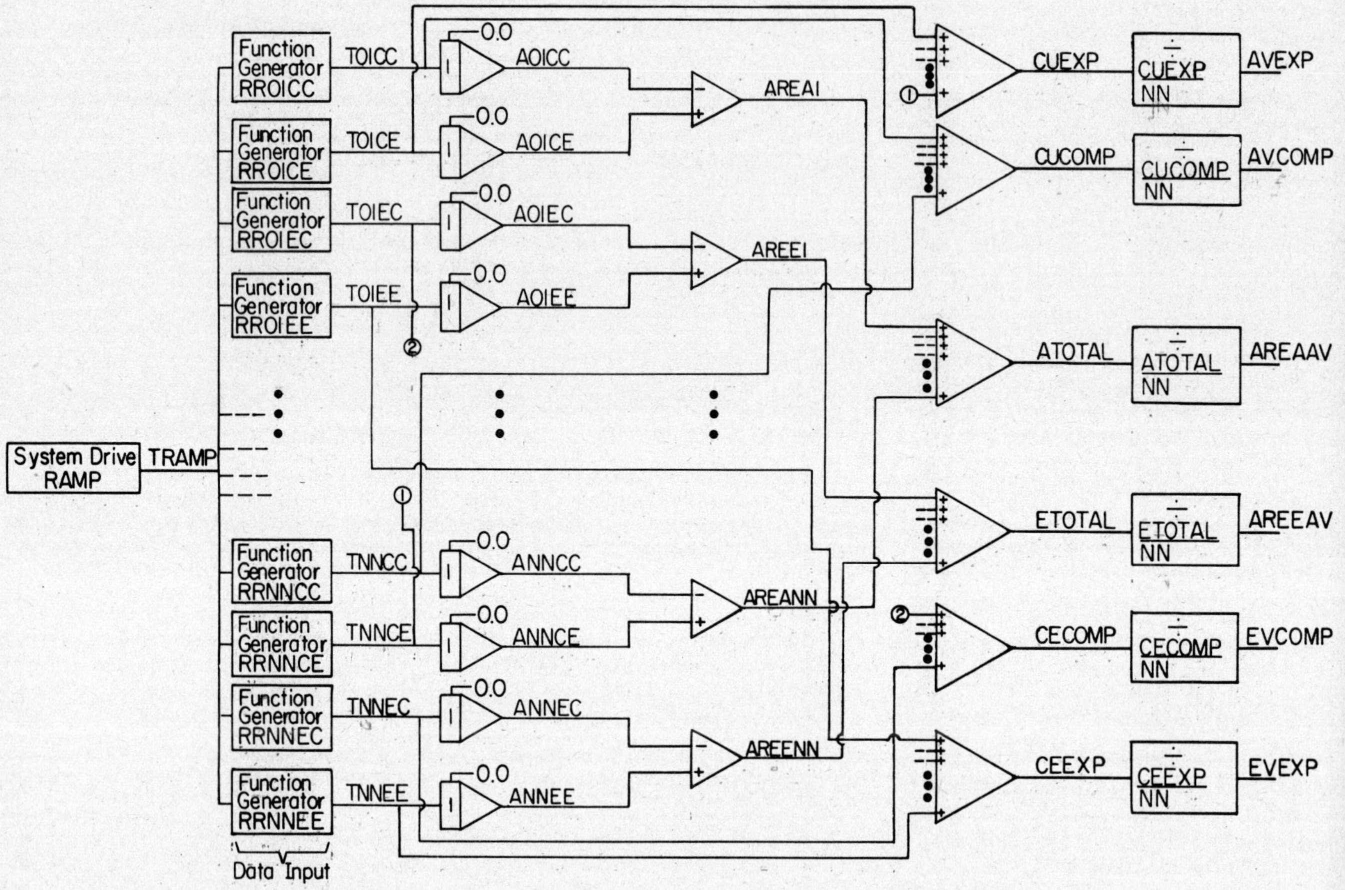

Fig 4.—Analog schematic of computer program for calculation of hysteresis area, average limbs, and average hysteresis areas.

tained on the surfactometer. The curves were split into compression and expansion limbs, and coordinates were picked from the various limbs and entered into the computer via the function generators. The program is intended to be flexible, and it allows a large number of curves to be processed simultaneously. In this particular case, 24 curves (12 experimental, 12 controls) were analyzed.

The coefficient of compressibility has been defined as[11]

$$C = -\frac{1}{A}\frac{dA}{d\gamma} \quad (1)$$

where

A = area in percent original area

C = coefficient and compressibility in centimeters per dyne

γ = surface tension in dynes per centimeter.

In this study, compressibility was computed (for the compression limbs only) by using the application program shown in block diagram form in Fig 5. This produced values of compressibility at room temperature and gave continuous plots of compressibility versus percent area.

Stability index, $\bar{S}$, which is used as an index of pulmonary surfactant and which was introduced and defined by Clements,[12] as

$$\bar{S} = \frac{\text{Change of tension}}{\text{Average tension}} = 2\,\frac{(\gamma_{max}-\gamma_{min})}{(\gamma_{max}+\gamma_{min})}, (2)$$

was also calculated for each curve.

Results

No significant difference in body weight between the experimental and control groups was observed following the 28-day exposure ($P >$ 0.05), although the lung weights of experimentals were significantly higher.

Surface tension-area measurements from both groups of alveolar wash gave marked hysteresis loops upon cyclic compression and expansion of the surface film (Fig 3). The effects of the nitrogen dioxide exposure on the surface tension properties demonstrated on the surface tension balance are shown in Table 1. The only measurement showing a significant variation between the control and nitrogen dioxide-exposed animals was the hysteresis-shape index, $\bar{\rho}$, discussed later.

Figure 6 shows the average surface tension-area curves for the experimental and control groups. These curves show some slight variation between the groups which is difficult to quantitate. The application program produced plots of compressibility for each individual surface tension-area curve, but little information could be extracted from the large number of

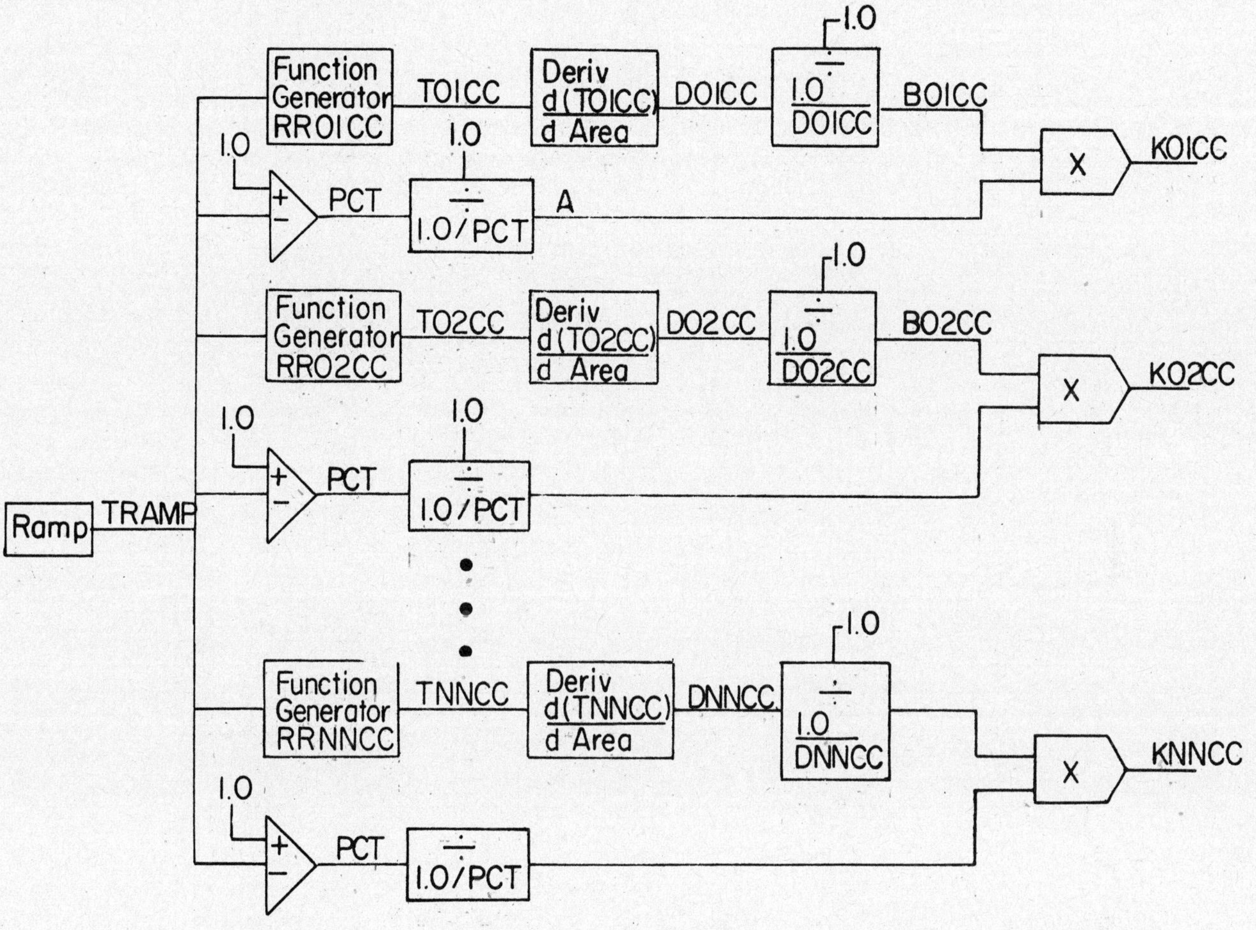

Fig 5.—Analog schematic of computer program for calculation of the coefficient of compressibility.

plots. Therefore, the compressibility of the average compression limbs (Fig 6) was calculated. Figures 7 and 8 show plots of the compressibility of the average compression limbs versus surface tension and percent area, respectively. These figures reveal that while there are slight compressibility variations between the control and nitrogen dioxide-exposed animals, meaningful conclusions about the extent of surface property alterations are difficult to deduce. This is largely because a criterion for drawing such conclusions based on the coefficient of compressibility has not been adequately formulated. Brown[11] states, however, that the minimum coefficient of compressibility roughly characterizes the type of surface film.

These results indicated that variations in the properties of pulmonary surfactant which are demonstrated on the surface tension balance are subtle. Figure 6 shows some (nonsignificant) hysteresis area variation and a slight shape difference in the

Table 1.—Surface Properties of Alveolar Wash for Control and Experimental Animals

Group	Average Valves ± SE (N = 12) γ_{min} (Dyne/cm)	γ_{max} (Dyne/cm)	$\bar{S}$	$\bar{\rho}$	Hysteresis Area (Dyne/cm)
Control (Filtered air)	3.04 ±0.43	39.74 ±1.31	1.72 ±0.04	0.498 ±0.021	795.83 ±46.1
Experimental (NO_2 exposed)	2.75 ±0.55	41.60 ±1.36	1.76 ±0.04	0.442 ±0.012	691.65 ±38.7

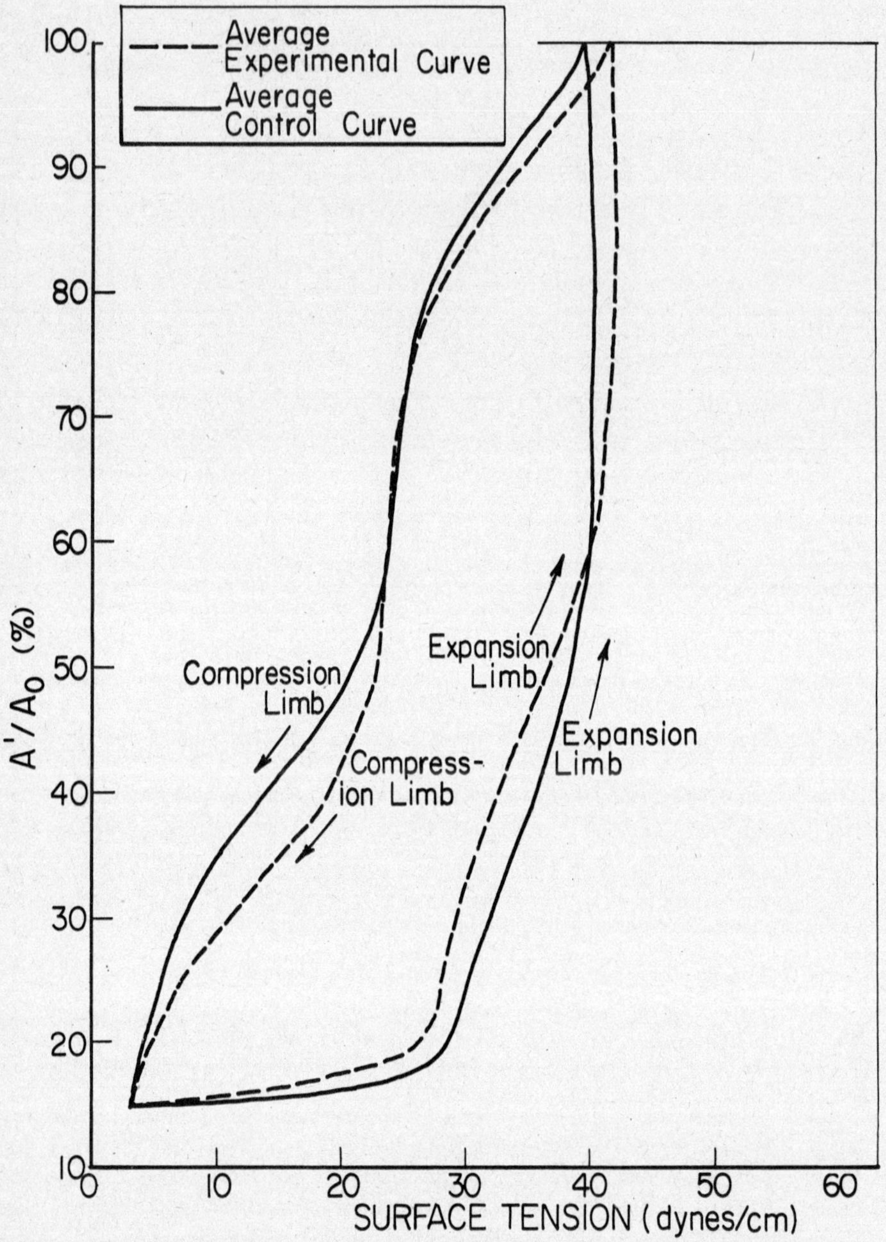

Fig 6.—Average surface tension-area curves for control and experimental animals.

average curves. An index which takes both of these measures into account might show significant variation. Such an index was developed[8] and is referred to here as the hysteresis shape index, $\bar{\rho}$. This dimensionless index is defined as the following:

$$\bar{\rho} = \frac{1}{k} \sum_{n=10}^{k} (1.0 - \gamma_c/\gamma_e) \quad \text{area} = [90-(n-1)70/(k-1)]\% \qquad (3)$$

where

K = number of increments to be used,

γ_c = the compression limb surface tension as a function of area, and

γ_e = the expansion limb surface tension as a function of area.

In this study, K = 8 was found to be satisfactory. The range of $\bar{\rho}$ is

$$0 \leq \bar{\rho} \leq 1 \qquad (4)$$

for typical surface tension-area hysteresis loops. As shown in Table 1, $\bar{\rho}$ did demonstrate significant ($P <$ 0.05) variation between the groups.

Table 2 summarizes the lipid analysis of the 20-ml surfactometer trough samples. It reveals that the nitrogen dioxide-exposed animals yielded more phospholipid with a significant 62.5% increase. Lecithin concentration was also significantly higher with a nearly identical percent increase in the nitrogen dioxide-exposed group. Since the percent lecithin was essentially the same for both groups, the proportional increase in total phospholipid appears to be largely because of the increase in lecithin.

Comment

Surface tension-area measurements obtained from lung washings demonstrated the characteristics of surface-active material believed to be the lining of the alveolar surface. Phospholipids are the principal agents which give rise to the film forming capacity, and lecithin is the primary component. Alteration in surface tension or phospholipids or both in lung washing would imply alteration in the surface-active material. Based on these assumptions, exposure to 15 ppm nitrogen dioxide for 28 days does not appear to significantly alter the surface active material. This conclusion is based on the observation that γ_{min}, γ_{max}, $\bar{S}$, and hysteresis area were not significantly different from the control. The only measurement which showed significant variation was the hysteresis-shape index, $\bar{\rho}$, which measures a more subtle variation in curve shape and hysteresis area.

The apparent discrepancy is the fact that washings from nitrogen

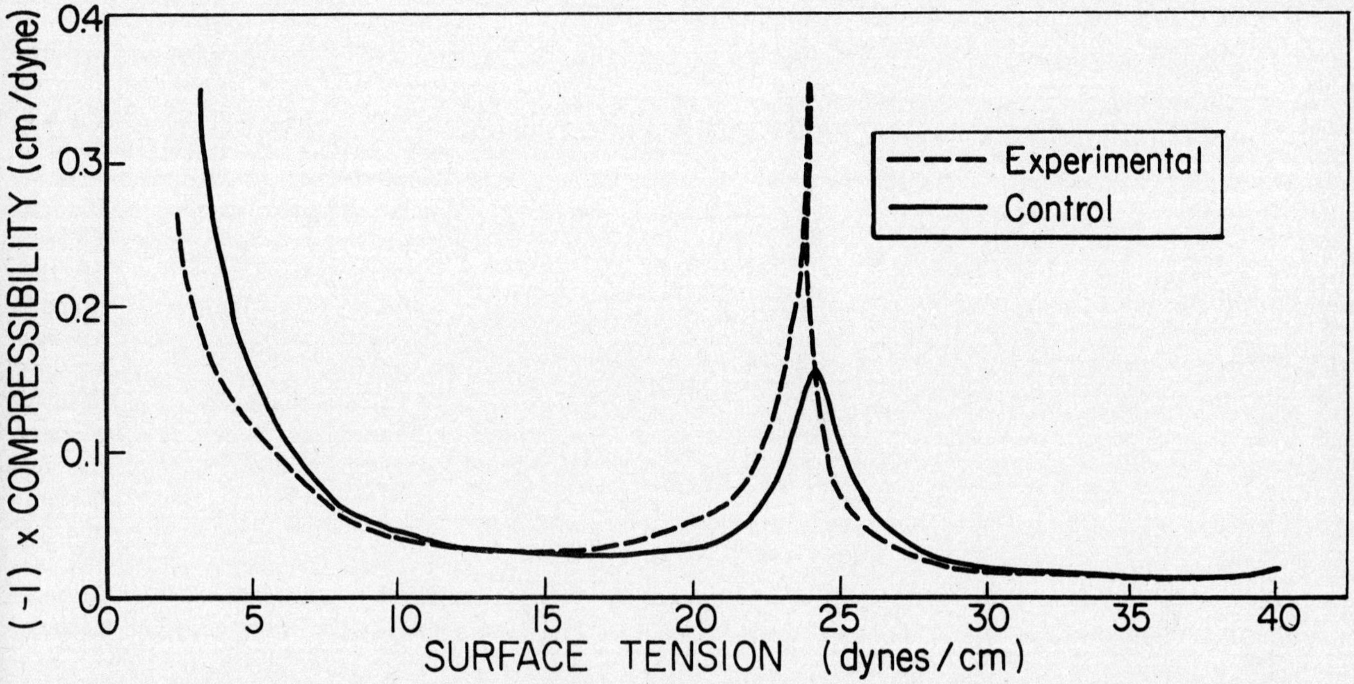

Fig 7.—Average coefficient of compressibility (compression limbs) versus surface tension for control and experimental animals.

Fig 8.—Average coefficient of compressibility (compression limbs) versus percent area for control and experimental animals.

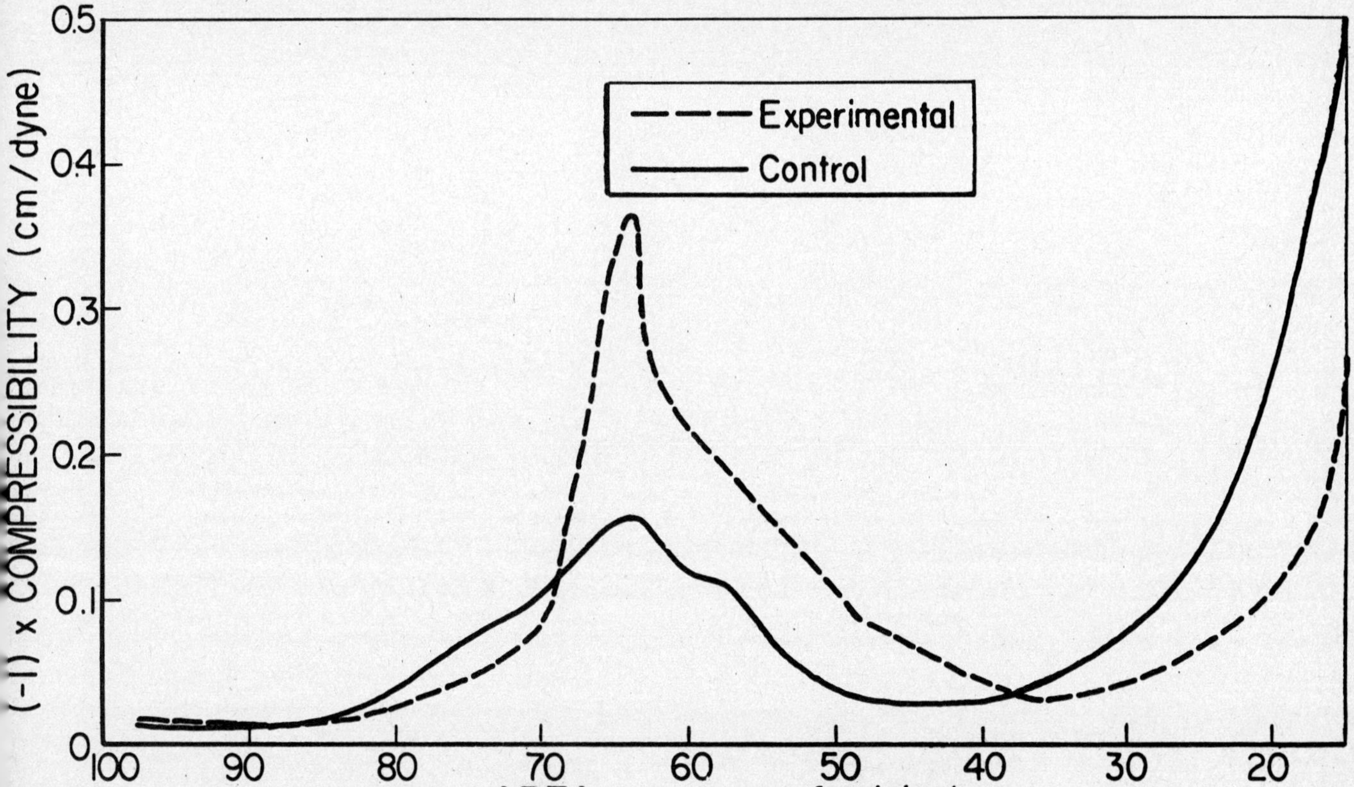

Table 2.—Phospholipid and Lecithin Variations Between Experimental and Control Animals

Group	Total Phospholipid (μg/ml)	Lecithin (μg/ml)	% Lecithin
	Values Based on 20-ml Samples Salvaged From Surfactometer Trough (N = 12)		
Control (Filtered air)	13.82 ±4.88 SD	10.22 ±3.99 SD	74.0
Experimental (NO_2 exposed)	22.46* ±5.95 SD	16.56* ±3.75 SD	73.7

* Significantly different from control value at the 5% level.

Table 3.—Average Values of Indexes Normalized to Average Lecithin Concentrations in Trough

Indexes		Experimentals	Controls	% Difference From Control
$\frac{\gamma_{min}}{\text{Lecithin}}$	$\left(\frac{\text{dyne/cm}}{\mu\text{g/ml}}\right)$	0.166	0.297	44.1
$\frac{\gamma_{max}}{\text{Lecithin}}$	$\left(\frac{\text{dyne/cm}}{\mu\text{g/ml}}\right)$	2.51	3.89	35.4
$\frac{S}{\text{Lecithin}}$	$(\mu\text{g/ml})^{-1}$	0.106	0.168	36.9
$\frac{\rho}{\text{Lecithin}}$	$(\mu\text{g/ml})^{-1}$	0.027	0.049	44.9
$\frac{\text{Hysteresis Area}}{\text{Lecithin}}$	$\left(\frac{\text{dyne/cm}}{\mu\text{g/ml}}\right)$	41.77	77.87	46.3

dioxide-exposed lungs contained significantly more phospholipid (specifically lecithin) and yet exhibited essentially normal surface tension properties. The subtle variations noted on the surface balance become more vivid if the mean indexes of the surface tension-area curves are normalized to the mean lecithin concentrations in the trough for each group. Such a comparison is shown in Table 3. These normalized indexes show rather large percent variation from the control values, and hence it appears that the surface activity of the experimental washings has been altered to some degree. However, the degree of alteration may not be as dramatic as Table 3 indicates since the relationship between lecithin concentration and the various indexes have not been well established. However, Rosenberg[15] has reported a correlation with concentration and $\bar{S}$, γ_{min} and to a lesser extent with hysteresis area.

Pulmonary damage at the alveolar level from nitrogen dioxide exposure has been reported by others.[3,13,14] Alveolar damage in most of these studies occurred at a lower nitrogen dioxide exposure dosage. The results of this study indicate that the surface properties of lecithin are altered to some extent by nitrogen dioxide exposure either by direct action on the material or because of contamination by components of the injured lung tissue. The question of how nitrogen dioxide initiates pulmonary damage remains open, but it appears that altered lecithin properties could play a role.

This investigation was supported in part by Public Health Service grants AP-00022-06 and ES-00335.

References

1. Clements JA, Brown ES, Johnson RP: Pulmonary surface tension and the mucus lining of the lungs: Some theoretical considerations. *J Appl Physiol* **12**(2):262-268, 1958.
2. Pattle RE: Surface lining of lung alveoli. *Physiol Rev* **45**:48-79, 1965.
3. Blair WH, Henry MC, Ehrlick R: Chronic toxicity of nitrogen dioxide: II. Effects on histopathology of lung tissue. *Arch Environ Health* **18**:186-192, 1969.
4. Pattle RE: Lung surfactant and its possible reaction to air pollution. *Arch Environ Health* **14**:70-76, 1967.
5. Scarpelli EM: *The Surfactant System of the Lung.* Philadelphia, Lea & Febiger, 1968, pp 34-43.
6. Hinners RG, Burkart SK, Punte CL: Animal inhalation exposure chambers. *Arch Environ Health* **16**:194-206, 1968.
7. Godish D, Rhoades RA: Quantitative recovery of phospholipids from alveolar wash. *Resp Physiol* **10**:396-404, 1970.
8. Williams RA: *Computer Analysis and Model of the Properties of Pulmonary Surfactant: Effects of Nitrogen Dioxide,* thesis. Pennsylvania State University, University Park, 1970.
9. Parsons JG: *A Study of Phospholipids of Cocoa Beans by Two-Dimensional Thin Layer Chromatography,* thesis. Pennsylvania State University, University Park, 1968.
10. Morrison WR: A fast, simple and reliable method for the microdetermination of phosphorus in biological materials. *Arch Biochem* **11**:218-224, 1964.
11. Brown ES, Johnson RP, Clements JA: Pulmonary surface tension. *J Appl Physiol* **14**(5):717-720, 1959.
12. Clements JA, Hustead RF, Johnson RP, et al: Pulmonary surface tension and alveolar stability. *J Appl Physiol* **16**(3):444-450, 1961.
13. Freeman G, Haydon GB: Emphysema after low level exposure to NO_2. *Arch Environ Health* **8**:125, 1965.
14. Wagner WD, Duncan BR, Wright PG, et al: Experimental study of threshold limit of NO_2. *Arch Environ Health* **10**:455-466, 1965.
15. Rosenberg E: Analysis of the properties of pulmonary surfactant using modified Wilhelmy balances. *Resp Physiol* **7**:72-87, 1969.

Alveolar Injury in Acute Carbon Tetrachloride Intoxication

Victor E. Gould, MD, and Edward A. Smuckler, MD, PhD, Seattle

Rats receiving orally 0.25 mg of carbon tetrachloride per 100 gm of body weight were killed after 1, 4, 8, 12, and 24 hours. Light microscopy disclosed focal perivascular edema, atelectasis, and hemorrhages. Ultrastructurally, earliest changes occurred in inclusions of granular pneumocytes with lamellar attenuation and decreased osmiophilia. Disruption of ribosomal aggregates, endoplasmic reticulum, and mitochondria and decrease in multivesicular bodies occurred at four hours. Small vesicles in granular pneumocytes, increased endothelial pinocytosis, and septal edema appeared later. Subsequently there was granular pneumocyte necrosis, endothelial sloughing, denudation of endothelial basal lamina, intracapillary platelet aggregation, formation of mural thrombi, and intraalveolar fibrin. Early changes are the result of pulmonary CCl_4 excretion, the latter substance acting as a lipid solvent upon elements of alveolar wall. Possible formation of a proximate toxin through a xenobiotic enzyme system remains speculative.

Carbon tetrachloride produces centrilobular liver necrosis when administered to a variety of animals.[1] More recently it has been recognized that this substance is associated with subtle alterations in other organs such as a sublethal injury to proximal renal tubules.[2] The lungs represent a major route of CCl_4 excretion and participate in the exchange of rather extensive quantities of this haloalkane.[3] Previous studies demonstrated an accumula-

Received for publication Oct 21, 1970; accepted April 5, 1971.

From the Department of Pathology, University of Washington School of Medicine, Seattle.

Read in part before the Tenth Annual Hanford Biology Symposium on Pollution and Lung Biochemistry, Richland, Wash, June 5, 1970, jointly sponsored by the Battelle Memorial Institute-Pacific Northwest Laboratories, National Air Pollution Control Administration, National Institute of Environmental Health Sciences, and the US Atomic Energy Commission.

Read in part before the International Academy of Pathology, San Francisco, March 11, 1969.

Reprint requests to BB218, University Hospital, Seattle 98105 (Dr. Gould).

tion of fatty droplets in the granular pneumocytes of guinea pigs following CCl_4 administration.[4] We wished to detail the structural alterations in rat lungs following CCl_4 ingestion, since these changes may represent cellular alterations related to the parent toxin and reflect the response of the lung to the presence of significant quantities of a lipid-solving agent. The chemical and physical similarity of CCl_4 and some other halogenated hydrocarbons used as anesthetics suggested that the pulmonary lesions may indeed represent a model system pertinent to other inhalants. A preliminary report on this investigation has been published.[5]

Materials and Methods

Adult male Sprague-Dawley pathogen free rats weighing between 200 to 250 gm were given by gastric intubation 0.25 ml of carbon tetrachloride per 100 gm of body weight dissolved in an equal volume of mineral oil. Control animals received mineral oil only. No anesthesia was used during intubation. The animals were fasted during 16 hours prior to the administration of the drug and subsequently were provided water ad libitum but no food. Groups of three animals were killed by cervical dislocation at 1, 4, 8, 12, and 24 hours.

Complete autopsies were performed on all animals. Tissues for light microscopy were fixed in 10% buffered formaldehyde solution, embedded in paraffin, and stained with hematoxylin-eosin. Fragments of lung which represented all lobes were fixed for electron microscopy in 1% osmium tetroxide buffered with s-collidine[6] at pH 7.4 at 0 C for two hours, then dehydrated in increasing concentrations of anhydrous alcohol and embedded in epoxy resin (Epon).[7] One-micron sections were stained with toluidine blue[8]; thin sections were cut with diamond knives, mounted on enamel (Formvar) and carbon-coated copper grids, and stained with uranyl acetate and lead hydroxide.[9] Sections were examined with an electron microscope (RCA 3G). Original magnifications ranged from 2,700 to 12,300;

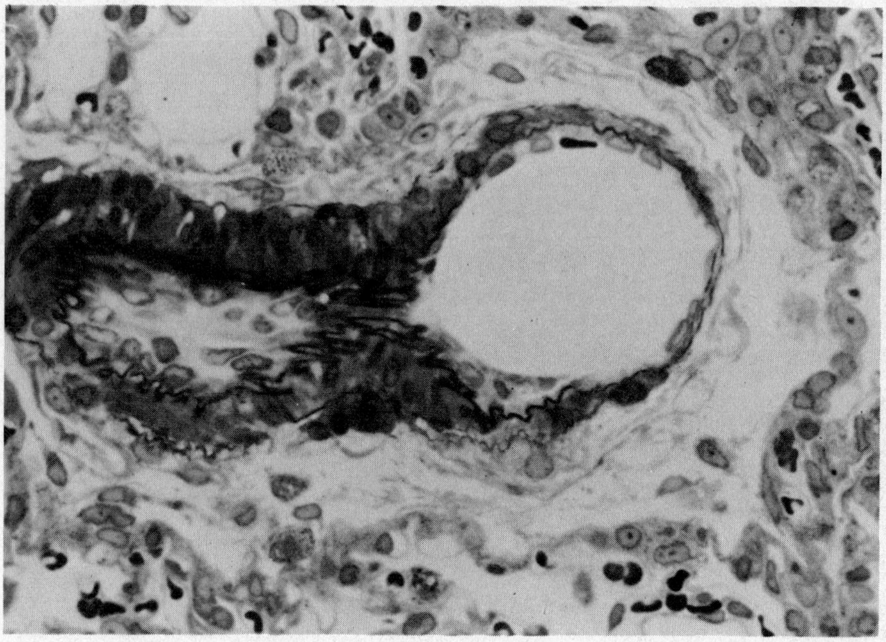

Fig 1.—Severe edema with scattered mononuclear cells seen around small pulmonary artery. One hour after CCl_4 administration; 1μ thick, epoxy resin embedded (toluidine blue stain, ×340).

Fig 2.—Normal alveolar architecture appears obliterated by collapse and confluent hemorrhages. Twelve hours after CCl_4 administration, 1μ-thick, epoxy resin embedded (toluidine blue stain, ×340).

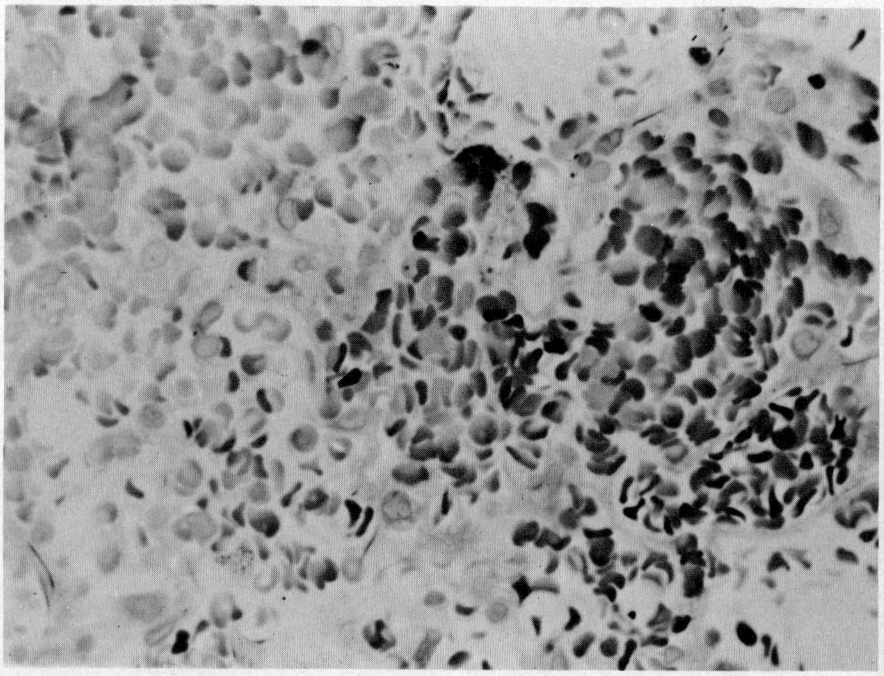

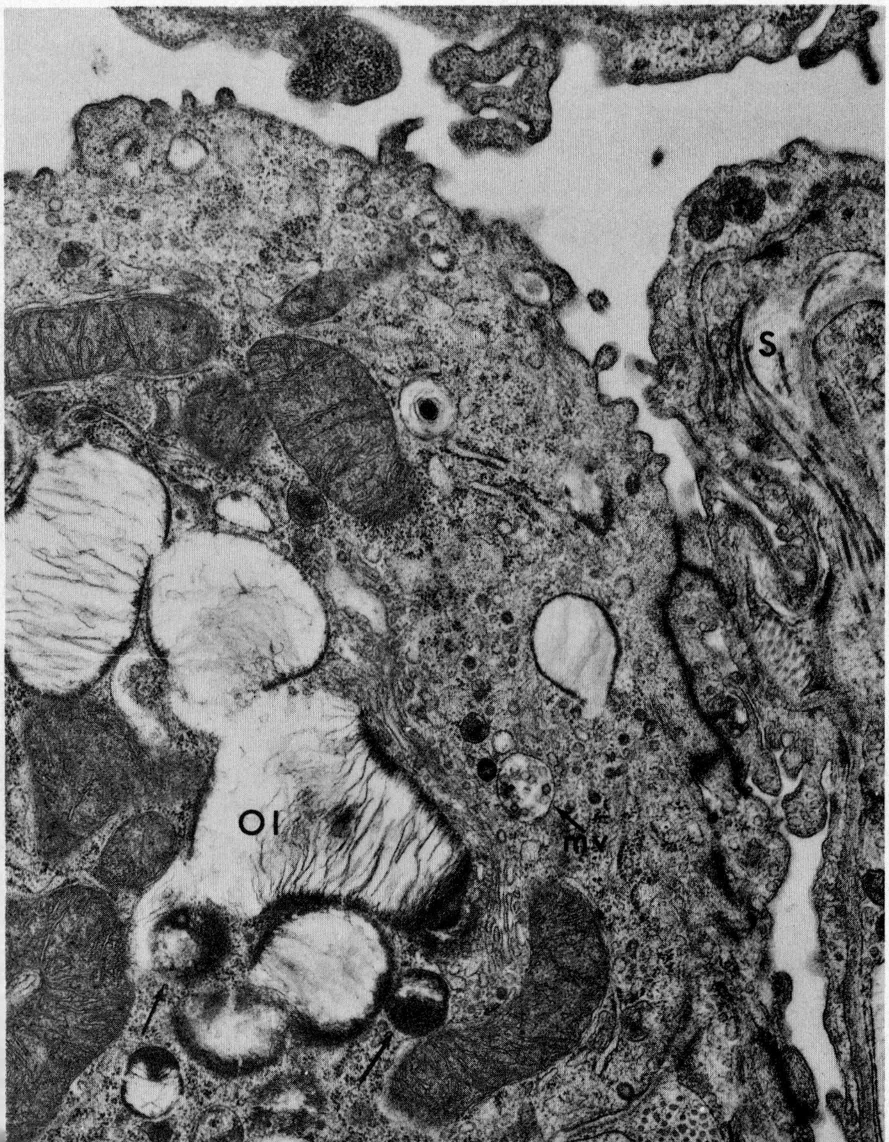

Fig 3.—Control granular pneumocyte. Notice the numerous osmiophilic inclusions (01); *abundant multivesicular bodies* (mv, arrow) *and several transitional forms* (arrows). *The thin septum* (S) *with rather compactly arranged fibers is readily apparent* (× 20,450).

from these photographic enlargements were prepared.

Results

At the dosage levels used and with pathogen free rats maintained in this laboratory, a mortality of less than 10% was observed in other experiments. No mortality was observed in these experiments. The animals showed little clinical response to CCl_4 until three to four hours following its administration, at which time piloerection and lassitude were noted. There was no significant change in appearance during the subsequent 20-hour period. In other experiments, intoxicated animals tend to eat less than the mineral oil-treated controls but changes in body weight were not statistically significant at 24 hours. In these experiments, no weight changes were noted.

Gross Description

The lungs of both treated and control animals were generally well expanded but patchy areas of apparent consolidation and hemorrhage were observed at eight hours following CCl_4 administration. These lesions became somewhat more evident at subsequent intervals but remained discrete.

Light Microscopy

Perivascular edema and mononuclear infiltration were noted in the first four hours after CCl_4 administration (Fig 1). These areas were focal in nature but were thought to involve at least 10% of the parenchyma examined. By 8 to 12 hours after administration areas of atelectasis and intraalveolar hemorrhages involved about 15% to 20% of the parenchyma in randomly taken sections (Fig 2). At subsequent intervals the involved areas increased but even in the most severely involved lungs, areas of apparently uninvolved tissue could be found. Control lungs showed no significant changes; no evidence of pneumonitis was found in control rats from this colony during the period of these experiments.

Electron Microcopy

A control granular pneumocyte plus a segment of an alveolar septum are depicted in Fig 3. One hour after CCl_4 administration the granular pneumocytes displayed swollen inclusions with decreased osmiophilia and attenuated lamellae (Fig 4); these changes became more severe four hours after administration. By four to eight hours after administration cytoplasmic edema, dislocation of dense ribosomal aggregates from the surface of the endoplasmic reticulum membranes, and mitochondrial disruption became apparent; multivesicular bodies were conspicuously decreased (Fig 5). At eight hours after administration some barely recognizable osmiophilic inclusions showed complete obliteration of their normal lamellar structure, the core ranging from moderately dense to "empty." In addition, numerous, small individual vesicles were seen while larger ribosomal aggregates again became apparent (Fig 6). While phagocytosed and severely injured granular pneumocytes were occasionally seen as early as four to eight hours after CCl_4 administration (Fig 7 and 8), frank necrosis was frequently found at 12 to 24 hours. Alveolar lumina contained extravasated erythrocytes and, occasionally, fibrin; multivesicular bodies did not appear to reconstitute.

Endothelial cells displayed markedly increased pinocytotic vesicles one hour after administration of

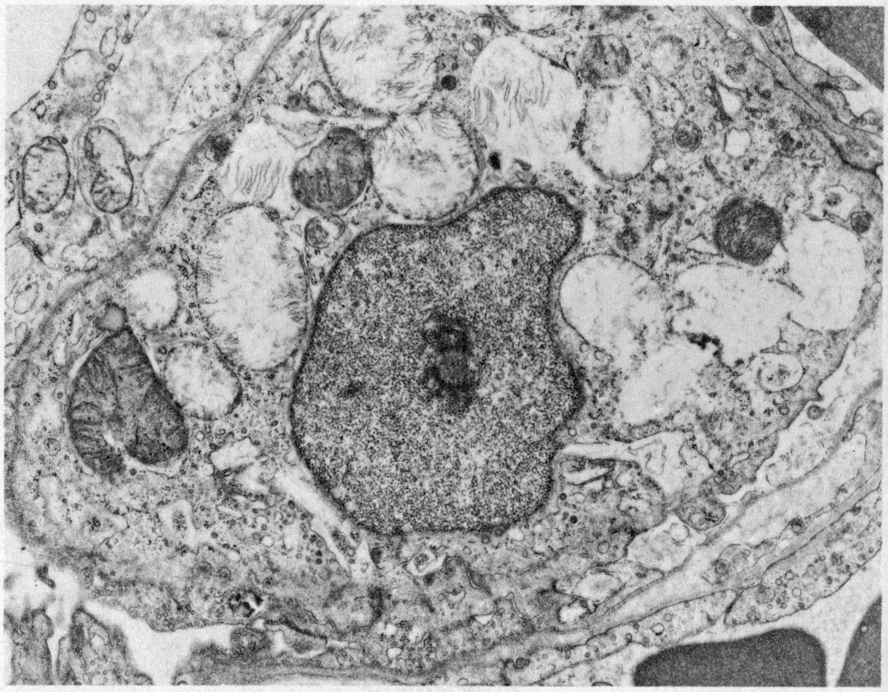

Fig 4.—Granular pneumocyte showing osmiophilic inclusion with decreased density and lamellar attenuation. One hour after CCl_4 administration (× 11,450).

Fig 5.—Inclusions display markedly decreased osmiophilia and attenuated lamellation. Also, notice decrease in overall cytoplasmic density, dislocation of dense ribosomal aggregates, and mitochondrial disruption (arrows). *Rare multivesicular* (mv, arrow) *can be detected. Four hours after CCl_4 administration (× 16,800).*

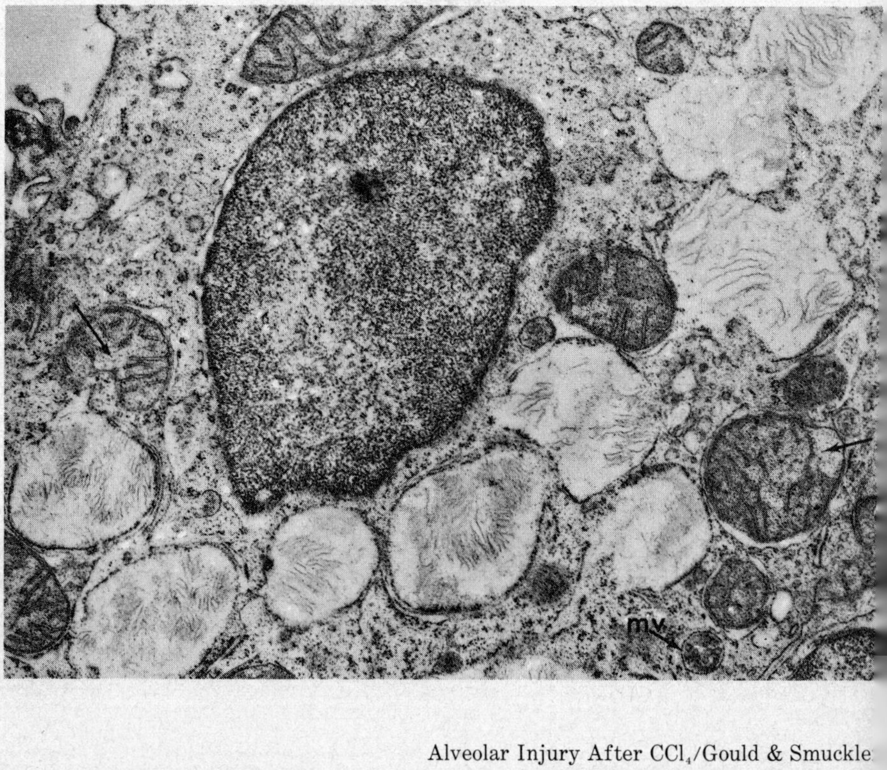

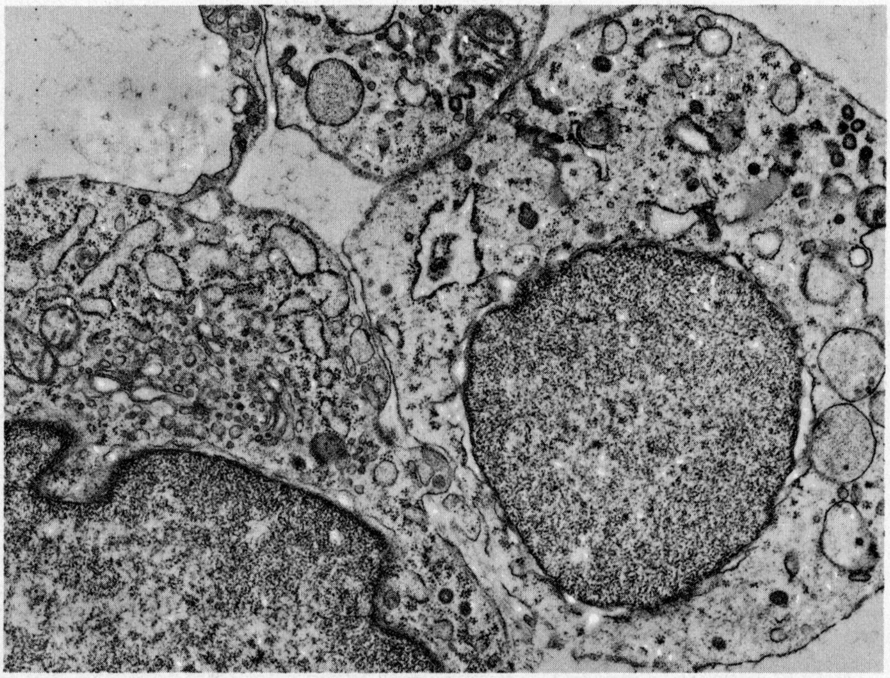

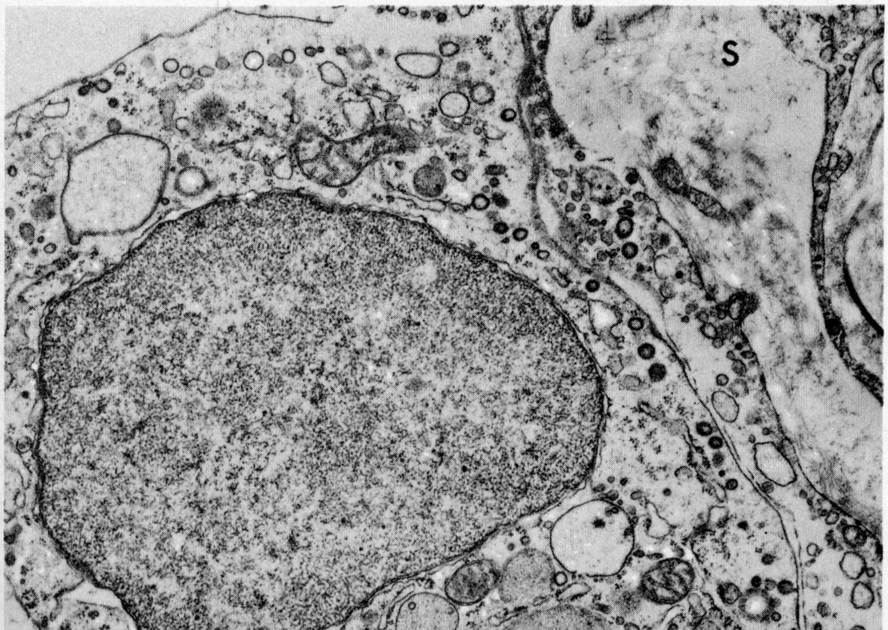

Fig 6.—Top and bottom, Granular pneumocytes lacking normal osmiophilic inclusions. There are numerous large single membrane limited "vacuoles" containing low density material and, occasionally, vesicles. Notice the abundant, small individual cytoplasmic vesicles, the cytoplasmic edema, and the reappearance on dense ribosomal aggregates. There are no recognizable multivesicular bodies. Septal edema is conspicuous (S). Eight and twelve hours after CCl_4 (×16,100 and 14,600 respectively).

CCl_4 (Fig 9). Focally, large cytoplasmic blebs and platelet aggregates were also evident (Fig 10 and 11). Edema of the septal ground substance and cells was found at four hours and progressed steadily thereafter (Fig 12). From eight hours after CCl_4 administration onwards, disruption of endothelial cells became severe; there were also increasing amounts of intracapillary platelets, dissolution and sloughing of endothelial cytoplasm, and mural platelet thrombi formation (Fig 13 and 14).

Comment

Carbon tetrachloride was employed originally as an anesthetic and subsequently as an antihelminthic; however, severe liver injury precluded continued therapeutic use. Administration of this haloalkane to various animal species by oral, subcutaneous, intraperitoneal, or respiratory routes results in centrilobular liver necrosis. Continued administration is associated with cirrhosis and, in some species, with hepatic neoplasms.[1,10] Despite the widespread interest evoked by this experimental model of cell death, altered regeneration, and carcinogenesis, the mechanism whereby cell injury is produced is not readily apparent. Current information suggests that the parent compound (CCl_4) is not injurious by itself to liver cells but that it is metabolized within those cells yielding a proximate toxin which causes cell damage.[11-17] The nature of this proximate toxin is not known but there is evidence to suggest that the dehalogenating mechanisms available to the hepatocyte are instrumental in its production. These findings imply that the original mechanism of injury predicated upon lipid solubility is not relevant to liver injury. However, other organs do respond to CCl_4 per se but with less marked structural changes than the liver; a sublethal proximal tubular injury occurs in the kidney.[2] This lesion affects primarily the mitochondria and cell surfaces and is associated with marked renal dysfunction. Chronologically, the renal lesion follows the hepatocyte change and occurs after peak blood levels during a time when the kidneys play a key role in CCl_4 excretion.[17] Recognition that the lungs are a major route of CCl_4 excretion[3] and the insufficient evidence to date to indicate that the lung possesses xenobiotic systems capable of metabolizing this haloalkane prompted us to investigate the effects of this agent on the lung structure.

The distal air spaces of the mammalian lungs are covered by an uninterrupted layer of epithelium consisting of two distinct cell types.[18-21] The smaller cell, type I or membranous pneumocyte, is regarded as a selective barrier to diffusion. The large, type II cell or granular pneumocyte, displays characteristic lamellated osmiophilic inclusions and is considered to be involved in the production of lipoprotein materials that modify alveolar surface tension.[22-27]

Following CCl_4 administration and occurring during the time of maximum blood levels and maximal excretion through the lungs, there are significant pulmonary changes. Focal atelectasis and hemorrhages are seen by light microscopy. Ultrastructurally, there is damage to all components of the alveolar wall with conspicuous changes in the granular pneumocyte, necrosis of both types of pneumocytes, septal edema, endothelial cell alterations, and the appearance of intracapillary platelet thrombi. This, together with the rec-

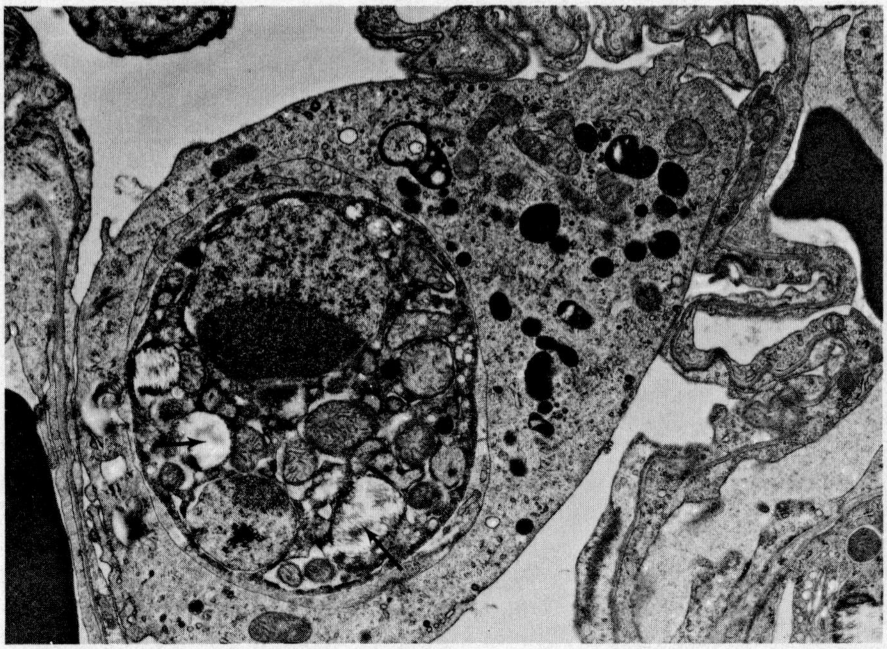

Fig 7.—Alveolar macrophage containing cell remnants recognizable as those of a granular pneumocyte; note the characteristic inclusions (arrows). *Four hours after CCl_4 administration (× 12,700).*

Fig 8.—Necrotic granular pneumocyte. Notice cytoplasmic fragmentation, nuclear pyknosis and incomplete detachment from the basement membrane. Twenty-four hours after CCl_4 administration (× 12,700).

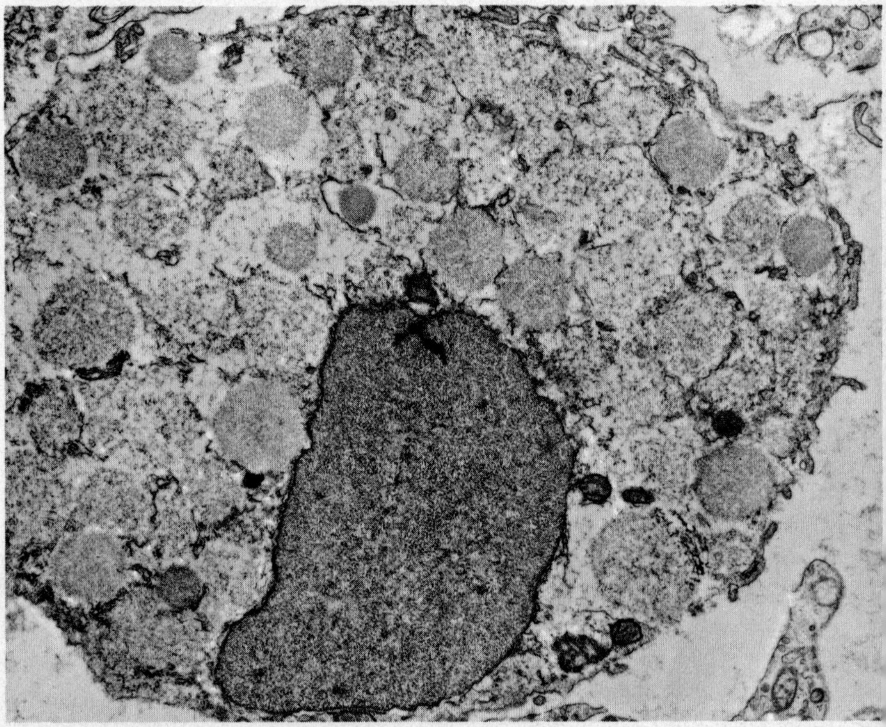

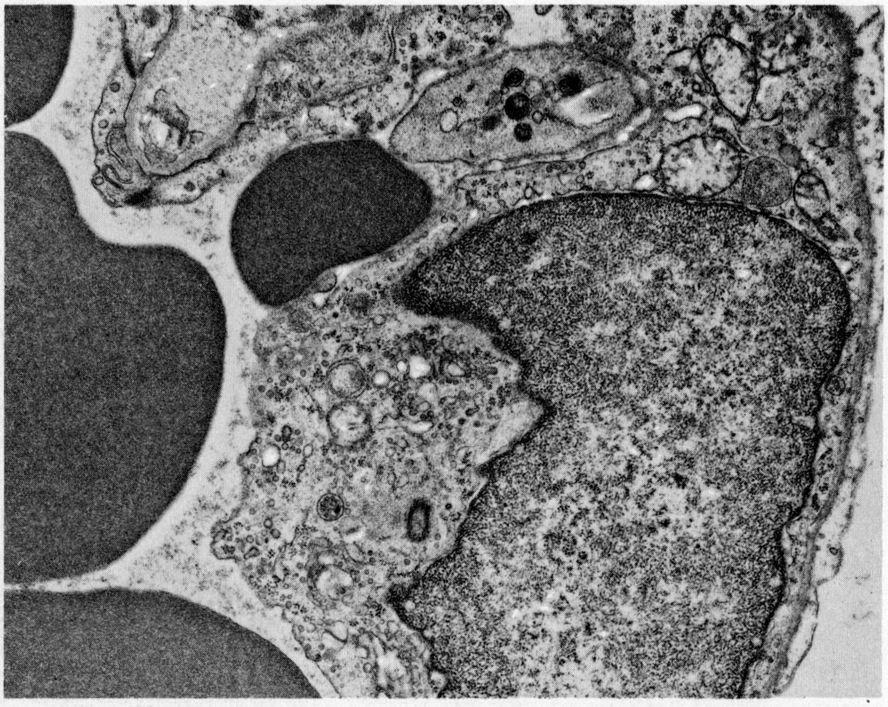

Fig 9.—Endothelial cell showing increased numbers of pinocytotic vacuoles. A platelet is seen within the capillary lumen. One hour after CCl_4 administration (×10,250).

Fig 10.—Segment of endothelium displaying confluence of pinocytotic vacuoles resulting in conspicuous cytoplasmic blebs. Four hours after CCl_4 administration (×16,800).

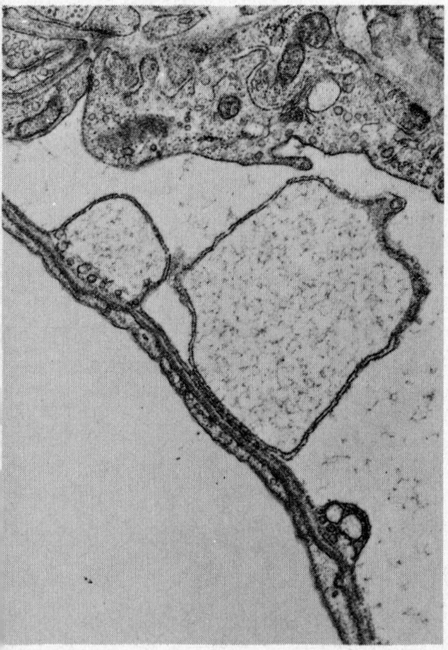

Fig 11.—Capillary lumen displaying several erythrocytes and a large platelet aggregate. Eight hours after CCl_4 administration (×6,700).

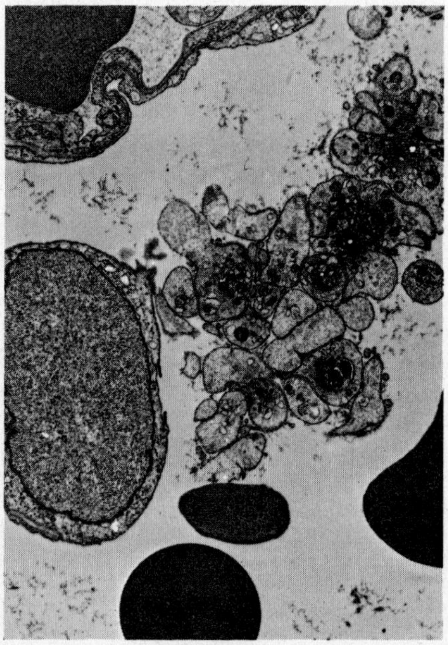

ognition of fibrin within alveoli point to significant alterations in vascular permeability. The lesions are focal in nature but seem to become more extensive following peak blood levels of CCl_4 (one to two hours).

The changes in the distal respiratory tree are not restricted to one layer. The endothelium must be the first recipient of CCl_4 in its passage from the blood to the air spaces; evidently CCl_4 or a byproduct thereof can cause significant changes as demonstrated by perivascular and septal edema and, eventually, leakage of fibrinogen into alveolar lumina. In addition, the presence of abundant intracapillary platelets was noted. Surprisingly, vascular changes in the liver and kidney are not conspicuous during these time periods. Platelet thrombi have been noted in the liver but the reticuloendothelial cells appear morphologically and functionally unimpaired.[28,29] It is possible that the focal nature of the pulmonary lesions, the ease of detecting the area, and the marked vascularity of this organ fortuitously allowed identification of these areas, whereas vascular lesions in other involved organs may not be so apparent.

The relationship between the described changes and CCl_4 is not readily apparent. The appearance of alveolar injury and altered vascular permeability is concomitant with peak blood levels of CCl_4. We interpret the earlier lesions to represent direct solvent effect of CCl_4; consistent with this notion are the morphological and functional changes in the lungs following the administration of various lipid solvent materials[30,31] as well as the known solubility of the osmiophilic inclusions in chloroform-methanol.[32] The changes occurring in the late stages of our experiments may be

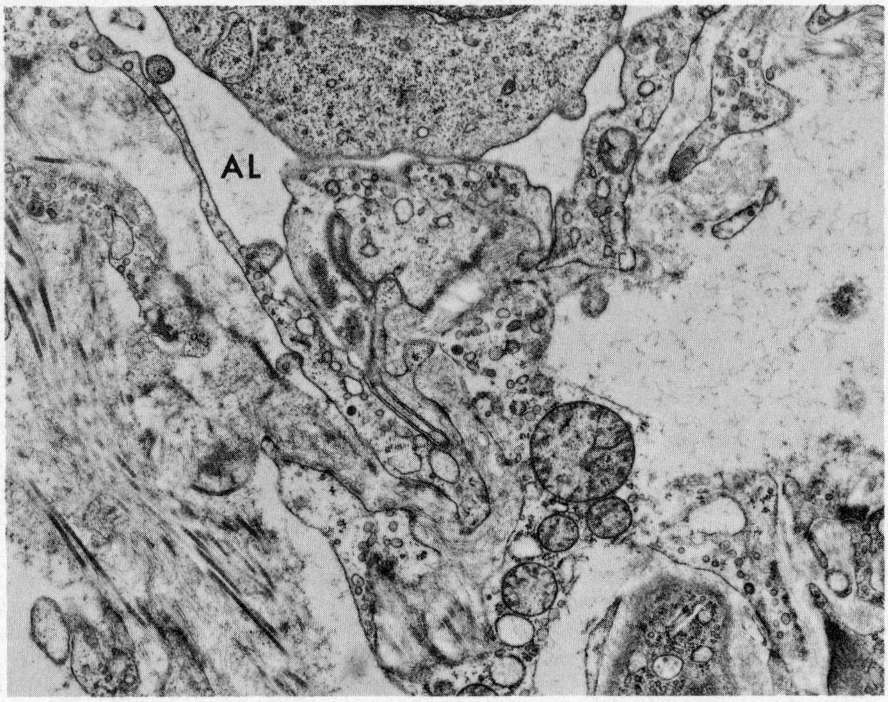

Fig 12.—Severe septal edema with disruption of ground substance fibers and septal cell cytoplasm. The alveolar lumen (AL) *contains a mononuclear cell. Eight hours after CCl_4 administration (× 12,700).*

Fig 13.—Segment of alveolar wall showing dissolution of endothelial cytoplasm and denudation of the basement membrane; several clumps of fibrin (arrows) *are apparent. Twelve hours after CCl_4 administration (× 13,150).*

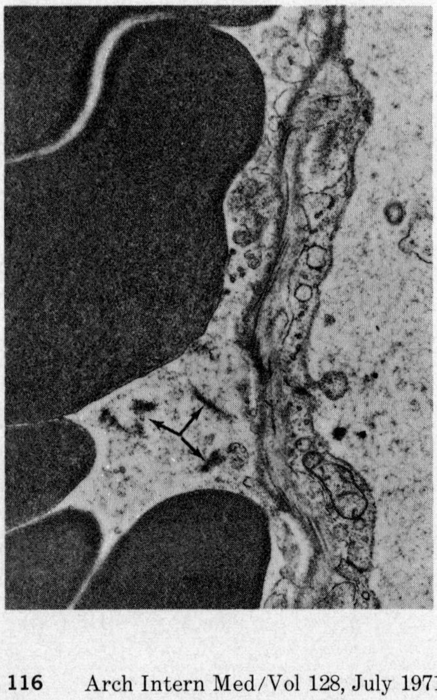

Fig 14.—Changes are similar to those of Fig 13; in addition, a mural thrombus composed of platelets is seen. Twenty-four hours after CCl_4 administration (× 13,150).

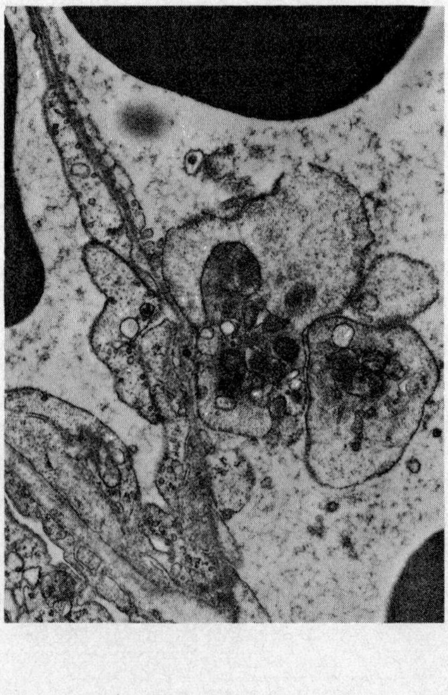

caused by a proximate toxin though definitive evidence is not available. Not all granular pneumocytes are fatally injured; those that escape the initial, massive damage show peculiar cytoplasmic changes. Significantly, remarkable numbers of small cytoplasmic vesicles appear during the later stages of our experiments. Since most recent investigations point to multivesicular bodies as the most likely origin of the osmiophilic inclusions,[32-36] one may suspect that the myriad of vesicles contained within granular pneumocytes represent an incompletely successful attempt at reconstituting the vital osmiophilic inclusions.

The basis for the focal nature of the pulmonary changes may be related to nonuniform alveolar function with resulting relative increase in specific alveolar CCl_4 concentration in some areas. It has been repeatedly suggested that not all alveoli are ventilated or perfused uniformly.[37-39] A direct consequence of this phenomenon would be the increase in CCl_4 not exchanged because of failure of dilution. The presence of this lipid active agent could affect alveolar status directly by injuring granular pneumocytes, indirectly through edema formation or by a combination of both mechanisms.

We believe that the pulmonary changes associated with experimental CCl_4 intoxication may represent a valuable model system for the study of a variety of alveolar changes particularly those following contact with lipid solvents which include furniture polish, kerosene and, possibly, halogenated hydrocarbon anesthetics.

This investigation was supported in part by Public Health Service grant AM-08686 and GM-13543 and by the US Tobacco Research Council.

Johsel Namkung prepared the photographs for publication.

References

1. Recknagel RO: Carbon tetrachloride hepatoxicity. *Pharmacol Rev* **19:**145-208, 1967.

2. Striker G, Smuckler EA, Kohnen PW, et al: Structural and functional changes in rat kidney during CCl_4 intoxication. *Amer J Path* **53:**769-789, 1968.

3. McCollister DD, Beamer WH, Atchison GJ, et al: The absorption, distribution and elimination of radioactive carbon tetrachloride by monkeys upon exposure to low vapor concentrations. *J Pharmac Exp Ther* **102:**112-124, 1951.

4. Valdivia E, Sonnad J: Fatty change of the granular pneumocyte in CCl_4 intoxication. *Arch Path* **81:**514-519, 1966.

5. Goldenberg VE, Smuckler EA: Pulmonary alveolar injury in acute carbon tetrachloride intoxication. *Lab Invest* **20:**583, 1969.

6. Bennett HS, Luft JH: s-Collidine as a basis for buffering fixatives. *J Biophys Biochem Cytol* **6:**113-114, 1959.

7. Luft JH: Improvements in epoxy resin embedding methods. *J Biophys Biochem Cytol* **9:**409-414, 1961.

8. Trump BF, Smuckler EA, Benditt EP: A method for staining epoxy sections for light microscopy. *J Ultrastruct Res* **5:**343-348, 1961.

9. Millonig GA: A modified procedure for lead staining of thin sections. *J Biophys Biochem Cytol* **11:**736-739, 1961.

10. Reuber EL, Glover EL: Cirrhosis and carcinoma in the liver of male rats given subcutaneous carbon tetrachloride. *J Nat Cancer Inst* **44:**419-427, 1970.

11. Smuckler EA: Structural and functional alterations of the endoplasmic reticulum during CCl_4 intoxication, in Gran F (ed): *Proceedings of the Fourth Annual Meeting of the Federation of the European Biochemical Society,* Oslo, Norway. London, Academic Press Inc, 1967, pp 13-55.

12. Smuckler EA: Studies on carbon tetrachloride intoxication: IV. Effect of carbon tetrachloride on liver slices and isolated organelles in vitro. *Lab Invest* **15:**157-164, 1966.

13. Slater TF: Necrogenic action of carbon tetrachloride in the rat: A speculative mechanism based on activation. *Nature* **209:**36-40, 1966.

14. Smuckler EA, Hultin T: Effects of SKF 525-A and adrenalectomy on the amino acid incorporation by rat liver microsomes from normal and CCl_4-treated rats. *Exp Molec Path* **5:**504-515, 1966.

15. Seawright AA, McLean AEM: The effect of diet on carbon tetrachloride metabolism. *Biochem J* **105:**1055-1060, 1967.

16. McLean AEM, McLean EK: Diet and toxicity. *Brit Med Bull* **25:**278-281, 1969.

17. Recknagel RO, Litteria M: Biochemical changes in carbon tetrachloride fatty liver: Concentration of carbon tetrachloride in liver and blood. *Amer J Path* **36:**521-531, 1960.

18. Low FN: The pulmonary alveolar epithelium of laboratory mammals and man. *Anat Rec* **117:**241-263, 1953.

19. Karrer HE: The ultrastructure of mouse lung: General architecture of capillary and alveolar walls. *J Biophys Biochem Cytol* **2:**241-252, 1956.

20. Policard A, Collet A, Pregermain S: Recherches au microscope electronique sur les cellules parietales alveolaires du poumon des mammiferes. *Z Zellforsch* **50:**561-587, 1959.

21. Schultz H: *Die Submikroskopische Anatomie und Pathologie der Lunge.* Berlin, Springer Verlag, 1959.

22. Macklin CC: The pulmonary alveolar film and pneumonocytes. *Lancet* **1:**1099-1104, 1954.

23. Buckingham S, Avery ME: Time of appearance of lung surfactant in the foetal mouse. *Nature* **193:**688-689, 1962.

24. Buckingham S, McNary WF Jr, Sommers SC: Pulmonary alveolar cell inclusions: Their development in the rat. *Science* **145:**1192-1193, 1964.

25. Bensch K, Schaefer K, Avery ME: Granular pneumonocytes: Electron microscopic evidence of their exocrine function. *Science* **145:**1318-1319, 1964.

26. Buckingham S, Heinemann HO, Sommers SC, et al: Phospholipid synthesis in the large pulmonary alveolar cell: Its relation to lung surfactants. *Amer J Path* **48:**1027-1041, 1966.

27. Kikkawa Y, Motoyama EK, Gluck L: Study of the lungs of fetal and newborn rabbits: Morphological, biochemical and surface physical development. *Amer J Path* **52:**177-209, 1968.

28. Smuckler EA, Arcasoy M: Structural and functional changes of the endoplasmic reticulum of hepatic parenchymal cells. *Int Rev Exp Path* **7:**305-418, 1969.

29. Monlux G, Smuckler EA: An autoradiographic study of protein synthesis in mouse liver parenchymal cells during CCl_4 intoxication. *Amer J Path* **54:**73-82, 1969.

30. Huxtable KA, Bolande RP, Klaus M: Experimental furniture polish pneumonia in rats. *Pediatrics* **34:**228-235, 1964.

31. Giammona ST: Effects of furniture polish on pulmonary surfactant. *Amer J Dis Child* **113:**658-663, 1967.

32. Sorokin SP: A morphologic and cytochemical study on the great alveolar cell. *J Histochem Cytochem* **14:**884-897, 1966.

33. Balis JU, Conen PE: The role of alveolar inclusion bodies in the developing lung. *Lab Invest* **13:**1215-1299, 1964.

34. Goldenberg VE, Buckingham S, Sommers SC: Pulmonary alveolar lesions in vagotomized rats. *Lab Invest* **16:**693-705, 1967.

35. Kuhn C III: Cytochemistry of pulmonary alveolar epithelial cells. *Amer J Path* **53:**809-833, 1968.

36. Goldenberg VE, Buckingham S, Sommers SC: Pilocarpine stimulation of granular pneumocyte secretion. *Lab Invest* **20:**147-158, 1969.

37. Wearn JT, Barr JS, German WJ: Behavior of arterioles and capillaries of the lung. *Proc Soc Exp Biol Med* **24:**114-115, 1926.

38. Leroy EP, Liebner EJ, Jensik RJ: The ultrastructure of canine alveoli after supervoltage irradiation of the thorax: I. Lesions of the latent period. *Lab Invest* **15:**1544-1558, 1966.

39. Goldenberg VE, Warren S, Chute R, et al: Radiation pneumonitis in single and parabiotic rats. Short term effect of supralethal total body irradiation. *Lab Invest* **18:**215-226, 1968.

Enzymic Mechanism of Metabolism of the Phosphorothionate Insecticides

Robert A. Neal, PhD, Nashville, Tenn

The insecticidal properties and, consequently, the toxic properties of the phosphorothionate insecticides results from their ability to phosphorylate and inactivate certain esteratic enzymes in insects and animals. The parent phosphorothionate itself is not capable of inhibiting these enzymes. However, it is metabolized by a mixed function oxidase enzyme in insects and animals to the phosphate analog which is capable of bringing about the inactivation. Further studies have revealed there is an additional product, formed by the action of what appears to be a different form of the mixed function oxidase enzyme. This is a product in which one of the ester bonds is cleaved to give the diester of phosphorothioic acid. Studies have shown that the rates of these two reactions are sensitive to change in the electronic environment about the phosphorus.

Recent administrative action in several states and by the federal government have affected the licensing, sale, and use of DDT and a few other chlorinated hydrocarbon insecticides. These steps indicate there will be a gradual phasing out of widespread use of the more persistent insecticides as represented by the chlorinated hydrocarbons. With the phasing out of these compounds more reliance will be placed on alternative methods of pest control. These include the use of predators and parasites of insects, the development of food or fiber plants which are resistant to insects, the application of bacteria or virus which infect the insect, the use of pheromones to attract insects to specific sites where they can be killed by various means, and the introduction of sterile males of a particular species into a geographic area. Currently, the most important of these alternatives is the use of nonpersistent chemicals such as the organophosphate and carbamate insecticides.

The first organophosphate in wide use as an insecticide was the compound tetraethyl pyrophosphate. This compound, marketed in Germany in 1944, was originally prepared by de Clermont in 1854, but was not recognized as an insecticide until 1938. The recognition of the insecticidal properties of tetraethyl pyrophosphate was an outgrowth of a long series of investigations by a group in Germany headed by Gerhard Schrader. These investigations led to the synthesis of many of the insecticidal phosphates in use today. The most notable of these is parathion.

The general formula for the organophosphate insecticides is shown in Fig 1.

These compounds may exist as esters of phosphoric, phosphonic, or phosphinic acid and their sulfur analogs, the phosphorothionates and the phosphonothionates. R_1 and R_2 may be widely varied but the normal substituent is an alkyl group or an amine. The X group is usually an acidic group and the P-X bond has some anhydride character.

The chemical basis for the toxic action of the organophosphate insecticides is the inhibition of certain esterase enzymes, and acetylcholinesterase in particular. The mechanism by which these organophosphates inhibit acetylcholinesterase is inherent in the mechanism by which the enzyme hydrolyzes its normal substrate acetylcholine. The reaction is as follows.

$$\text{Enzyme + Acetylcholine} \rightleftharpoons \text{Enzyme–Acetylcholine} \longrightarrow \text{Acetylated Enzyme + Choline} \xrightarrow{H_2O} \text{Acetate + Enzyme}$$

The reaction consists of the interaction of enzyme and acetylcholine to form an enzyme substrate complex which undergoes a reaction to yield choline and acetylated enzyme in which the acetate is covalently bound to a serine hydroxyl group in the enzyme. The final step in the re-

Received for publication Oct 21, 1970; accepted April 23, 1971.

From the Department of Biochemistry, Division of Toxicology, Vanderbilt University School of Medicine, Nashville, Tenn.

Read in part before the Tenth Annual Hanford Biology Symposium on Pollution and Lung Biochemistry, Richland, Wash, June 5, 1970, jointly sponsored by the Battelle Memorial Institute-Pacific Northwest Laboratories, National Air Pollution Control Administration, National Institute of Environmental Health Sciences, and the US Atomic Energy Commission.

Reprint requests to Department of Biochemistry, Division of Toxicology, Vanderbilt University School of Medicine, Nashville, Tenn 37203 (Dr. Neal).

action is the hydrolytic deacetylation of the enzyme to give acetate and regenerate the enzyme. The cholinergic organophosphates react with the enzyme in an analogous manner in which the organophosphate reacts with the enzyme to give an enzyme phosphate complex which reacts to form a phosphorylated enzyme and generate a free X group. In this case the phosphorylated enzyme hydrolyzes to phosphate and enzyme so slowly as to render that molecule of enzyme unavailable for further reaction with acetylcholine or another molecule of the organophosphate.

$$\text{Enzyme} + R_1R_2P(O)X \rightleftharpoons \text{Enzyme–}R_1R_2P(O)X \rightarrow \text{Enzyme}\bullet P(O)R_1R_2 + X \xrightarrow[\text{SLOW}]{H_2O} \text{Enzyme} + R_1R_2P(O)OH$$

When about 50% to 80% of the total acetylcholinesterase in the nervous tissue or effector organs is inactivated in this way, symptoms of poisoning are noted.[1]

The symptoms of poisoning by these compounds are those that might be expected from an inhibition of acetylcholinesterase and a buildup of acetylcholine. Thus, poisoning by these compounds results in excessive salivation, lacrimation, vomiting, and violent contractions of the gastrointestinal tract and bladder, all caused by accumulation of acetylcholine at the junctions of these organs with the parasympathetic nerve endings. Muscular twitching and paralysis are also seen. Death usually occurs as a result of respiratory failure brought about by both peripheral and central nervous system effects of the accumulation of acetylcholine.

In addition to supportive therapy, treatment for organophosphate poisoning consists of the administration of both atropine to counter the effects of the accumulated acetylcholine and some strong nucleophilic reagent to aid in the displacement of the phosphorus diester from the inhibited acetylcholinesterase. The nucleophil most widely used is pralidoxine chloride.

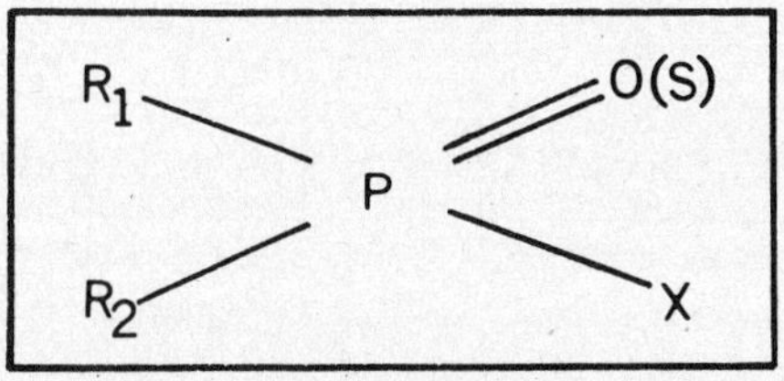

Fig 1.—The general formula for the organophosphate insecticides.

Some idea of the magnitude of the problem of poisoning by the organophosphate insecticides is given in data collected by the California Department of Public Health.[2] In California during the period 1951-1965, 25 accidental deaths from organophosphates were reported; most were among children. An additional number of suicides involved use of these compounds. There were also some 2,400 reported cases of nonfatal systemic poisonings by the organophosphate insecticides during a similar period. To give some idea of the difference in toxicity of the chlorinated hydrocarbon as compared to that of the organophosphate insecticides, during this same period only 140 cases of systemic poisoning from chlorinated hydrocarbons were reported. Thus the organophosphates present a much greater acute toxic hazard than do the chlorinated hydrocarbons.

Most of the organophosphate insecticides used commercially are triesters of phosphorothioic acid. These compounds are not good inhibitors of

Table 1.—Comparison of Enzyme Activity Toward Parathion in Various Tissues of the Rat*

Tissue	Amount of Metabolite Formed (μmol/hr/gm Tissue): Diethyl Phosphorothionate	Paraoxon
Liver	291	363
Lung	9	16
Kidney	13	34

* This experiment was conducted with the microsomes plus supernatant fraction (9,000 × g supernatant) from the various tissues. The procedures for incubation and for isolation and measurement of the quantities of metabolite are described in reference 5. The values shown for paraoxon represent the sum of paraoxon and diethyl phosphate formed during the incubation. From Fig 2 it can be seen that diethyl phosphate is derived from paraoxon by the action of an esterase.[5]

Table 2.—Effect of Various Enzyme Inhibitors on the Metabolism of Parathion*

Experiment, No.	Metabolite Formed (μmol/hr/gm of Liver): Diethyl Phosphorothionate	Paraoxon	Ratio of Paraoxon: Diethyl Phosphorothionate
1, None	194± 4	466±14	2.53±0.09
Bathophenanthroline (1.0 millimolar)	39± 6 (0.005)	101±18 (0.005)	2.64±0.15 (NS)
2, None	243±10	651±12	2.69±0.16
8-Hydroxyquinoline (3.0 millimolar)	160±14 (0.005)	278±13 (0.005)	1.76±0.15 (0.010)
PCMB† (0.05 millimolar)	175± 9 (0.005)	374±20 (0.005)	2.15±0.16 (0.050)
Proadifen hydrochloride (3.0 millimolar)	141± 9 (0.005)	326±22 (0.005)	2.33±0.23 (NS)

* The incubation procedures are described in reference 5. The values for each experiment are the means ± SD of the means of three separate determinations, carried out simultaneously with microsomes isolated from the same pooled sample of male rat livers. The *P* values, in parentheses, indicate the significance of differences between mean results of incubations in the presence and absence of inhibitors; NS, not significant.[6]

‡ PCMB signifies *p*-chloromercuribenzoate.

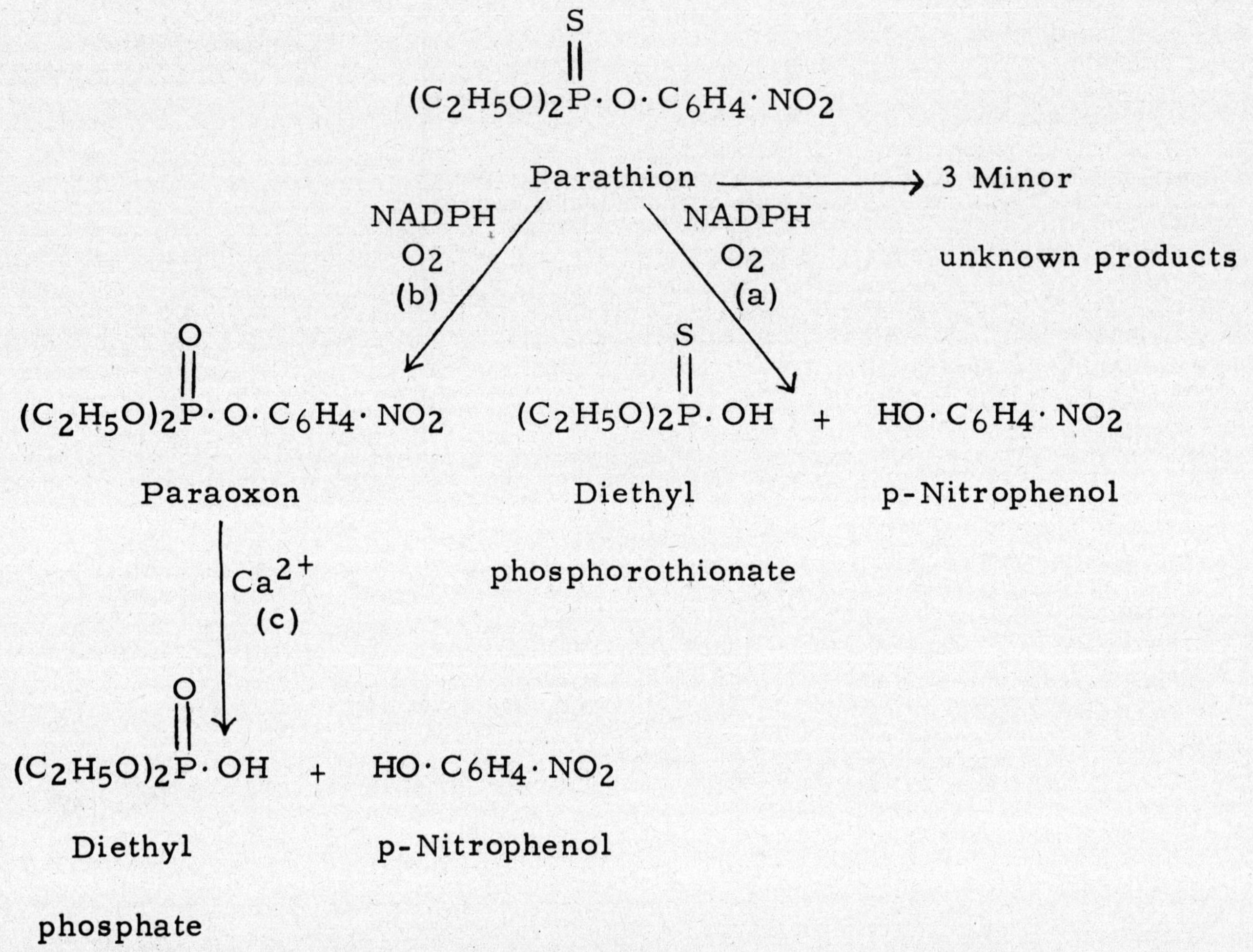

Fig 2.—The metabolism of parathion by rat liver microsomes in vitro. Reactions (a) *and* (b) *require NADPH and oxygen for activity. Reaction* (c) *is catalyzed by an esterase which requires only* Ca^{++} *for optimum activity.*[6]

acetylcholinesterase but are metabolized by enzymes in insect and animal tissues to the corresponding phosphates which are potent inhibitors of this enzyme. For example, the compund, diethyl *p*-nitrophenyl phosphorothionate (parathion), is in itself a poor inhibitor of acetylcholinesterase, but it is converted in insects and mammals to its oxygen analog, diethyl *p*-nitrophenyl phosphate (paraoxon), which is a very potent inhibitor of the enzyme. This enzymatic reaction appears to convert a reasonably nontoxic compound, parathion, to a very toxic compound, paraoxon. Thus, the animal appears to be metabolically responsible for its own death. The in vivo conversion of parathion to its toxic oxygen analog, paraoxon, was first shown by Diggle and Gage.[3] A few years ago we undertook a study of the metabolism of parathion by liver microsomes isolated from various animal species.[4] In these studies we were interested in knowing the nature and location of the enzymes and cofactors involved in the various reactions leading to the oxidative metabolism of the phosphorothionates. Initial experiments indicated the microsomes as the location of the enzymes. Using techniques such as thin-layer chromatography and infrared spectroscopy,[5] we identified the major metabolites of parathion in the microsomal preparations to be paraoxon, diethyl phosphorothionate, diethyl phosphate, and *p*-nitrophenol (Fig 2). Other minor metabolites are detectable but the sum of these represents somewhat less than 5% of the total metabolism. Our early studies indicated that the metabolism of parathion to these four metabolites required the presence of reduced nicotinamide adenine dinucleotide phosphate (NADPH) and molecular oxygen. The requirement for NADPH and molecular oxygen coupled with the fact that the metabolism of parathion was strongly inhibited by carbon monoxide clearly indicated that these oxidative reactions were catalyzed by the mixed function oxidase enzymes.

The kinetics of the appearance of the various metabolites of parathion with time in various animal species is shown in Fig 3. Note that there are some quantitative differences in the metabolism of parathion by the various animal species; eg, the adult female rat displays a generally lower overall activity toward parathion than any other animal examined. The other major quantitative difference is the greater accumulation of paraoxon and concomitant lower accumulation of diethyl phosphate in the adult male guinea pig as compared with other animals studied. Lower overall appearance of the metabolites in the female rat is due to less mixed function oxidase activity as compared to most other animal species. Only in the rat, however, is the sex difference in mixed function oxidase enzyme activity seen. The young weanling rat displays an enzyme curve similar to the adult female rat. Lower accumulation of diethyl phosphate in the adult male guinea pig is a result of less esteratic enzyme that metabolizes paraoxon to *p*-nitrophenol and diethyl phosphate.

Comparison of the oxidative activity toward parathion in liver, lung, and kidney of the rat is shown in

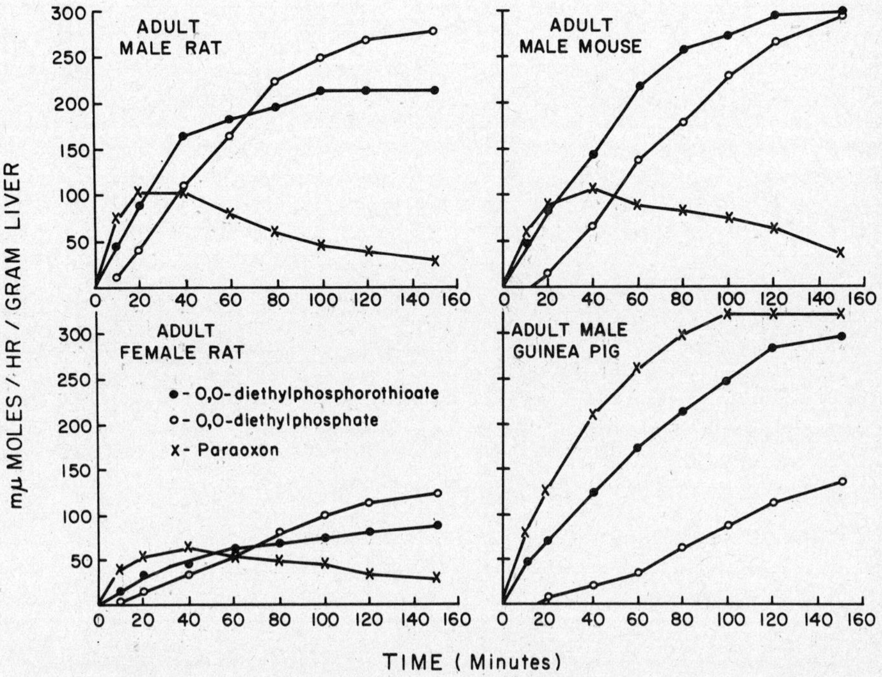

Fig 3.—Metabolism of parathion by various animal species. Microsomes isolated from the pooled livers of four each adult male rats, adult female rats, adult male mice, and adult male guinea pigs were incubated with parathion.[5]

Table 1. Note that the predominant activity is in the liver. The metabolism of parathion to these same products also occurs in the intestine and heart but to a lesser extent than in the liver, lung, and kidney. There is also some indication of an extremely small amount of metabolism of parathion to paraoxon in the brain of rats. Since the usual cause of death from poisoning by the organophosphate insecticides is respiratory paralysis, metabolism of parathion to paraoxon in the lung is the most significant reaction from a toxicological standpoint. However, most of the studies of the metabolism of these compounds reported in the literature utilize liver as the source of the enzyme because of the greater specific activity.

In Fig 2, reactions (*a*) and (*b*), an enzyme system is acting on the phosphorus atom of a single compound to yield two different products. In one case we have sulfur as the leaving group to form paraoxon, and in the other case, *p*-nitrophenol is the leaving group to form diethyl phosphorothionate.

We next undertook studies[6] to determine if reactions (*a*) and (*b*) were catalyzed by one or two enzyme systems. We approached the problem by examining the effect of various enzyme inhibitors or stimulators on the ratios of paraoxon and diethyl phosphorothionate seen on incubating microsomes with parathion and these various compounds.

Table 2 shows the effect of various enzyme inhibitors on the metabolism of parathion. In Table 2 we have designated as paraoxon the sum of paraoxon and diethyl phosphate. Figure 2 shows that diethyl phosphate is derived from paraoxon by the action of an esteratic enzyme. Therefore,

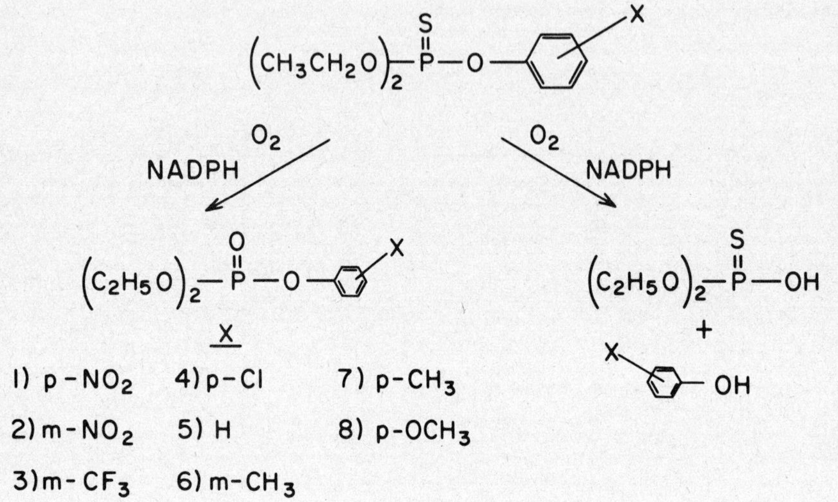

Fig 4.—General scheme for the oxidative metabolism of diethyl aryl phosphorothionates.

the sum of these two metabolites is the true measure of the amount of paraoxon that has been formed. The last column of Table 2 shows the ratio of paraoxon to diethyl phosphorothionate formed in the incubation in the presence and absence of various inhibitors. Note that in the first experiment, the metal binding agent, bathophenanthroline, strongly inhibited the metabolism of parathion to both diethyl phosphorothionate and paraoxon. Note also that the amount of inhibition of the formation of paraoxon is about the same as the inhibition of the formation of diethyl phosphorothionate, as evidenced by the fact the ratio of these two mebolites formed in the presence of inhibitors was not significantly different than the ratio of these two metabolites in the absence of inhibitor. The chelating agent, 8-hydroxyquinoline, also inhibits the metabolism parathion to the same products. However, this compound inhibited the metabolism of parathion to paraoxon more than to diethyl phosphorothionate, as shown by the decrease of the ratio of these two metabolites in comparison to the control. The sulfhydryl reagent, *p*-chloromercuribenzoate (PCMB), also inhibited the metabolism of parathion to paraoxon more strongly than to diethylphosphorothionate. The compound proadifen hydrochloride (SKF525-A), which is a well known inhibitor of the mixed function oxidase enzymes, was an inhibitor in this system; but the inhibition of diethyl phosphorothionate formation was of the same order of magnitude as the inhibition of paraoxon formation.

The metabolism of parathion by the mixed function oxidase systems in liver microsomes is stimulated by compounds containing reduced sulfur (Table 3). Note that in the case of all of these reduced sulfur compounds, the production of diethyl phosphorothionate and paraoxon are enhanced, but the formation of the diethyl phosphorothionate is considerably more stimulated than is the formation of paraoxon, as evidenced by the markedly different ratios of the two metabolites obtained.

Table 4 shows the effects of various organic electron acceptors on the metabolism of parathion. Riboflavin inhibits the formation of both diethyl phosphorothionate and paraoxon. However, the inhibition of diethyl phosphorothionate formation is greater than the inhibition of the formation of paraoxon, as evidenced by the ratios of the two metabolites. With menadione and methylene blue, the formation of dialkyl phosphorothionate was actually stimulated, whereas the formation of paraoxon was inhibited and, as a result, the ratio of the two metabolites is markedly different from that seen in the absence of these two compounds.

Table 5 shows the results of studies in which the metabolism of parathion by hepatic microsomes isolated from adult male rats pretreated with phenobarbital and with benzo[*a*]pyrene were compared. Phenobarbital stimulated the overall metabolism of parathion to diethyl phosphorothionate and to paraoxon to about the same degree. In contrast, benzo[*a*]pyrene stimulated the metabolism of parathion to paraoxon to a much greater extent than to diethyl phosphorothionate as indicated by the paraoxon:diethyl phosphorothionate ratio. Sladek and Mannering[7] have reported that administration of benzo[*a*]pyrene, 3-methylcholanthrene, or phenobarbital to male rats stimulated the *n*-demethylation of 3-methyl-4-methylaminoazobenzene by the mixed function oxidase enzyme in hepatic microsomes, but only phenobarbital stimulated the *n*-demethylation of ethylmorphine. A possible interpretation of our results and those of

Sladek and Mannering is there are two forms of cytochrome P-450 in rat liver microsomes, one of which is preferentially induced by administration of 3-methylcholanthrene and benzo[*a*]pyrene. It is probably this cytochrome which is responsible for catalysis of the reaction leading to the formation of paraoxon from parathion. The presence of two forms of the terminal cytochrome is also supported by the data on the effect of inhibitors, stimulators, and alternate substrates on the metabolism of parathion.

We next undertook a study of the effect of structure on the metabolism of diethyl aryl phosphorothionates. In these studies we determined the effect of alteration of the electrophilicity of the phosphorus atom on the rate of the two major oxidative reactions which these compounds undergo. Figure 4 shows these two oxidative reactions. In these studies we synthesized a number of diethyl aryl phosphorothionates labeled with ^{32}P, as described previously.[5] In the synthesis of these compounds the X-group shown in Fig 4 was varied from strong electronic withdrawing to strong electron donating. The substituents attached to the aryl group are listed at the bottom of Fig 4 in order of decreasing electron withdrawing power. These eight different diethyl aryl phosphorothionates were incubated with microsomes and NADPH and the Michaelis-Menten constant (K_m) and maximal velocities (V_{max}) for the formation of the two oxidative metabolites were calculated. The apparent K_m values for formation of each of these two metabolites from each substrate were found to vary slightly, but in no predictable manner. The V_{max} values, however, were found to vary predictably when the log V_{max} was compared with the Hammett substituent constant sigma.

Table 3.—Effect of Compounds Containing Reduced Sulfur on the Metabolism of Parathion*

Addition	Metabolite Formed (μmol/hr/gm of Liver): Diethyl Phosphorothionate	Metabolite Formed (μmol/hr/gm of Liver): Paraoxon	Ratio Paraoxon:Diethyl Phosphorothionate
None	257±11	604± 5	2.36±0.12
Mercaptoethanol (1.0 millimolar)	440± 5 (0.005)	732±11 (0.005)	1.67±0.04 (0.005)
Dithiothreitol (1.0 millimolar)	553± 3 (0.005)	820±12 (0.005)	1.48±0.02 (0.005)
1-Phenylthiourea (1.0 millimolar)	458±21 (0.005)	682±13 (0.005)	1.49±0.04 (0.005)
Sodium sulfide (1.0 millimolar)	323± 4 (0.005)	485±13 (0.005)	1.50±0.05 (0.005)

* The experimental conditions and statistical analyses were as in Table 2. The values for each experiment are the means ± SD of the means of three separate determinations, carried out simultaneously. The *P* values are in parentheses.[6]

Table 4.—Effect of Various Electron Acceptors on the Metabolism of Parathion*

Addition	Metabolite Formed (μmol/hr/gm of Liver): Diethyl Phosphorothionate	Metabolite Formed (μmol/hr/gm of Liver): Paraoxon	Ratio of Paraoxon: Diethyl Phosphorothionate
None	220± 5	584±16	2.65±0.07
Riboflavin (0.2 millimolar)	109± 8 (0.005)	367±37 (0.005)	3.37±0.18 (0.010)
Menadione (5 μmolar)	262±19 (0.050)	445±25 (0.005)	1.70±0.05 (0.005)
Methylene blue (1 μmolar)	258± 5 (0.005)	445± 8 (0.005)	1.73±0.06 (0.005)

* The experimental conditions and statistical analyses were as in Table 2. The values for each experiment are the means ± SD of the means of three separate determinations, carried out simultaneously. The *P* values are in parentheses.[6]

This comparison of the maximal rate of metabolism of the various substituted diethyl aryl phosphorothionates with the quantitative electron withdrawal or donation of the substituents on the aryl group indicated the following: (*a*) Both electron withdrawal and donation by the aryloxy group stimulated the rate of metabolism of the diethyl aryl phosphorothionates to diethyl phosphorothionate. The minimal rate was exhibited by the compound which had trifluormethyl as the substituent in the meta position of the aryl group. (*b*) Both electron withdrawal and donation by the aryloxy group stimulated the metabolism of the diethyl aryl phosphorothionates to the corresponding diethyl aryl phosphate. The minimal rate of this reaction was also exhibited by the compound which had trifluormethyl as the substituent in the meta position of the aryl group. The product of this reaction, diethyl *m*-trifluormethylphenyl phosphate, is a rather poor inhibitor of acetylcholinesterase in vitro.[8] In contrast, the compound with a nitro group in the para position, paraoxon, is a very potent inhibitor of acetylcholinesterase in vitro. Thus, the maximal rate of metabolism of the diethyl aryl phosphorothionates to

Table 5.—Oxidative Enzyme Activity Toward Parathion in Livers of Untreated, Phenobarbital-Treated, and Benzo[*a*]pyrene-Treated Adult Male Rats*

Treatment	Amount of Metabolite Formed (μmol/hr/gm of Liver)		Ratio of Paraoxon: Diethyl Phosphorothionate
	Diethyl Phosphorothionate	Paraoxon	
None	165±10	273± 5	1.65
Phenobarbital	283±13 (0.005)	465± 3 (0.005	1.62 (NS)
Benzo[*a*]pyrene	241± 8 (0.005)	627± 9 (0.005)	2.60 (0.005)

* Microsomes isolated from pooled livers of four rats in each of the treatment groups were incubated with parathion as described in reference 5. The phenobarbital-treated animals received a dose (80 mg/kg) of phenobarbital dissolved in 0.9% sodium chloride by intraperitoneal injection daily for four days and were killed 24 hours after the last injection. The benzo[*a*]pyrene-treated animals received a dose (20 mg/kg) of benzo[a]pyrene dissolved in corn oil by intraperitoneal injection daily for three days and were killed 24 hours after the last injection. The animals used in this experiment were from a single shipment and were of approximately the same size (± 2 days). All animals used in this experiment were killed on the same day. The results are given as the means ± SD of the means of four separate incubations.[5]

the toxic diethyl aryl phosphates favors the formation of the more toxic metabolite.

Comment

The metabolism of the dialkyl aryl phosphorothionates to their two major oxidative products has been examined. One of these metabolites is the oxygen analog of the parent compound in which sulfur has been replaced with oxygen, and the other is a compound in which the aromatic side chain has been displaced again by oxygen. Both of these reactions are oxidative, require NADPH and molecular oxygen, and are carried out by what appears to be two separate mixed function oxidase enzyme systems or a single mixed function oxidase system with two different forms of the terminal cytochrome. The rates of these reactions are sensitive to change in the electronic environment about the phosphorus; this change of rate of metabolism is predictable according to the electron withdrawing of electron donating properties of the aromatic group.

Although it appears the mixed function oxidase systems in the liver are converting a rather nontoxic compound, the sulfur analog, into the more toxic oxygen analog, this particular reaction in the liver is probably an overall detoxication reaction because of the presence of esterases in liver, blood, and other tissues that hydrolyze the toxic oxygen compound (paraoxon, in the case of parathion). The rate of metabolism of paraoxon by these esteratic enzymes far surpasses the rate of formation of paraoxon from parathion catalyzed by the mixed function oxidase enzymes in the liver. Therefore, it is rather doubtful that any of the paraoxon formed in the liver gains access to the brain or nerve endings where the fatal inhibition of the acetylcholinesterase occurs. The toxic reaction is probably the metabolism to the toxic oxygen analog in tissue at or near the nerve endings. In this way the acetylcholinesterase is inhibited before the compound is hydrolyzed by the esteratic enzymes.

Data from studies of this type should be useful in predicting the rate of metabolism in vivo of various dialkyl aryl phosphorothionates which have application commercially as insecticides. Since the toxicity of these compounds should be a function of how rapidly they are metabolized, information from studies of this type should be useful in predicting the toxicicity of a particular phosphorothionate. The phosphorothionates should also prove valuable as substrates in further studies of the mechanisms of action of the mixed function oxidase enzymes.

This study was supported by Public Health Service grants ES 00075 and ES 00267.

References

1. Koelle GB: Histochemical demonstration of reversible anticholinesterase action at selective cellular sites in vivo. *J Pharmacol Exp Ther* **120**:488-503, 1957.

2. West I: Pesticide-induced illness. *Calif Med* **105**:257-261, 1966.

3. Diggle WM, Gage JC: Cholinesterase inhibition in vitro by O, O-diethyl O-p-nitrophenyl thiophosphate (Parathion, E 605). *Biochem J* **49**:491-494, 1951.

4. Neal RA, DuBois KP: Studies on the mechanism of detoxification of cholinergic phosphorothioates. *J Pharmacol Exp Ther* **148**:185-192, 1965.

5. Neal RA: Studies on the metabolism of diethyl 4-nitrophenyl phosphorothionate (Parathion) in vitro. *Biochem J* **103**:183-191, 1967.

6. Neal RA: Studies of the enzymic mechanism of the metabolism of diethyl 4-nitrophenyl phosphorothionate (Parathion) by rat liver microsomes. *Biochem J* **105**:289-297, 1967.

7. Sladek NE, Mannering GJ: Induction of drug metabolism: I. Differences in the mechanisms by which polycyclic hydrocarbons and phenobarbital produce their inductive effects on microsomal N-demethylating systems. *Molec Pharmacol* **5**:174-185, 1969.

8. Fukuto TR, Metcalf RL: Structure and insecticidal activity of some diethyl substituted phenyl phosphates. *J Agr Food Chem* **4**:930-935, 1956.

Enzymatic Conversion of Benzo[*a*]pyrene

Hydroxylation vs DNA-Binding

Irene Y. Wang, PhD; Harvey S. Marver, MD; Ronald E. Rasmussen, PhD; and T. Timothy Crocker, MD, San Francisco

Hydroxylating and DNA-binding activity is increased in lung and liver microsomes after induction of enzyme activity by injecting benzo[*a*]pyrene (BaP) into intact rats. Overall enzymatic activity increases more in liver than in lung, and DNA-binding increases more than hydroxy product formation in microsomes from liver as compared to lung. Three major metabolites, detected by chromatography of a hexane-acetone extract after incubation of BaP labeled with tritium with preinduced liver microsomes, are reduced sharply by hematin at 5×10^{-5}M, and eliminated by 2.5×10^{-4}M. The greatest reduction was of a peak identical with a standard sample of 3-hydroxy-BaP. Hematin reduced DNA-binding to a greater degree than metabolite production. This suggests that hematin interferes with metabolic conversion of BaP to a DNA-binding product. The latter product may be a precursor of 3-OH-BaP since both DNA-binding and 3-OH-BaP production are similarly suppressed.

It is generally accepted that metabolic activation is a prerequisite for covalent binding of polycyclic hydrocarbons to cellular components including DNA.[1,2] The capacity of the individual hydrocarbons to undergo such activation correlates well with their carcinogenicity and cytoxicity. Since the ring hydroxylated derivatives of polycyclic hydrocarbons are relatively inert, it has been suggested, with some experimental support, that epoxides are the reactive intermediates in this process.[3] There is conflicting evidence regarding the question of whether or not carcinogenic epoxide and inert hydroxy derivatives represent successive intermediates in the same metabolic sequence. That epoxidation is not a proximal intermediate in hydroxylation is suggested by in vivo studies[4] and experiments employing cultured cells[5] which indicate that induction of microsomal hydroxylation protects against the toxicity of polycyclic hydrocarbons. Conflicting evidence in cell culture (Diamond et al[6]) has shown that there is correlation between the capacity of certain cells to hydroxylate polycyclic hydrocarbons and to undergo carcinogen-induced cytotoxicity. Moreover, the studies of Jerina and co-workers suggested that arene oxides are obligate intermediates in aromatic hydroxylation.[7] A method for resolving this problem has recently been provided independently by Gelboin[8] and by Grover and Sims.[9] These investigators demonstrated that polycyclic hydrocarbons could be converted to compounds capable of covalently binding to DNA if the hydrocarbons were incubated with liver microsomes and reduced nicotinamide adenine dinucleotide phosphate (NADPH) in the presence of atmospheric oxygen. Since ring hydroxylated derivatives do not bind to DNA, this suggests that the Grover and Sims method[9] or Gelboin method[8] provides an indirect assay for the enzymatic conversion of polycyclic hydrocarbons to carcinogenic intermediates, probably epoxides. In the past, some of the metabolites of BaP were identified by Falk et al[10] and many other workers[11] in in vivo systems and by Sims[12,13] in in vitro studies.

We sought the dissociation of enzymatically mediated DNA-binding of BaP from its hydroxylation in induced liver and lung enzyme systems. The distribution of active intermediate metabolites of BaP capable of binding to DNA, between microsomal membranes and the supernatant of the incubation mixture of microsomes with BaP was investigated. Profiles of metabolic products of BaP from cell and tissue cultures were compared with that from the incubation system of microsomes. These studies have indicated that hydroxylation of BaP and binding of BaP to DNA may be separable functions. Thus, it may be possible to encourage the production of relatively less toxic hydroxy products while inhibiting the binding of BaP to biologically important molecules.

Received for publication Oct 21, 1970; accepted April 5, 1971.

From the Cancer Research Institute and the Department of Medicine, University of California School of Medicine, San Francisco.

Read in part before the Tenth Annual Hanford Biology Symposium on Pollution and Lung Biochemistry, Richland, Wash, June 5, 1970, jointly sponsored by the Battelle Memorial Institute-Pacific Northwest Laboratories, National Air Pollution Control Administration, National Institute of Environmental Health Sciences, and the US Atomic Energy Commission.

Reprint requests to Cancer Research Institute, University of California, San Francisco 94122 (Dr. Wang).

Table 1.—The Effect of the Concentration of Liver Microsomes on the Hydroxylation of ³H-BaP and Its Binding to DNA in Vitro*

Microsomes (ml)	Binding of ^{3}H-BaP to DNA (cpm† mg DNA)	Hydroxylation of ^{3}H-BaP (cpm)†
0.0	0	0
0.1	18	156
0.3	70	487
0.5	81	532

* Rats were pretreated with BaP one day before preparation of microsomes. Specific activity of ^{3}H-BaP was 1.3×10^4 dpm/mμmol.
† Signifies counts per minute.

Table 2.—Binding of ³H-BaP to DNA and Hydroxylation of ³H-BaP*

Microsomes	Binding of ^{3}H-BaP to DNA (cpm/mg DNA)	Hydroxylation of ^{3}H-BaP (cpm)
Liver		
Phenobarbital†	38	3,030
Control	19	625
BaP‡	2,178	22,726
Control	13	1,268
Lung		
BaP‡	21	477
Control	4	203

* In vivo induction of enzyme activities for ^{3}H-BaP hydroxylation in vitro and for binding of ^{3}H-BaP to DNA in vitro. Incubation systems were as described in the text. Specific activity of ^{3}H-BaP was 2.6×10^5 dpm/mμmole.
† Rats pretreated with phenobarbital 8 mg/100 gm of body weight for four days before preparation of microsomes; control rates injected with saline only.
‡ Rats injected with 0.5 ml sesame oil containing benzo[a]pyrene 2 mg/100 gm of body weight one day before preparation of microsomes; control rats injected with sesame oil only.

Table 3.—Binding of ³H-BaP to DNA in Preincubated Reaction*

DNA incubated with	Binding of ^{3}H-BaP to DNA (cpm/mg DNA)
^{3}H-BaP, boiled microsomes, and NADPH	6
Supernatant of incubation mixture of ^{3}H-BaP, microsomes, and NADPH	25
Mixture of preincubated ^{3}H-Bap, microsomes, and NADPH	609

* Detection of the presence of DNA-binding metabolites of ^{3}H-BaP in the supernatant of preincubated reaction mixture of ^{3}H-Bap, liver microsomes from rates pretreated with BaP, NADPH as described in the last section of materials and methods. DNA was purified with sodium lauryl sulfate. Specific activity of ^{3}H-BaP was 2.6×10^5 dpm/mμmol.

Materials and Methods

Hydroxylation of Benzo[*a*]pyrene Labeled With Tritium and Its Binding to DNA Catalyzed by Microsomes.—Microsomes from female Sprague-Dawley rats were used. In general, rats were fasted overnight before a single intraperitoneal injection of BaP (2 mg/100 gm of body weight); control rats were injected with the sesame oil vehicle only. After 24 hours, rats were decapitated and livers or lungs removed. Microsomes were prepared by a modification of the fractionation method of Schneider.[14] Microsomes were suspended in 0.05M tromethamine (Tris), 0.25M potassium chloride, 0.005M magnesium chloride, 0.25M sucrose (TKM-sucrose buffer) at pH 7.4, in a volume equivalent to 1 gm wet liver per milliliter or 1.5 gm wet lung per milliliter, respectively. The final incubation system contained 10 mg DNA, 2.5 mg NADPH, 0.5 ml microsomes, 0.6μmol ^{3}H-BaP in 0.3 ml methanol (specific activity, 1.3×10^4 to 2.6×10^5 disintegrations per minute [dpm] per mμmol) in a total volume of 17.5 ml in saline-citrate buffer at pH 7.4 (0.14M sodium chloride, 0.015M sodium citrate), unless otherwise specified. Incubations were carried out under yellow light. The reaction was initiated by the addition of microsomes to the other components of the incubation mixture. Immediately after mixing, a 1 ml aliquot was removed and added to 2 ml cold acetone to serve as zero-time value for hydroxylation. This value was found to be the same as the value obtained when boiled microsomes were used for incubation. The mixture of zero-time reactant and acetone was extracted with 6 ml hexane[15] for 30 minutes. Four milliliters of the hexane layer was extracted with an equal volume of 0.25N potassium hydroxide in 50% ethyl alcohol[16] for 30 minutes. One milliliter of the aqueous layer, which contained alkaline-extractable metabolites of ^{3}H-BaP, was counted in 15 ml of a scintillation solution (0.25 gm 1,4-bis-2-(5-phenyloxazolyl)-benzene [POPOP], 13 gm 2,5- diphenyloxazole [PPO], 130 gm naphthalene, 600 ml anhydrous ethyl alcohol, 1 liter dioxane, and 1 liter toluene).

The major volume of the reaction mixture was incubated at 37 C for 20 minutes. At the end of the incubation, 1 ml of the incubation mixture was pipetted into 2 ml cold acetone; hexane and alkaline extractions and counting of the alkaline-extractable metabolites were performed as previously described. The rest of the reaction mixture was washed three times with cold ethyl ether to remove unreacted BaP. Denatured microsomal proteins were removed by centrifugation in stainless steel tubes at 46,000 g for 60 minutes. DNA was precipitated with two volumes of 95% ethyl alcohol, soaked in 70% ethyl alcohol overnight, redissolved in citrate buffer, and purified with sodium lauryl sulfate (Duponol).[17] Deoxyribonucleic acid was precipitated again with 95% ethyl alcohol, washed with acetone, air dried, and weighed on an electron balance. The weighed DNA was digested with deoxyribonuclease and counted in the scintillation solution previously described.

Chromatography of Metabolities of ³H-BaP.—Hexane extracts of a microsomal incubation mixture or hexane-acetone (3:1) extracts of organ or cell culture materials incubated with ^{3}H-BaP, were concentrated under nitrogen gas, then chromatographed on thin layer chromatography sheets of glass microfiber impregnated with silica gel with a solvent system of hexane saturated with *N,N*-dimethyl

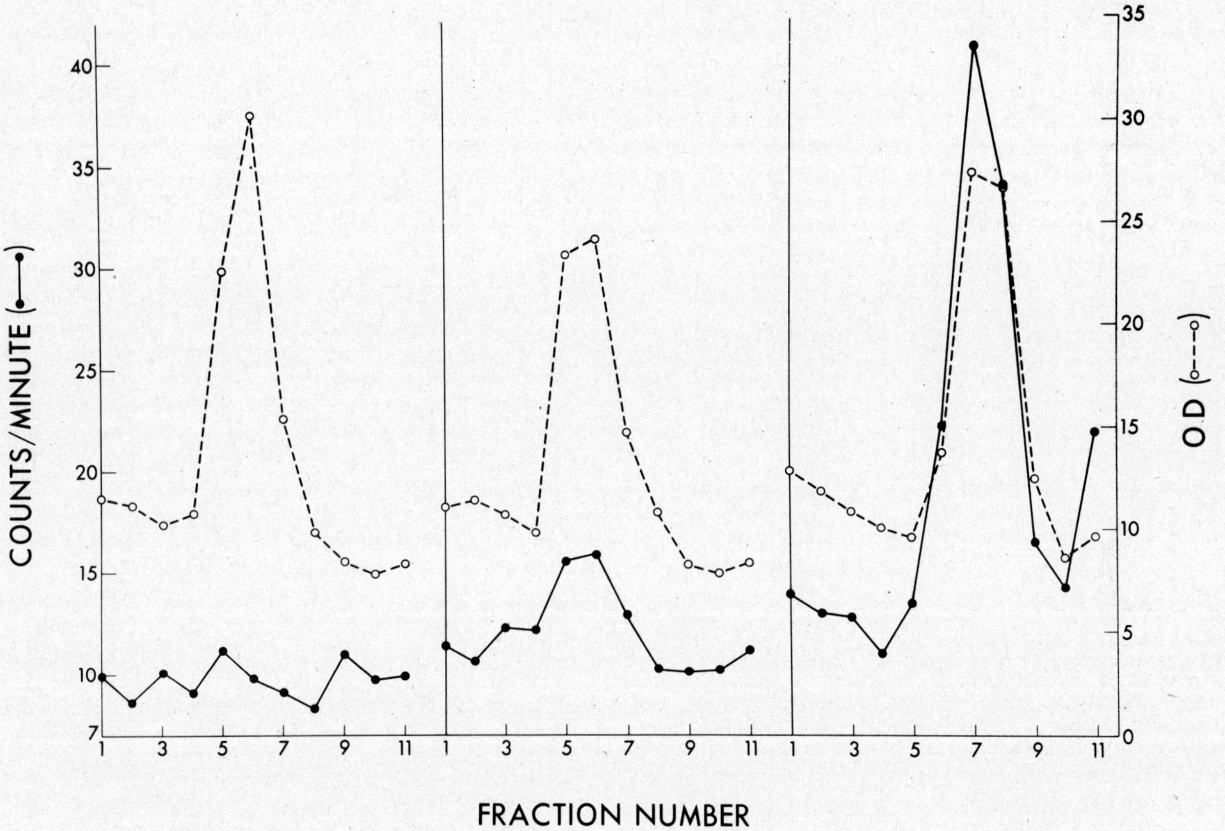

Fig 1.—Fraction from CsCl gradient of DNA incubation mixture. Radioactivities and optical density of the fractions were measured as described in the last section of the text on materials and methods. At left, DNA incubated with killed microsomes and ³H-BaP. At center, DNA incubated with supernatant of mixture of microsomes preincubated with ³H-BaP. At right, DNA incubated with mixture of microsomes preincubated with ³H-BaP.

formamide.

The distribution of radioactivity on the chromatogram was determined by cutting the chromatogram into 1 cm segments which were dropped into the liquid scintillation solution previously described for counting of products released into medium.

Detection of Active Intermediate Metabolite(s) of ³H-BaP.—One and eight-tenths micromol ³H-BaP of specific activity 2.6 × 10^5 dpm/mμmol was preincubated for 15 minutes with 1.5 ml of liver microsomes from BaP pretreated rats, and NADPH in a final volume of 15 ml of saline-citrate buffer solution. The reaction mixture was chilled and microsomes were sedimented at 100,000 g for 60 minutes at 0 C. Five milliters of the supernatant was added to 10 ml of saline-citrate buffer containing 10 mg DNA and incubated for another 15 minutes. An "active control" reaction system was prepared and processed in the same way as the foregoing system except that it was chilled at 0 C during the 60-minute period of centrifugation of microsomes. When 5 ml of supernatant from the centrifugation was added to 10 ml of buffer solution containing DNA, the same volume of the complete, chilled, active control preparation was incubated with a parallel DNA solution.

At the end of the incubation, 5 ml of 0.4% sodium lauryl sulfate solution was added to the incubation mixture. One third of the reaction mixture composed of this supernatant incubated with DNA underwent cesium chloride gradient centrifugation (average density of CsCl solution, 1.7 gm/ml) at 100,000 g for 70 hours. The gradient was collected at 30 drops per fraction. A 10μliter aliquot of each fraction was spotted on a small piece of paper (Whatman No. 3), air dried, and washed successively with 5% trichloroacetic acid, 70% ethyl alcohol, and acetone. The filter paper pieces were added to 5 ml of scintillation solution for counting. The optical density of each fraction was read at 260 mμ wavelength after dilution (1:50). From the remaining two thirds of the reaction mixture composed of DNA and the supernatant from preincubation of microsomes and ³H-BaP, DNA was purified with sodium lauryl sulfate, weighed, and counted as previously described.

Detection of Metabolites in Cell and Organ Culture.—Cell cultures of adult hamster tracheal epithelium were obtained by exposing the lumens of excised tracheas

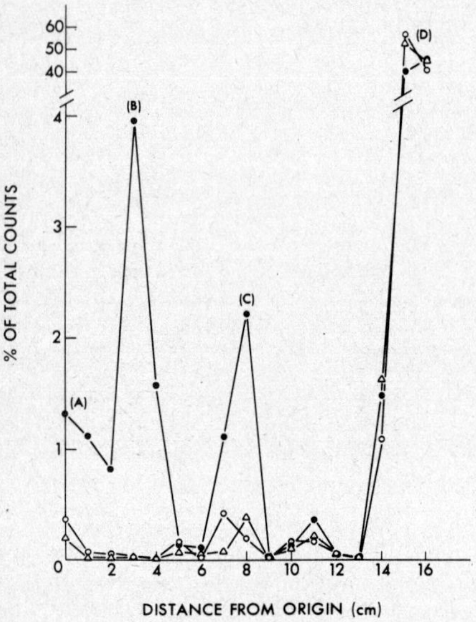

Fig 2.—Comparison of the chromatographic profiles of metabolic products of ^{3}H-BaP produced by microsomes of BaP-pretreated rats and of control rats. Specific activity of ^{3}H-BaP was 2 × 10^5 dpm/mμmol. Chromatograms were run as described in the text. Black circle *signifies BaP-pretreated rats, 20-minute incubation.* Open triangle *signifies BaP-pretreated rats, zero time.* Open circle *signifies control rats, 20-minute incubation.*

to 0.25% trypsin for four successive periods of 15 minutes. The trypsin solutions were pooled, the cells washed free of trypsin with Tyrode's solution, and planted in plastic Petri dishes (50 mm) in Eagle's minimum essential medium containing 15% calf serum. When the cell layer became confluent, the cells were subcultured.

These secondary cell cultures were tested for heterogeneity of cell type by plating at 300 or 1,000 cells per 50 mm plastic culture dish. Colonies present after ten days of incubation were fixed with methanol, stained with Giemsa stain, and all were found to be epithelial in type with a plating efficiency of 2% to 6%.

To test for the production of metabolites of ^{3}H-BaP by the secondary, epithelial cell cultures, plastic Petri dishes were seeded with 2 × 10^5 cells, and, after five days' growth, fresh medium containing ^{3}H-BaP, 0.25mμmol/ml (specific activity 1.7^8 × 10^7 dpm/mμmol) was supplied. After 24 hours, the medium was removed and extracted with an equal volume of hexane-acetone (3:1). The organic phase was taken nearly to dryness in a stream of N_2, and this concentrate was then chromatographed as previously described.

Organ cultures of 3-month-old female hamster tracheas were prepared by cutting the excised tracheas into approximately 2 mm × 2 mm plaques which were placed, epithelial surface up, on rayon mesh supported by the stainless steel grid of the organ culture dish (Falcon Plastic). Immediately after preparation of the cultures, the medium described by Pallekar et al,[18] containing ^{3}H-Bap, 1.25 mμmol/ml (specific activity as previously described) was added and the cultures incubated for two days. At this time, the tissue fragments were washed with phosphate-buffered saline and frozen for later processing. To test for the presence of metabolites of ^{3}H-BaP in the tissue, the fragments were thawed, homogenized with a probe sonifier, and the homogenate extracted with an equal volume of hexane-acetone (3:1). The organic phase was then concentrated and chromatographed as for cell culture media.

Results

The extent of binding to DNA and the yield of metabolic products increased with microsome concentration as shown in Table 1. Molecular oxygen and NADPH are essential both for DNA-binding and hydroxylation of BaP, catalyzed by microsomes under in vitro conditions.

The enzyme systems for DNA-binding and hydroxylation of BaP are inducible in vivo. The inducing effect of pretreatment of rats with phenobarbital or with BaP is shown in Table 2, where it can be seen that the enzyme activities for DNA-binding and hydroxylation of ^{3}H-BaP were induced to different degrees. Lung microsomal enzyme activity with respect to DNA-binding increased fivefold while hydroxy product formation increased less than 2.5-fold.

The presence of intermediate metabolites of BaP, which persist and bind to DNA after removal of microsomes, was detected in the supernatant of the mixture of ^{3}H-BaP preincubated with microsomes and NADPH (Fig 1). DNA containing covalently bound ^{3}H-BaP was isolated on a CsC1 gradient. Similar results were obtained when the DNA in the supernatant was purified with sodium lauryl sulfate (Table 3). While considerably more ^{3}H-BaP was bound to DNA in the presence of microsomes than in the presence of the supernatant from the microsome-BaP incubation mixture, the degree of binding by the supernatant metabolite, which was stable for at least 60 minutes at low temperature during sedimentation of microsomes is appreciable.

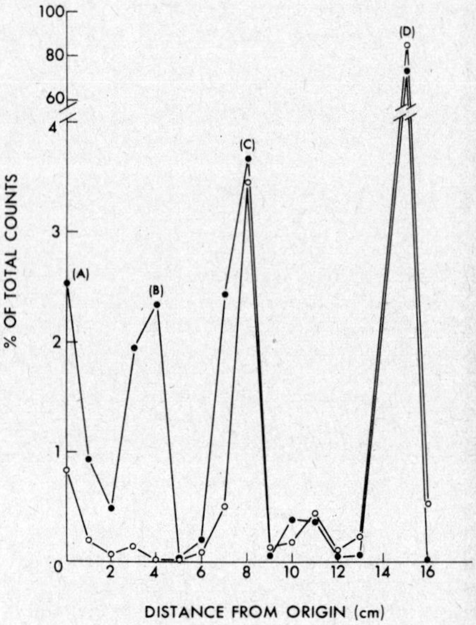

Fig 3.—The effect of 5 × 10^{-5}M hematin added to the incubation mixture on the chromatographic profile of metabolic products of ^{3}H-BaP. Microsomes from rats pretreated with BaP were used. Specific activity of ^{3}H-BaP was 1.3 × 10^4 dpm/mμmol. Black circle *signifies no hematin, 30-minute incubation.* Open circle *signifies 5 × 10^{-5}M hematin, 30-minute incubation.*

In chromatograms of metabolites of ^{3}H-BaP produced by rat liver microsomes, three regions of the chromatograms contained the major metabolites (Fig 2). Liver microsome

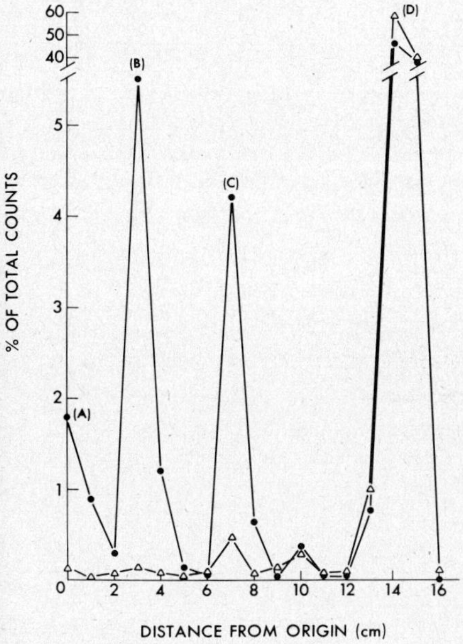

Fig 4.—The effect of 2.5 × 10^{-4}M hematin added to the incubation mixture on the chromatographic profile of metabolic products of ^{3}H-BaP. Incubation systems were as in Fig 3. Note progressive reduction in peaks near the origin (at left) where the more polar metabolites would be expected. Black circle *signifies no hematin, 30-minute incubation.* Open triangle *signifies 2.5 × 10^{-4}M hematin, 30-minute incubation.*

isolated from rats pretreated with BaP produced a metabolite that was not detectable (peak B) when microsomes from untreated animals were used.

Hematin diminished BaP hydroxylation in vitro (Figs 3, 4). The metabolite at peak B was greatly reduced at 5 × 10^{-5}M hematin concentration. At 2.5 × 10^{-4}M hematin concentration, the heights of peak A and peak C were also greatly reduced as is shown in Fig 4. Benzo[*a*]pyrene labeled with tritium was concentrated at peak D. Peak B was very likely 3-hydroxy-BaP, as was evidenced by the R_f value and its fluorescence compared with those of a 3-OH-BaP standard which was run on the same chromatogram.

The chromatographic profiles obtained with extracts of cell and organ cultures of hamster tissues were different from those of rat liver microsomes (Fig 5). The relative yield of polar metabolites was lower in the hamster systems (Figs 2, 5). The two hamster systems produced metabolites giving similar chromatographic profiles in which the major metabolites were near the origin (most polar) rather than located at intermediate points in the chromatogram as in the rat microsomal system. The organ culture medium was processed as in the case of the cell culture medium, but the concentration of metabolites was too low for chromatographic study in the present system.

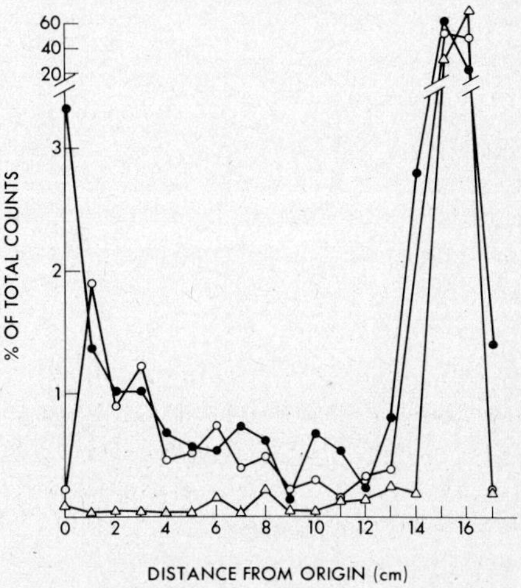

Fig 5.—Chromatographic profiles of BaP metabolites produced in cell and organ cultures. Black circle *signifies tracheal tissue extract.* Open circle *signifies cell culture medium extract.* Open triangle *signifies extract of medium incubated without cells but with ^{3}H-BaP.*

Comment

The processes of BaP hydroxylation and its binding to DNA in vitro are closely correlated, as can be seen from the data in Tables 1 and 2. Moreover, the fact that microsomal enzymes, NADPH, and molecular oxygen are required for the two processes indicates that microsomal mixed function oxidation[19] is an obligatory step for both. Binding to DNA and hydroxylation are increased following pretreatment of animals with BaP. However, the two processes were induced to different degrees. This, together with additional data (eg, our studies with hematin indicating disproportional effects on hydroxylation and DNA binding[20]) suggest the possibility that the metabolic steps involved are dissociable. Thus, while BaP must first undergo oxidative transformation, subsequent steps in its conversion determine the ratio of toxic and nontoxic intermediates.

The present results demonstrate that the DNA-binding intermediates produced in the microsomal enzyme system are sufficiently stable to permit identification in the supernatant following sedimentation of the microsomes. This may indicate that the reactive intermediates of BaP which may bind to DNA are most stable when complexed with microsomal membranes. The present incubation system was compared to that of Gelboin, isolating DNA both by CsCl isopycnic sedimentation and by deproteinization with sodium lauryl sufate. It was found that, in the present system, the apparent covalent binding of BaP to DNA was much greater (130:1) than in Gelboin's system. This difference may be due to the fact that the present system employs a higher concentration of NaCl and sodium citrate in lieu of edetic acid (EDTA) as an inhibitor of DNases. EDTA has been reported to be an inhibitor of the microsomal hydrocarbon hydroxylase system[15] and may interfere with the generation of DNA-binding intermediates as well. The stabilizing effect of DNA of increased sodium concentration and the efficacy of citrate as a nuclease inhibitor were suggested by the fact that DNA was recovered from the incubation mixtures as a fibrous precipitate that could be collected on a glass rod.

Further evidence supporting dissociation of the production of polar metabolites of BaP from that of reactive intermediates which bind to DNA is offered by studies in which hematin was used as an inhibitor of the microsomal hydroxylases. While hematin suppressed both in vitro hydroxylation of BaP and its binding to DNA, the inhibition of DNA binding was significantly greater.[20] Inhibition of BaP hydroxylation by hematin was seen to affect the metabolites migrating to the central region of the chromatograms (Figs 3 and 4, peaks B and C). That the production of metabolites of BaP was not suppressed uniformly with increasing concentrations of hematin may indicate that BaP is metabolized by a number of independent enzymatic pathways of differing susceptibility to heme. Another possibility is that BaP may be acted upon in a stepwise manner with certain steps inhibited to a greater degree by heme. Although the data presented do not allow a choice between these alternatives, it is clear that it may be possible to direct the metabolism of BaP in such a way that the involvement of a vital molecule, in this case DNA, can be avoided.

The chromatographic profiles of metabolic products found in extracts of cell and tissue cultures were different from those observed in the microsomal system. This may be due to cell or tissue-specific metabolism of BaP. Alternatively, it is possible that the metabolites with intermediate polarity produced in the microsomal system are also produced in intact cells but become covalently bound to cellular components and, therefore, would not be extractable with the organic solvent used in this study. Nevertheless, these results emphasize the complexity of the metabolism of BaP, and, because of its very complexity, encourage the search for modifiers of its carcinogenic action.

While the lung is a target organ for carcinogenesis by BaP, the induced hydroxylase activity in the liver is much higher than in the lung. The absence of a correlation between hydroxylase activity and susceptibility to carcinogenesis when comparing different tissues suggests that additional aspects of BaP-cell interactions are also significant determinants of the response to potential carcinogens.

This work was supported in part by the University of California Cancer Research Fund, the Christine L. Webster Cancer Research Fund; a fellowship grant from the Bank of America-Giannini Foundation to Dr. Ronald E. Rasmussen; Porphyria grant AM-11296, and Research Career Development award 1 K04 AM14301-01 to Dr. Marver.

The 3-hydroxy-BaP standard was provided by H. V. Gelboin, PhD.

References

1. Brooks P, Lawley PD: Evidence for the binding of polynuclear aromatic hydrocarbons to the nucleic acids of mouse skin: Relation between carcinogenic power of hydrocarbons and their binding to deoxyribonucleic acid. *Nature* **202**:781-784, 1964.

2. Goshman LM, Heidelberger C: Binding of tritium-labeled polycyclic hydrocarbons to DNA of mouse skin. *Cancer Res* **27**:1678-1688, 1967.

3. Boyland E, Sims P: Metabolism of polycyclic compounds: The metabolism of 9,10-epoxy-9,10-dihydrophenanthrene in rats. *Biochem J* **95**:788-792, 1965.

4. Wattenberg LW, Leong JL: Effects of phenothiazines on protective systems against polycyclic hydrocarbons. *Cancer Res* **25**:365-370, 1965.

5. Alfred L, Di Paolo J: Protection of cultured hamster embryonic cells from DMBA cytotoxicity following induction of benzpyrene hydroxylase. *Proc Amer Assoc Cancer Res* **9**:2, 1968.

6. Diamond L, Sardet C, Rothblat GH: The metabolism of 7,12-dimethylbenz(A)anthrecene in cell cultures. *Int J Cancer* **3**:838-849, 1968.

7. Jerina D, Daly J, Witkop B, et al: Role of the arene oxide-oxepin system in the metabolism of aromatic substrates: 1. In vitro conversion of benzene oxide to a premercapturic acid and a dihydrodiol. *Arch Biochem* **128**:176-183, 1968.

8. Gelboin HV: A microsome-dependent binding of benzo(a)pyrene to DNA. *Cancer Res* **29**:1272-1276, 1969.

9. Grover PL, Sims P: Enzyme-catalyzed reactions of polycyclic hydrocarbons with deoxyribonucleic acid and protein in vitro. *Biochem J* **110**:159-160, 1968.

10. Falk HL, Kotin P, Lee SS, et al: Intermediary metabolism of benzo(a)pryene in the rats. *J Nat Cancer Inst* **28**:699-724, 1962.

11. Williams RT: *Detoxication Mechanisms*, ed 2. New York, John Wiley & Sons Inc, 1959, pp 222-225.

12. Sims P: The Metabolism of benzo(a)pyrene by rat-liver homogenates. *Biochem Pharmacol* **16**:613-618, 1967.

13. Sims P: Metabolism of some aromatic hydrocarbons by mouse embryo cell cultures. *Biochem Pharmacol* **19**:285-297, 1970.

14. Schneider WC: Intracellular distribution of enzymes: III. The oxidation of octanoic acid by rat liver fractions. *J Biol Chem* **176**:259-266, 1948.

15. Nebert DW, Gelboin HV: Substrate-inducible microsomal aryl hydroxylase in mammalian cell culture: 1. Assay and properties of induced enzyme. *J Biol Chem* **243**:6242-6249, 1968.

16. Silverman DA, Talalay P: Studies on the enzymic hydroxylation of 3,4-benzpyrene. *Molec Pharmacol* **3**:90-101, 1967.

17. Kay ERM, Simmons NS, Dounce AL: An improved preparation of sodium deoxyribonucleate. *J Amer Chem Soc* **74**:1724-1726, 1952.

18. Palekar L, Kuschner M, Laskin S: The effect of 3-methylcholanthrene on rat trachae in organ culture. *Cancer Res* **28**:2098-2104, 1968.

19. Gillette JR: Biochemistry of drug oxidation and reduction by enzymes in hepatic endoplasmic reticulum. *Advances Pharmacol* **4**:219-261, 1967.

20. Wang IY, Marver H, Crocker T: Enzymatic conversion of benzo(a)pyrene (BaP) to an ultimate carcinogen: Hydroxylation vs DNA binding. *Clin Res* **18**:476, 1970.

Lysosomes and the Toxicity of Particulate Pollutants

A. C. Allison, MD, Harrow, Middlesex, England

The pathogenesis resulting from inhaled particulate pollutants centers around their effects upon the macrophage. An analysis of pathogenesis must proceed in two stages: first, determining how particles kill macrophages, and second, determining how this relates to fibrogenesis. Silica (silicon dioxide) alters the secondary lysosomal membrane, making it permeable to the contained lysosomal enzymes. Silica surfaces alter the lysosomal membrane through hydrogen bonding. Asbestos produces similar effects but not to the extent shown by silica. Fibrogenesis occurs through macrophage damage and release of as yet unknown factors.

Many particles inhaled into the lung are more or less innocuous, eg, the carbon particles that remain in macrophages for long periods. However, some inhaled particles, especially silica and asbestos, stimulate a severe fibrogenic reaction, and there are indications that these and other particles also represent an important portal of introduction of carcinogens such as benzo[a]pyrene into the pulmonary tissues. I have been concerned with silica and asbestos, and wish to describe experiments on the cytotoxic effects of these particles. It is necessary, however to begin with a brief description of the materials themselves.

Silicon and oxygen are the commonest elements by weight in the lithosphere; they can exist as silica (silicon dioxide) or in combination with other elements in the form of silicates such as asbestos, mica, kaolin, or talc. Silica is composed of tetrahedra in which a silicon atom lies centrally and four oxygen atoms are each shared with a neighboring atom of silicon. Differences in the spatial relationships of the tetrahedra, as shown by the x-ray diffraction pattern, account for the various physical forms of silica. If the pattern is irregular, the silica is termed amorphous, as in the case of quartz glass (vitreous silica), obtained by melting; and diatomaceous earth (kieselguhr). Each type of crystalline silica has a characteristic regular array of tetrahedra in three dimensions. Quartz is the stable crystal at atmospheric pressure, whereas two other crystal types, tridymite and cristobalite, formed at higher temperatures than quartz, are metastable. Two further types of crystalline silica, coesite and stishovite, are formed at very high temperatures and pressures. Both have been synthesized[1] and isolated as natural

Received for publication Oct 20, 1970; accepted Jan 29, 1971.

From the Clinical Research Center, Harrow, Middlesex, England.

Read in part before the Tenth Annual Hanford Biology Symposium on Pollution and Lung Biochemistry, Richland, Wash, June 5, 1970, jointly sponsored by the Battelle Memorial Institute Pacific Northwest Laboratories, National Air Pollution Control Administration, National Institute of Environmental Health Sciences, and the US Atomic Energy Commission.

Reprint requests to Clinical Research Center, Harrow, Middlesex, England (Dr. Allison).

minerals from Meteor Crater, Ariz. Stishovite is unique in not having the usual tetrahedral form; it has, instead, an octahedral structure in which six shared oxygen atoms are attached to each atom of silicon, a disposition found also in the rutile variety of titanium dioxide.[3] Stishovite has the highest density, then coesite, then the low pressure forms, with tridymite and cristobalite having more open structures than quartz.

The name "asbestos" is applied to minerals that break down into fibers when crushed or processed. This property results from a molecular structure in which the units are linked together most strongly in one direction. A number of fibrous mineral silicates differing in chemical composition show the properties of asbestos. These include two main mineral groups: (1) pyroxenes–chrysotile, and (2) amphiboles–crocidolite, amosite, anthophyllite, tremolite, and actinolite. Chrysotile, or white asbestos, is the most common type, making up more than 90% of that used commercially. Extensive deposits are mined in many parts of the world, especially Canada, Russia, and Rhodesia. Chrysotile is a hydrated magnesium silicate in the form of scrolls or tubes which vary in diameter from 150 to 400 angstroms (Fig 1). The mineral forming these tubes is crystalline; that in the hollow centers and between the tubes is amorphous. The tubes do not adhere together very strongly, and this accounts for the ease with which chrysotile can be broken down into very fine fibers. The tubes are formed from two layers, the inner a continuous network of hexagonally arranged silica units, which is interlocked with the second layer, a brucite-like sheet of octagonal magnesium hydroxide. The spacing of the silica sheet is tighter than required for a perfect fit with the brucite layer, and this accounts for the contortion into tubes or scrolls with the magnesium hydroxide layer on the outside.

The other commercially important asbestos minerals are members of the amphibole group; the molecular structure is essentially the same, with individual types characterized by variations in the composition of the cation chains. The smallest fibers (usually between 800 and 1,000 A in diameter) are solid and coarser than the finest fibers of chrysotile. The structure of the amphiboles is well established.[4] They consist of octahedral cation oxide units arranged in narrow strips and sandwiched between corresponding strips of hexagonally arranged silica tetrahedra. Since the strips are loosely bonded to each other along the edges and faces, fibrous cleavage readily occurs. Of the amphiboles, crocidolite (blue asbestos) is also commercially important. It is sodium ferroso-ferric silicate, mined in South Africa and other countries, and was the first form shown to be carcinogenic. It is very resistant to acid. Another amphibole is amosite, ferrous magnesium silicate, in the form of long brownish-yellow fibers mined in South Africa and used in asbestos cement and heat-insulating products. A third amphibole used commercially on a small scale is anthophyllite, fibrous magnesium silicate. Two other varieties of amphibole asbestos–tremolite (calcium magnesium silicate) and actinolite (calcium magnesium iron silicate)–have less commercial use.

Study of the biological properties of asbestos is complicated by several factors, including the presence of many varieties, the variable contamination of the basic minerals by other materials which may be biologically important, and the fact that biological effects are markedly dependent on fiber size. The longest asbestos fibers normally encountered may be 2 inches or more in length, but the attrition that is unavoidable in separating asbestos fiber from nonfibrous rock results in the presence of fibers so short that the length is hardly greater than the diameter. The finest fibers are always present to a considerable extent in asbestos dust, and these are too small to be resolved in an optical microscope.

Particle size and shape is important in relation to likelihood of inhalation into the lungs, site of deposition, and probability of clearance. This is a complex problem beyond the terms of reference of this article, but it will be obvious that smaller particles have a greater chance of remaining suspended in respired air, penetrating to the alveolar ducts, and so being retained in the lungs, than larger particles. Shape can also be important; highly asymmetric asbestos particles, especially when they are curved (as in the case of chrysotile) are less likely to penetrate deep into the lung than nearly isometric particles, such as silica, of comparable weight. On the other hand, the asymmetry may hinder phagocytosis, and this may account for the fact that asbestos particles reach the pleural mesothelium; this seldom, if ever, happens with silica particles, which are engulfed by alveolar macrophages.

Effects of Toxic Particles on Macrophages

It is generally accepted that the initial event in silicosis is the phagocytosis of silica particles by alveolar macrophages and consequent death of the cells. The particles so released are taken up by other macrophages which are, in turn, killed. In this way death of macrophages continues and stimulates collagen synthesis by fibroblasts in the neighborhood. Analysis of pathogenesis must therefore proceed in two stages: first determining how silica particles kill macrophages, and, second, determining how this is related to fibrogenesis.

As Marks[5] showed, the cytotoxic effects of silica can be conveniently reproduced in cultures of peritoneal or alveolar macrophages, and the relative toxicity of different forms of silica, and of different dusts, on cell cultures agrees with the pathogenicity and fibrogenic activities of the dusts in vivo.[6,7] When my colleagues (T. Nash, J. Harrington, and M. Birbeck) and I began working on this problem in 1964, there was no satisfactory explanation of silica toxicity. King, is his well-known "solubility" theory, suggested that silicic acid liberated into the tissues from silica particles brings about deposition of collagen. Later observations did not support this interpretation, as King[8] himself pointed out. Curran and Rowsell[9] showed that silica particles implanted into the peritoneum in diffusion chambers do not induce any fibrogenic reaction, although silicic acid is liberated from the chambers. Vigliani and Pernis[10] formulated an autoimmune theory of silicosis, but several workers were unable to obtain experimental evidence in support of this interpretation.[11]

We, therefore, made a detailed study of the effects of toxic and nontoxic particles on cultures of macrophages, using time-lapse phase-contrast cinephoto-micrography, histochemistry, and electron microscopy.[12] Particles of silica, diamond dust, and other materials were rapidly included in phagosomes surrounded by single membranes. Lysosomes became attached to the phagosomes and discharged their enzymes into the phagosomes. So far, there was no difference between the toxic and nontoxic particles. After about 18 hours' incubation, however, clear differences were apparent. The nontoxic particles and associated enzymes were still enclosed in secondary lysosomes, whereas many of the toxic particles and associated lysosomal enzymes had escaped into the cytoplasm. The macrophages that had ingested nontoxic particles were fully extended and moving about freely, whereas many of those exposed to toxic particles were rounded and immobile. Thus, it was evident that silica particles, unlike nontoxic particles, can react with lysosomal membranes and make them permeable. Histochemical studies showing release of peroxidase taken up into lysosomes of macrophages after treatment with silica, confirming our observations with acid phosphatase, have been published by Nadler and Goldfischer.[13]

Conventional biochemical studies of the redistribution of lysosomal enzymes from the particulate to the supernatant fraction could not be carried out because homogenization of normal macrophages in the presence of silica particles showed disruption of lysosomes. Hence, an indirect measure of enzyme release which follows such redistribution after phagocytosis of bacteria[14] was used. We found that several lysosomal enzymes were released into the medium after exposure of macrophages to silica, whereas this was not seen in control cells incubated with nontoxic dusts or silica coated with a protective material, poly-2-vinyl-pyridine-*N*-oxide (PVPNO). The release of lysosomal enzymes into the medium preceded release of the cytoplasmic enzyme lactic dehydrogenase and cell death as determined by several criteria (trypan blue staining, tetrazolium reduction, and fluorescein ester cleavage). Thus, the lysosomal enzyme release appears to precede rather than follow cell death.

Our observations have been confirmed repeatedly. Silica particles taken up in culture[15,16] or following inhalation exposure[17,18] are initially in membrane-bound vacuoles or secondary lysosomes but are later observed free in the cytoplasm; the latter coincides with morphological signs of damage to mitochondria and other cell organelles. Ingested coal[19] or kaolin[20] produced only minimal cytological changes. The effects of inhaled silica on macrophages progress more slowly than in culture, in which the number of particles or aggregates per cell is higher, but the sequence of events is essentially the same.[18] Release of acid phosphatase and other lysosomal enzymes from macrophages exposed to silica into the medium, and its prevention by PVPNO, has been confirmed by Comolli,[21] Sakabe and Koshi[22] and Beck.[16]

Interaction of Silica With Biological Membranes

The observations which have been described focus attention on the capacity of silica particles, in contrast to those of many other particles, to react with lysosomal membranes and make them permeable. Silica particles can, in fact, interact with a variety of biological membrane systems. The simplest demonstration is provided by mixing washed erythrocytes with suspensions of silica particles or with silicic acid preparations.[23,24] The erythrocytes are quite rapidly lysed by several fibrogenic forms of crystalline silica, whereas one form which is not fibrogenic (stishovite), and several other types of nonfibrogenic dust of comparable size and surface area, produce very little hemolysis. We have presented reasons[24] for believing that the toxicity of silica is due to the fact that the particles are easily ingested and by interaction with water form on their surface silicic acid which can act as a powerful hydrogen bonding agent.

There are two classes of hydrogen bonding compounds. The larger class comprises hydrogen acceptors such as ethers and ketones with active lone-pair electrons on oxygen or nitrogen. The smaller class comprises hydrogen donors of which only the phenols are important among organic compounds and silicic and some other very weak acids among inorganic compounds. Compounds of one class interact with those of the other, so that it is not surprising that in one class (the former), the members are compatible with living cells, sometimes in very high concentration, whereas those of the other class are damaging.

Model experiments showed that hydrogen bonding of phenolic hydroxyl groups, of the type present in silicic acid, occurs with secondary amide groups of proteins, and this can lead to protein denaturation. However, the interaction with phospholipids is stronger, and we have presented evidence that this is more important in interactions with biological membrane systems.

In view of the interaction with membranes and lysis of erythrocytes, the question arises whether silica particles can kill macrophages or other target cells by interaction with their outer membranes. If relatively large amounts of silica (>100μg/ml) are added to macrophages in a saline medium lacking protein, such rapid killing by cell membrane lysis is observed. Oxygen consumption falls rapidly, within one hour there is considerable leakage of lactate dehydrogenase and other cytoplasmic proteins into the medium, and within two or three hours most of the cells are dead, as shown by the lack of fluorescein diacetate hydrolysis using the method of Rotman and Papermaster[25] and other criteria. However, this is a completely unphysiological situation, and if silica is added to cells in a medium containing serum protein or bronchial washings, this type of surface interaction does not occur. The silica particles are coated with serum protein, even after repeated washing, as can be shown by agglutination with antibody of appropriate specificity staining with fluorescein-labeled antibody. The particles coated in this way are taken up into lysosomes, and it is only when this coating is digested away after some hours (as shown by the disappearance of staining around the particles by fluorescein-labeled antibody) that the underlying silica surface is exposed to interact with the lysosomal membrane.

Since most forms of silicic acid in solution are less damaging than silica particles, even though the former have hydrogen-bonding groups, it seems that the rigid structure of the quartz, with many hydrogen-bonding groups arranged in a regular and immovable order on its surface, must be important in damaging cells. Presumably, the formation of multiple bonds distorts the membrane structure and so leads to the breakdown of the membrane.

Prevention of Silica Toxicity by Polyvinylpyridine-N-Oxide (PVPNO)

Evidence in support of the interpretation that hydrogen bonding is important in silica toxicity comes from experiments with PVPNO. It was found by Schlipköter et al[26] that this polymer markedly reduces the amount of fibrous tissue formed after intravenous injection of silica. Other experiments on the inhibition of quartz fibrosis by PVPNO were summarized by Schlipköter[27]; although silica and PVPNO did not have to be given together, they had to be administered in such a way that they reached the same sites. The protective action of PVPNO in animals has been confirmed by numerous other workers and the compound has also been shown to protect cells in vitro against the damaging effects of silica particles.[12,28] Comparisons between protection of cell cultures in vitro and of whole animals in vivo against silica toxicity of fibrogenicity by various polymers[29] led to the conclusion that compounds ineffective in tests on cultured cells would also be ineffective in animals, whereas some polymers which protect macrophages against quartz in cultures are ineffective in animals. This is understandable if some compounds fail to reach or persist in secondary lysosomes of cells in which silica is taken up in vivo, because the compounds are rapidly metabolized or for some reason other than rapid metabolism.

Allison et al[12] reported that PVPNO is taken up by pinocytosis and concentrated in secondary lysosomes in the same way as dextran, povidone (polyvinylpyrrolidone), and other polymers.[30] The uptake of PVPNO into lysosomes of macrophages and other cells has been confirmed by Grundmann,[31] Bruch,[17] Beck and Boje,[32] Bairati and Castano,[33] and others; these observations have been made by histochemistry, electron microscopy, and cell fractionation and autoradiography using labeled polymer. Nash et al[24] pointed out that PVPNO has oxygen atoms which can readily form hydrogen bonds with phenolic hydroxyl groups, so that the polymer can preferentially interact with silicic acid on the surface of silica particles before the latter can attack lysosomal membranes. In support of this interpretation, Dehnen and Fetzer[34] reported that PVPNO protected rat liver lysosomes from damage by quartz.

In 1966 Nash and I synthesized another compound, polyvinylpyridinioacetic acid, which has even greater hydrogen bonding capacity than PVPNO and very efficiently protects macrophages from silica toxicity. This protection was confirmed by Sakabe and Koshi,[22] who also showed that it prevents the increase in acid phosphatase in macrophages following exposure to silica. Holt et al[35] also reported that some poly(2-vinylpyridinium) salts prevented quartz toxicity in cultures. Thus the presence of hydrogen-accepting groups (either *N*-oxides or pyridinium groups) is frequently associated with protection, although other factors may also be involved. Thus, Holt et al[35] found a difference between the protective effect of syndyotactic and isotactic PVPNO, polymers that differ only in the spatial arrangement of the structural units.

These two facts are sufficient to explain why silica is so toxic to macrophages: the particles are taken up into lysosomes and readily damage lysosomal membranes through hydrogen-bonding interactions. Various secondary reactions may occur. Thus, Munder et al[36] have found a considerable increase in the concentration of lysolecithin, as compared with lecithin, in macrophages damaged by quartz. This could follow activation of the enzyme phospholipase A, which catalyses the reaction lecithin → lysolecithin and which is known to be lysosomal. However, the fact that silica lyses erythrocytes (membranes of which do not contain demonstrable amounts of phospholipase A) suggests that this process is unnecessary for interaction of silica with membrane systems, although the formation of surface-active lysolecithin could well accelerate damage induced by silica in macrophages.

Suspensions of silica particles readily release enzymes from isolated liver lysosomes in vitro, as Dehnen and Fetzer's[34] experiments and our own have shown; the relatively low temperature coefficient for this release suggests that physicochemical rather than enzymic reactions are involved.

The second question remains: how is macrophage damage related to fibrogenesis. An interesting lead has been obtained by Heppleston and Styles.[37] They found that macrophages incubated in culture with silica particles released into the supernatant fraction a factor which, when added to fibroblast cultures, stimulated collagen formation as judged by synthesis of hydroxyproline. This stimulation appeared to be due to a specific product of the macrophage-silica interaction. It was not seen in normal macrophages or in macrophages exposed to nontoxic particles (titanium dioxide, ie, anatase) or to silica in the presence of sufficient PVPNO. The nature of the stimulating factor is still unknown, but it seems likely that no direct interaction of particulate silicate with fibroblasts is involved.

Potentiation by Silica of Tuberculous Infections

All published studies of silicotic human subjects have shown a much higher incidence of tuberculosis than in nonsilicotic subjects from the same areas.[38] Before drugs were introduced, tuberculosis was reported as the main cause of death in classical silicosis.[39] The response to chemotherapy of tuberculous infections in patients with pneumoconiosis is also less satisfactory than in subjects without the latter.[40] Moreover, since the work of Cesa-Bianchi[41] it has been recognized that infections with *Mycobacterium tuberculosis* in experimental animals are aggravated by injections or inhalations of silica dust. Such potentiation has been observed with a substrain of BCG in guinea-pigs and with a virulent strain of *M tuberculosis* in rats[38,42] and also with *M kansasii*, a human pathogen, in guinea-pigs.[43] The potentiation by silica is demonstrable in several ways, including establishment of infections with fewer organisms than are required to produce lesions in the absence of silica particles, higher counts of recovered organisms, spread from subcutaneous inoculation sites to the lungs, and fatal outcome of infection only in animals exposed to silica dust.

These results show that in both human subjects and experimental animals that growth and spread of tubercle bacilli are increased by concomitant exposure to silica dust. There is no evidence that silica interferes with immune responses to *M tuberculosis*. Indeed it has been found that animals exposed to silica or silicate actually have greater humoral and cell-mediated immune re-

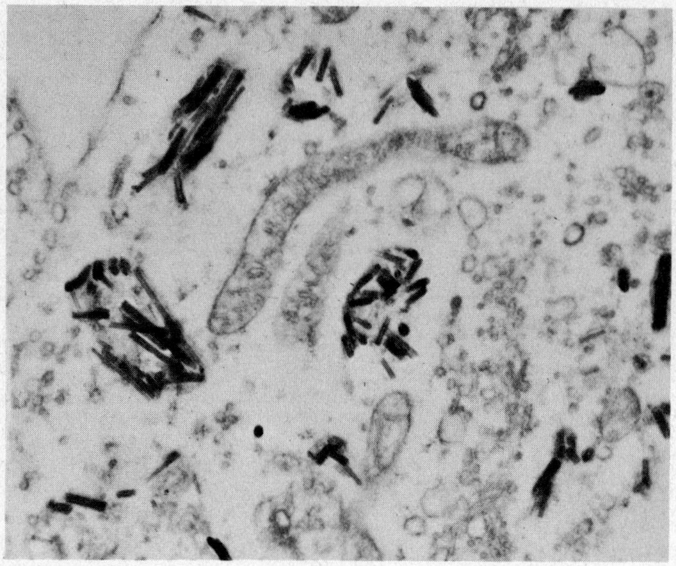

Fig 1.—Electron micrograph of a macrophage that has ingested short fibers of chrysotile (×20,000). The asbestos fibers are seen in secondary lysosomes.

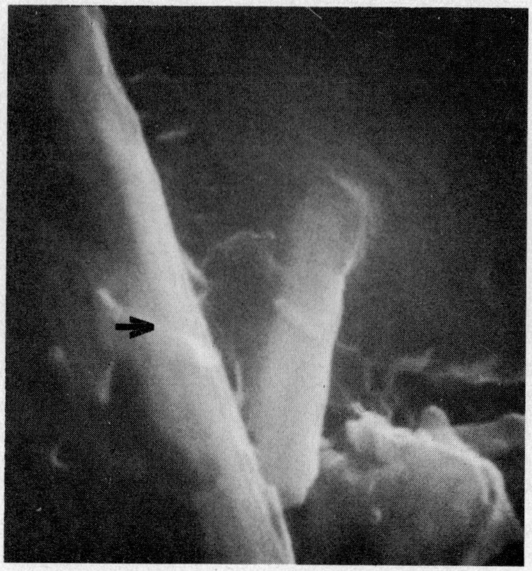

Fig 2.—Stereoscan electron micrograph of a macrophage that has incompletely ingested asbestos fibers (×50,000). The plasma membrane is reflected at the point marked by the arrow. The parts of the fibers below this point are enveloped by invaginated plasma membrane and cytoplasm; the upper parts of the fibers are free.

sponses than in the absence of silica or silicate.[44,45] Vaccination with BCG was ineffective in preventing the increased growth of tubercle bacilli in silicotic guinea-pigs,[42] and allergic reactions to tuberculin are greater in infected silicotic animals than in infected controls.[38,42,43]

Hence, it seems that some factor other than conventional immunity must be involved in the potentiation by silica of the growth of tubercle bacilli. One possibility is that the response of macrophages to intracellular *M tuberculosis* is altered in the presence of silica. The role of macrophages in protection against tuberculous and other intracellular infections has been extensively discussed by Mackaness.[46] "Activation" of macrophages by infection can increase resistance against apparently unrelated organisms, which helps to illustrate the key role of macrophages in overcoming such infections. Since both intracellular infective organisms and silica particles are present in secondary lysosomes of macrophages, it seemed that the latter might potentiate the growth of tubercle bacilli. To test this possibility Hart and I examined the effect of sublethal doses of silica on the multiplication of *M tuberculosis* in macrophages from normal mice cultured in the absence of immune serum. In such a closed system general effects on host resistance would be excluded and specific effects on macrophages revealed.

We found[47] that growth of a relatively virulent strain of *M tuberculosis* (H37RV) in cultures of macrophages was potentiated by the addition of sublethal doses of silica. Macrophages treated with silica showed earlier multiplication of organisms, and the cells were released from their glass support into the medium sooner than control macrophages, both infected without silica or treated with silica alone. Mycobacteria are released mainly by death and dissolution of the macrophages in which they grow. There is little doubt that if these two factors—faster multiplication and earlier release from host cells—operate also in vivo they would greatly facilitate the growth and spread of organisms in the presence of silica particles. This may be sufficient to account for the well-documented aggravation of tuberculous infections in both man and experimental animals by exposure to silica dust.

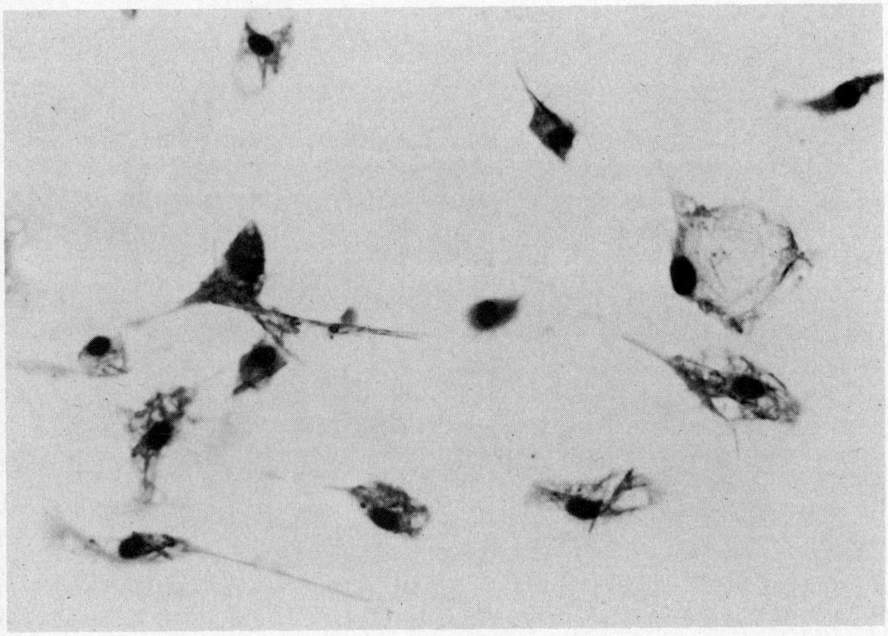

Fig 3.—Macrophage culture two days after exposure to chrysotile asbestos, showing vacuolation of some cells and dense-staining cytoplasm of others.

Effects of Asbestos Particles on Cells

Exposure of humans and experimental animals to asbestos has three main consequences: (1) the development of asbestos bodies, in which the typical particles are found, surrounded by iron-containing pigment which on electron microscopy is seen to contain ferritin and hemosiderin; (2) the fibrogenic response characteristic of asbestos (this may be marked, although it is less severe than that produced by comparable amounts of silica); and (3) development of tumors in the lung. These tumors include a high proportion of mesotheliomas arising from the layer of cells lining the pleura (or occasionally the peritoneum)—a type of tumor that is extremely rare in individuals not exposed to asbestos.

Although the presence of many mineral forms of asbestos, variety of sizes, and variability of results depending on experimental conditions makes it difficult to draw general conclusions about effects of asbestos on cells, some overall points are beginning to emerge. The first is that certain types of asbestos can certainly interact with cell membranes. This is shown by the hemolytic effects of asbestos described by Macnab and Harington[48] and Secchi and Rezzonico.[49] Both groups of authors found chrysotile is at least as hemolytic as silica, but Macnab and Harington reported that PVPNO and aluminum oxide, which markedly reduced hemolysis by silica, had less effect on chrysotile hemolysis. Ethylenediaminetetraacetate or simple phosphates markedly reduced chrysotile hemolysis, which is not surprising since the crystal structure of chrysotile is such that the surface consists of magnesium hydroxide. Chrysotile was found by Secchi and Rezzonico to adsorb the erythrocyte membrane enzyme acetylcholinesterase strongly but the cytoplasmic enzyme lactate dehydrogenase only weakly. They suggested that the highly hemolytic activity of chrysotile is related to the adsorptive capacity of the dust for erythrocyte membrane components. Crocidolite, amosite, and anthophyllite were only weakly lytic.

There are apparent discrepancies between descriptions by various authors of effects of asbestos on macrophages and other cells in culture. On the one hand, there is a report by Parazzi et al[50] that crocidolite and chrysotile are very toxic to guinea pig macrophages, crocidolite being more toxic than chrysotile or tridymite dust used for comparison; fibers were more damaging than particles. On the other hand, the cellular changes found by Beck et al[15] and Davis[51] on exposure of organ cultures to chrysotile were relatively slight.

My co-workers and I have examined the effects of various asbestos dusts (International Union Against Cancer [IUCC] standard samples) on cultures of mouse peritoneal macrophages, prepared as previously described,[12] and on organ cultures of mouse peritoneum in the same medium. The peritoneum is lined by mesothelial cells which are involved in asbestos malignancies, so that their reaction to asbestos was worth studying. This preparation was of interest for several reasons—fibroblasts quickly grew out and were found to take up and be affected by asbestos particles much less than mesothelial cells. The first experiment concerned the capacity of cells to take up asbestos fibers of different lengths. Fractions containing high and low percentages of long fibers were added to cells in medium 199 containing 10% fetal calf serum. Independently of the asbestos type, short fibers ($<5\mu$) were readily and completely taken up by phagocytosis, whereas long fibers ($>30\mu$) were not.

The cells were closely attached to or enveloped the ends of the latter, as shown by ordinary and stereoscan electron micrographs (Fig 2), but part of the asbestos fibers remained outside the cell. This was confirmed by phase-contrast cinephotomicrographs. With very long fibers, two or more cells could be seen closely attached to a single fiber, sometimes with apparent continuity of cytoplasm; such attachment may favor syncytium formation. Cells attached to long fibers in the presence of serum in the medium remained healthy for at least a week in culture.

In contrast, when asbestos fibers were added to macrophages in buffered saline medium lacking serum, marked cytotoxic effects rapidly occurred. Thus, when mouse macrophages were exposed to 100μg/ml medium of IUCC standard chrysotile, 90% of cells had lost the capacity to split fluorescein diacetate within two hours. Release from cells of protein, including the cytoplasmic enzyme lactate dehydrogenase, was marked within one hour of exposure to asbestos, whereas release of acid phosphatase and β-glucuronidase was delayed until later. Cinephotomicrography showed sudden cessation of movement and sometimes blebbing of the cell membrane. Hence, it seems highly probable that this type of rapid cytotoxic reaction is due to a direct interaction of asbestos fibers with cell membranes, analogous to hemolysis. The analogy is strengthened by the observation in my experiments that chrysotile is the most effective of all the IUCC samples in early cytotoxicity, followed by crocidolite, amosite, and anthophyllite in that order. This is in contrast to the rather surprising report of Parazzi et al[50] that the rapid early cytotoxic reaction of crocidolite is greater than that of chrysotile.

In any case, it is doubtful whether the rapid cytotoxic reation produced by asbestos fibers in media lacking serum or bronchial washings has much physiological relevance. I have, therefore, examined the long-term effects on macrophages and mesothelial cells of exposure to fibers that are mostly of ingestible size in medium containing 10% fetal calf serum. Such fibers are taken up into vacuoles that become secondary lysosomes, as shown by acid phosphatase and other marker enzymes. It is already clear that all types of asbestos dusts are much less toxic .to macrophages and other cells than are silica dusts. However, it would be wrong to conclude that asbestos dusts are entirely devoid of cytotoxic potential. Macrophages exposed to chrysotile (20 to 50μg/ml IUCC standard) often show after two or three days in culture very large lightly staining vacuoles in their cytoplasm (Fig 3). Some cells show pyknotic cytoplasm and nuclei and about 20% are no longer viable. Hence, there was certainly some cytotoxic reaction, as well as other abnormalities. One of the most striking was the development in mesothelial cells, and to a lesser extent in macrophages, of brown pigmented autofluorescent granules in the cytoplasm; this was greatly accentuated after ingestion of asbestos, especially crocidolite. Perhaps the iron favors lipid peroxidation.

Apart from formation of iron-containing pigment, already mentioned, the most striking ultrastructural change in asbestos-treated cells is the development of an electron-dense matrix surrounding the asbestos particles in secondary lysosomes. This is not seen in silica-treated cells and could provide a protective layer between the asbestos particles and the vulnerable membrane surrounding the secondary lysosome. This may, in fact, explain why asbestos is less toxic than would be expected from its capacity to react with membranes, as shown by hemolysis.

Although much remains to be learned about the effects of asbestos on cells, certain important differences from effects of silica are already apparent. One is the failure of ingestion of many asbestos fibers because they are too long. Another is the obviously weaker cytotoxicity of asbestos than silica, although some forms of asbestos, especially chrysotile, are certainly more toxic than inert dusts such as anatase or diamond dust. The slowly progressive damage to macrophages so produced may be an important factor in the fibrotic reaction to asbestos. Also observed in asbestos-treated cells is lipid peroxidation and accumulation in vacuoles or iron-containing pigment; this contributes to the formation of asbestos bodies in vivo.

References

1. Stishov SM, Belov NV: Crystal structure of a new dense modification of silica. *Dokl Akad Nauk SSSR* **143**:951, 1962.

2. Bohn E, Stover W: Isolation of coesite and stishovite as natural minerals. *Neues Jb Miner Mb* **5**:89, 1966.

3. Preisinger A: Structure of stishovite, high density SiO_2. *Naturwissenschaften* **49**:345, 1962.

4. Deer WA, Howie RA, Zussman J: *Rock-Forming Minerals.* London, Longmans Green & Co Ltd, 1962.

5. Marks J: The neutralization of silica toxicity in vitro.

Brit J Industr Med **14**:81, 1957.
6. Marks J, Nagelschmidt G: Study of the toxicity of dust with use of the in vitro dehydrogenase technique. *Arch Industr Health* **20**:383-389, 1959.
7. Vigliani EC, Pernis B, Monaco L: Study of the action of quartz particles on macrophages in vitro, in Davies CN (ed): *Inhaled Particles and Vapours*. London, Pergamon Press Inc, 1961, p 348.
8. King EJ: Volubility theory of silicosis. *Occup Med* **4**:26, 1967.
9. Curran RC, Rowsell EV: The application of the diffusion-chamber technique to the study of silicosis. *J Path Bact* **76**:561, 1958.
10. Vigliani EC, Pernis B: Immunological aspects of silicosis. *Adv Tuberc Res* **12**:230, 1963.
11. Voisin GA, Collet A, Martin JC, et al: Propriétes immunologigues de la silice et de composés du beryllium: Les formes solubles comparées aux formes insolubles. *Rev Franc Etud Clin Biol* **9**:819, 1964.
12. Allison WC, Harington JC, Birbeck M: An examination of the cytotoxic effects of silica on macrophages. *J Exp Med* **124**:141, 1966.
13. Nadler S, Goldfischer S: The intracellular release of lysosomal contents in macrophages that have ingested silica. *J Histochem Cytochem* **18**:368, 1970.
14. Cohn Z, Hirsch JG, Wiener E: Lysosomes-endocytosis: Cytoplasmic granules of phagocytic cells and the degradation of bacteria in De Reuck AVS, Cameron MP (eds): *Lysosomes: Ciba Foundation Symposium*. Boston, Little Brown & Co, 1963, p 126.
15. Beck EG, Bruch J, Sack J: Beobachtungen über die Morphologie der Staubphagozytose in vitro. *Ergebn Unters Geb Staubund Silikosekek Steinkohlenbergbau* **6**:131, 1967.
16. Beck EG: Die Reaktion in vitro gezuchter Zellen auf partikelformige Luftverunreinigungen und hochpolymere Stoffe. *Forschungsberichte Landes Nordrhein-Westfalen* No 2083, pp 125.
17. Bruch J: Ein elektronenmikroskopischer Beitrag zum Frühstadium der Silikose. *Fortschr Staublungensforsch* **2**:249, 1967.
18. Bruch J, Otto H: Electronenmikroskopische Beobachtungen an Alveolarmakrophagen in der Rattenlunge nach Quartzstaubinhalation. *Ergebn Unters Geb Staub-Silikosekek Steinkohlenbergbau* **6**:141, 1967.
19. Collet A, Martin JC, Norman-Reuet C, et al: Recherches infra-structurales sur l'evolution des macrophages alveolaries et leurs reactions aux poussieres minerales, in Davies CN (ed): *Inhaled Particles and Vapours*. Davies Pergamon Press Inc, 1967, vol 2, p 155.
20. Ruttner JR, Grieshaber E, Vogel A, et al: Phagozytoze und Fibrillogenese im peritonealen Staubknotchen electronen mikroskopische befunde bei Kaolin-induzierten knotchen. *Fortschr Staublungensforsch* **2**:89, 1967.
21. Comolli R: Cytotoxicity of silica and liberation of lysosomal enzymes. *J Path Bact* **93**:241, 1967.
22. Sakabe H, Koshi K: Preventative effect of polybetaine on the cell toxicity of quartz particles. *Industr Health* **5**:181, 1967.
23. Stalder H, Stober W: Haemolytic activity of suspensions of different silica modifications and inert dusts. *Nature* **207**:874, 1965.
24. Nash T, Allison AC, Harington JS: Physicochemical properties of silica in relation to its toxicity. *Nature* **210**:259, 1966.
25. Rotman B, Papermaster BW: Membrane properties of living mammalian cells as studied by enzymatic hydrolysis of fluorogenic esters. *Proc Nat Acad Sci USA* **55**:134, 1966.
26. Schlipköter HW, Dolgner R, Brockhaus A: Ein Beitrag zur Therapie der experimentellen Silikose. *German Med Monthly* **8**:509, 1963.
27. Schlipköter HW: Die Wirkung von Polyvinylpyridin-N-oxid (P204) im Tierexperiment. *Arbeitsmed Sozialmed Arbeitshyg* **4**:133, 1967.
28. Beck EG, Bruch J, Brockhaus A: Alteration of the cytotoxic effect of quartz on mouse fibroblasts (strain L) by polyvinylpyridine-N-oxide. *Z Zellforsch* **49**:568, 1963.
29. Schlipköter HW, Beck EG: Observations on the relation between quartz cytotoxicity and fibrinogenicity while testing the biological activity of synthetic polymers. *Med Lavoro* **56**:485, 1965.
30. de Duve C, Wattiaux R: Functions of lysosomes. *Ann Rev Physiol* **28**:435, 1966.
31. Grundmann E: Experimentelle Untersuchungen über die zellulare Speicherung des Polyvinyl-pyridin-N-oxid. *Fortschr Staublungensforsch* **2**:223, 1967.
32. Beck EG, Boje H: Zytologische Untersuchungen über die Wirkung vol Poly-(2)vinylpyridin-N-oxid in der Zellkultur. *Fortschr Staublungensforsch* **2**:231, 1967.
33. Bairati A, Castano P: Studio al microscopio elettronico della localizzazione, nel fegato dei topi, di polimeri sintetici citoprotettivi nei confronti della silice (poli-vinipriridino-N-ossido e poli-p-dimetilamminostirolo-N-ossido). *Med Lavoro* **59**:81, 1968.
34. Dehnen W, Fetzer J: Über die Wirkung von Polyvinylpyridin-N-Oxid (P204) au die Stabilitat isolieter Ratten leberlysosomen. *Ergebn Unters Geb Staub-und Silikosekek in Steinkohlenbergbau* **6**:161, 1967.
35. Holt PF, Lindsay H, Beck EG: Some derivatives of polyvinylpyridine 1-oxides and their effect on the cytotoxicity of quartz in macrophage cultures. *Brit J Pharmacol* **38**:192, 1970.
36. Munder PG, Modolell M, Ferber E, et al: Phospholipids in quartz-damaged macrophages. *Biochem Z* **344**:310, 1966.
37. Heppleston AG, Styles JA: Activity of a macrophage factor in collagen formation by silica. *Nature* **214**:521, 1967.
38. Vorwald AJ, Delahant AB: The influence of silica on the natural and acquired resistance of the tubercle bacillus. *Amer Rev Tuberc* **38**:347, 1938.
39. Hart PDA, Aslett EA: Chronic pulmonary disease in South Wales coalminers: I. Medical studies. *Med Res Counc Spec Rep Series* **243**:186, 1942.
40. *Miners' Chest Diseases Treatment Centre Report*. London, Medical Research Council, 1967.
41. Cesa-Bianchi D: Staubinhalation und Lungen Tuberculose. *Z Hygiene Infektionskrank* **73**:166, 1963.
42. Vorwald AJ, Dworski M, Pratt PC, et al: BCG vaccination in silicosis. *Amer Rev Tuberc* **62**:455, 1950.
43. Policard A, Gernez-Rieux C, Taquet A, et al: Influence of pulmonary dust load on the development of experimental infection by *Mycobacterium kansasii*. *Nature* **216**:177, 1967.
44. Pernis B, Paronetto P: Adjuvant effect of silica (tridymite) on antibody production. *Proc Soc Exp Biol Med* **110**:390, 1962.
45. Wilkinson PC, White RG: The role of mycobacteria and silica in the immunological response of the guinea-pig. *Immunology* **11**:229,1966.
46. Mackaness G: Cellular immunity, in van Furth R (ed): *Mononuclear Phagocytes*. Oxford, Blackwell Scientific Publications, p 461, 1970.
47. Allison AC, Hart PDA: Potentiation by silica of the growth of *Mycobacterium tuberculosis* in macrophage culture. *Brit J Exp Path* **49**:465, 1968.
48. Macnab G, Harington JS: Haemolytic activity of asbestos and other mineral dusts. *Nature* **214**:522, 1967.
49. Secchi GC, Rezzonico A: Hemolytic activity of asbestos dust. *Med Lavoro* **59**:1, 1968.
50. Parazzi E, Pernis B, Secchi GC, et al: Studies on "in vitro" cytotoxicity of asbestos dust. *Med Laboro* **59**:561, 1968.
51. Davis JMG: The effects of chrysotile asbestos dust on lung macrophages maintained in organ culture: An electron-microscope study. *Brit J Exp Path* **48**:379, 1967.

Introduction

Premature Ventricular Beats

Douglas P. Zipes, MD, Utica, NY, and
Charles Fisch, MD, Indianapolis

This monthly series of electrocardiograms (ECG) for physicians interested in electrocardiography will be presented to demonstrate basic electrocardiographic and electrophysiologic principles. Initial issues will provide a foundation upon which we shall build as more complex arrhythmias are discussed. Occasionally, we will include pertinent references and briefly mention therapy when appropriate.

The *ladder diagram* will be employed frequently to depict depolarization and conduction schematically. Straight lines drawn on a tiered framework beneath an ECG trace represent electrical events occurring in the various cardiac structures (Fig 1).

Certain features of the ladder diagram need further explanation. Since the ECG, and, therefore, the ladder diagram, record electrical activity against a time base, conduction is indicated by the sloping lines of the ladder diagram in a left to right direction. A less steep line depicts slower conduction; a short bar drawn perpendicular to a sloping line represents blocked conduction (Fig 2).

On occasion, activity originating in an ectopic ventricular site, or produced by an artificial pacemaker, may be indicated in another tier drawn beneath V. In general, ectopic atrial, A-V junction (nodal), or ventricular activity will be diagrammed to begin in the appropriate tier (Fig 3).

It is important to remember that the standard ECG fails to record depolarization or repolarization of most of the structures in the specialized conducting system: the sinus node

Received for publication Feb 17, 1971.

From the Masonic Medical Research Laboratory, Utica, NY (Dr. Zipes) and the Indiana University Medical Center, Krannert Institute of Cardiology, Indianapolis (Drs. Fisch and Zipes).

Reprint requests to 1100 W. Michigan St, Indianapolis 46202 (Dr. Zipes).

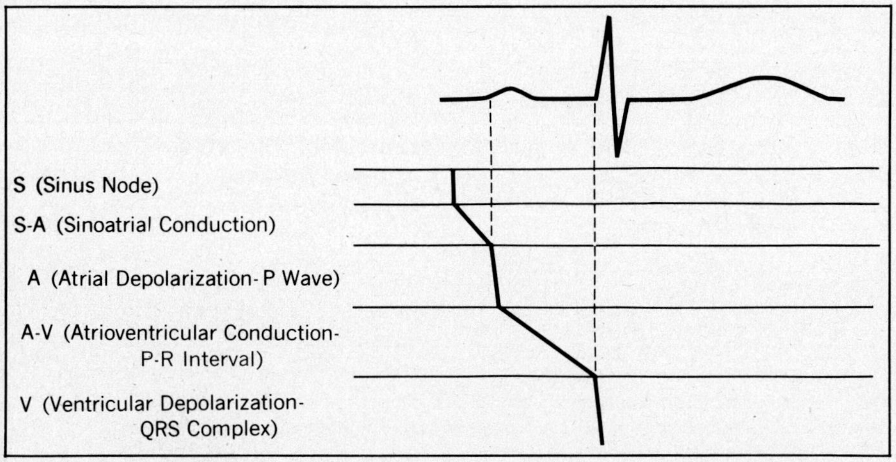

Fig 1.—Ladder diagram construction. A straight or slightly sloping line beginning with P wave or QRS complex indicates atrial or ventricular depolarization. Point at which sinus node discharges and duration of sinoatrial conduction cannot be measured in the surface ECG and are, therefore, assumed. Sloping line connecting A and V represents A-V conduction.

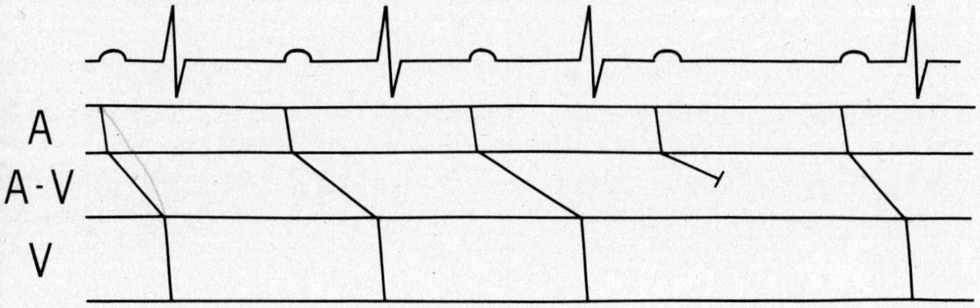

Fig 2.—A-V Wenckebach. In diagrammatic example of A-V Wenckebach (T waves are not drawn) the P-R interval lengthens progressively until finally the fourth P wave fails to reach the ventricles. As P-R interval prolongs, note decreasing slope of line representing A-V conduction, until fourth P wave blocks.

Fig 3.—Ectopic beats. Normal sinus, ectopic atrial, A-V junctional, and ventricular beats are drawn in A-D with appropriate ladder diagrams beneath. Retrograde atrial conduction is inscribed for latter two beats (T waves omitted). As with sinus node, exact discharge time of the A-V junctional focus and conduction time from that point to the ventricles and atria are assumed.

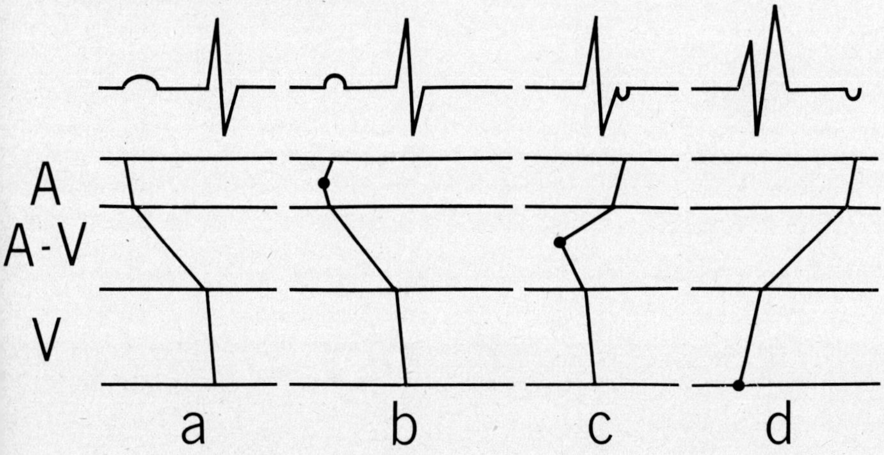

and sino-atrial (S-A) conduction, specialized internodal or interatrial tracts, A-V node, His's bundle, bundle branches or Purkinje system. Ventricular and atrial depolarization, ventricular and sometimes atrial repolarization are all that are recorded. A catheter technique allows recording of His's bundle and sometimes bundle branch activity and will be discussed at length at a later time. Therefore, sinus node discharge and conduction, and under certain circumstances, A-V junctional discharge and conduction, can only be assumed, and will be diagrammed when they play an important role in the interpretation of the arrhythmia.

Premature Ventricular Beats

When ectopic ventricular beats interrupt sinus rhythm, the heart rate, coupling interval, and the speed of A-V conduction determine the events which occur in the wake of the premature ventricular contraction (PVC). The following examples recorded from a 45-year-old asymptomatic man illustrate these aftereffects (Fig 4).

A compensatory pause—defined as a pause, following a premature beat, of sufficient duration to make the P-P interval between the two normal beats flanking the premature beat twice the basic P-P interval—occurs most frequently. As seen in tracing A, antegrade A-V conduction prevents retrograde ventricular conduction from reaching, depolarizing, and prematurely resetting the timing of atrial (sinus node) discharge. The nonconducted P wave lies buried in the ST-T wave of the PVC. Minimal sinus slowing makes the interval between the second and fourth beats slightly longer than twice the P-P interval in this example.

In tracing B, a slower sinus rate

Fig 4.—Premature ventricular beats. Events following premature ventricular beats in these examples are described in the text.

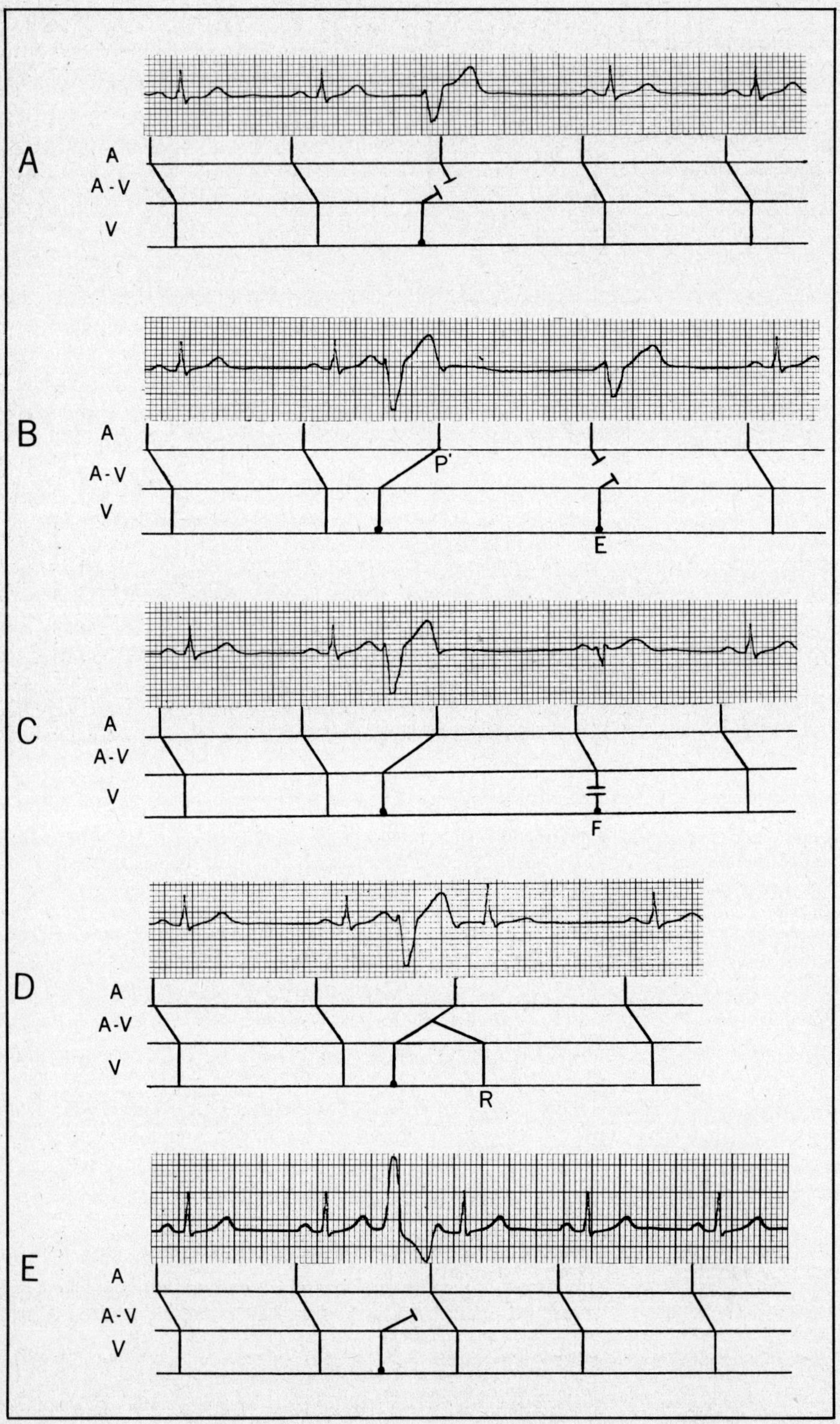

and a PVC occurring earlier in the cycle combine to permit retrograde atrial excitation (P′). The sinus node is reset, and makes the next sinus cycle begin from that point. The pause is therefore noncompensatory. However, before the normal, sinus-initiated P wave which follows the retrograde P can conduct to the ventricle, a ventricular escape beat occurs (E).

Tracing C is the same as tracing B except for a slightly faster sinus rate. This permits the P wave, following the PVC and retrograde P wave, to partially depolarize the ventricles at the same time the ventricular escape beat occurs, which results in a ventricular fusion beat (F). The simultaneous activation of one chamber by two foci produces a fusion beat, which then represents a blend of the characteristics of the normally conducted beat and the beat originating ectopically.

In tracing D, the impulse propagating retrogradely to the atrium reverses its direction after a delay, and returns to reexcite the ventricles (R). This is called a ventricular echo, and is a form of reentrant excitation.

In tracing E, obtained from a different patient, retrograde conduction by the PVC retards but does not block conduction from the following P wave. The P-R interval of this beat lengthens because the impulse travels over pathways discharged by the PVC and not yet fully recovered. When the P wave following the PVC conducts to the ventricles the PVC is said to be interpolated.

These tracings demonstrate that the timing of the electrical events and the capability of A-V conduction determine whether a compensatory pause, a noncompensatory pause, or other phenomena follow a premature ventricular beat.

The Funding of Graduate Education

The funding of intern and residency training is now becoming a major consideration of executive faculties and hospital administrators as they attempt to plan for the future. There are two views of this economic issue—and one might have anticipated that the positions involved related to whether or not you are the payee or the payor. The house staff would like to have higher salaries; the administrators are reluctant to increase the costs of health care in their institutions. Also involved, however, is the broader question of the specific purposes of graduate medical education and of the balance of elements that must be struck between what are the educational goals and responsibilities of the training physician and what are his or her needs and expectations as a young man or woman in our aspiring society.

The central point of discussion is the level of salary for a house officer. At many institutions the house officers have formed an association (there is now also a national house officer's association) which, in effect, has begun to act as a union organization quite analogous to the unions of industry. These groups have asked to sit down with the director of the hospital to discuss salary scales and to consider possible "fringe" benefits, ie, malpractice insurance, disability insurance, longer paid vacations, life insurance policies, family health insurance policies, and paid-for scientific conference attendance (including travel expenses).

At these meetings between house officers and administrators the generation gap can be most conspicuous in that the men who are serving as medical directors and executive faculties had their own house staff training during a period when $25 per month was considered a standard house officer's wage. The principle of deferred income was woven into the standards of that period of some 25 years ago, and the notion of having the hospital facility or a medical center provide anything more than a meal and a room while on duty was not entertained. The immediate "gut" response of the hospital director who was so raised in his own career is to listen in amazement and irritation; but such an attitude is as unrealistic as hoping that 5 cent bus fares will return. The fact of the matter is that house officers are now a cadre of people who are not wedded to the notion of prolonged latent periods, who feel strongly that young professionals are to be viewed first as professionals without any undue emphasis on the fact of being young, and that the development of families—most often begun in undergraduate college years—requires the same financial and security considerations for a physician as it does for a young stock broker, engineer, advertising executive, or beginning industry employee.

Once the hospital director and/or executive faculty reset their sights as to what is expected by the house officers and once they set about the task of meeting these requests, they run into the very hard question of how to finance the programs that are being requested. The total amount of money available in the health care system to pay personnel does have some finite limit. Just how much that limit is may not as yet be settled, but we may be very near the ceiling level now, particularly as community organizations and governmental units enter into the negotiation to insuring people for health care. One of the critical questions to be asked is how much of the money now being invested in the total physician manpower pool is to be absolutely increased, and how much simply redistributed?

For a moment let us step back and take a wide-angle, low-power view of a physician's earning curve during his total career. Over his entire professional life, which we may consider to span approximately 40 years (age 25 through 65) he will earn a total income of between 1 to 1½ million dollars. At the present time, the shape of that curve is one which is skewed to the right: there is a relatively low annual income during the early years, then a gradual peak rise to the late middle period, and then a moderate decline towards the final years. What the young physicians are requesting is that the low rate of annual income for the early years be increased. There has been no discussion of whether or not the other portions of the curve are to be modified. In order to accomplish that objective, therefore, there are but two possibilities: either add to the total amount of money that a physician earns over his entire career (raise the level of the early part of the curve and leave the remainder unchanged) or redistribute the total amount of monies earned for the entire period. The two alternative paths are clearly different.

Three components will most likely play a role in determining the final pattern of resource utilization for both the period of house officer training and for the total career of a physician. First, there will be the effect of the almost universal academic-mantling of all residency training programs. The recent decision of the American Medical Association's House of Delegates to no longer accredit any free-standing internship means that graduate education will become part of the university medical center's responsibility and will link directly into the medical school curricula. Of course, not all residency training will take place in the university medical centers, but all residency programs will most likely be *affiliated* in some shape or form with universities so that there will be a purposeful continuity between undergraduate and graduate education. It will mean that there will be more rigorous supervision and monitoring of the substantive content of graduate education. This will create a greater degree of responsibility and obligation for the house officer. Moonlighting activities—such as doing unsupervised admission histories and physicals at small private hospitals for the practitioners in those facilities—will be viewed as flagrantly irrelevant and distracting from the singular educational task of a graduate trainee. Unsupervised training can be the most self-deluding and erosive factor in a career program that is otherwise designed to develop excellence. By eliminating this form of income-generation, the trainee will be constrained to stay firmly inside the academic range. That means there will be greater pressure upon the university medical center and the affiliated programs to provide all the income that the house officer deems is minimally necessary to maintain his family.

Second, the scale of salaries and accompanying benefits for house officers—graduate students—will become universally increased as it has for graduate trainees in all other areas of our society. The responsibility for families, the earlier degree of social maturation, the increased degree of mobility will also be important determinants in the level of support. The necessary and significant contributions that graduate students make to the health care delivery system will be clearly identified and recognized, and this will be given a monetary value certainly equal to graduate trainees in engineering, merchandising, legal counseling, and other areas of the community.

Third, there will be specific, negotiated arrangements (agreements, contracts, charters, and such) between the people who need health care and the health care professionals who will deliver it. These agreements will spell out in detail how health care will be dispensed and financed. The government will play a major role as both a designer of these contracts and as an underwriter of the cost of the health care activities. Nongovernmental groups and agencies (insurance companies, industries, community health councils) will also figure into the brokering of these contracts between the providers of health care and the people. And all members of the health care system—residents, nurses, therapists of all kinds, clerks, full professors, individual practitioners—will come under the cover of these contracts. A reasonable balance and a governed supervision will be the guidelines determining the distribution of the resources. Into those contractual arrangements the value and worth of graduate training will be designated. In the final analysis, the community will negotiate with the health professions what it is willing to pay for the growth, development, and maintenance of its health professionals. As we enter upon these negotiations we must realize that there is a continuum of career evolution and that the needs of the young are as important as the accomplished excellence of the old.

Thus the stipends to be paid the house staff will be determined by this interplay of factors—educational, cultural, and contractual—and the eventual levels to be settled upon will require a satisfactory fulfillment of the needs of all components. The negotiation will no longer be conducted on a two-party basis—house staff vis a vis hospital administration. The participation of the university and of the community units means that the educational and service activities will be very carefully cost-accounted and the appropriate assessment of how a house officer spends his day will become part of an institutional audit. In the long run this should lead to a more clearly defined curriculum of training and to a more precise allocation of service activities. For the short term, there may be inadvertent inequities for which all parties will have to bear some responsibility: if the participating groups—house staff, administration, faculty, communities—can work through the transition period with poise, it is certain that the eventual goal of both the clinical competence and the funds paid for such competence will be significantly increased.

M.D.B

AMA Drug Evaluations

A Praiseworthy Venture

The past decade has witnessed a rising groundswell of concern regarding many of the circumstances which surround the evaluation, marketing, and prescription of drugs within the United States. This concern has arisen from increasingly varied sources and, in turn, it has led to a barrage of frequently legitimate criticism toward the current practices, policies, and attitudes of governmental regulatory agencies, the pharmaceutical industry, hospitals, medical schools, physicians, etc. Under-manned regulatory agencies have been said to be too autocratic, inflexible, and generally unprepared to deal squarely and simultaneously with the special needs of industry, research, and the consumer; the pharmaceutical industry has been accused of gross commercialism, misleading and superabundant advertising, and inadequate evaluation of drug safety and efficacy; hospitals and medical schools have been brought to task for the provision of too little instruction in clinical pharmacology for students and house officers; physicians themselves have been said to be too susceptible to the salesmanship of the pharmaceutical industry, too unfamiliar with the clinical, physiological, and pharmacological consequences of the drugs that they prescribe, too indiscriminate in their use of drugs in general, and too unresponsive to the savings in cost that might accrue to the consumer through the adoption of different attitudes toward drug selection and prescription. Criticism of the events that surround the prescription of drugs for legitimate illness has been sharpened further by an increased awareness of the magnitude of drug abuse among consumers whose use of drugs has been neither prescribed by the physician nor required for physical or mental illness. By now, it should be obvious to all that the problems which envelop the development, evaluation, distribution, and accessibility of drugs are national in scope, and that their solutions must eventually require effective interaction between all strata of our society. Responsible solutions are always achieved with much more difficulty than the identification of problems; the road ahead cannot be traveled easily . . . but we must begin.

Physicians, as the primary dispensers of legitimate drugs, should and must assume a leading role in the search for viable solutions to the problems that swirl about us. But first, we must feel confident that our own house has been set in order; we must assure ourselves that we are familiar with the mechanisms of action, indications, benefits, and potential adverse effects of the drugs that we prescribe, we must concern ourselves with the relative cost of different drugs that might be used with equal effectiveness for the same complaint, and we must tidy up our prescribing habits while asking ourselves if this or that drug is of proven benefit or truly necessary. Unnecessary chemical pollution of the body's internal environment should not be condoned beneath the guise of well-intentioned psychotherapy.

Education and innovative rejuvenation of training exercises in clinical pharmacology offer at least one long-term approach to the establishment of improved prescription habits among practitioners, house officers, and students. For that reason, the medical profession should welcome the recent publication and nationwide distribution of the 1970 first edition of *AMA Drug Evaluations*, a 1,040 page compendium of useful clinical pharmacology that has been prepared under the supervision of the AMA Council on Drugs. Its conception, compilation, and publication is a laudable and noble effort whose self-declared purpose is "to give the practicing physician the most important information to help in his prescribing practices." It is both editorial and reportorial in its approach to the description of available drugs, their uses, side effects, and dosages. It does not hesitate to declare that certain drugs are "not recommended" for specific conditions and, when indicated, it has made an honest and commendable effort to include statements as to the relative efficacy of certain drugs. Perhaps most important, it represents the first broad-based effort to compile a useful book on clinical pharmacology that can be said to have arisen solely from within the medical and scientific community itself. Over 300 professional consultants contributed to its compilation and publication, a feat that in itself was four years in the making. Thus, it can be said to have arisen free of any constraints, real or imagined, that might have been imposed by collaboration or association with either the pharmaceutical industry or governmental regulatory agencies. Hopefully, in the hands of the practitioner, it and subsequent revisions will serve to take the place of the long-familiar *Physicians Desk Reference* or "PDR." Such a compendium, if used, can be viewed as an important national attempt on the part of the profession itself to improve its own prescription practices.

The Council on Drugs is also well aware that all will not agree with its opinions, "particularly on controversial matters." Furthermore, it is equally aware of the responsibility that is imposed by editorial comment and opinion in areas where facts may be conflicting and controversial. This sense of awareness is imparted by the content of a 15-page section of "General Information" which explains and justifies the "ground rules" which underlay many of the judgments, opinions, and approaches that were adopted. Nevertheless, the fragility and well-recognized vulnerability of editorial opinion cannot be used as an excuse for factual error or a misstatement of general opinion. In several instances, the surety of the volume is marred by either simple misstatement or universally accepted fact, or by editorial opinion which is not representative of either acceptable practice or opinion of the best talent available. For example, as nephrologists with a long interest in the site and mechanism of action of diuretic drugs, we could not help but be drawn immediately to the section on "Diuretics." Within this chapter, we were surprised to find that furosemide and ethacrynic acid had been assigned to a smallish section entitled "Miscellaneous Diuretics." Certainly, as implied by the editorial commentary, few or none of our university-based colleagues would relegate either of these potentially potent and important drugs to a secondary role in the management of edema. Either drug can be used most properly as a first-line agent in the control of edema, and indeed, the wide dose-response curve of furosemide and ethacrynic acid may even be said to have simplified diuretic therapy by permitting the physician to adjust the dose of drug to the specific need and clinical condition of his patient. A small dose of either of these agents will be effective of a diuresis of no greater magnitude than that achieved with other agents such as the organomercurials or thiazides. Insofar as the management of edema is concerned, the physician can thus restrict his knowledge of diuretic drugs to a single agent—if he so chooses.

Undoubtedly, at least some of the shortcomings and bias of this particular section, and perhaps others as well where we feel less qualified to comment, can be attributed to an undue delay between composition and publication during a period when rapid advances were underway in specific areas of therapy. Nevertheless, the overall objective of the volume contains such great merit that we can only hope that the Council on Drugs will continue to exert a concerted effort to obtain broad, meaningful, and the most effective participation by the best available talent as it compiles its next edition. Constructive criticism of the first edition must be sought actively by the Council, and means must be identified to insure that revision and review occur annually at least. Inclusion of a section on the identification of tablets, capsules, etc, would be helpful to practitioners, and information of the relative cost of different agents would be welcome. In at least some instances, clear acknowledgement of the existence of legitimate differences of opinion might be preferable to the arbitrary exercise of value judgment. And finally, more careful editing and review of final versions by ad hoc study *groups* outside the Council on Drugs is almost mandatory. Insofar as possible, compositional objectives should include reasoned anticipation of the state of the art at the time of publication, and not at the time of actual writing. The success of the venture will depend upon the compilation of dependable facts in a practical format that is useful to the practitioner, speedy revision, and the factual validity of the selected content—a function of the quality of scientific input. The venture is praiseworthy; we hope that it will not fail.

Roscoe R. Robinson, MD
James R. Clapp, MD
Durham, NC

Easing the Pain

To the Editor.—Your news item "Easing the Pain" in the February issue (*Arch Intern Med* **127**:200, 1971) is inaccurate in two important details. Neither open surgical cordotomy nor percutaneous cordotomy deprives a patient of his sense of touch. What is lost is the perception of pain, heat, and cold.

Further, I doubt that injecting any amount of "normal saline" in the patient's lumbar subarachnoid space will relieve pain. The original work that was done on this procedure involved injecting the supernatant of iced saline. In actual fact of the matter, the supernatant ends up being hypertonic saline because of the crystallization out of water and the concentration of the hypertonic saline is somewhere between 3% and 5%. The problem of midline, lower back, and bilateral lower extremity pain in patients who have had extensive cobalt therapy and surgery for malignancies in the pelvis is a most difficult one. The bilaterality of the pain requires that any surgical cordotomy procedure be bilateral. Phenol injection is sometimes a temporary expedient in relieving pain in the perineum following a combined abdominal perineal operation but has not been adequate in my experience for patients whose pain is located in the limbs.

French neurosurgeons have performed a procedure called a commissural myelotomy that consists of dividing the anterior commissure of the spinal cord in the lumbar and sacral segments. This essentially divides the crossing spinothalamic tracts with their pain fibers and theoretically at least leaves untouched the corticospinal tracts and the other sensory modalities. This, however, requires a thoracic and lumbar laminectomy to perform and suffers from the same drawback that open cervical cordotomy suffered from, that is, the necessity of performing a major operation for pain relief in a debilitated patient. For this reason alone, it is doubtful that this will ever be a very popular procedure.

I have seen or known three of four patients who have had intrathecal hypertonic saline injections—a most painful procedure—and the results are a rather mixed group of good and poor.

JOHN L. SEYMOUR, MD
Minneapolis

Books

Current Dermatologic Management. Edited by Stuart Maddin, MD. Price, $38.75. Pp 330, with 116 illustrations, including 76 full-color plates. CV Mosby Co, 3207 Washington Blvd, St. Louis 6310, 1970.

We do not have a dermatologist on our island, so the internists are obliged to see a multitude of vexing dermatologic problems. For those oriented toward cardiology, hematology, etc, the sudden requirement to deal with unfamiliar skin things sends one scurrying nervously to the library on frequent occasions. There are abundant tomes available, but many are out of date, others are laden with ponderous microscopic morphology and pathology, some lack worthwhile colored photographs, and most seem reluctant to deal with the nuts and bolts of management.

Now comes a book which seems to fill the bill. It is the first multi-authored (would you believe 176!) text on treatment. It is packed with 76 excellent color photographs of common and uncommon dermal perturbations, and the discussions of treatment are current, feasible and comprehensive.

There are three major divisions: (1) dermatologic procedures (including hair transplantation procedures, hypnotherapy, topical treatment, cytotoxic agents and intralesional therapy); (2) therapeutic management (which is remarkably comprehensive, including dermatologic manifestations of systemic diseases, malignancies, and the vast area of skin woes from acne to yaws); and (3) a drug index in which pharmacist T. H. Brown provides formulas, drug descriptions, modes of action, and adverse reactions. This section is a most valuable adjunct to the text.

The various subjects, each written by one or two authors, vary in quality; some are brief to the point of being terse, others are quite detailed. Each discussion, regardless of brevity, is attended by several references, some as recent as 1968; others cite classic papers (such as Rendu, 1896). Pertinent editor's notes are sprinkled throughout the text adding small gems of current information. It is a book for scanning and spot reading for specific information. It does not seem designed for cover to cover study.

I was intrigued by "tree-woods, lichens, and liverwarts, problems arising from contact with" (which reminded me of Thurber's great-aunt who died of the oak blight or was it Sequoisis?); I was charmed by the presentation describing the cultivation of hair on previously barren slopes, impressed with the detailed presentation of dyslipidoses, and pleased with the first person style of several of the authors.

The only disquieting note was a contradiction in the Preface. Dermatologist-editor Stewart Maddin says "Considerable effort has been expended in making available not only specific and detailed information concerning the therapeutic agents of choice, but also the methods of detecting and preventing untoward side affects that may occur." And this most laudible undertaking brought cheers from the gallery. But on the very next page under Notice he says, "Care has been taken that the dosage schedules are those recommended by the manufacturers."

Zounds! This would imply that not one of Maddin's 176 stalwart, free-thinking coauthors disagreed with the anonymous authors of package inserts! That would be an amazing coincidence, I did not check it out, but I hope it is not so.

Despite this distressing sign of the times, Maddin's book emerges as the best reference source on management of dermatologic problems that has crossed my desk in recent recollection. I predict the sturdy binding will get a rigorous test in years to come, since "Maddin" should become a worthy addition to the pivot and reach the shelf of every working, would-be dermatologist.

ROBERT H. MOSER, MD
Wailuku, Hawaii

Communications to this Department may be sent directly to Robert H. Moser, MD, the Maui Medical Group, Maui Professional Center, Wailuku, Maui, Hawaii 96793, or to the Chief Editor for transmittal to him.

Antimicrobial Agents and Chemotherapy—1969. Proceedings of the Ninth Interscience Conference on Antimicrobial Agents and Chemotherapy, Washington, DC, 27-29 October 1969. Edited by Gladys L Hobby. Price $15. Pp 510. American Society for Microbiology and Williams & Wilkins Co, Baltimore, 1970.

Although this volume is featured as the Transactions of the Ninth Annual Conference on Antimicrobial Agents and Chemotherapy held under the sponsorship of the American Society for Microbiology, it is, in fact, part of a longer continuous series of similar conferences, having the same general objectives, involving similar groups of participants and dating back to 1953. In that year, the First Antibiotic Symposium was held in Washington on October 28 to 30 under the chairmanship of Henry Welch, Director of the Division of Antibiotics of the Food and Drug Administration, and under the joint sponsorship of that agency and of the journal *Antibiotics and Chemotherapy* which was jointly edited and published by Welch with Felix Marti-Ibanez. The transactions of that symposium were published in a volume entitled *Antibiotics Annual 1953-1954* with the same editors and publishers. Similar conferences were held under the same auspices in October of each year for the next seven years, the last one, in 1959, being recorded in *Antibiotics Annual 1959-1960*.

As a result of some internal problems within the FDA, the sponsorship of the conference in 1960 was assumed by the Society of Industrial Microbiology, and it was organized and held that year under the chairmanship of Lloyd G. Herman of the National Institute of Health. The transactions of that conference were published by the sponsoring Society under the title *Antimicrobial Agents–1960.* In the following year the American Society for Microbiology assumed the sponsorship of the annual symposiums under the title *Interscience Conference on Antimicrobial Agents and Chemotherapy* (commonly referred to as ICAAC) and its transactions were published in the volume entitled *Antimicrobial Agents and Chemotherapy–1961.*

Since then the ICAAC conferences have been held annually under the same sponsorship, and the first day of that conference has been sponsored jointly with the Infectious Diseases Society of America, which has held its meeting on the preceding two days. The editors of the new series of the annual volumes of *Antimicrobial Agents and Chemotherapy* are appointed by the editorial committee of the American Society for Microbiology, and they are charged with maintaining the high quality and scientific and literary standards demanded of all publications of the Society.

The editor of *Antimicrobial Agents and Chemotherapy–1969* is Gladys L. Hobby, and this is the fifth consecutive annual volume for which she has served in this capacity. Throughout these years Hobby has taken full advantage of a large editorial board of authorities in various scientific disciplines and she has not hesitated to call on many outside consultants to review the manuscripts. The papers are required to conform to the style of the other publications of the American Society for Microbiology. As a result, these well-edited and printed volumes, handsomely bound in hard covers, represent a useful and authoritative contribution to the scientific literature. Although published annually they are recognized as offering primary scientific papers and have been indexed and abstracted along with general scientific and medical periodicals.

In the opening communication at the First Antibiotic Symposium in 1953, Marti-Ibanez noted that this was the first time that research workers from various disciplines, including clinicians, academicians, chemists, and bacteriologists got together with the single purpose of studying antibiotics from various points of view, thus marking it as an event of historic significance. The conferences have continued to bring together scientists from universities, hospitals, industrial laboratories, and also clinicians interested in the development and application of antimicrobial agents for the therapy of infections and neoplastic diseases, thus truly justifying the title of the conferences.

E. M. Foster, then president of the American Society for Microbiology, in the preface to the current volume, points out that when the society assumed the sponsorship of these interdisciplinary conferences it was a new venture for that society. But they soon recognized the need for a mechanism through which microbiologists, chemists, geneticists, physiologists, clinicians and, in fact, all scientists with an interest in antimicrobial agents and chemotherapy could meet and exchange information. This need, and the fact that it has become recognized is attested by the fact that the average attendance at the conferences has more than doubled in the past nine years. The proceedings of these conferences have become a valuable repository of information on the latest developments in the field in this country, and to some extent also in foreign countries, and have thus served a very valuable purpose.

As in previous volumes, the present one includes some general reviews and communications, (91 in number) dealing with specific antimicrobials including antiviral agents, their action in vitro and in experimental infections, their pharmacokinetics, mechanisms of action, and of resistance at the molecular level and reports of their clinical application in the control of infections in humans. The first communication is the presidential address by Albert B. Sabin on the "Control of Infectious Diseases," a thoughtful and concise review of the current status and of the prospects for the future. This is followed by four papers dealing with various aspects of the use of "Antibiotics as Probes to Elucidate Cell Biochemistry" by Vernon Bryson and his coworkers; Bernard B. Davis; P. J. F. Henderson and H. A. Lardy; and Berton C. Pressman. The individual communications that follow include new findings about well established antimicrobials and detailed presentations of totally new agents some of which were soon to become available and others of general interest but not likely to achieve important therapeutic status.

This reviewer, who has participated actively in nearly all of the antibiotic conferences since the first one in 1953, considers these volumes of their transactions a most valuable source of information because they contain the primary reports on nearly all the important aspects of the origin, development, properties, potential uses, and early clinical reports of nearly all of the new and important antimicrobial agents.

The present volume is of superior quality, for which its hard working editor deserves most of the credit. It is strongly recommended as a useful and reliable sourcebook to all scientists and clinicians interested in infectious diseases and in the basic information concerning the development, properties, and uses of the major specific antimicrobial agents and chemotherapeutic agents for managing these diseases.

MAXWELL FINLAND, MD
Boston

Annual Review of Pharmacology, vol 10. By Henry W Elliott, editor; Windsor C Cutting, Robert H Dreisbach, associate editors. Price, $10. Pp 505. Annual Reviews Inc, 4139 El Camino Way, Palo Alto, Calif 94306, 1970.

The tenth annual issue of this fine series, *Annual Review of Pharmacology*, vol 10, 1970 is a feast with several prize courses. I can single out only a few of the 24 courses or chapters in this short review. My choice of which of the chapters upon which to comment corresponds to my own bias of what I think is important.

If this were a wholly clinically oriented text I would choose to comment on chapter subjects on an existential basis, what can help a reader here and now in his daily work. The approach in this series is designed primarily to report what has been recently done in an area from a pharmacological standpoint and also, by extrapolation on what the future may hold. However, the *Annual Review of Pharmacology* is nonetheless of use or interest to the clinician.

Drug metabolism is a dynamic, viable study, subject to change due to discovery of new facts and what is as important, new views or interpretations. There are three separate chapters on drug metabolism in this book. Schreiber's chapter, "The Metabolic Transformation of Drugs" clearly points to the fact that in a drug's trek through the body biotransformation takes place. For that—among other reasons—radioactivity of a drug as measured in tissues or as excreted is not necessarily the same substance as introduced into the body. Biotransformations of several substances are briefly brought out in this chapter, as for example, diazepam (Valium), chlordiazepoxide hydrochloride (Librium), norepinephrine and epinephrine, mescaline, perazine (Taxilan), and diethylpropion hydrochloride (Tenuate). The study of biotransformation often shows relationships and contradistinctions between or among drugs, and at times it becomes possible to draw correlations in their action.

Lasagna's chapter, "Challenges in Drug Evaluation in Man" cites some of current concepts. One example: it is not so much a question if a drug has a therapeutic effect, but rather how does that effect compare to that of similar drugs or placebos. The chapter recounts some of the ways that these evaluations are done, offers notions in this activity as well as criteria relevant to these questions, and also, what variables in a study may contribute to results. A corollary to this is an evaluation of toxicity, immediate or deferred. Biotransformation is implicit here too.

While we emphasize that species difference is an important aspect in evaluating a drug, nonetheless, we frequently refer to the effect of a drug on man, when actually the study done was on rats. Then, to refine techniques, we add several other species of animals. But this does not solve the problem, the effects of a drug in ten species does not entitle us to extrapolate ten times as validly on the effect of that drug in man. It is not a question of discarding animal data on drugs but of knowing the differences. It is gratifying therefore to find Hucker's chapter, "Species Differences in Drug Metabolism."

That chapter recites the findings in various animals of a number of drugs, such as imipramine hydrochloride (Tofranil), chloroquine, aminopyrine, phenylbutazone (Butazolidin), amines as amphetamine, diphenhydramine hydrochloride (Benadryl); also atropine, aspirin, indomethacin (Indocin), procaine. The fact remains that due to species difference the predictive effect in man, from data derived in animals, is not reliable. Hucker points out that this predictive facility must await better understanding of metabolism.

Possibly the most engrossing chapter is Breckenridge's "Cyclic AMP (Adenosine Monophosphate) and Drug Action." Perhaps no other substance is as protean in its distribution and function. Formed from ATP—the energy source in which thousands of reactions are involved—it is a fact that hardly a tissue or a biochemical event can be said to be outside of the scope of ATP. This chapter presents a broad but not comprehensive review of the subject.

Other chapters among the 24 in this book which deserve mention include nonsteroid antifertility agents which comprises discussion of inflammation and methods of testing those agents, L-asparaginase metabolism, antifertility agents, and particularly inhibitors of adrenal steroid biosynthesis, the uses and the agents. As usual in previous volumes, Chauncey Leake's "Review of Reviews" lends focus and proportion to the advances in pharmacology. I wish, however, that trade names would have accompanied the generic names, as most drugs are often better known by their trade names.

ERWIN DI CYAN, PhD
New York

The Coronary Care Unit. By WJ Grace, V Keyloun. Price, not given. Appleton-Century-Crofts Inc, Meredith Corp, 35 W 32nd St, New York, 1970.

This book is a guide to the operation of a coronary care unit based on the practice and the experiences of the authors. The format is excellent. It opens with a description of the natural history of patients with acute myocardial infarction and closes by emphasizing the necessity for an intermediate coronary care unit. In between these two chapters, the major problem areas in management of patients with myocardial infarction are considered.

Although the authors make a laudable plea for avoiding the use of new terms that contribute little or nothing to a better understanding of fundamental mechanisms (page 148), they descend to terms such as "coronoid," "coronette" and "mitral madness." The example chosen to illustrate pulsus alternans, is not the classic form. Throughout the book there is unnecessary repetition which detracts from this otherwise concise volume.

The book is intended as a guide for those just starting a new coronary care facility. It could have been of greater value if many of the organizational problems had been dealt with in greater depth. Overall, this work should prove to be of particular help to interns and residents assigned to a coronary care unit.

SHAHBUDIN H. RAHIMTOOLA, MD
Chicago

The Reticuloendothelial System. By AE Stuart. Price, $19.50. Pp 255, with 185 figures, 66 in color. Williams & Wilkins Co, 428 E Preston St, Baltimore 21202, 1970.

With the recent developments in immunology, particularly the immunology of tissue transplantation and cellular interaction, there is a real need for a thorough and lucid discussion of the reticuloendothelial system (RES). It is intended to provide basic text for beginners; it is certainly a welcome addition to the medical literature. The nine chapters deal with the anatomy, physiology, and responses to stimulation and depression of the reticuloendothelial system. The two chapters concerning anatomy and responses to stimulation and depression of the RES are particularly well written. The quality of the color plates is excellent. Vital staining technics are used throughout to identify and trace the reticuloendothelial cells to study the functions of the RES in lipid metabolism, experimental infections and immunologic reactions.

The book, however, is written largely from a histologist's point of view. A good part of the text and most of the pictures deal primarily with tissue changes of the RES rather than cytologic changes of the macrophages. The dynamic character of the macrophage is not well pointed out. Since the trend of present research on RES has moved from tissue to cell, ie, the macrophages, a dynamic discussion of these cells should have been more prominent. Undoubtedly, this is a good reference book for those interested in problems of the RES; however, individuals more interested in the biology of macrophages will find themselves in need of additional source material.

LUNG T. YAM, MD
Boston

Handbook of Legal Medicine. By Alan R Moritz, MD; R Crawford Morris, LLB. Price, $8.75. Pp 238. CV Mosby Co, 3207 Washington Blvd, St. Louis 63103, 1970.

To paraphrase: here is almost everything you wanted to know about medical jurisprudence (. . . but were afraid to ask because no one ever mentioned such things during medical training). Although the book is titled a *Handbook of Legal Medicine*, the title is somewhat misleading. Legal medicine usually refers to medical knowledge applied to the administration of justice; medical jurisprudence, on the other hand, pertains to legal principles affecting medical practice. It is the latter, at the present time, which commands the great interest of the medical profession. While the book contains some information seemingly slanted more toward the legal profession (eg, some very basic definitions of medical terms), just about all the data of value to the lawyer is, in reality, even more helpful and practical for the medical practitioner.

Within a little more than 200 pages of text, there are 43 fact-packed chapters (some no more than one page long, yet encompassing a wealth of pragmatism). The book is divided into two major subdivisions. The first is headed "Scientific Medicolegal Investigation," and begins with the "Physician's Responsibility in Cases of Death by Violence or From Unexplained Causes." From there on the topics include the identity of the dead person, how to determine the time of death, bullet wounds, and the battered child syndrome, to mention only a few chapters.

The second half is called "Physician and Patient—Physician and the Law." Here, nearly all aspects of how the law may impose itself on the physician-patient relationship, as well as on the physician's relationship with his hospital, government officials, and subordinates are discussed. The gamut runs from "A" (abortion, adoption, artificial insemination) to "W" (workman's compensation, wrongful death actions), in alphabetical order. In between, practical, pertinent, topics are found: physician liability for the acts of others, judicial interpretation of patient consent to diagnostic procedures, as well as treatment, and the role of the medical society under the law.

Now that the essence of this excellent book has been outlined, it is only right to look at a few topics with a more meticulous eye. One of the shortest chapters (inversely proportional to its practical importance) is entitled "Proximate Cause"; it is a subject about which most physicians are quite unaware. Simply put, if a patient's act causes harm or damage to himself, and it can be shown that physician was in any way (no matter how slight) negligent in allowing that patient to cause harm or damage, then the physician can be made partially or totally responsible for his patient's actions. Although this book does not detail any specific cases, only recently two physicians from opposite ends of the mainland United States were forced to make tremendous financial restitution to victims of their patient's destructive acts. In both instances, remarkably similar, the patients had epilepsy, and the physicians did not report the fact to their state authorities as required by law. When the patients were involved in auto accidents which resulted in deaths as well as damages, their physicians were considered to be the "proximate cause" of the accidents and were held financially responsible. In California, this year, a statute was proposed that would have made physicians proximately liable for accidents caused by drivers, where the physician was aware that the drivers could be considered alcoholics and did not report same to state officials. While that proposed law was not passed, it should offer adequate warning of the "handwriting on the wall." California already requires physicians to report patients who might suffer "lapse of consciousness" while driving no matter what the etiology.

Another chapter on being a medical witness and the limits that can be imposed on a physician's testimony should set many a mind at ease. Although reported statistics vary, it is said that nine out of every ten physicians are so subpoenaed to testify in court at some time during their active years. Because there is more than an even chance that someday you will be required to offer your opinions about the medical aspects of a lawsuit, the book's brief "cookbook style" advice on what you can and cannot be made to testify about, what support you may rely on (textbooks, models, diagrams, records, etc) and how you might well be "tricked" while testifying, are of great value before a court appearance.

Such obvious endorsement of this book is not meant to imply that there are no errors within its pages. One example can be found where it is stated that a hospital, as such, does not practice medicine. The Supreme Court of Illinois has already reversed this attitude (*Darling vs Charleston Community Memorial Hospital, 33 Ill, 2d 326*). And to carry this even further, the Court of Appeals of the state of New York has now placed "proximate liability" on physicians where hospitals are considered to be practicing medicine (*Toth vs Community Hospital at Glen Cove, 239 NE 2d 368)*.

But the most flagrant error of all is to be found in the book's foreword, where it is printed that criminal justice needs truth and that such truth can be supplied through psychiatric analysis for criminal intent. Contrast this unscientifically founded presumption with the words of John M. Suarez, assistant professor of psychiatry in residence at the University of California in Los Angeles School of Medicine. In a talk before the American Psychiatric Association (*J Forensic Sci* **12**:172, 1967), Suarez states: "The moment that a psychiatrist is pressed to give his opinion [in court], which is nothing more than his personal guess or his moral conviction, there appears something "tangible" and "scientific" [about his testimony]." A physician's "personal guess" or "moral conviction" does not provide the "truth" needed by criminal justice. Suarez went on to say: "Under the guise of science, part or all of the [law's] responsibility is handed over to the psychiatrist." And then he blatantly admits that: "Psychiatry, whether from ignorance, insecurity, or grandiosity, accepted this Trojan Horse unreluctantly." While the book's propagation of such false and misleading information tends to diminish the overall merit of this work, it does cite the need for a more comprehensive work on psychiatric testimony, and, all too clearly, points out the "black sheep" within legal medicine.

Still, it is not unfair to say that the application of the few hours required to read this handbook could markedly reduce the present-day malpractice problem facing the medical profession. It's real value is in the prevention of misunderstanding between physicians and their patients, as well as between physicians and those on the legal side of the fence. Facts have shown that it is misunderstanding more than actual negligence that causes so many lawsuits against physicians. Since it seems impossible to make patients understand all the ramifications of medical practice, it is only right that physicians devote more of their time to the problem as a preventive, rather than defensive, measure.

EDWARD R. PINCKNEY, MD, LLB
Beverly Hills, Calif

BOOKS RECEIVED

Recent Advances in Neurology. By F Plum, MD. Price, $8. Pp 264, with 35 illustrations. FA Davis Co, 1915 Arch St, Philadelphia 19103, 1969.

Ophthalmic Plastic Surgery, ed 14. By SA Fox, MS, MD, FACS. Price, $29.75. Pp 590. Grune & Stratton Inc, 757 Third Ave, New York 10017, 1970.

The Earlier Gain and the Later Loss of Cortical Bone: In Nutritional Perspective. By SM Garn, PhD. Price, $12. Pp 146, with illustrations. Charles C Thomas Publisher, 301-327 E Lawrence Ave, Springfield, Ill 62703, 1970.

Symposium on Ocular Anti-Inflammatory Therapy. Edited by HE Kaufman, MD. Price, $19. Pp 272, with 75 illustrations. Charles C Thomas Publisher, 301-327 E Lawrence Ave, Springfield, Ill 62703, 1970.

Allergic Contact Dermatitis in the Guinea Pig. By B Magnusson, MD, AM Kligman, PhD, MD. Price, $17.50. Pp 141. Charles C Thomas Publisher, 301-327 E Lawrence Ave, Springfield, Ill, 1970.

Proceedings of the First National Conference on Electronics in Medicine. By Electronics Management Center. Price, $14.50. Pp 211, with many figures. McGraw-Hill Book Co Inc, 330 W 42nd St, New York 10036, 1969.

Human Nutrition and Dietetics. By Sir S Davidson, MD; R Passmore, MD. Price, $20. Pp 899, with few illustrations. Williams & Wilkins Co, 428 E Preston St, Baltimore 21202, 1969.

Häufige Internistische Notfälle. By RH Salter, MB, BS, MRCP. Price, not given. Pp 156. FK Schattauer Verlag, New York, 1970.

ERRATUM

In the Original Article entitled "Australia Antigen and Viral Hepatitis in Drug Abusers" by Alton I. Sutnick, MD, and co-workers which appeared in the May issue of the ARCHIVES (**127**:939-941, 1971), the following errors appeared: In Table 1, under *P*, the first brace should apply to a comparison between lines 1 and 2, Drug abusers and Multiply transfused patients. The second brace applies to lines 1 and 3 and is correct. Similarly, in Table 2, the first brace under *P* should apply to lines 1 and 2, Hepatitis in drug abusers and Posttransfusion hepatitis. The second brace applies to items 1 and 3 and is correct.

Internal medicine at large

Myocardial perfusion

San Diego investigators are applying a technique used to examine circulation in the lung to the study of myocardial perfusion.

The diagnostic technique is based on the principle of capillary blockade. Particles of macroaggregated albumin of less than 80μ in diameter were labelled with 99m technetium or iodine 131 and injected into 29 patients. One patient had a saphenous vein bypass graft, and the other 28 patients were suspected of having coronary artery disease.

Allan L. Simon, MD, of the University Hospital of San Diego County, reported the study at the Association of University Radiologists meeting in Durham, NC. He said that this technique seems better than other types of radionuclide coronary angiography because:

- multiple views can be seen with a single injection
- various coronary branches can be examined by using different radionuclides
- the image can be controlled well by selective catheterization, and
- background radiation is all but eliminated.

Scintograms of at least three, and usually four views of the heart were taken. "Large myocardial perfusion defects were found in six patients that correlated well with areas of ischemia and localized ventricular wall motion abnormalities associated with coronary atherosclerosis, with or without major vessel occlusion," said Dr. Simon to the medical audience.

Two radionuclides were injected into 13 patients, and the investigator said he found this technique valuable for studying regional myocardial perfusion.

The investigator said the particles disappear within 24 hours and that there is no danger to the patient if fewer than 800,000 of the tiny particles are injected.

Another investigator disagreed, however, and said that the procedure could not be called safe without more extensive testing. Herbert L. Abrams, MD, chairman of the Department of Radiology at Harvard Medical School, said that too few patients have been studied, and that while 17 dogs had also been tested by the San Diego investigators, the animals had no preexisting circulatory complications. Dr. Abrams also said there is a need for more data on circulatory function before and after scanning.

"It's perfectly clear that sooner or later, if you have knocked out 800,000 vessels of 80μ size or less, one may come across individuals who are at a threshold level–individuals who have a severely impaired coronary circulation. I don't think you can say, unequivocally, this is a safe procedure under these conditions," Dr. Abrams said.

Dr. Simons replied that the dogs had received up to 30 times the equivalent clinical dose without any adverse effects, and that all 29 patients apparently were unharmed by the procedure. "Electrocardiograms and continuous arterial pressure recording taken during and after the injections showed no changes," Dr. Simon said.

Highlights This Month

Children born to drug-addicted mothers may be protected against excess bilirubin accumulation . . . page 186.

New York investigators look into the relationship between alcohol and liver disease . . . page 187.

Cryosurgery is described as the preferred treatment for chronic rhinitis . . . page 192.

Internists in the news . . . pages 193 and 196.

Internal medicine at large

Bilirubin levels

Opiates passed from the addicted mother to the infant may enhance transferase activity in the addicted newborn and prevent excess bilirubin accumulation, New York investigators believe.

A group at Montefiore Hospital and Medical Center, New York City, were surprised to find that an infant born to a heroin-addicted mother had normal bilirubin levels. This was true even though the child was undergoing withdrawal, and had pneumonia, anemia, and a positive Coombs test. The highest bilirubin level found, on the fourth day of life, was 4.2 mg/100 ml.

Gerald Nathenson, MD, and his coworkers, Michael I. Cohen, MD, Helen McNamara, MD, and Iris F. Litt, MD, conducted more studies after this case. Dr. Nathenson told the American Pediatric Society in Atlantic City, NJ, that in a review of 52 infants born with heroin addiction and treated with paregoric, "the clinical observation of significant jaundice occurred only twice, and few bilirubin determinations were considered indicated in this group of newborns."

Next the team began a prospective study comparing 18 addicted and 35 normal newborns. They found that although the mean birth weight of the addicted infants was 2,380 gm compared to 3,146 gm for normal infants, bilirubin levels were similar. Four infants were premature in the addicted group, and six other babies of low birth weight were dysmature.

In a control study comparing 51 mice addicted to morphine sulfate with 58 mice given comparable amounts of saline, the investigators found that the addicted mice produced significantly greater amounts of bilirubin glucuronide. Similar increases of glucuronidated salicylamide were found in the urine of two addicted infants compared to two normal newborns.

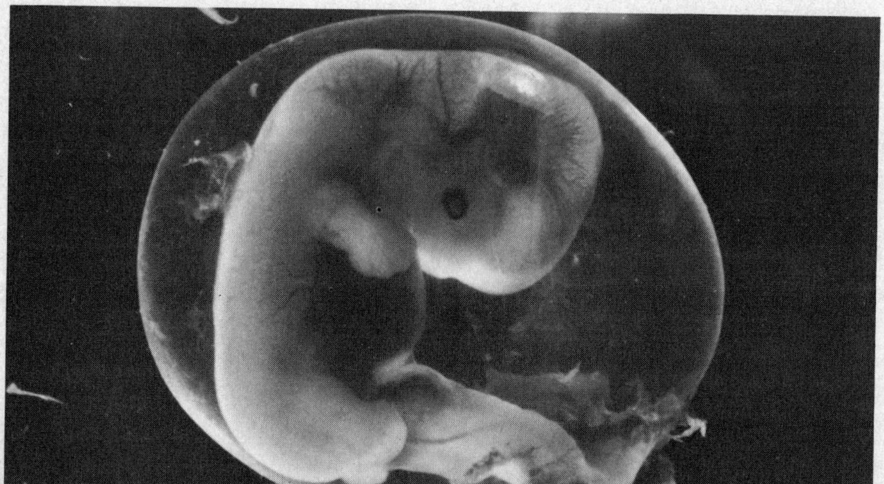

"12 mm Human Embryo" received honorable mention in Medical Photography: Student/House Staff Division, 1971 SAMA Medical Art Competition. Milton M. Rowley, MD, photographer.

Febrile disorders

Mathematical computations are being combined with a dye test to aid in a differential diagnostic problem: Fever of uncertain origin.

"There's nothing magic about this," says Ralph D. Feigin, MD, who—along with colleagues at St. Louis Children's Hospital—developed the formulas.

"It's a tool, a guide. You still need a detailed history and a thorough physical examination. This doesn't obviate the need for a physician."

However, properly used in connection with a complete history, physical findings, and laboratory results, the computations should help provide an accurate diagnosis in febrile disorders, Dr. Feigin and colleagues feel.

The test uses nitroblue tetrazolium dye, which has been proposed for detecting chronic granulomatous disease in children and for differentiating between bacterial and nonbacterial disease. (Byunghak Park, MD, of the University of Minnesota Medical School, and colleagues, noted that an increased number of neutrophils—phagocytizing leukocytes—from children with bacterial infections would reduce nitroblue tetrazolium dye in vitro.) The pale yellow powder is reduced to a blue-black formazan pigment when taken up by the cell.

Using the nitroblue tetrazolium (NBT) dye test, the St. Louis researchers determine the percentage of leukocytes from the patient's blood sample which have taken up the powder and reduced it to formazan. They also count the absolute number.

These two values then are plotted on a nomogram with the percentage of NBT-positive cells on the abscissa and the absolute number of NBT-positive cells as the ordinate. According to the point where the two values intersect, the patient is categorized as:

- Normal (usually controls).
- Suffering from viral infection, partially treated bacterial infection, or non-infectious febrile illness.
- Suffering from untreated bacterial infection.
- Suffering from ineffectively treated bacterial infection.

There is no correlation between the percentage of NBT-positive cells, and the patient's white blood cell count or temperature at the time the test is performed, emphasizes Dr. Feigin. The technique now has been used with approximately 500 patients, and correlation of categorization with subsequent patient history so far shows an accuracy of better than 70%.

The test requires only an hour, compared with two or three days for many laboratory tests. Dr. Feigin and his colleagues see possible applications also as a guide to efficacy of therapy, especially in bacterial fevers.

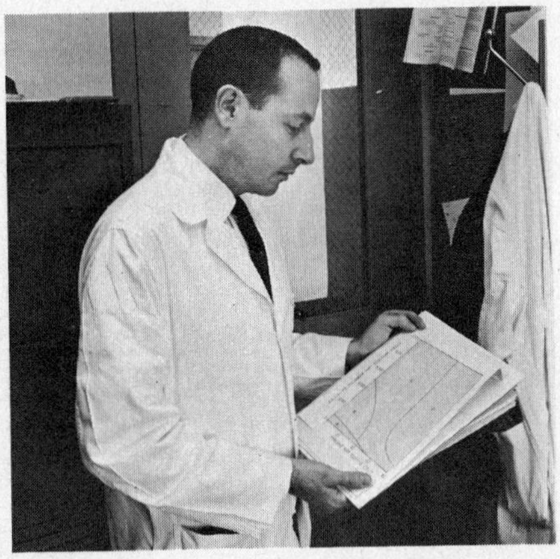

Dr. Feigin studying a nomogram.

Working with Dr. Feigin, who is assistant professor of pediatrics at Washington University School of Medicine, are Penelope G. Schackelford, MD, and Sung C. Choi, PhD.

Alcohol and the liver

Liver disease in alcoholics may have nothing to do with poor dietary habits, a study in baboons indicates.

Baboons on a high-protein, low-fat diet with plenty of vitamins and minerals quickly developed hepatic damage if 36% of their calories were supplied by ethanol. This percentage of alcohol consumption is lower than that of many alcoholics who take in as much as 50% of their calories in ethanol, according to the investigator, Charles S. Lieber, MD, professor of medicine at Mt. Sinai School of Medicine, New York City, and chief of the Section on Liver Diseases and Nutrition, Bronx VA Hospital.

Dr. Lieber and co-workers controlled the diets of seven pairs of baboons for two years. Caloric consumption in the control animals of each pair consisted of 20% protein, 14% fat, and 66% carbohydrate. The other seven test animals were given the same high-protein, low-fat regimen, but carbohydrates were reduced to 30% of caloric intake, and 36% of the calories were given in the form of ethanol.

The liver damage which developed in the test group soon after the diets were started included a ten-fold increase in triglycerides after three to five months; a 25-fold increase within 15 to 19 months; steatosis; enlarged, distorted mitochondria; and endoplasmic reticulum changes.

When another group of animals was placed on a low-protein diet, their livers remained normal until the time that ethanol was added. They then displayed hepatic abnormalities similar to the seven animals in the previous test group.

Chinese journalism

Long before anyone ever heard of ping pong diplomacy, a unique medical journal kept a communication channel open between Red China and the West.

The journal contained articles and summaries, translated to English, from the Chinese Medical Association's journal and other Chinese medical publications.

That channel closed abruptly two years ago and there is no indication whether the apparent mild thaw in the relations between the United States and Communist China may bring about a reappearance of the Peking-produced publication.

Even should the journal's circulation in the West resume, months may

continued

Internal medicine at large

Journalism continued

pass before American medical librarians become aware of its re-appearance. In the past, the monthly (titled *Chinese Medical Journal* until its October 1966 name change to *China's Medicine*) rarely reached American medical libraries until about six months after publication.

The December 1968 issue arrived in mid-1969, and after that *China's Medicine* simply stopped coming. The reason for this has never been explained. A clue to why the journal was produced and distributed in the first place may perhaps be found in Fu Lien-chang's presidential address to the Chinese Medical Association in July 1956:

"The subscription of the (then) *Chinese Medical Journal* in English also has increased, and it has exchange relations with 270 journals abroad, an important factor in our country's international interchange of information and research in medicine."

In announcing the name change to *China's Medicine* in 1966, the Chinese Medical Association reiterated that it would "welcome subscriptions and exchange." Among other things, the announcement said, the journal would report on:

- "Experience in medical research and clinical practice guided by the invincible thought of Mao Tse-tung."
- "Advances in the synthesis of modern medicine and traditional Chinese medicine."
- "New people and new things on the medical front resulting from the creative study and application of Mao Tse-tung's thought."

The last issues of *China's Medicine* that reached the United States contained articles on subjects in which medical interest has been rekindled with the recent slight opening of Communist China's door to Americans—acupuncture, rejoining of severed limbs, public health measures, and the "barefoot doctors" in rural areas. But half to two-thirds of the journal's fewer than 100 pages were usually filled by ideological articles.

These ideological articles occupied the front of the journal, following a photo of Mao on the frontispiece. The back of the journal contained articles with some bearing on medicine. But even these supposedly scientific articles were heavily flavored with ideology.

A report from a Shantung hospital (no individual authors listed) on a "Boy's Severed Arm Successfully Rejoined" in the November 1968 issue explains: "Our successful re-implantation of a completely amputated arm of a 7-year-old child once again testifies eloquently that Mao Tse-tung's thought is a spiritual atom bomb of infinite power."

The anonymous authors continued: "Since the report of the first case of successful clinical salvage of a completely amputated forearm in 1963, many hospitals, big and small, have successfully performed similar operations. These achievements are all victories of Mao Tse-tung's thought."

Mao's thought also played a part in medical education. Describing freshmen in a three-year medical training program, an anonymous author said

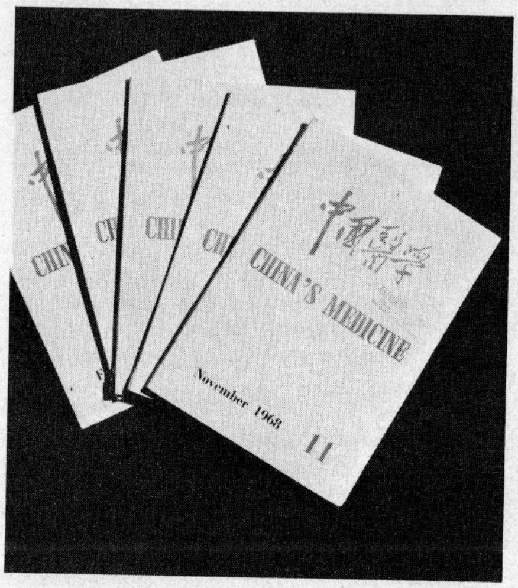

in the May 1968 issue:

"They can correctly prescribe many widely used drugs and can do acupuncture therapy for some 40 diseases, being familiar with more than 80 acupuncture points . . . peasants praise them as good students of Chairman Mao. . ."

Occasionally, *China's Medicine* offered space for rebuttals, as in August 1968 after a report of "successful Removal of a 45 kg Retroperitoneal Neurofibroma" from a 37-year-old woman living in a commune.

The original description of the 12-hour surgical procedure was critical of "so-called specialists and authorities" at a larger hospital who almost four years earlier had declined to operate on the woman. The follow-up article responded to criticism, that apparently had been voiced through the Soviet news agency TASS. "The Soviet revisionist renegade clique ranted that our 'reliance on Mao-Tse-tung's thought for carrying out the operation' was 'a matter of sheer absurdity.' This in itself unmasked your shameless betrayal of Marxism-Leninism," the retort stated.

In its last years, the journal emphasized the need for cooperation between physicians trained in traditional Chinese medicine and those with modern Western training. The final issues stressed the importance of semi-trained "barefoot doctors" and their right to prescribe drugs, which apparently, at least for a time in some places, was challenged by those with more medical training.

Recent reports from some observers who have visited Communist China suggest that venereal disease—an increasing health problem in many areas of the world—is under control there. As far back as October 1966, Ma Hai-teh of the Chinese Academy of Medical Sciences, Peking, wrote that China "in less than 15 years conquered venereal disease and eradicated it from almost the whole country."

As a result of overruling Soviet medical experts who wanted to continue using arsenicals in treating VD, and continued public health efforts, Ma Hai-teh predicted in that issue of *China's Medicine*, venereal disease in China "will be completely eradicated."

Herpesvirus

Although a direct link between herpesviruses and cancer has not been established, recent experiments show that the viruses may "transform" normal hamster embryo cells.

Furthermore, when these transformed embryo cells were subjected to a number of cell passages, and were then injected into newborn hamsters, one-third of the animals developed tumors.

Some of these hamster tumor cells were transplanted into another group of weanling hamsters, producing tumors in all of the animals within two weeks. The tumor cells differed morphologically from normal hamster embryo cells, and they showed no contact inhibition—a common property of cancer cells. The chromosomes of the tumor cells were broken and dislocated in much the same way as other kinds of hamster and human cells when they are exposed to herpes simplex virus.

The study, conducted at the Pennsylvania State University College of Medicine, was described at a meeting of the American Society for Microbiology in Minneapolis. Ronald Duff, PhD, assistant professor of microbiology, and Fred Rapp, PhD, professor and chairman of the Department of Microbiology at the medical school were co-workers on the project.

The investigators isolated the viruses from human cells and exposed them to ultraviolet irradiation. Irradiation eliminated the lethal activity of the viruses, which usually kill any cells they infect.

By preventing destruction of the infected cells, the investigators were able to study other effects the viruses produced besides causing cell destruction.

While the investigators could not isolate any virus from the tumor cells, they found herpesvirus antigen was present in a few of them. The researchers also found that when they mixed sera from the tumor-bearing animals with herpesvirus, the viral activity was reduced or neutralized for rabbit kidney cells.

It is often difficult to find evidence of virus in a cancer caused by that virus, and it is also possible that the irradiation made the cells incapable of proper reproduction, it was explained.

According to Drs. Rapp and Duff, the evidence is not conclusive that the herpesvirus actually transformed the normal cells to cancer cells. It is possible, they said, that the cells could have changed spontaneously, while the DNA from the herpesvirus became a part of these cells.

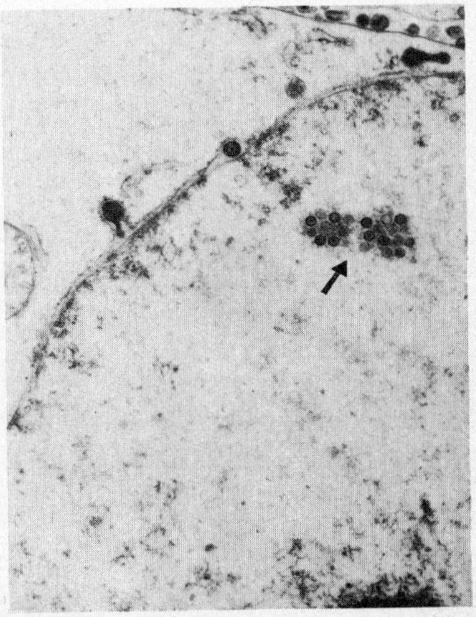

Electronmicrograph above illustrates a cluster of herpes simplex particles (arrow) in the nucleus of a human cell. Two particles can be seen leaving the cell's nucleus.

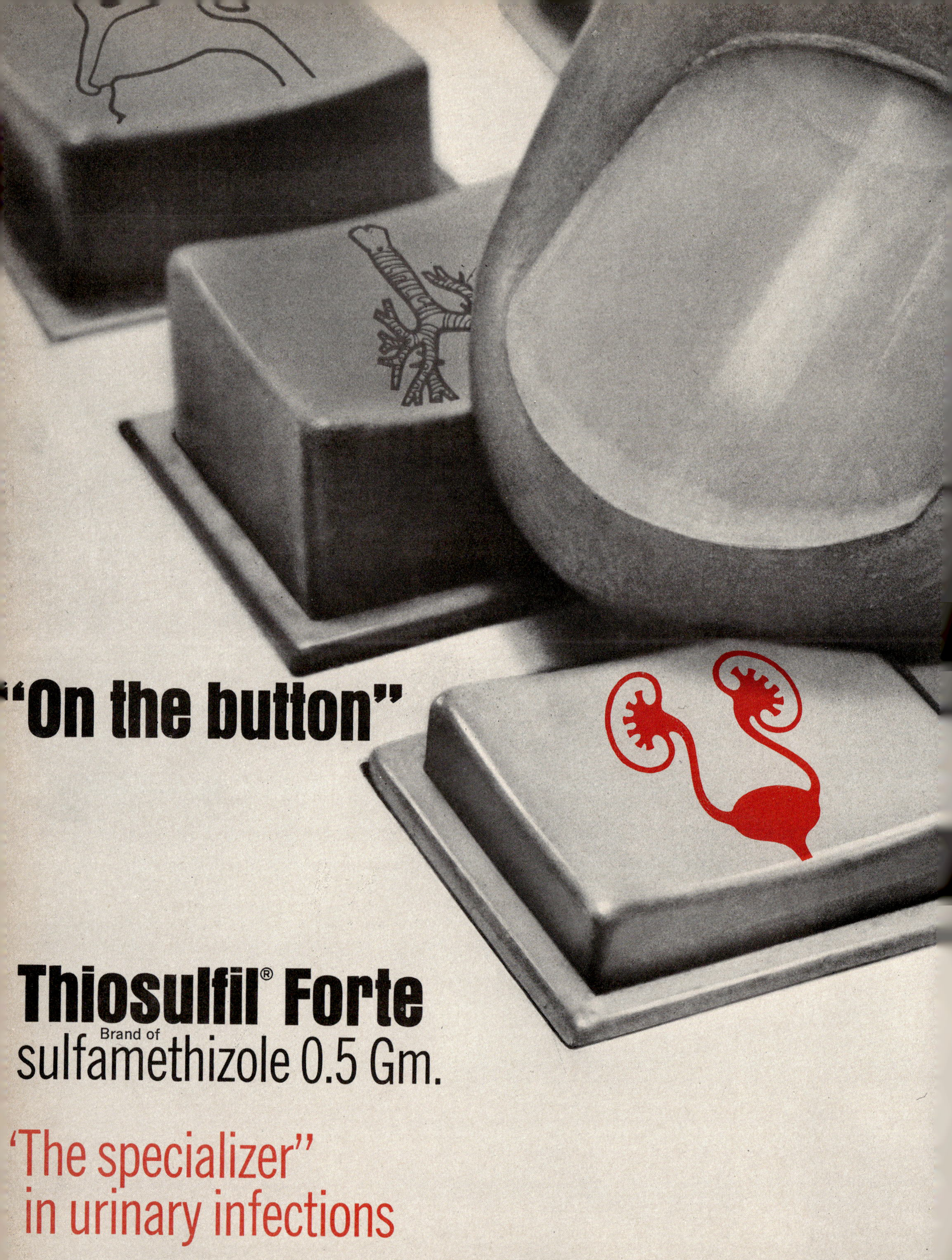
"On the button"
Thiosulfil® Forte
Brand of
sulfamethizole 0.5 Gm.
'The specializer"
in urinary infections

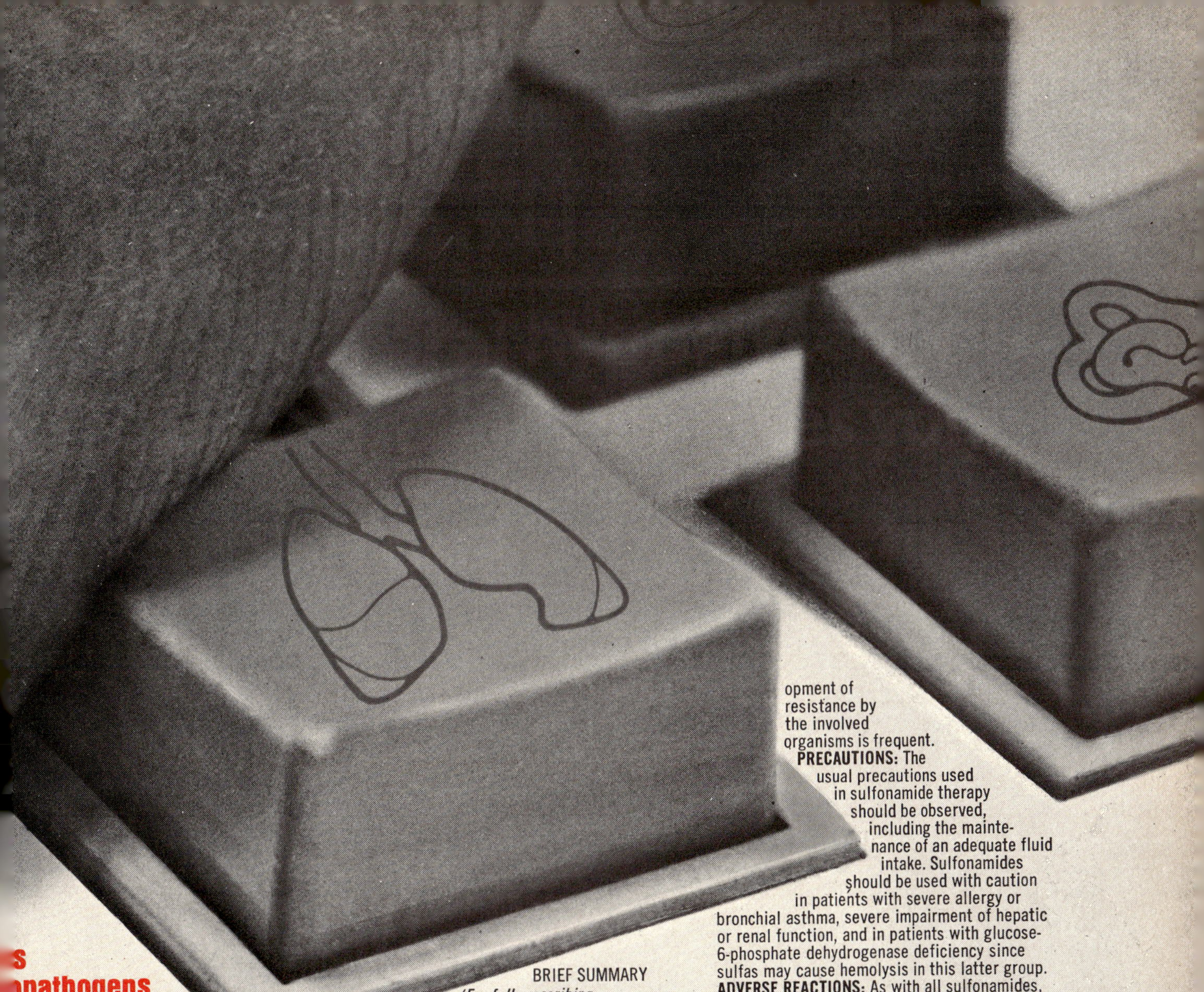

s
›pathogens
ere they live...
ard and fast!

A *true specific* in cystitis...
a *true specific* in pyelitis.
In fact, THIOSULFIL Forte
lfamethizole 0.5 Gm.) accumu-
›s so *little* in the respiratory
:t and other tissues that it has
y one indication—urinary
:t infections due to susceptible
anisms.
Rapidly absorbed and excreted,
IOSULFIL Forte delivers its
ent antibacterial action *locally*.
hin eight hours, about 80
cent of the drug is in the
ıary tract in free, active form—
ight the infection where it is.
The patient on THIOSULFIL
te uses less sulfonamide...
; more action for his money.
l there's no need for excessive
ling or priming doses.

BRIEF SUMMARY
(For full prescribing information, see package circular.)

THIOSULFIL® Forte (sulfamethizole 0.5 Gm.)
Bacteriostatic agent for use in Urinary Tract Infection (due to susceptible organisms)

INDICATIONS: THIOSULFIL is indicated in the treatment of acute and chronic urinary tract infections—cystitis, urethritis, prostatitis, pyelonephritis, and pyelitis—caused by susceptible bacteria, normally *Escherichia coli, Klebsiella aerobacter, Staphylococcus aureus, Proteus mirabilis,* and less frequently, *Proteus vulgaris.* As with most antibiotics and all antimicrobials, THIOSULFIL is most effective in acute, uncomplicated urinary tract infections. **CONTRAINDICATIONS:** Sulfonamides should not be used in patients hypersensitive to sulfa drugs. They should not be used in infants less than two months of age, in pregnancy at term, and during the nursing period because sulfonamides pass the placenta and are excreted in the milk and may cause kernicterus. **WARNINGS:** Sulfonamides should not be used to treat group A streptococci infections or their sequelae. The occurrence of sore throat, fever, pallor, purpura, or jaundice during sulfonamide administration may be an early indication of serious blood dyscrasias. Frequent blood counts and renal function tests should be carried out during sulfonamide treatment, especially during prolonged administration. Microscopic urinalyses should be done once a week when a patient is treated for longer than two weeks. Urine cultures should be made to confirm eradication of bacteriuria. (Para-aminobenzoic acid must be added to the culture media while the patient is on sulfonamide.) Because sulfonamides are bacteriostatic, development of resistance by the involved organisms is frequent. **PRECAUTIONS:** The usual precautions used in sulfonamide therapy should be observed, including the maintenance of an adequate fluid intake. Sulfonamides should be used with caution in patients with severe allergy or bronchial asthma, severe impairment of hepatic or renal function, and in patients with glucose-6-phosphate dehydrogenase deficiency since sulfas may cause hemolysis in this latter group. **ADVERSE REACTIONS:** As with all sulfonamides, the possibility of the following reactions exists: agranulocytosis, aplastic anemia, thrombocytopenia, leukopenia, hemolytic anemia, purpura, hypoprothrombinemia, methemoglobinemia, erythema multiforme (Stevens-Johnson Syndrome), generalized skin eruptions, exfoliative dermatitis, anaphylactoid reactions, periorbital edema, conjunctival and scleral injection, photosensitization, arthralgia, allergic myocarditis, drug fever, chills, toxic nephrosis with oliguria and anuria, periarteritis nodosum, L. E. phenomenon, hepatitis, pancreatitis, stomatitis, nausea, emesis, abdominal pains, diarrhea, anorexia, headache, peripheral neuritis, mental depression, convulsions, ataxia, hallucinations, tinnitus, vertigo, and insomnia. The sulfonamides bear certain chemical similarities to some goitrogens, diuretics (acetazolamide and the thiazides), and oral hypoglycemic agents. Goiter production, diuresis, and hypoglycemia have occurred rarely in patients receiving sulfonamides and cross-sensitivity may exist with these agents. However, the incidence of severe reactions following the use of THIOSULFIL (sulfamethizole) has been very low. **HOW SUPPLIED:** THIOSULFIL Forte—No. 786—Each tablet contains sulfamethizole 0.5 Gm. (scored), in bottles of 100 and 1,000. Also in unit dose package of 100. THIOSULFIL—No. 785—*Tablets*—Each tablet contains sulfamethizole 0.25 Gm. (scored), in bottles of 100 and 1,000. No. 914—*Suspension*—Each 5 cc. (teaspoonful) contains sulfamethizole 0.25 Gm., in bottles of 16 fluidounces.

Ayerst. AYERST LABORATORIES
New York, N.Y. 10017

7128

Internal medicine at large

Cryosurgery for rhinitis

Cryosurgery seems preferable to other surgical and non-surgical methods for treating patients with chronic rhinitis, a Yale physician reports.

James M. Ozenberger, MD, professor of otolaryngology at Yale University School of Medicine, told an audience at the Miami meeting of the Society for Cryosurgery that the freeze technique also appears useful for dealing with nasal tumors, polyps, or epistaxis. The cryoprobe lessens bleeding, makes the polyps easier to manage, and is not as irritating to the patient as electrocoagulation and electrocautery instruments, he said.

Dr. Ozenberger has found that oral decongestants, silver nitrate cautery, "painting" with phenol, surgical resection, and submucosal repository steroids and electrocautery are less effective than cryosurgery in treating chronic, non-allergic, rhinitis.

Cryosurgery causes the diseased mucosa of the inferior turbinate and surrounding tissue to die and then slough off in about three to five days. The tissue is replaced by more normal tissue within four to eight weeks. The investigator said that in treating 145 patients with the technique he always found the airways improved following surgery. In addition there was less secretion in most patients. The nasal mucosa has remained normal for up to two years after treatment.

The nose seems to reflect emotional stress in some people, Dr. Ozenberger said. During periods of anxiety, the parasympathetic nervous system stimulates secretion through the vidian nerve and causes the nasal "erectile" tissue to swell. Some people notice that in a stressful situation they sneeze more, or experience nasal congestion and increased secretion.

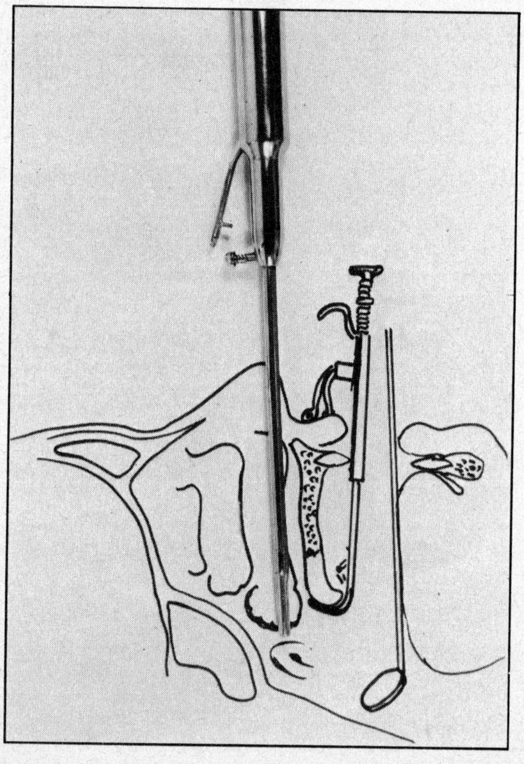

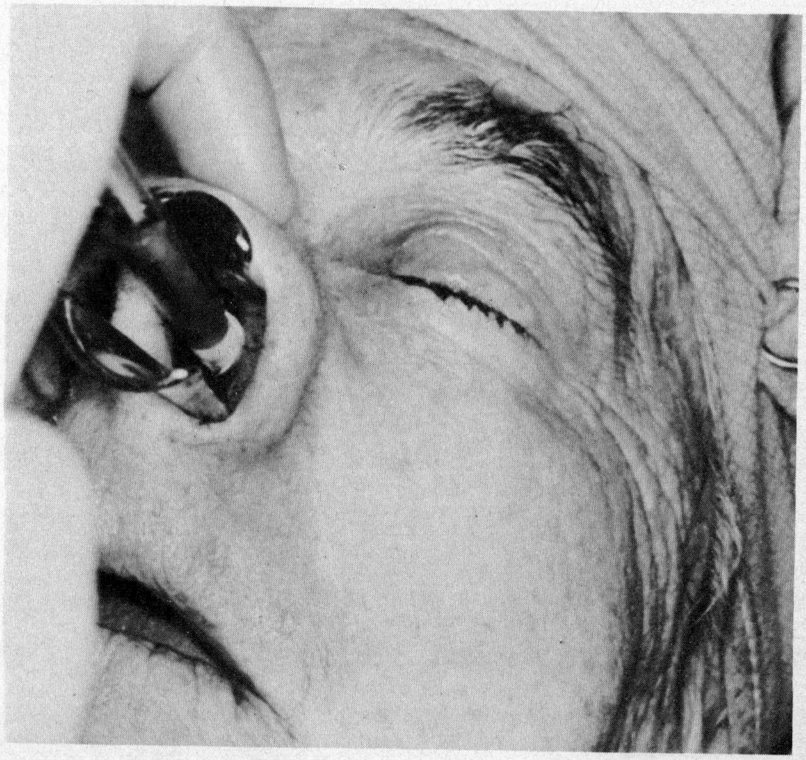

Diagram at left shows position of cryoprobe in patient's nose. The soft palate is retracted so that the physician can monitor the placement of the probe. Photograph shows treatment with Freon cryoprobe.

Jerry I. Newman, MD, will assume the position of associate dean of the Peoria School of Medicine where he will also be associate professor of medicine. The medical school was created by the University of Illinois College of Medicine, Chicago.

Sydney Stillman, MD, has become president of the Arthritis Foundation's American Rheumatism Association Section. He is also director of the Arthritis Clinical Research Center at Robert B. Brigham Hospital, Boston; associate clinical professor of medicine, Harvard Medical School; consulting physician in arthritis, West Roxbury VA Hospital, Mass; and associate visiting physician at Boston City Hospital.

John L. Decker, MD, has been named president-elect of the Arthritis Foundation's American Rheumatism Association Section. Dr. Decker serves as head of the Arthritis and Rheumatism Branch of the National Institute of Arthritis and Metabolic Diseases of the National Institutes of Health, and is a consultant in internal medicine at the Walter Reed Army Medical Center in Washington, DC, and at the National Naval Medical Center in Bethesda, Md.

The 1971 **ASPET Award for Experimental Therapeutics** was presented to **Elliot S. Vesell**, MD, at the meeting of the American Society for Experimental Therapeutics held in Chicago. Dr. Vesell is professor and chairman of the Department of Pharmacology at the Milton S. Hershey Medical Center of The Pennsylvania State University.

Samuel B. Guze, MD, will assume the position of vice-chancellor for medical affairs at the Washington University School of Medicine in St. Louis. The physician is also professor of psychiatry at the university and associate psychiatrist at Barnes and Renard Hospitals. **William H. Danforth**, MD, who was the previous vice-chancellor has now become chancellor for medical affairs.

Christopher C. Fordham III, MD, who has been dean of the school of medicine at the Medical College of Georgia, Augusta, for the past two years, will become dean of the University of North Carolina School of Medicine in September. **Isaac M. Taylor**, MD, the present dean of the North Carolina medical school, will return to teaching in the Department of Medicine.

David J. Albert, MD, has been chosen to head the Department of Urology at the Roswell Park Memorial Institute, the New York State Department of Health cancer research and treatment center in Buffalo.

The American Urological Association's annual **Hugh Hampton Young Award** was presented to **Grayson Carroll**, MD, who received the award for his contributions to the study and treatment of urinary tract infection. Dr. Carroll is clinical professor emeritus of St. Louis University School of Medicine, director of urology at St. John's Mercy Hospital, and a consultant to Jewish Hospital and St. Louis Hospital. The award carries with it a plaque and a $2,000 grant from Bristol Laboratories.

Maynard Merle Dewey, PhD, will become chairman of the anatomy department at the State University of New York at Stony Brook. Dr. Dewey was chairman and professor of anatomy at the Medical College of Pennsylvania previous to his recent appointment.

James A. Pittman, Jr., MD, has been named head of the Veterans Administration medical research and education program. **Lyndon E. Lee**, Jr., MD, who previously held the position, is now ACMD for Professional Services.

The American Electroencephalographic Society and **The American Society of EEG Technologists** (ASET) will hold their **annual meetings** Sept. 13-18 at the Hotel Radisson South in Bloomington, Minn. The scientific sessions will be Sept. 16-18, with special workshops on the evening of Sept. 16. The program includes a Symposium on Psychological Correlates of the EEG and another Symposium on Generalized versus Focal Electroencephalographic Seizure Activity. ASET will present a one-day course on Fundamentals of EEG Technology on Sept. 16, with general sessions on the next two days. Further information on both meetings is available from Mrs. **Margaret H. Henry**, Executive Secretary, The American EEG Society, 36391 Maple Grove Road, Willoughby Hills, Ohio, 44094.

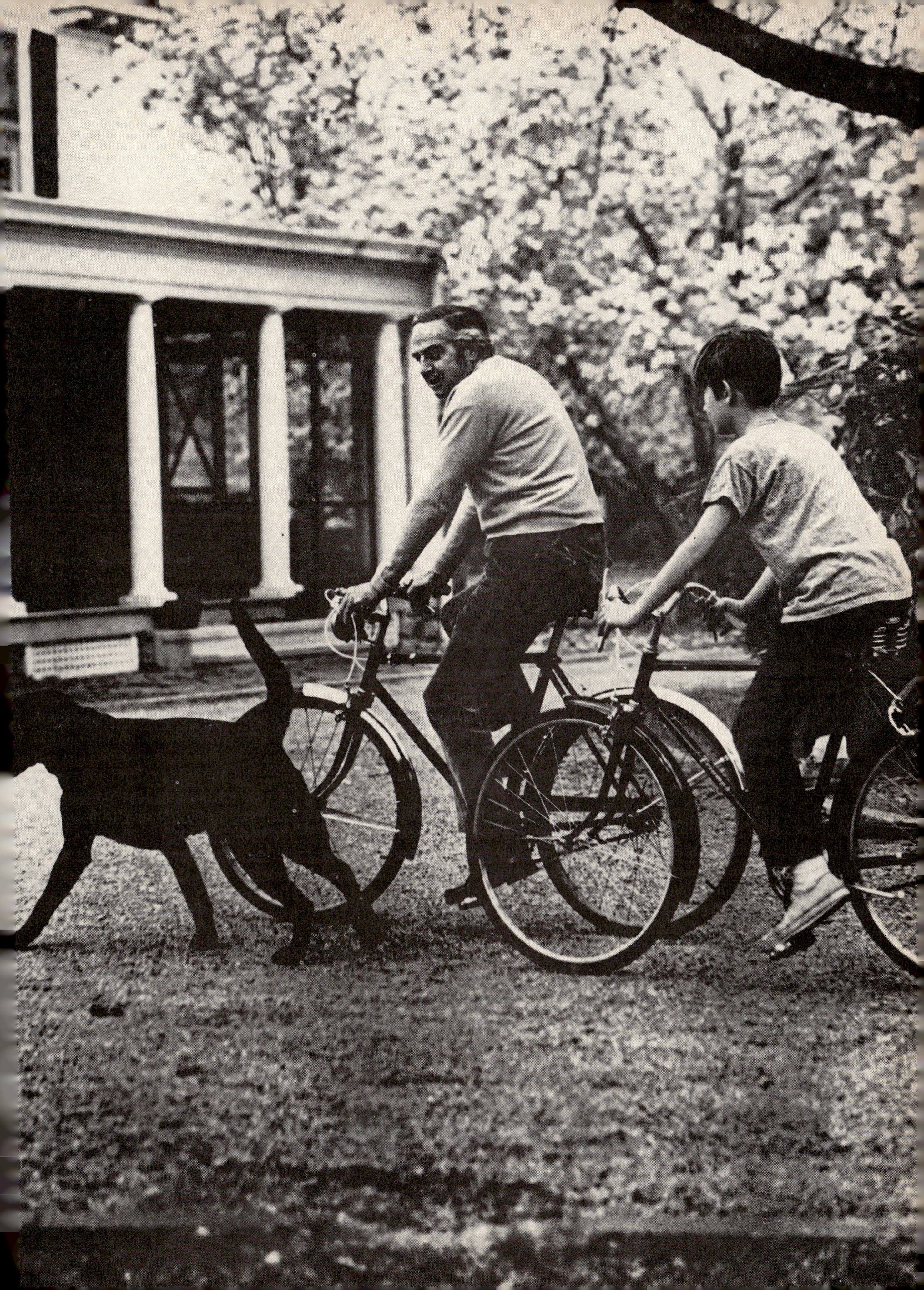

Internal Medicine at large

The President's Committee on Employment of the Handicapped has named **Kenneth D. Arn**, MD, **"Physician of the Year."** Dr. Arn, of Dayton, Ohio, is director of the Department of Internal Medicine at Miami Valley hospital, and a member of the staff at Kettering hospital.

Alfred I. Kaplan, MD, has been named to the Pulmonary Physiology Section of the Leonard Morse Hospital in Natick, Mass. He is assistant chief of the pulmonary section of the Boston Veterans Administration Hospital and assistant professor of medicine at Boston University School of Medicine.

> The new Medical School of the University of Missouri-Kansas City plans to develop its permanent teaching staff around **Docents**—visiting physician-teachers who would join the faculty for 3 to 12 months. The Docents' duties will be related entirely to teaching the students and their contribution to the curriculum will be coordinated through a Council of Docents. The compensation for Docents will be $2,000 a month and the school hopes to attract the participation of academicians of all ages, whether on sabbatical leave or in retirement.
>
> Further information is available from the Council of Docents, School of Medicine, University of Missouri-Kansas City, Kansas City, Mo, 64110.

Julius B. Richmond, MD, has become head of the Department of Preventive and Social Medicine at Harvard Medical School. He will also continue in his past positions as professor of child psychiatry and human development at the medical school, and director of the Judge Baker Guidance Center and psychiatrist-in-chief at the Children's Hospital Medical Center. Dr. Richmond was the first director of Project Head Start in the Office of Economic Opportunity.

The new president of the Association of University Radiologists is **James H. Scatliff,** MD, chairman of the Department of Radiology at the University of North Carolina School of Medicine. **Elliott C. Lasser,** MD, chairman of the Department of Radiology at the University of California, San Diego, School of Medicine, was chosen president-elect of the association.

Erwin O. Hirsch, MD, director of medical education at the Princeton, NJ, Hospital, has been appointed the successor of **Gerald A. Weichmann,** PhD, as associate dean of student affairs at the Medical College of Wisconsin. Dr. Hirsch was also named associate professor of medicine at the school.

Grant W. Liddle, MD, has been presented the first Distinguished Leadership Award in Endocrinology by the Endocrine Society. He is professor and chairman of the Department of Medicine, and director of the Endocrinology Division at Vanderbilt University.

Joseph Newall, MD, has been appointed professor of radiology at the New York University School of Medicine.

Solomon A. Berson, MD, and **Rosalyn S. Yalow,** MD, were 1971 co-recipients of the **Howard Taylor Ricketts Award** of the University of Chicago. The investigators developed a radioimmunoassay for peptide hormones in the blood. Dr. Berson is the Murray M. Rosenberg Professor and chairman of the Department of Medicine, Mt. Sinai School of Medicine, and director of the Department of Medicine of Mt. Sinai Hospital, New York City. Dr. Yalow is chief of the nuclear medicine service of the Bronx VA Hospital, and research professor of medicine in the Mt. Sinai School of Medicine.

Thomas H. Kirschbaum, MD, professor of obstetrics and gynecology at the University of California Los Angeles School of Medicine, has been named the first chairman of the new Department of Obstetrics, Gynecology and Reproductive Biology at Michigan State University College of Human Medicine.

Peter A. Ward, MD, has been named recipient of the 15th annual **Parke Davis Award** of the American Society for Experimental Pathology. Dr. Ward is chief of the Immunology Branch of the Armed Forces Institute of Pathology, and will become associate professor of pathology at the University of Connecticut School of Medicine and Dental Medicine in Hartford.

Volume 128, Number 2, August 1971

Archives of Internal Medicine

Original Articles

Mortality and Coronary Heart Disease Among Men Studied for 23 Years

Ancel Keys, PhD; Henry Longstreet Taylor, PhD; Henry Blackburn, MD; Josef Brozek, PhD; Joseph T. Anderson, PhD; and Ernst Simonson, MD, Minneapolis

Twenty-year coronary heart disease (CHD) incidence is analyzed for 279 men, CHD-free at the ages of 47 through 57 years and characterized by three examinations before 20 annual follow-up examinations. Sixty men developed CHD, 42 dying or suffering infarction. Among 20 entry characteristics, three had major predictive power, especially for CHD death or infarction: cold pressor test, a high level of serum cholesterol, and systolic blood pressure. Smoking and relative weight seemed unimportant. Major CHD incidence was proportional to cholesterol to the 3.4 power. Five-variable multiple logistic analysis permitted placement of men into deciles of estimated risk differing more than tenfold in CHD incidence. The combination of only cholesterol and systolic pressure was nearly as good. The multiple logistic coefficients applied to five-year data on 1,287 men among whom 182 CHD developed in 182 yielded satisfactory agreement between observed and predicted distributions of CHD cases in classes of estimated risk.

In 1947 a group of middle-aged business and professional men living in the Twin Cities of Minneapolis and St. Paul and suburbs were enrolled in a program of annual examinations with the purpose of attempting to identify some characteristics predisposing to the development of coronary heart disease (CHD).[1] We have reported on the 15-year follow-up of 281 of those men who were CHD-free when examined in January to March 1948.[2] Four men whose entry examinations were delayed until 1948 and 1949 were not included in that report.

Here we report on 20 years of experience of that group beginning with the completion of the third round of annual examinations in March 1950, the follow-up continuing through the spring of 1970. During the two years following the entry examinations in January through March 1948, there were no deaths but CHD developed in two men. Consequently, the 20 years of observations beginning in 1950 start with 283 CHD-free men, including four late entrants in 1948 and 1949 noted above and a loss for the analysis of only two men, both with angina pectoris diagnosed in 1949. A 1950 starting date allows much better characterization of the men at the start of follow-up because several interesting items of test and measurement were added to the examinations in 1949 and 1950. In addition, an average of measures from three visits more reliably characterizes the men at entry in respect to such items as blood pressure, resting pulse rate, serum cholesterol concentration, and relative body weight.

Finally, three men who died of accidents and one of suicide have been excluded from the present report. Accordingly, this report concerns 5,580 man-years of 279 men, accounted for as follows: the 281 men previously reported plus 4 men added in 1948 and 49, less 2 men who developed CHD be-

Received for publication Dec 7, 1970; accepted March 5, 1971.

From the Laboratory of Physiological Hygiene, School of Public Health, University of Minnesota, Minneapolis. Dr. Brozek is now with Lehigh University, Bethlehem, Penn.

Reprint requests to Laboratory of Physiological Hygiene, School of Public Health, University of Minnesota, Minneapolis 55455 (Dr. Keys).

tween 1948 and 1950, less the 4 men who died violently.

Subjects

The method of recruitment of the subjects has been described.[1,2] Among 1,000 men whose names were on an eligibility roster compiled by the personnel officers of local business firms, 916 men agreed to participate. After giving priority to the most overweight men and to some men certified as being unusually zealous in physical activity programs, the invited cohort was made up to 300 men by random choice among the volunteers. For public relations reasons, invitations to join the group were extended to 34 men prominent in the community or in the University of Minnesota.

Among the 334 men on the provisional roster, 11 proved to be outside the prescribed age range of 45 through 55 years at entry, 23 were excluded initially for medical reasons, three men withdrew at the end of the first examination, and 11 declined to return for the second examination. Later, one man was dropped from the cohort for analysis because a history of CHD, previously concealed, was discovered. Among the men in the final cohort, a few were of modest means and position but the majority had highly responsible positions. This study, then, concerns men in the upper socioeconomic class in a midwestern metropolis.

Methods and Examination Procedure

For the most part, the examination procedure and methods have been described in a previous report.[2] The men came to the laboratory by appointment in the morning without breakfast. Parking space provided a few steps from the laboratory entrance helped the men to follow the instruction to avoid any vigorous activity before the examinations. After undressing and resting quietly at least ten minutes, the blood pressure and pulse rate were recorded three times during rest in the supine position. A 12-lead electrocardiogram was recorded in supine rest; a venous blood sample was taken, avoiding stasis; a six-foot posteroanterior chest roentgenogram was made; and a urine sample was obtained. A detailed interim medical history was recorded and a physical examination was made by an internist with special experience in cardiology. In recent years the subjects have, at each examination, filled out standard medical questionnaires which included the cardiovascular questionnaire on chest pain of the London School of Hygiene.[3]

Other tests and measurements were included in the examinations from time to time. In 1949 the cold pressor test was administered, according to the procedure prescribed by Hines and Brown.[4] The hand was immersed in ice water for 60 seconds and blood pressure was recorded by the auscultatory method in the opposite arm before immersion, at 30 seconds, and in the last 10 to 15 seconds of immersion. Forced expiratory volume (vital capacity) was measured with a low resistance spirometer.

In the blood, hemoglobin was measured in a colorimeter as the ammonia hemochromogen, calibration being done with oxygen capacity. Serum cholesterol was estimated by Bloor's method in the first examination and later by our modification[5] of the method of Abell et al.[6] The application of both methods to duplicate serum samples from all men showed very high correlation but it was necessary to multiply the Bloor values by 0.85 to correspond with the values from the method of Abell et al. Cholesterol values referred to here are in Abell terms. Serum protein-bound iodine was measured by the method of Barker[7] as modified by Tucker and Keys.[8]

Several methods were used to evaluate relative body weight and obesity. Here, relative body weight means the percentage of the average weight for given height and age as given in the medico-actuarial tables published by Davenport[9] and widely republished. We have published those weight-height-age tables after converting them to the metric system.[10] In many respects the relative body mass index, the weight divided by the square of the height, is a better measure of relative weight, so analyses were also made with the use of that measure.

Relative weight or body mass index does not distinguish between the tissues of the body and is not a good indicator of obesity, or relative fatness, except at the extremes. Here, two measures more directly related to the proportion of the body that is made up of fat were used. Skinfold thickness was recorded with constant pressure calipers over the triceps muscle and over the tip of the scapula, the sum of these two, Σ-skinfolds, being the measure used for analysis. Body density was determined by weighing under water with simultaneous estimation of residual air by the method of nitrogen washout. Rather than estimating the fat percentage of the body from density, which requires assumptions that cannot be tested, the density itself, with volume corrected for residual air, was used in the present analyses.

Follow-Up and Diagnostic Criteria

The great majority of the survivors have been examined each year. However, these men, now from 67 to 77 years of age, find it increasingly difficult to report for examination every year. By 1970, 49 men were living outside the state of Minnesota; while many of them return from time to time, the period between visits is lengthening. In the first half of 1970, only nine of the 49 nonresidents returned for examination. Physical disability hinders the return of some men to the laboratory. A few men have lost interest in our examination because they are getting regular check-up examinations more conveniently elsewhere. Some men tend to come in every other year. In 1968, 168 out of 221 living subjects were examined; in 1969 the figure was 151 out of 215 alive; in 1970, 153 members of the 212 living members of the cohort came for examination.

So far no one has been lost to follow-up. Information about health status is periodically obtained from correspondence with the men, their wives, or their personal physicians, or all three. In cases of death, diagnosis has been made on the basis of the official death certificates, communications with the family and the physicians concerned, and hospital reports, which include the autopsy when performed, with interpretation aided by the extensive medical histories on file in the laboratory.

The criteria for the diagnosis of CHD are those used in the International Cooperative Study of Cardiovascular Epidemiology, coordinated by this laboratory, and described recently.[11] The Minnesota Code[3,12] has been applied to the classification of the ECGs. In decreasing order of diagnostic reliability and medical importance, the diagnoses are death from CHD, nonfatal myocardial infarction, classical angina pectoris, and other CHD. In the present analysis, these diagnoses are mutually exclusive, each man being classified only to the highest category in this hierarchy that is applicable. "Other CHD" requires clinical judgment of *definite* heart disease plus etiology specified as myocardial infarct by history (without diagnostic ECG evidence) *or* clinical judgment of *possible* CHD by history plus any of the major Minnesota ECG codes 1.2, 1.3, 5.1, 5.2, 6.1, 6.2, 7.1, 7.2, 7.4, or 8.3 in the follow-up examinations. Criteria for other CHD were met in only seven cases.

Complete diagnostic accuracy cannot be guaranteed, of course, but specified rules, objectively applied with established end points, have been maintained. One postoperative death listed CHD as the immediate cause of death on the death certificate was *not* charged to CHD here because of coding rules which give priority to major malignancies. The diagnosis of myocardial infarction has also been conservative, the requirements being major Q waves in the ECG (Minnesota code 1.1), or lesser Q waves plus major T-wave changes (Minnesota codes 1.2 + 5.1 or 5.2), or clinical judgment of heart disease *and* etiology specified as myocardial infarct by history and any of Minnesota codes 1.2, 1.3, 5.1, 5.2, 6.1, 6.2, 7.1, 7.2, 7.4, or 8.3 (clinical infarction with confirmatory ECG changes). Angina pectoris, based entirely on symptoms, is more troublesome. Only *definite* diagnoses are considered here. Conservatism in this regard is indicated by the fact that only 11 cases of angina pectoris as the sole indication of CHD are included in the present total of 60 cases of CHD.

Most of the analyses in the present report distinguish between "hard" criteria CHD–death from CHD or myocardial infarction–and all CHD, which includes angina pectoris and

Table 1.—Characteristics of the CHD-Free Cohort at the Start of Follow-Up*

Item	47-48	49-50	51-52	53-54	55-57
N, men	53	51	71	53	51
Systolic blood pressure (median)	123	124	124	126	127
Diastolic blood pressure (median)	71	74	74	73	73
Weight/height² (median)	23.8	24.8	24.9	25.6	25.0
Rest pulse rate/min (median)	66	68	66	67	66
Cholesterol (mg/dl) (median)	219	214	215	215	222
Hemoglobin (gm/100 ml) (median)	14.7	14.9	14.5	14.6	14.6
Σ-skinfolds (mm) (median)†	31	36	32	30	32
Cold pressor (median)‡	16	15	14	16	15
N, systolic blood pressure >140	4	8	3	11	13
N, systolic blood pressure >160	0	2	0	2	6
20-year events					
N, deaths	12	8	14	18	23
N, CHD	11	8	15	9	14
CHD, % of men	21	16	21	17	27

* Characteristics of the CHD-free cohort, classified by age at start of the 20-year follow-up, and 20-year "events." Four men who later died violently, are excluded. Averages for each man at examinations in 1948, 1949, and 1950 are used to characterize blood pressure, resting pulse rate, serum cholesterol concentration, and body mass index (weight in kilograms divided by square of height in meters). "Cold pressor" is millimeter rise in systolic blood pressure at end of one minute with hand in ice water. "N", is number of men.

† Three men without data.

‡ Thirty-nine men without data.

Table 2.—Cigarette Smoking at Entry and Subsequent Incidence of CHD*

			Smoking Habit (Cigarettes/Day)				
Age	No. of Men	Item	Never	Stopped	<10	10 to 19	20+
47, 48	53	% with habit	23	19	9	19	30
49, 50	51	% with habit	33	14	14	10	29
51, 52	69	% with habit	17	25	14	14	30
53, 54	53	% with habit	36	28	8	13	15
55 to 57	51	% with habit	24	35	8	16	17
47 to 57	277	No. of men	82	39	62	41	53
		Hard CHD rate (%)	12.2	25.6	4.8	17.1	22.6
		Hard CHD rate (SE)	±3.6	±7.0	±2.7	±5.9	±5.7
		All CHD rate (%)	22.0	35.9	8.1	19.5	28.3
		All CHD rate (SE)	±4.6	±7.7	±3.4	±6.2	±6.2

* Cigarette smoking habits, by age at start of the 20-year follow-up, 20-year incidence rates (per 100 men), and standard errors (SE) of the rates. "Hard CHD" = CHD death and myocardial infarcts. "All" includes angina pectoris and other CHD diagnoses. "Deaths" are from all causes except violence.

Table 3.—Incidence of CHD in 20 Years Among Men Classified by 18 Variables at Entry*

Item	Age (Yr)			Height			Weight/Height[2]		
	47 to 49	50 to 52	53 to 57	Low	Mid	High	Low	Mid	High
No.	88	87	104	93	93	93	93	93	93
Hard CHD	12	14	16	15	14	13	9	13	20
All CHD	16	21	23	20	21	19	14	21	25
	Hard X^2=0.22		P=0.90	Hard X^2=0.17		P=0.92	Hard X^2=5.21		P=0.07
	All X^2=0.96		P=0.62	All X^2=0.22		P=0.89	All X^2=3.95		P=0.14

Item	Relative Body Weight			Σ-Skinfolds			Body Density		
	Low	Mid	High	Low	Mid	High	Low	Mid	High
No.	93	93	93	92	92	92	86	87	86
Hard CHD	11	14	17	8	15	19	18	12	9
All CHD	16	20	24	14	20	26	24	19	13
	Hard X^2=1.51		P=0.47	Hard X^2=5.50		P=0.06	Hard X^2=3.84		P=0.15
	All X^2=2.04		P=0.36	All X^2=4.60		P=0.10	All X^2=4.62		P=0.10

Item	Resting Pulse Rate			Basal Metabolism/kg			Blood Hemoglobin		
	Low	Mid	High	Low	Mid	High	Low	Mid	High
No.	93	93	93	64	64	64	93	93	93
Hard CHD	11	13	17	10	8	7	9	19	14
All CHD	15	21	23	13	13	13	15	25	20
	Hard X^2=1.58		P=0.45	Hard X^2=0.64		P=0.73	Hard X^2=4.20		P=0.12
	All X^2=2.24		P=0.33	All X^2=0		P=1.00	All X^2=3.18		P=0.20

Item	Systolic Blood Pressure			Diastolic Blood Pressure			Serum Cholesterol		
	Low	Mid	High	Low	Mid	High	Low	Mid	High
No.	93	93	93	93	93	93	93	93	93
Hard CHD	7	15	20	11	13	18	7	15	20
All CHD	17	16	27	18	19	23	11	26	23
	Hard X^2=7.23		P=0.03	Hard X^2=2.19		P=0.34	Hard X^2=7.23		P=0.03
	All X^2=4.71		P=0.10	All X^2=0.89		P=0.64	All X^2=8.03		P=0.02

Item	Fasting Blood Sugar			Residual Air			Vital Capacity (ml/m of Height)		
	Low	Mid	High	Low	Mid	High	Low	Mid	High
No.	86	86	86	80	80	80	84	85	84
Hard CHD	15	13	12	15	15	9	18	12	9
All CHD	21	21	16	20	20	15	22	19	16
	Hard X^2=0.41		P=0.82	Hard X^2=2.20		P=0.33	Hard X^2=3.86		P=0.15
	All X^2=1.11		P=0.57	All X^2=1.18		P=0.55	All X^2=1.23		P=0.54

Item	Blood Protein-Bound Iodine			Cold Pressor Rise		Smoking Habit	
	Low	Mid	High	<20 mm	≥20 mm	<10 Cigarettes/Day	10+ Cigarettes/Day
No.	91	91	91	198	67	183	94
Hard CHD	18	11	12	22	18	22	20
All CHD	27	14	19	37	21	36	27
	Hard X^2=2.47		P=0.29	Hard X^2=9.70	P=0.002	Hard X^2=4.13	P=0.04
	All X^2=5.75		P=0.06	All X^2=4.69	P=0.03	All X^2=0.57	P=0.32

* Twenty-year incidence of CHD among men classified by single variable characteristics at entry. "Hard CHD" = CHD death or myocardial infarction. "All CHD" adds angina pectoris and other CHD diagnosis. "Low," "Mid," and "High" refer to the parts of the distribution of the variable. "N" = all men for whom data are available.

other CHD. Among the 279 men CHD-free at the outset, in 20 years 60 men became cases of CHD of which 42 were hard CHD.

Characteristics of the Men at Entry

Table 1 summarizes some characteristics of the men, classified by age, at entry and shows the distribution by age of the 60 men who later developed CHD and of the 75 men who died of nonviolent causes in the 20-year period of follow-up. Note that three-visit averages were used here to characterize each man in regard to systolic and diastolic blood pressure, resting pulse rate, the body mass index (weight in kilograms divided by the square of the height in meters), and the concentration of cholesterol in the blood serum.

Besides indicating the center of the distributions for each of the variables listed, Table 1 shows that over the 11-year age range, 47 through 57 years, most of the variables show no indication of being related to age. One exception is the prevalence of hypertension. Though in Table 1 there was very little age trend in the median systolic blood pressure and none at all in the median diastolic pressure, there is a clear tendency for the prevalence of hypertension to increase with greater age. For example, among 148 men aged 47 through 51 years, 14 men had resting systolic pressure of 140 mm or more, or a prevalence of hypertension by that criterion of 9.5%; among 131 men aged 52 to 57, 25, or 19.1%, were in that category. The difference is associated with $\chi^2 = 5.35$ and $P =$ approximately 0.02. There is a similar difference when pressure of 160 mm is the criterion of hypertension.

Table 1 fails to show that susceptibility to subsequent CHD is age-related in the range concerned here. However, the age trend in deaths from any cause (except violence) is striking in Table 1. This point must be borne in mind in any analysis of the relationship of death rate to blood pressure. An analysis of all-causes deaths in this cohort will be published separately.

At entry, the men in the present study might be judged to have been, on the average, somewhat less at risk than men of corresponding age in some other prospective studies in the United States. In regard to arterial blood pressure and serum cholesterol level, comparison can be made with data from five other studies summarized in Appendix Table 4 in monograph 29 of the American Heart Association.[11(p204)] In all of those other studies hypertension by any criterion was considerably more common than in this Minnesota cohort. Men with a diagnosis of hypertensive disease at first examination were not admitted into the present cohort. More important may be the fact that basal metabolic conditions at the examination were maintained in the present study but not in the other studies noted.

In the other studies about half of the men had serum cholesterol values of greater than or equal to 250 mg/deciliter; only a third of the men in the present study had such high values in the first three examinations. This difference cannot be attributed to the examination conditions. It is well known that serum cholesterol level is relatively independent of time of day and time since the previous meal.[13-15]

Comment may be called for about the relative body mass index. While that index seems to be particularly suitable in evaluating relative weight, until now it has not often been used in medical publications. It can be stated here, in respect to this index, that the present Minnesota cohort was similar, at entry, to the railroad employees in the northwestern part of the United States reported by Taylor and others.[16] They were also similar to the railroad men in relative body weight.

In this Minnesota cohort heavy cigarette smoking was somewhat less common reported from some surveys of American men of similar age. Their cigarette smoking habits at the start of the 20-year follow-up are summarized in Table 2. Thirty percent of these men had never smoked cigarettes and another 26% of them had stopped before the start of the present study; 19% of them were smoking 20 or more cigarettes daily at entry. In contrast, among the US railroad employees referred to already,[16] 25% of the executives had never smoked and 28% of them were smoking 20 or more cigarettes daily at comparable age.

Table 2 shows that the smoking habits at entry were to some extent age-related. In the short range of 11 years of age, there was a marked increase of smokers who had stopped smoking and a decrease in the relative frequency of heavy smoking. Among 88 men aged 47 through 49 years, 18, or 20%, smoked 30 or more cigarettes per day; among 109 men 50 to 53 years old, 8, or 7%, smoked that much; among 104 men aged 53 to 57, only 3, or 4%, were such heavy smokers. The lesson is plain; where morbidity and mortality rates are closely related to age, great care must be exercised in the analysis of the relationship of sickness and death to smoking habits. Standardizing by decades of age is too coarse a method to avoid attributing to smoking habits some effects more properly charged to age.

Twenty Years of Follow-Up

Single Variables.—Besides showing the distribution of smoking habits at the onset of the 20-year follow-up, Table 2 summarizes the relationship between those habits and the 20-year incidence of CHD. While the incidence rates were higher among heavy smokers—20 or more cigarettes daily—than among men who had never smoked, the men who had stopped smoking tended to be the most CHD-prone of the categories in regard to smoking. On the other hand, the very light smokers, those never smoking as many as ten cigarettes a day, were much less susceptible to CHD than the men in the other smoking categories. The difference is highly significant statistically ($P < 0.001$).

The 20-year CHD experience of the cohort in respect to 18 characteristics at entry, considered one at a time, is summarized in Table 3. None of the measures of relative weight or body fatness was found to show a statistically significant relationship to subsequent CHD incidence, though the body mass index and the sum of the skinfolds are close to meeting the requirement of showing a difference that would occur no more than one out of 20 trials ($P \leq 0.05$). Diastolic blood pressure failed to be important but systolic blood pressure was highly significant, as was the concentration of cholesterol in the blood serum. Smoking habit could not be shown to be important with any single cutting point for quantity per day but cutting the distribution at ten cigarettes a day, as in Table 3, gave the nearest approach to significance—$P = 0.09$. The rate of CHD incidence among nonsmokers was not significantly lower than the rate among smokers but the peculiarity of the light smokers, mentioned above, must be noted.

The most significant single variable for CHD prediction proved to be the rise of diastolic blood pressure in the cold pressor test. The relative risk ratio for CHD death or myocardial infarction of the hyper-reactor group was 2.4 times that of the men who showed a rise of less than 20 mm in diastolic pressure in the test. Among 198 men with a rise of less than 20 mm in the cold pressor test, 22 subsequently died from CHD or suffered a definite infarction. Those 198 men amounted to 74.72% of all the men at risk, so, if the cold pressor test had no discriminating power, among the total of 40 men who later developed hard CHD, $0.7472 \times 40 = 29.887$ would be the expected number of cases in the group with only a small cold pressor response. Accordingly, the ratio of observed to expected cases in that group was $O/E = 22/29.887 = 0.736$. For the men with a more positive cold pressor response, the expected number was $40 \times 67/265 = 10.113$ but 18 cases were observed: $O/E = 18/10.113 = 1.780$. The cold pressor hyper-reactors were $1.780/.736 = 2.4$ times more prone to hard CHD than the other men.

Among the other variables considered in Table 3, all are very far from having a statistically significant relationship to CHD incidence. The closest approach to a distribution significantly different from zero is blood hemoglobin concentration. But interest in the hemoglobin level wanes when it is noted that the distribution peculiarity for CHD vs hemoglobin level is that it shows a hump or inverted "u." It seems unreasonable to propose that the risk of developing CHD is less in relative anemia and relative polycythemia than in the middle of the hemoglobin range.

Serum Cholesterol—An Exponential Relationship

In an analysis of CHD experience of men in the Framingham Study[18] and in an earlier report on this Minnesota cohort[2] it was noted that the relationship between incidence of CHD and the serum cholesterol level

Table 4.—Incidence of CHD in 20 Years Among Men Classified by Axillary Hair at Entry*

Hair Weight Distribution	Hard CHD No	Hard CHD Yes	No CHD	Any CHD	No CHD	Soft CHD
Lower half	86	19	81	24	81	5
Upper half	92	12	82	22	82	10
All men	178	31	163	46	163	15
	$\chi^2=1.78$		$\chi^2=0.08$		$\chi^2=1.47$	
	$P=0.18$		$P=0.77$		$P=0.77$	

* Experience of 209 men during 18 years following measurement of weight of axillary hair. "Hard" = CHD deaths and infarcts; "Any" = Hard + angina pectoris and other CHD; "Soft" = Any − Hard. Entries are numbers of men.

was curvilinear. With increasing cholesterol the risk rose more than in linear proportion. For the Minnesota cohort it was indicated that the risk rose by something like the square or the cube of the cholesterol level.[2] For the Framingham material it was suggested that the cholesterol raised to the 2.66 power might be a good measure of risk.[17]

With the present material, this question was examined again. With the model, $y = ax^b$, where y = incidence rate and x is serum cholesterol concentration, the question is to find the best value for the exponent b. By trial and error iteration, a value of more than $b = 3$ was indicated for the incidence of hard criteria CHD. For all CHD diagnoses a value of more than $b = 2$ was indicated.

A simple, direct approach to the solution of the exponential equation involves classifying men into deciles of the distribution of serum cholesterol level—28 men in each decile class except decile 5 which was given 27 men. The incidence rates for those decile classes were then ascertained so that for each decile there was a rate, y, and a median cholesterol value, X, for the exponential equation. Taking natural logarithms (base e) there were then ten sets of data in the form:

$$\ln y = \ln a + b \ln X,$$

which could then be solved for linear regression by the ordinary method of least squares.

For CHD deaths and infarcts, the result was $b = 3.35$ and the correlation between ln cholesterol (median) and ln incidence (rate) was $r = 0.823$. For all CHD incidence, the corresponding figures were $b = 2.24$ and $r = 0.734$. As noted above, in the analysis of Framingham data a value of $b = 2.66$ was suggested.[17] That was for the incidence of all diagnoses of CHD—no analysis was reported on only hard criteria CHD or any specific diagnostic category. In other reports on Framingham material,[18] it is clear that angina pectoris incidence was less closely related to cholesterol level than was myocardial infarction. In a longitudinal study of men at the Hawthorn Works in Chicago of the Western Electric Company[19] and in a study of Los Angeles civil servants,[20] it was also indicated that the incidence of angina pectoris was less closely related to serum cholesterol level than was the incidence of infarct and CHD death.

In the present material there was no significant relationship between the serum cholesterol level and the incidence of soft criteria CHD, angina pectoris, and other CHD as defined earlier. Note that in the tertiles of the cholesterol distribution in Table 3, the incidence of soft criteria CHD was 4, 11, and 3 cases in the low, mid, and high tertiles, respectively. The numbers are too small to warrant speculation about the meaning of that curious distribution.

Physical Activity

Almost all business and professional men are physically relatively

Table 5.—Coefficients of Correlation Between the Variables Taken Two at a Time

	Age	Weight Height²	Density	Vital Capacity/ Height	Resting Pulse	Systolic Blood Pressure	BMR (kg)	Choles- terol	Smok- ing
Weight/height²	0.05								
Density	−0.15	−0.65							
Vital capacity height	−0.13	−0.05	0.13						
Resting pulse	−0.08	−0.02	−0.06	−0.10					
Systolic blood pressure	0.15	0.02	−0.23	−0.24	0.32				
Basal metabolic rate	−0.10	−0.66	0.48	0.07	0.21	−0.08			
Cholesterol	0.05	0.08	0.09	−0.05	0.04	−0.04	−0.14		
Smoking	−0.11	−0.01	−0.06	−0.14	0.08	−0.01	0.13	0.14	
Cold Pressor	0.00	−0.01	0.03	−0.10	−0.09	0.13	0.01	0.11	0.08

inactive on the job and the present cohort was not exceptional in this respect. Queried about their activity habits, it was obvious that the word "sedentary" carried a derogatory connotation to most of the men and few of them would so describe themselves. They emphasized the frequency of leaving the desk, the "brisk" walks between offices and to luncheon places, and such items as snow-shoveling in the winter, tending to the lawn in the summer, and odd jobs around the house throughout the year. However, in general it did not seem possible to estimate actual energy expenditure reliably from the responses to questions about physical activity in those respects.

Some men regularly participated in activity programs at the local athletic clubs and YMCAs and in the period 1948 through 1950 claimed to spend from half an hour to two hours a week in calisthenics, playing volley ball, and swimming. When the cohort was organized in 1947, it was thought that some 50 of the men could be considered as unusually active in this respect. Further inquiry by our colleague, Austin Henschel, PhD, indicated, however, that only 34 men actually merited that description. Dr. Henschel classified another 31 men as being remarkably sedentary.

Those two groups of men differed little in their measured characteristics at entry, the least active and the most active being characterized, respectively, by mean values: age, 51.8 vs 52.0 years; correlation between body density and body mass index, weight/height² (Wt/Ht²), 24.16 vs 26.25; systolic blood pressure, 124.7 vs 124.6; vital capacity, 2,323 vs 2,501; serum cholesterol concentration, 219.3 vs 217.7; and resting pulse rate 66.87 vs 63.90. None of the differences is statistically significant.

These two small groups contrasting in physical activity at entry showed no significant differences in incidence of CHD or of death from all causes in the 20-year follow-up. Among 34 least active men, four developed CHD while 5.23 was the expected number; among 31 most active men, six developed CHD, 4.77 being expected. The χ^2 value is only 0.717 and $P = 0.60$. Similarly, comparing the least active with the rest of the men in the cohort failed to suggest any real difference. For deaths from all causes, three least active men died while the expected number was 2.8; the χ^2 value was only 0.017. The number of men classified with certainty as to physical activity in this cohort was too small to attach any weight to these negative findings.

Axillary Hair

It has been suggested that the amount of growth of axillary hair is a secondary sex characteristic tending to be related to maleness or androgen activity.[21] Since susceptibility to CHD is greater in men than in women, at least before old age, it might be argued that susceptibility to CHD is related to maleness and androgen activity. On the other hand, a better argument would seem to be that susceptibility to CHD is reduced by femaleness and estrogen activity, which is not simply the other side of the coin of the androgen argument. In any case, at the urging of James B. Hamilton, MD, the axillary hair was clipped from 212 of the men of this cohort at the annual examinations in January through March 1952. The "crop" from each man was sent to Dr. Hamilton who reported the weight as measured under standardized conditions in his laboratory.

Table 4 summarizes the analysis of the data on axillary hair weight and the subsequent 18-year experience of CHD. When the men were classified into the lower and upper halves of the distribution of hair weights the men

Table 6.—Coefficients for the Logistic Equation Relating CHD Incidence to Multiple Variables*

Criteria-Item	α	Systolic Blood Pressure	Cholesterol	Cold Pressor	Weight/Height²	Smoking Habit
Hard CHD						
5 variables	−9.9901	0.0065	0.0182	0.0352	0.1013	0.6067
1.96 SE	±0.1272	±0.1054	±0.0254	±0.0107	±0.0405	±0.7158
4 variables	−9.7860	0.0061	0.0194	0.0337	0.0947	Omit
1.96 SE	±0.3974	±0.0249	±0.0106	±0.0401	±0.1043	Omit
3 variables	−8.1548	0.0123	0.0195	0.0313	Omit	Omit
1.96 SE	±0.3834	±0.0222	±0.0103	±0.0398	Omit	Omit
3 variables	−9.2362	0.0074	0.0192	Omit	0.0893	Omit
1.96 SE	±0.3918	±0.0255	±0.0105	Omit	±0.1041	Omit
2 variables	−7.8286	0.0139	0.0194	Omit	Omit	Omit
1.96 SE	±0.3873	±0.0222	±0.0104	Omit	Omit	Omit
Any CHD						
5 variables	−6.6219	−0.0025	0.0131	0.0059	0.1031	0.2534
1.96 SE	±0.3142	±0.0231	±0.0089	±0.0352	±0.0902	±0.6234
4 variables	−6.5983	−0.0023	0.0136	0.0054	0.1006	Omit
1.96 SE	±0.3137	±0.0230	±0.0088	±0.0351	±0.0897	Omit
3 variables	−5.1083	0.0058	0.0139	0.0034	Omit	Omit
1.96 SE	±0.3039	±0.0202	±0.0086	±0.0348	Omit	Omit

* The constant, α, and the coefficients from the Walker-Duncan method for the multiple logistic equation using five, four, three, and only two variables for the probability of developing CHD. "Hard" = CHD death or infarction; "Any" CHD includes also angina pectoris and "other CHD." Approximate 95% confidence limits of the coefficients are indicated by ± 1.96 standard error of the mean.

Table 7.—Relation of CHD Incidence to Entry Characteristics Estimated From Three Examinations vs a Single Examination*

Variable	Class	N at Risk	Classed by Three Exams			Classed by One Exam		
			Cases	X^2	P	Cases	X^2	P
Systolic blood pressure	1	93	7	7.23	0.03	9	3.57	0.17
	2	93	15			15		
	3	93	20			18		
Cholesterol	1	93	7	7.23	0.03	8	5.51	0.06
	2	93	15			14		
	3	93	20			20		

* Incidence of CHD death or myocardial infarct in 20 years among men classified by systolic blood pressure and by serum cholesterol level from the average of three examinations and from one examination (the second of the three examinations).

in the lower half had a nonsignificant tendency (P = 0.18) to be more prone to infarction and CHD death than the "hairier" members of the cohort. In contrast, the men in the upper half of the hair weight distribution had a nonsignificant tendency (P = 0.2) to be more prone to angina pectoris and other soft criteria CHD. For all CHD diagnoses combined there was not the slightest suggestion of a difference in susceptibility between the men contrasting in axillary hair weight.

In the course of examining the question of the relevance of the axillary hair mass, its relationship to some other characteristics of interest were anlayzed. No significant correlations were discovered. The coefficients of correlation between axillary hair mass and other variables were: weight/height², r = −0.08; Σ-skinfolds, r = −0.05; systolic blood pressure, r = −0.16; serum cholesterol concentration, r = −0.06; and age, r = 0.

Multivariate Analysis

It is widely agreed that, to quote Oglesby Paul, MD, the picture of CHD "is clearly that of a multifactorial disease."[19] In other words, a number of factors or variables contribute to susceptibility or resistance to the disease. Those factors are commonly depicted as being additive though searching examination of the relationships, with adequate numbers of incidence cases well characterized before onset of CHD, has not been made. The known and suspected risk factors cannot truly be isolated except in animal experiments that have only dubious relevance to the incidence of the disease in man; but with material such as reported here, it is possible to apply statistical methods to learn how several variables can be effectively combined to separate persons who will become victims of CHD from their fellows who will not have that destiny—in a specified period of time following the measurement of those variables.

When the relationship is examined of CHD incidence to single variables one at a time, as in Table 3, important questions about intercorrelations between the variables must be answered before drawing final conclusions about the significance of the individual variables. For example, recently it has been shown in several studies that most of the excess risk of developing CHD that has been attributed to overweight is accounted for by a correlation between hypertension and overweight,[22] or between serum cholesterol value and overweight.[20] As a preliminary to multivariate consideration it is useful to inspect the correlations between the variables taken two at a time. Table 5 summarizes the findings for ten variables in the present material.

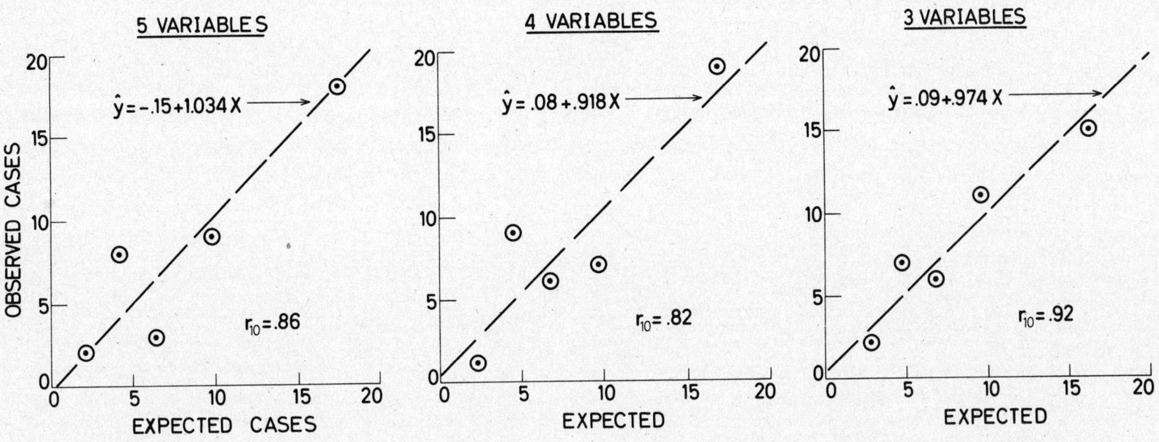

Fig 1.—Coronary heart disease death and myocardial infarctions observed and expected in quintile classes of risk probability. The five variables are systolic blood pressure, serum cholesterol, cold pressor rise, body mass index, and smoking. The four variables omit smoking. The three variables omit body mass index also.

Among the 45 correlations in Table 5, not many are statistically significant and few promise to be important for the present analysis. For N = 253 to N = 279, as in this material, significance at the 5% and the 1% levels is attained by about r = 0.12 and 0.16, respectively. However, with r = 0.12 the relationship between the two variables is exceedingly tenuous and accounts for only 1.44% of the variance. As expected, there is a fairly high correlation between body density and the body mass index, Wt/Ht^2, but the correlation coefficient of r = −0.65 means that only 42% of the variance is accounted for. More interesting is the negative correlation between basal metabolic rate per kilogram of body weight and the body mass index and the positive correlation between the basal metabolic rate (BMR) measure and the body density. But these findings have no obvious implication for the present analysis.

The relative independence from each other of most of the variables that appeared to be of interest in Table 3 suggests that no great reservations need be attached to most of the indications in Table 3 about the relative importance of the single variables. However, the correlations of systolic blood pressure with density, vital capacity, and with resting pulse rate call for thought in interpreting the relevant parts of Table 3. Such data emphasize the desirability of an analysis that considers a number of risk variables simultaneously in order to assess their joint contribution to the total risk.

Among various methods of multivariate analysis that could be applied to such material as the present, cogent arguments have been made in favor of the multiple logistic.[23,24] As in the more common discriminant function, the contributions of the several variables to the total estimated risk are assumed to be linearly additive but in the logistic the contributions are linearly added in an exponential expression:

$$\hat{y} = 1/[1 + e^{-(\alpha + \beta_1 x_1 \ldots\ldots + \beta_n x_n)}]$$

where $\hat{y}$ is the estimated probability of the individual developing the disease, $x_1 \ldots\ldots x_n$ are the values of the several variables for that individual, $\beta_1 \ldots . \beta_n$, are the coefficients to be applied to those variables, α is a constant, and e is the base of natural logarithms (= 2.781 . . . .). By definition the value of $\hat{y}$ for the individual is between 0 and 1 and, for any set of data on a sample of individuals to be analyzed, the sum of the $\hat{y}$ values of the individuals equals the total number of cases of the disease observed in the sample.

Truett et al[23] developed a method for obtaining, for any given set of data, the constant and the coefficients for the logistic equation and applied it to data on entry characteristics and 12-year follow-up experience of CHD of people in Framingham, Mass. Their method depends on assumptions about the character of the distributions—multivariate normal, with equal variances and covariances but different means—that can be rarely justified. But the prac-

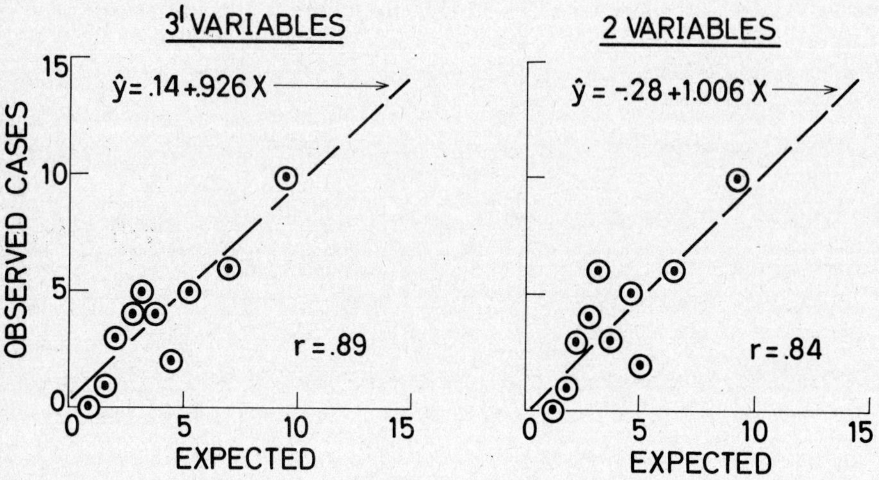

Fig 2.—Same as Fig 1 but showing decile class numbers from the three variables of systolic blood pressure, serum cholesterol, and body mass index and two variables omitting body mass index.

tical result was good in the only application made with the method. The results showed great power in "predicting" the probability in that sample of developing CHD or, more precisely, in distinguishing after the fact, those who did and those who did not develop CHD. With the constant and coefficients reported for Framingham men, we found a reasonably good agreement, with r = 0.83, between the estimated average *relative* risks in 13 population samples and the actual *relative* incidence rates observed in a five-year follow-up.[24]

Walker and Duncan[25] developed an iterative or recursive method of solving the multiple logistic equation without the assumptions made by Truett et al. Their method requires a very large computer and the program is relatively costly in computer time because six to eight iterations in the computer are needed to arrive at a stable set of coefficients. The theoretical superiority of the Walker-Duncan method led us to choose it for the present material.

Table 6 gives the coefficients obtained by the method of Walker and Duncan for estimating the probability of developing CHD, either by the hard criteria, CHD death, myocardial infarction, or by any criterion of CHD. The data in Tables 3 and 4 provided guidance in selecting the variables that seemed to be most closely related to subsequent CHD: systolic blood pressure, serum cholesterol concentration, rise of diastolic pressure in the cold pressor test, the body mass index, and smoking habit, the latter being graded zero for men smoking fewer than ten cigarettes daily (including those who never smoked and those who stopped smoking) and one for men smoking ten or more daily. The rationale of that code for smoking is indicated in Tables 2 and 3 and the associated discussion.

Missing data for one or another of these variables required exclusion of 15 subjects, so the multivariate analysis was based on 264 rather than 279 men. Among the 15 excluded men were two who had developed CHD (meeting hard criteria) between 1950 and 1970.

It should be noted that the coefficients in Table 6 are applied as multipliers to variables that differ widely in magnitude, the mean values and standard deviations for the 264 men at the start of the follow-up being as follows: systolic blood pressure, 125.4 mm Hg (SD = 14.9); cold pressor rise, 15.31 (SD = 8.45); body mass index, 24.8 (SD = 2.63); and smoking, 0.337 (SD = 0.474).

It will be noted that the omission of smoking habit, cold pressor test, or body mass index does not have great effect on the coefficients for the other variables except in the case of systolic blood pressure when body mass index is omitted. That reflects the fact that systolic pressure and body mass index are significantly correlated (r = 0.29).

Table 6 also gives values for 1.96 times the standard errors of the coefficients, thereby indicating the approximate 95% confidence limits of the coefficients. Inspection of Table 6, with these values in mind, shows that most of the individual coefficients are indicated to have at least one chance in 20 of being 0 or of opposite sign to the sign shown in the table. Further, attention to the confidence limits leads to the conclusion that it would be unjustifiable to draw many conclusions about the relative strength of the several variables as discriminators. Only serum cholesterol concentration is consistently indicated to be a significant discriminator, and with the same sign, in every analysis. In any combination of variables and with either hard or any CHD criteria, cholesterol is indicated to be a discriminator with $P < 0.005$.

But questions about the probable values of the coefficients that would be obtained from further random samples of the same population are less useful than the question as to how well the several *sets* of coefficients discriminate between those men who did and those who did not develop CHD. How well, in fact, does the multiple logistic equation perform with this material?

The effectiveness of the multiple logistic equation in discriminating between men in their probability of developing CHD can be appraised in several ways, one of the most straightforward and easiest to visualize being illustrated in Fig 1, 2, and 3. With the constant and the coefficients obtained by the Walker-Duncan method, the total risk probability, *P*, is computed for each man with the use of his values for the variables. The men are then arrayed in order from the lowest to the highest values of *P* and grouped into appropriate classes. The sum of the calculated risk probabilities for the men in each class gives the expected or predicted number of cases, these numbers then being compared with the numbers of cases observed in the class. With the present material we have used decile classes of *P*, the numbers of men in them being, from decile 1 to 10, respectively, 26, 27, 26, 27, 26, 26, 27, 26, 27, 26. For Fig 1, decile classes were combined into quintile classes because of the small number of cases of hard CHD. However, the regression equations and correlation coefficients in Fig 1 were calculated from the decile classes.

For hard criteria CHD the discrimination is reasonably good using five, four, or three variables and there is no notable difference in discrimination when any of the four sets of variables is used. The average of the four sets shows 1.5 cases in the lowest and 16.75 cases in the top quintile, a ratio of 11 to 1.

Figure 2 also refers to CHD deaths and infarcts but uses the three variables, systolic blood pressure, serum cholesterol concentration, and Wt/Ht^2, in the multiple logistic. The discrimination is not shown to be inferior to that obtained using the variables covered in Fig 1. Finally, Fig 2 shows the results of the analysis with only the two variables, systolic blood pressure and serum cholesterol concentration. The loss in discriminatory power in going from five to two variables is slight.

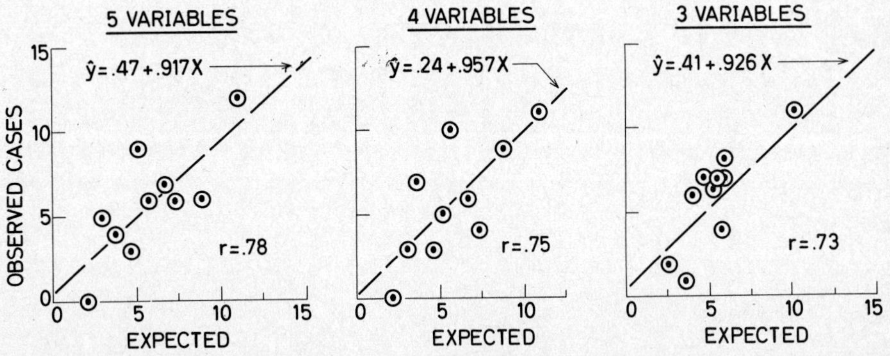

Fig. 3.—All CHD diagnoses observed and expected in decile classes of risk probabilities from the same five, four, and three variables as in Fig 1.

Discrimination is less impressive when *any* diagnosis of CHD is considered. Whereas the correlation coefficients between observed and expected numbers of cases in each decile class range from r = 0.82 to r = 0.92 for hard CHD, the range for any CHD is from r = 0.73 to r = 0.75. This finding reinforces the conclusion from other studies as well as from Table 3 here, that there is only a very weak relationship of angina pectoris and other CHD with the risk variables considered here.

Repeated Baseline Examinations

In the present study an attempt was made to reduce misclassification of the subjects by averaging the results of three examinations made before the start of the follow-up period. Table 7 compares results from men classified on the basis of data in a single examination with the results from the same men classified by the measurements in three examinations.

When average values from three examinations were used to classify each subject into the tertile classes of systolic blood pressure and of serum cholesterol concentration, the distributions of 42 CHD deaths or myocardial infarctions in those classes showed a significant relationship of the disease development to the characteristic before development of the disease for both variables; the probability of chance explanation is only 3%. But when data from only one examination, the middle of the sequence of three, were used to classify the men the relationship between the characteristic before development of the disease and the disease, itself, was much less clear. For serum cholesterol concentration, the indication was that the finding has a 6% chance of being fortuitous. The conclusion from data limited to one examination would be that systolic blood pressure might actually be unimportant; the tendency for the disease to occur more often with increasing blood pressure could happen by chance in about one out of six trials.

Body Mass Index vs Relative Body Weight

For discriminating between men who developed CHD from those who

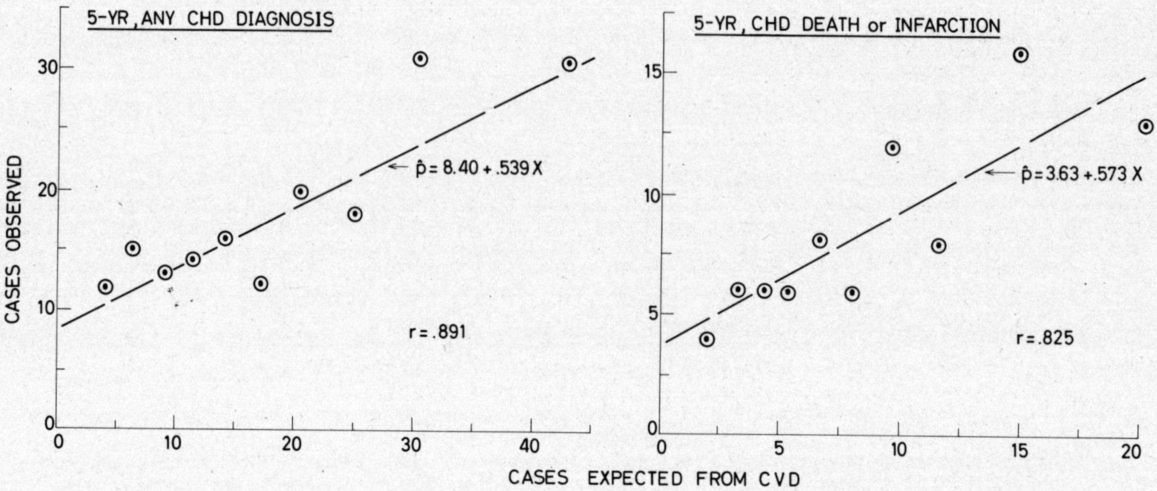

Fig 4.—Coronary heart disease cases among US railroad men followed five years after examination at the age of 50 to 59 years vs those predicted from the coefficients in the multiple logistic equation found for the 20-year incidence of CHD in the Minnesota business and professional men.

did not, in this study the body mass index proved to be considerably better than the long popular "relative body weight." This finding reinforces the conclusion from other considerations that the time is overdue to abandon weight-height-age-sex tables and the associated arguments about standards for relative body weight, their change with age and, at the same age, their change over time and from population to population. No doubt, people will still insist on asking what is "normal" and insurance companies will continue to issue pronouncements about "ideal" and "desirable" weight. However, reporting the body mass index in medical publications would prevent a good deal of confusion and misunderstanding, and, unlike all of the standard relative weight tables, the definition and meaning of the body mass index is clear and unchangeable.

Cold Pressor Test

One of the major surprises in the present analysis was the discovery of the value of information from the cold pressor test. The original publications about the cold pressor test and its significance[26,27] left much to be desired in respect to controls, follow-up results, and the analysis of such data as were reported. Hines and Brown tried to emphasize the cold pressor test as a means of detecting "prehypertension" but their own data in support were largely anecdotal. Two of the men with the greatest prestige in the field of hypertension, Sir George Pickering and Sir Horace Smirk, in their respective books on that subject,[28,29] dismissed the cold pressor test as being unreliable in predicting hypertension. Since that time interest in the test evaporated, but no one looked at the question of what other significance the cold pressor test might have. The application of the test in the present study considerably antedated the pronouncements of Pickering and Smirk. The fact is that whatever may be the defects of the test for predicting hypertension, the cold pressor test seems to have some value in estimating the probability of development of CHD.

Diastolic Blood Pressure

We have remarked that CHD incidence by any criterion was not significantly related to the diastolic blood pressure at rest in the entry examinations. In part this may be related to the fact that men with a diagnosis of hypertensive disease were not admitted into the cohort. Still, 18 men had three-year averages, 1948 through 1950, of 90 mm Hg or more in diastole and the absence of cases of hypertensive disease at entry did not prevent the finding that CHD incidence is highly related to systolic blood pressure.

In this material systolic blood pressure proved to be far more important than the diastolic reading but it may still be asked whether the diastolic blood pressure adds anything to the information provided by the systolic blood pressure. This question has been examined by several systems of cross classifications with consistent results. In regard to the future health of these men, the diastolic blood pressure could not be shown to add any significant information beyond that provided by the systolic blood pressure.

Ballistocardiogram

Beginning in 1951 both high-frequency and low-frequency (critically damped) ballistocardiograms were recorded with the subjects of this study. The results will be reported separately.

Comparison With Other Follow-Up Studies

Comment has already been made that the present subjects came from a segment of society, or socioeconomic class, that may have only minor representation in the samples of men in most other prospective studies on CHD reported so far. It would not be surprising, then, if the findings were discrepant in some respects. Actually, however, for comparably measured variables, the discrepancies are few, the most interesting being in regard to smoking habits.

In the studies at Framingham and Albany, NY, the men who had stopped smoking were reported to be almost as free from CHD in the follow-up as the men who had never smoked.[30,31] In this Minnesota cohort there was no suggestion that the men who had stopped smoking approached those who had never smoked in freedom from CHD in the follow-up; if anything, the Minnesota smokers who had stopped smoking tended to be more prone to CHD than the men in any other smoking category. Almost all of the Minnesota smokers who had stopped had quit many years before the start of the study and had quit without being advised that they were especially prone to CHD.

The other peculiarity in respect to smoking of this Minnesota cohort concerns the very light smokers, the men who smoked only occasionally or who smoked regularly but never as many as ten cigarettes a day. Those men were less prone to CHD than the men in any of the other smoking classes, which included the men who had never smoked. No such lack of susceptibility of men with similar smoking habits has been reported from other studies.

Another, but less marked discrepancy between the present results and those reported from other major follow-up studies in the United States concerns relative body weight. We have commented on the difficulty of comparing data on relative body weight in different studies; at least four different tables of "standards" have been used. However, it appears that overweight, reported by whatever was the favored criterion, tended to be a risk factor in most other US studies. In those studies the penalty of overweight tended to vanish when blood pressure was taken into account. In the present study no such attention to confounding variables is needed to arrive at the conclusion that relative body weight was unimportant for the risk of future CHD of this sample. This, as well as the discrepancy in regard to the significance of smoking habits, is unexplained; it is appropriate to remark on the limited numbers of subjects as well as differences in socioeconomic class.

In spite of these discrepancies, there is good agreement on several major points, notably in regard to blood pressure and serum cholesterol concentration. There seems to be unanimous agreement that systolic is more important than diastolic blood pressure and no one has reported that the prognostication from blood pressure in these epidemiological studies is improved when diastolic blood pressure is added to the information from the systolic blood pressure alone. There also seems to be agreement that susceptibility to CHD death and myocardial infarction is more closely related to serum cholesterol concentration than are angina pectoris and soft criteria diagnoses of CHD, and, from the limited detailed data available from other studies, it would seem that there is agreement with the finding here that the risk of CHD rises more steeply with serum cholesterol concentration than with systolic blood pressure.

The present data indicate that the risk of CHD death or infarction is proportional to cholesterol raised to about the 3.3 or 3.4 power. In similar exponential terms, the risk of such events is proportional to the systolic blood pressure raised to approximately the 1.5 power. With Framingham data on all CHD diagnoses, Jerome Cornfield[17] found the risk to rise slightly less than in proportion to the cube of the cholesterol level.

The coefficients for the multiple logistic equation given in Table 6 describe the 20-year experience of this particular sample of men. Due caution should be observed in attempts to apply them to other periods of follow-up and to other samples of men. It must be remarked, too, that age was omitted in the equation because in the small age range in this Minnesota cohort, no clear relationship of CHD incidence to entry age could be shown. Certainly age could not be ignored, however, in a sample with ages extending over a range of 15 or more years.

Still, as Fig 4 shows, the solutions to the multiple logistic equation may be useful for estimating the relative risk of men in other samples followed for much less time. With the coefficients in Table 6 relating the probability of CHD death or infarction to the three variables of systolic blood pressure, serum cholesterol concentration, and body mass index, incidence probabilities were calculated for each of 1,287 US railroad men aged 50 to 59 years at entry who were followed for five years.[16] The sum of the probabilities was 327.47, but the total cases of hard criteria CHD and of any diagnosis of CHD were 85 and 182, respectively. Accordingly, the probabilities calculated for hard criteria CHD and for any CHD were multiplied by the ratios 85/327.47 = 0.2596 and 182/327.47 = 0.5558, respectively.

Figure 4 summarizes the results when these railroad men were classified into deciles of the individual probabilities of developing CHD calculated from the fourth set of coefficients in Table 6. The least-squares regression of observed on predicted numbers of cases in the decile classes does not pass through the origin and its slope is far from being 45° in both diagnostic categories, but the correspondence between observed and expected cases is still impressive.

This investigation was supported in part by Public Health Service grants H-10 and continuations and HE 04997 and continuations. During early years of the follow-up, aid was also received from the American Heart Association and from the Winton Companies Fund, Minneapolis.

Austin Henschel, PhD, and Olaf Mickelsen, PhD, participated in the initial planning. Gunnar Blomquist, MD; B. Bronte-Stewart, MD (deceased); Rafael Carmena, MD; Carleton Chapman, MD; James Dahl, MD; Patrick Daly, MD; Fredrick de la Vega, MD; A.S. Dontas, MD; Thomas Gibbons, MD; Francisco Grande, MD; Burt Hamrell, MD; Gottfried Härtel, MD; Bruce Hatfield, MD; William Maloney, MD; Mario Mancini, MD; Yoshiyuki Ohno, MD; Thomas Puchner, MD; Sven Punsar, MD; Pentti Rautaharju, MD; Thomas Strasser, MD; Cesar Vasquez, MD; Djordje Vukadinović, MD; H.C. Walker, MD; and Paul Winchell, MD, performed physical examinations and supplied medical histories.

Olaf Mickelsen, PhD, supervised chemical analyses. Nedra Foster and Angie Sturgeon Skinner had charge of schedules and supervised the staff of technicians.

Prof Strother Walker and Richard B. McHugh provided The Walker-Duncan program. Norris Schultz, R. Willis Parlin, Jakko Kihlberg, PhD (deceased), Rosemarie Wirtz Hilk, and Mary Ann O'Brien assisted with data processing. E.S. Fletcher, PhD, helped with the annual interviews for nine years.

References

1. Keys A, Taylor HL, Simonson E, et al: The C.V.D. research program of the Laboratory of Physiological Hygiene: An explanation and a "letter to guinea pigs." *Lancet* **81**:291-295, 1961.
2. Keys A, Taylor HL, Blackburn H, et al: Coronary heart disease among Minnesota business and professional men followed 15 years. *Circulation* **28**:381-395, 1963.
3. Rose GA, Blackburn H: Cardiovascular survey methods. *WHO Monogr Ser* **56**:172, 1968.
4. Hines EA, Brown GE: A standard test for measuring the variability of the blood pressure: its significance as an index of the prehypertension state. *Ann Intern Med* **7**:209-217, 1933.
5. Anderson JT, Keys A: Cholesterol in serum and lipoprotein fractions: Its measurement and stability. *Clin Chem* **2**:145-159, 1956.
6. Abell L, Levy B, Brodie B, et al: A simplified method for the estimation of total cholesterol in serum and the demonstration of its efficacy. *J Biol Chem* **195**:357-366, 1962.
7. Barker SB: Determination of protein-bound iodine. *J Biol Chem* **173**:715-724, 1948.
8. Tucker RG, Keys A: Concentration of serum protein-bound iodine in normal men. *J Clin Invest* **30**:869-873, 1951.
9. Davenport CB: *Body Build and Its Inheritance*, Publication 329. Carnegie Institute, 1923, 1-176.
10. Keys A, et al: Epidemiological studies related to coronary heart disease: Characteristics of men aged 40-59 in seven countries. *Acta Med Scand*, suppl 460, p 392, 1967.
11. Keys A, et al: Coronary heart disease in seven countries. *Amer Heart Assoc Monograph* **29**, abstracted. *Circulation* **41, 42** (suppl 1): 211, 1970.
12. Blackburn H, Keys A, Simonson E, et al: The electrocardiogram in population studies: A classification system. *Circulation* **21**:1160-1175, 1960.
13. Collen MF, DeKruif D, Geier F: Plasma cholesterol concentration following ingestion of 5 grams of cholesterol in patients with coronary artery disease. *Permanente Found Med Bull* **7**:60-66, 1949.
14. Keys A: The relation in man between cholesterol levels in the diet and in the blood. *Science* **112**:79-81, 1950.
15. Keys A, Anderson JT, Mickelsen O: Serum cholesterol in men in basal and non-basal states. *Science* **123**:29, 1956.
16. Taylor HL, Blackburn H, Keys A, et al: Coronary heart disease in seven countries: IV. Five-year follow-up of employees of selected U.S. railroad companies. *Circulation* **41** (suppl 1):20-39, 1970.
17. Cornfield J: Joint dependence of risk of coronary heart disease on serum cholesterol and systolic blood pressure: A discriminant function analysis. *Fed Proc* **21**:58-61, 1962.
18. *The Framingham Study: An Epidemiological Investigation of Cardiovascular Disease.* Section 12 US Government Printing Office, 1968.
19. Paul O, Lepper MH, Phelan WH, et al: A longitudinal study of coronary heart disease. *Circulation* **28**:20-31, 1963.
20. Chapman JM, Massey FJ: The interrelationship of serum cholesterol, hypertension, body weight, and risk of coronary heart disease: Results of the first ten years' follow-up in the Los Angeles Heart Study. *J Chronic Dis* **17**:933-949, 1964.
21. Hamilton JB: Patterned loss of hair in man: Types and incidence. *Ann New York Acad Sci* **53**:708-728, 1951.
22. Van Buchem FSP: Coronary heart disease in seven countries: VIII. Zutphen, a town in the Netherlands. *Circulation* **41,42**(suppl 1):76-86, 1970.
23. Truett J, Cornfield J, Kannel W: Multivariate analysis of the risk of coronary heart disease. *J Chronic Dis* **20**:511-524, 1967.
24. Keys A: Coronary heart disease in seven countries: XIII. Multiple variables. *Circulation* **41,42** (suppl 1):138-144, 1970.
25. Walker SH, Duncan DB: Estimation of the probability of an event as a function of several independent variables. *Biometrika* **54**:167-179, 1967.
26. Hines EA Jr, Brown GE: The cold pressor test for measuring the reactibility of the blood pressure: Data concerning 571 normal and hypertensive subjects. *Amer Heart J* **11**:1-9, 1936.
27. Hines EA Jr: Vascular reactivity and hypertensive disease, in *Hypertension—A Symposium.* University of Minnesota Press, Minneapolis, 1950, pp 331-341.
28. Pickering GW: *High Blood Pressure.* London, J&A Churchill Ltd, 1955, p 549.
29. Smirk FH: *High Arterial Pressure.* Oxford, England, Blackwell Scientific Publications, 1957.
30. Doyle JT, Dawber TR, Kannel WB, et al: The relationship of cigarette smoking to coronary heart disease. *JAMA* **190**:886-890, 1964.
31. Doyle JT, Dawber TR, Kannel WB, et al: Cigarette smoking and coronary heart disease: Combined Framingham and Albany experience. *New Eng J Med* **266**:796-801, 1962.

Glutethimide Intoxication

A Prospective Study of 70 Patients Treated Conservatively Without Hemodialysis

Joseph A. Chazan, MD, and Serafino Garella, MD, Providence, RI

A prospective study of 70 patients admitted to the Rhode Island Hospital and treated for glutethimide intoxication conservatively, without hemodialysis, was undertaken. The diagnosis was confirmed in each case by elevated blood glutethimide levels; mixed intoxications with barbiturates were excluded by negative blood levels. Although only 1 patient died, 31 were unresponsive on admission and had complicated clinical courses associated with significant morbidity. Blood and cerebrospinal fluid glutethimide levels obtained on admission and subsequently were poorly correlated with duration of coma or morbidity. We conclude that (1) plasma glutethimide values are needed to confirm the diagnosis but are of little prognostic significance; (2) conservative treatment is associated with a very low mortality, although frequent and significant morbidity does occur among comatose patients; and (3) hemodialysis would appear to be needed rarely in the treatment of patients with glutethimide intoxication.

Many patients seen each year because of acute overdosage with glutethimide (Doriden) have life-threatening intoxication. It is generally agreed that the primary therapy should be directed towards providing adequate ventilation and tissue perfusion; when possible, unabsorbed drug should be removed from the gastrointestinal tract.[1-6] Forced diuresis is of little value since absorbed glutethimide is metabolized to the inactive glucuronide and only insignificant quantities of active drug are excreted in the urine.[7] Hemodialysis, either aqueous[2,3,8-10] or lipid,[11] has been proposed as a valuable adjunct in the treatment of patients severely intoxicated with glutethimide. Unfortunately, the amount of drug removed with hemodialysis is small, and studies of comparably intoxicated patients treated without hemodialysis are not available for comparison.

Since the use of hemodialysis per se remains of questionable value, especially in view of previous observations which failed to demonstrate any beneficial effects of this procedure,[6] we undertook a prospective study to evaluate the effects of conservative treatment in patients with acute glutethimide intoxication. The clinical course, morbidity, mortality, and prognostic indicators of 70 consecutive, unselected patients with well-documented glutethimide intoxication admitted to the Rhode Island Hospital during a three-year period are described. Thirty-one of these patients were moderately or severely intoxicated and, although pulmonary complications were frequent among these patients, only one died. On the basis of these observations we conclude that the use of hemodialysis is rarely, if ever, indicated in the treatment of glutethimide intoxication.

Received for publication Nov 30, 1970; accepted Feb 26, 1971.

From the Department of Medicine, Division of Renal Diseases, Rhode Island Hospital; and the Division of Biological and Medical Sciences, Brown University, Providence, RI.

Reprint requests to Division of Renal Diseases, Rhode Island Hospital, Providence, RI 02903 (Dr. Chazan).

Methods

All patients admitted to the Rhode Island Hospital during a three-year period from May 1967 to April 1970 with documented glutethimide intoxication were studied. The diagnosis of glutethimide intoxication was documented by history as well as by the presence of an elevated blood glutethimide level determined by a chemical method[12] which is both reproducible and specific for glutethimide and which measures total glutethimide. Although newer methods are available for the determination of glutethimide, this method is satisfactory for clinical purposes, since in our laboratory it has been found to be reproducible within ±5% and unaffected by the presence of barbiturates. In each patient blood barbiturate levels were determined and only patients with negative levels were included in this study.

The patients were classified according to their state of consciousness on admission to the hospital and the presence or absence of hypotension during the first few hours in the hospital. Patients were considered to be mildly intoxicated if they were responsive to painful stimuli, moderately intoxicated if they were unresponsive to painful stimuli but not hypotensive, and severely intoxicated if they were both unresponsive to painful stimuli and hypotensive (systolic blood pressure < 100 mm Hg). All of the moderately and severely intoxicated patients were seen by one of us in consultation early during their hospital course. Therapy was directed towards providing adequate ventilation, supporting blood pressure when necessary, and removing unabsorbed drug from the gastrointestinal tract. Endotracheal intubation, tracheostomy, and mechanical support of ventilation were instituted when hypoxia or hypercapnia were detected. Appropriate antibiotics and ventilation therapy were provided at the earliest indication and vasopressors, metaraminol bitartrate (Aramine) or levarterenol (Levophed Bitartrate), were administered to severely hypotensive patients. Gastric intubation and lavage along with the induction of diarrhea with sorbitol and castor oil were employed in most comatose patients. We did not measure the quantity of drug removed by these procedures.

The patients were subsequently followed-up closely with frequent reevaluation of their state of consciousness and blood glutethimide levels until complete recovery from the intoxication occurred. In addition, cerebrospinal fluid glutethimide levels were measured on admission in 24 patients and again at 24-hour intervals for as long as coma persisted in 16 of these patients.

Table 1.—Total Number, Sex Distribution, and Age of All Patients Studied

	No.	Males	Females	Age (yr) Range	Age (yr) Mean
Mild intoxication	39	15	24	9-78	37
Moderate intoxication	18	8	10	14-59	35
Severe intoxication	13	8	5	22-61	41
Total	70	31	39		37

Table 2.—Duration of Coma and Pulmonary Complications in All Patients With Moderate and Severe Intoxications

	Duration of Coma (hr)		Pulmonary Complications			
	Mean	Range	Endotracheal Intubation	Pneumonia	Tracheostomy	Ventilatory Failure
Moderate (n = 18)	14	4-32	11 (61%)	9 (50%)	1 (6%)	1 (6%)
Severe (n = 13)	38	12-100	10 (77%)	8 (62%)	1 (8%)	9 (69%)

Results

A total of 70 patients with glutethimide intoxication were evaluated: intoxication was mild in 39, moderate in 18, and severe in 13. All three groups were comparable with regard to sex and age distribution (Table 1).

Clinical Course and Morbidity.—*Mild Intoxications (39 Patients).*—The only clinical signs of intoxication in these patients were drowsiness or lethargy. All recovered without significant morbidity; 24 were alert and responsive when first seen and, therefore, were either not admitted to the hospital at all or were discharged within 24 hours.

Moderate Intoxications (18 Patients) (Table 2).—These patients were unresponsive to painful stimuli but not hypotensive (systolic blood pressure always >100 mm Hg) on admission or during their hospital course. Although none of these patients died, coma persisted for an average of 14 hours (range 4 to 32 hours) and pulmonary complications occurred frequently—11 (61%) required endotracheal intubation, 9 (50%) developed pneumonia, and 1 (6%) had evidence of respiratory failure and required supportive ventilation.

Severe Intoxications (13 Patients).—All of these patients were both unresponsive to painful stimuli and hypotensive (systolic blood pressure < 100 mm Hg) on or shortly after admission to the hospital. Most had no reflexes along with widely dilated pupils which did not react to light. The duration of hypotension ranged between 12 and 100 hours (mean 38 hours) and in five patients was considered to be severe enough by the attending physician so that vasopressor therapy (metaraminol or levarterenol) was instituted. Although these patients were hypotensive, the urine output remained adequate, skin was warm and dry, and none developed evidence of acute tubular necrosis. The morbidity was significant—ten patients (77%) required endotracheal intubation, eight (62%) developed pneumonia, and nine (69%) required supportive ventilation for up to 90 hours (mean 34 hours). One died suddenly and unexpectedly while eating lunch approximately 36 hours after he had recovered from the direct effects of the intoxication and was completely alert. Unfortunately, no necropsy was performed.

Correlation of Blood Glutethimide Levels With Clinical Course.—Blood glutethimide levels at admission to the hospital for all 70 patients are shown in Fig 1. As can be seen, there is marked overlap among the three groups, although the mean blood glutethimide level in the mildly intoxicated patients is significantly lower ($P < 0.01$) than the mean levels for the moderately and severely intoxicated patients. Blood glutethimide levels below 5 mg/100 ml occurred frequently in all three groups, whereas levels above 5 mg/100 ml occurred almost exclusively among

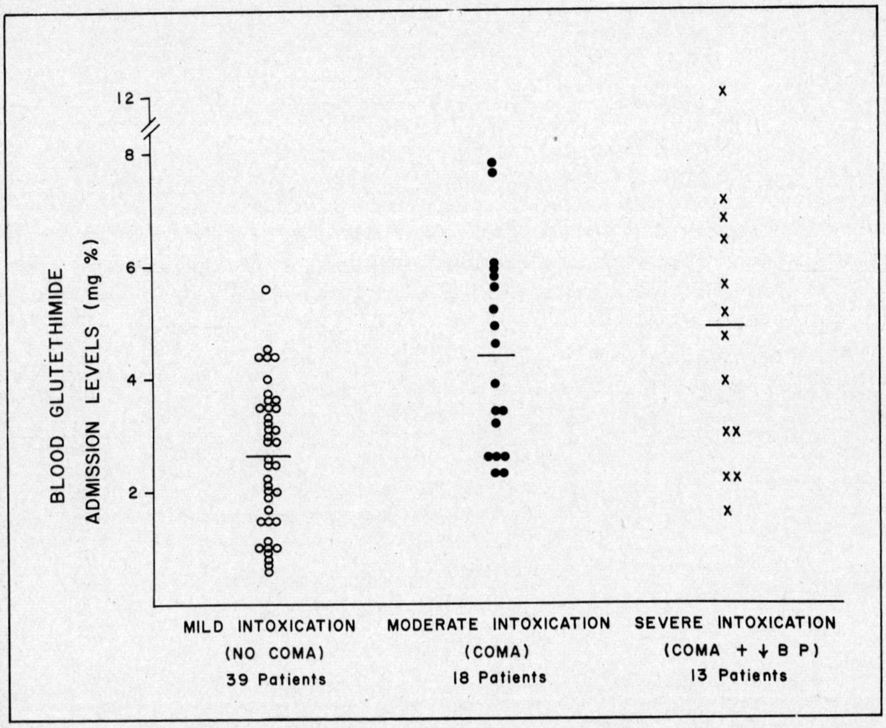

Fig 1.—Blood glutethimide levels for all 70 patients on admission. The horizontal line represents the mean value for each group. The mean of the mildly intoxicated patients is significantly lower ($P < 0.01$) than that for the other two groups; however, there is no statistical difference between the mean of the moderately and severely intoxicated groups.

Fig 2.—The blood glutethimide levels at admission have been plotted against the duration of coma for all patients with moderate and severe intoxications. There is no correlation between the initial levels and the duration of coma.

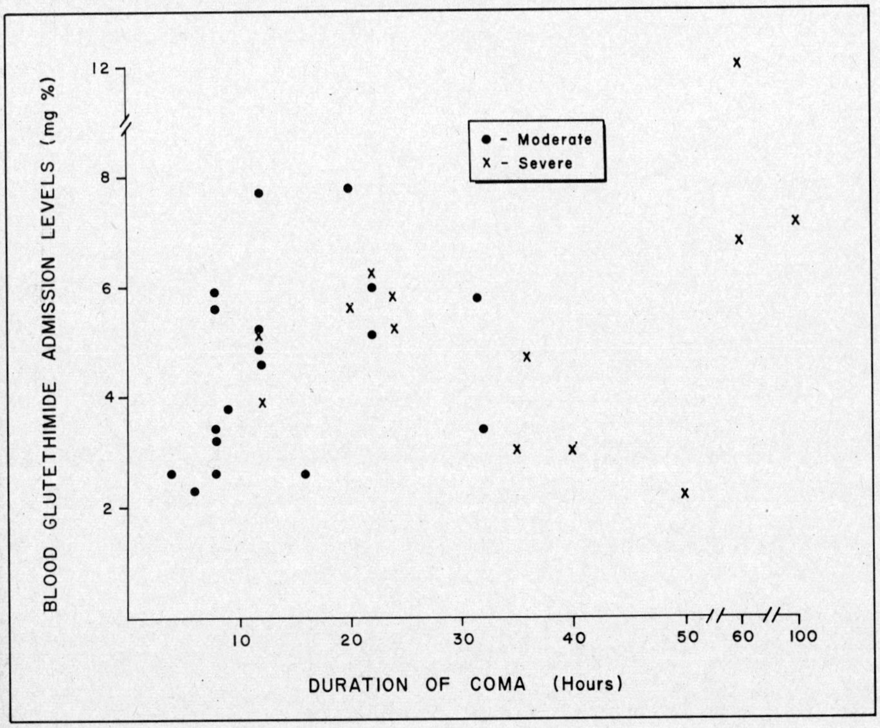

moderately or severely intoxicated patients. The apparent lack of relationship between blood glutethimide levels and clinical course is further elucidated by the data presented in Fig 2 and 3. Figure 2 depicts the relationship between blood glutethimide levels and duration of coma and Fig 3 shows the changes in blood glutethimide levels between admission values and those at the end of the comatose period. As can be seen, an apparent relationship was not observed between duration of coma and blood glutethimide levels on admission, or between the state of consciousness and subsequent changes in blood levels. In fact, in ten patients the blood level at the end of the comatose period was equal to or greater than the admission value, in 17 the level at the end of the comatose period was greater than 50% of the admission value, and in only 4 patients was there a fall in the blood glutethimide level to below 50% of the admission value before the patient awoke.

Cerebrospinal Fluid Glutethimide Levels.—In an attempt to find a more useful prognostic indicator, cerebrospinal fluid glutethimide levels along with blood glutethimide levels were measured in 8 mildly, 12 moderately, and 4 severely intoxicated patients at admission and again at 24-hour intervals for as long as they remained in coma (Fig 4). Unfortunately, cerebrospinal fluid levels were linearly correlated, with blood glutethimide levels being approximately 60% of the blood values over a wide range and were, therefore, not better correlated with the clinical course than the blood levels.

Comment

The severity of the overdosage among our 70 patients ranged from only minimal drowsiness to prolonged coma of up to 100 hours. The severity

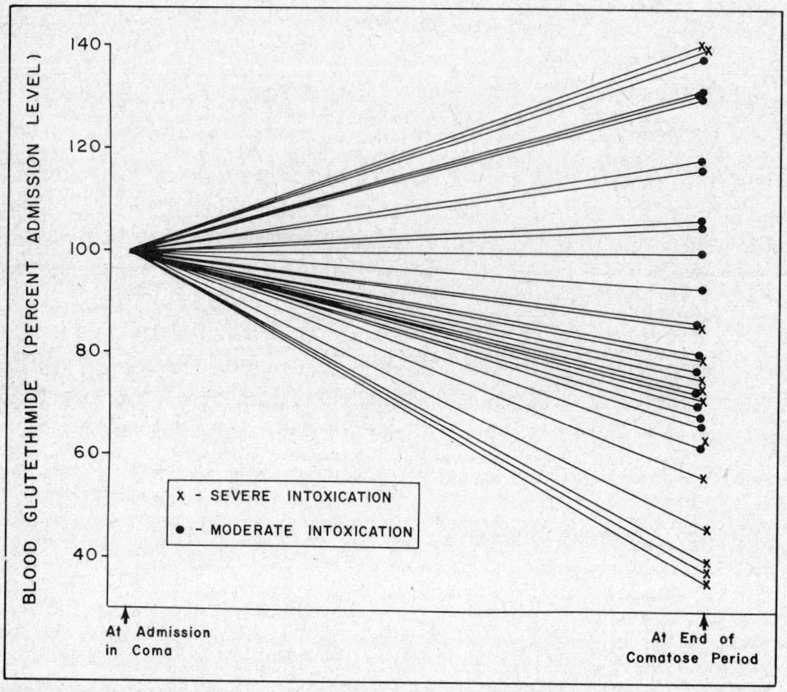

Fig 3.—Percent change of blood glutethimide levels at admission and at the end of the comatose period for all patients with moderate and severe intoxications. The greatest majority of the patients became responsive while blood glutethimide levels were still > 50% of admission levels. All four patients who remained in coma until the blood levels fell below 50% of admission values were severely intoxicated patients who were in coma for prolonged periods of time.

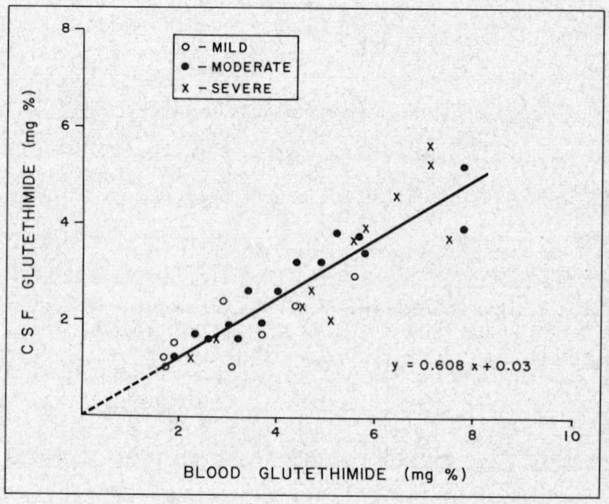

Fig 4.—Relationship between levels of cerebrospinal fluid glutethimide and blood glutethimide. Cerebrospinal fluid values were linearly correlated with the blood values over a wide range of blood glutethimide levels.

of the clinical course was difficult to predict on the basis of the amount of ingested drug, since this information was often unobtainable or unreliable. The clinical presentation of patients with acute glutethimide intoxication is difficult to distinguish from the clinical presentation of patients who have ingested other sedatives or hypnotics. The findings of markedly dilated, unreactive pupils and gastrointestinal atony, although frequently observed during glutethimide intoxication, are not specific but are related to the parasympatholytic activity of the drug, a property shared by other hypnotics as well. Although determination of blood glutethimide levels is necessary to confirm the diagnosis, it appears to be of no prognostic value (Fig 1-3). This lack of relationship between the blood glutethimide level and the clinical course has several possible explanations: (1) The amount of glutethimide free to circulate in the blood stream is only a small and probably unrepresentative fraction of the total in the body; since glutethimide is quite lipid soluble, most of the absorbed drug is deposited in the body tissues. (2) The chemical determination used for the detection of glutethimide measures active as well as inactive drug, a better clinical correlation might be obtained if only active drug were identified. (3) Patients who have been ingesting glutethimide over a long period might have adapted to the drug and thus be expected to have fewer toxic symptoms at the same blood values than patients who had not adapted to the drug.

It is worth noting that blood glutethimide levels > 6 mg/100 ml which were observed in seven of our patients have generally not been observed in other reports.[1-4,8-10] This discrepancy may reflect the fact that in our study blood was drawn in all patients immediately on their arrival at the hospital and the determinations were done promptly. Plasma glutethimide levels may be reduced by either a delay in performing the determination (Martin HF, unpublished data) or by the administration of fluid therapy which can lead to volume expansion and dilution. The failure of other reports to demonstrate such high blood glutethimide levels may reflect the fact that these reports include patients who had been referred from other hospitals where fluid therapy had already been administered and also that there may have been a delay in the determination of the plasma glutethimide level.

In the present study neither blood nor cerebrospinal fluid glutethimide levels were of prognostic value and, therefore, the patients were classified according to their state of consciousness on admission and the presence or absence of hypotension (systolic blood pressure < 100 mm Hg) during their hospital course. This clinical classification was of prognostic value for each group. None of the patients with mild intoxication had significant morbidity, whereas many of the patients with moderate and most of the patients with severe intoxication had significant morbidity (Table 2). The duration of coma was longer and the need for support of ventilation was more frequent in this latter group, the only observed death occurred in a severely intoxicated patient.

It seems unlikely that the mortality rate in this series could have been significantly modified by the use of hemodialysis, since the only patient who died did so after he had recovered from the direct consequences of the glutethimide intoxication. Of course, it is not possible to exclude that dialysis might have significantly reduced the morbidity; however, our previous experience tends to refute this possibility. In that study a comparison of two groups of comparably intoxicated patients failed to show that hemodialysis shortened the duration of coma or lessened the complications.[6]

It is tempting to speculate that our conclusions regarding the conservative treatment of patients with acute glutethimide intoxication may be applicable to patients intoxicated with other forms of hypnotic or tranquilizer drugs. The value of hemodialysis per se in the treatment of drug intoxication can be proven only when data are available from either a well-controlled series or when it is demonstrated that large amounts of pharmacologically active forms of the drug in question are removed in the dialysate. It is possible that the beneficial effects previously attributed to hemodialysis in the treatment of intoxication with ethchlorvynol (Placidyl)[13] and methyprylon (Noludar)[14] among others, reflect improvement in the general medical care of these patients rather than in the use of hemodialysis, since neither data from controlled series nor measurements of pharmacologically *active* drug in the dialysate have been reported.

At the present time we feel that therapy of patients intoxicated with glutetimide should be directed towards providing an airway, supporting ventilation, treating pulmonary infection, maintaining tissue perfusion, and, when possible, removing unabsorbed drug from the gastrointestinal tract either by gastric suction or by induced diarrhea. It would appear that hemodialysis is rarely if ever indicated in the treatment of such patients, although it is possible that with the advent of newer dialytic techniques, hemodialysis may become of greater value in the future.

This study was supported in part by the Sergi S. Zlinkoff Memorial Fund.

References

1. Schreiner GE, Berman LB, Kovach R, et al: Acute glutethimide (Doriden) poisoning: The use of bemegride (Megimide) and hemodialysis. *Arch Intern Med* **101**:899-911, 1958.

2. Maher JF, Schreiner GE, Westervelt FB Jr: Acute glutethimide intoxication: Clincial experience (22 patients) compared to acute barbiturate intoxication (63 patients). *Amer J Med* **33**:70-81, 1962.

3. McDonald DF, Greene WM, Kretchmar L, et al: Experiences in acute glutethimide (Doriden) intoxication: Superiority of extracorporeal dialysis over peritoneal dialysis. *Invest Urol* **1**:127-133, 1963.

4. Irvine ROH, Montgomerie JZ, Spence M: Assisted respiration, noradrenaline infusion and the artificial kidney for glutethimide ("Doriden") poisoning. *Med J Aust* **2**:277-279, 1963.

5. *Acute Overdosage of Doriden (Glutethimide): Suggested Treatment* Summit, NJ, Ciba Pharmaceutical Company, 1968.

6. Chazan JA, Cohen JJ: Clinical spectrum of glutethimide intoxication: Hemodialysis reevaluated. *JAMA* **208**:837-839, 1969.

7. Keberle H, Hoffmann K, Bernhard K: The metabolism of glutethimide (Doriden ®). *Experientia* **18**:105-111, 1962.

8. Maher JF, Schreiner GE: Acute glutethimide poisoning: II. The use of hemodialysis. *Trans Amer Soc Artif Intern Organs* **7**:100-106, 1961.

9. Lubash GD, Ferrari MJ, Scherr L, et al: Sedative overdosage and the role of hemodialysis. *Arch Intern Med* **110**:884-887, 1962.

10. DeMyttenaere M, Schoenfeld L, Maher JF: Treatment of glutethimide poisoning: A comparison of forced diuresis and dialysis. *JAMA* **203**:885-887, 1968.

11. Ginn HE, Matter BJ, Shinaberger JH, et al: Clinical experience with lipid dialysis. *J Clin Invest* **47**:40a, 1968.

12. Goldbaum LR, Williams MA, Koppanyi T: Determination of glutethimide in biological fluids. *Anal Chem* **32**:81-84, 1960.

13. Teehan BP, Maher JF, Carey JJH, et al: Acute ethchlorvynol (Placidyl) intoxication. *Ann Inter Med* **72**:875-882, 1970.

14. Yudis M, Swartz C, Onesti G, et al: Hemodialysis for methyprylon (Noludar) poisoning. *Ann Inter Med* **68**:1301-1304, 1968.

Cardiac Performance Three to Eight Weeks After Acute Myocardial Infarction

Shahbudin H. Rahimtoola, MB, MRCPE; Michael M. DiGilio, MD; M. Ziad Sinno, MD; Henry S. Loeb, MD; Kenneth M. Rosen, MD; and Rolf M. Gunnar, MS, MD, Chicago

When cardiac performance was assessed three to eight weeks after uncomplicated acute myocardial infarction (AMI) in patients not in clinical cardiac failure, abnormalities of left ventricular (LV) function were demonstrated in 22 of 27 patients who, by clinical criteria, were recovering satisfactorily. Left ventricular end-diastolic pressure (LVEDP) was measured in 24 patients. It was elevated in 19, ranged from 14 to 20 mm Hg in 13, and was > 20 mm Hg in 6. Patients comprised three groups: group 1—5 patients with normal LVEDP, cardiac index (CI), stroke index (SI), and preejection period (PEP) to left ventricular ejection time (PEP/LVET) ratio; group 2—12 patients with elevated LVEDP (14 to 24 mm Hg) but normal CI, SI, and PEP/LVET ratio and; group 3—10 patients with elevated LVEDP (14 to 30 mm Hg), reduced CI and SI (< 2.5 liters/min/sq m and < 30 ml/sq m), and increased PEP/LVET ratios (> 0.381).

Occlusion of a major coronary artery in the experimental animal rapidly results in a bulge of the ischemic area of the myocardium during systole.[1-3] There is reduction of cardiac output (CO), systemic arterial pressure[4,5] and, depression of left ventricular (LV) function.[1-6] In man, following an acute myocardial infarction (AMI), there is a similar reduction of cardiac output,[7-12] increase of left ventricular end-diastolic pressure (LVEDP),[13-16] and impairment of left ventricular function.[15,16]

There is incomplete recovery of ventricular function one week after experimental myocardial infarction[6] and, at the end of four to eight weeks, residual increases of LVEDP have been attributed to an alteration of ventricular distensibility.[17] In man, reported changes in CO three to eight weeks after AMI have followed no consistent pattern.[10,18]

This study assesses left ventricular function in man during the early convalescent phase after AMI. It demonstrates that impairment of LV performance in the first three to eight weeks after AMI is frequent.

Received for publication Dec 1, 1970; accepted March 3, 1971.

From the Department of Adult Cardiology and the Hektoen Institute for Medical Research, Cook County Hospital; and the Department of Medicine, Abraham Lincoln School of Medicine, University of Illinois College of Medicine, Chicago.

Reprint requests to Department of Adult Cardiology, Cook County Hospital, 1825 W Harrison St, Chicago 60612 (Dr. Rahimtoola).

Material and Methods

Hemodynamic studies were carried out in 27 patients who had recently sustained an AMI. There were 18 men and 9 women patients and their ages ranged from 44 to 85 years (mean 62.2 years).

Patients were selected for study on the basis of (1) documented recent AMI, (2) informed consent being obtained, and (3) the absence of significant complications, such as severe arrhythmias and congestive heart failure. Thus, the patients did not have paroxysmal nocturnal dyspnea, orthopnea, and they were not dyspneic. Further, they did not have edema, elevated jugular venous pressure, liver enlargement, or rales at the lung bases. The diagnosis of AMI was based on the history of ischemic cardiac pain, appropriate changes in the serum enzymes (serum glutamic oxaloacetic transaminase [SGOT], lactic dehydrogenase [LDH], and

Table 1.—Clinical Data of the Patients*

Patient No.	Age (yr)	Time of Study (Days After AMI)†	Extent of AMI	Angina	Physical Examination: Cardiac Enlargement	S_3†	S_4†	SM†	Chest Roentgenogram: CTR†	Pulmonary Ventricular Congestion	Therapy: Digoxin	Diuretics
1	65	30	TM†	0	0	0	+†	0	—	—	+	+
2	45	35	NTM†	0	0	0	+	+	—	—	0	0
3	61	24	TM	0	0	0	+	0	0.49	—	+	0
4	68	25	NTM	0	0	0	+	0	0.63	—	0	+
5	52	21	TM	0	0	0	+	0	0.54	—	0	0
6	52	30	TM	0	0	0	+	0	0.50	0	0	0
7	65	23	TM	0	0	0	+	0	—	—	0	0
8	65	20	TM	0	0	0	+	0	—	—	0	0
9	44	28	TM	0	0	0	+	0	0.45	0	+	+
10	64	20	TM	0	+	0	+	+	0.58	0	0	0
11	58	26	TM	0	0	±†	+	0	0.46	0	0	0
12	69	28	TM	0	0	±	0	+	0.44	0	0	+
13	53	34	TM	0	0	0	0	+	0.45	0	0	0
14	67	22	NTM	0	0	0	+	+	0.45	0	0	0
15	62	32	NTM	+	0	0	+	+	0.59	0	0	0
16	64	26	TM	0	0	+	+	0	0.54	0	0	0
17	59	32	NTM	+	0	0	+	+	0.48	0	0	+
18	60	22	TM	0	0	0	+	0	—	—	+	+
19	75	60	TM	+	+	0	+	+	0.60	±	+	+
20	62	32	TM	0	0	0	+	0	0.46	0	0	0
21	55	21	NTM	+	±	±	+	+	0.58	±	0	0
22	85	41	NTM	0	0	0	+	+	—	—	0	0
23	73	53	NTM	0	0	0	+	0	—	—	0	0
24	68	30	TM	0	0	0	+	+	—	—	+	0
25	52	27	NTM	0	0	0	+	0	0.54	0	0	0
26	61	26	TM	0	0	0	+	+	0.45	0	0	0
27	76	22	TM	0	0	+	+	0	0.56	0	+	0

* No patient had orthopnea, paroxysmal nocturnal dyspnea, peripheral edema, or raised jugular venous pressure.

† AMI = acute myocardial infarction, TM = transmural, NTM = nontransmural, S_3 = diastolic gallop, S_4 = presystolic gallop, SM = systolic murmur, CTR = cardiothoracic ratio, + = present, O = absent, — = not available for review at the present time, and ± = uncertainty about its presence.

Fig 1.—The chest roentgenograms (PA view) of two patients with impairment of LV function. Left, *Patient 20; the cardiothoracic ratio (CTR) is 0.46. There is no pulmonary venous congestion.* Right, *Patient 10; the CTR is 0.58.*

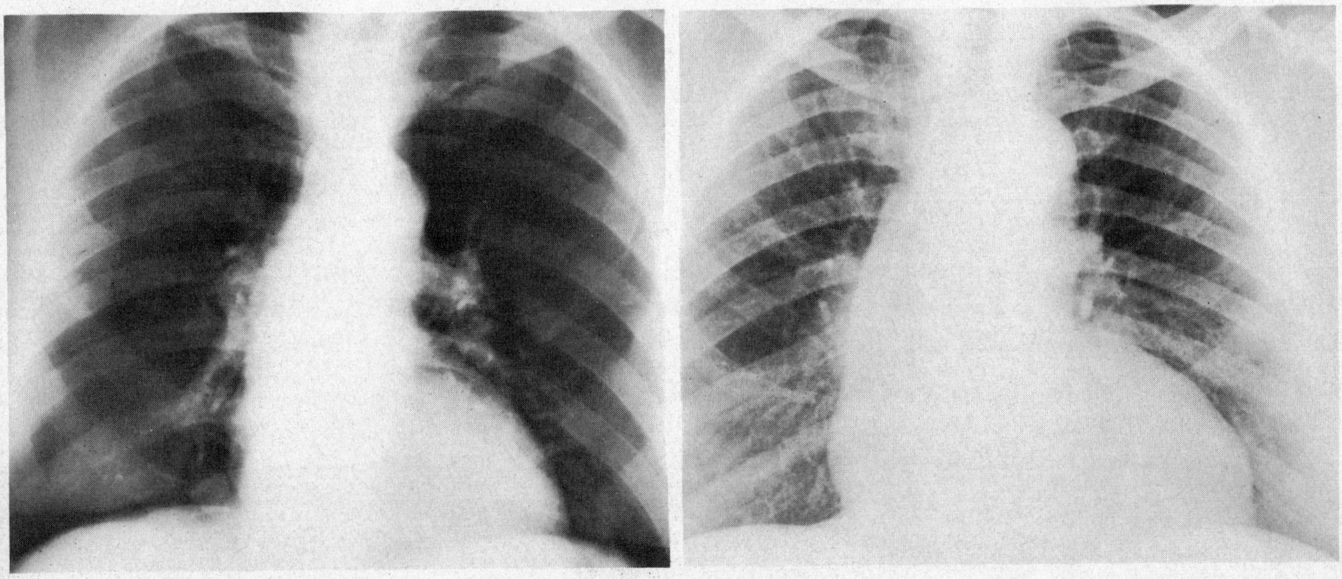

Table 2.—Hemodynamic Data and Systoli

Patient No.	Aorta (mm Hg)	LV (mm Hg)	Right Atrial or CVP (mm Hg)	CO (Liters/min)	CI (Liters/min/sq m)	SI (ml/sq m)	Heart Rate (Beats per Minute)	QS_2 (msec)	LVET (msec)	PEP (msec)
1	156/75	156/0-8	4	4.1	2.9	46	63	348	263	85
2	162/96	162/4-12	3	5.1	2.9	58	50	398	295	103
3	120/83	115/1-10	6	6.4	3.4	36	96	293	226	67
4	140/71	140/0-12	2	5.5	2.9	54	54	414	326	88
5	174/95	154/4-10	0	4.6	2.9	28	102	349	238	111
6	118/70	118/2-14	3	4.9	2.9	31	95	329	240	89
7	194/82	194/10-24	3	5.2	2.8	41	69	389	292	97
8	148/80	148/0-20	4	5.9	3.3	39	84	376	275	100
9	130/84	130/0-18	2	4.8	2.6	31	85	365	265	100
10	194/88	194/7-20	...	6.6	3.1	39	80	385	280	105
11	158/77	158/1-30	4	7.5	3.8	58	65	419	324	95
12	168/80	168/4-14	4	5.5	3.1	57	54	...	...	...
13	155/99	158/1-15	5	4.5	2.9	54	54	420	314	106
14	182/92	182/4-21	6	3.8	2.5	38	66	422	324	98
15	196/76	196/5-20	7	7.1	3.8	63	60	425	359	66
16	170/85	170/6-21	6	5.4	3.9	40	96	368	289	79
17	186/102	186/4-14	6	9.5	4.9	71	70	384	311	73
18	130/76	128/17-28	3	4.1	2.3	26	90	331	230	101
19	194/100	192/4-16	1	3.1	2.0	27	75	386	276	110
20	90/63	90/10-33	2	3.2	1.6	18	87	310	196	114
21	135/96	135/0-19	0	4.5	2.3	26	88	378	256	122
22	185/82	...	1	3.6	2.3	35	66	413	273	140
23	136/76	...	1	3.7	2.0	20	102	314	284	110
24	156/86	...	1	2.9	1.9	20	96	312	209	103
25	114/96	114/7-15	6	4.3	2.3	31	75	354	200	154
26	154/75	154/5-20	12	2.2	1.3	15	84	412	257	155
27	147/70	147/8-14	3	3.2	1.8	22	81	...	...	...

Table 3.—Patients Grouped on the Basis of Cardiac Index (CI) and Left Ventricular End-Diastolic Pressure (LVEDP)

Group	Patients		Extent of Infarct*		LVEDP	CI	SI	PEP/LVET
	No.	%	TM	NTM	>12 mm Hg	<2.5	<30	>0.381
1	5	19%	3	2	0	0	1	1
2	12	44%	8	4	12	0	0	0†
3	10	37%	7	3	7‡	10	8	9†

* TM = transmural, NTM = nontransmural.
† Not measured in one patient.
‡ Only measured in seven patients.

Table 4.—Left Ventricular Diastolic Pressures

Group	Prior to Atrial Contraction		End-Diastole	
	Mean	Range	Mean	Range
1	7	4-10	10	8-12
2	9	6-15	19	14-24
3	12	7-16	20	14-33

creatine phosphokinase [CPK]),[19] and characteristic alterations of the electrocardiogram.[20,21] Eighteen patients were judged to have a transmural AMI because of the presence of pathological Q waves on the ECG, and the rest (nine patients) were considered to have a nontransmural AMI. Twenty-four patients were studied three to five weeks after AMI. Three patients were studied on the 41st, 53rd, and 60th day, respectively, after the episode of AMI.

The patients were investigated in the diagnostic cardiac catheterization laboratory. Central venous or right atrial pressure was recorded with 16-gauge radiopaque catheters (Intracath); left ventricular and aortic pressures were recorded via 5 F polytef (Teflon) catheters with the use of strain gauges (Statham P23Db). The catheters were introduced percutaneously by the Seldinger technique[22] into brachial artery, femoral artery, and an antecubital vein. In some patients a catheter (No. 6 Goodale Lubin) was introduced with use of a percutaneous catheter introducer and advanced to the pulmonary artery (PA) and PA wedge positions. One of the arterial catheters was advanced retrograde across the aortic valve into the left ventricle. In three patients the left ventricle could not be entered easily and thus left ventricular pressures were not obtained. Mean pressures were obtained by electrical damping. Heart sounds were recorded using a contact crystal microphone. All the variables including indicator dilution curves were recorded on photographic paper with the use of a recorder (Electronics for Medicine, model DR 16). Normal values for left ventricular diastolic pressures were ob-

s of All Patients

PEP/LVET Ratio	PEP_c (msec)	$LVET_c$ (msec)	QS_{2c} (msec)
0.323	110	370	480
0.349	123	380	503
0.296	107	394	501
0.266	110	420	520
0.468	152	401	563
0.371	127	402	529
0.332	125	409	534
0.362	134	418	552
0.377	134	410	544
0.375	137	416	553
0.293	121	435	556
...	...	...	...
0.337	159	411	540
0.302	124	434	559
0.184	91	466	557
0.273	115	440	555
0.234	107	457	564
0.439	137	383	520
0.399	140	404	544
0.582	149	344	493
0.477	157	406	563
0.513	166	385	551
0.539	151	377	528
0.493	141	372	513
0.735	182	321	503
0.603	189	402	591
...	...	...	...

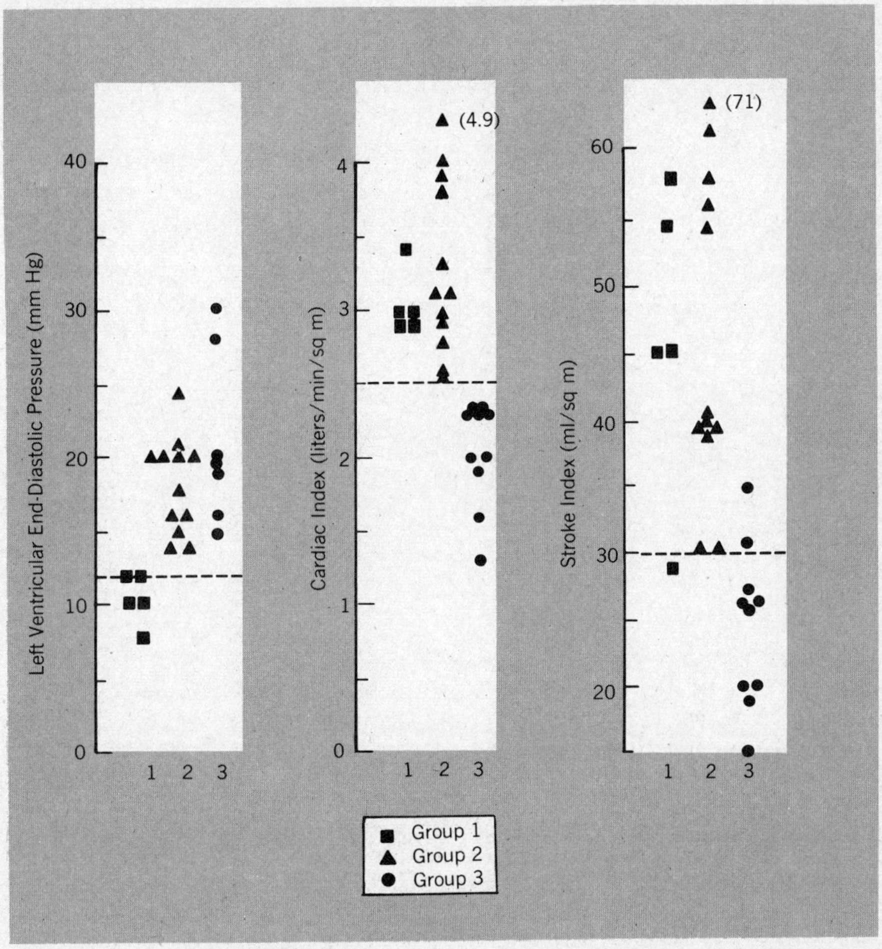

Fig 2.—Graph showing the distribution of left ventricular end-diastolic pressure (left panel), cardiac index (center panel), and stroke index (right panel). The patients were divided into three groups—1 (squares), *2* (triangles), *and 3* (circles).

tained from the studies of Braunwald and co-workers.[23]

Cardiac output was determined by the indicator dilution technique (IDC) according to the method of Hamilton and associates.[24] Indocyanine green was injected into the right atrium and sampled in the central aorta. With the use of a withdrawal infusion pump, blood was withdrawn at a constant rate of 15 to 30 ml/min past a densitometer (Waters Corp., model D400) and the change in optical density associated with the passage of dye was amplified and recorded. The densitometer was calibrated using the patients' blood. Heart rate was obtained from the ECG. Cardiac output was divided by the body surface area in square meters to give the cardiac index (CI). Normal values for CI ($\geqq$ 2.5 liters/min/sq m) and stroke index (SI) (mean ± SD = 46 ml/sq m ± 8) were taken from the data of Barrat-Boyes and Wood.[25]

Systolic time intervals (STI) in milliseconds were determined from the phonocardiogram, ECG, and aortic pressure pulse with the use of the method described by Weissler et al.[26] The QS_2 is the time from the onset of the Q wave of the ECG to the first high frequency vibrations of the second heart sound and represents electromechanical systole, LVET is the left ventricular ejection time obtained from the aortic pressure pulse and, PEP (preejection period) is the time from the Q wave of the ECG to the onset of ventricular ejection (obtained by subtracting LVET from QS_2). The PEP/LVET ratio was computed. The STI were corrected for heart rate (PEP_c, $LVET_c$, and QS_{2c}) by the regression equation obtained from data for normal people as given by Weissler et al.[26] Normal values used for STI were (mean ± SD) PEP_c = 131 ± 13 and $LVET_c$ = 413 ± 10;[26] PEP/LVET = 0.345 ± 0.036.[27]

Isometric exercise was performed on nine patients by hand grip on a dynamometer. The day before the study the maximal voluntary contraction (MVC) was determined for each patient. The patients performed isometric exercise at 30%, 50%, and 100% of their MVC. All three levels of exercise were not obtained in all patients.

One patient, on a regimen of anticoagulants, required exposure of the brachial artery and one stitch in the artery to obtain hemostasis. There was an atheromatous plaque at the site of entry of the catheter. Another patient had a transient episode of dysphasia from which she recovered fully. There were no other complications.

Clinical Status of Patients.—All the patients were making an uncomplicated recovery from their recent acute myocardial infarction (Table 1). Four patients were having occasional anginal pain. Slight cardiac enlargement was considered to be present in two patients. Twenty-five patients had an atrial gallop (S_4 heart sound) and in three patients a diastolic gallop (S_3 heart sound) was

Table 5.—Effect of Isometric Exercise (Hand Grip) on Left Ventricular Function

	Aorta (mm Hg)		LV (mm Hg)	Mean Right Atrial (mm Hg)	CO (Liters/min)	SV (ml)	Heart Rate (Beats per Minute)	PEP (msec)	LVET (msec)	QS_2 (msec)
Group 1										
Patient 2										
Control	162/96	(118)*	162/4-12	3	5.2	85	50	103	295	398
30% of MVC†	178/94	(122)	178/4-15	3	...	...	67	107	286	393
100% of MVC	188/112	(137)	188/8-18	6	...	...	81	100	268	368
Patient 4										
Control	140/71	(92)	140/0-12	2	5.5	102	54	88	326	414
50% of MVC	198/96	(152)	198/3-18	7	7.0	97	72	83	326	409
Group 2										
Patient 9										
Control	130/84	(99)	130/0-14	2	4.8	66	78	100	265	365
100% of MVC	148/92	(111)	148/2-21	2	...	...	87	110	255	365
Patient 13										
Control	155/99	(128)	158/1-15	5	5.5	102	54	106	314	420
50% of MVC	176/108	(138)	176/8-17	6	7.3	122	60	107	310	417
Patient 15										
Control	208/78	(124)	208/10-24	9	7.0	117	60	63	378	441
50% of MVC	253/103	(170)	253/16-35	10	9.0	115	78	46	352	398
Group 3										
Patient 18										
Control	130/76	(94)	128/17-28	3	4.1	44	90	101	230	331
50% of MVC	150/112	(125)	150/32-45	2	...	...	124	108	216	324
Patient 20										
Control	90/63	(75)	90/10-30	2	3.2	39	82	118	203	321
30% of MVC	96/72	(80)	96/16-36	2	3.4	38	85	118	200	318
50% of MVC	110/80	(90)	110/20-46	2	3.0	30	99	124	184	308
Patient 25										
Control	114/96	(102)	114/7-15	6	4.3	57	75	154	200	354
50% of MVC	143/104	(126)	143/6-23	8	4.5	50	90	131	226	357
Patient 27										
Control	147/70	(108)	147/8-14	3	3.2	40	81	86	263	349
50% of MVC	164/78	(123)	164/8-19	...	4.1	44	93	95	291	386

* Values in parentheses are mean values. † MVC = maximum voluntary contraction.

Fig 3.—Left ventricular (LV) diastolic pressure and pulmonary artery (PA) wedge pressure in one patient. Atrial contraction elevates the LV diastolic pressure to a high level at end-diastole (33 mm Hg, left panel) without a proportionate rise in mean PA wedge pressure (18 Hg, right panel).

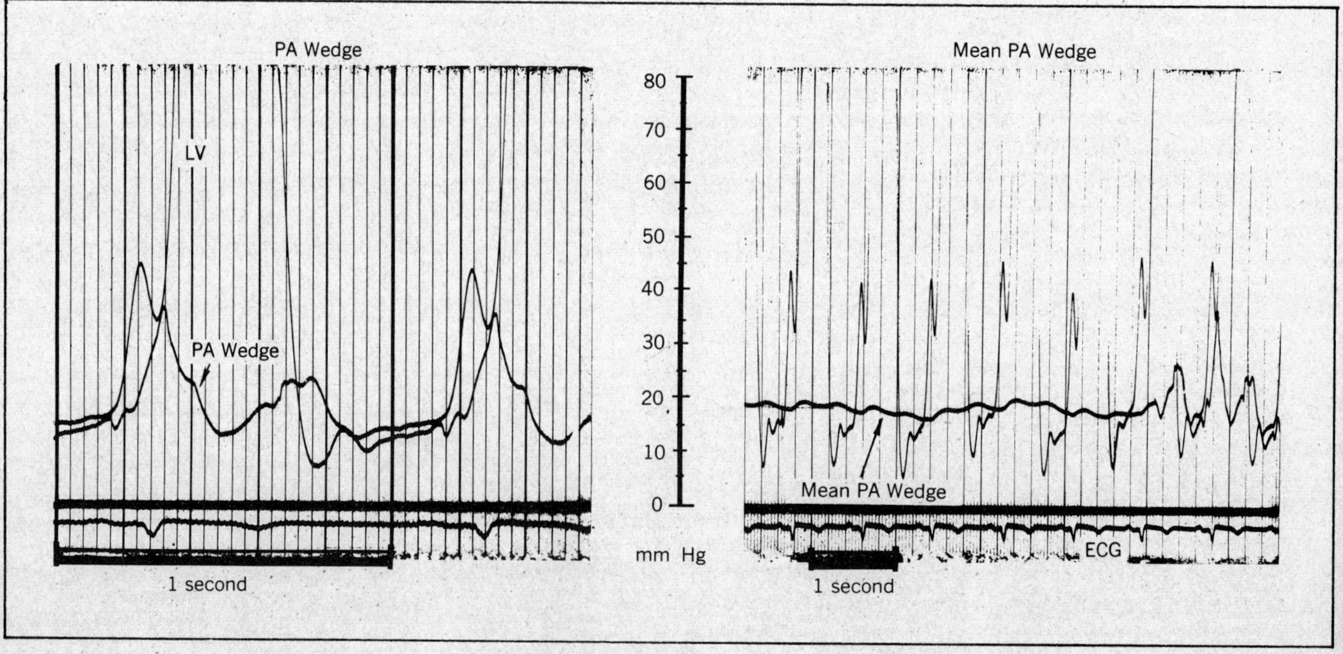

PEP/LVET Ratio	PEP_c (msec)	$LVET_c$ (msec)	QS_{2c} (msec)
0.349	123	380	503
0.374	134	400	534
0.373	132	406	538
0.266	110	418	528
0.255	111	445	556
0.377	134	410	544
0.431	145	403	548
0.337	128	406	534
0.345	129	405	534
0.167	87	478	565
0.131	78	490	568
0.439	137	383	520
0.500	158	427	584
0.581	151	342	493
0.580	150	345	497
0.673	164	352	516
0.770	184	327	511
0.580	167	379	546
0.327	118	401	519
0.326	128	430	558

heard. Two patients had apical holosystolic murmurs (grade 1/6) and ten others had ejection systolic murmurs (grade 1 to 2/6). All patients were in normal sinus rhythm. At the time of this report the chest roentgenogram was available for review in 19 patients. The heart size was normal (cardiothoracic ratio < 0.50) in ten (Fig 1) and in nine patients there was cardiomegaly. Four patients were receiving digitalis and diuretics, two were receiving digitalis alone, and another three were only receiving diuretics.

Results

The LVEDP was measured in 24 patients and was elevated in 19 (> 12 mm Hg). The LVEDP was between 14 and 20 mm Hg in eight patients, > 20 mm Hg in three, and was normal in five patients (Table 2). The CI was low (< 2.5 liters/min/sq m) in ten patients and the SI was low (< 30 ml/sq m) in nine patients. Right atrial or central venous pressure was normal in 26 patients and, thus, did not reflect the elevated LVEDP.

The PEP_c was reduced (< 118 msec) in six patients and was increased (> 144 msec) in eight patients. The $LVET_c$ was decreased (< 391 msec) in eight patients and was elevated (> 435 msec) in three patients. The PEP/LVET ratio was < 0.309 in six patients and was > 0.381 in ten patients.

On the basis of CI and LVEDP the patients have been divided into three groups (Fig 1 and 2). Patients with a CI of < 2.5 have been placed in group 3. Patients with a CI of 2.5 or more have been further divided into groups 1 and 2 on the basis of LVEDP. Those with a LVEDP of > 12 mm Hg have been placed in group 2 and the remainder in Group 1. Thus, the findings in these patients were (Table 3) as follows:

Group 1.—Five patients (1 to 5) had normal LVEDP (≦ 12 mm Hg) and normal CI. The SI was normal in four. The mean values ± the standard error of the mean for PEP_c and $LVET_c$ were 120.4 ± 7.5 and 393.0 ± 7.7, respectively. The mean values were normal. The mean ± the standard error of the mean for the PEP/LVET ratio was 0.340 ± 0.030. The PEP/LVET ratio was < 0.381 in all but one patient. Patient 5 had systemic hypertension which was associated with a reduced SI and a prolonged PEP that resulted in an abnormally prolonged PEP/LVET ratio. Three patients had a transmural AMI.

Group 2.—Twelve patients (6 to 17) had a normal CI and an elevated LVEDP (14 to 24 mm Hg). The SI's were normal. In one patient the systolic time intervals (STI) were not interpreted as the patient had an intraventricular conduction defect. The mean values ± the standard error of the mean for PEP_c and $LVET_c$ were 124.9 ± 5.0 and 427.1 ± 6.0, respectively. The mean values were normal. However, the PEP_c was prolonged in one and reduced in three patients and the $LVET_c$ were prolonged in three patients. The mean ± the standard error of the mean of the PEP/LVET ratio was 0.312 ± 0.018. PEP/LVET ratios were not increased (< 0.381). Eight patients had a transmural AMI.

Group 3.—Ten patients had a reduced CI. The LVEDP was elevated in all seven patients in whom it could be determined and ranged from 14 to 33 mm Hg. The SI were low (< 30 ml/beat/sq m) in eight patients. The mean values ± the standard error of the mean for PEP_c and $LVET_c$ were 156.9 ± 5.9 and 377.1 ± 9.0, respectively. The mean value for PEP_c was increased and that for $LVET_c$ was reduced. The PEP_c was increased in seven patients and $LVET_c$ was reduced in six patients. The PEP/LVET ratio was > 0.381 in nine patients (mean ± the standard error of the mean = 0.530 ± 0.031). The STI were not measured in one patient because of an inadequate quality of the phonocardiographic recording. Six patients had a transmural AMI.

Thus, 81% of the patients (groups 2 and 3) had abnormalities of LV function. In over half of these patients abnormalities of LV function could not be determined by measurement of CO or STI but only by measurement of LV pressure. An example of LV diastolic and pulmonary artery (PA) wedge pressures in one patient are shown in Fig 3. The PA wedge pressure is a damped and delayed representation of the left atrial pressure[28] and thus accounts for the small differences seen between LV diastolic pressure and PA wedge pressure (left panel). The LVEDP ("z" point) is 33 mm Hg, the mean PA wedge pressure is 18 mm Hg (right panel). Atrial contraction elevated the LV diastolic pressure to a

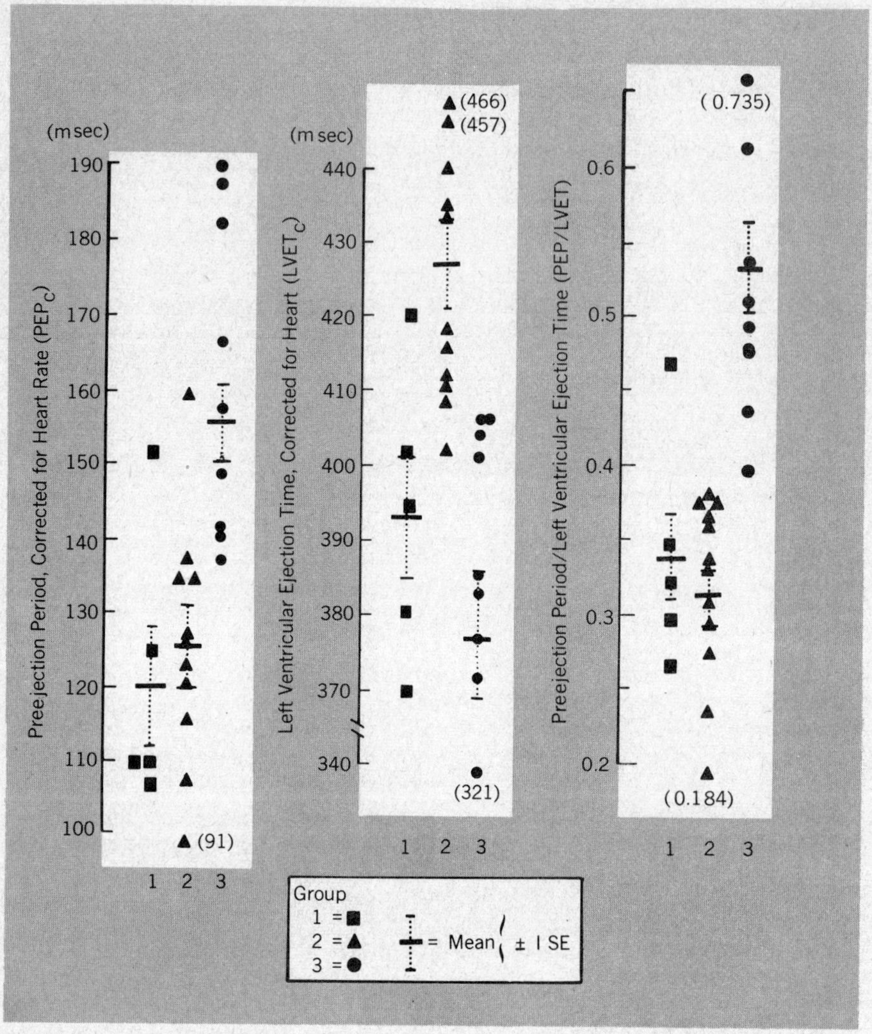

Fig 4.—Graph showing the distribution of corrected preejection period (left panel), corrected left ventricular ejection time (center panel), and the ratio of preejection period to left ventricular ejection time (right panel). The patients were divided into three groups—1 (squares), *2* (triangles), *and 3* (circles). *The mean ± standard error of the mean of the values are also shown.*

high level at end-diastole (left panel) without a proportionate rise in the mean PA wedge pressure (right panel). The mean PA wedge pressure appears to be more closely related to LV diastolic pressure just prior to atrial contraction. The LV diastolic pressures prior to atrial contraction and at end-diastole are shown in Table 4. Powerful atrial contraction made a significant contribution to elevating LV diastolic pressure at end-diastole in the patients in groups 2 and 3.

The effects of isometric exercise were different in patients in group 3 as compared with patients in groups 1 and 2 (Table 5). Patients in groups 1 and 2 (2, 4, 9, 13, and 15) had a small increase or no change in LVEDP, PEP_c, $LVET_c$, QS_{2c}, and PEP/LVET ratio and in many of these patients the STI continued to remain in the normal range. Two patients in group 3 (25 and 27) had an increase of LVEDP, increase of $LVET_c$ and QS_{2c}. The PEP_c was increased in one patient and reduced in the other. The PEP/LVET ratio was unchanged in one and decreased in the other. The other two patients in group 3 (18 and 20) had large increase in left ventricular early diastolic and end-diastolic pressures, PEP_c and PEP/LVET ratio; there was a small increase of QS_{2c}. The right atrial pressure was not significantly changed. With isometric exercise the cardiac output in the patients in groups 1 and 2 and one patient in group 3 increased, while the cardiac output in the other two patients in group 3 showed no significant change.

Comment

Impairment of left ventricular function was frequently demonstrated in the early recovery period following a clinically uncomplicated acute myocardial infarction. Varying states of ventricular performance were present: (1) There were five patients in whom all measured indexes of ventricular function were essentially normal (group 1). (2) In 12 patients who had an elevated left ventricular-end-diastolic pressure, the output of the heart and STI were normal (group 2). (3) Ten patients had an elevated LVEDP and the CO and STI were also abnormal (group 3).

An elevated LVEDP signifies an abnormality of LV function and may result from an alteration of ventricular distensibility, an increased ventricular end-diastolic volume (and thus myocardial fiber-length) or from a combination of both factors.[29,30] Since we have not measured ventricular volumes in our patients we cannot elucidate which mechanism is operative. In animals recovering from experimental myocardial infarction the increased LVEDP has been shown to be associated with a normal LV end-diastolic volume, thus implicating an alteration of ventricular distensibility.[17]

The left ventricle can alter its performance by one of two adjustments[31]: (1) changes in length-tension relationship (Frank-Starling mechanism)[32,33] and, (2) shifts of the force-velocity curve. If the increased LVEDP seen in our patients was associated with an increased end-diastolic volume then the left ventricle would appear to be utilizing the Frank-Starling mechanism to cope with the recent severe injury it had sustained (ie, AMI). Utilizing this compensatory mechanism the left ventricle could maintain a normal output in only half of the patients.

Powerful atrial contraction can increase ventricular end-diastolic pressure without a proportionate increase in mean atrial pressure[34]—this has been called the "booster pump action" of the atrium.[35] The ability of the atrium to perform such a function has the advantage of increasing the force of contraction of an impaired LV (end-diastolic pressure being a determinant of the force of contraction) without an associated increase of mean left atrial pressure (Fig 4) and, thus, avoiding the ill effects of a high pulmonary venous pressure.[36] Atrial contraction contributed significantly to the elevation of LVEDP (Table 4). If, as illustrated in Fig 4, mean PA wedge (indirect left atrial) pressure corresponds more closely to LV diastolic pressure prior to atrial contraction than to LVEDP, then, this may explain the lack of the symptoms of pulmonary venous hypertension in the presence of a high LVEDP and may also explain the lack of pulmonary venous congestion on the chest roentgenogram.

The systolic time intervals can be obtained by noninvasive techniques and are related to the performance characteristics of the heart and left ventricle.[37-39] In heart failure, PEP is prolonged, LVET is abbreviated[26,40,41] and the PEP/LVET ratio is increased.[27] The PEP/LVET ratio has been related to the ejection fraction[42] and by implication to myocardial performance, since myocardial performance is an important determinant of the ejection fraction.[43,44] Of the nine patients in group 3 (Fig 4) in whom STI were measured, seven had a lengthening of PEP_c, six had a reduction of $LVET_c$ and the PEP/LVET ratio was increased in all nine. Systolic time intervals therefore suggest impairment of LV performance of patients in group 3 but by this method we were unable to demonstrate abnormalities of ventricular performance of patients in groups 1 and 2.

It has been shown that areas of LV asynergy are found in zones of myocardial ischemia and asynergy can occur in the absence of cardiac enlargement.[45] We have not performed LV angiograms and thus cannot assess the contribution of LV asynergy to the impairment of LV function. Areas of LV asynergy may lead to abnormalities of STI which we were able to demonstrate only in patients in group 3.

Isometric exercise in normal subjects results in an increased aortic pressure, heart rate and cardiac output; the stroke volume remains unchanged.[46] Patients in groups 1 and 2 had changes that can be expected from an increased afterload that occurs with isometric exercise. On the other hand, patients in group 3 had a great increase of left ventricular diastolic pressures, lengthening of PEP_c, and increased PEP/LVET ratio or lengthening of $LVET_c$. The CO showed no change or a small increase (Table 4). The increased LV diastolic pressures were not caused by the patients inadvertently performing the Valsalva maneuver as the right atrial pressure was not significantly altered. The myocardial oxygen requirements[47] can be expected to increase with this form of exercise. In two of the three patients in group 3 in whom flow was measured, the cardiac output remained unchanged and the stroke volume fell. Isometric exercise magnified the abnormalities of LV function of patients in group 3 but did not bring out evidence of impaired LV function of the two patients in groups 1 and 2. The findings also suggest that isometric exercise is potentially hazardous in patients convalescing after AMI.

Clinically, our patients were considered to be making a satisfactory recovery from an uncomplicated acute myocardial infarction. However, abnormalities of LV function were demonstrated in 22 of the 27 patients (81%). In ten of these patients abnormality of LV function could be demonstrated by measurement of CO and STI, and in over half of the patients (12 of 22) alteration of LV function was only demonstrated by measuring LV pressure.

This investigation was supported in part by Public Health Service research grant HE-08834-07 from the National Heart and Lung Institute.

References

1. Tennant R, Wiggers CJ: The effect of coronary occlusion on myocardial contraction. *Amer J Physiol* **112**:351-361, 1935.

2. Prinzmetal M, Schwartz LL, Corday E, et al: Studies on the coronary circulation: VI. Loss of myocardial contractility after coronary artery occlusion. *Ann Intern Med* **31**:429-449, 1949.

3. Tatooles CJ, Randall WC: Local ventricular bulging after acute coronary occlusion. *Amer J Physiol* **201**:451-456, 1961.

4. Wegria R, Frank GW, Misrahy GA, et al: Immediate hemodynamic effects of acute coronary occlusion. *Amer J*

Physiol **177**:123-127, 1954.

5. Agress CM, Glasser HF, Binder MJ, et al: Hemodynamic measurements in experimental coronary shock. *J Appl Physiol* **10**:469-475, 1961.

6. Kumar R, Hood WB Jr, Joison J, et al: Experimental myocardial infarction: II. Acute depression and subsequent recovery of left ventricular function: Serial measurements in intact conscious dogs. *J Clin Invest* **49**:55-62, 1970.

7. Gilbert RP, Aldrich SL, Anderson L: Cardiac output in acute myocardial infarction. *J Clin Invest* **30**:640, 1951.

8. Murphy GW, Glick G, Schreiner BF Jr, et al: Cardiac output in acute myocardial infarction: Serial determination by precordial radioisotope dilution curves. *Amer J Cardiol* **11**:587-593, 1963.

9. MacKenzie GJ, Flenley DC, Taylor SH, et al: Circulatory and respiratory studies in myocardial infarction and cardiogenic shock. *Lancet* **2**:825-832, 1964.

10. Malmcrona R, Varnauskas E: Hemodynamics in acute myocardial infarction. *Acta Med Scand* **176**(suppl 417):1-54, 1964.

11. Shillingford J, Thomas M: Hemodynamic effects of acute myocardial infarction in man. *Progr Cardiovasc Dis* **9**:571-593, 1967.

12. Gunnar RM, Loeb HS, Pietras RJ, et al: Hemodynamic measurements in a coronary care unit. *Prog Cardiov Dis* **11**:29-44, 1968.

13. Kirby BJ, McNichol MW, Tattersfield AE: Left ventricular pressures in two patients with myocardial infarction. *Lancet* **1**:944-946, 1968.

14. Cohn JN, Khatri IM, Hamosh P: Diagnostic and therapeutic value of bedside monitoring of left ventricular pressure. *Amer J Cardiol* **23**:107, 1969.

15. Hunt D, Potanin C, Pombo J, et al: Left ventricular function in clinically uncomplicated myocardial infarction. *Clin Res* **18**:313, 1970.

16. Gunnar RM, Sinno MZ, Loeb HS, et al: Left ventricular performance during first two days after acute myocardial infarction. *Circulation* (suppl 3):3-162, 1970.

17. Weisse AB, Saffa RS, Levinson GE, et al: Left ventricular function during early and late stages of scar formation following experimental myocardial infarction. *Amer Heart J* **79**:370-383, 1970.

18. Nager F, Thomas M, Shillingford J: Changes in cardiac output and stroke volume during first four months after cardiac infarction. *Brit Heart J* **29**:859-870, 1967.

19. Cohen L: Contributions of serum enzymes and isozymes to the diagnosis of myocardial injury. *Mod Conc Cardiovasc Dis* **36**:43-47, 1967.

20. Massie E, Walsh TJ: *Clinical Vectorcardiography and Electrocardiography.* Chicago, Year Book Publishers Inc, 1960, p 592.

21. Gunnar RM, Pietras RJ, Blackaller J, et al: Correlation of vectorcardiographic criteria for myocardial infarction with autopsy findings. *Circulation* **35**:158-171, 1967.

22. Seldinger SI: Catheter replacement of the needle in percutaneous arteriography: A new technique. *Acta Radiol* **39**:368-376, 1953.

23. Braunwald E, Brockenbrough E, Frahm CJ, et al: Left atrial and left ventricular pressures in subjects without cardiovascular disease: Observations in 18 patients studied by transseptal left heart catheterization. *Circulation* **24**:267-269, 1961.

24. Hamilton WF, Moore JW, Kinsman JM, et al: Studies on the circulation: IV. Further analysis of the injection method and of changes in hemodynamics under physiological and pathological condition. *Amer J Physiol* **99**:534-551, 1932.

25. Barratt-Boyes BG, Wood EH: Cardiac output and related measurements and pressure value in the right heart and associated vessels, together with an analysis of the hemodynamic response to the inhalation of high oxygen mixtures in healthy subjects. *J Lab Clin Med* **51**:72-90, 1958.

26. Weissler AM, Harris WS, Schoenfeld CD: Systolic time intervals in heart failure in man. *Circulation* **37**:149-159, 1968.

27. Weissler AM, Harris WS, Schoenfeld CD: Bedside techniques for the evaluation of ventricular function in man. *Amer J Cardiol* **23**:577-583, 1969.

28. Connolly DC, Tomkins RG, Lev R, et al: Pulmonary artery wedge pressures in mitral valve disease: Relationship to left atrial pressures. *Proc Staff Meet Mayo Clin* **28**:72-78, 1953.

29. Braunwald E, Ross J Jr: The ventricular end-diastolic pressure: An appraisal of its value in the recognition of ventricular failure in man. *Amer J Med* **34**:147-150, 1963.

30. Jones JW, Rackley CE, Bruce RA, et al: Left ventricular volumes in valvular heart disease. *Circulation* **24**:887-891, 1964.

31. Braunwald E, Ross J Jr, Sonnenblick E: *Mechanisms of Contraction of the Normal and Failing Heart.* Boston, Little Brown & Co, 1968, p 43.

32. Frank O: Zur dynamik des herzmuskels. *Z Biol* **32**:370, 1895.

33. Starling EH: The Linacre lecture on the law of the heart. *Brit Med J* **1**:122, 1918.

34. Gesell RA: Auricular systole and its relation to ventricular output. *Amer J Physiol* **29**:32-63, 1911.

35. Mitchell JH, Gilmore JP, Sarnoff SJ: The transport function of the atrium: Factors influencing the relation between mean left atrial pressure and left ventricular end-diastolic pressure. *Amer J Cardiol* **9**:237-247, 1962.

36. Braunwald E, Frahm CJ: Studies on Starling's law of the heart: IV. Observations on the hemodynamic functions of the left atrium in man. *Circulation* **24**:633-642, 1961.

37. Frank O: in Chapman CB, Wasserman E (trans): On the dynamics of cardiac muscle. *Amer Heart J* **58**:282-317, 467-478, 1959.

38. Wiggers CJ: Studies on the consecutive phases of the cardiac cycle: II. The laws governing the relative duration of ventricular systole and diastole. *Amer J Physiol* **56**:439-459, 1921.

39. Katz LN, Feil HS: Clinical observations on the dynamics of ventricular systole: I. Auricular fibrillation. *Arch Intern Med* **32**:627-696, 1923.

40. Blumberger K: Die untersuchung der dynamik des herzens beim menschen. *Ergebn Inn Med Kinderheilk* **62**:424-531, 1942.

41. Jezek V: Clinical value of the polygraphic tracing in the study of the sequence of events during cardiac contraction. *Cardiologia* **43**:298-316, 1963.

42. Gerrard CJ Jr, Weissler AM, Dodge HT: The relationship of alterations in systolic time intervals to ejection fraction in patients with cardiac disease. *Circulation* **42**:455-462, 1970.

43. Miller GAH, Kirklin JW, Swan HJC: Myocardial function and left ventricular volumes in acquired valvular insufficiency. *Circulation* **31**:374-384, 1965.

44. Dodge HT, Baxley WA: Hemodynamic aspects of heart failure. *Amer J Cardiol* **22**:24-34, 1968.

45. Herman MV, Gorlin R: Implications of left ventricular asynergy. *Amer J Cardiol* **23**:538-547, 1968.

46. Donald KW, Lind AR, McNicol GW, et al: Cardiovascular responses to sustained (static) contractions. *Circ Res* **20**(suppl 1):1-15, 1967.

47. Braunwald E: The determinants of myocardial oxygen consumption. *Physiologist* **12**:65-93, 1969.

Evaluation of Equilin 3-Monosulfate and Other Estrogens

Comparison by Study of Urinary Gonadotropins in Women

R. Palmer Howard, MD, and E. Corinne Keaty, PhD, Oklahoma City

Previous clinical studies rarely provided quantitative evaluations of the relative potency of estrogens. Eight oophorectomized and seven other amenorrheic women with elevated urinary gonadotropins (HPG) were selected, and HPG responses followed during estrogen treatment and withdrawal. The effects of the daily administration of the purified 3-monosulfates of equilin, estrone, rarer components of conjugated estrogens, and diethylstilbestrol were compared. Because of differing sensitivities between individuals, comparative effects were determined in subjects independently. The majority of the comparisons between estrogens were obtained in three oophorectomized women and the remainder from three additional oophorectomized and four other amenorrheic subjects. Diethylstilbestrol and equilin 3-monosulfate were more potent than conjugated estrogens. Estrone 3-monosulfate and other components were less potent than conjugated estrogens. The relative effects may be similar when these are prescribed in various clinical conditions.

The purpose of this work was to demonstrate a quantitative comparison of the biological effects of estrogens in the human. Orally active compounds related to estrone, such as those in conjugated estrogens (Premarin), have been prescribed often in clinical practice.

The relative potency of estrogens in women has been determined by objective methods only infrequently. Some workers[1-3] followed the induction of uterine bleeding after estrogen administration to amenorrheic women. Others[4,5] studied changes in the vaginal smear. In the present study satisfactorily quantitative comparisons were obtained by following the level of urinary gonadotropins (HPG) during estrogen administration to women with deficient ovarian function. Consequently, this method was chosen for the evaluation of a number of orally active estrogens isolated from the urine of pregnant mares, which are constituents of conjugated estrogens.

This mixture, conjugated estrogens, has been widely used, not only in women with estrogen deficiency, but also in men, for example, survivors of myocardial infarctions. Thus, further knowledge of the actions of the constituents of conjugated estrogens in the human would be useful as background information for comparisons with estrone and other estrogens in clinical trials. Finally, the study of estrone-related steroids might reveal one with unexpected potency in man.

Methods

Subjects.—The subjects were 15 women with amenorrhea associated with elevated urinary HPG. They were otherwise in good health and well nourished. Eight women (subjects 1 through 8) between 22 and 48 years of age had undergone bilateral oophorectomy and hysterectomy for diagnoses other than cancer, four (subjects 9 through 12), aged 55 to 81 years, had experienced a natural menopause and three, (subjects 13 through 15), aged 17 to 33 years, had Turner's syndrome.

Urine Collection.—The more than 1,600 timed (usually 24 hour) urine specimens were kept refrigerated or iced during collection. Creatinine was determined as an index of completeness of the 24 hour collection.

Bioassay Method.—The level of urinary gonadotropins was assayed according to the "nondialysis" method of Klinefelter et al[6] with minor modifications. Female white mice 21 to 23 days old, weighing 6 to 9 gm, were obtained in 50 to 100 lots once a week. The strain is called NL Jax by the producer (National Laboratory Animal Co.), because it was derived originally from a Jackson Memorial Laboratory strain. Four to five saline-injected mice were included as controls with each bioassay. The mean uterine weight was 7.1 ± 0.7 mg for the control mice (mean and standard deviation were determined on the first 100 control mice and confirmed repeatedly). Occasionally, the mean uterine weight of the controls was 8.0 mg or more; in such cases the whole bioassay was rejected. A test animal was considered stimulated when the uterus weighed more than 9 mg, ie, exceeded by more than 2 standard deviations the mean of the controls.

According to the method used[6] the amount of gonadotropin in the urine specimens was expressed in mouse uterine units (MU) per 24 hours. Portions of urine corresponding to 180 minutes were extracted with 8 volumes of alcohol and assayed at levels of 48 to 384 MU/24 hr, using two mice at 48 MU and three at higher levels. The smallest fraction of a 24 hour urine collection which caused a significant (>2 SD) enlargement of the mice uteri was determined. The reciprocal of this fraction expressed the result in MU per 24 hours. For example, if 1/96 of a 24 hour urine specimen, or its equivalent, resulted in uterine stimulation, the specimen was reported to contain more than 96 MU/24 hr, while if 1/192 of the

Received for publication Jan 21, 1970; accepted Oct 15.

From the cardiovascular and the endocrinology and metabolism sections, Oklahoma Medical Research Foundation, and the Department of Medicine, University of Oklahoma Medical Center, Oklahoma City.

Reprint requests to 825 NE 13th St, Oklahoma City 73104 (Dr. Howard).

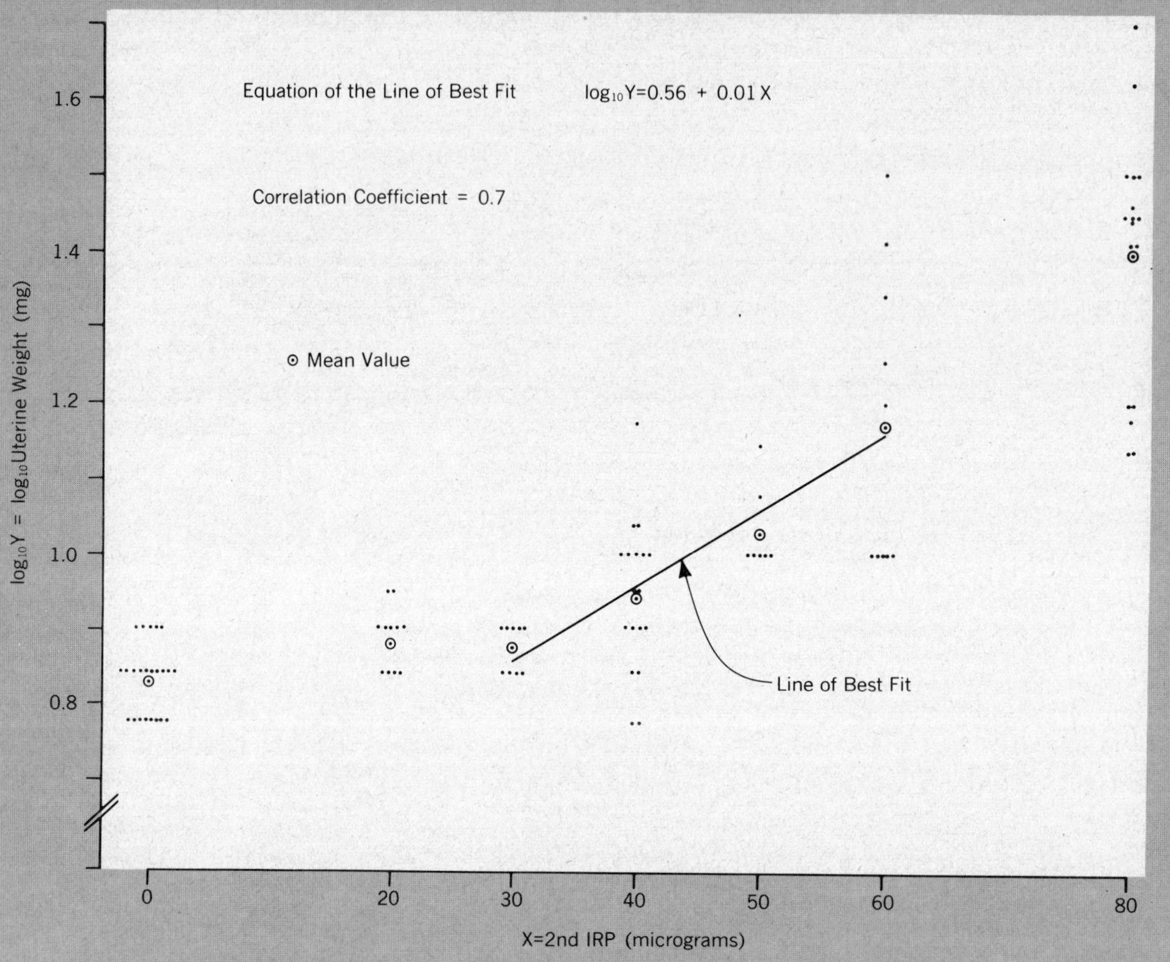

Scattergram for $\log_{10}Y$ (mouse uterine weight) plotted against second IRP. The least squares method[8] was used to determine the line of best fit between 30μg and 60μg. An analysis of variance revealed that the regression mean square was significant ($P < 0.005$). The deviation from linearity mean square was not significant ($P > 0.05$). The correlation coefficient 0.68 is significant for $n = 44$.

Table 1.—Time Required for Suppression of Urinary HPG in Seven Oophorectomized Women by Intensive Daily Estrogen Administered Orally*

Days of Administration	Total: No. of Subjects	Total: (No. of Assays)	HPG >192 MU/24 hr: No. of Subjects	HPG >192 MU/24 hr: (No. of Assays)	HPG >96<192 MU/24 hr: No. of Subjects	HPG >96<192 MU/24 hr: (No. of Assays)	HPG <96 MU/24 hr: No. of Subjects	HPG <96 MU/24 hr: (No. of Assays)
Control	7	(44)	7	(44)	0	(0)	0	(0)
1 through 7	5	(22)	5	(20)	2†	(2)	0	(0)
8 through 14	7	(22)	5	(8)	4	(8)	5‡	(6)
15 through 21	7	(13)	1	(1)	3	(6)	6	(6)
22 or more	4	(18)	0	(0)	1	(1)	4	(17)

* Conjugated estrogens (equine) 10 mg daily.

† The sum of the number of subjects represented at the three HPG assay levels may exceed the total number of subjects tested at any period of time because of gradual responses in individuals.

‡ Results by the 14th day are significantly lower ($P < 0.01$), as determined by the Friedman two-way analysis of variance by ranks.[9]

Table 2.—Time Required for High Levels of Urinary HPG to Reappear in Seven Oophorectomized Women After Previous Suppression by Estrogen Administration

Days After Withdrawal of Estrogen	Total		HPG >192 MU/24 hr		HPG >96<192 MU/24 hr		HPG <96 MU/24 hr	
	No. of Subjects	(No. of Assays)	No. of Subjects	(No. of Assays)	No. of Subjects	(No. of Assays)	No. of Subjects	(No. of Assays)
Control	7	(28)	0	(0)	0	(0)	7	(28)
1-7	4	(7)	0	(0)	1	(1)	3	(6)
8-14	7	(14)	4*	(5)	3	(3)	3†	(6)
15-21	4	(8)	3	(6)	1	(2)	0	(0)
22 or more	6	(32)	6	(31)	1	(1)	0	(0)

† The sum of the number of subjects represented at the three HPG assay levels may exceed the total number of subjects tested at any period of time because of gradual responses in individuals.

* Results by the 14th day are significantly lower ($P<0.01$), as determined by the Friedman two-way analysis of variance by ranks.[9]

specimen resulted in no uterine stimulation the result was expressed as less than 192 MU/24 hr.

Standardization of Bioassay With the Second International Reference Preparation of Human Menopausal Gonadotropin (WHO/BS/723; Sept 23, 1964) (Second IRP).—The sensitivity of the mouse strain was semiquantitatively established with an international preparation of chorionic gonadotropin initially, and thereafter, at intervals, confirmed with a commercially available preparation. In order to quantitate the responsiveness of the mice to a standard gonadotropin preparation, an ampule containing 5 mg of second IRP was used. The characteristics of this standard have been discussed by Rosemberg.[7]

During four experiments with the standard preparation, the 23 saline-injected control mice had uterine weights between 6 to 8 mg. The 72 test mice were divided into groups of four or five. Quantities of second IRP between 20μg and 80μg were injected into each animal. Assays at some levels were repeated. When 20μg and 30μg were injected the uterine weights were not significantly increased (Figure). At the 40μg test level, however, the mean uterine weight from 18 mice was 9.1 mg. At the 50μg to 80μg test levels each uterus weighed at least 10 mg and the mean weights were progressively greater.

It was concluded from the standardization that one mouse unit approximated 40μg of second IRP. Therefore, for example, a urine specimen assayed at more than 192 MU/24 hr might be expressed as containing approximately 7.68 mg of second IRP/24 hr. The bioassay results obtained in previous clinical studies were not recalculated in terms of the standard.

Clinical Studies

Estrogens.—In addition to the usual pharmaceutical tablets of diethylstilbestrol (0.5 mg) and conjugated estrogens (0.3 to 2.5 mg), the substances studied were specially-prepared tablets containing 0.3 to 2.5 mg chemically pure sodium 3-monosulfates of estrone, estradiol-17β, estradiol-17α, equilin, dihydroequilin-17α, or dihydroequilenin-17α. Similar tablets containing no estrogens were also available.

Control State.—When the eight oophorectomized subjects were studied before, or more than a month after, estrogen administration, the level of urinary HPG was greater than 384 MU/24 hr in 66 of 97 assays and greater than 192 MU/24 hr in 100 of 102 tests. Thus, the latter level was taken to indicate the absence of estrogen effect on HPG. The degree of cornification of the vaginal epithelium and the frequency of hot flashes were recorded but these criteria of estrogen effect were not used in the evaluation for the present study.

Estrogen Effects on HPG Levels.—Extensive preliminary studies were required to establish the time relationships between initiation and discontinuation of the daily oral administration of estrogens and urinary HPG levels. Suppression of HPG excretion in some women did not occur within five weeks when doses of conjugated estrogens smaller than 10 mg/day were employed. In seven oophorectomized-hysterectomized women receiving conjugated estrogens (10 mg/day), a total of 75 urine specimens were collected during the first five weeks of treatment. The HPG level was very high during the first week (days 1 through 7), became progressively and significantly lower[9] during the second and third weeks, and was consistently below 192 MU/24 hr after day 22 of treatment (Table 1).

Effect of Withdrawal of Estrogen Therapy.—A total of 61 assays was performed during the five weeks following cessation of intensive estrogen therapy. The HPG level was still low during the first week, significantly higher[9] than the control level during the second week, and high in the third week (Table 2). These time relations were indicated in a preliminary report.[10]

Plans of Clinical Evaluation.—*Maintenance of HPG Suppression.*—Most of the studies were designed to establish the minimal amount of each estrogen necessary to maintain urinary HPG excretion at less than 96 MU/24 hr, as determined by four or more assays of urine obtained between day 15 and 28 of estrogen administration. Since four-week periods of intensive estrogen therapy (conjugated estrogens, 10 mg/day) always suppressed HPG excretion from the high levels found in oophorectomized women, such suppressive periods were alternated with test periods of a selected estrogen. For each test period, smaller or larger doses of estrogen were given in order to establish (*a*) the lowest dose which maintained the state of HPG suppression, and (*b*) an adjacent but smaller amount which failed to maintain HPG suppression. These two amounts defined the responsiveness of the subject to one estrogen and could be compared with the responsiveness to another estrogen.

Suppression Method.—Studies of two or more estrogens were conducted in each of ten untreated women with high urinary HPG excretion. In these subjects the diagnoses included natural menopause, Turner's syndrome, and oophorectomy. Estimates of the comparative potency of various estrogens were made by noting whether or not consistent suppression of the HPG titer to less than 192 MU/24 hr (based on at least three urine samples) occurred by the fourth week of daily oral administration of the selected amount. For each estrogen tested in an individual the least amount necessary to suppress HPG was determined. The result could be compared with the finding for another estrogen in the same subject.

The daily medication was usually given after eating, in three or four divided doses. Tests at low medication levels required only one or two tablets during the day. Tablets containing no estrogen were given as placebos, in the same number as the previous medication, during intervals between test estrogens.

Results

Studies by the Maintenance of Suppressed HPG Levels.—The relative potencies on a milligram per day basis of the estrogens in respect to the maintenance of previously suppressed urinary HPG in three oophorectomized women are presented in Table 3. Individuals have different sensitivities to estrogens but are consistent (in subject 3 approximately twice as much equilin sulfate, conjugated estrogens, or estrone sulfate was required as in subjects 1 or 2).

In the three women diethylstilbestrol appeared equivalent to, or slightly more potent than, equilin sulfate when compared on a milligram per day basis. However, equilin sulfate was twice as potent as conjugated estrogens and four to eight times as potent as estrone sulfate. Three trials with 17α-dihydroequilin sulfate, four with 17α-estradiol sulfate and two with 17α-dihydroequilenin sulfate at various doses between 5 to 15 mg daily for four weeks failed to maintain HPG excretion at low levels.

Studies of HPG Responses in Untreated Women.—The results of 64 trials to suppress high HPG levels with various daily dosages of these estrogens provided several comparisons among conjugated estrogens, equilin sulfate, and estrone sulfate (Table 4). Unfortunately, it was not possible with some estrogens to make comparisons of estrogenic potency by this method. In the amounts selected, diethylstilbestrol (1.5 to 5 mg/day), 17α-estradiol sulfate (5 mg/day), and equilin sulfate (1.2 to 10 mg/day) were always suppressive, so distinctions could not be drawn among them.

17α-Dihydroequilin sulfate was

Table 3.—Amounts of Estrogens Administered Daily Necessary for Maintenance During at Least Four Weeks of Low Urinary Gonadotropins Previously Suppressed by Higher Dosages for Four Weeks

Estrogen (mg/day)	Total Trials	Subject No. 1	Subject No. 2	Subject No. 3
Diethylstilbestrol	4	0.5;0.25*	0.5;X†	0.5;X
Equilin 3-monosulfate	10	0.6;0.3	0.6;0.3	1.2;0.6
Conjugated estrogens	15	1.2;0.6	1.2;0.6	2.4;1.2
Estrone 3-monosulfate	10	2.4;1.2	5;2.5	7.5;5
17α-Dihydroequilin 3-monosulfate	3	Y‡;10	Y;10	Y;5
17α-Estradiol 3-monosulfate	4	Y;15	Y;5	—•
17α-Dihydroequilenin 3-monosulfate	2	Y;10	Y;10	—•

* The figures given are the lowest adequate amount for maintenance and the highest amount tested which failed to maintain.

† X signifies test conducted at a lower amount, but the amount shown was adequate for maintenance.

‡ Y signifies test conducted at a higher amount, but the amount shown was inadequate for maintenance.

Table 4.—Amounts of Estrogens Administered Daily for Four Weeks Necessary for the Suppression of Previously Elevated Urinary Gonadotropins

Estrogen (mg/day)	Total Trials	Subject No. 2	Subject No. 3	Subject No. 4	Subject No. 5	Subject No. 6	Subject No. 9	Subject No. 13	Subject No. 14	Subject No. 15
Diethylstilbestrol	3							1.5;X*	2.0;X	
Equilin 3-monosulfate	19			2.5;X	2.5;X	5;X	3.7;X	1.2;X	1.2;X	2.5;X
17β-Estradiol 3-monosulfate	2				5;X		5;X			
Conjugated estrogens	18	5;2.5†	5:3.7	3.7;X		10;5		2.5;X	10;1.2	10;X
Estrone 3-monosulfate	8				10;X	Y‡;5	7.5;X	3.7;2.4		
17α-Dihydroequilin 3-monosulfate	5	20;X		25;X	25;X		25;X			
17α-Estradiol 3-monosulfate	6			50:25			50;X			Y;10
17α-Dihydroequilenin 3-monosulfate	3				Y;25		Y;50			Y;10

† The figures given are the lowest adequate amount for suppression and the highest amount tested which failed to suppress.

* X signifies no test conducted at lower amount, but the amount shown was adequate for suppression.

‡ Y signifies no test conducted at higher amount, but the amount shown was inadequate for suppression.

more effective than 17α-estradiol sulfate in subject 4, and more effective than 17α-dihydroequilenin sulfate in subjects 5 and 9. 17α-Estradiol sulfate was more effective than 17α-dihydroequilenin sulfate in subject 9. The data on subjects 4, 5, 6, 9, 13, 14, and 15 indicate that equilin sulfate was more effective for suppression of HPG than at least one other estrogen.

Different degrees of HPG-responsiveness were manifest in different women given the same estrogen. Thus, the minimal amount of conjugated estrogens observed to suppress HPG excretion in nine subjects varied from 2.5 to 10 mg/day. However, in only four of these nine subjects was a lower dose tested and found inadequate for HPG suppression. In one subject 5 mg/day suppressed while 3.7 mg did not; in another subject 10 mg/day suppressed but 5 mg did not. Accordingly, the comparisons between estrogens shown in Table 4 must be evaluated separately for each subject.

Evaluation of the Comparative Potency of the Estrogens.—These orally administered estrogens were evaluated from their effects on suppressing the HPG level in untreated amenorrheic women (Table 4), and from their effects on the maintenance of low HPG levels which had been previously suppressed (Table 3). Conjugated estrogens was arbitrarily assigned an activity of 1.0. The comparative activities of estrogens tested in individual subjects were expressed on the basis of conjugated estrogens (X/conjugated estrogens). For each estrogen a mean was calculated from all values relative to conjugated estrogens which had been obtained in individuals. For example, estrone sulfate was assigned values ranging from 0.25 to 0.66 in the individual comparisons of minimal effective doses (Tables 3 and 4); the mean activity for estrone sulfate was 0.4 (in terms of conjugated estrogens). In this manner the following approximations were deduced in relation to the activity of conjugated estrogens (1.0).

Estrogen	Ratio
Diethylstilbestrol	2.5
Equilin 3-monosulfate	2.0
Estrone 3-monosulfate	0.4
Dihydroequilin-17α, 3-monosulfate	0.12
Estradiol-17α, 3-monosulfate	0.06
Dihydroequilenin-17α, 3-monosulfate	0

No ratio of activity for estradiol-17β, 3-monosulfate was derived, since it was always active in the doses tested.

Comment

The alcohol method for extraction of HPG from urine was criticized by Albert[11] because of the inability to detect small titers and because of the uncertain recovery, which was substantially lower during subsequent dialysis. The detection of the low HPG levels characteristic of young women and men was not a major concern in this investigation of ovarian deficient women, so dialysis was not used. Klinefelter and associates[6] obtained good recoveries by the nondialysis method with or without alcohol extraction.

Rosemberg et al[12] indicated the feasibility of using HPG preparations of urine from postmenopausal subjects, or estrone, as standard reference materials in the mouse uterine weight assay. Quantitation of each bioassay could have been obtained had such reference standards been used throughout the present studies.

Miescher[13] concluded that differences in intestinal absorption and the rate of liver inactivation may be reasons for the variable activity of certain natural and synthetic estrogens in animals and man. Therefore, the comparison of the effectiveness in man must be based solely on studies in man. Individual variability remains, whether due to the above or other metabolic factors.

The relative therapeutic activities of administered estrogens depend upon the route of administration, solubility of pure or modified steroids, frequency of dosage, and type of clinical assay. Previous observations have included effects on menopausal symptoms, vaginal epithelium, endometrial bleeding, and the urinary HPG levels. Although androgens may also suppress gonadotropin production, no clinical androgenic effects were noted with any of the compounds administered in the present study.

Turner et al[1] found the administration orally of conjugated estrogens (incorrectly termed sodium estrone sulfate) and stilbestrol to be approximately equivalent for the production of hormone withdrawal uterine bleeding in amenorrheic women. On the other hand, Allen[2] found conjugated estrogens to be about one-fifth, and pure estrone, one-tenth, as active as stilbestrol when each was given orally. Bishop et al,[3] however, using uterine bleeding in a larger series, described the relative potency as diethylstilbestrol, 1.0; conjugated estrogens, 0.49; equilin (pure), 0.37; and estrone (pure), 0.05. The differences between the results of Bishop and co-workers and those of the present study might be attributable to the fact that they used pure equilin and estrone, whereas we used the sodium 3-monosulfates, which are more readily absorbed. However, the results are quite similar, despite the different methods of clinical evaluation. The relative potencies of estrogens using vaginal smear changes can not be readily compared with those by our method, in part because the authors also used different estrogenic compounds.[4,5] In this regard, Bradbury and Long[14] noted that a lower daily amount of equilin by mouth caused vaginal smear changes than that necessary for withdrawal bleeding or urinary HPC suppression.

Although equilin is not secreted in humans it is noteworthy that it is more potent than estrone in man. In a large mixture of mare's urine the proportions of estrogens by chemical analysis were 51% sodium estrone sulfate, 22% sodium equilin sulfate, 16% sodium 17α-dihydroequilin sulfate, and smaller amounts of the sodium sulfates of equilenin, 17α-dihydroequilenin and 17α-estradiol. Small amounts of related "nonestrogenic" steroids were also present.[15] Since in respect to HPG suppression in women the activity of equilin sulfate appears to be approximately five times that of estrone sulfate, and since none of the other major components of conjugated estrogens is as potent, equilin sulfate is probably responsible in large measure for the therapeutic efficacy of conjugated estrogens.

The influence of equilin sulfate, conjugated estrogens, and other estrogens on the serum lipids and lipoproteins has been reported from this laboratory,[16,17] and similar effects of various estrogens have been reported by other investigators. Stamler and associates[18] reported the effectiveness of conjugated estrogens therapy in a long-term survey of survivors of myocardial infarction. Recently, however, the Coronary Drug Project Research Group has reported adverse effects from a higher dosage schedule of estrogens in such survivors.[19] Interest continues in the use of estrogens for the treatment of selected individuals with serum lipid disorders, as well as in their use for many other clinical conditions.

Conclusions

The serial determination of urinary HPG provides a suitable means for the comparative evaluation of estrogens in the human subject. The method, however, is time-consuming and is dependent on the selection of hypergonadotropic individuals, each of whom must respond consistently to the administration or withdrawal of estrogen. Based on other measurements of estrogenic activity, different schedules of estrogen administration would be effective. An appreciation of the relative activities in respect to HPG of these estrogenic substances, however, should be valuable in interpreting their effects in clinical conditions.

This investigation was supported in part by Public Health Service grant A-179 from the National Institute of Arthritis and Metabolic Diseases, and grants H-1429, H-1694, and H-2528 from the National Heart Institute; and by the Oklahoma Heart Association, and the Ayerst Laboratories, New York.

The diethylstibestrol used in this investigation was supplied through A. Scribner, MD, of Winthrop Laboratories, New York. John Jewell, MD, Ayerst Laboratories, New York, supplied the tablets of placebos, conjugated estrogens—equine (Premarin), and the pure steroidal sulfates which were prepared by W. L. Glen, PhD, and R. Gaudry, PhD, Ayerst Laboratories, Montreal.

E. C. Reifenstein, Jr., MD, contributed to the initial planning of this work, and E. N. Brandt, Jr., MD, J. R. Assenzo, PhD, and J. P. Costiloe of the Biostatistical Unit, University of Oklahoma Medical Center, did the statistical evaluation.

References

1. Turner VH, Davis CD, Hamblen EC: Oral therapy with sodium estrone sulfate: I. Induction of bleeding and cycle regulation in functional amenorrhea. *J Clin Endocr* **3**:453-454, 1943.

2. Allen WM: The biological activity of various estrogens. *Southern Med J* **37**:270-280, 1944.

3. Bishop PMF, Richards NA, Perry WLM: Stilboestrol sulphate, oestrone, and equilin: Further observations on the potency and clinical assessment of oestrogens. *Lancet* **1**:818-820, 1951.

4. Stoddard FJ, Metzger I: A clinical comparison of three commercial estrogenic preparations. *J Clin Endocr* **2**:209-212, 1942.

5. Brown WE, Bradbury JT: The use of the human vaginal smear in the assay of estrogens. *J Clin Endocr* **9**:725-735, 1949.

6. Klinefelter HF Jr, Albright F, Griswold GC: Experience with a quantitative test for normal or decreased amounts of follicle stimulating hormone in the urine in endocrinological diagnosis. *J Clin Endocr* **3**:529-544, 1943.

7. Rosemberg E: Use of standards: General considerations, in Rosemberg E (ed): *Gonadotropins 1968.* Los Altos, Calif, Geron-X Inc, 1968, pp 383-391.

8. Steel RGD, Torrie JH: *Principles and Procedures of Statistics.* New York, McGraw-Hill Book Co Inc, 1960, chap 9.

9. Siegel S: *Nonparametric Statistics for the Behavioral Sciences.* New York, McGraw-Hill Book Co Inc, 1957, pp 166-172.

10. Howard RP, Keaty C, Reifenstein EC Jr: The consistency of urinary gonadotropin levels in castrate women, and their time relationships to estrogen therapy. *Clin Res Proc* **2**:17, 1954.

11. Albert A: Human urinary gonadotropin, in Pincus G (ed): *Recent Progress in Hormone Research.* New York, Academic Press Inc, 1956, vol 12, pp 227-301.

12. Rosemberg E, Lewis W, Russell E: Performance control of preparations which could be used as reference material for the estimation of urinary gonadotropins in the mouse uterine weight method. *J Clin Endocr* **22**:953-958, 1962.

13. Miescher K: On the relation of activity to constitution in the sexogens, with special reference to the doisynolic acids, in Pincus G (ed): *Recent Progress in Hormone Research.* New York, Academic Press Inc, 1948, vol 3, pp 47-69.

14. Bradbury JT, Long RC: Equilin, an orally active estrogen in women. *Amer J Physiol* **163**:700-701, 1950.

15. Gaudry R, Glen WL: Sur la fraction stéroide de l'urine de jument gravide, in *Extrait du Compte Rendu du XXXI Congrès International de Chimie Industrielle.* Liège, Belgium, September, 1958.

16. Furman RH, Howard RP, Norcia LN, et al: The influence of androgens, estrogens and related steroids on serum lipids and lipoproteins; observations in hypogonadal and normal human subjects. *Amer J Med* **24**:80-97, 1958.

17. Furman RH: Gonadal steroid effects on serum lipids, in Salhanick HA, Kipnis DM, Vande Wiele RL (eds): *Metabolic Effects of Gonadal Hormones and Contraceptive Steroids.* New York, Plenum Pub Corp, 1969, pp 246-264.

18. Stamler J, Pick R, Katz LN, et al: Effectiveness of estrogens for therapy of myocardial infarction in middle-age men. *JAMA* **183**:632-638, 1963.

19. The Coronary Drug Project Research Group: The coronary drug project: Initial findings leading to modification of its research protocol. *JAMA* **214**:1303-1313, 1970.

Variations in Motor Nerve Conduction Velocity in Normal and Uremic Patients

Namiko Kominami, MD; H. Richard Tyler, MD;
Constantine L. Hampers, MD; and John P. Merrill, MD, Boston

Ulnar nerve conduction velocity (NCV) was measured daily using surface electrodes and achieving reproducibility within 2 meters/sec in each patient on a given day. Five normal subjects had a mean NCV of 56.9 meters/sec ± 4.0 (SD). The NCV varied daily during a ten-day period and the percent difference between the slowest and most rapid measurements of NCV averaged 17.8% (range 24.6% to 12.4%). Seven uremic patients had a mean NCV of 49.6 meters/sec ± 7.0. The average percent difference in NCV was 16.6% (range 24.9% to 8.4%). The NCV variation was unrelated to other chemical and clinical features, including the electroencephalogram in two patients. It is concluded that because of variation, the NCV is an unreliable tool for following uremic patients unless the changes are marked. It is necessary to determine the degree of daily variation in NCV from one period to another.

With the advent of long-term hemodialysis, polyneuropathy has become one of the major complications of uremia interfering with patient rehabilitation.[1-7] In the early days of maintenance hemodialysis therapy, many patients developed disabling neuropathy while on a once weekly dialysis schedule. It is now widely accepted that this complication can be improved or prevented with more frequent dialysis. However, once neuropathy appears, it requires over a year with frequent dialysis for its reversal.[8]

Received for publication Aug 28, 1970; accepted Oct 12.

From the departments of medicine (Drs. Kominami, Hampers, and Merrill) and neurology (Dr. Tyler), Peter Bent Brigham Hospital, and Harvard Medical School, Boston. Dr. Kominami is now with the Straub Clinic, Honolulu.

Reprint requests to Dialysis Facilities, Peter Bent Brigham Hospital, 721 Huntington Ave, Boston 02115 (Dr. Hampers).

Jebsen et al[9] found that the peripheral nerve conduction velocity (NCV) was abnormally prolonged in uremic patients with clinically manifest neuropathy. It was also demonstrated to be prolonged in some patients who had no clinical signs of nerve damage.[8,10-12] The appearance of prolonged NCV is not well correlated with the severity of uremia. It is seldom noted in patients with serum creatinine levels below 5 mg/100 ml, whereas prolonged NCVs were more frequent among patients with creatinine levels above 7 mg/100 ml.[9] Not all patients with high creatinine concentrations, however, have abnormal NCVs or clinical neuropathy.[9] Once developed, it will persist for a long time, regardless of the therapy. Moreover, severe clinical neuropathy may develop suddenly in neurologically asymptomatic patients with prolonged NCVs.[12]

Just as in other forms of therapy, the primary dictum in chronic hemodialysis is prevention. Early hemodialysis, before the onset of neuropathy, is clearly desirable. However, life independent of dialyzer is so much more preferable that an indiscriminately early beginning must be guarded against. Some objective methods are therefore necessary to judge the time for the commencement of chronic hemodialysis therapy. Jebsen and co-workers[9] propose NCV as a sensitive and objective index of peripheral nerve function and have measured it periodically as a guide to the adequacy of dialysis. Since it is not known whether the NCV has any short-term variability, it is difficult to evaluate results obtained from measurements taken over long periods of time, unless one knows how accurate the tests are.

Accordingly, the present study was designed to ascertain the day-to-day stability of the NCV, and to evaluate its usefulness in assessing the need for treatment of uremic patients.

Materials and Methods

Nerve conduction velocity measurements were performed in uremic and normal subjects daily for eight to ten days.

Seven uremic patients were studied. Three of them were not yet treated by dialysis, three were, and one was in the immediate posttransplant stage. Five normal subjects were also tested. Four of the five normal subjects underwent the study together during the same ten-day period (Table 1 and 2). Two of the seven uremic patients also underwent daily electroencephalograms, neurological and mental examinations, and blood analyses for Na^+, Cl^-, K^+, $HCO_3^=$, Ca^{++}, PO_4^+, Mg^{++}, blood urea nitrogen (BUN), and creatinine.

One of us (N.K.) performed two to three separate measurements on the right ulnar nerve daily on each subject by the surface electrode method.[13,14] The subjects remained in the recording room at an ambient temperature of about 72 F for at least ten minutes before measurements were carried out. A silver disk recording electrode was attached to the skin over the abductor digiti quinti manus muscle after the skin was cleaned with alcohol. The nerve was stimulated at the elbow and at the wrist. The recording electrode was removed and reattached to the skin after the NCV measurement was taken and the whole procedure repeated once or twice more; the mean of these velocities was recorded as the value for a given day.

Table 1.—Right Ulnar NCV in Uremic Patients (meters/sec)

Patient/Age (yr)/Sex	Serum Creatinine Range (mg/100 ml)	Dialysis	Days 1	2	3	4	5	6	7	8	9	10	Mean	SD	Fastest-Slowest	Difference/Fastest (%)
1/19/F	8.2- 9.2	No	57.5	58.1	57.5	61.0	58.5	61.2	62.2	60.0	59.0	62.8	59.8	2.3	5.3	8.4
2/40/F	3.0-15.0	Yes	50.8	55.4	50.8	56.2	46.3	51.9	54.8	56.9	52.9	. . .	53.0	3.3	10.6	18.6
3/30/M	5.3- 5.4	No	47.9	47.6	52.2	47.9	48.9	48.0	48.0	56.8	44.9	52.3	49.5	3.4	11.9	21.0
4/48/M	12.3-12.9	No	46.9	47.3	42.6	48.0	46.9	51.0	50.0	47.9	. . .	. . .	47.6	2.6	8.4	16.5
5/22/M	6.0-15.0	Yes	34.7	46.2	39.5	41.7	43.8	44.1	37.5	45.3	43.3	. . .	41.8	4.0	10.6	24.9
6/48/F	3.0-12.0	Yes	47.2	48.0	44.6	45.5	51.3	46.2	50.5	50.0	51.4	. . .	48.3	2.8	6.8	13.2
7/20/M	6.0-18.0	Yes	40.5	41.0	39.3	42.0	42.7	39.5	44.0	39.5	44.9	. . .	41.4	2.0	5.6	12.5
												Group mean =	49.6	7.0	8.5±2.6	16.6

Clinical neuropathy appears in the lower extremities before it becomes apparent in the upper extremities, and so the selection of the ulnar nerve, alone, in the present study merits explanation. Honet et al[15] have shown that the ratio of the average NCVs in the posterior tibial and peroneal nerves to those in the ulnar and median nerves did not differ significantly among the normal and uremic patients with and without neuropathies. The ulnar nerve is the most accessible, most easily stimulated; hence, conduction measurements are possible in all patients in contrast to the difficulties sometimes encountered with the peroneal nerve.

Nerve conduction velocity measurements, EEG recordings, blood samples, and neurological examinations were performed at about 3 PM each day on two patients. One patient (subject 1) came for the test after attending school each day. The other patient (subject 2) was in the hospital for the initiation of hemodialysis. She underwent dialysis on the first, second, and eighth day of the study. The studies were performed immediately before the first dialysis and after the second and eighth dialyses. Blood urea nitrogen, creatinine, and electrolyte determinations were carried out by standard methods with an autoanalyzer; EEG tracings were obtained in the routine manner in the hospital laboratory.

Results

The individual values for daily NCVs are listed in Table 1 and 2. The mean difference in the NCVs measured on a particular subject each day was 0.99 meters/sec ± 1.29 (SD).

Normal Subjects.—The NCV varied to some degree in the daily measurements in all five subjects tested. The mean NCV for the group was 56.9 meters/sec ± 4.0 (SD). In the subject (patient 3) who demonstrated the greatest variation in measurements, the NCV ranged from 48.7 to 64.6 meters/sec. The difference between the slowest and the fastest NCV in normal subjects over a ten-day period ranged from 7.8 to 15.9 meters/sec with a group mean of 11.1 meters/sec ± 2.97 (SD). The percentage difference ranged from 12.4% to 24.6% of the fastest NCV. The group mean percentage variation was 17.8%.

Uremic Subjects.—As in the normal subjects, the NCVs varied to some degree daily whether or not they were being dialyzed. Subject 1 had a NCV that varied daily, but within the established normal range.[16-18] Subjects 2, 3, 4, and 6 had NCVs that were usually within this normal range, but occasionally had days in which the NCVs were slower than normal. Subjects 5 and 7 had NCVs consistently slower than normal. Their NCVs, however, varied daily just as in the other uremic patients and normal subjects. The mean NCV for the uremic subjects was 49.6 ± 7 meters/sec. The difference between an individual's fastest and slowest NCV ranged from 5.3 to 11.9 meters/sec with a mean variation for the uremic group of 8.5 meters/sec ± 2.64 (SD). The group mean percent variation was 17%.

The two patients who underwent daily EEG and electrolyte studies in addition to the daily NCV measure-

Table 2.—Right Ulnar NCV in Normal Subjects (meters/sec)

Patient/Age (yr)/Sex	Days 1	2	3	4	5	6	7	8	9	10	Mean	SD	Fastest-Slowest	Difference/Fastest (%)
1/24/M	56.7	64.1	57.9	54.1	63.4	64.2	62.2	65.0	65.0	55.5	60.7	10.9	10.9	16.8
2/21/F	58.5	50.0	60.0	58.5	58.5	54.4	57.8	55.6	60.0	58.5	57.2	3.0	10.0	16.7
3/32/M	64.6	55.2	55.3	53.3	48.7	56.0	53.0	54.0	56.9	57.3	54.9	3.3	15.9	24.6
4/48/F	55.4	53.1	53.7	53.8	53.7	48.9	54.8	60.0	53.5	52.4	53.9	2.7	11.1	18.5
5/20/F	57.5	55.0	62.8	60.0	55.0	56.1	55.0	57.5	59.7	55.0	57.4	2.7	7.8	12.4
										Group mean =	56.9	4.0	11.1±2.97	17.8

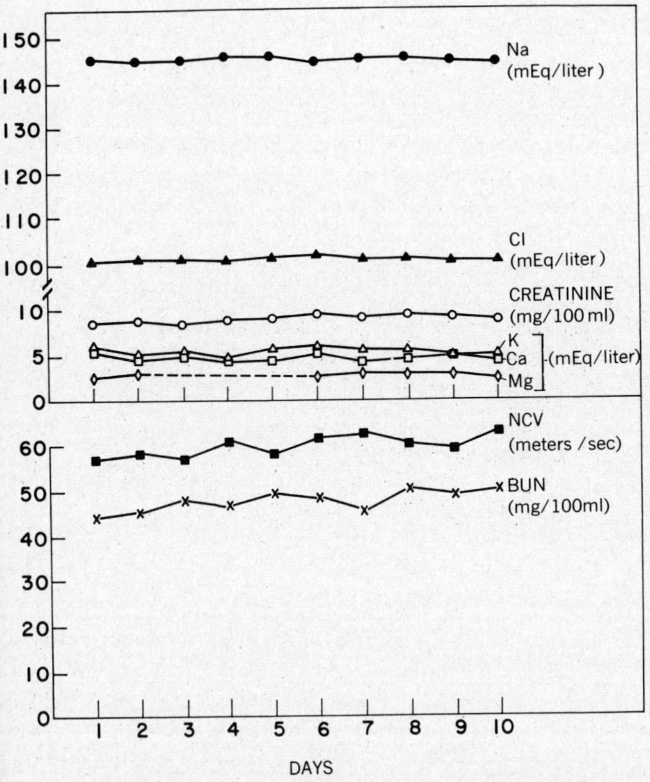

Fig 1.—Laboratory data on subject 1. No correlation between changes in any factors tested and variation in NCV.

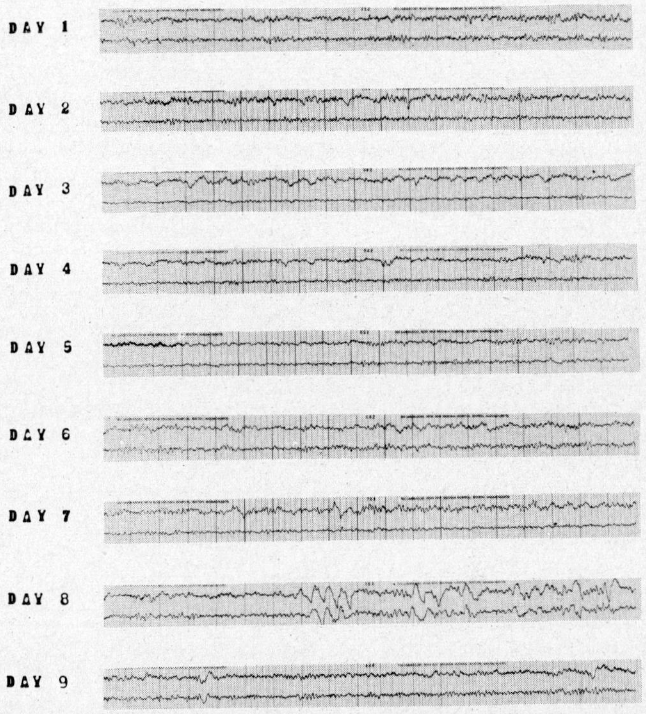

Fig 2.—EEG taken on subject 1. Right-sided bipolar leads taken from frontal and frontal-cerebral areas on consecutive days of studies. There are significant changes in day-to-day recordings independent of mental status or chemistries.

ment are reported in further detail.

Subject 1.—This 19-year-old patient, not yet on dialysis, had daily BUN levels that ranged from 44 to 50 mg/100 ml with a mean of 48 mg/100 ml ± 2. The mean creatinine value was 8.9 mg/100 ml ± 3. The electrolytes did not vary significantly from day to day, except for potassium (Fig 1). The EEG on the first day showed slight slowing and rare paroxysmal discharges. On the second day the record was worse with an increase in 4 to 6/sec activity and more paroxysmal high voltage bursts. The record was better on the third and fourth days. Slight slowing increased on the fifth day, but the record was markedly improved on the sixth and seventh days. The records showed some slowing again on the eighth and ninth days, which was less obvious on the tenth day (Fig 2). These EEG changes were not accompanied by clinical symptoms or changes in neurological examination. Furthermore, there was no relationship among the NCV, EEG, BUN, creatinine, and electrolyte concentrations.

Subject 2.—This 38-year-old woman had a BUN level of 101 mg/100 ml and a creatinine level of 15 mg/100 ml on the first day. Electrolytes were within normal limits, and the NCV was 50.8 meters/sec. She complained of bifrontal headache and had mild mental changes. The EEG was mildly and diffusely abnormal with excessive 4 to 6/sec slowing underneath the regular rhythm. The EEG was stable to the third day, when there was less paroxysmal slowing but more flatness and instability of baseline. Slowing increased in the sixth day and on the eighth day, following dialysis, the record was severely deranged with marked slowing and paroxysmal features. She was dialyzed for three hours on the first day after the initial NCV study, and again for six hours on the following morning. The NCV and other measurements on the second day, therefore, were obtained after a total of nine hours of hemodialysis. The BUN level had dropped to 11 mg/100 ml

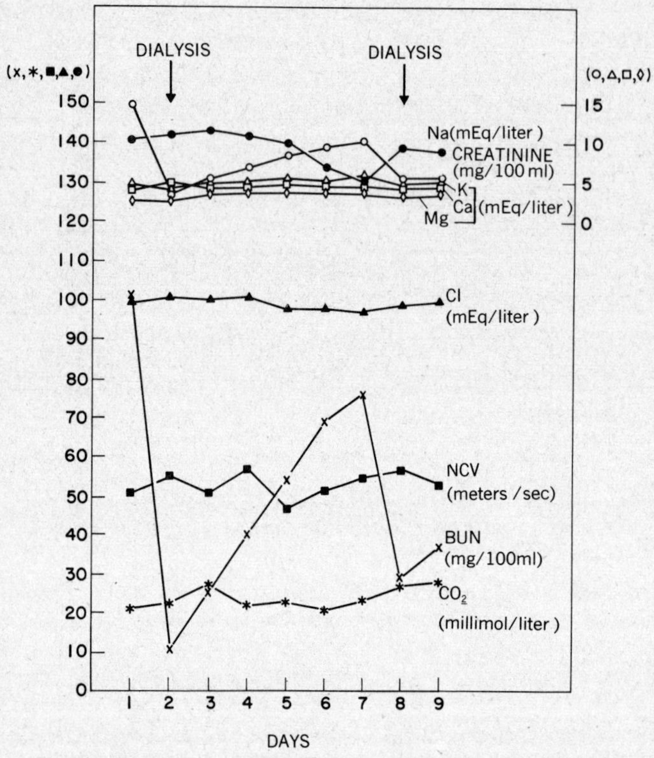

Fig 3.—Laboratory data on subject 2. Variations in NCV were independent of other factors studied.

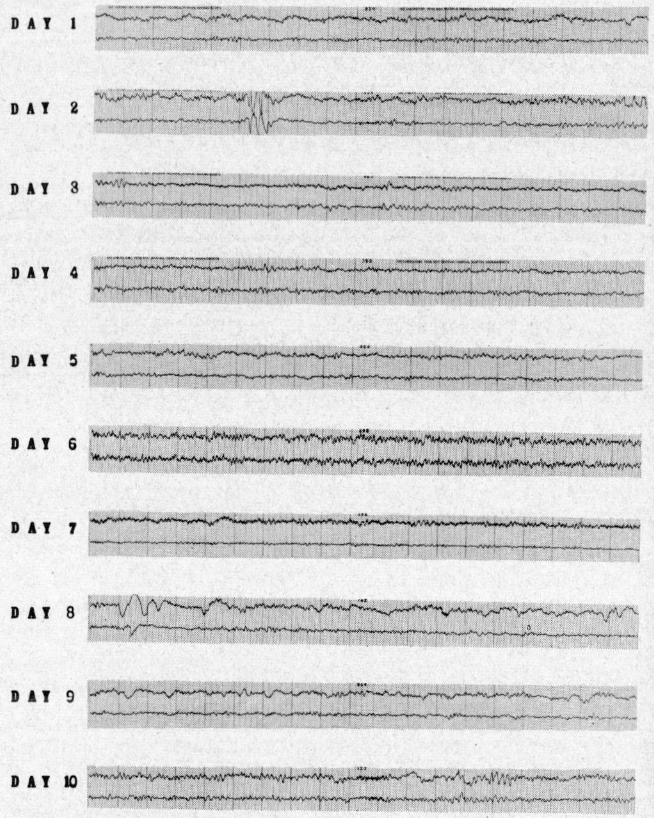

Fig 4.—Sequential EEGs on subject 2 (see legend for Fig 2).

and creatinine level to 3.1 mg/100 ml, potassium was down from 4.8 to 3.7 mEq/liter, calcium had increased slightly from 4.6 to 5.0 mEq/liter, and phosphorus from 2.3 to 2.9 millimol/liter. There was no asterixis, but no significant improvement in mentation was observed. The NCV was 55.4 meters/sec and the EEG was unchanged.

On the four subsequent days, both the BUN and creatinine concentrations increased predictably; potassium also increased, while sodium gradually decreased in concentration (Fig 3). The patient felt very well on the third day and showed improvement of mentation. As the BUN and creatinine levels increased, however, she began to experience weakness and generalized malaise, and by the sixth day, asterixis had reappeared together with a slowing of cerebration. Despite clinical improvement, the EEG was only slightly better on the third day, and became worse on the subsequent days. The NCV was the slowest on the fifth day and became more rapid on subsequent days, with similar daily variations to those seen in the other subjects. She underwent another six-hour hemodialysis on the eighth day and her postdialysis BUN level was 29 mg/100 ml and the creatinine level was 5.4 mg/100 ml. As would be expected and reported previously,[19] the EEG (Fig 4) shortly after dialysis deteriorated further and remained so the following day. Asterixis persisted, although the patient had mentally improved after the dialysis.

Again, daily variations in NCV could not be correlated at all with the changes in BUN, creatinine, and electrolyte concentrations resulting from dialysis, and similarly could not be correlated with the manifest clinical state of the patient. Improvement in the EEG lagged behind the improvement in the blood chemistry pattern and the general clinical state.

Available data on BUN, creatinine, and electrolytes on the other subjects also showed no correlation with variations in their daily NCVs.

Comment

There are certain inherent limitations in the accuracy of the NCV measurements. For example, the surface stimulating electrode may not be directly over the nerve segment being stimulated. The measurement of the distance between the stimulating electrode placement is approximate and gross. Furthermore, the method gives information about the most rapidly-conducting motor fibers which are the largest; the status of the slower conducting fibers remains unknown. Moreover, the NCV has been shown to vary with age (becoming slower with advancing age)[14,20] and with temperature of the extremities.[21] In spite of these limitations, the reproducibility of the measurements during any one recording session was satisfactory enough to consider the test useful in assessment of state of the most rapidly conducting motor nerve fibers in a given nerve.

In our study of both normal and uremic patients, the maximum variation in NCV was as much as 9.6 meters/sec ± 2.99. This would suggest that caution should be employed in interpretation of the meaning of a single reading if major clinical decisions are to be based on it. Certainly, differences between single NCV determinations carried out days or months apart may not be useful. On the other hand, the mean of multiple NCVs can be more meaningfully compared with the mean of a similar series conducted at another time, if major therapeutic decisions are to be based on this laboratory finding. We were unable to determine the etiology of the daily variation in NCV in the two patients studied. As noted, it could not be correlated with our clinical impressions of the patients, the EEG changes, nor with the blood chemistry changes measured. In particular, no clear-cut explanation of NCV variation can be made on the basis of membrane potential changes due to the observed changes in extracellular electrolyte concentrations.

We conclude that neither NCV measurements nor EEG recordings are useful objective tools in determining the day-to-day status of uremic patients. The NCV can be of possible usefulness in a long-term follow up of a uremic patient, if proper consideration is given to the "normal" daily variation.

This investigation was supported by Public Health Service contract 4-403-AM39599-02.

References

1. Barker ND, Nakamoto S, McCormack LJ, et al: Pathologic anatomy of 13 patients after prolonged periodic hemodialysis. *Trans Amer Soc Artif Intern Organs* **9**:21-27, 1963.

2. Gonzalez FM, Pabico RC, Brown HW, et al: Further experience with the use of routine intermittent hemodialysis in chronic renal failure. *Trans Amer Soc Artif Intern Organs* **9**:11-17, 1963.

3. Hegstrom RM, Murray JS, Pendras JP, et al: Two year's experience with periodic hemodialysis in the treatment of chronic uremia. *Trans Amer Soc Artif Intern Organs* **8**:266-280, 1962.

4. Heron JR, Konotey-Ahulu FID, Shaldon S, et al: Nerve conduction in chronic renal failure treated with dialysis. *Trans Europ Dial Transpl Assoc* **2**:138-143, 1965.

5. Lindholm DD, Burnell JM, Murray JS: Experience in the treatment of chronic uremia in an outpatient community hemodialyses center. *Trans Amer Soc Artif Intern Organs* **9**:3-10, 1963.

6. Preswick G, Jeremy D: Subclinical polyneuropathy in renal insufficiency. *Lancet* **2**:731-732, 1964.

7. Konotey-Ahulu FID, Baillod R, Comty CM, et al: Effect of periodic dialysis on the peripheral neuropathy of end-stage renal failure. *Brit Med J* **2**:1212-1215, 1965.

8. Tenckhoff HA, Boen FST, Jebsen RM, et al: Polyneuropathy in chronic renal insufficiency. *JAMA* **192**:1121-1124, 1965.

9. Jebsen RH, Tenckhoff H, Honet JC: Natural history of uremic polyneuropathy and effects of dialysis. *New Eng J Med* **277**:327-333, 1967.

10. Funck-Bretano JL, Vantelon J: Les polinevrites des uremies chroniques traitee par hemodialyses repetees, *Proceedings of the First International Congress on Nephrology*. Amsterdam, Excerpta Medica Foundation, 1964.

11. Versaci AA, Olsen KJ, McMain PR, et al: Uremic polyneuropathy and motor nerve conduction velocities. *Trans Amer Soc Artif Intern Organs* **10**:328-329, 1964.

12. Tenckhoff HA, Jebsen RH, Honet JC: The effect of long-term dialysis treatment on the course of uremic neuropathy. *Trans Amer Soc Artif Intern Organs* **13**:58-61, 1967.

13. Hodes R, Larrabee MG, German W: The human electromyogram in response to nerve stimulation and the conduction velocity of motor axon: Studies on normal and on injured peripheral nerves. *Arch Neurol Psychiat* **60**:340-365, 1948.

14. Wagman IH, Less H: Maximum conduction velocities of motor fibers of ulnar nerve in human subjects of various ages and sizes. *J Neurophysiol* **15**:235-244, 1952.

15. Honet JC, Jebsen RH, Tenckhoff HA, et al: Motor nerve conduction velocity in chronic renal insufficiency. *Arch Phys Med* **47**:647-652, 1966.

16. Johnson EW, Olsen KJ: Clinical value of motor nerve conduction velocity determination. *JAMA* **172**:2030-2035, 1960.

17. Mayer RF: Nerve conduction studies in man. *Neurology* **13**:1021-1030, 1963.

18. Thomas PK, Sears TA, Gilliatt RW: The range of conduction velocity in normal motor nerve fibers to the small muscles of the hands and foot. *J Neurol Neurosurg Psychiat* **22**:175-181, 1959.

19. Hampers CL, Doak PB, Callaghan MN, et al: The electroencephalogram and spinal fluid during hemodialysis. *Arch Intern Med* **118**:340-346, 1966.

20. Norris AH, Shock NW, Wagman IH: Age changes in maximum conduction velocity of motor fibers of human ulnar nerves. *J Appl Physiol* **5**:589-593, 1953.

21. Hendriksen JD: *Conduction Velocity of Motor Nerves in Normal Subjects and Patients With Neuromuscular Disorders*, thesis. University of Minnesota, Minneapolis, 1956.

The mechanisms controlling glucose dynamics and insulin secretion of nine patients with symptomatic postprandial hypoglycemia following subtotal gastrectomy were studied. Following oral administration of glucose, the patients showed early hyperglycemia and late hypoglycemia. Insulin secretion was exaggerated; plasma insulin and glucose responses to intravenously administered glucose, tolbutamide sodium, secretin, and glucagon were either low or normal compared to control subjects. Intravenously administered glucose followed by glucagon also given intravenously 25 minutes later caused an exaggerated insulin secretion and delayed hypoglycemia. In two patients, carbohydrate restriction for several months resulted in unchanged early plasma glucose curves, absent later hypoglycemia, and markedly decreased insulin secretion following oral administration of glucose. Carbohydrate refeeding of one patient reestablished postprandial hypoglycemia and exaggerated insulin secretion. The data suggest that postgastrectomy hypoglycemia is caused by an inducible gastrointestinal factor which potentiates glucose-mediated insulin release.

Mechanism of Postgastrectomy Hypoglycemia

Kirkwood T. Shultz, MD; Francis A. Neelon, MD;
Laurance B. Nilsen, MD; and Harold E. Lebovitz, MD, Durham, NC

Although surgical intervention is frequently necessary or desirable in treatment of peptic ulcer disease of the gastrointestinal tract, the postoperative course may be complicated by the appearance of new and distressing symptoms: the so-called postgastrectomy syndromes. These symptom complexes are classified[1] by their temporal relation to the preceding meals. Early symptoms (neurovascular and gastrointestinal) appear within 30 minutes after eating and have been the subject of numerous clinical and experimental studies[2]; however, the pathophysiology and etiology remain unclear.

Late symptoms appear two to three hours after eating and have long been known to be due to hypoglycemia. In 1933 Lapp and Dibold noted that oral glucose tolerance was altered by gastrectomy[3] and, in the same year, Beckermann described postprandial hypoglycemia in gastrectomized patients.[4] By 1949 Muir,[5] in discussing postgastrectomy hypoglycemia (PGH) considered only two etiological mechanisms as plausible: (1) an excessive insulin output in response to an initial hyperglycemia; and (2) an increased responsiveness to normal levels of circulating insulin. Despite the development of insulin radioimmunoassay techniques clearly capable of distinguishing between these two possibilities, only two studies of insulin secretion in PGH have been published. Roth and Meade[6] noted excessive insulin secretion during the early (hyperglycemia) phase of the oral glucose tolerance test in patients with PGH and postulated that the prolonged hyperglycemic phase, per se, resulted in insulin hypersecretion ultimately leading to hypoglycemia. Holdsworth et al[7] published similar findings but differed in their interpretations, preferring to postulate that insulin hypersecretion was due to the release of an intestinal "hormone factor" which, in turn, augmented pancreatic insulin secretion.

Our studies were undertaken to elucidate the mechanism controlling glucose dynamics and insulin secretion in patients with PGH.

Materials and Methods

Nine patients were selected for study on the basis of documented postprandial hypoglycemia following previous subtotal gastrectomy (subsequently referred to as PGH patients). No patient had personal or family history of diabetes mellitus, and body weights were stable. The patients were hospitalized in the clinical research unit of Duke Hospital for the duration of studies. All were on unrestricted diets containing at least 300 gm of carbohydrate per day, prior to and during tests, except as noted. Control data were obtained in normal subjects matched in age and weight and free from personal or family history suggesting disorders of carbohydrate metabolism. All tests were performed in the morning after an overnight fast and with the patient recumbent in bed. All samples were collected through an indwelling needle placed in the antecubital vein. The procedures for the studies were as follows:

Oral glucose tolerance test: 100 gm of glucose in 400 ml of lemon juice was administered over 15 to 20 minutes. Samples for glucose and insulin were withdrawn at times indicated in the appropriate figure.

Intravenous glucose tolerance test: 25 gm of glucose (50% solution) was administered intravenously over one to two min-

Received for publication Oct 6, 1970; accepted Dec 4, 1970.

From the Division of Endocrinology, Department of Medicine, Duke University Medical Center, Durham, NC. Dr. Shultz is now at Malcolm Grove Hospital, Andrews Air Force Base, Washington, DC. Dr. Nilsen is now in private practice in Phoenix, Ariz.

Reprint requests to Department of Medicine, Duke University Medical Center, Durham, NC 27706 (Dr. Lebovitz).

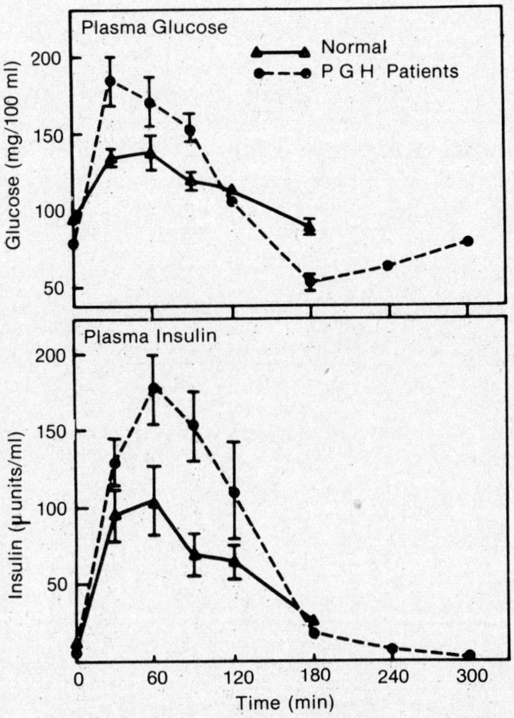

Fig 1.—Mean ± standard error of the mean (SEM) plasma glucose and insulin response to 100 gm of orally administered glucose in 11 normal subjects and 9 PGH patients. The PGH patients show significant elevation of glucose at 30 and 90 minutes ($P<0.01$) and significant lowering at 0 and 180 minutes ($P<0.01$). Insulin is significantly elevated in PGH patients at 60 ($P<0.05$) and 90 ($P<0.01$) minutes.

Fig 2.—Plasma insulin response to intravenously administered glucose in normal subjects and PGH patients. K represents the glucose disposal constant. The mean plasma glucose ± SEM 10 minutes and 60 minutes after glucose administration was 198±5 and 100±6, respectively, for the normals and 242±16 and 139±9, respectively, for the PGH patients.

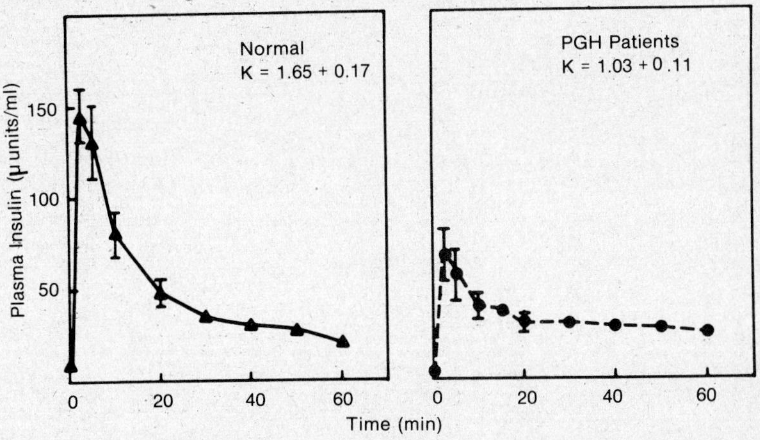

utes. Samples for glucose and insulin determinations were withdrawn from the opposite arm at 5 minute intervals for 60 minutes. Additional samples were drawn at 2½ and 90 minutes.

Intravenous tolbutamide test: 1 gm of tolbutamide sodium was administered intravenously over one to two minutes.

Response of Four Patients With Postgastrectomy Hypoglycemia to Intravenously Administered Secretin (1 unit/kg)*

Time (min)	Plasma Glucose (mg/100 ml)	Plasma Insulin (μunit/ml)
0	86±5.1	8±2.0
5	83±3.9	55±5.8
10	88±3.8	21±5.3
15	81±2.4	12±2.7
20	80±3.3	9±0.9
25	82±2.1	9±1.9
30	81±3.2	9±0.9
35	82±3.4	15±4.1
40	81±3.5	9±1.7
45	82±3.7	7±2.5
50	88±4.8	10±2.6
55	94±7.9	11±5.6
60	92±6.6	11±3.0

* Data represent mean ± SEM.

Samples for glucose and insulin determinations were drawn at 0, 2½, 5, 10, 15, 20, 30, 45, 60, and 90 minutes.

Glucagon test: 1 mg of commercial pancreatic glucagon was administered intravenously over two to three minutes. Samples for glucose and insulin determinations were drawn at times indicated on the appropriate figure.

Secretin test: 1 unit/kg of commercial secretin was administered intravenously over one to two minutes in four patients. Blood for glucose and insulin determinations was withdrawn at five minute intervals for one hour.

Magnesium sulfate test: 25 gm of magnesium sulfate (300 ml of a 0.4M solution) was given orally to two patients and blood for glucose and insulin determinations was withdrawn at 0, 15, 30, 60, 90, 120, 240, and 300 minutes.

Intravenous glucose-glucagon test: 25 gm of glucose was given intravenously over one to two minutes at the start of the test. Twenty-five minutes after the glucose had been given, 1 mg of glucagon was administered intravenously over one to two minutes. Blood for glucose and insulin determinations was withdrawn at the intervals indicated on the appropriate figures.

Plasma insulin was measured by a radioimmunoassay technique previously described.[8] Plasma glucose was measured by an automated ferricyanide technique.[9]

Results

The glucose and insulin dynamics following the administration of 100 gm of glucose by mouth to the PGH patients is shown in Fig 1. For comparison, the three-hour oral glucose tolerance test response of a group of normal subjects is included. During the early phase of the test, the PGH patients had glucose values which were significantly higher than the control subjects ($P<0.01$ at 30 and 90 minutes). At 180 minutes there was a pronounced fall to frankly hypoglycemic levels. Insulin response was significantly exaggerated (as compared to normals) at 60 and 90 minutes but returned to fasting levels with the onset of hypoglycemia.

Figure 2 depicts glucose and insulin responses to intravenous glucose in

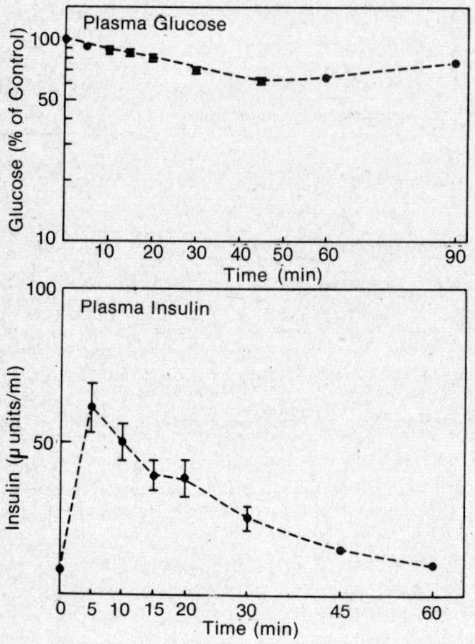

Fig 3.—Plasma glucose and insulin response to intravenously administered tolbutamide in nine PGH patients (mean ±SEM).

the same nine PGH patients. Glucose response is recorded as K, the glucose disposal constant, which represents the percent fall in plasma glucose per minute.[10] The mean K value for the PGH patients was significantly less than that for the normals ($P<0.01$). Four PGH patients had glucose disposal constants in the diabetic range ($K<0.9$), while four had values in the normal range ($K>1.1$). The insulin response to intravenously administered glucose was significantly lower in the PGH patients as compared to the normals at 0, 2½, 5, and 10 minutes. The data thus indicate that for a comparable intravenous glucose load, the PGH patients secrete less insulin than the normals during an intravenous glucose tolerance test.

Figure 3 shows the glucose and insulin response in PGH patients to intravenously administered tolbutamide. When compared to published normal values[11,12] and our own unpublished data, this represents low normal insulin secretion and a somewhat blunted glucose response.

The data from the intravenous glucose and tolbutamide studies indicated that the exaggerated insulin secretion noted during the oral glucose tolerance test could not be accounted for by a general hyperresponsiveness of the pancreatic β cell. However, a number of prior observations[13-15] have shown that the gastrointestinal tract plays an active role in the insulin (and hence the glucose) response to oral glucose loads, apparently through the elaboration of an insulin secretagogue. To assess the possibility that PGH patients might hypersecrete insulin in response to hormonal factors of gastrointestinal origin, the glucose and insulin response to intravenously administered secretin was measured over 120 minutes (Table). Secretin had no significant effect on blood glucose but did cause a transient rise in plasma insulin levels, a response identical to that reported for normals.[16,17]

Another series of intestinal agents that could potentially influence insulin secretion and glucose utilization are the gastrointestinal glucagon-like materials.[18] Since these are not available for human administration and since pancreatic glucagon mimics their effect on insulin secretion, the response of the PGH patients to intravenous pancreatic glucagon was studied (Fig 4). Both the glucose rise and insulin increase following glucagon administration to the PGH patients were the same as has been reported for normal subjects by several investigators.[16,19]

Machella had reported in 1949[20] that nonnutritive hypertonic solutions could produce early dumping syndrome symptoms in gastrectomized patients. The possibility that hypertonicity might influence glucose and insulin dynamics was investigated. Two PGH patients were given oral hypertonic magnesium sulfate solutions. No detectable insulin or glucose changes were noted over the five hours that these were observed.

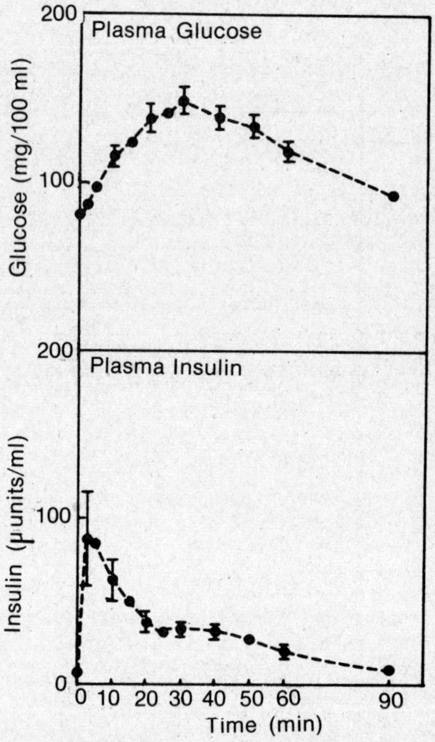

Fig 4.—Plasma glucose and insulin response to intravenously administered glucagon in 9 PGH patients. (Mean ±SEM).

Since none of the intravenous insulinogenic stimuli were capable of causing exaggerated insulin secretion in PGH patients, as noted in the oral glucose tolerance test, an attempt was made to simulate the sequence of events which might be expected to occur following oral glucose ingestion. The four PGH patients with essentially normal glucose ($K=1.03$ to 1.22) and insulin responses to intravenously administered glucose were selected for study to determine the effect of sequential stimulation with

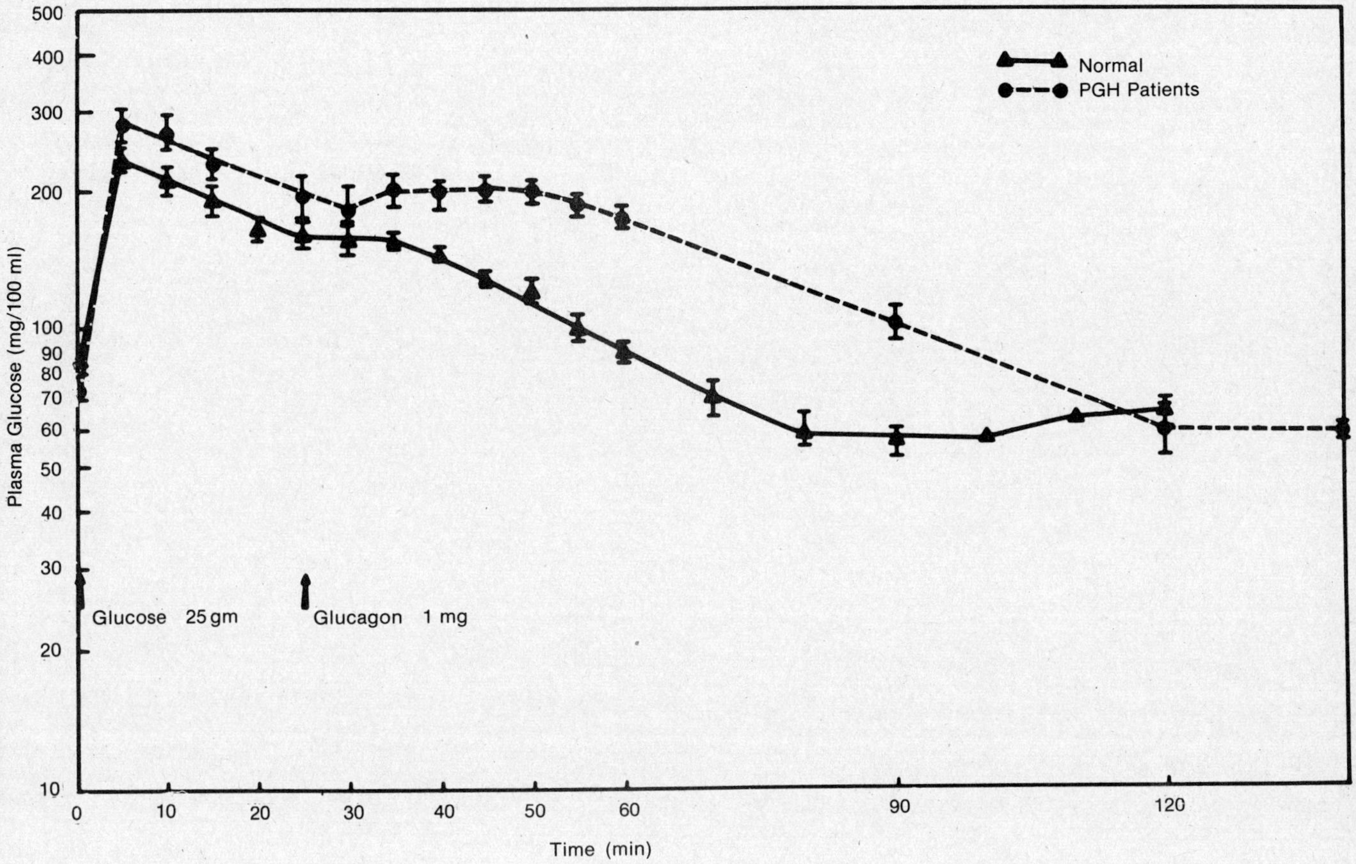

Fig 5.—Plasma glucose response to a combination of intravenously administered glucose and glucagon in five normal subjects and four PGH patients (mean ± SEM).

glucose and glucagon administered intravenously. Five normal subjects underwent the same study for comparison. The results (Fig 5 and 6) show that the plasma glucose in PGH patients rose to a slightly higher value after the glucose load, but the initial rate of glucose utilization (K) was identical to that of normals, as was expected since they were selected on the basis of normal glucose utilization. The plasma glucose response to glucagon, however, showed a more sustained plateau in the PGH patients. Subsequently, glucose fell to hypoglycemic levels (55 to 60 mg/100 ml) in both groups. The insulin response (Fig 6) to the glucose stimulus was identical in both groups. However, the insulin response of both groups to glucagon was markedly augmented (Fig 4) by the preceding glucose load. In addition, though the PGH patients secreted considerably more insulin after glucagon administration than did the controls, the blood glucose fall was delayed. This study suggests glucose administered intravenously plus glucagon stimulated the glucose and insulin responses seen following the oral glucose tolerance test in PGH patients.

Muir[5] pointed out that PGH symptoms do not appear until several months postoperatively, in contrast to neurovascular and gastrointestinal symptoms which may appear with the first postoperative meal. Numerous authors[5,21,22] have advocated low carbohydrate diet in treatment of these symptoms but usually without adequate explanation or experimental proof of efficacy. To assess the effect of limited carbohydrate ingestion on glucose and insulin responses, two PGH patients were placed on a 50 gm carbohydrate, 2,500 calorie, 6 feedings diet for several months. On this regimen both patients gained weight and had a striking amelioration of their hypoglycemic symptoms. Oral glucose tolerance tests before and after these restricted carbohydrate diets are shown in Fig 7 and 8. The remarkable decrease in insulin output despite insignificant change in glucose dynamics (except for the absence of symp-

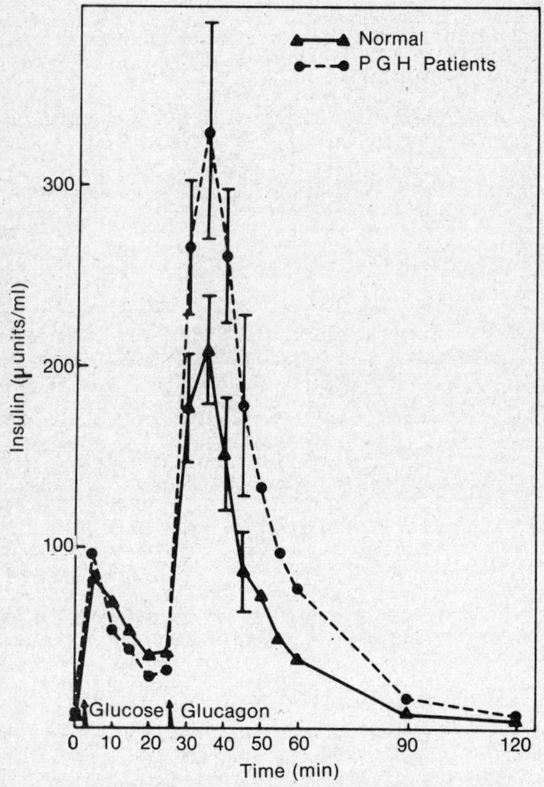

Fig 6.—Plasma insulin response to a combination of intravenously administered glucose and glucagon in five normal subjects and four patients PGH (mean ± SEM).

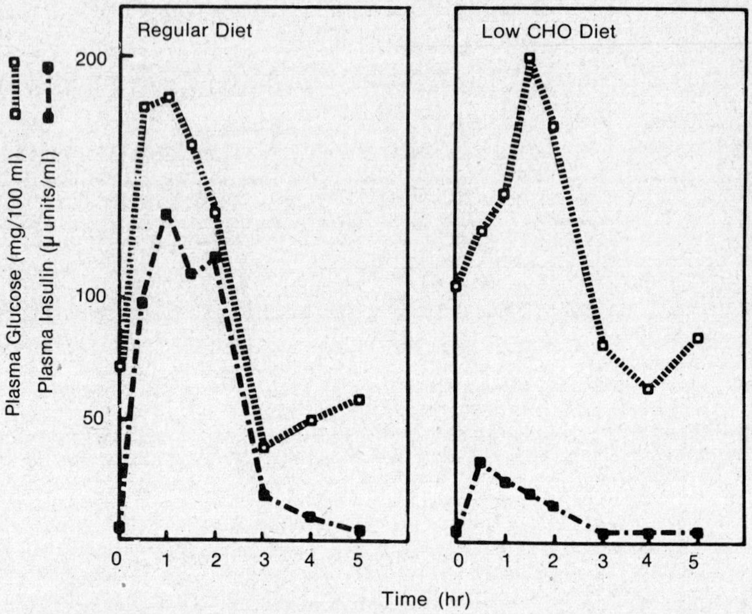

Fig 7.—Plasma glucose and insulin response to 100 gm of orally administered glucose in patient 1 on a regular diet and after several months on a restricted carbohydrate (CHO) diet.

Fig 8.—Plasma glucose and insulin response to 100 gm of orally administered glucose in patient 2. The first study (regular diet) was prior to carbohydrate restriction; she was having severe hypoglycemic symptoms. The second study (low carbohydrate diet) was done after several months on a carbohydrate restricted diet, and she was asymptomatic. The third study (high carbohydrate diet) was done several months after a high carbohydrate diet had been reinstituted and she had again developed hypoglycemic symptoms.

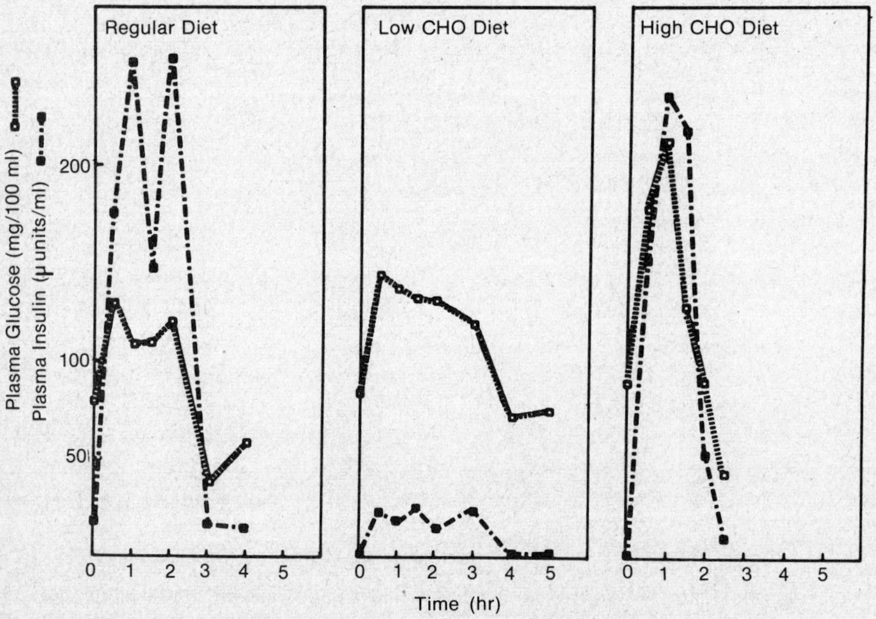

tomatic hypoglycemia) is apparent. One patient voluntarily resumed a high carbohydrate diet. After several months on this program her hypoglycemic symptoms reappeared and the oral glucose tolerance test at that time is shown in Fig 8. Although the initial hyperglycemia was more pronounced than with the previous studies, the reappearance of insulin hypersecretion with concomitant hypoglycemia was striking. Indeed, the test had to be discontinued at 150 minutes due to the patient's symptomatic state. Subsequently, she has returned to a low carbohydrate diet with amelioration of her symptoms once more.

Comment

In 1965, Roth and Meade[6] demonstrated that PGH was due to the hypersecretion of insulin. The question then became what drives the insulin secretion to excess? Roth and Meade concluded that the prolonged hyperglycemic phase, which they noted during the first two hours of the oral glucose tolerance test in PGH patients, was responsible. That is, the pancreas, in some unspecified manner, was being stimulated to insulin oversecretion in response to the elevated blood glucose itself. This explanation seems unlikely since intravenous injection of glucose produces blood glucose levels even higher than those seen after oral loads, but does not result in subsequent hypoglycemia (Fig 2). Holdsworth et al came to similar conclusions for similar reasons.[7] Even more compelling is the observation (Fig 8) that the late hypoglycemia can occur during glucose tolerance testing in PGH patients despite the absence of early hyperglycemia.

Since a number of studies[23,24] have implicated various gastrointestinal hormones in the modulation of the insulin secretory response to oral glucose, it seems likely that alterations in such hormonal factors may be involved in the PGH syndrome. Two alternate hypotheses are plausible explanations for such a mechanism: (1) PGH occurs in that population of postgastrectomy patients whose pancreases are exceptionally sensitive to various insulin releasing stimuli. (2) The anatomical alteration of the gastrointestinal tract somehow produces excessive quantitative release of the insulin secretory hormone(s) and, in some patients, this reaches such magnitudes that hypoglycemia results. Our experiments seem to preclude excessive sensitivity of the pancreas to insulin secretory stimulation since the responses of all the patients to intravenously administered glucose, tolbutamide, secretin, and glucagon were normal or slightly depressed. The excessive elaboration of some intestinal insulin secretory factor in postgastrectomy patients as the cause of PGH seems most plausible. Samols et al[25] have demonstrated that postgastrectomy patients have a significantly greater rise in plasma immunoreactive glucagon-like material following orally ingested glucose than do normal individuals. The majority of this material was thought to be released from the small bowel. The combined intravenous glucose-glucagon administration performed in the present study clearly demonstrates that high glucagon levels occurring while the blood glucose is moderately elevated will lead to markedly excessive insulin secretion with a resultant hypoglycemia.

The results (Fig 5 and 6) demonstrate the first instance in our study of excessive response by PGH patients to any stimulus other than orally ingested glucose. Figure 5 shows the glucose response in both normal and PGH patients. In both instances, there is an eventual hypoglycemic phase which was not seen when either glucose or glucagon were given independently. However, the hypoglycemic nadir in PGH patients is displaced temporally due to the more prolonged hyperglycemic plateau in these patients as compared to normal individuals. Figure 6 shows that the insulin secretion to the initial glucose bolus is identical in both groups. However, the PGH patients hypersecrete insulin after the glucagon as compared to normal controls. While it might be argued that the insulin secretion in the PGH patients outstrips that of the normal subjects due to the more prolonged glucose response in these patients (Fig 5), this explanation seems unlikely since the insulin excess was apparent within five minutes after the glucagon was administered, at a time when the plasma glucose had not begun to plateau. However, there is no definitive means, at present, of excluding this possibility. In any case, intravenous administration of glucagon in the setting of a preinduced hyperglycemia, results in a marked insulin secretion with subsequent hypoglycemia in both normal and PGH patients. We infer from these data that the hypersecretion of an insulin releasing gastrointestinal factor akin to glucagon could explain the oral glucose tolerance test results seen in PGH and postulate the following sequence: loss of pyloric modulation allows rapid influx of carbohydrate into the small intestine with resultant hyperglycemia. There is concomitant hypersecretion of the gastrointestinal insulin secretagogue which, in the setting of preinduced hyperglycemia, results in late hypoglycemia.

The observation that normal individuals will become hypoglycemic after a combination of intravenous glucose and glucagon indicates that the abnormality in PGH patients is probably an exaggeration of the normal gastrointestinal regulation of insulin secretion and not of the action of insulin. The hyperresponsiveness of the PGH patients to this intravenous combination suggests that the system is constantly overstimulated and therefore hyperresponds to the stimulus.

The response to dietary carbohydrate restriction (Fig 7 and 8) was most striking and appears to demonstrate that the insulin hyperresponsiveness of PGH is "inducible" (at least in a generic sense). This inductive process appears to take several months as demonstrated by the response of the patient shown in Fig 8 and accounts for the clinical observation that hypoglycemic symptoms are not seem in the early postoperative period.[5] Pertinent here are the findings of Grey et al[26] who studied the insulin response to orally ingested glucose before and after fasting in rats. They found that a 48-hour fast markedly reduced the insulin response to glucose. The insulin response could be restored by refeeding a carbohydrate containing diet but not by an isocaloric, carbohydrate-free diet. They further demonstrated that there is a glucose mediated, inducible insulin secretory mechanism in the pancreatic β cell which decays rapidly in the absence of carbohydrate. If these studies are applicable to humans, the response of our patients to carbohydrate restriction could be interpreted as a loss of the ability of the pancreas to respond to the gastrointestinal stimulus. It seems likely to us, however, that the gastrointestinal secretagogue itself is inducible, explaining the months-long delay in onset of symptoms following surgery or the reintroduction of the high carbohydrate diet. A similar ability of the intestinal tract to modify its functional capabilities in response to the intraluminal stimuli presented to it, has been noted in connection with absorptive functions by Nunn and Ellert.[27]

The striking decrease in insulin secretion following carbohydrate restriction provides evidence for the mechanism of efficacy of low carbohydrate diets in PGH. In most instances diet therapy has been considered indicated where various digestive or absorptive capabilities were lacking, eg, lactase deficiency or pancreatic insufficiency.[28] Our observations demonstrate that dietary restriction is beneficial in preventing the induction of certain functional capacities of the small intestine which in the present instance leads to a syndrome of excessive insulin secretion with resultant hypoglycemia.

This study was supported by Public Health Service grant M 01 FR30 from the Clinical Research Center Branch, Division of Research Facilities and Resources; and by grants AM-01324, 5T1 AM-5074, and K3 AM-17,954 from the National Institute of Arthritis and Metabolic Diseases.

References

1. Woodward ER: *The Postgastrectomy Syndromes.* Springfield, I11, Charles C Thomas Publisher, 1963, pp 1-56.

2. Fenger JH: Clinical and experimental studies of dumping disposition. *Acta Chir Scand* supp 371, pp 1-128, 1967.

3. Lapp FW, Dibold H: Blutzuckerablauf in seiner Bezeihung zum resezierten Magen. *Klin Wschr* **12**:547-548, 1933.

4. Beckermann F: Über spontanae Hypoglykämie nach Magenoperationen. *Deutsche Med Wschr* **59**:683-684, 1933.

5. Muir A: Postgastrectomy syndromes. *Brit J Surg* **37**:165-178, 1949.

6. Roth DA, Meade RC: Hyperinsulinism-hypoglycemia in the postgastrectomy patient. *Diabetes* **14**:526-528, 1965.

7. Holdsworth CD, Turner D, McIntyre N: Pathophysiology of postgastrectomy hypoglycemia. *Brit Med J* **4**:257-259, 1969.

8. Horton ES, Johnson C, Lebovitz HE: Carbohydrate metabolism in uremia. *Ann Intern Med* **68**:63-74, 1968.

9. Hoffman WS: A rapid photoelectric method for the determination of glucose in blood and urine. *J Biol Chem* **120**:51-55, 1937.

10. Silverstone FA, Brandfonbrener M, Shock NW et al: Age differences in the intravenous glucose tolerance tests and the response to insulin. *J Clin Invest* **36**:504-514, 1957.

11. Rojas L, Soeldner JS, Gleason RE, et al: Offspring of two diabetic parents: Differential serum insulin responses to intravenous glucose and tolbutamide. *J Clin Endocr* **29**:1569-1579, 1969.

12. Samols E, Marks V: Evaluation of the intravenous tolbutamide test in the recognition and differential diagnosis of spontaneous hypoglycemia, in Butterfield WJH, Westering WV (eds): *International Congress Series.* New York, Excerpta Medica Foundation, 1967, No. 149, pp 147-156.

13. Ebrick H, Stimmler L, Hlad Jr CJ, et al: Plasma insulin response to oral and intravenous glucose administration. *J Clin Endocr* **24**:1076-1082, 1964.

14. Dupré J, Beck JC: Stimulation of release of insulin by an extract of intestinal mucosa. *Diabetes* **15**:555-559, 1966.

15. Perley MJ, Kipnis DM: Plasma insulin responses to oral and intravenous glucose: Studies in normal and diabetic subjects. *J Clin Invest* **46**:1954-1962, 1967.

16. Deckert T: Stimulation of insulin secretion by glucagon and secretin. *Acta Endocr* **57**:578-584, 1968.

17. Dupré J, Rojas L, White JJ, et al: Effects of secretin on insulin and glucagon in portal and peripheral blood in man. *Lancet* **2**:26-27, 1966.

18. Unger RH, Ohneda A, Valverde I, et al: Characterization of the responses of circulating glucagon-like immunoreactivity to intraduodenal and intravenous administration of glucose. *J Clin Invest* **47**:48-65, 1968.

19. Samols E, Marri G, Marks V: Interrelationship of glucagon, insulin and glucose: The insulinogenic effect of glucagon. *Diabetes* **15**:855-866, 1966.

20. Machella TE: The mechanism of the postgastrectomy "dumping" syndrome. *Ann Surg* **130**:145-159, 1949.

21. Oberhelman Jr HA: *Physiological Principles of Gastric Surgery.* Springfield, Ill, Charles C Thomas, Publisher, 1968, p 78.

22. Barnes CG: Hypoglycemia following partial gastrectomy. *Lancet* **2**:536-539, 1947.

23. Dupré J, Curtis JD, Unger RH, et al: Effects of secretin, pancreozymin or gastrin on the response of the endocrine pancreas to administration of glucose or arginine in man. *J Clin Invest* **48**:745-757, 1969.

24. Dupré J: An intestinal hormone affecting glucose disposal in man. *Lancet* **2**:672-673, 1964.

25. Samols E, Tyler J, Rege VP, et al: The possible role of glucagon (pancreatic and extrapancreatic), in Östman J, Milner RDG (eds): *Insulin Secretion: Diabetes. Proceedings of VIth Congress of the International Diabetes Federation.* Amsterdam, Excepta Medica Foundation, 1969, pp 446-454.

26. Grey NJ, Goldring S, Kipnis DM: The effect of fasting, diet and actinomycin D on insulin secretion in the rat. *J Clin Invest* **49**:881-889, 1970.

27. Nunn Jr AS, Ellert MS: Absorption and electrolyte changes of intestinal mucosa following substrate induction. *Amer J Physiol* **212**:711-716, 1967.

28. Ingelfinger FJ: The dietotherapy of gastrointestinal complaints. *Viewpoints Digestive Dis* **1**:3, 1969.

Serratia marcescens Bacteremia

Clinical Observations and Studies of Precipitin Reactions

Jackson G. Crowder, MD; Gareth H. Gilkey, MD; and Arthur C. White, MD, Indianapolis

Sixteen cases of *Serratia marcescens* bacteremia were seen in three hospitals. Most patients had severe underlying disease and had been treated with antibiotics prior to development of bacteremia. Five patients had organisms other than *S marcescens* isolated from blood. Portals of entry included intravenous cannulas and pulmonary, urinary, peritoneal, and wound infections. Sera from eight of nine patients tested contained precipitating antibodies against an ultrasonic extract of *S marcescens* in gel diffusion plates. All sera tested more than seven days after onset of bacteremia contained precipitins. All blood culture isolates tested were sensitive to gentamicin, and isolates from five patients were sensitive to gentamicin alone. Two of three patients treated with gentamicin were cured. Three patients with a urinary portal of entry survived, despite treatment with antibiotics to which their organisms showed in vitro resistance.

Serratia marcescens, a gram negative bacillus and member of the family Enterobacteriaceae, was previously considered to be nonpathogenic for man. In the past two decades, however, the organism has been isolated with increasing frequency from patients and has been incriminated as the causative agent of a variety of infections. Infections produced by *S marcescens* include urinary tract infection,[1-3] pneumonia,[4] pleural empyema,[5] lung abscess,[6] wound infection,[7,8] meningitis,[9] omphalitis and balanitis,[10] peritonitis,[11] osteomyelitis,[12] and suppurative arthritis.[13]

Fields and associates,[14] in reviewing the literature three years ago, could find only 15 reported cases of *S marcescens* bacteremia, adding three of their own. Since then, reports of *S marcescens* bacteremia in large numbers of patients from several institutions have appeared.[15-17] Coinciding with the increased incidence of *S marcescens* bacteremia has been an increase in the reports of *Serratia* endocarditis. Whereas prior to 1969 there had been five reports of this entity,[18-22] in the past year, four additional cases have been reported.[23-25]

Serratia marcescens is a well established cause of nosocomial infection. Genitourinary infections have been associated with urinary instrumentation.[1,2] Pulmonary infections have been traced to contamination with *S marcescens* of intermittent positive-pressure breathing machines[26] and ultrasonic nebulizers.[5] Meningitis has followed lumbar puncture,[9] and peritonitis has followed peritoneal dialysis.[11] Umbilical cord colonization in a newborn nursery was found to be due to contaminated saline used to moisten the umbilical cord.[10]

Although the organism may produce a red pigment, prodigiosin, the majority of strains isolated at present are nonpigmented.[14,16,27]

Sixteen cases of *S marcescens* bacteremia have been encountered by the authors in the past year. The purposes of the present report are to describe the clinical characteristics of these cases, the antibiotic susceptibilities of these and other *Serratia* isolates, and the results of serum precipitating antibody determinations in nine of the 16 patients.

Materials and Methods

The 16 patients were seen by the authors in three general hospitals of Indiana University Medical Center in the past year. Five patients were in one hospital, five in another hospital, and the remainder in the third hospital. All patients, except one, had two or more positive blood cultures.

Identification.—*Serratia marcescens* was identified by standard procedures described by Edwards and Ewing.[27] The majority of isolates were nonpigmented.

Precipitin Tests.—Precipitating antibodies to *S marcescens* were studied by

Received for publication April 16, 1970; accepted Oct 2.

From the Department of Medicine, Indiana University Medical Center, Indianapolis.

Reprint requests to Department of Medicine, Indiana University Medical Center, 1100 W Michigan St, Indianapolis 46202 (Dr. Crowder).

means of double diffusion in agar gel plates. An antigen extract was prepared by disruption of one volume of a washed suspension of *S marcescens* in four volumes of 0.9% saline. The suspension was treated with ultrasonic vibration for two hours in a batch model U-20 cooled with circulating water at 4 C. After ultrasonic disruption, the debris was removed by centrifugation at 15,000 g for 30 minutes, and the supernatant fluid stored at −20 C until used for testing.

Gel diffusion plates were prepared with 0.9% Noble agar.[28] The inner well was filled with undiluted *Serratia* extract and the outer wells with serial twofold dilutions of serum. The plates were kept at 37 C and examined daily for five days for the presence of precipitin lines.

Antibiotic Sensitivity Studies.—Disk sensitivity tests were performed on Mueller-Hinton medium measuring diameters of zones of inhibition for each antibiotic.[29]

Tube dilution sensitivity studies were performed using a 10^{-2} dilution of an overnight culture of the organism in heart infusion broth.

Results

Clinical Findings.—The clinical findings in all 16 patients were similar to those found in other gram negative bacteremias.[30] Maximum temperature varied from 101 F to 106 F (38.3 to 41.1 C). Only two patients had a maximum temperature of less than 102 F (38.9 C), and both of these patients were uremic. Significant hypotension with systolic blood pressures of less than 80 mm Hg occurred in nine patients. Maximum peripheral blood leukocyte counts ranged from 11,100/cu mm to 51,200/cu mm. Ten patients had leukocyte counts of 20,000/cu mm or greater.

Further clinical findings are shown in Table 1. Four patients were uremic. Two had rheumatic heart disease and three, arteriosclerotic heart disease. Two patients had pulmonary emphysema, one had superimposed *Serratia* pneumonia. Two patients had severe trauma with multiple fractures. Ten of the patients had had a recent surgical procedure. Six patients had diabetes mellitus and four had received adrenal corticosteroids prior to developing *Serratia* bacteremia.

Five patients had an additional organism isolated from the blood. Patient 8 was being treated with colistin sulfate for *Pseudomonas* bacteremia when he developed *Serratia* bacteremia. Later in his course, peptostreptococci and *Serratia* were present in multiple blood cultures. Patient 16 had *Candida albicans* fungemia prior to her *Serratia* bacteremia. Patient 3, 13, and 15 had an additional organism isolated concomitantly with *S marcescens* in multiple blood cultures.

Eleven patients had received intermittent positive pressure breathing, including the four with a pulmonary portal of entry. Cultures of the respirator were obtained in only one of these four patients with negative results.

The portal of entry could be clearly documented in 12 patients by evidence of disease and the isolation of *S marcescens* at the suspected portal. Three patients had the urinary tract as portal of entry. Two had indwelling Foley catheters and one of these had had recent cystoscopy. All four patients with a pulmonary portal of entry had pneumonic infiltrates.

The portal of entry was peritoneal in two patients. One had had resection of a colonic polyp followed by leakage and peritonitis. The other patient developed peritonitis during peritoneal dialysis.

In two patients, the only evidence for a portal of entry was by an intravenous cannula. Both of these patients improved promptly when the infected cannula was removed and chemotherapy administered. Three additional patients had *S marcescens* cultured from the tip of an intravenous cannula. In one, patient 3, the cannula was inserted after onset of his bacteremia. The second, patient 13, had, in addition, pneumonia with *S marcescens* in sputum cultures. The third, patient 14, had, in addition, pneumonia and empyema with *S marcescens* isolated from pleural fluid and from abdominal fluid during peritoneal dialysis. In the latter two cases, it was impossible to determine the portal of entry with certainty. Only two patients, patient 15 and 16, had no cultural evidence to suggest a portal of entry.

Eleven patients had received antibiotics prior to their bacteremia. The most frequently used antibiotic had been cephalothin sodium.

Precipitin Tests.—Sera from seven of nine patients with *S marcescens* bacteremia contained detectable antibodies to a *Serratia* extract when initially tested (Table 2, Fig 1 and 2). From one to four precipitin lines were produced between the extract and various sera. In addition, serum of patient 8, which was negative on initial testing, was positive 24 days later. Sera of the remaining seven patients were not available for study.

The antigen extract used was obtained from the organism isolated from patient 1. Only one of 55 sera from noninfected individuals gave a precipitin line against this *Serratia* extract.

All sera obtained eight or more days after onset of bacteremia contained precipitins. Positive sera were obtained from 8 to 38 days after onset of bacteremia with the exception of patient 13, whose serum was positive on the day of onset of her bacteremia. In this patient, *Serratia* bacteriuria had been present several months prior to her bacteremia, so that the antibodies detected probably represented a response to previous *Serratia* infection. Antibodies could not be detected in two sera, obtained four and five days after onset of bacteremia. In addition, precipitins could not be detected in serum of patient 9, obtained five days after onset of bacteremia, against an extract of his own infecting organism or the standard *Serratia* extract.

Long term follow-up was obtained only on patient 8, whose serum did not contain detectable antibody five months after infection was cured.

Antibiotic Studies.—The antibiotic sensitivities of the *S marcescens* isolated from blood cultures of these patients, the therapy, and results are shown in Table 3. Seven patients (44%) died of their infection. Two additional patients died later in their hospitalization, after their infection had been cured, giving an overall mortality of 56%. Six of the nine patients treated with an antibiotic, to which their organism showed in vitro sensitivity, survived the infection. Three of seven patients treated with an antibiotic, to which their organism demonstrated in vitro resistance, survived. All three of the survivors in the latter group had the urinary tract as portal of entry.

All isolates tested were sensitive to gentamicin in vitro by the disk method. Five of the 16 isolates were sensitive only to gentamicin or gentamicin and nalidixic acid. *Serratia marcescens* organisms isolated from seven of these patients were tested by tube dilution methods and all were inhibited by 3.9μg/ml or less of gentamicin. Bacteremia was cleared in five days in two patients treated with gentamicin. Bacteremia continued in one patient for 21 days, despite excessively high peak serum gentamicin levels (32μg/ml). *Serratia* and peptostreptococcal bacteremia cleared promptly when the gentamicin dosage was reduced and chloramphenicol added.

To further determine antibiotic sensitivities of *S marcescens*, the disk sensitivities were tabulated of all isolates excluding blood in one of our hospitals (Table 4). There were 92 isolates obtained from 50 patients. The majority of the isolates were from sputum or urine. All 28 isolates tested were sensitive to gentamicin. The next most effective antibiotics were kanamycin sulfate followed by chloramphenicol. Eighty-two (89%) of the isolates were sensitive to either chloramphenicol, kanamycin, or both.

Fig 1.—Gel diffusion plate demonstrating precipitin lines between serratia extract (S) *and serum dilutions of patient 5, nine days after onset of bacteremia. Human γ-globulin is in uppermost well.* Inner line *is present with 1:2 dilution;* outer line, *with undiluted serum.*

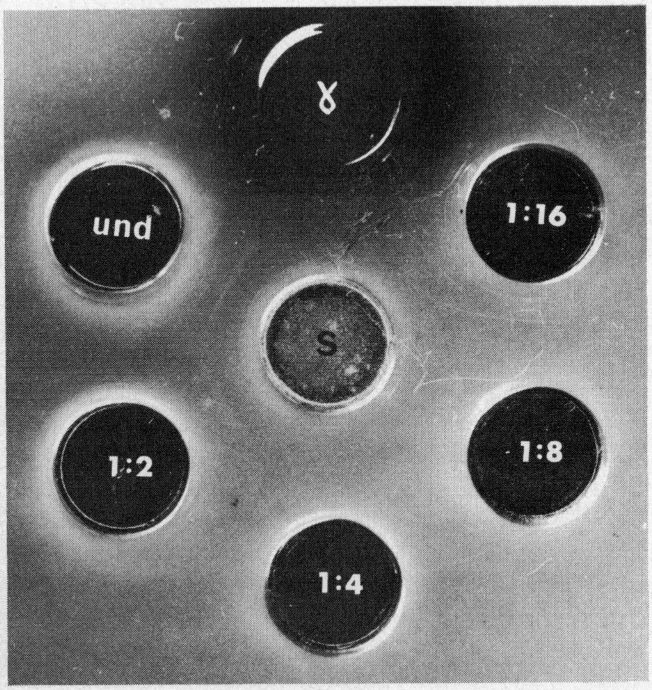

Fig 2.—Plate demonstrating precipitin lines between extract and serum dilutions of patient 5 at 16 days after onset of bacteremia. Outer line *has become thicker and now extends to a 1:2 dilution of serum.*

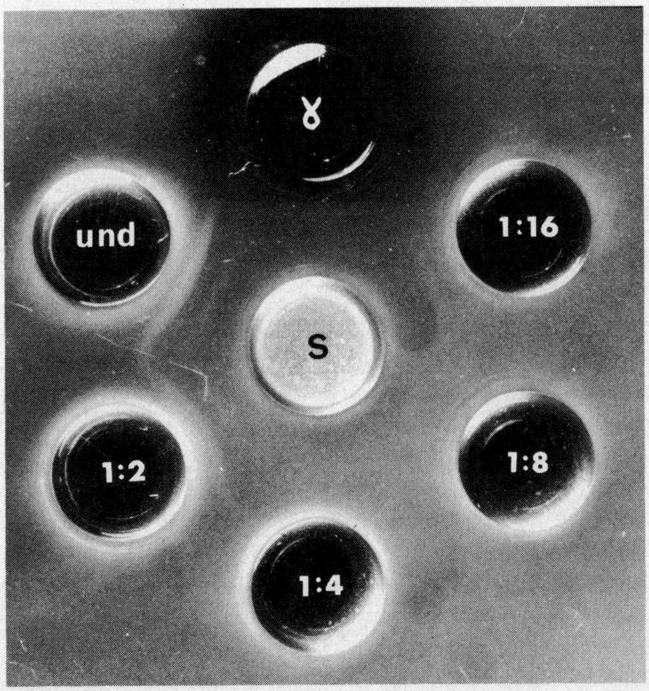

Table 1.—Clinical Findings in *S marcescens* Bacteremia

Patient	Age	Sex	Underlying Disease	Portal of Entry	Antibiotic at Time of Acquisition	Comment
1	62	M	Aortic insufficiency, congestive failure, prostatic hypertrophy, cystoscopy, uremia	Urinary	Cephalothin	No evidence of endocarditis
2	62	M	Diabetes mellitus, emphysema, *Serratia* bacteriuria	Urinary	None	Hypotensive
3	48	M	Alcoholism, cirrhosis	Urinary	None	Hypotensive, *Proteus* and enterococci in blood
4	69	M	Diabetes mellitus, rheumatic heart disease, congestive failure, emphysema, subdural hematoma	Pulmonary	None	
5	39	M	Diabetes mellitus, marsupialization of pancreatic pseudocyst	Pulmonary	None	Hypotensive followed by cardiac arrest and resuscitation
6	45	F	Multiple fractures, fat embolism, steroid therapy	Pulmonary	Cephalothin	
7	50	M	Multiple fractures	Pulmonary	Penicillin, streptomycin, cephalothin	
8	60	M	Peritonitis after colon resection	Peritoneal	Kanamycin, cephalothin, colistin	Hypotensive, also *Pseudomonas* and peptostreptococcal bacteremia
9	47	M	Malignant nephrosclerosis, uremia, peritonitis after dialysis	Peritoneal	Cephalothin	
10	65	M	Aortic valve replacement, mediastinitis, wound infection, steroid therapy	Wound	Lincomycin	
11	49	M	Diabetes mellitus, myocardial infarction, embolectomy for aorto-femoral thromboembolism	Intravenous cannula	None	
12	50	M	Small bowel intussuception and resection of necrotic bowel	Intravenous cannula	Penicillin, streptomycin	Hypotensive
13	55	F	Chronic pyelonephritis, uremia, bleeding ulcer, cholecystectomy	Intravenous cannula or pulmonary	Cephalothin	Hypotensive, also *Aerobacter* in blood
14	54	F	Diabetes mellitus, hypertension, congestive failure, acute renal failure, uremia, steroid therapy	Intravenous cannula, pulmonary, or peritoneal	Cephalothin, kanamycin, polymyxin	Hypotensive
15	77	F	Infected Aust-Moore prosthesis right hip	Undetermined	Cephalothin, kanamycin	Hypotensive, also *Pseudomonas* in blood
16	72	F	Diabetes mellitus, peptic ulcer, gastrocolic fistula, steroid therapy	Undetermined	Ampicillin, cephalothin, kanamycin	Hypotensive, *Candida* preceding fungemia

Table 2.—Precipitin Tests in *S marcescens* Bacteremia

Patient	Days After Onset Serum Obtained	No. of Precipitin Lines	Reciprocal of Titers
1	8	4	und* 2, 4, 4
3	11	1	2
5	9	2	und, 2
	16	2	2, 2
	20	2	2, 2
7	18	1	8
	38	3	2, 4, und
8	4	None	None
	28	1	2
10	11	3	4, 4, 2
12	20	1	2
13	1	1	2
9	5	None	None

* Und indicates undiluted serum.

Table 3.—Antibiotic Disk Sensitivities of *S marcescens* Isolates From Blood in Relation to Therapy and Outcome

Patient	Antibiotics to Which Organism was Sensitive	Antibiotic Therapy	Outcome
1	NA, G	P, Sm	S
2	Ch, K, G, NA	P	S
3	G	Ce, K	S
4	Ch, T*	Ce, K	D
5	Ch, Sm, K, G	Ce, G	S
6	NA, G	Co	D
7	G	Ce, G	S
8	Ch, Sm, T, K, G	Ch, G	S
9	Ch, K, G	K	D
10	T, Am, Sm, K, G	Ch, K	D
11	Ce, Sm, T, K, G	Ce, K	S
12	Ch, K, G	K	S
13	Ch, K, T, Sm*	K	S
14	G	Ce, K, P	D
15	Ch, Sm, K, T*	Ce, K	D
16	None*	Amph	D

Abbreviations are as follows: NA indicates nalidixic acid, G, gentamicin; P, penicillin; Sm, streptomycin; Ch, chloramphenicol; K, kanamycin; T, Tetracycline; Ce, cephalothin; Am, ampicillin; Amph, amphotericin B. S, survived; D, died.
* Not tested against gentamicin.

All but one isolate was sensitive to nalidixic acid. More than 50% of the isolates were resistant to each of the remainder of the antibiotics tested. Although five of 16 patients in this series had bacteremia with an organism resistant to all antibiotics tested except gentamicin and nalidixic acid, only one isolate from sources other than blood cultures showed this pattern of resistance.

Comment

The clinical setting for these cases is similar to that previously described for *S marcescens* infection in that severe underlying disease was usually present, instrumentation or surgery had been performed, and prior antibiotic therapy had been given.[2,5,7,15,16] Six patients had diabetes mellitus. The association of diabetes mellitus and *S marcescens* infection has been previously noted,[4,14] as has the association with steroid therapy which had been given in four patients in this series.[15]

In five of our 16 patients, *Serratia* bacteremia occurred in combination with bacteremia due to another organism. *Serratia marcescens* as part of multiple species bacteremia was noted in only two of 62 positive blood cultures by Dodson[15] in his study of 16 cases and in only four of 39 cases of *S marcescens* bacteremia by Wilfert and associates.[16] Multiple species bacteremia is most frequently seen in patients with severe underlying disease and has a higher mortality than that due to a single species.[30,31]

Forty-four percent of our patients died of their infection. This mortality is similar to that of 40% reported by Altemeier and associates[17] and 36% reported by Wilfert and associates.[16]

The portals of entry in our patients were diverse. The patients with the urinary tract as portal of entry as of interest since their bacteremias cleared despite the administration of an antibiotic to which their organisms showed in vitro resistance. It is possible that the high urinary levels of streptomycin and kanamycin obtained were sufficient to suppress the focus seeding the blood stream despite in vitro resistance by the usual criteria.

Intravenous cannulas have received emphasis as important sources of hospital acquired bacteremia.[32,33] They have also been documented as a source of *S marcescens* bacteremia. Wilfert and associates[16] found that an indwelling polyethylene catheter had been used in 17 of their 39 patients and that in 7 of these patients, the catheter appeared to be the only portal of entry. Altemeier and associates[17] found intravenous catheters a source of bacteremia in 15 of their 42 patients with *S marcescens* bacteremia.

Limited epidemiologic study in our patients has not revealed evidence of how the organisms were transmitted to these patients. However, since these cases occurred in three different hospitals and there were multiple portals of entry, it seems

Table 4.—Antibiotic Sensitivities of *Serratia* Isolates From Sputum and Urine

Antibiotic	No. of Isolates	% Sensitive	% Intermediately Sensitive	% Resistant
Gentamicin	28	100	0	0
Kanamycin	92	83	4	13
Chloramphenical	92	72	1	27
Streptomycin	92	41	7	52
Tetracycline	91	16	9	75
Colistin	92	18	2	80
Ampicillin	92	7	8	85
Cephalothin	92	4	0	96
Nitrofurantoin	26	8	4	88
Nalidixic acid	27	96	0	4

unlikely that there was a single source for all of these patients.

Previous studies have showed elevated agglutinin titers in patients with *S marcescens* infection[1,6,8,18,19] and in laboratory workers exposed to an aerosol of *S marcescens*.[34] In this study a precipitin response was found in all sera obtained seven days or more after onset of bacteremia.

The detection of precipitating antibodies to group antigens by means of double diffusion in agar gel plates has been useful in the diagnosis of other bacterial infections. Antibodies to staphylococcal teichoic acids or type specific antigens can be detected by this method in the majority of patients with staphylococcal infections, but not in nasal carriers of staphylococci or in normal individuals.[35,36] Precipitins to *Pseudomonas aeruginosa* were detected in sera of 64% of patients with a variety of *Pseudomonas* infections, but were not detected in sera of patients with upper respiratory tract colonization by *Pseudomonas* without infection or in normal individuals.[37] Often, when *S marcescens* is isolated from sputum or urine, it is difficult to determine whether the organism is responsible for disease. In this study, precipitins were detectable in sera of patients with well documented *Serratia* bacteremia but were not demonstrable in sera of normal individuals. We have recently detected precipitins in serum of a patient with well documented *Serratia* pulmonary infection and in another patient with well documented *Serratia* urinary tract infection, both without bacteremia. Thus it appears that demonstration of precipitins in agar-gel diffusion studies may be helpful in distinguishing serratial disease from colonization as has previously been demonstrated for *Staphyloccus aureus* and *P aeruginosa*.

The protective effect of *Serratia* precipitins is unknown. Seven of eight patients with detectable precipitins survived their infection. The development of an adequate antibody response may have been a factor in their survival; however, other factors may have been of more importance and allowed survival long enough for a precipitin response to become manifest.

The treatment of *S marcescens* infections has been unsatisfactory due both to the severe underlying disease in the patients and to the resistance of the organism to most antibiotics.

Kanamycin or the combination of chloramphenicol and kanamycin have been suggested as the most effective therapeutic regimen in the past.[1,2,4,15,17] Although the majority of isolates from sputum and urine in the present study were sensitive to either chloramphenoicol or kanamycin, organisms resistant to this combination were isolated from blood in 38% of the patients in this study.

It would appear that gentamicin is presently the drug of choice for at least the initial therapy of serious *S marcescens* infection. All of the isolates tested in the present study were sensitive to gentamicin. Two of the three patients treated with gentamicin showed a satisfactory response. The third had peptostreptococcal bacteremia in addition and neither infection cleared until chloramphenicol was added.

Other studies have demonstrated in vitro sensitivity of *S marcescens* isolates to gentamicin. Wilfert et al[16] found that all 180 isolates tested by the replica plate method were sensitive to gentamicin. Edmondson and Sanford[38] reported 14 isolates sensitive to less than 10μg/ml. Thornton and Andriole[39] found that all 34 isolates tested were inhibited by 1.5μg/ml or less.

Although the majority of isolates tested by disk methods demonstrated sensitivity to nalidixic acid, the effectiveness of this drug would appear to be limited in the treatment of severe *S marcescens* infection by the diffculty in achieving adequate tissue levels and the development of resistance to nalidixic acid during therapy.[40]

This investigation was supported by grant TOI-AI343 and AI-07902 from the National Institutes of Health.

Sue Miller and Theodore Stein gave technical assistance.

Nonproprietary and Trade Names of Drugs

Gentamicin sulfate—*Garamycin.*
Cephalothin sodium—*Keflin.*
Ampicillin—*Penbritin.*
Amphotericin B—*Fungizone.*

References

1. Lancaster LJ: Role of *Serratia* species in urinary tract infections. *Arch Intern Med* **109**:536-539, 1962.
2. Clayton E, von Graevenitz A: Nonpigmented *Serratia marcescens. JAMA* **197**:1059-1064, 1966.
3. Allen SD, Conger KB: *Serratia marcescens* infection of the urinary tract: A nosocomial infection. *J Urol* **101**:621-623, 1969.
4. Bernard LA, Sutton WC: Infection due to chromobacteria. *Arch Intern Med* **105**:311-315, 1960.
5. Ringrose RE, McKown B, Felton FG, et al: A hospital outbreak of *Serratia marcescens* associated with ultrasonic nebulizers. *Ann Intern Med* **69**:719-729, 1968.
6. Elston HR, Magnuson CW: Lung abscess caused by nonchromogenic *Serratia marcescens. Amer Rev Resp Dis* **92**:624-631, 1965.
7. Gale D, Sonnenwirth AC: Frequent human isolation of *Serratia marcescens. Arch Intern Med* **109**:414-421, 1962.
8. Graber CD, Tumbusch WT, Rudnicki RP, et al: Generalized Shwartzman-like reaction following *Serratia marcescens* septicemia in a fatal burn. *Surg Gynec Obstet* **110**:443-450, 1960.
9. Graber CD, Higgens LS, Davis JS: Seldom-encountered agents of bacterial meningitis. *JAMA* **192**:956-960, 1965.
10. McCormack RC, Kunin CM: Control of a single source nursery epidemic due to *Serratia marcescens. Pediatrics* **37**:750-755, 1966.
11. McCracken AW, Lipscomb FE: *Serratia marcescens* infection complicating peritoneal dialysis. *Brit Med J* **1**:1536-1537, 1965.
12. Derian PS, Fisher LC III, Adkins J: Acute osteomyelitis from *Serratia marcescens. Amer J Orthop* **8**:96-98, 1966.
13. Atlas E, Belding ME: *Serratia marcescens* arthritis requiring amputation. *JAMA* **204**:167-169, 1968.
14. Fields BN, Uwaydah MM, Kunz LJ, et al: The so-called "paracolon" bacteria: A bacteriologic and clinical reappraisal. *Amer J Med* **42**:89-106, 1967.
15. Dodson WH: *Serratia marcescens* septicemia. *Arch Intern Med* **121**:145-150, 1968.
16. Wilfert JN, Barrett FF, Kass EH: Bacteremia due to *Serratia marcescens. New Eng J Med* **279**:286-289, 1968.
17. Altemeier WA, Culbertson WR, Fullen WD, et al: *Serratia marcescens* septicemia: A new threat in surgery. *Arch Surg* **99**:232-238, 1969.
18. Wheat RP, Zuckerman A, Rantz LA: Infection due to chromobacteria: Report of 11 cases. *Arch Intern Med* **88**:461-466, 1951.
19. Howe AJ, Hughes MH: Bacterial endocarditis due to *Chromobacterium prodigiosum. Brit Med J* **1**:968-970, 1954.
20. Reissell P, Jansson E: *Serratia marcescens* septicemia: A case report. *Acta Med Scand* **176**:253-256, 1964.
21. Denny JD, Kaye D, Hagstrom JWC: Endocarditis due to *Serratia marcescens. New Eng J Med* **276**:1362, 1967.
22. Amoury RA, Bowman FO Jr, Malm JR: Endocarditis associated with intracardiac prostheses: Diagnosis, management, and prophylaxis. *J Thorac Cardiovasc Surg* **51**:36-48, 1966.
23. Alexander RH, Reichenbach DD, Merendino KA: *Serratia marcescens* endocarditis. *Arch Surg* **98**:287-291, 1969.
24. Quintiliani R, Gifford RH: Endocarditis from *Serratia marcescens. JAMA* **208**:2055-2059, 1969.
25. Alexander R, Holloway GA Jr, Honsinger RW Jr: Surgical debridement for resistant bacterial endocarditis. *JAMA* **210**:1757-1759, 1969.
26. Cabrera HA: An outbreak of *Serratia marcescens*, and its control. *Arch Intern Med* **123**:650-655, 1969.
27. Edwards PR, Ewing WH: *Identification of Enterobacteriaceae*, ed 2. Minneapolis, Burgess Publishing Co, 1962, chap 11.
28. Rinker G, White A: Quantitative studies of antibodies against Jensen's antigen A in human sera, in Hobby GL (ed): *Antimicrobial Agents and Chemotherapy 1964*. Bethesda, Md, American Society for Microbiology, 1965, pp 672-676.
29. Petersdorf RG, Sherris JC: Methods and significance of in vitro testing of bacterial sensitivity to drugs. *Amer J Med* **39**:766-779, 1965.
30. McCabe WR, Jackson GG: Gram-negative bacteremia: II. Clinical, laboratory, and therapeutic observations. *Arch Intern Med* **110**:856-864, 1962.
31. DuPont HL, Spink WW: Infections due to gram-negative organisms: An analysis of 860 patients with bacteremia at the University of Minnesota Medical Center, 1958-1966. *Medicine* **48**:307-332, 1969.
32. Smits H, Freedman LR: Prolonged venous catheterization as a cause of sepsis. *New Eng J Med* **276**:1229-1233, 1967.
33. Bentley DW, Lepper MH: Septicemia related to indwelling venous catheter. *JAMA* **206**:1749-1757, 1968.
34. Paine TF: Illness in man following inhalation of *Serratia marcescens. J Infect Dis* **79**:226-232, 1946.
35. Daugharty H, Martin RR, White A: Antibodies against staphylococcal teichoic acids and type-specific antigens in man. *J Immun* **98**:1123-1129, 1967.
36. Daugharty HD, Martin RR, White A: Reactions of sera and nasal secretions with staphylococcal antigens. *J Lab Clin Med* **73**:1011-1018, 1969.
37. Crowder JG, White A: A serologic response in human *Pseudomonas* infection. *J Lab Clin Med* **75**:128-136, 1970.
38. Edmondson EB, Sanford JP: The *Klebsiella-Enterobacter (Aerobacter) Serratia* group: A clinical and bacteriological evaluation. *Medicine* **46**:323-340, 1967.
39. Thornton GF, Andriole VT: Antibiotic sensitivities of nonpigmented *Serratia marcescens* to gentamicin and carbenicillin. *J Infect Dis* **119**:393-394, 1969.
40. Ronald AR, Turck M, Petersdorf RG: A critical evaluation of nalidixic acid in urinary-tract infections. *New Eng J Med* **275**:1081-1089, 1966.

Prolonged *Salmonella* Bacteremia in Patients With *Schistosoma mansoni* Infection

Heonir Rocha, MD, Salvador, Brazil, and John W. Kirk and Charles D. Hearey, Jr., MPH, New York

Eleven cases of prolonged *Salmonella* bacteremia (2 to 12 months) occurred in patients with Manson's schistosomiasis. Blood cultures were found to be a very reliable diagnostic method if at least three blood samples from each patient were inoculated into both bile broth and trypticase soy broth and observed for 15 days. Bile broth was found superior to trypticase soy broth in isolating *Salmonella* organisms from the blood. Stool, urine, and bile cultures, and Widal agglutination tests were poor indicators. Patients responded equally well to parenterally administered ampicillin sodium and orally administered chloramphenicol. No relapses were noted. The pathogenesis of prolonged *Salmonella* bacteremia is discussed, especially in regard to the controversial role played by the underlying *Schistosoma mansoni* infection in producing an altered state of human resistance.

Since 1959, Brazilian and Chinese investigators have been describing a new clinical picture of *Salmonella* infection characterized by prolonged (1 to 24 months) intermittent fever and bacteremia in patients with intercurrent *Schistosoma mansoni* or *Sch japonicum* infections.[1-5] Although initially designated "prolonged typhoid fever"[2] at least 12 *Salmonella* species have now been implicated as causative agents[4] in this entity, the clinical picture of which is quite distinct from classic enteric fever. The present report relates our experience with 11 cases of prolonged *Salmonella* bacteremia, describing the clinical manifestations, some important bacteriologic findings, and the response to parenterally administered ampicillin sodium. Additional comments regarding pathogenesis are made especially with reference to the controversial role played by the underlying *Sch mansoni* infection.

Materials and Methods

Patients included in this report were studied on the medical service of the Hospital Prof Edgard Santos of the Federal University of Bahia, Salvador, Brazil, between 1965 and 1969. Inclusion in the study depended on a history of prolonged fever, isolation of a *Salmonella* species from the blood, and the presence of an active infection with *Sch mansoni* as revealed by viable eggs in the stool. In addition to routine clinical workup, including basic laboratory procedures, multiple blood cultures were drawn in all cases and patients were further studied with cultures of stool (eight cases), urine (two cases), and bile (two cases) and with Widal agglutination tests. All temperatures were taken by the axillary method.

Blood samples were inoculated into both bile broth (BB) and trypticase soy broth (TSB) and observed with frequent subcultures for 15 days. Urine was cultured by standard quantitative method in blood agar base, and 1 ml was inoculated in trypticase soy and bile broth media. Stool samples were plated initially on *Shigella* and *Salmonella,* eosin-methylene-

Received for publication May 27, 1970; accepted July 28.

From the Department of Medicine, Faculty of Medicine of the University of Bahia, Salvador, Brazil (Dr. Rocha) and Cornell University Medical College, New York (Mr. Kirk and Mr. Hearey).

Reprint requests to Hospital Prof Edgard Santos, Salvador, Bahia, Brazil (Dr. Rocha).

Table 1.—Clinical Data in Patients With *Sch mansoni* Infection and Prolonged *Salmonella* Bacteremia

Case No.	Duration of Fever (mo)	Age, Sex	Abdominal Pain	Diarrhea	Epistaxis	Cough	Pulse Rate (Beats/min)	Edema	Petechiae	Adenopathy	Ascites	Hepatomegaly	Splenomegaly
1	8	19, M	+	+	+	+	112	+	+	+	0	+	+
2	2	12, M	+	+	+	0	80	+	+	+	0	+	+
3	2	5, M	+	+	+	+	140	0	0	+	+	+	+
4	7	17, M	+	+	0	+	88	+	0	+	+	+	+
5	3	12, F	0	0	+	0	100	0	0	0	0	+	+
6	12	15, M	+	+	0	0	110	0	0	0	0	+	+
7	4	7, F	+	+	+	+	148	0	0	+	0	+	+
8	6	17, F	+	+	0	0	90	0	+	0	0	+	+
9	8	10, M	+	+	+	0	88	0	0	+	0	+	(0) Splenectomy
10	9	21, F	+	+	0	0	110	0	0	+	0	+	0
11	3	10, M	+	0	+	0	112	0	0	+	0	+	+

* + signifies positive; 0, negative.

blue, and Selenite media. Identification of bacteria was done according to standard technique.

Results

The most important clinical findings of the 11 cases studied are found in Tables 1 and 2.

Only two *Salmonella* species were isolated in this series, *Sal typhi* (four cases) and *Sal choleraesuis* (seven cases).

A total of 26 blood cultures were performed diagnostically in the 11 patients, with 23 positive and only 3 negative results. Out of the 23 positive blood samples, bile broth was positive in 22 of them, trypticase soy broth in only 14. In eight instances then, BB was positive while TSB was negative, while the reverse was true only once (Table 3). Further comparison of the two media revealed that BB usually turned positive before TSB, but even in BB, five out of 22 cultures turned positive later than 7 days after inoculation, one of these after 14 days (Table 4). This underscores the need of observing all cultures for at least 15 days to prevent false-negative results.

Stool, urine, and bile cultures on the other hand, and even Widal agglutination tests, were found to be poor indicators of this type of *Salmonella* infection. Only three of eight patients studied with stool cultures had stools positive for *Salmonella*, and of the two urine cultures and two bile cultures, none was positive. Widal agglutination tests were done in nine cases, being negative in six and showing titers of only 1/160 to 1/200 against H or O antigen in the other three cases.

Comment

The most constant and striking clinical feature of this form of salmonellosis is the prolonged fever, from 2 to 12 months in this series, and up to 24 months in other series.[4] The fever pattern was irregular in most cases, but assumed a quotidian regularity in others, and was frequently accompanied by chills. It is notable that the patients tolerated the long intervals of infection remarkably well during most of the course.

Among the other features of the disease, significant hepatosplenomegaly was particularly prominent and almost universal, while abdominal pain, diarrhea, epistaxis, generalized lymphadenopathy, anemia, eosinophilia, and elevated serum globulin levels were present in the great majority of cases (Tables 1 and 2). Although the importance of the *Salmonella* infection in producing each aspect of this clinical picture is hard to define in the presence of intercurrent schistosomiasis and varying degrees of other parasitic infections and nutritional deficiency, treatment solely of the salmonellosis has repeatedly been observed to result in significant regression of hepatosplenomegaly, reduction of serum globulin levels, and improvement of anemia along with general clinical improvement.[3]

Although some previous reports have indicated that blood cultures are not reliable in isolating the organism in prolonged salmonellosis[1] our present experience has shown that with the proper bacteriologic techniques blood cultures are an extremely reliable diagnostic tool. Bile broth was by far a superior medium to TSB for the isolation of *Salmo-*

Table 2.—Laboratory Data and Therapeutic Regimen in Patients With *Sch mansoni* Infection and Prolonged *Salmonella* Bacteremia

Case No.	*Sch mansoni* Eggs in Feces	Hgb/gm/100 ml	WBC/cu mm × 10^3	Eosinophils (%)	Bilirubin (mg/100 ml)	Albumin: Globulin	Widal (H or O Antigen)	Stool Culture	Urine Culture	*Salmonella* Isolated From Blood	Antibiotic Therapy
1	+	4.4	4.8	7	1.2	1.4:4.8	0	0	. . .	C_1	Ampicillin
2	+	7.4	8.8	9	0.9	3.0:4.0	0	0	. . .	*Sal typhi*	Ampicillin
3	+	. . .	8.4	9	. . .	4.0:4.1	0	0	0	C_1	Chloramphenicol
4	+	6.6	5.4	1	4.3	2.2:1.6	0	0	0	C_1	Ampicillin
5	+	10.0	. . .	. . .	. . .	3.3:4.8	0	+	0	C_1	Ampicillin
6	+	10.8	9.0	20	0.8	2.8:4.5	1/200	0	. . .	C_1	Ampicillin
7	+	11.5	8.2	25	. . .	3.3:5.1	. . .	. . .	0	C_1	Chloramphenicol
8	+	8.3	14.2	15	0.8	2.1:7.0	1/200	+	. . .	*Sal typhi*	Ampicillin
9	+	12.0	16.6	13	0.5	2.4:7.0	1/160	. . .	. . .	*Sal typhi*	Ampicillin
10	+	10.0	9.0	9	9.2	3.2:3.1	. . .	. . .	0	*Sal typhi*	Chloramphenicol
11	+	10.0	8.2	14	0.4	4.2:4.1	0	+	0	C_1	Ampicillin

* + signifies positive; 0, negative.

nella species from blood, as previously reported.[6] Another important conclusion from this series rests on the observation that although one blood sample inoculated into both BB and TSB made the diagnosis in 81.8% of our cases (nine of 11), and two samples effectively diagnosed 90.9% (ten cases), three blood samples were required to produce 100% diagnosis.

It is of interest that even though other reports have shown somewhat better correlation between Widal titers and the presence of *Salmonella* infection, the diagnostic reliability of Widal testing in this type of salmonellosis had been generally poor.[1-4] Modified host response and late reduction of agglutination titers in prolonged infection have been offered as hypothesis[1] but there is no definitive data available to explain this finding.

Patients in this series received 14-day courses of either intramuscularly administered ampicillin (seven cases) or orally administered chloramphenicol (four cases). Patients on both regimens showed prompt afebrile responses, generally by the second day of therapy. In spite of remission of

Table 3.—Results of 23 Positive Pretreatment Blood Cultures in 11 Cases of Prolonged *Salmonella* Bacteremia*

Culture	No.
Total positive blood cultures	23
Positive in BB	22
Positive in TSB	14
Positive simultaneously in TSB and BB	13
Positive in BB and negative in TSB	9
Positive in TSB and negative in BB	1

* BB signifies bile broth; TSB, trypticase soy broth.

fever, however, two patients receiving ampicillin (cases 4 and 11) had positive blood cultures after initiation of therapy and one patient receiving chloramphenicol (case 8) had a positive stool culture during therapy. Still, there were no treatment failures and no relapses reported in periods of follow-up, supporting other reports of the effectiveness of parenterally administered ampicillin as compared to chloramphenicol in the treatment of *Salmonella* infections.[7]

The pathogenesis of this prolonged

Table 4.—Time Required for Growth in Positive Blood Cultures in BB and TSB*

Time Interval (Days)	No. of Positive Cultures	
	BB	TSB
1	8	1
2	3	0
3	1	1
4	2	2
5		2
6	3	2
7		1
8	1	
9	1	1
10		
11	2	2
12		1
13		
14	1	1
Total	22	14

* BB signifies bile broth; TSB, trypticase soy broth.

course of *Salmonella* infection remains unexplained, but there is no doubt that the relationship between the infecting organisms and the human host is altered from that seen in other kinds of *Salmonella* infection. The long duration of the bacteremia and the surprising tolerance of the patient to it suggest either an altered pathogenicity of the *Salmonella* or an altered state of human reactivity, or both, resulting in an unusual balance between patient and infecting organism. Further suggestion of the altered relationship can be seen in the failure of even *Sal choleraesuis*, usually an extremely invasive species, to localize in the course of this prolonged bacteremia.

We have no evidence that the biliary tract was the site of *Salmonella* multiplication and seeding of the bloodstream. Most of the patients in our series had no signs or symptoms of biliary disease, the great majority of stool cultures were negative, both bile cultures performed were negative, and all the patients showed rapid clinical and bacteriological response to antibiotics. Even the two patients in this series with jaundice (case 10 with choledocholithiasis and cholelithiasis; case 4 with an apparently normal biliary tract) had negative stool cultures and showed satisfactory response to antibiotics.

Whatever the nature of the altered *Salmonella* host relationship, the most controversial problem remains the role of the underlying *Sch mansoni* infection. It has been shown that white mice infected with *Sch mansoni* had significantly decreased resistance to subsequent inoculation with *Sal typhimurium* relative to a control group. This decreased resistance was manifested by increased mortality, increased multiplication of organisms in liver and spleen, and greater bacteremia.[8] These data suggested that the reticuloendothelial cells initially trapping the *Salmonella* were unable to kill the bacteria, and even allowed the *Salmonella* to multiply within them, resulting in blood stream invasion.

In human studies it has been shown that the serum of patients with hepatosplenic schistosomiasis has reduced anti-*Salmonella* activity compared to a control group,[9] and that there is a delayed and inhibited leukocytic migration, as demonstrated by the skin window technique, in patients with hepatosplenic schistosomiasis.[10] Each of these studies suggests a different mechanism for the altered resistance to *Salmonella* infection in patients with schistosomiasis and none yet provides a definitive explanation for the apparently very specific susceptibility to, and yet remarkable tolerance for, the protracted *Salmonella* bacteremia. It seems extremely likely, however, that the schistosomes will eventually be implicated quite directly in the pathogenesis of this type of salmonellosis.

Recently it has been observed that when various gram-negative organisms are injected into animals parasitized by schistosomes, the bacteria can penetrate the schistosomes, multiply within their ceca, and kill them.[11] Although this discovery was initially of interest because it suggested a new approach to the biological control of schistosomiasis, it also suggests that the site of *Salmonella* multiplication and seeding of the bloodstream in prolonged salmonellosis could be the schistosomes themselves.[12] This conjecture could explain an earlier report of the cure of ten cases of prolonged salmonellosis with therapy only for the intercurrent *Sch mansoni* infection.[13] In our attempts to elucidate the pathogenesis of prolonged *Salmonella* bacteremia in patients with *Sch mansoni* infection this possibility merits further investigation.

Nonproprietary and Trade Names of Drug

Ampicillin sodium—*Amcill-S, Alpen-N, Omnipen-N, Penbritin-S for injection, Polycillin N for injection, Principen/N, Totacillin-N.*

References

1. Teixeira R: Typhoid fever of protracted course. *Rev Inst Med Trop S Paulo* **2**:56-70, 1960.

2. Teixeria R: Estudo clínico de casos de febre tifoide prolongada, thesis. Salvador, Brazil, 1959.

3. Tai TY, Hsu CY, Chang HC, et al: Typhoid and paratyphoid fevers occurring in cases of schistosomiasis. *Chin Med J* **76**:426-435, 1958.

4. Neves J, Martins NRLL: Long duration of septicemic salmonellosis: 35 cases with 12 implicated species of *Salmonella*. *Trans Royal Soc Trop Med Hyg* **61**:541-552, 1967.

5. Neves J: Salmonelose septicemica prolongada. *J Bras Med* **15**:247-259, 1968.

6. Kaye D, Palmieri M, Rocha H: Effect of bile on the action of blood against *Salmonella*. *J Bact* **91**:945-952, 1966.

7. Kaye D, Rocha H, Eyckmans L, et al: Comparison of parenteral ampicillin and parenteral chloramphenicol in the treatment of typhoid fever. *Ann NY Acad Sci* **145**:423-428, 1967.

8. Rocha H, Castilho EA, Barreto AC, et al: Características da infecção por *S. typhimurium* em camundongos infectados com *S. mansoni*. *Gaz Med Bahia* **68**:6-18, 1968.

9. Rocha H, Magnavita M, Teles ES, et al: Atividade antibacteriana do sôro de pacientes com forma hepatosplênica da esquistossomose mansônica. *Rev Inst Med Trop S Paulo* **10**:364-369, 1968.

10. Fernandes DJ, Rocha H: Características da reação inflamatória em pacientes com forma hepatosplênica da esquistossomose mansônica e calazar. *Rev Inst Med Trop S Paulo* **9**:129-133, 1967.

11. Ottens H, Dickerson G: Bacterial invasion of schistosomes. *Nature* **223**:506-507, 1969.

12. Biological control of schistosomiasis, editorial. *Lancet* **2**:477-478, 1969.

13. Neves J, Marinho RP, Martins NRLL, et al: Prolonged septicemic salmonellosis: Treatment of intercurrent schistosomiasis with Niridazole. *Trans Royal Soc Trop Med Hyg* **63**:79-84, 1969.

Ascending Aorta Synchronized Pulsation

A New Form of Circulatory Assist for Treatment of Cardiogenic Shock

Tzu-Wang Lang, MD; Eliot Corday, MD; Samuel Meerbaum, MS; Jose R. Lozano, MD; Hugo Carrasco, MD; and Herbert Gold, MD, Los Angeles

Ascending aorta synchronized pulsation (AASP) was found to be simple and effective method of counterpulsation directed at the root of the aorta. It provided excellent mechanical assistance for the treatment of severe cardiogenic shock following coronary artery ligation. Because the proximal site of counterpulsation requires low stroke pump volumes, only minimal hemolysis resulted. The AASP counterpulsation was performed for periods up to 90 minutes in ten dogs. After two minutes a significant increase in coronary flow and reduction in systolic pressures were observed, and after 90 minutes of continued AASP counterpulsation, pressures and flows increased from shock levels toward normotensive control levels and hemodynamic indices improved. These improvements persisted after AASP pumping was stopped in nine dogs, which proved AASP reversed the cardiogenic shock state.

Localized myocardial ischemia resulting from occlusion of a coronary artery may induce cardiogenic shock and precipitate remote hemodynamic metabolic disturbances which, in turn, generate vicious feedback mechanisms. These tend to aggravate and perpetuate the shock state. Feedback mechanisms, which include hypotension, hypoxemia, and lactic acidemia, retard metabolism and contractility of the remaining viable myocardium and result in further failure of the heart as a pump.

If the nutrition of the viable, noninfarcted myocardium can be improved while at the same time the workload of the heart is reduced the myocardial metabolism and contractility will be restored and the shock state reversed. No pharmacologic agents have yet been able to provide such combined benefits. Therefore, we have looked for temporary circulatory assist systems, relatively simple to apply, which would not cause gross destruction of the formed elements of the blood or other tissues of the body. Our biological engineers have now developed assist devices which might satisfy

Received for publication Oct 12, 1970; accepted March 3, 1971.

From Cedars-Sinai Medical Center and the Department of Medicine, University of California at Los Angeles School of Medicine, Los Angeles.

Read before the Section on Diseases of the Chest at the 119th annual convention of the American Medical Association, Chicago, June 24, 1970.

Reprint requests to 4751 Fountain Ave, Los Angeles 90029 (Dr. Corday).

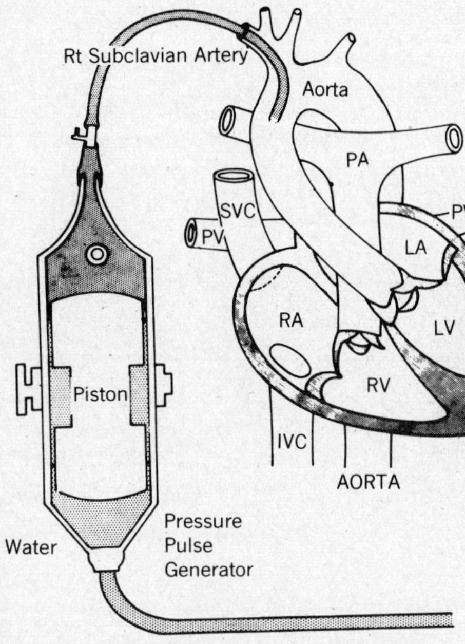

Fig 1.—Schematic diagram of AASP with catheter inserted into the ascending aorta and connected to the pressure pulse generator for synchronized counterpulsation. Blood is withdrawn from the root of the aorta to reduce systolic pressure and pumped back during diastole.

Fig 2.—Simultaneous recording of ECG, LAD coronary flow, and central aortic and left ventricular pressures during cardiogenic shock after 15 and 90 minutes of AASP and 10 minutes after counterpulsation stopped. Aortic pressure increased coronary flow, reduced myocardial afterload effectively, and reversed the shock state. Both S-T segment elevation and heart rate diminished.

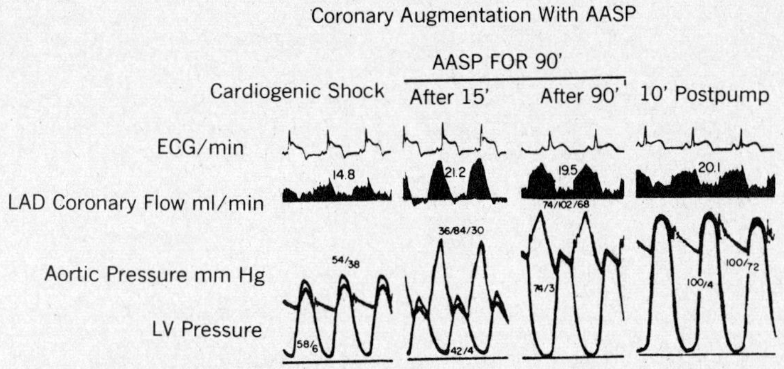

the two most important basic physiologic requirements[1]: (1) reduction of myocardial energy expenditure in systole, and (2) provision of supplementary energy through an augmented aortic pressure wave which would propel blood into the myocardium during diastole to supply necessary nutrients and remove metabolites of the heart.

Many bypass circulatory assist techniques have been developed, but they usually required pumping of large stroke volumes, and this necessitated blood priming. When an oxygenator had to be used in conjunction, as is the case in veno-arterial bypass, it often caused excessive destruction of formed blood elements. Most circulatory assistance techniques are so complicated that they require insertion of many large cannulae and the services of a large team of experts.

Previous experience with arterial-arterial counterpulsation revealed that rapid displacement of a volume of blood from the femoral arteries all the way up to the ascending aorta was accompanied by considerable energy dissipation before reaching the coronary ostia and therefore required a large pumped volume displacement.[2,3] Therefore, we postulated that fluid counterpulsation, directly into the root of the aorta and in the vicinity of the coronary ostia, could provide blood perfusion energy at the most meaningful location with a minimum pump displacement and little energy dissipation.[4]

In a search for a simple technique, we adapted the arterial-arterial counterpulsation system to provide "augmentation" of pressure in diastole and "sink" in systolic pressure directed at the root of the aorta.

Method

Ten morphine (2 mg/kg intramuscularly) and pentobarbital (Nembutal) (12 mg/kg intravenously) anesthetized mongrel dogs weighing 25 to 30 kg (56 to 66 lb) were used in the experiments. Respiration was controlled via tracheal intubation and respiration pump. The chest was opened through an incision in the fourth intercostal region and a short midline abdominal incision for installation of instruments to measure flow and pressure. Pulsed field electromagnetic flow probes were positioned on the ascending aorta, left anterior descending (LAD) coronary artery, and carotid and renal arteries. Left ventricular pressure and its rate of rise (dp/dt) was measured by transapical catheter connected to a transducer (Statham P-23 Gb) and special differentiator for dp/dt, ascending aortic pressure with a catheter introduced via the right brachial artery and connected to a transducer (Statham P-23 Db). Central venous pressure was measured in the right atrium with the use of a transducer (P-23 BB). An electrocardiogram was obtained by applying a standard lead II. Hematocrit, hemoglobin, and plasma microhemoglobin values were measured every 30 minutes.

A semirigid, thin-wall, wire-reinforced F 16 catheter of 3.5 mm internal diameter, with three large side openings at its tip, was introduced through the left subclavian artery and advanced into the ascending aorta (Fig 1). This catheter was connected to the pulse pressure generator (PPG) of a hydraulic unit. The PPG was triggered from the R wave of the ECG.

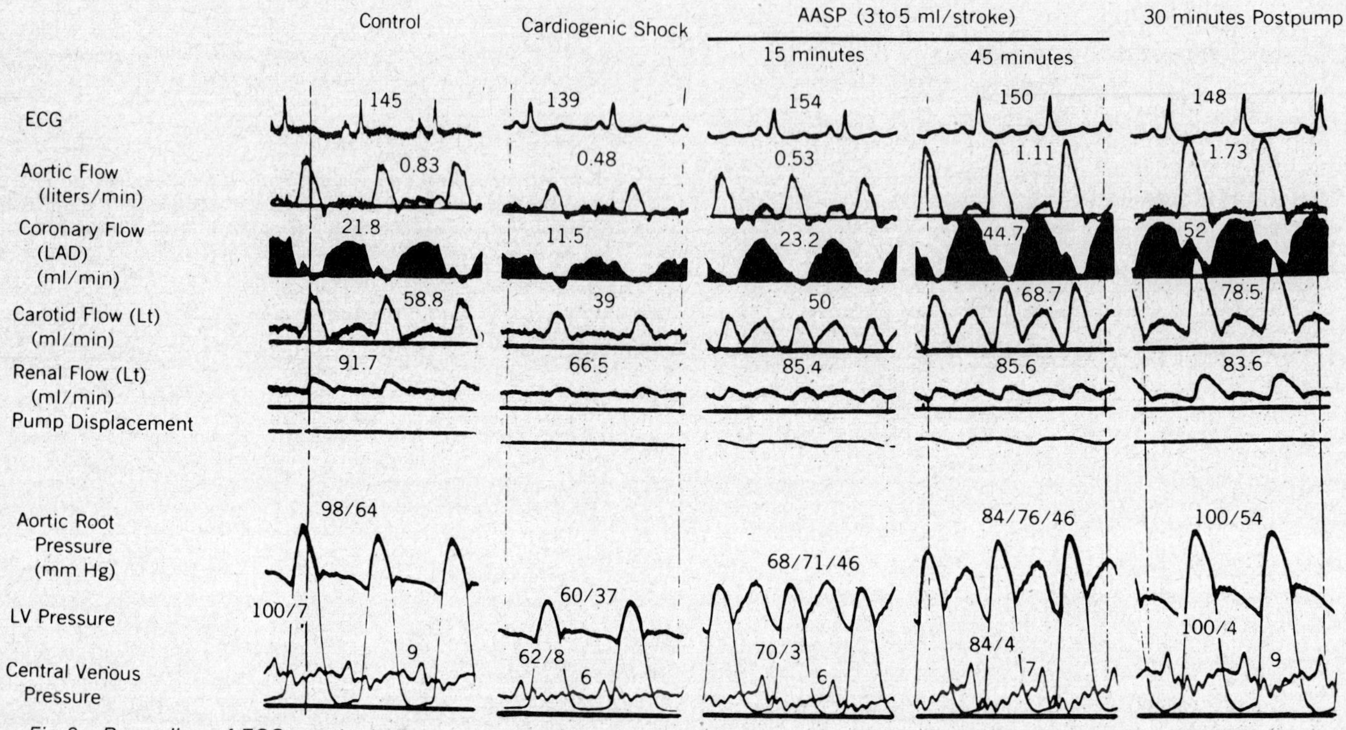

Fig 3.—Recording of ECG, aortic, LAD coronary, carotid, and renal flows, pump displacement, aortic root pressure, left ventricular, pressure and central venous pressure during control period, cardiogenic shock, and AASP pumping, 15 minutes and 45 minutes, respectively, and 30 minutes after AASP.

Specific pump volumetric displacement and rates of counterpulsation suction and injection could be preset in the electric programmer (SIMAS).

Following attachment of all instruments, two measurements were recorded within a 15-minute interval to act as the postsurgical control. These included flows from the ascending aorta, LAD coronary, and carotid and renal arteries; pressures from the right atrium, ascending aorta, and left ventricle (with rate rise [dp/dt] computation), pump displacement, and magnified left ventricular end-diastolic pressure (LVEDP).

Cardiogenic shock was induced by progressive ligation of branches of the left circumflex coronary artery until the blood pressure fell and remained below a level of 80 mm Hg systolic for a period of 30 minutes. Recordings were made every ten minutes during the shock control period. Counterpulsation through the catheter, whose distal tip rested in the ascending aorta, was then instituted, displacing 3 to 10 ml per stroke for a 60- to 90-minute period. Hemodynamic measurements were recorded before, 2 minutes after initiation of counterpulsation, then every 15 minutes during pumping, immediately after pumping was stopped, and then 10 to 30 minutes later (Fig 2 and 3). Toward the end of the counterpulsation the total pump displacement was gradually reduced by either pumping alternate beats or reducing the pulse pressure generator stroke volume.

Blood pH, P_{CO_2}, and P_{O_2} were constantly monitored during control, shock, pumping, and postpump periods. All dogs were killed at the end of the experiment.

Results

Averages of hemodynamic measurements which are summarized in Table 1 and the percentage changes plotted in Fig 4 include heart rate, aortic flow, cardiac stroke volume, LAD coronary artery flow, left carotid artery flow, left renal artery flow, LVEDP, peak aortic systolic pressure, maximum left ventricular isometric contraction ($[dp/dt]_{max}$) and tension-time index per minute (TTI). The aortic flow does not represent complete cardiac output because it does not include the coronary flow. Similarly, the term stroke output computed from measured aortic flow and heart rate is slightly less than the actual stroke.

Hemodynamic Measurements in the Shock State.—In the ten animals used, the shock state was characterized by a reduction in aortic flow to 60% of control. Average shock values compared to control levels were as follows: systolic pressure, 110 vs 73 mm Hg ($P<0.001$); aortic flow, 1.03 vs 0.6 liters/min ($P<0.01$); LAD coronory flow, 22 vs 14.2 ml/min ($P<0.02$); left carotid flow, 36 vs 28 ml/min; and left renal flow, 103 vs 79 ml/min. Left ventricular diastolic pressure increased from 5.7 to 7.4 mm Hg.

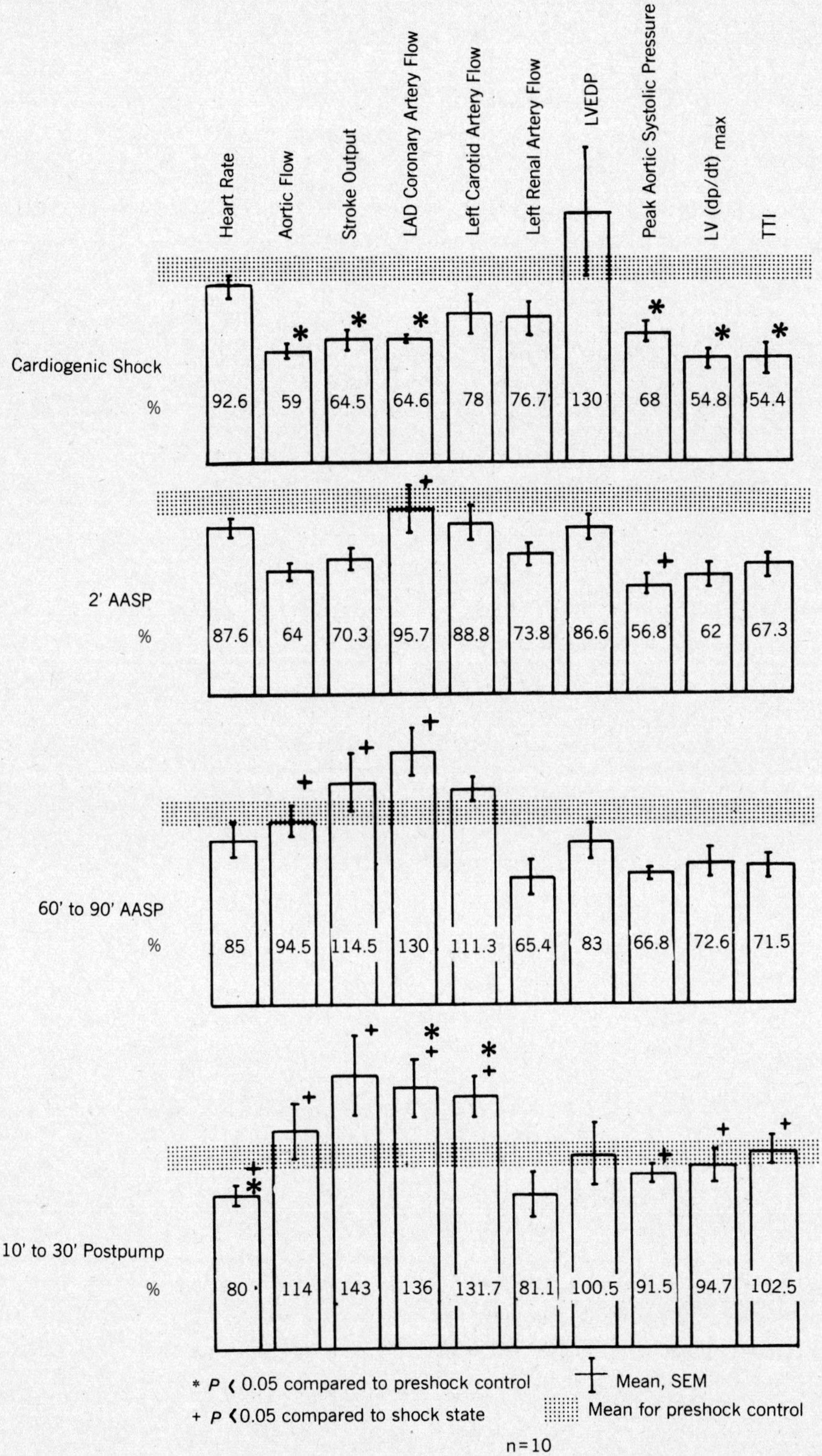

Fig 4.—Bar graph of average measurements of heart rate, aortic flow, stroke output, LAD coronary artery flow, left carotid artery flow, left renal artery flow, LVEDP, peak aortic systolic pressure, left ventricular $(dp/dt)_{max}$, and TTI during cardiogenic shock: 2 and 60 to 90 minutes of AASP; and 10 to 30 minutes after counterpulsation stopped. Gray line represents control levels.

There was no significant alteration in central venous pressure.

Effect of AASP on Pressure and Regional Flow.—*After two Minutes of AASP.*—During the initial two minutes of counterpulsation, the sink in aortic pressures lowered the peak aortic systolic pressure by 16% from shock levels of 73 mm Hg to 61 mm Hg ($P < 0.01$). At the same time diastolic augmentation increased the peak diastolic aortic root pressure by 79%, from 48 to 70 mm Hg. Other alterations included reduction of LVEDP from 7.4 to 4.9 mm Hg; slightly increased mean aortic flow, from 0.6 to 0.66 liters/min; a 50% increase in LAD coronary flow, from 14 to 21 ml/min ($P<0.05$); and an 8% rise in carotid flow, from 28 to 32 ml/min. Mean renal flow remained essentially constant. All *P* values used analyzing AASP data related to the shock state.

After 90 Minutes of AASP.—The mean of the central aortic peak systolic pressure increased slightly to 72 mm Hg, while diastolic pressure was augmented to 76 mm Hg. Aortic flow was resorted almost to its control value of 0.97 liters/min ($P<0.005$). The LAD coronary flow increased 104% to 28.6 ml/min ($P<0.001$) and carotid flow, 43% to 40 ml/min ($P<0.02$). Renal flow decreased slightly to 67.4 ml/min. Stroke volume increased above normal preshock control to 8.6 ml ($P<0.01$).

After Discontinuance of AASP.—All hemodynamic measurements improved or returned to preshock control values after AASP, which indicated reversal of the shock state by counterpulsation. Systolic pressure was restored to 99 mm Hg compared to 108 mm Hg in the preshock control state. Aortic flow increased to 1.17 liters/min, compared with 1.03

Effects of AASP on Regional Hemodynamics in Cardiogenic Shock

		Shock State		Two Minutes After Initiation of AASP		60-90 Minutes After AASP		15-30 Minutes After Pumping		
	Control	Values	P to Control	Values	P to Shock	Values	P to Shock	Values	P to Control	P to Shock
Heart Rate (beats per minute)	148 ± 6.5	137 ± 7.8		130 ± 4.5		126 ± 7.5		119 ± 8.4	<0.02	<0.02
Aortic Flow (liters/min)	1.03 ± 0.13	0.6 ± 0.04	<0.01	0.66 ± 0.07		0.97 ± 0.12	<0.005	1.17 ± 0.15		<0.005
Stroke Volume (ml/beat)	7.5 ± 0.9	4.8 ± 0.3	<0.01	5.3 ± 0.4		8.6 ± 1.3	<0.01	10.7 ± 1.6		<0.001
LV peak systolic pressure (mm Hg)	110 ± 4	74 ± 5	<0.001	65 ± 5	<0.02	73 ± 4		99.3 ± 3		<0.005
LV diastolic pressure	5.7 ± 1.6	7.4 ± 1.9		4.9 ± 0.4		4.7 ± 0.5		5.9 ± 1.0		
Aortic systolic pressure	108 ± 4	73 ± 6	<0.001	61 ± 5	<0.01	72 ± 3		99 ± 4		<0.005
Aortic end-diastolic pressure	79 ± 5	48 ± 5		45 ± 5		49 ± 3		64 ± 3		
Peak aortic diastolic pressure (augmentation)				70 ± 4		76 ± 4				
Mean CVP	9.8 ± 1.4	10.3 ± 1.1		8.8 ± 0.8		9.7 ± 1.1		11.8 ± 1.0		
LAD coronary artery flow (ml/min)	22 ± 2.8	14.2 ± 0.3	<0.02	21 ± 2.9	<0.05	28.6 ± 3.2	<0.001	30 ± 3.5	<0.001	<0.001
Left carotid artery flow (ml/min)	36 ± 5.4	28 ± 3.3		32 ± 5.5		40 ± 3.6		47.8 ± 4.1	<0.05	<0.005
Left renal artery flow (ml/min)	103 ± 11	79 ± 9.2		76 ± 6.5		67.4 ± 9.8		84 ± 14		
LV (dp/dt) max (mm Hg/sec)	1,669 ± 481.6	915 ± 124.1	<0.02	1,034 ± 124.4		1,212 ± 141		1,580 ± 161.4		<0.01
Tension time per minute (mm Hg/sec)	1,848 ± 704	997 ± 142	<0.02	1,215 ± 441		1,316 ± 480		1,810 ± 665		<0.01

liters/min; LAD coronary flow to 30 ml/min, compared with 22 ml/min; and carotid flow to 47.8 ml/min, as compared with 36 ml/min in the control period. Renal flow was partially restored to 83.6 ml/min, compared with 103 ml/min. Cardiac stroke volume increased to 10.7 ml which was markedly higher than the control value of 7.5 ml/stroke. The heart rate was slowed to a mean of 119 beats per minute as compared with 148 beats per minute in the control period.

Effects of AASP on Myocardial Contractility.—Indices of myocardial contractility are derived by computing dp/dt and the tension-time integral of aortic pressure per minute. During the shock state $(dp/dt)_{max}$ had dropped from a control value of 1,669 mm Hg/sec to 915 mm Hg/sec ($P<0.02$). At the initiation of AASP, $(dp/dt)_{max}$ increased to 1,035 mm Hg/sec and improved gradually during counterpulsation to 1,212 mm Hg/sec at the time of termination of AASP. Ten to 30 minutes after discontinuation of AASP, $(dp/dt)_{max}$ had risen to 1,580 mm Hg/sec ($P<0.01$) which was near the preshock level.

Computed TTI was reduced in the shock state from 1,848 mm Hg/sec (control) to 997 mm Hg/sec ($P<0.02$). Two minutes after initiation of AASP, TTI increased to 1,215 mm Hg/sec and then gradually to 1,316 mm Hg/sec at the time of termination of AASP. Ten to thirty minutes after discontinuation of AASP, TTI returned to control levels.

Comment

Clauss et al[5] and Birtwell et al[6] reported that synchronous arterial-arterial counterpulsation should be able to pump a column of blood via the femoral arteries up to the coronary ostia in diastole to nourish the failing myocardium. However, Mulder et al,[7] Hahnloser et al,[8] Goldstein et al,[9] Tanaka et al,[10] Sugg et al,[11,12] and ourselves,[1-3] noted that the arterial-arterial technique was not able to augment the coronary flow appreciably. Because of this, and failure of clinical trials,[11] we searched for other counterpulsation techniques. We adapted the synchronized arterial-arterial counterpulsation system to provide a veno-arterial pulsatile partial bypass (VAPPB). Venous blood was drawn through an oxygenator and with blood priming provided adequate circulatory assist through two femoral cannulae.[2] The increased energy wave could then be forced upwards to the ascending aorta in diastole. We were able to demonstrate excellent augmentation of the coronary circulation with the larger pump displacements of 20 to 30 ml.[2] The VAPPB reversed the shock state in nine out of ten animals and augmented all regional circulations except that of the kidney.[3] In clinical trials, systemic pressure was restored in two patients with severe cardiogenic shock after a period of two to four hours of VAPPB.[1] This period of pumping did not cause a significant destruction of the formed elements of the blood, even though a bubble oxygenator was inserted into the circuit.

Jacobey et al[13] used a pneumatic pump to provide arterial-arterial counterpulsation, via a double-lumen catheter inserted into the ascending aorta through the left subclavian artery, in a series of four patients in cardiogenic shock. He stated results of such pumping were unsatisfactory, and he did not report hemodynamic data. Jacobey also applied this arterial-arterial counterpulsation to patients with chronic coronary artery disease to try to improve the collateral coronary circulation. He experienced some technical complications with this procedure during clinical trials.

The intraaortic balloon counterpulsation first reported by Moulopoulos et al[14] and later popularized by Kantrowitz et al[15,16] has been used with some clinical success. However, reports of experimental studies in the animal reveal great variability in results, mainly due to improper synchronization.[1] The potential benefits of intraaortic balloon counterpulsation as follows are: (1) It tends to propel blood in both cephalad and caudad directions within the aorta during inflation of the balloon in diastole, the principal period of coronary flow in the left ventricle. This should increase coronary perfusion pressure and augment myocardial nutrition. (2) Rapid deflation of the balloon should cause a sink in aortic pressure late in diastole and in systole to reduce the systolic pressure and workload of the heart. However, uniform sink and diastolic augmentation waves which might provide beneficial results cannot be consistently generated with the balloon. Programming must be exquisitely phased to ensure the wave of augmentation does not occur during systole and thus increase cardiac work; and also the sink in presystolic pressure must not occur too soon, because it might reduce the diastolic coronary perfusion period. It is difficult to adjust the augmenting wave characteristics of intraaortic balloon counterpulsation to accommodate changing physiological states. Other drawbacks to this form of counterpulsation include the difficulty of fitting the balloon to the aorta to prevent obstructive phenomena or improper inflation and deflation.

We theorized that we should be able to provide the desired effects of sink and augmentation more effectively by a simple catheter inserted into the ascending aorta through the axillary artery.[1-4] In contrast to other conventional femoral artery counterpulsation techniques, the AASP system does not require displacement of large volumes of blood to achieve effective augmentation and sink characteristics. Thus, both the need for large external energy sources for blood displacement and blood hemolysis are minimized. We were able to achieve all the potential benefits of intraaortic balloon counterpulsation consistently in dogs weighing up to 35 kg using only small blood volume displacements of 3 to 10 ml via a simple single-lumen catheter. We found that such pump displacements through a counterpulsation catheter of 3.5 mm internal diameter caused little blood trauma. This small energy wave was able to improve the nutrition of the ischemic myocardium within a 15-minute period and at the same time reduce the workload of the heart. We anticipate we will require pump displacements of 10 to 20 ml per stroke in treatment of the human with cardiogenic shock.

The AASP corrected the cardiogenic shock state in nine out of ten dogs within 90 minutes (Table and Fig 2, 3, and 4). In contrast, results of another series of five dogs in cardiogenic shock induced by identical procedures of serial ligation of branches of the circumflex coronary artery and no treatment indicate rapid deterioration and no survivals. Four of the five dogs died within 30 to 60 minutes, and one dog died after a period of 100 minutes subsequent to the initiation of hypotensive shock (unpublished data). In another series of nine dogs in similarly induced cardiogenic shock, the only treatment employed over one hour was a 300-ml fluid loading of 5% dextrose in water. No improvement comparable to that found with counterpulsation was observed with preloading treatment.[17]

Our new AASP technique provides an effective aortic pressure sink which starts at the end of diastole and extends into systole. This accomplishes a reduction of cardiac workload and oxygen demands. The counterpulsation significantly augments aortic pressure during diastole when there is least impedance to coronary flow in the left ventricle. This combined approach restores myocardial nutrition as exemplified by improved coronary flow and contractile function demonstrated by dp/dt and tension-time index.

The beneficial physiological effects of 90 minutes of AASP are exhibited as averages in ten dogs with severe cardiogenic shock: (1) The heart rate gradually slowed from 137 to 119 beats per minute while the elevated S-T segment injury current gradually disappeared. (2) Aortic flow increased from 0.6 to 1.17 liters/min. (3) Cardiac stroke volume increased from 4.8 to 10.7 ml/min. (4) Peak left ventricular pressure rose from 74.0 to 99.3 mm Hg. (5) Maximum aortic diastolic pressure was augmented from 48 to 76 mm Hg during AASP. (6) The AASP generated an initial drop of 12 mm Hg in peak systolic pressures. (7) Left anterior descending coronary flow increased from 14.2 to 30 ml/min. (8) Carotid flow increased from 28 to 47.8 ml/min. (9) The $(dp/dt)_{max}$ rose from 915 to 1,580 mm Hg/sec to signify improved contractility. (10) The TTI returned to normal after pumping, while during pumping it increased as cardiac stroke output improved, but remained at 67% to 71% of the preshock control level, which was found nonsignificant relative to the shock state. Tension time index increases significantly after pumping is discontinued (Fig 4). The AASP pumping increases, which may be considered as an index counter-pulsation effectiveness, and indicates an improvement in oxygen supply relative to oxygen demands. Renal flow did not increase during the pumping.

The plasma microhemoglobin levels measured in five dogs during four hours of AASP did not increase appreciably, which indicates that AASP counterpulsation did not injure the red blood cells[18] because it used small pump volume displacements.

The AASP technique is well suited to gradual reduction of the counterpulsation; this avoids secondary rebound phenomena which result from sudden stoppage of counterpulsation.

These encouraging results suggest that AASP is capable of restoring systemic pressures and cardiac output because it improved myocardial contractility. The workload of the heart was reduced during counterpulsation. The benefits persisted into the postpump period.

The AASP technique appears to provide all the potential benefits of aortic balloon pumping more consistently with lower volume displacements. It is more simple to control.

Conclusion

Sixty to ninety minutes of arterial-arterial counterpulsation with a single-lumen catheter in the root of the aorta restored myocardial function and corrected the shock state in nine out of ten dogs in extreme cardiogenic shock. The technique is practical because it can be simply applied and does not cause destruction of the formed blood elements.

This study was supported in part by Public Health Service contract PH 43-68-1333 from the National Heart Institute and by research grants from the John A. Hartford Foundation, Inc., Mrs. Anna Bing Arnold, Mrs. Isabel Kaufman, Mr. Norman Levin, the Abe and Muriel Lipsey Charitable Foundation Fund, and the Jules Stein and Hal Wallis Foundations.

References

1. Corday E, Swan HJC, Lang TW, et al: Physiologic principles in the application of circulatory assist for the failing heart: Intra-aortic balloon circulatory assist and veno-arterial phased partial bypass. *Amer J Cardiol* **26**:595-602, 1970.

2. Goldman A, Boszermenyi E, Utsu F, et al: Veno-arterial pulsatile partial bypass for circulatory assist. *Dis Chest* **50**:633, 1966.

3. Lang TW, Rosselot E, Gold H, et al: Effect of veno-arterial pulsatile partial bypass (VAPPB) on the coronary, renal and mesenteric circulations in cardiogenic shock. *Amer J Cardiol* **27**:41-45, 1971.

4. Lang TW, Meerbaum S, Lozano J, et al: Optimum site for aortic counterpulsation, abstracted. *Circulation* **41-42**(suppl 3):76, 1970.

5. Clauss RH, Birtwell WC, Albertal G, et al: Assisted circulation: The arterial counterpulsator. *J Thorac Cardiov Surg* **41**:447, 1961.

6. Birtwell WC, Soroff HS, Wall M, et al: Assisted circulation: Improved method for counterpulsation. *Trans Amer Soc Artif Intern Organs* **8**:35, 1962.

7. Mulder OG, Frank CG, Nozaki M, et al: Cardiac assist pump: Hemodynamic observations in the experimental animal. *Ann Thorac Surg* **3**:337, 1967.

8. Hahnloser PB, Gallo E, Schenk WG Jr: The hemodynamics of counterpulsation. *J Thorac Cardiov Surg* **51**:366, 1966.

9. Goldstein JD, Dormandy JA, Kirpke DC, et al: Coronary sinus blood flow in counterpulsation. *Surg Forum* **18**:150, 1970.

10. Tanaka S, Rassman W, Lande A, et al: Cardiovascular responses of the failing dog heart to counterpulsation. *J Thorac Cardiov Surg* **58**:112, 1969.

11. Sugg WL, Rea MJ, Webb WR, et al: Cardiac assistance (counterpulsation) in ten patients: Clinical and hemodynamic observations. *Ann Thorac Surg* **9**:1, 1970.

12. Sugg WL, Martin LF, Webb WR, et al: Influence of counterpulsation on aortic, right and left coronary blood flow following ligation of the left circumflex coronary artery. *J Thorac Cardiovasc Surg* **59**:345-351, 1970.

13. Jacobey JA, Craddock LO, Kolf PS, et al: Clinical experience with counterpulsation in coronary artery disease. *J Thorac Surg* **56**:33, 1968.

14. Moulopoulos SD, Topaz S, Kolff WJ: Diastolic balloon pumping (with carbon dioxide) in the aorta: A mechanical assistance to the failing circulation. *Amer Heart J* **63**:669, 1962.

15. Kantrowitz A, Tjonneland S, Freed PS, et al: Initial clinical experience with intra-aortic balloon pumping in cardiogenic shock. *JAMA* **203**:135, 1968.

16. Kantrowitz A, Krakauer JS, Rosenbaum A, et al: Phase-shift balloon pumping in medically refractory cardiogenic shock. *Arch Surg* **99**:739-743, 1969.

17. Lozano JR, Carrasco HA, Lang TW, et al: Pharmacodynamic application of L-Dopa for the treatment of cardiogenic shock. Read before the 20th convention of American College of Cardiology, Washington DC, 1971.

18. Lang TW, Meerbaum S, Lozano JR, et al: New concepts in temporary circulatory assist for treatment of cardiogenic shock. *Geriatrics*, to be published.

Spontaneous Reestablishment of Renal Function After Complete Occlusion of a Renal Artery

Saul J. Dobrzinsky, MD; Erich Voegeli, MD; Harry A. Grant, MD;
Albert R. Christlieb, MD; Herbert L. Abrams, MD; and Roger B. Hickler, MD, Boston

Renal artery stenosis does not necessarily cause hypertension in man.[1,2] Even stenosis of over 50% of the luminal diameter has been found in normotensive patients. On the other hand total renal arterial occlusion is associated with renal ischemia and is considered capable of producing renovascular hypertension. We have recently examined a patient who suddenly became hypertensive in 1966 and in whom a nonfunctioning left kidney was shown by urography. A subsequent arteriogram demonstrated a complete left renal artery occlusion. One and one half years later sufficient collateral circulation had developed to permit good function in the diseased kidney and a normal intravenous pyelogram. The hypertension improved markedly, and renal vein renin activity was normal.

Patient Summary

A 47-year-old black housewife was referred to the Peter Bent Brigham Hospital in 1968 for evaluation of hypertension of 1½ years' duration. She gave a history of recurrent edema of the face, hands, and feet since 1953. In 1963 she had been admitted to another hospital for evaluation of her edema. She was not hypertensive at that time and had no abnormal physical findings other than edema. Findings of routine laboratory examination, including blood urea nitrogen value and intravenous pyelogram, were normal (Fig 1).

In 1967 the patient saw a physician because of malaise and easy fatigability. Her blood pressure was 200/105 mm Hg. No edema was noted. An intravenous pyelogram at that time disclosed a normal right kidney and a nonfunctioning left kidney. On aortography the left renal artery was completely occluded (Fig 2). The patient declined the recommended renal surgery. She was maintained on a regimen of bendroflumethiazide (Benuron), 5 mg twice a day (bid) and hydralazine (Apresoline), 25 mg bid, with four recorded blood pressures over the following nine months which averaged 180/105 mm Hg. During the subsequent eight months her fatigability gradually diminished, her blood pressure decreased to 146/100 (mean of three readings) despite a reduction in antihypertensive medication to hydralazine (10 mg bid), and she had no other complaints.

When she was first seen at the Peter Bent Brigham Hospital in July of 1968, her blood pressure was 130/80 mm Hg while taking hydralazine, 10 mg bid. She was asymptomatic. Physical examination revealed a young-looking woman without any significant physical findings. The blood urea nitrogen value was 22 mg/100 ml, serum creatinine was 1.0 mg/100 ml, and creatinine clearance was 60 ml/min. Other laboratory findings were normal. A rapid-sequence intravenous pyelogram showed a 1.2 cm discrepancy in kidney size (left kidney, 11.5 cm; right kidney, 12.7 cm), but there was no disparity in the nephrogram with the nephrogram seen equally on the one, two, and three minute films. Concentrating ability was equal bilaterally with good concentration of the dye in the calyces and pelves at five minutes (Fig 3). An aortorenal arteriogram confirmed the presence of total occlusion of the left renal artery. No intrarenal arterial branches filled although the nephrogram was of normal density. Some enlarged periureteric and capsular arteries were shown to function as collaterals (Fig 4).

The renal veins were selectively catheterized and renal vein blood samples were drawn for renin activity according to the method of Boucher as modified by Hickler.[3] There was no significant difference in renal vein renin activity, the right being 569 ng/100 ml and the left being 750 ng/100 ml. In this laboratory, a renal vein renin ratio of 2.5 for the involved kidney/uninvolved kidney is considered indicative of a significant renal artery stenosis.[4]

From July 1968 until February 1970, seven recorded blood pressures have averaged 138/88 mm Hg with the patient taking hydralazine, 10 mg bid, and triamterene, 25 mg, plus hydrochlorthiazide, 25 mg (Dyazide), one tablet daily.

Comment

This case reemphasizes the need to evaluate function as well as structure in suspected cases of renovascular hypertension. Renal artery disease in a patient with hypertension may be coincidental or at

Received for publication March 11, 1970; accepted March 22, 1971.

From the departments of medicine and radiology, Harvard Medical School and Peter Bent Brigham Hospital, Boston.

Reprint requests to Research Editors, Department of Radiology, Peter Bent Brigham Hospital, Boston 02115 (Mrs. Sally Ann Edwards).

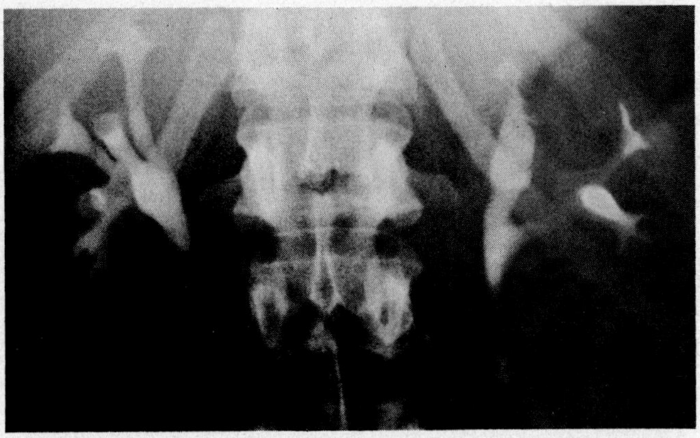

Fig 1.—Intravenous pyelogram (1963). Normal function and morphology.

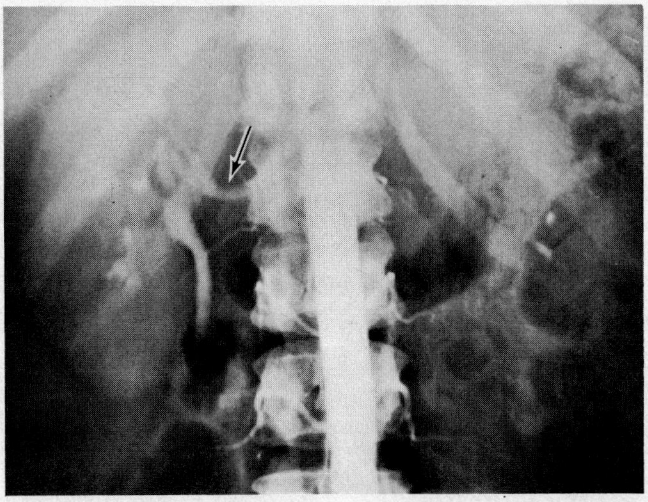

Fig 2.—Mainstream aortogram (1966). The opacification of the right renal artery is faint due to low catheter position. The left renal artery is completely occluded. Opacification of the collecting system of the right kidney is from a technically unsatisfactory first run. Arrow indicates right renal artery.

least not of prime etiologic importance.

In one third of 20 patients studied by Lawrence et al,[5] the functional pattern of renal ischemia was absent in spite of unequivocal radiologic evidence of renal artery stenosis. In some series surgical success has been higher when the functional importance of the renal arterial stenosis, as measured by divided ureteral urine studies or differential renal-vein renin activity assay, was used to select patients for surgery.[4,6] Reliance on arteriography alone may result in a lower cure rate.[7]

Bookstein[8] has discussed one of the reasons for this apparent discrepancy between the anatomic and physiologic data: the measurement of pressure gradients across stenoses of renal arteries explored at surgery suggests that the narrowing must be quite severe to cause an appreciable pressure drop. Cannon has shown that the pressure gradient and the percent reduction in arterial flow rise significantly only after a 90% reduction in lumen size.[9]

The initial functional significance of the original occlusion in the present case was indicated by the appearance of hypertension associated with a nonfunctioning kidney by intravenous pyelogram and complete left renal artery occlusion by arteriography. Subsequently, such effective collaterals developed that renal perfusion rose enough to sustain a functioning kidney, although the function was compromised as manifested by a creatinine clearance of 60 ml/min. This is not an unknown event. Brolin[10] has reported cases in which the collateral circulation associated with renal artery occlusion maintained normal renal size and function.

In acute occlusion of the main renal artery collateral avenues develop within 60 minutes.[11] When occlusion

Fig 3.—Intravenous pyelogram (1968). Bilateral normal function and morphology.

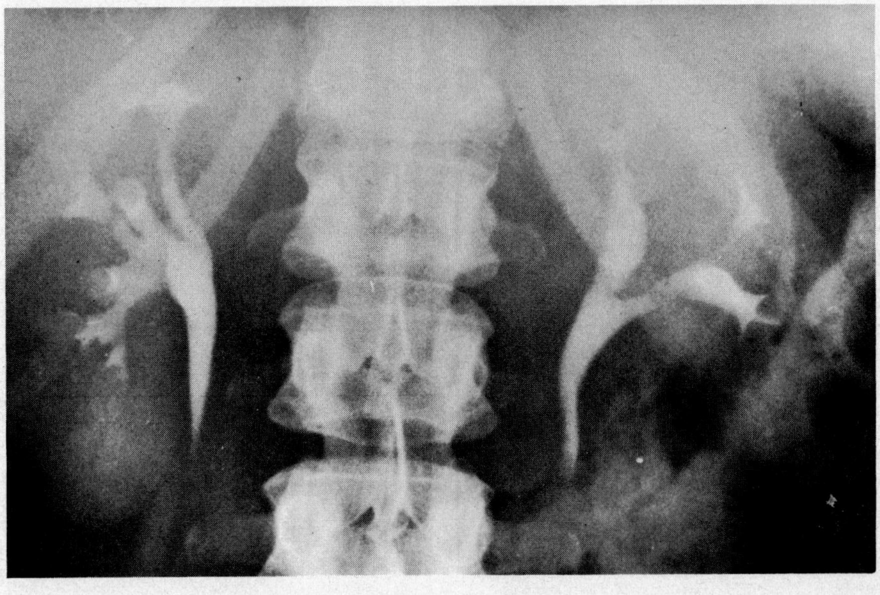

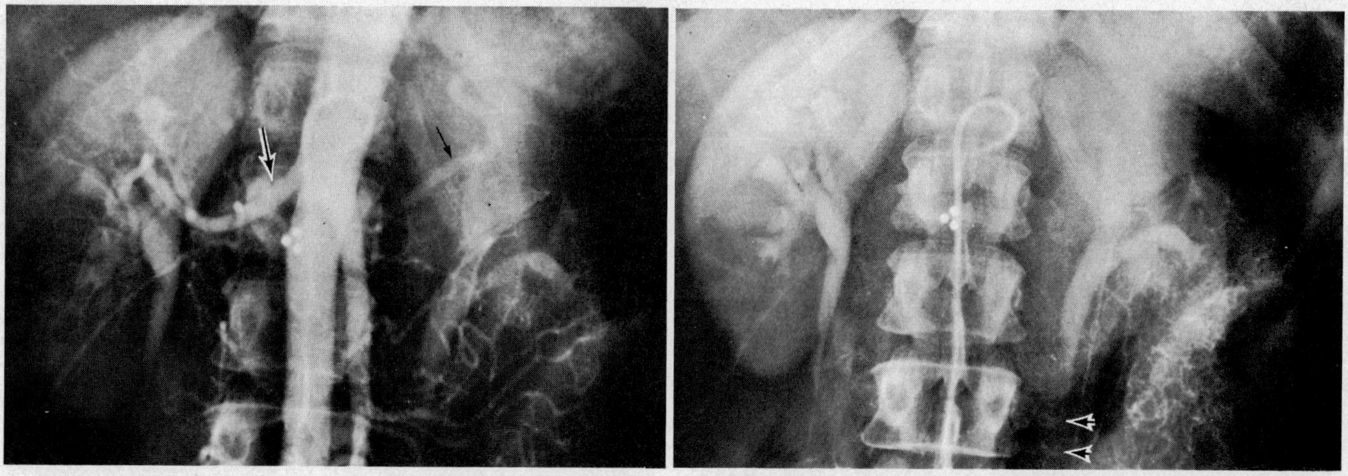

Fig 4.—Mainstream aortogram (1968). Left, *Early phase: Normal, single renal artery on right side* (open arrow). *Splenic artery* (black arrow). Right, *Late phase: Periureteric artery on left side visualized participating in the collateral circulation supplying the left kidney* (arrows).

occurs gradually, the collateral circulation may become extremely rich.[12] The collateral sources available to the ischemic kidney are the lumbar, peripelvic, periureteric, capsular, and adrenal arteries.[13] Only the periureteric and capsular vessels were seen in the present case, but this does not rule out the participation of other arteries. The collateral arteries are frequently difficult to demonstrate angiographically. They may at times produce the characteristic ureteral notching on the intravenous pyelogram, but this was not seen in our patient.

These findings support the hypothesis that this patient initially had renovascular hypertension related to occlusion of the left renal artery and that the subsequent development of a collateral circulation reduced or eliminated the renal ischemia. The hypertension virtually disappeared and the kidney, no longer ischemic, produced normal quantities of renin.

Summary

A 47-year-old housewife was known to have normal renal function in 1963. She later developed hypertension and in 1967 had a nonfunctioning left kidney and total occlusion of the left renal artery. She refused nephrectomy and was managed medically with improvement of her hypertension. By 1968, although the renal artery remained totally occluded, revascularization through collateral channels were so effective that an intravenous pyelogram gave no indication of occlusion. Renal vein renin activity was equal and normal on both sides. Parallel with the functional improvement, her hypertension became mild and easy to control.

This work was supported in part by Public Health Service grants 9377-3, HE03043, and HE11668 and by the John A. Hartford Foundation, Inc.

References

1. Eyler WR, Clark MD, Garman JE, et al: Angiography of the renal areas including a comparative study of renal stenoses in patients with and without hypertension. *Radiology* **78**:879-891, 1962.

2. Holley KE, Hunt JC, Brown AL, et al: Renal artery stenosis: A clinical-pathological study in normotensive and hypertensive patients. *Amer J Med* **37**:14-22, 1964.

3. Blaufox MD, Birbari AE, Hickler RB, et al: Peripheral plasma renin activity in renal-homotransplant recipients. *New Eng J Med* **275**:1165-1168, 1966.

4. Amsterdam EA, Couch NP, Christlieb AR, et al: Renal vein renin activity in the prognosis of surgery for renovascular hypertension. *Amer J Med* **47**:860-868, 1969.

5. Lawrence JR, Doig A, Knight JCS, et al: Renal artery stenosis without renal ischemia. *Lancet* **1**:62-65, 1964.

6. Michelakis AM, Foster JH, Liddle GW, et al: Measurements of renin in both renal veins. *Arch Intern Med* **120**:444, 1967.

7. Schreiber MH: Renal artery-parenchyma ratios in the diagnosis of reno-vascular hypertension. *Amer J Roentgen* **96**:877-886, 1966.

8. Bookstein JJ: Appraisal of arteriography in estimating the hemodynamic significance of renal artery stenosis. *Invest Radiol* **1**:281-294, 1966.

9. Cannon JA, Lobpreis EL, Herrold G, et al: Experience with a new electro-magnetic flow meter for use in blood flow determinations in surgery. *Ann Surg* **152**:635-647, 1960.

10. Brolin I, Stener I: Collaterals in obstruction of the renal artery. *Acta Radiol (Diagn)* **4**:449-462, 1966.

11. Love L, Bush IM: Early demonstration of renal collateral arterial supply. *Amer J Roentgen* **104**:296-301, 1968.

12. Habighorst LV, Kössling FK, Albers P: Die perirenalen Arterien und der Kollateralkreislauf der Niere im postmortalen Angiogramm. *Forschr Roentgenstr* **105**:35-48, 1966.

13. Abrams HL, Cornell SH: Patterns of collateral flow in renal ischemia. *Radiology* **84**:1001-1012, 1965.

Erosive Osteoarthritis and the Main en Lorgnette Deformity

(Opera Glass Hand)

Robert L. Swezey, MD, and Stanley J. Alexander, MD, Los Angeles

The opera glass hand or main en lorgnette deformity has been recognized since the term was coined by Marie and Leri in 1913.[1] They described the telescoped phalanges with overlying infolded skin caused by extensive reabsorption of the phalangeal articular bone.[1] Reports of main en lorgnette deformity have been given under other titles such as arthritis mutilans, absorptive arthritis, and resorptive osteopathy.[2-4] These terms have usually been used to describe a destructive rheumatoid arthritis, or a variant thereof, which affects the hands as well as other joint areas. In 1953 Silver and Steinbrocker mentioned resorptive arthropathy in degenerative joint disease,[3] and Crain, in 1961, described a resorptive, inflammatory arthritis involving the terminal interphalangeal joints without evidence of rheumatoid disease. Some of Crain's patients had been receiving intraarticular steroids into the affected joints.[5] An appreciation of the extensive juxtearticular erosion in the distal interphalangeal (DIP) joints in cases of severe osteoarthritis was not general until the reports of Kidd and Peter and Peter et al.[6,7] They described radiographic and pathological changes in erosive osteoarthritis and stressed its differentiation from rheumatoid arthritis. In one of their patients (case 5) changes suggestive of the main en lorgnette syndrome are present.[7]

A recent observation of one 92-year-old woman with main en lorgnette deformity who had no evidence by history or clinical examination of joint disease other than osteoarthritis and two additional cases of erosive osteoarthritis suggested that, with the passage of time, the initial destruction of erosive osteoarthritis may proceed to the stage of a main en lorgnette deformity.

Received for publication March 24, 1970; accepted April 16, 1971.

From the Department of Physical Medicine and Rehabilitation and the Section of Rheumatic Disease and Clinical Immunology, Department of Medicine, University of Southern California School of Medicine, Los Angeles.

Reprint requests to Los Angeles County-University of Southern California Medical Center, 1200 N State St, Box 723, Los Angeles 90033 (Dr. Swezey).

Patient Summaries

Patient 1.—A 92-year-old white woman was referred because of a chronic joint deformity of both hands. The patient gave a history of having had an onset of generalized aching at approximately the age of 35 to 40 years with pain in her fingers and hands which subsided over a period of five years. Since that time she has had residual and apparently slightly progressive deformities of the hands. However, because of some memory loss, details of this are obscure. She does complain from time to time of arthralgia in the shoulders, knees, and in her feet and states that she recalls a swelling of about a month's duration on the dorsum of the left foot about eight years previously. She does not recall whether or not this was associated with trauma or inflammation.

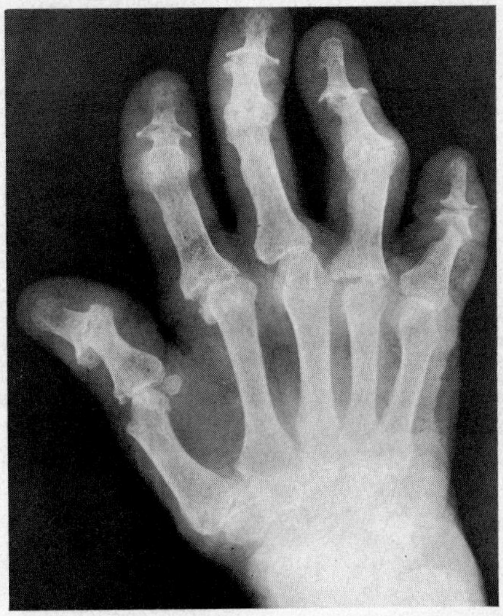

Fig 1.—Ninety-two-year-old woman. Note prominent distal interphalangeal destruction and relative sparing of metacarpophalangeal joints and wrist except for trapeziometacarpal joint.

The past history is unremarkable with the patient specifically denying psoriasis or other chronic dermatitis.

The patient was an elderly, blind, white woman with a glass prosthesis in the right eye. Her vital signs were normal. The left cardiac border was in the anterior axillary line. No subcutaneous nodules were felt. Significant findings were as follows: the

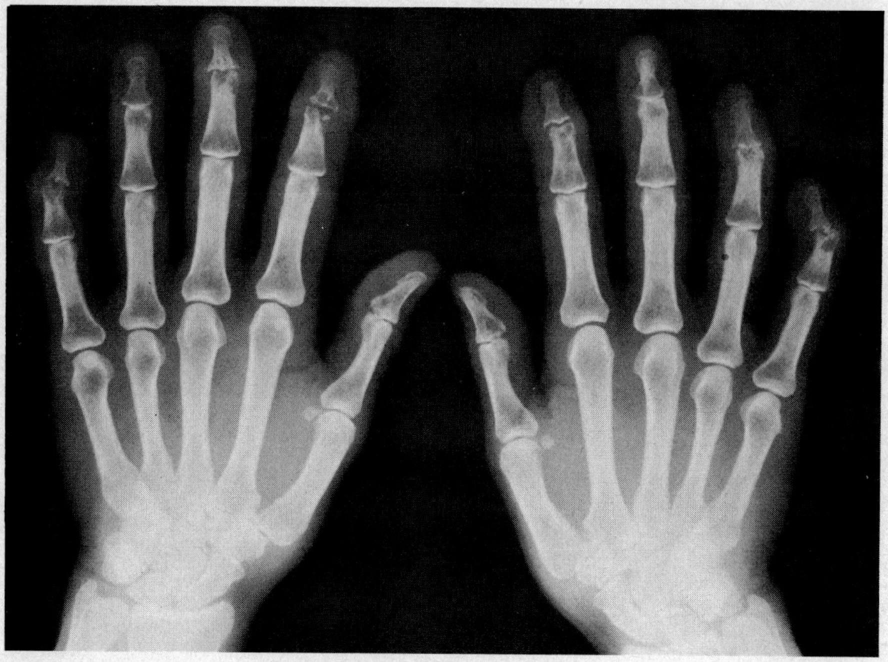

Fig 2.—Forty-two-year-old woman. Erosive changes are limited to distal interphalangeal joints.

hands had the typical appearance of degenerative arthritis with Heberden's nodes and, in addition, evidence of bony reabsorption in all fingers was demonstrable with marked hypermobility of the joints of the hands and particularly of the little fingers bilaterally. These fingers showed the typical "doigt" (finger) en lorgnette deformity characterized by the infolded skin over the areas of bony reabsorption. Some pain was elicited at the extremes of motions of the elbows and shoulders, but the range of motion was normal in those joints as well as all other joints except for the hands. There were no skin changes nor nail changes of psoriasis.

Urine was normal; hemoglobin value was 11.5 gm/100 ml (serum iron value was 72μg/100 ml with an iron binding capacity of 432μg/100 ml); white blood cell count (WBC) was 6,000/cu mm with 71% polymorphonuclear leukocytes; 27% lymphocytes, 1% eosinophils, and 1% monocytes. The Venereal Disease Research Laboratory (VDRL) test was negative; serum uric acid value was 4.2 mg/100 ml; latex fixation test (Singer and Plotz) for rheumatoid factor was negative; sulfobromophthalein sodium (BSP) dye retention was 5.4%; serum creatinine value was 1.1 mg/100 ml; and two-hour postprandial blood glucose value was 121 mg/100 ml. Findings of serum protein electrophoresis were normal and antinuclear antibodies (fluorescent technique) were not present. The chest roentgenogram was consistent with pulmonary fibrosis. Roentgenograms of the hands are shown in Fig 1.

PATIENT 2.—A 42-year-old married white woman was seen because of "floppy" finger joints. Nine years previously she had the onset of acute joint pain, swelling, and stiffness of the hands, elbows, shoulders, and knees which cleared with prednisone therapy in a maximum dose of 20 mg a day tapered off over a few months. Since that time, she had persistent swelling of the distal interphalangeal joints. In the past three to four years these joints have become hypermobile but have remained asymptomatic. There has been an occasional drainage of mucus from a cyst over the third left distal interphalangeal joint. There was no generalized stiffness, gel phenomenon, nor limitation of motion noted during examination nor described by the patient whether on or off steroid therapy.

The patient gave a history of a Coomb's positive hemolytic anemia which predated the arthritis and was associated with hepatosphenomegaly. For the preceding five years this patient has required 12 to 15 mg daily of prednisone for control of the anemia. The patient has worked as a typist and has also operated a cash register. There was no family history of arthritic disease, anemia, or related disorders.

Significant findings on examination revealed that the second through the fifth DIP joints of the hands were deformed by Heberden's nodes, and this was associated with hypermobility of these joints. All other joints appeared normal. No subcutaneous nodules or skin abnormalities were present.

The following values were obtained: hemoglobin, 10.2 gm/100 ml; hematocrit, 29%; WBC, 11,400/cu mm; polymorphonuclear leukocytes, 69%; segmented neutrophils, 5%; lymphocytes, 24%; monocytes, 2%; sedimentation rate (Wintrobe), 15 mm/hr; serum bilirubin–direct, 0.4 mg/100 ml, indirect, 2.3 mg/100 ml; serum glutamic oxaloacetic transaminase (SGOT), 13 units (normal, 8 to 40 units); serum alkaline phosphatase, 1.3 units/100 ml (normal 1 to 3 units/100 ml); and serum uric acid, 4.8 mg/100 ml. The lupus erythematosus (LE) preparation, and results of serum protein electrophoresis and tests for rheumatoid factor and antinuclear antibodies were normal.

Roentgenograms revealed marked narrowing of the distal interphalangeal joints bilaterally with destruction, irregularity, and fragmentation of articular margins and advanced periarticular cystic changes with mild to moderate dorsal spurring. Minor narrowing of the proximal interphalangeal (PIP) joints and the trapeziometacarpal joint with mild cystic changes of the latter joint were also noted. The remaining metacarpophalangeal (MCP) joints were spared (see Fig 2).

PATIENT 3.—A 61-year-old white woman was evaluated because of inability to use her hands. She stated that about five years ago she had the onset of progressive painful arthritis in her hands. This has been associated with morning stiffness in the hands for about 15 minutes daily. There has been some swelling and increasing deformity in the fingers, and except for occasional shooting pain in the low back and aching in the elbows, there have been no other articular complaints.

For the past year since suffering from "a nervous breakdown," she has been unable to use her hands to sew, cut meat, or pick up coins. She further states that she suffered a nervous breakdown five years previously, at the age of 18 years, and at the age of 9. The latter episode was also said to be "the St. Vitus dance."

Her current antirheumatic therapy has consisted of indomethacin, 25 mg daily, and 1,200 to 1,800 mg of buffered aspirin daily. She states that she previously had taken a corticosteroid preparation three times daily for three months, but steroids had not been administered intra-articularly. Her other medications were thyroid, 163 mg (2½ grains) daily, and trifluoperazine hydrochloride (Stelazine).

There was no other history of arthritic disorders, rheumatic fever, psoriasis, sun sensitivity, or diabetes. The patient's father and one sister have been diagnosed as having osteoarthritis, the latter suffering from erosive osteoarthritis.

The physical examination showed a well developed, moderately obese woman who was alert, pleasant, and cooperative. Her height was 154.9 cm (5 ft 1 in); weight, 76.7 kg (169 lb); blood pressure, 170/90 mm Hg; and pulse rate, 80 beats per minute and regular. The significant extra-articular findings were slight anisocoria, forearm vitiligo, and a soft palpable liver edge felt one fingerbreadth below the costal margin.

The musculoskeletal examination disclosed minimal limitation of lumbar motion. There were no subcutaneous nodules, nor tophi. There was no dermatitis and no fingernail pitting. Heberden's nodes were present on all distal interphalangeal joints. Distal phalanges of the left second and the right second through fifth fingers were deviated radially. Ulnar deviation, instability, and boney irregularity were present in the third through fifth PIP joints bilaterally. The skin overlying these joints was loose and infolded.

A complete blood cell count (CBC), sedimentation rate, and findings of urine analysis were within normal limits. The latex fixation test for rheumatoid factor was negative.

Roentgenograms showed extensive destruction and resorption of the right first and second, and left second and fifth DIP joints. Similar destructive changes of the right third and fifth, and the left third, fourth, and fifth PIP joints were present. There were marked hypertrophic changes in both trapeziometacarpal joints. The MCP and wrist joints were normal except for a generalized demineralization of all osseous structures in the hands and wrists (Fig 3). The lumbar spine showed mild demineralization and minimal hypertrophic changes. No abnormalities of the sacroiliac joints or elbows were noted.

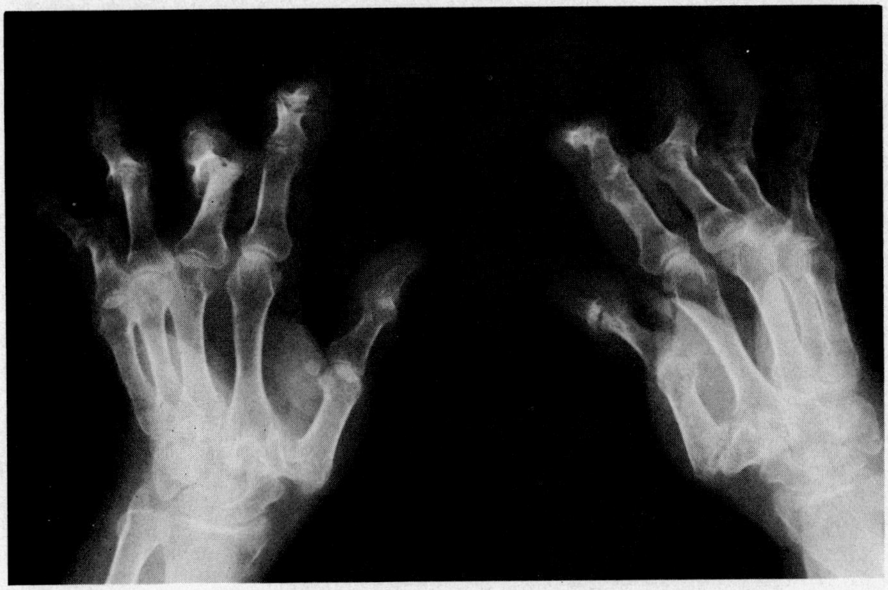

Fig 3.—Sixty-one-year-old woman. Note prominent erosions of distal interphalangeal and proximal interphalangeal joints with sparing of metacarpal joints and wrists except for the trapeziometacarpal joints.

Comment

Concepts of osteoarthritis as a purely degenerative process have been challenged by several authors in recent years.[8-11] The distribution of primary generalized osteoarthritis affecting predominantly the DIP joints has been thoroughly discussed by Kellgren[8] and by Stecher.[11] The erosive inflammatory nature of a particularly virulent variety of this disorder designated as erosive osteoarthritis by Kidd and Peter and Peter et al is now well accepted.[6,7] A characteristic distribution of osteoarthritis joints involving primarily the DIP joints by Bouchard's nodes and in addition, the carpal metacarpal joint of the thumb is well recognized.[12] At least one of the cases of Peter et al had apparent greater destruction of the PIP than the DIP joints.[7]

The pattern of distribution of involved hand joints in rheumatoid arthritis is characterized by severe involvement of the PIP joints with sparing of the DIP joints.[13] McCarty in a recent paper stressed that involvement of the DIP joints can occur more commonly than is usually recognized in rheumatoid arthritis.[14] In rheumatoid arthritis the region of the wrist in relationship to the ulna is usually most heavily involved while the carpal metacarpal joint of the thumb is often spared. The converse is true in osteoarthritis. In psoriasis the terminal interphalangeal joint may be severely involved with erosive changes with or without involvement in other more proximal joints, and this is usually associated with psoriatic nail changes.[15]

Rheumatoid arthritis and psoriasis with arthritis are the most common diseases complicated by the main en lorgnette deformity.[3,15,16] The disorder has also been seen with scleroderma and in reticulohistiocytosis (lipoid dermatoarthritis).[2,17,18]

In ankylosing spondylitis a severe boney resorptive process has been described involving the hips and shoulders, but not the hands.[3] A number of other entities causing resorptive arthropathy which may mimic main en lorgnette deformity include syringomyelia, Hansen's disease, syphilis, thromboangiitis obliterans, diabetes mellitus, hematoporphyrinuria, ainhum, madura mycosis, blastomycosis, sarcoidosis, and mycobacterial infection.[19-22] These disorders can be readily differentiated on the basis of the localization of the osseous lesions, their nonarticular manifestations, as well as by histological and pathological examinations.

In the first patient presented the

details of the history are obscured by an impaired memory of a 92-year-old. The possibility that the swelling in her left ankle represented a manifestation of rheumatoid arthritis cannot be excluded.

The distribution of her destructive joint changes being generally most severe in the DIP joints, slightly less severe in the proximal interphalangeal joints, and least severe at the metacarpophalangeal joints is most compatible with a primary osteoarthritic process even though, rarely, cases with rheumatoid arthritis have impressive DIP erosions.[16,23]

Involvement of the metacarpophalangeal joints in osteoarthritis is well documented,[24,25] but severe destructive changes as seen in patient 1 have not been reported. Because destructive changes have been noted in the metacarpophalangeal joints in hemachromatosis,[26] serum iron and iron binding capacity tests were performed, and the serum iron was at the lower limits of normal. Involvement of the carpal metacarpal joint of the thumb with sparing of the remainder of the wrist is also most consistent with osteoarthritis.[13]

In the second patient the administration of systemic steroids for a hemolytic anemia in the initial phase of her arthritic involvement may have contributed to the severe destructive process.[14] That a similar destructive terminal interphalangeal joint process can occur without steroid therapy is certainly well documented.[6,7] The concurrence of Coomb's positive hemolytic anemia and arthritis raises a question of a related collagen disorder. Systemic LE is characterized by the relative lack of destructive joint disease. Secondary gout must be considered in the presence of a hemolytic process, but no evidence to support this was seen, and gouty involvement of all of the terminal phalangeal joints of the fingers with relative sparing of other areas would be most unusual.

All three cases present features consistent with primary, generalized osteoarthritis. In the first case the inference is that with the passage of time and accompanying generalized osteoporosis of old age, destruction has progressed to the point of an arthritis mutilans primarily involving the DIP joints, and to the least extent, the MCP joints of the fingers.

The addition of another possible etiology to the list of disorders manifesting main en lorgnette deformity emphasizes the importance of a careful study of this symptom complex. The importance of delineating erosive osteoarthritis from rheumatoid as well as other disorders stems from the prognostic and therapeutic considerations that follow.[6,7]

Summary

Three women had severe destructive osteoarthritis involving primarily the DIP joints. One patient, a 92-year-old white woman, had typical main en lorgnette deformity. None of these patients had evidence of rheumatoid arthritis, psoriasis, gout, or other destructive forms of arthritis. Possibly erosive osteoarthritis may lead to destructive main en lorgnette deformity.

This investigation was supported in part by a grant from the Southern California Arthritis Foundation and the National Arthritis Foundation.

References

1. Marie P, Leri A: Une variete rare de rheumatisme chronique: La main en lorgnette. *Bull Soc Med Hop Paris* **36**:104-107, 1913.

2. Nielsen B, Snorrason E: Arthritis mutilans (main et doigt en lorgnettes). *Acta Radiol* **27**:607-616, 1946.

3. Silver W, Steinbrocker O: Resorptive osteopathy in inflammatory arthritis ("absorptive arthritis," "opera glass hand"). *Bull Hosp Joint Dis* **14**:211-222, 1953.

4. Soloman WM, Stecher RM: Chronic absorptive arthritis or opera-glass hand. *Ann Rheum Dis* **9**:209-220, 1950.

5. Crain DC: Interphalangeal osteoarthritis. *JAMA* **17**:1049-1053, 1961.

6. Kidd KL, Peter JB: Erosive osteoarthritis. *Radiology* **86**:640-647, 1966.

7. Peter JB, Pearson CM, Marmor L: Erosive osteoarthritis of the hands. *Arthritis Rheum* **9**:365-388, 1966.

8. Kellgren JH, Moore R: Generalized osteoarthritis and Heberden's nodes. *Brit Med J* **1**:181-187, 1952.

9. Sokoloff L: Experimental studies of degenerative joint disease. *Bull Rheum Dis* **14**:317-318, 1963.

10. Moskowitz RW, Klein L, Mast WA: Current concepts of degenerative joint disease (osteoarthritis). *Bull Rheum Dis* **17**:459-463, 1967.

11. Stecher RM: Heberden's nodes, a clinical description of osteoarthritis of the finger joints. *Ann Rheum Dis* **14**:6-10, 1955.

12. Lawrence JS, de Graaff R, Laine AI: Degenerative joint disease in random samples and occupational groups, in *The Epidemiology of Chronic Rheumatism I.* Oxford, England, Blackwell Scientific Publications, 1963, pp 98-121.

13. Calabro J: Chronic arthritides. *J Amer Phys Ther Assoc* **44**:584-591, 1964.

14. McCarty DJ, Gatter RA: A study of distal interphalangeal joint tenderness in rheumatoid arthritis. *Arthritis Rheum* **9**:325-336, 1966.

15. Avila R, Pugh DG, Slocumb CH: Psoriatic arthritis: A roentgenologic study. *Radiology* **75**:691-702, 1960.

16. Smyth CJ: Bone absorption in rheumatoid arthritis, in *Rheumatic Diseases.* Philadelphia, WB Saunders Co, 1952, pp 196-208.

17. Johnson HM, Tilden IL: Reticulohistiocytic granulomas of the skin associated with arthritis mutilans. *Arch Derm* **75**:405-417, 1957.

18. Warin RP, Evans DC, Hewitt M, et al: Reticulohistiocytosis (lipoid dermatoarthritis). *Brit Med J* **1**:1387-1391, 1957.

19. Brailsford JP: *The Radiology of Bones and Joints.* Baltimore, Williams & Wilkins Co, 1948, pp 57-58.

20. Patterson DE, Job DK: *Leprosy in Theory and Practice*, ed 2. Baltimore, Williams & Wilkins Co, 1964, pp 425-434.

21. Klinenberg JR, Grimley PM, Seegmiller JE: Destructive polyarthritis due to a photochromogenic mycobacterium. *New Eng J Med* **272**:190-193, 1965.

22. Stead EA Jr, Castleman B: Sarcoidosis of 52 years' duration. *New Eng J Med* **281**:375-383, 1969.

23. Simon G: *Priniciples of Bone X-Ray Diagnosis*, ed 2. Philadelphia, FA Davis Co, 1960, p 170.

24. Kellgren JH, Lawrence JS: Radiological assessment of osteoarthritis. *Ann Rheum Dis* **16**:494-502, 1957.

25. Swezey RL, Peter JB, Evers PL: Osteoarthritis of the metacarpophalangeal joint: Hook-like osteophytes. *Arthritis Rheum* **12**:405-410, 1969.

26. Schumacher HR: Hemachromatosis and arthritis. *Arthritis Rheum* **7**:41-50, 1964.

Lactic Acidosis and Associated Hypoglycemia

Ramon Medalle, MD; Robert Webb, MD; and Christine Waterhouse, MD, Rochester, NY

Lactic acidosis has elicited considerable clinical interest since 1961 when Huckabee[1,2] drew attention to it as a clinical entity. Waters et al[3] listed the etiologies of excess lactic acid production as follows: no known cause (idiopathic, spontaneous), diabetes mellitus, phenformin hydrochloride, shock, acute anoxia, exercise, extracorporeal circulation, liver glycogen storage disease, and epinephrine injection. Only in the cases of glycogen storage disease[4-8] has the association of hyperlactacidemia with hypoglycemia been noted and the necessity of glucose administration been stressed. Among the reported cases of well documented lactic acidosis not associated with glycogen storage disease, four patients had concomitant hypoglycemia[9-12] but the authors failed to mention the role of hypoglycemia in those patients. Johnson and Waterhouse[11] did, however, point out the need of glucose and insulin in their report of lactic acidosis in a diabetic patient receiving phenfromin. This communication describes three patients with lactic acidosis and concomitant hypoglycemia, which we believe are etiologically related, and directs attention to the necessity of glucose replenishment in this situation.

Received for publication July 28, 1970; accepted Nov 25.

From the Department of Medicine, University of Rochester (NY) School of Medicine and Dentistry.

Reprint requests to 260 Crittenden Blvd, Rochester, NY 14620 (Dr. Waterhouse).

Methods

The pyruvate and lactate determinations were done by the enzymatic method of Rosenberg and Rush.[13] Serum electrolyte and glucose levels were determined by automatic chemical analysis and arterial pH and blood gasses by pH-carbon dioxide pressure (P_{CO_2}) meter system. Serum carbon dioxide determination was done by the Van Slyke manometric method,[14] and oxygen saturation (satn) by an oximeter. Plasma insulin level was determined by immunoassay.[15]

Patient Summaries

PATIENT 1.—A 60-year-old white man had proven aortic stenosis and mild aortic insufficiency secondary to rheumatic heart disease. With increasing cardiac decompensation, the patient was admitted to the hospital for aortic valve replacement on March 3, 1969.

On admission, the vital signs were blood pressure, 138/60 mm Hg; pulse rate, 90 beats per minute; and temperature, 98.6 F (37 C). Positive physical findings included marked cardiomegaly with a grade 4/6 aortic systolic ejection murmur, a grade 1-2/6 holosystolic murmur at the apex, and S-3 gallop; hepatomegaly; and 2-3+ pitting edema. Initial laboratory values were as follows: hematocrit, 35%; white blood cell count (WBC), 8,750/cu mm; reticulocyte count, 3.9%; normal results of urinalysis: blood urea nitrogen (BUN), 71 mg/100 ml; two-hour postprandial blood glucose 152 mg/100 ml; serum creatinine, 2.0 mg/100 ml; serum sodium 135 mEq/liter; potassium, 3.6 mEq/liter; chloride, 96 mEq/liter; CO_2, 24 millimols/liter; alkaline phosphatase, 4 Bodansky units (BU); total bilirubin, 2.0 mg/100 ml; and serum glutamic oxaloacetic transaminase (SGOT), 44 Karmen units (KU). The electrocardiogram and x-ray film of the chest revealed an enlarged left ventricle and atrium.

While the patient was being prepared for open-heart surgery he was found to be depressed. He complained that he was constantly nauseated and refused to take his food. On March 24, 1969, the patient was found to be somnolent and tachypneic although there was no apparent change in his cardiac status. On March 25, a wide "anion gap" was noted (Table 1), and on the afternoon of March 26, the arterial pH was 7.30.

The diagnosis of lactic acidosis was subsequently verified by a blood lactate level of 9.1 mEq/liter and pyruvate level of 0.22 mEq/liter. The blood glucose level determined at the same time was 31 mg/100 ml. Infusion of 10% dextrose was started and the patient was given additional glucose by mouth during a 12-hour period. On March 27, 1969, the blood glucose level was 202 mg/100 ml and arterial pH was 7.50. The blood lactate and pyruvate levels had dropped to 1.8 mEq/liter and 0.08 mEq/liter, respectively. During the next three days, the serum CO_2 value ranged from 23 to 26 millimols/liter with blood glucose value ranging from 98 to 206 mg/100 ml. A fasting plasma insulin level was less than 1 microunit/ml when the blood glucose level was 98 mg/100 ml. On March 31, 1969, the patient was found to have slurred speech, and was confused and somnolent. The blood glucose level was 17 mg/100 ml and the serum CO_2 value had dropped to 17 millimols/liter. Glucose administration rapidly corrected the symptoms and the following day the CO_2 value had risen to 23 millimols/liter. A similar episode occurred on April 15, 1970. Further episodes of lactic acidosis did not occur after initiation of forced feeding and maintenance of normal blood glucose

Table 1.—Blood Chemistries of Patient 1

	mEq/Liter											
	L*	P†	Na	K	Cl	CO_2, Millimols/Liter	pH	P_{CO_2}, mm Hg	O_2 Satn, %	Blood Glucose, mg/100 ml	SGOT, KU	Comments
3/6/70 10 AM			135	3.6	91	24				152‡	44	← 3/24 somnolent, tachypneic, BP 140/60 mm Hg
3/25/70 8:55 AM			134	4.2	87	17						
3/26/70 8 AM			132	4.9	90	12						
2:45 PM						7	7.31	13	97		38	
8 PM	9.1	0.22	131	5.0	86	9	7.30	13	93	31		
												← 3/26 9 PM-3/27 7 AM 25 gm glucose, 40 gm glucose postoperatively with clearing of symptoms
3/27/70 8 AM			122	4.3	86	23	7.51	27	96	202	13	
3:40 PM	1.8	0.08	126	4.0	90	26				206	25	← Alert
3/29/70 8:30 AM			131	4.1	90	23				158		
3/31/70 8:30 AM			132	4.7	92	17				17		← Confused, slurred speech relieved by glucose given intravenously
4/1/70 9 AM			122	4.8	89	23				134		

* L = lactate.
† P = pyruvate.
‡ Two-hour postprandial.

levels. Subsequently, the patient developed staphylococcal pneumonia and sepsis, and died.

Postmortem examination showed acute bacterial endocarditis (mitral valve), rheumatic heart disease with mitral insufficiency and aortic stenosis, pulmonary embolism, chronic passive congestion and centrolobular necrosis of the liver, and focal glomerulitis.

Patient 2.—A 59-year-old white woman was admitted to the hospital on July 27, 1969, with signs of increasing right sided heart failure and appearance of a harsh systolic murmur. She had suffered a myocardial infarction two months previously.

On admission, the patient appeared depressed. Pertinent physical findings were blood pressure, 112/82 mm Hg; pulse rate, 76 beats per minute; respiration rate, 14 per minute; temperature, 97.5 F (36.4 C); distended neck veins; cardiomegaly with a grade 5/6 harsh systolic murmur over the whole precordium and transmitted to the left axilla and back, accentuated pulmonic second sound and frequent ventricular extrasystoles; crepitant rales at both lung bases; hepatomegaly; ascites; and 1-2+ pretibial pitting edema.

Initial laboratory findings were hematocrit, 50%; WBC, 8,800/cu mm; trace proteinuria with normal urine sediment; BUN, 33 mg/100 ml; serum creatinine, 1.5 mg/100 ml; blood glucose, 106 mg/100 ml; serum sodium, 137 mEq/liter; potassium, 4.6 mEq/liter; chloride, 93 mEq/liter; CO_2, 25 millimols/liter; serum protein, 6.4 gm/100 ml; albumin, 3.7 gm/100 ml; SGOT, 19 KU; and alkaline phosphatase, 16 BU. The ECG showed an old diaphragmatic myocardial infarct, right bundle branch block, and multifocal ventricular extrasystoles. X-ray film of the chest revealed left atrial and left ventricular enlargement, and pulmonary congestion.

In the days following admission, dietary intake was markedly inadequate. On July 30, 1969, the patient was found stuporous and disoriented. The blood pressure was unobtainable. The serum electrolytes showed a wide "anion gap" and arterial pH was 7.35 (Table 2). The patient was given a total of 132 mEq of sodium bicarbonate during the next two hours, but arterial pH dropped further to 7.25. The blood lactate level was 9.6 mEq/liter and pyruvate level was 0.16 mEq/liter. The blood glucose level determined at the same time was 34 mg/100 ml. In the ensuing four hours, 50 gm of glucose and an additional 88 mEq of $NaHCO_3$ were given intravenously. At the end of this period the blood glucose level rose to 254 mg/100 ml, and arterial pH rose to 7.40. The blood lactate and pyruvate levels had dropped to 7.36 mEq/liter and 0.20 mEq/liter, respectively. During the next 36 hours, with maintenance of near normal blood glucose level and without further bicarbonate therapy, the blood lactate level decreased to 1.98 mEq/liter and arterial pH rose to 7.59. No further episodes of acidosis were observed following maintenance of adequate blood glucose levels. On Aug 1, 1969, following the demonstration of a large ventricular septal defect by cardiac catheterization, open-heart surgery was performed with excision of the infarcted myocardium and closure of the ventricular septal defect. On Aug 3, 1969, the patient died of cardiac failure.

Postmortem examination revealed a myocardial infarct secondary to coronary thrombosis, and acute hepatic and generalized visceral congestion.

Patient 3.—A 62-year-old white man with a Starr-Edwards ball valve prosthesis for rheumatic aortic stenosis was admitted to the hospital on Dec 31, 1969, with a one-day history of chills and fever.

On admission, vital signs were blood pressure, 108/54 mm Hg; pulse rate, 96

Table 2.—Blood Chemistries of Patient 2

	mEq/Liter											
	L*	P	Na	K	Cl	CO_2, Millimols/Liter	pH	P_{CO_2}, mm Hg	O_2 Satn, %	Blood Glucose, mg/100 ml	SGOT, KU	Comments
7/28/69 8 AM			137	4.6	93	25				106	19	← BP 110/80
												← 7/30 4 AM stuporous, BP unobtainable, 5-7:45 AM 132 mEq $NaHCO_3$ intravenously
7/29/69 1:05 PM			132	4.2	88	20						
7/30/69 5:30 AM			137	6.1	91	7	7.35	12	98		125	
9 AM	9.6	0.16	137	5.8	87	10	7.25	24	82	34	188	← 9:15 AM 50 gm glucose intravenously
												← 10-11 AM 88 mEq
1:25 PM			133	4.4	85	16	7.40	27	81	254	500	$NaHCO_3$ intravenously, glucose 5%, 50 ml/hr, by continuous infusion
3 PM	7.4	0.20				22	7.48	32	78			
7/31/70 11 AM			135	2.8	82	34				137	43	
2:40 PM						39	7.56	45	90			
11:30 PM			132	4.2	88	35				124		
8/1/69 10:40 AM	2.0	0.21				36	7.59	37	90			
												← 6 PM open-heart surgery
8/2/69 10 AM			131	3.2	89	23	7.52	29	97	282		

* See footnotes for Table 1.

beats per minute; respiration rate, 16 per minute; and temperature, 100.6 F (38.1 C). Pertinent findings on examination were engorged neck veins; bilateral basilar rales; minimal cardiomegaly with a grade 2/6 systolic murmur at the apex and grade 2/6 diastolic murmur at the left sternal border; hepatomegaly; splenomegaly, and no peripheral edema.

Initial results of laboratory studies were hematocrit, 37%; WBC, 10,300/cu mm with 86% segmented cells and 10% bands, reticulocyte count, 6.1%; normal results of urinalysis; two-hour postprandial blood glucose, 143 mg/100 ml; BUN, 23 mg/100 ml; serum sodium, 130 mEq/liter; postassium, 3.3 mEq/liter; chloride, 100 mEq/liter; CO_2, 20 millimols/liter; SGOT, 867 KU; alkaline phosphatase, 6 BU; total bilirubin, 4.8 mg/100 ml, and direct bilirubin, 1.6 mg/100 ml. The ECG showed left ventricular and atrial enlargement with wandering atrial pacemaker, and the x-ray film of the chest showed pulmonary congestion without any infiltrate. Serial blood cultures grew *Staphylococcus aureus* sensitive to penicillin.

The patient initially improved on intravenously administered penicillin but on Jan 1, 1970, *Klebsiella* and *Aerobacter* pneumonia developed and treatment was started with kanamycin sulfate and chloramphenicol. On the night of Jan 13, 1970, the patient was found to be markedly dyspneic. Blood gasses drawn at this time were P_{CO_2}, 32 mm Hg, oxygen saturation, 94%; and CO_2, 14 millimols/liter, and arterial pH was 7.26 (Table 3). The patient was believed to be in metabolic acidosis and during the ensuing two hours received 178 mEq of $NaHCO_3$ which corrected the pH to 7.41. Six hours later arterial pH was found to be 7.29 and the blood glucose level was 42 mg/100 ml. An additional dose of 132 mEq of $NaHCO_3$ was given which increased the arterial pH to 7.38. At this time the diagnosis of lactic acidosis was finally entertained and confirmed by a blood lactate level of 7.4 mEq/liter and pyruvate level of 0.19 mEq/liter. In the next four hours 75 gm of glucose was given by both intravenous and oral routes. The lactate and pyruvate levels after the glucose administration dropped to 4.0 mEq/liter and 0.17 mEq/liter respectively. The arterial pH rose to 7.45. Subsequently, the patient maintained normal blood pH although no further alkali was given. The patient died of cardiac failure on Jan 15, 1970.

Postmortem examination revealed marked biventricular hypertrophy, pneumonia, and centrolobular necrosis of the liver.

Clinical Findings

The three patients described had many clinical features in common. They all had excess lactate with systemic acidosis. The lactate levels at the time of diagnosis exceeded 7.0 mEq/liter with a range of 7.4 to 9.6 mEq/liter. The pyruvate levels were slightly elevated with a range of 0.16 to 0.22 mEq/liter. The lactate increase was disproportionate to the pyruvate increase, giving a lactate: pyruvate (L:P) ratio ranging from 39 to 60. The arterial pHs ranged from 7.25 to 7.30. The patients fulfilled the criteria for the diagnosis of lactate

Table 3.—Blood Chemistries of Patient 3

	mEq/Liter L*	P	Na	K	CL	CO2, Millimols/Liter	pH	P_{CO_2}, mm Hg	O_2 Satn, %	Blood Glucose, mg/100 ml	SGOT, KU	Comments
12/31/69 7:30 PM			130	3.3	100	20				143	867	
1/13/70 8 PM			130	5.0	102	22	7.44	33	92			
11 PM						14	7.26	32	84			← Marked dyspnea, BP 134/50 mm Hg
												← 12:45-2:30 AM 178 mEq $NaHCO_3$ intravenously
1/14/70 3 AM						16	7.41	24	93			
9 AM			141	6.4	95	13	7.29	29	94	42	1,950	
12:15 PM	7.4	0.19				18	7.38	32	95	50		← 11:30 AM 132 mEq $NaHCO_3$ intravenously
12:50 PM										40		← 12:30 PM 25 gm glucose intravenously
4:30 PM	5.8	0.17	141	7.1	94	17	7.31	32	96	142		← 3:30 PM 50 gm glucose postoperatively, 88 mEq $NaHCO_3$ IV intravenously
9:15 PM			143	6.4	93	26	7.41	42	95	216	3,750	← 6 PM-2 AM (1/15) continuous glucose intravenously and glucose by nasogastric tube
1/15/70 1:15 AM			142	5.8	95	30	7.45	43	94	214		
9:45 AM	4.0	0.17	144	6.4	93	25	7.45	35	93	96	6,420	
10:50 AM												← Cardiacasystole

* See footnotes for Table 1.

acidosis as defined by either Tranquada et al[9] or Oliva.[16]

Hypoglycemia was present in all the patients. The blood glucose levels determined at approximately the same time as the initial blood samples for lactate and pyruvate determinations ranged from 31 to 42 mg/100 ml.

The patients all had congestive heart failure but none were hypoxic initially. Arterial O_2 saturation ranged from 94% to 98%.

Hepatic dysfunction was evident in all patients. All had hepatomegaly. The alkaline phosphatase and SGOT levels were elevated in patients 2 and 3, although the SGOT level in patient 2 began to rise on the day she developed acidosis. The serum total bilirubin level was increased in patients 1 and 3 but hemolysis was also present. Both had high reticulocyte counts. At postmortem examination, patients 1 and 3 had centrilobular necrosis of the liver and patient 2 had marked hepatic congestion.

Inadequate caloric intake prior to the lactic acidosis was well documented in two of the patients and in all the patients the need for glucose in correcting the acidosis was evident. Effectiveness of glucose was exemplified by patient 1 who received no alkali therapy. In patients 2 and 3 "refractory acidosis" became more amenable to alkali therapy.

This group of patients reemphasizes the serious prognostic implication of lactic acidosis. All eventually succumbed to their primary disease, even though recovery from lactic acidosis was achieved in each patient.

Comment

Most of the known causes of lactic acidosis can be eliminated in the patients described. Shock or circulatory insufficiency appeared unlikely since the widening of the "anion gap" occurred long before the episodes of hypotension. More significantly, hyperlactatemia was corrected without attendant attempts to improve circulation. The initial O_2 saturation was greater than 93% in all patients and ruled out acute hypoxia as a cause of lactic acidosis. Huckabee[17] has shown in human beings than excess lactate due to acute hypoxia did not occur until O_2 saturation dropped below 74%. The patients were probably not diabetic although patients 1 and 3 had slightly elevated two-hour postprandial blood glucose levels. In the past, both patients had normal fasting and two-hour postprandial blood glucose levels during elective admissions but had slightly elevated blood glucose levels during acute illnesses. Allison et al[18,19] have shown that patients who are not diabetic may develop abnormal glucose tolerance when subjected to nonspecific stresses. The patients were not receiving phenformin.

The maintenance of normal blood glucose levels involves many factors. The blood glucose level, however, is ultimately dependent upon the rate of glucose produced from exogenous carbohydrate, hepatic glycogenolysis and glyconeogenesis on one hand, and the rate of glycolysis on the other. Hypoglycemia results from either diminished glucose production, increased rate of glycolysis, or both. Patients 1 and 2 had documented inadequate caloric intake for several days prior to their hypoglycemia, and liver glycogen was probably depleted in both. The elevated lactate and pyruvate levels in all patients suggest inadequate hepatic uptake of these substrates. Berry,[20] extrapolating animal liver perfusion data to man, concluded that the normal liver is capable of handling the maximal lactate production from the total carbohydrate stores of the body. Marliss et al[21] demonstrated striking elevation of plasma amino acids in patients with lactic acidosis which suggests impaired hepatic uptake of amino acids. The impaired hepatic handling of lactate, pyruvate, and probably amino acids in our patients indicated that glyconeogenesis from these substances was also inadequate.

The small amount of glucose needed to correct hypoglycemia, and the ease with which the patients became hyperglycemic speak against an increased rate of glycolysis. Studies with tagged glucose in human beings estimated normal glucose turnover rates to range from 4.8 to 12.3 gm/hr.[22-24] With the rate of glucose administered as a very gross index, we estimated glucose turnover rates in our patients to be within normal limits. For example, in patient 1 the blood glucose level rose from 31 to 202 mg/100 ml after administration of 65 gm of glucose in ten hours as an average rate of 6.5 gm/hr. The development of hyperglycemia would indicate that glucose turnover rate was less than or approximated the rate of glucose administration, if endogenous glucose production was not considerable.

There were several mechanisms by which hypoglycemia could have contributed to hyperlactatemia in our patients. DiSalvo et al[25] demonstrated hyperlactatemia during insulin hypoglycemia, and blunting of the rise of the blood lactate level by adrenergic blocking agents, which suggest that epinephrine released during hypoglycemia was the mediator of the lactate rise. Bearn et al[26] showed that epinephrine acts by increasing lactate production in extrahepatic tissues. However, infusion of 0.17μg of epinephrine/kg/min for 50 minutes in human beings achieved lactate levels of only 2 to 4 mEq/liter.[25] Epinephrine released during hypoglycemia in our patients may have been partially responsible for the increased lactate levels.

Hypoglycemia superimposed on previously damaged livers may have resulted in gross impairment of hepatic handling of lactate in our patients. Although lactic acidosis has been reported in patients with cirrhosis in precoma or coma,[27] it was not likely that hepatic damage alone was directly the cause of the hyperlactacidemia in our patients. On administration of glucose, hyperlactacidemia decreased markedly but hepatic function, exclusive of the ability to handle lactate, did not change significantly. In fact, the SGOT values in patients 2 and 3 continued to rise when lactate levels were decreasing. Furthermore, difficulties with lactate metabolism have not been universally observed in all cases of liver disease. It would appear that in the setting of liver dysfunction, a critical amount of glucose is needed as an energy source for normal hepatic uptake of lactate.

In a more specific liver disorder, von Gierke's disease, hypoglycemia causes hyperlactatemia by stimulating hepatic glycogenolysis and outpouring of lactate instead of glucose due to a deficiency of glucose-6-phosphatase.[5,6,28] This mechanism appears unlikely because our patients' medical history and the microscopic features of the patients' livers were not suggestive of von Gierke's disease. However, hepatic glucose-6-phosphatase activity was not assayed and its deficiency cannot be entirely ruled out.

It is suggested that a vicious cycle involving principally hypoglycemia and impaired hepatic uptake of lactate was operating in our patients. The initiating event is not clear but taking hypoglycemia as the starting point we can conceive the cycle as follows: hypoglycemia in the presence of hepatic damage → impaired hepatic uptake of glucose precursors including lactate (hyperlactacidemia) → impaired glyconeogenesis → hypoglycemia, etc. It is also apparent from the patients' clinical response that glucose could break the cycle, correcting not only the hypoglycemia but lactic acidosis as well. Whether glucose is effective in patients with lactic acidosis but without hypoglycemia is not known. Alpert[29] has shown in eviscerated animals that insulin administration improves lactate utilization. Johnson and Waterhouse[11] successfully corrected lactic acidosis in a diabetic patient on a regimen of phenformin by administration of glucose and insulin. Our patients were not given insulin because it was felt that endogenous insulin response would be adequate. Whether or not insulin, either endogenous or exogenous, in conjunction with glucose is necessary for the correction of hyperlactacidemia remains a question.

Summary

The clinical course of three patients with lactic acidosis and concomitant hypoglycemia are described. The first patient was treated with glucose alone, and the second and third patients were treated with glucose and minimal alkali therapy. Blood lactate levels returned to normal or near normal levels in all patients.

It seems likely that the hypoglycemia in these patients was produced by inadequate caloric intake associated with impaired glyconeogenesis. We feel that hypoglycemia contributes to the maintenance of hyperlactacidemia.

It is suggested that hypoglycemia should be looked for in cases of lactic acidosis, especially in the face of hepatic insufficiency and inadequate caloric intake. If these factors are present, glucose administration appears to be the therapy of choice with or without additional alkali therapy.

This investigation was supported by Public Health Service research grant RR-00044 from the Division of Research Facilities and Resources.

Nonproprietary and Trade Names of Drug

Phenformin hydrochloride–*DBI, DBI-TD.*

References

1. Huckabee WE: Abnormal resting blood lactate: I. The significance of hyperlactatemia in hospitalized patients. *Amer J Med* **30**:833-839, 1961.
2. Huckabee WE: Abnormal resting blood lactate: II. Lactic acidosis. *Amer J Med* **30**:840-848, 1961.
3. Waters WC III, Hall JD, Schwartz WB: Spontaneous lactic acidosis. *Amer J Med* **35**:781-793, 1963.
4. Manson HH, Sly GE: Blood lactic acid in liver glycogen disease. *Proc Soc Exp Biol Med* **53**:145-147, 1943.
5. Manson HH, Andersen DH: Glycogen disease of the liver (von Gierke's disease) with hepatoma: Case report with metablic studies. *Pediatrics* **16**:785-700, 1955.
6. Sokal JE, Lowe CH, Sarcione EJ, et al: Studies of glycogen metabolism in liver glycogen disease (von Gierke's disease): Six cases with similar metabolic abnormalities and responses to glucagon. *J Clin Invest* **40**:364-374, 1961.
7. Oei TL: Hexose monophosphate, pyruvate and lactate in the peripheral blood in glycogen-storage disease. *Clin Chim Acta* **7**:193-198, 1962.
8. Howell RR, Ashton DM, Wyngaarden JB: Glucose-6-phosphatase deficiency glycogen storage disease. *Pediatrics* **29**:553-565, 1962.
9. Tranquada RE, Grant WJ, Peterson CR: Lactic acidosis. *Arch Intern Med* **117**:192-202, 1966.
10. Perrett CL, Hopf MA, Frei J: Spontaneous lactic acidosis. *Helv Med Acta* **33**:16-21, 1966.
11. Johnson HK, Waterhouse C: Lactic acidosis and phenformin. *Arch Intern Med* **122**:367-370, 1968.
12. Oliva PB, Schwartz HA: Survival of a patient with spontaneous lactic acidosis. *Ann Intern Med* **71**:587-591, 1969.
13. Rosenberg JC, Rush BF: An enzymatic-sphectrophotometric determination of pyruvic and lactic acid in blood: Methodologic aspects. *Clin Chem* **12**:299-307, 1966.
14. Van Slyke DD, Neill JM: The determination of gasses in blood and other solutions by vacuum extraction and manometric measurement. *J Biol Chem* **61**:523-572, 1924.
15. Morgan CR, Lazarow A: Immunoassay of insulin: Two antibody system. *Diabetes* **12**:115-126, 1963.
16. Oliva PB: Lactic acidosis. *Amer J Med* **48**:209-225, 1970.
17. Huckabee WE: Relationship of pyruvate and lactate during anaerobic metabolism: III. Effect of breathing low oxygen gases. *J Clin Invest* **37**:264-271, 1958.
18. Allison SP, Hinton P, Chamberlain MI: Intravenous glucose tolerance, insulin, and free fatty acid levels in burned patients. *Lancet* **11**:1113-1116, 1968.
19. Allison SP, Tomlin PJ, Chamberlain MI: Some effects of anaesthesia and surgery on carbohydrate and fat metabolism. *Brit J Anaesth* **41**:588-593, 1969.
20. Berry MN: The liver and lactic acidosis. *Proc Roy Soc Med* **60**:52-54, 1967.
21. Marliss EB, Aoki TT, Felig P, et al: Altered amino acid metabolism in lactic acidosis. *Diabetes* **19**(suppl 1): 355, 1970.
22. Reichard GA Jr, Moury NF Jr, Hochella NJ, et al: Quantitative estimation of the Cori cycle in the human. *J Biol Chem* **238**:495-501, 1963.
23. Cahill GF Jr, Herrera MG, Morgan AP, et al: Hormonefuel interrelationship during fasting. *J Clin Invest* **45**:1751-1769, 1966.
24. Waterhouse C, Keilson J: Cori cycle activity in man. *J Clin Invest* **48**:2359-2366, 1969.
25. DiSalvo RJ, Bloom WL, Brust AA, et al: A comparison of the metabolic and circulatory effects of epinephrine, norepinephrine, and insulin hypoglycemia with observations on the influence of autonomic blocking agents. *J Clin Invest* **35**:568-577, 1956.
26. Bearn AG, Billing B, Sherlock S: The effect of adrenaline and noradrenaline on hepatic blood and splanchnic carbohydrate metabolism in man. *J Physiol* **115**:430-441, 1951.
27. Mulhausen R, Eichenholz A, Blumentals A: Acid-base disturbance in patients with cirrhosis of the liver. *Medicine* **46**:185-189, 1967.
28. Havel RJ, Balasse EO, Williams HE, et al: Splanchnic metabolism in von Gierke's disease (glycogenosis type I). *Trans Assoc Amer Physicians* **82**:305-323, 1969.
29. Alpert NR: Lactate production and removal and regulation of metabolism. *Ann NY Acad Sci* **119**:995-1012, 1965.

Portal Hypertension in a Patient With Osteopetrosis

A Case Report With Discussion of the Mechanism of Portal Hypertension

Edward K. Denison, MD; Robert L. Peters, MD; and Telfer B. Reynolds, MD, Los Angeles

Portal hypertension without cirrhosis of the liver has been described in several hematological conditions.[1-15] Though there may be thrombosis of the portal, splenic, or hepatic veins in cases of the myeloproliferative syndromes,[13-15] many cases have been described in which these veins were patent.[1-8,13] The etiology of portal hypertension in these patients with patent venous systems has not been clearly elucidated. Alternative explanations include increased portal flow secondary to splenomegaly, the "forward flow" theory,[2,3,8] and increased hepatic resistance from infiltrative lesions in portal tracts and sinusoids.[7,13]

Portal hypertension without cirrhosis also occurs in tropical splenomegaly[16] and systemic-portal arteriovenous fistulae.[17,18] Investigations in these patients have also suggested that increased portal blood flow may cause portal hypertension in the absence of cirrhosis.[16,17]

The case described here represents an example of hematological portal hypertension. Bone marrow obliteration led to hepatosplenomegaly from extramedullary hematopoesis. Portal hypertension became obvious when a large epigastric collateral vein appeared. This patient is unique in that this is the first reported case of portal hypertension in a patient with osteopetrosis.

Patient Summary

A 56-year-old white woman (LAC-USCMC 178-78-53) with osteopetroasis was referred to the hepatic service of the Los Angeles County-University of Southern California Medical Center (LAC-USCMC) for evaluation of hepatosplenomegaly with a large abdominal collateral vein. She was the second of three children and her parents were first cousins. An older brother died at the age of six years and is said to have had paraplegia, a large head, and normal intelligence. A younger brother is living and has no evidence of osteopetrosis. There was no known family history of osteopetrosis. The patient was born in Germany in 1912 and immigrated to the United States in 1923. The diagnosis of osteopetrosis had been made when the patient was four years of age following fracture of the right femur. She has had multiple fractures involving long bones, ribs, and the pelvis, throughout her life. Exophthalmus began during childhood. Blindness of the left eye, oculus sinister (OS), occurred at the age of twelve years. Progressive loss of vision of the right eye, oculus dexter (OD), resulted in blindness at approximately 50 years of age. Development of her deciduous teeth is not known but the permanent teeth had crumbled or decayed by the age of 14 years. A draining sinus of the left maxilla developed at the age 25 years and has persisted to the present time. There has been progressive auditory impairment and dysosmia since the age of 30 years.

The patient was first seen at the LAC-USCMC at the age of 20 years for a spontaneous fracture of the right femur. The diagnosis of osteopetrosis was confirmed by x-ray films of the skull, pelvis, and long bones. The red blood cell count was 4,690,000/cu mm.

She was next seen at LAC-USCMC in 1957, at the age of 45 years, and was hospitalized for a fractured humerus. Pertinent findings at that time included: bilateral exophthalmus, blind OS, tunnel vision OD, pallor of both optic disks, thoracic asymmetry secondary to multiple previous rib fractures, draining sinus of the left maxilla, and bilateral pes cavus deformities. The liver and spleen were not palpable. X-ray films of the skull, chest, pelvis, and long bones revealed typical changes of osteopetrosis (Fig 1). Laboratory data included hemoglobin level, 11.5 gm/100 ml; white blood cell (WBC) count, 3,300/cu mm; reticulocytes, 3.7%; serum albumin level, 4.9 gm/100 ml; serum

Received for publication July 29, 1970; accepted Sept 10.

From the departments of medicine and pathology, University of Southern California School of Medicine and John Wesley County Hospital, Los Angeles.

Read before the Southern California Society of Gastroenterology, May 26, 1970, Los Angeles.

Reprint requests to 550 Washington St, Suite 123, San Diego, Calif 92103 (Dr. Denison).

globulin level, 2.0 gm/100 ml; alkaline phosphatase activity, 1.4 Bessey-Lowry (B-L) units/ml; and acid phosphatase activity, 16 King-Armstrong units/ml.

There were two hospitalizations in 1958 for Naffzinger decompressions of the optic nerves. The level of hemoglobin was unchanged and a total of 8 units of blood was transfused during the surgical procedures. Progressive visual impairment OD and blindness OS were not affected.

In June 1965, the liver was palpable 5 cm blow the right costal margin, and the spleen 6 cm blow the left costal margin. The hemoglobin level had fallen to 6.6 gm/100 ml. The following values were normal: albumin, globulin, calcium, phosphorus, cholesterol, serum iron, protein-bound iodine and urinary ketogenic steroids. The following values were obtained: plasma ^{59}Fe clearance following administration of ferric chloride Fe 59, 25 minutes (normal 60 to 120 minutes); ^{51}Cr, red blood cell survival following administration of chromic chloride Cr 51, 20 days (normal, $>$ 28 days); ^{51}Cr splenic-precordial ratio, 2.4 (normal, $<$ 1.5); ^{51}Cr spleen-liver ratio, 2.8 (normal, $<$ 2.0; ^{59}Fe splenic uptake, elevated; and ^{59}Fe hepatic uptake, normal.

The patient was admitted to the hepatic service in May 1969. In addition to the previously mentioned findings; there was bilateral horizontal nystagmus, blindness OU, and bilaterial ophthalmoplegia. Anosmia and moderate nerve deafness were present. There was a dilated tortuous epigastric vein with a thrill and continuous Cruveilhier-Baumgarten (C-B) murmur (Fig 2). The liver was palpable 4 cm below the right costal margin and was firm and slightly tender. The spleen was palpable to the level of the iliac crest and was quite firm. Laboratory values included serum albumin level, 2.3 gm/100 ml; serum globulin level, 4.3 gm/100 ml; total bilirubin, 0.8 mg/100 ml; alkaline phosphatase activity, 2.6 B-L units/ml, glutamic oxalacetic transaminase (SGOT) activity, 9 Karmen units/ml; glutamic pyruvate transaminase (SGPT) activity, 16 Karmen units/ml; prothrombin activity, 100%; hematocrit value, 18%; WBC count 5,100/cu mm; reticulocyte count, 4.3% platelets, 75,000/cu mm; and sodium sulfobromophthalein (Bromsulphalein) retention, 3% at thirty minutes.

Wedged hepatic vein pressure (WHVP) and abdominal collateral vein pressure were measured simultaneously. The WHVP was 9 mm Hg greater than inferior vena cava (IVC) pressure and wedging of the catheter was confirmed by contrast media injection. The pressure in the abdominal collateral vein was 12 mm Hg $>$ IVC pressure. The abdominal vein was then occluded cephalad of the point of pressure measurement so that equilibration with portal pressure could occur. During this maneuver, the WHVP increased to 11 mm Hg $>$ IVC pressure; the abdominal vein pressure, measured simultaneously, increased to 21 mm Hg $>$ IVC pressure. Estimated hepatic blood flow (EHBF) was measured with indocyanine green (ICG) by comparing arterial and hepatic venous plasma ICG disappearance curves after injection of ICG 0.5 mg/kg body weight.[19] Half-time for ICG clearance was 3.2 minutes (normal 3 $\pm$ 0.5), the K value was 0.216, and the extraction rate was 0.606. Estimated hepatic blood flow was 1,440 ml/min (normal 1,200-1,800). Estimated blood volume was 4,000 ml.

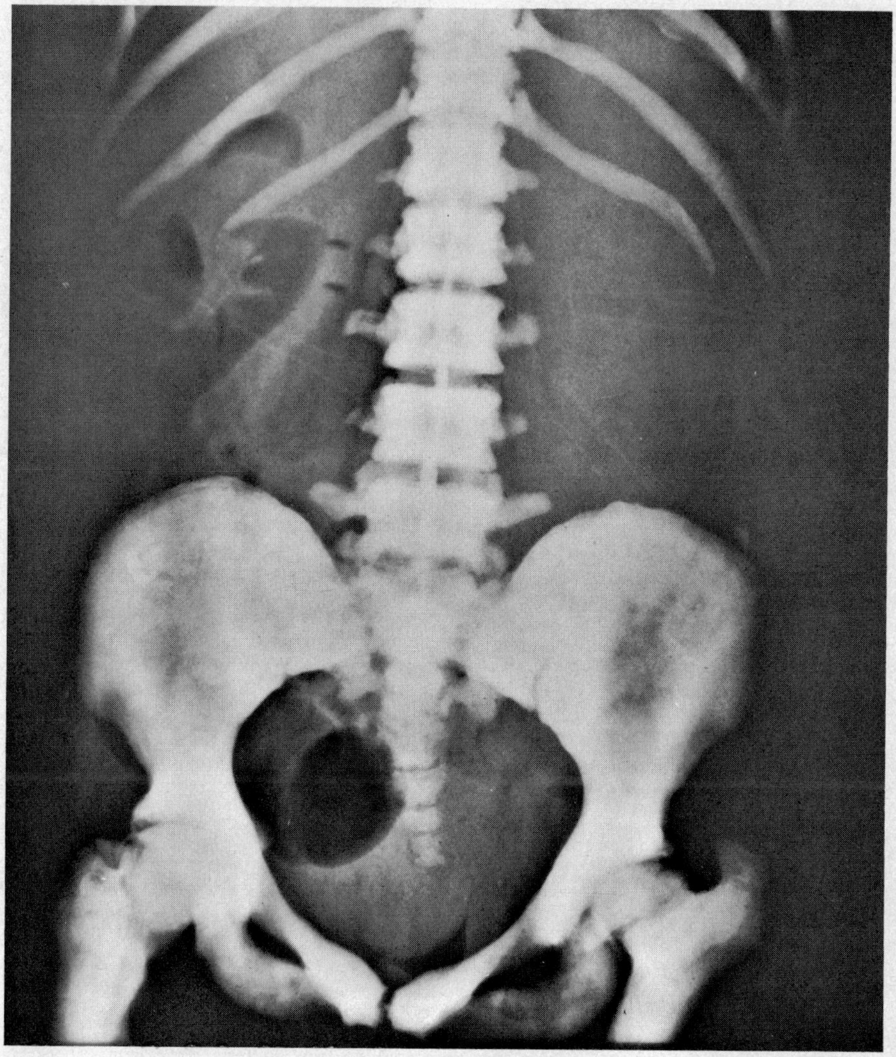

Fig 1.—X-ray film of kidneys, ureterers, and urinary bladder taken in 1969, showing diffuse osteosclerosis, splenomegaly, and rib and femur fractures.

Nine months later the patient was readmitted to the hospital. Physical findings were unchanged. Laboratory values were not significantly changed and sulfobromophthalein retention was again 3% at thirty minutes. Hepatitis-associated (Australia) antigen and smooth-muscle antibodies were not detectable. Microscopic examination of a liver biopsy specimen taken on Feb 4, 1970 (Fig 3 and 4) revealed that the lobular architecture was maintained with central and portal areas

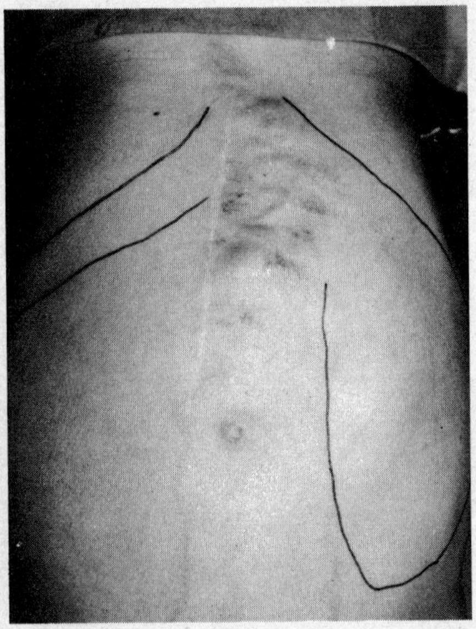

Fig 2.—Patient's abdomen in 1969, showing abdominal collateral veins. Liver and spleen have been outlined.

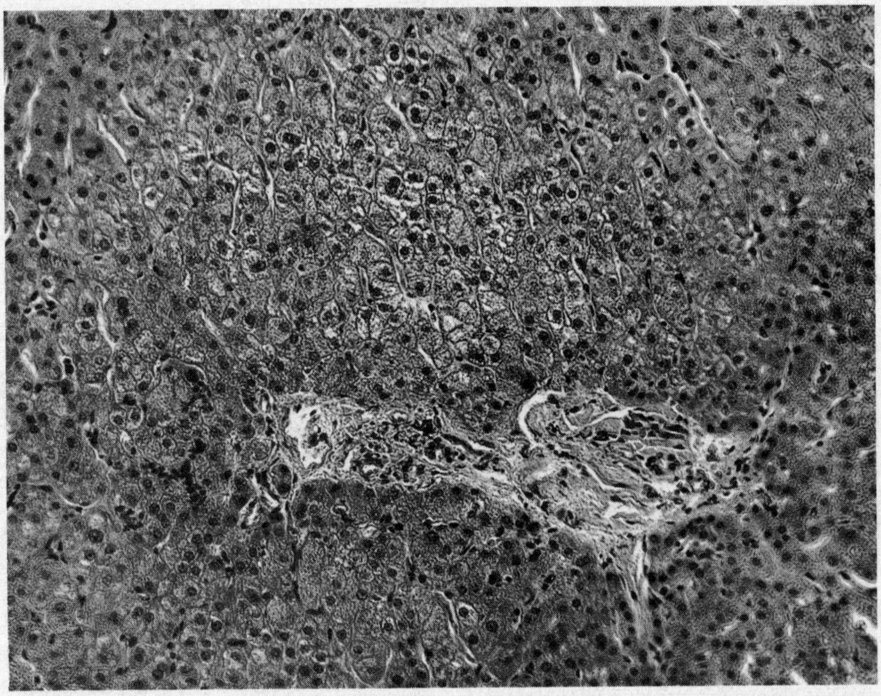

Fig 3.—Liver biopsy specimen showing an intact portal area and extramedullary hematopoiesis. Regular cord pattern is evident (hematoxylin-eosin stain ×100).

in a proper relationship to one another; there was no fibrosis or nodularity. The portal regions were small; the portal vein was identifiable and was not thickened. The collagen in the portal area was somewhat more dense than usual but did not extend beyond the limiting plates. Cholangioles and arteriolar structures were not remarkable. Within the liver, there was modest extramedullary hematopoiesis with megakaryocytes and islands of erythromyelopoiesis throughout the lobules. There was a faint eosinophilic thickening of the sinusoidal walls which, on Masson stain for connective tissue, gave a staining reaction for collagen. The sinusoids, however, were not obliterated or occluded by the collagenous material. Congo red and thioflavine T staining of the liver showed no staining for amyloid.

Comment

To our knowledge, this patient is unique in that hers is the first reported case in which portal hypertension accompanied osteopetrosis. There are other unique features of her illness which also merit brief discussion.

Osteopetrosis is divided into two types: the dominantly inherited, clinically benign form, and the recessively inherited, clinically malignant form.[20-24] The number of cases of each type reported in the literature is almost equal.[20] In the benign form of the disease, hepatosplenomegaly and anemia do not occur. Fractures and bone pain are common, and cranial nerve palsy, osteomyelitis, and exophthalmus may be present infrequently.[20] Approximately 50% of patients with the benign form are asymptomatic. In a review of the features of 50 patients with the recessive malignant disease, Johnston et al found optic atrophy in 78%, splenomegaly in 62%, and hepatomegaly in 48%.[20] They state that death from anemia or infection usually occurs early in life and that no reported cases have survived beyond age 20. Our patient has developed all of the most common features of the malignant form of this disease and is still alive at the age of 57 years. It is of interest that anemia and hepatosplenomegaly did not appear until the fifth and sixth decade respectively. The family history is notable in that consanguinity existed between her parents and a sibling died at an early age with a large head. A large head is said to be present in 22% of those with the recessive disease.[20] It would be unusual for two of three siblings to be affected by a recessive trait.

The presence of portal hypertension is confirmed by the elevated WHVP and by the high pressure in the abdominal collateral vein. The difference in these two pressure levels suggests that the portal hypertension is predominantly presinusoidal in nature. The presence of a dilated abdominal vein and C-B murmur confirm patency of the portal vein since these collaterals are known to arise from the intrahepatic portion of the left branch of the portal vein. Parenchymal hepatic disease as the cause of portal hypertension seems to be exluded by the

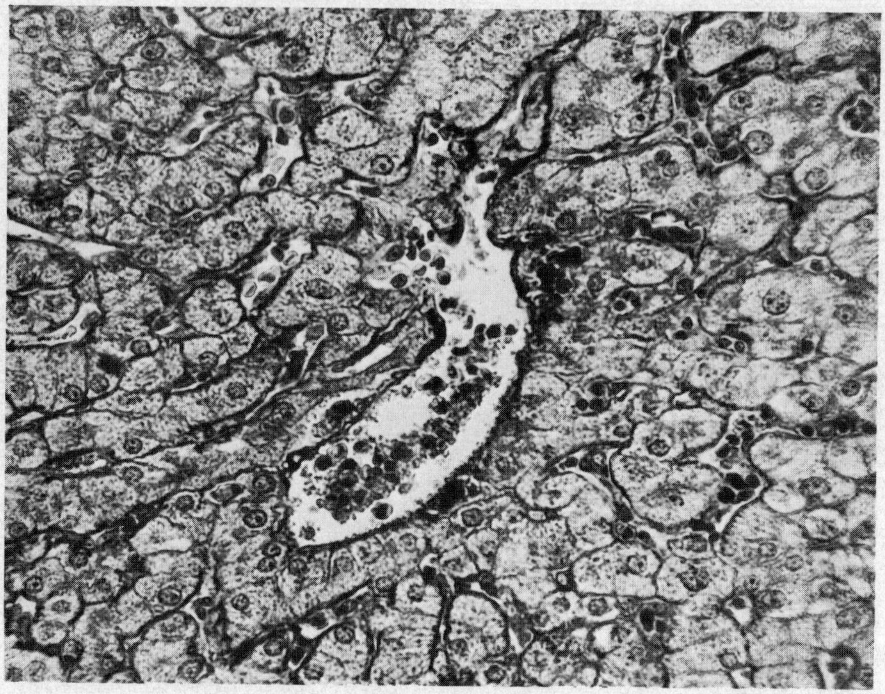

Fig 4.—Liver biopsy specimen showing sinusoidal wall thickening and patent sinusoidal lumina in a centrilobular area (Masson stain ×210).

normal hepatic tests, except albumin, normal sulfobromophthalein retention, and the lack of significant pathological condition in the liver biopsy specimen. The EHBF is within the normal range. The question to be considered is the mechanism of development of portal hypertension in this setting.

In an attempt to explain the development of "hematological portal hypertension" in certain patients, the forward flow theory has been advanced.[2,3] The reasoning has been that increased portal flow occurs secondary to splenomegaly, and that this flow results in increased pressure according to the laws of fluids in motion. Hemodynamic data on patients with hematologic portal hypertension is limited. Three patients studied by Shaldon and Sherlock[7] had patent portal systems, portal hypertension, and normal EHBF. All had either portal fibrosis or infiltrative lesions in portal tracts, and all had elevated serum alkaline phosphatase activity. Splenic-WHVP gradient suggested presinusoidal obstruction to blood flow. The authors concluded that in their patients there was no evidence to support the forward flow theory. Rosenbaum et al[8] studied five patients with myeloproliferative disorders. Four of their patients had elevated WHVP; the other had splenomegaly but no proof of portal hypertension. The EHBF was normal in one case and elevated in three. Alkaline phosphatase activity and sulfobromophthalein retention were abnormal in most patients. Hepatic histological study was available in one patient and showed moderate periportal fibrosis. The authors felt that increased portal flow may cause portal hypertension when hepatic disease prevents hepatic vascular distensibility. Dal Palu et al[13] studied a patient with chronic lymphocytic leukemia and portal hypertension. Splenic-WHVP gradient and EHBF were normal. Portal spaces and centrolobular zones contained extensive lymphocytic infiltrates. It was concluded that the infiltrative lesions caused increased vascular resistance and portal hypertension.

Blendis et al[25] studied 20 patients with hematological disorders and splenomegaly. Thirteen had portal hypertension and all had increased splenic blood flow. Most of the patients had abnormal liver histology. However, five patients with portal hypertension had normal liver biopsy specimens and the only explanation found for portal hypertension was increased splenic blood flow.

Williams et al[16] studied 15 patients with idiopathic tropical splenomegaly. Portal hypertension, when present, was predominantly presinusoidal. Estimated hepatic blood flow was elevated in ten of 11 patients. Splenic blood flow was elevated in all seven patients whose total splenic weight was determined. In one patient EHBF fell from 1,170 to 670 ml/min sq mm after splenectomy. The authors felt that portal hypertension was caused by increased splenic blood flow.

Donovan et al[17] studied two patients with systemic-portal arterioventricular (AV) fistulas, portal hypertension, and bleeding esophageal varices. Hemodynamic studies in one patient revealed normal EHBF and portal hypertension that was predominantly presinusoidal. Liver biopsies in both patients showed highly vascularized, slightly widened portal spaces with thickened intrahepatic portal vein radicals. It was felt that these abnormalities were a consequence of increased hepatic blood flow and that portal hypertension was secondary to these vascular changes. The authors felt that the hepatic vasculature had responded to excess flow by changes which increased intrahepatic presinusoidal resistance. This caused portal hypertension and diminution of hepatic blood flow. Stone et al,[18] in reviewing the literature on systemic portal AV fistulas, noted symptoms during the first year compatible with acute congestive changes in the viscera, followed by two or three years of minimal symptoms, then followed by symptoms of bleeding esophageal varices. Donovan et al[17] suggest that bleeding varices occur only after increased resistance has developed in the hepatic vasculature.

No definite conclusion can be made regarding the etiology of portal hypertension in our patient. The EHBF was within our normal range and the portal hypertension was predominantly presinusoidal. The normal EHBF does not indicate normal portal blood flow since an unknown amount of blood is diverted through portal collaterals. Hepatic function was well preserved. Liver biopsy specimen was normal except for extramedullary hematopoiesis and the collagen deposition along the sinusoidal walls. The etiology of this collagen deposition and its relationship to osteopetrosis is unknown.

We believe it likely that splenomegaly can cause increased portal flow, and that the liver vasculature can respond to increased flow by increasing intrahepatic resistance. This response would tend to reduce hepatic blood flow toward normal and would result in portal hypertension with collateral vessel development to divert part of the portal flow around the liver. Such patients do not usually come to attention until these changes are present and the available studies reflect the situation after hepatic compensatory developments have occurred.

Summary

A patient had osteopetrosis and portal hypertension which was evident clinically by the findings of a dilated epigastric vein, Cruveilhier-Baumgarten murmur, and a thrill. Osteopetrosis was manifest by severe anemia, hepatosplenomegaly, blindness, deafness, maxillary osteomyelitis, typical roentgenographic bone changes, and a lifelong history of many fractures. Hepatic hemodynamic studies confirmed the presence of portal hypertension and the liver biopsy excluded the usual hepatic causes of elevated portal pressure. Portal hypertension is attributed to extramedullary hematopoiesis with increased splenic blood flow and the subsequent development of increased intrahepatic vascular resistance.

References

1. Fauvert R, Hartmann L: La mesure de la vitesse de la circulation portale et les explorations combinées transpléniques. *Rev Hepatol* **5**:695-704, 1955.
2. Paraf A, Chalut J, Caroli J, et al: Manométrie splénique et splénoportographie dans les affection du systeme hemopoietique, les pyléphlébitis, les cirrhoses due foie. *Rev Hepatol* **5**:617-660, 1955.
3. Hunt AH: *A Contribution to the Study of Portal Hypertension.* London, E & S Livingstone Ltd, 1958.
4. Oishi N, Swisher SN, Stormont JM, et al: Portal hypertension in myeloid metaplasia: Report of a case without apparent portal obstruction. *Arch Surg* **81**:80-86, 1960.
5. Weinberg T: Observation on the occurrence of varices of the oesophagus in routine autopsy material. *Amer J Clin Path* **19**:554-557, 1949.
6. Levitan R, Diamond HD, Craver LF: Esophageal varices in Hodgkin's disease involving the liver. *Amer J Med* **27**:137-143, 1959.
7. Shaldon S, Sherlock S: Portal hypertension in the myeloproliferative syndrome and the reticuloses. *Amer J Med* **32**:758-764, 1962.
8. Rosenbaum DL, Murphy GW, Swisher SN: Hemodynamic studies of the portal circulation in myeloid metaplasia. *Amer J Med* **41**:360-368, 1966.
9. Lima JP, Von Eye G, Delima CP, et al: Portal venous pressure in Hodgkin's disease with hepatic involvement and esophageal varices. *Amer J Med* **32**:618-620, 1962.
10. Pitcock JA, Reinhard EH, Justus BW, et al: A clinical and pathological study of 70 cases of myelofibrosis. *Ann Intern Med* **57**:73-84, 1962.
11. Nakai GS, Craddock CG, Figueroa WG: Agnogenic myeloid metaplasia: A survey of 29 cases and a review of the literature. *Ann Intern Med* **57**:419-440, 1962.
12. Aufses AH Jr: Bleeding varices associated with hematologic disorders. *Arch Surg* **80**:655-659, 1960.
13. Dal Palu CD, Ruol A, Belloni G: Postsinusoidal portal hypertension in a patient with chronic lymphatic leukemia. *Amer J Digest Dis* **8**:845-851, 1963.
14. Burris MB, Arrosmith WR: Vascular complications of polycythemia vera: A study of 68 cases. *Surg Clin N Amer* **33**:1023-1028, 1953.
15. Fountain JR: Hemorrhagic thrombocythaemia: Report of two cases treated with radioactive phosphorus. *Brit Med J* **2**:126-130, 1958.
16. Williams R, Parsonson A, Somers K, et al: Portal hypertension in idiopathic tropical splenomegaly. *Lancet* **1**:329-333, 1966.
17. Donovan AJ, Reynolds TB, Mikkelsen WP, et al: Systemic-portal arteriovenous fistulas: Pathological and hemodynamic observations in two patients. *Surgery* **66**:474-482, 1969.
18. Stone HH, Jordan WD, Acker JJ, et al: Portal arteriovenous fistulas. *Amer J Surg* **109**:191-196, 1965.
19. Caesar J, Shaldon S, Chiandussi L, et al: The use of indocyanine green in the measurement of hepatic blood flow and as a test of hepatic function. *Clin Sci* **21**:43-57, 1961.
20. Johnston CC Jr, Lavy N, Lord T, et al: Osteopetrosis: A clinical, metabolic and morphologic study of the dominantly inherited, benign form. *Medicine* **47**:149-167, 1966.
21. Harnapp GO: Zum Bilde der Marmorknochenkrankheit: Die familiare, gutartige Form der diffusen Osteosklerose. *Mschr Kinderheilk* **69**:1-46, 1937.
22. McPeak CN: Osteopetrosis: Report of eight cases occurring in three generations of one family. *Amer J Roent* **36**:816-829, 1936.
23. Nussey AM: Osteopetrosis. *Arch Dis Child* **13**:161-172, 1938.
24. Schinz HR: Erbtypen and Formen bei Marmorknochenerkrankung (Morbus Albers-Schonberg). *Der Erbatz* **12**:33, 1944.
25. Blendis LM, Banks DC, Ramboer C, et al: Spleen blood flow and splanchnic haemodynamics in blood dyscrazia and other splenomegalies, abstracted. *Gastroenterology* **58**:280, 1970.

Diabetes Mellitus of Juvenile Onset With 40 Years' Survival and No Gross Damage

In-depth Study of and by a 50-Year-Old Physician

Glen R. Shepherd, MD, Newport Beach, Calif

Insulin was first used for human diabetics in 1922. Not until 1959 would it be likely that any cases of 40 years' survival of insulin-dependent diabetics could be reported. A thorough search of the world medical literature back through 1959 reveals only two cases of juvenile onset insulin-dependent diabetics with 40 years' undamaged survival reported, both in the nonabstracted literature by Blöch and Korp[1] in 1963. One case, also in the German literature, of a maturity onset (age 26) insulin-dependent diabetic, was reported in 1967 by von Csapo and Hobi[2] as having survived without complications for more than 40 years. Although White passingly reported 19 patients surviving 40 to 45 years,[3] there was no discussion of those extraordinary patients in that article or subsequently, nor was there any implication they were not damaged. In response to specific inquiry about those patients, White did not claim lack or relative lack of physical damage in them (personal communication, 1969).

The following case report is, therefore, apparently the first in the English literature, the third in the world literature about such undamaged survival, and possibly the first in-depth report of such a case by a physician who is also the patient. The case is presented in the third person with the patient referred to as G.R.S.

There are at least three common denominators among the two cases reported by Blöch and Korp which are discussed under Comment and that of G.R.S. These could have significance in further investigations as well as in the outlook for present juvenile onset diabetics.

Except for the recent status, laboratory data (1925 to 1953) will not be given because records of the early data have disappeared or have been destroyed by the physicians then involved. The patient, G.R.S., made no effort to collect and preserve the early data because he did not expect to survive remarkably long, based on prognoses published in the 1930's. Similar flat negative prognoses have been published as recently as 1963, 1967, and 1968.[4-6]

In instances of indirect or hearsay information about the early life of the patient rather than direct recorded or clearly remembered first-hand information, such indirect data is labeled as to source.

Patient Summary

In the winter of 1965 to 1966, after 40 diabetic years, G.R.S., a white male unmarried physician nearly 46 years old, had his usual annual clinical and laboratory examinations. There were only two positive findings, as follows: asteroid hyelosis of the left vitreous (since 1962), and five peripheral microaneurysms in the fundi. There was, otherwise, no clinically detectable angiopathy, retinopathy, lenticular changes, renopathy, or neuropathy. Laboratory findings, exercise electrocardiogram, and chest roentgenogram were all normal.

Vitreous asteroid hyelosis is not regarded as damage related to diabetes mellitus on the basis of the existing literature which seems to show lack of relationship.[7-9]

The five peripheral, not posterior, very small retinal microaneurysms had appeared first in 1953 after 27 to 28 diabetic years. They had remained unchanged since that time until their disappearance in 1969. They were not the source of the right perimacular hemorrhage six months later. For these reasons, as well as the literature references cited in the Comment section, the peripheral retinal findings are not regarded as "damage" in this patient.

Therefore, for the first 40 diabetic years, this patient clinically appeared to be physically undamaged.

This did not continue. After 40+ diabetic years, three newly developed right perimacular larger microaneurysms bled superfically, interfering with right macular vision. The first bleeding occurred overnight in July 1966, and the second and third perimacular hemorrhages occurred overnight in December 1966. These reduced right eye vision with glasses to 20/100.

The treatment used was avoidance of lifting or other exercise that might increase intraocular pressure, increase of ascorbic acid intake from 0.5 to 3 gm daily, and continuing efforts to maintain diabetic control within physiological limits.

By April 1967, oculus dexter (OD) vision had returned to 20/25–, with all macular landmarks restored except the foveal reflex. By May 1969, OD vision was 20/25+ and the right macula showed no residual evidence of hemorrhage. There were three small perimacular aneurysms but none peripherally.

A bulging microaneurysm in the left perimacular area was noted in December 1966, but it had disappeared without a trace and without bleeding by or before December 1968.

However, by December 1968, urine volume had perceptibly increased. Colorimetric determination (Albutest) showed a

Received for publication July 29, 1970; accepted Oct 23.

From the Department of Medicine, College of Medicine, University of California, Irvine.

Reprint requests to Department of Medicine, College of Medicine, University of California, Irvine 92664 (Dr. Shepherd).

trace of protein. Quantitative studies by a competent laboratory showed the following 24 hour urine findings: January 1969, 24 hour volume, 6,400 ml, 259 mg total protein, 36 gm total glucose; February 1969, 24 hour volume, 6,698 ml, 234 mg total protein, 11 gm total glucose; and March 1970, 24 hour volume, 6,490 ml, 200 mg total protein, 32 gm total glucose.

Those laboratory findings indicate that after almost 43 years of diabetes mellitus, there is beginning clinical evidence of renopathy, although with a remarkable lack of progression in the 14 months after apparent onset.

As of the last complete clinical and laboratory examination in 1969, the only other physical or laboratory abnormalities are a slightly increased systolic sitting blood pressure in both arms (140/80 mm Hg) and a slight lessening of malleolar vibratory sense (tuning fork) bilaterally. Previous systolic sitting pressures since medical student days had been lower consistently, in the 105 to 120 mm Hg range. The exercise ECG continued to be normal, pedal pulses are present, and the toes appear entirely normal.

Table 1 presents the daily routine G.R.S. currently follows and that, except for insulin dosage, has been requisite for the past ten years because of the increasing lability or "brittleness" of the diabetes. His diet, insulin, timing, and seven to ten urine tests daily are followed rigorously on a strict self-imposed schedule designed to maintain as biochemically physiological a state as is feasible.

Whether or not there is overnight glycosuria, there is often a positive tablet (Acetest) reaction for ketones in the overnight urine, but this disappears within one half to one hour after breakfast. Overnight slight ketonuria even in the absence of glycosuria has become a frequent occurrence only since 1969, the past year, although it appeared occasionally in the previous five years. Ketonuria does not appear in daytime or evening specimens even on the rare occasions of heavy glycosuria. The appearance of glycosuria correlates with any of the following: (1) upper-respiratory tract infection (rare); (2) more carbohydrate than necessary for impending insulin reaction; (3) cyclic changes in carbohydrate tolerance preceding adjustment of insulin dose by 1 or 2 units; and (4) emotional stress. Treuting[10] in 1962 reported this role of emotion.

Table 2 shows the present diet, which

Table 1.—Daily Schedule

Time	Activity
8:15 AM	Arise, void overnight urine, test
8:30	Inject 24 units unmodified insulin subcutaneously
9:30	Breakfast (see Table 2 for meal values)
12:30	Void, test urine for sugar and acetone
1:00 to 1:25 PM	Lunch after voiding for testing 2nd specimen
4:30	Void and test
5:00	Void and test this 2nd specimen. Food as required
5:30	Inject 14 to 16 units unmodified insulin
6:00 to 6:40	Drink 2 to 3 oz. Scotch whiskey with water
6:45 to 6:55*	Begin dinner in restaurant catering to G.R.S. diet
11:00	Void, test for sugar
12:00 to 12:30	Void, test 2nd specimen for sugar. Take food in accord with result of test (8 oz skim milk + sugar)
1:00 AM	Retire for night after making sure there are no symptoms of insulin reaction

* Dinner must begin less than 11 hours after morning insulin and less than 1½ hours after predinner insulin, to avoid insulin reaction. Similarly, lunch must be begun (with orange juice) less than 5 hours after morning insulin.

Table 2.—Present Diet of G.R.S.

	Estimated Grams*			
	Carbohydrates	Protein	Fat	Calories
Breakfast†	47	8	5	265
Lunch†	59	40	3	423
Predinner	11	...	1	53
Dinner	75	50	59	1,031
Bedtime	30	2	...	128
Scotch whisky (3 to 4 oz)‡	...	...	...	210 to 280
Totals	222	100	68	2,110 to 2,180

* All computations rounded to whole numbers.
† Each meal is exactly the same daily, to reduce variables.
‡ Total amount averaged daily, taken predinner and bedtime. Alcohol appears to have a mild antiketogenic effect and does not appear to require insulin for its utilization.

Table 3.—Numerical Data on G.R.S. for 17 Years

Date	Weight,* lb	Blood Pressure, mm Hg	Insulin, Units AM	PM	Total	Serum Cholesterol, mg/100 ml	Total Serum Lipids, mg/100 ml
3/23/53	150½	115/75	42	24	66	...	...
10/27/55	146	130/80	Not recorded			...	...
8/31/56	143	120/70	30	26	56	173	...
4/12/58	146	120/74	30	20	50	...	...
12/26/58	138	115/80	24	18	42	155	...
12/28/59	128½	125/85	Not recorded			155	595
12/27/60	137½	120/80	26	16	42	132	...
12/28/61	145	115/75	26	18	44	155	...
12/27/62	141	125/80	24	18	42	...	...
8/19/64	129	...	24	18	42	...	...
11/64	134½	...	24	19	43	180	502
1/65	137	104/70	25	19	44	194	...
2/2/66	145½	104/70	26	20	46	160	541
4/12/68	150½	115/70	26	20	46	180	568
2/69	152	140/80	24	19	43	178	...

* Weights given are in office, dressed but without shoes or jacket. These weights are about 5 lb more than stripped weight.

has been followed generally for the past six years. It is essentially a low fat, high carbohydrate (for a diabetic), and normal protein diet. Except for a lower caloric intake coincident with retiring from full time career work, the relative proportions of carbohydrate, protein, and fat have been much the same throughout adult life. No meals may be skipped or delayed. Exercise almost daily consists of walking 1.3 to 3 miles.

Recent History.—Table 3 presents a summary for the past 17 years of body weights, blood pressures, insulin doses, and serum cholesterol and total serum lipid values. Fractional blood sugar values have been used solely to validate second specimen (fractional) urine sugars, ie, to establish that a negative tablet (Clinitest) test represents a momentary (Folin) blood sugar of 150 mg/deciliter or less. Second specimen urine sugars provide convenient immediately available data many times daily, unlike blood sugars.

Diabetic control was considered good (as discussed in Comment) during this period, as it had been during the preceding 27+ years, although there have been greater swings in glycosuria since 1960 due to hyperlability.

The patient, G.R.S., had not had to be hospitalized for any reason since his middle teen years. He had continued, without significant interruption, school from the sixth grade through high school, college, medical school, internship, private practice in a preceptorship with a board certified internist, faculty position in a medical school, and, from 1955 until July 1960, a staff position with a national medical association.

Due to a combination of circumstances, diabetic control steadily worsened during the winter of 1959 to 1960. The patient left his full time position for a less stressful temperate climate where he could set his own insulin, meal, and exercise schedules and control his diet better than the duties of his salaried position had permitted.

After three years, during most of which G.R.S. had good diabetic control, he returned to full time salaried staff work in Chicago. However, it became apparent after seven months that the meal and schedule irregularities required by such a full time position were incompatible with the brittle diabetes G.R.S. obviously now had. Therefore, he resigned and returned to Southern California in October 1964 to concentrate on perfecting his diabetic control. This was achieved in several months and continues to date.

Past History.—The patient was a full term normal infant normally delivered in a hospital Feb 26, 1920, with a birth weight of 3.9 kg (8½ lb). Breast fed for the first ten months, according to the mother, the baby showed normal weight gain. It was 12.7 kg (28 lb) at the age of 1 year and 21.3 kg (47 lb) by the fourth year of age. No early behavioral, feeding, or physical problems were reported by the mother.

At the age of approximately 5½ years (in 1925), according to the mother, G.R.S. had a severe case of scarlet fever, with temperature rising to 106 F (41.1 C) for at least several hours. The treatment used was ice packs. Physicians in attendance, according to the mother, warned the parents that there might be serious sequelae of such a severe highly febrile infection.

Immediately after recovery, G.R.S. was, according to his mother, markedly underweight and feeble, in contrast to his robust good health preceding the scarlet fever. Within a now indeterminate period of days to a month, G.R.S. showed the classical diabetic signs of polyphagia, polydipsia, and polyuria. Hospitalization and appropriate tests established the diagnosis of diabetes mellitus. No other sequelae, such as carditis, were found.

The onset of diabetes thus appeared when G.R.S. was between 5½ and 6 years of age, just 3½ to 4 years after insulin had first been used in human diabetes mellitus.

Insulin had not been adopted generally by practitioners in the midwestern area then. Therefore, the initial treatment, according to the mother, was a starvation (Wilson) diet. Within the year following diabetes onset, that is in 1926 to 1927, G.R.S. was taken to the local medical school hospital where insulin administration was begun, in a small amount twice daily, with continued stringent dietary restriction. The parents began keeping a daily record of urine tests for sugar, insulin administered, and weight of all foods as planned each day and as eaten by G.R.S.

Late in 1928, according to the mother, G.R.S. became comatose from pneumonia and ketoacidosis. He was hospitalized under the care of an internist specializing in diabetes; his insulin was increased and, later, the diet.

No other episodes of hospitalization for ketoacidosis are known.

All food was still weighed as planned, as it had been since the initial diagnosis and continued to be until 1934.

In September 1932, when G.R.S. was 12, he began regular attendance at a small public school, in the sixth grade. He had been unable or not permitted to attend the first five grades, having been tutored at home. Thus, the first daily social contacts with his peers began in his 12th year. Even then, he did not play with other children during school recess, at his parents' and the physician's request, from fear of insulin reactions during exercise. For the same reason, he was excused from physical education classes in high school. He ate all meals at home, only three blocks from both the grade and high schools.

Although his intellectual development had proceeded unimpaired and possibly had been aided by the opportunities for omniverous reading, his social and emotional development had been retarded severely at a crucial period of maturation (ages 6 to 12 years). The patient fitted exactly the personality and emotional profile of the diabetic child so well described by Swift[11] in 1967 and by Birkbeck et al in 1968.[12]

In the summer of 1934, at the age of 14, G.R.S. first was taken to a Wisconsin medical clinic catering to diabetics. Physicians there believed that diabetes should be treated by a relatively high carbohydrate, relatively low fat, and normal protein diet with sufficient insulin for normal weight for age, height, and build. After validation of urine sugars by repeated blood sugar tests, both second specimen ante cibcum and 24 hour quantitative urine sugar levels were used to judge diabetic control. Both total food and total insulin were increased, when G.R.S. was entering the growth spurt of puberty.

For the first time, he was given some major responsibility for his treatment in terms of insulin self-administration, urine testing, and diet choice, which thereafter was estimated by household portions rather than by being weighed. The major factor was that he received adequate food and sufficient insulin for normal growth. It was, in a sense, a pre-Tolstoi regimen.

In 1936, at the age of 16 years, G.R.S. was one of a group of patients in whom the then experimental long-acting protamine insulin suspension was tried in the hospital, where he received his annual checkup. It was not successful for G.R.S. Except for the overnight period, he could be well controlled with thrice daily doses of regular (unmodified) insulin. However, while taking protamine insulin, he alternated between hyperglycemia with ketoacidosis and hypoglycemia. (This statement is based on finger-tip blood samples taken every two hours throughout the waking hours during the trial, as well as on frequent urine examinations, signs, and symptoms.)

By the age of 21 years, he had just entered medical school. He had increased the unmodified insulin dose to 30 units before each of the three major meals, a total of 90 units daily, with a diet increased calorically and relatively normal for distribution of carbohydrate, fat, and protein. There was a concommitant weight gain to 77.1 kg (170+ lb), which was excessive for his height of 69½ (176.5 cm) inches and his relatively slight frame.

Diabetic control continued generally good, as it had been throughout, in the sense of avoiding ketonuria and in maintaining a feeling of well-being and a productive life. He continued, as he had from the outset, to have overnight glycosuria, often 4+ or 2% but without ketonuria.

The errors of diabetic control, except for the overweight and the overnight glycosuria, were on the side of hypoglycemia during the waking hours.

The patient adjusted his insulin dose and total food intake downward during medical school so that body weight became and remained a more ideal 68 kg (150 lb).

In 1952, when G.R.S. was 32 years old, he began having severe daily insulin reactions in mid-afternoon. He then eliminated the prelunch insulin, and he was able thenceforth to the present to maintain fair to good control (except in early 1960 and in 1964) on two doses daily of unmodified insulin—one before breakfast and the second before dinner, without major alteration of diet except for a decrease in lunch calories and increase in bedtime food. Simultaneously with dropping the prelunch insulin, the overnight urine became aglycosuric, indicating that there had been an increase in the duration of activity of the unmodified insulin from its usual seven to eight hours to as much as 14 to 15 hours. (This was confirmed with blood sugar examinations at appropriate times.) Indeed, it then became necessary to take a midnight "meal" to prevent insulin reactions during sleep.

From at least high school age onward until late 1959 (age 39), G.R.S. had a relatively broad plateau of control between hyperglycemia-ketoacidosis on the one side and hypoglycemia-insulin shock on the other. Therefore, he was successful in managing his diabetes with a relatively casual attention. This permitted full time study and work until the onset of a more brittle diabetes at the age of 40 years.

Family History.—It is definitely known that there was no symptomatic diabetes mellitus in the parents, brother (at least to present age 56), three grandparents, or consanguinous uncles, aunts, and cousins. The maternal grandfather died prematurely in his sixth decade from a perforated appendix. All other consanguinous relatives (except the brother and cousins who are still in their fifth and sixth decades) lived into their eighth and ninth decades without developing overt diabetes. Insofar as is known, no glucose tolerance tests were done an any of them, except the brother.

The causes of most deaths were various forms of cancer, rather than cardiovascular, renal, or liver diseases.

Comment

The notable features of the G.R.S. case are as follows: (1) acute onset of diabetes mellitus followed severe infection with high fever at the age of 5½ years, with lack of diabetic genetic background; (2) the 40 years of diabetes with only a few peripheral tiny retinal microaneurysms after 27 to 28 diabetic years without other demonstrable changes in the following 13 years except for vitreous asteroid hyelosis unilaterally; (3) the use solely of unmodified insulin throughout the diabetes, except for three weeks at the age of 16 years of experimental trial of protamine insulin; (4) fair to good but less than ideal diabetic control during 18 hours of the day during the first 26 diabetic years, and throughout the 24 hour day thereafter except for two periods of several months each at the ages of 40 and 44 calendar years; (5) increased prolongation of activity of unmodified insulin after its multiple daily use for 26 years, permitting for the first time better 24 hour control of glycosuria thereafter; (6) development of a more labile or "brittle" form of diabetes after 35 years of the disease; (7) the lasting effects on emotional and social development following the early and continuing rigid control efforts and isolation from peers in childhood; (8) high fat low carbohydrate diet during the first eight diabetic years without apparent adverse vascular effects subsequently; and (9) development after 42+ diabetic years of proteinuria, indicating clinical renopathy, though with a surprising lack of progression in the following 14 months.

Some of these points warrant discussion in relation to recent medical literature on juvenile onset insulin-dependent diabetes.

MacLean and Ogilvie[13] in 1959 in a report on the pancreatic islet tissue of young diabetic subjects mentioned infection as a cause. John's review in 1949 of 500 juvenile onset diabetics also alludes to the role of infection in etiology.[14] Baumslag and Yodaiken[15] in 1968 emphasized the role of infection in diabetes etiology.

The common denominators among the two cases of 40 years' survival without complications of Blöch and Korp and the G.R.S. case are as follows: (1) prepubertal onset of diabetes; (2) strict, continuous, and generally successful attempts to control the diabetes from the onset; and (3) use of unmodified insulin continuously, begun shortly after onset.

In a case of diabetes of adult onset with 40 years' survival without complications reported by von Csapo and Hobi,[2] unmodified insulin was also used continuously from onset at the age of 26 years (1924) until the age of 63 years (1961) when therapy with protamine zinc insulin suspension was begun. He had also been strictly controlled with no coma, although acidosis and hypoglycemia appeared in the history. These authors wrote, "It is interesting that our patient until the recent few years used only unmodified insulin as did the patients of Blöch and Korp. The other 30 year diabetic without complications in our series also used only unmodified insulin."

It is noteworthy that of four cases, including G.R.S., of 40+ year diabetes survival without gross physical damage, all had at least fairly strict metabolic control and all used unmodified (regular) insulin. A case of 30 year survival with no complications[2] also used only unmodified insulin.

It is possible that lack of daily injection of a possible occult antigenic foreign protein in unmodified insulin could be an important factor for extreme longevity without damage in the diabetics cited. It seems entirely possible that daily introduction parenterally into the human body of a fish protein (protamine) or other foreign protein such as globin could, over a period of one to three decades (the usual interval in which diabetic angiopathies and neuropathies appear), produce some of the organ damage which has been attributed to the diabetic state itself. The reaction of the human organism to foreign protein even of another human is now well documented. What then of the body's reaction to tiny daily amounts of even more foreign a protein over decades of time? It appears to be a question worthy of further research at the cellular, macromolecular, and biochemical levels rather than merely in terms of retrospective case studies.

Belmonte[4] raised this question in 1963, when he wrote, ". . . some workers today fear that protamine itself may be related to the vascular complications through a hypersensitivity mechanism."

Cahill[16] in 1966 rather incidentally raised the same question when he wrote,

The author uses the lente type of insulin solely, but for the present primarily on theoretical grounds that the less antigen injected, the better. Therefore, according to theory, it is preferable to avoid immunizing adjuvants such as protamine or globin.

It does appear that a greater possibility exists for long survival of juvenile onset diabetics than one would infer from the literature on diabetes mellitus to date. For instance, Belmonte wrote in 1963,

Under optimum conditions, life expectancy of the juvenile onset diabetic is still only two thirds normal; within 20 years of the onset of diabetes, despite the best control, vascular complications begin to appear in the retina and kidneys.[4]

Davidson wrote as recently as 1968,

Life expectancy after diagnosis is three fourths normal life span. The rare patient lives 45 years; some have lived to age 60. Life expectancy is shortened for the juvenile diabetic by 20 to 25 years. The median age for death is 32 years.[6]

It is strange that in the 35 years since similar negative prognoses were published, there has been no general improvement. Perhaps the general use of protamine and globin modified insulins has not been harmless.

Continuous effort to maintain good metabolic control was offered as one of the common denominators in the long survivals without physical damage. Regarding the degree and efficacy of control by diet, insulin, and other regimentation, there first must be considered what constitutes good to excellent control. According to Joslin Clinic "Measures of Control," a mimeographed sheet accompanying White's 1969 letter to me, good chemical control consists of the following: normal blood glucose before meals, elevated blood glucose after meals, postcibal glycosuria but no more than 5% to 10% glucose in 24 hours in terms of dietary carbohydrate, zero to trace acetonemia, zero to trace acetonuria, normal lipids values, normal growth, normal endurance, and no symptoms.

Under these criteria, G.R.S.'s control would vary from good to fair. Except for not having a normal glucose level before breakfast and often excreting more than 10% of dietary carbohydrate in grams per 24 hour urine, G.R.S.'s control would qualify as good.

If, however, one adopts a more pragmatic attitude that good to excellent diabetic control permits normal adolescent growth, maintains body weight within reasonable limits of the normal in adulthood, prevents ketoacidotic coma as well as severe hypoglycemic episodes, and permits normal education and career activity, G.R.S. had such control. He had it during the first seven diabetic years except for school attendance, and after the 34th year to the present except for continuation of his full-time career.

Since his 35th diabetic year, G.R.S. has of necessity built his life around maintaining as closely as possible a physiological metabolic control. The resolution of the retinal hemorrhages after 1966, lack of progression of retinopathy since then, and lack of progression of proteinuria from January 1969 to March 1970 seem to justify this.

One might argue that the results themselves justify calling the more pragmatic definition good to excellent diabetic control, or one could speculate that the genetic endowment of G.R.S. (and of the other cases cited) made organ damage unlikely with almost any degree of diabetic control that maintained life.

In the G.R.S. case, the three tiny peripheral right retinal microaneurysms or scars and two similar left retinal lesions first seen in 1953 after 27 to 28 diabetic years were not regarded as "damage" because they remained unchanged until their disappearance in 1969. None of those seen previously were the site of retinal hemorrhage in 1966, after 40+ years of diabetes.

Several investigators have published information about retinal aneurysms in nondiabetic subjects.[17-19]

The increased duration of activity of unmodified (regular) insulin in G.R.S. beginning in 1952 (his 26th to 27th diabetic year) and continuing without interruption to date is a puzzle. The following might be considered as possible explanations: (1) slowed absorption from overuse of the same injection sites; (2) a change in the composition of the insulin, such as an increase in its zinc content, which could prolong its activity; (3) a change in the insulin standard unit; (4) decrease in need for exogenous insulin because of dietary changes, increased exercise, lessening of anxieties, aging, or other life style changes (but none of these apply in G.R.S.); and (5) greater serum protein binding as well as hepatic and tissue binding of the exogenous insulin with its subsequent slow release to the active form after the usual seven to eight hour period of activity of normal unmodified insulin.

None of these hypotheses are credible except possibly the fifth, and that cannot now be confirmed or refuted because there were no serum protein insulin binding studies in G.R.S. before the change in duration of insulin activity for comparison with subsequent studies.

Regarding the first hypothesis, the prolonged insulin activity continues to date despite repeated change of injection sites to virgin areas into which a needle has never entered, such as the inner aspects of the thighs and the abdominal fat below the umbilicus.

The second hypothesis was exploded by one drug company, whose regular insulin G.R.S. has used continuously since the late 1930's. A search by the company of their manufacturing records revealed that although a different method of crystallization had been initiated in 1951, it actually resulted in less total zinc content in the insulin than had been the case in the years 1945 to 1951.

The third hypothesis is refuted by Lacey[20] in a 1968 paper regarding lack of change in the international insulin standard.

The fourth and fifth hypotheses have been commented upon.

As for the increasing lability or "brittleness" in G.R.S.'s diabetes since early 1960, I have no explanation. Despite repeated appropriate laboratory examinations, there has at no time been evidence of any other endocrine disturbance, such as in thyroid or adrenal secretion, which could be a factor. Although some authors suggest overly zealous insulin therapy as a cause, that has not been the case in G.R.S., whose insulin dose declined appreciably in the 1956 to 1960 period (Table 3) preceding the increased lability. Molnar[21] and Gastineau[22] have written excellent papers about diabetic hyperlability.

Although there was a coincidental emotional depression in G.R.S. at the time of onset of increased lability, one cannot thereby establish a cause and effect relationship. The positive interrelationship of emotional factors and diabetic control has been remarked, perhaps best by Treuting.[10]

However, Molnar does not credit psychological factors as causes of lability. He wrote, in part, "We do not believe that lability is psychogenic but brittleness certainly can be aggravated as much by emotional oscillations and swings in mood as by all the physical stresses of life."[21]

The preceding comments about emotional factors leads into the final aspect of this paper. It is the impaired emotional and social growth of a child and adolescent diabetic by overrestrictive, too protective, and too anxious parents and physicians. The parents, in their natural desire to follow doctor's orders and to protect the child against the dangerous consequences of unexpected hypoglycemia away from home, literally isolated the child from play and school socialization opportunities with his normal peers. This happened almost completely with G.R.S. until the age of 12 years and to a greater rather than a lesser extent for some years beyond. Apparently in consequence, emotional and social maturity were delayed greatly as compared to intellectual maturity.

Although vicarious emotional and social experience of sorts may be acquired from reading, books cannot teach the many modes of nonverbal communication that children acquire unconsciously and without effort in play and schoolroom. Acceptable and nonacceptable offers and responses, as well as the range of normal responses, are learned by informal socializing with one's peers. Further, there may be critical ages for the easiest acquisition of such "common sense."

To a certain extent, the deprivation may not be entirely replaceable or repairable beyond these critical years. At least, that has been the experience of G.R.S.

This aspect of early juvenile onset diabetes, although not entirely neglected, has received far less attention than have the more tangible biochemical aspects. It is easy for the busy physician, especially one who is not especially interested in the emotional and social aspects of his patients' illnesses, to concentrate on the biochemical-physiological factors in his child diabetics, with little or no attention to the social and emotional immaturities he may be fostering by the restrictions imposed or by anxieties his remarks foster in the parents.

A few papers reveal some insight into the emotional aspects from the child's point of view, such as those by Treuting,[10] Swift,[11] and Pond.[23]

More than psychiatric attention, sympathetic counseling, and socialization episodes in summer diabetic camps may be required to prevent the social and emotional crippling which can occur in a diabetic child. In order for the child to achieve complete growth in all respects, some compromises with ideal diabetic dietary, insulin, and exercise restrictions appear to be not only defensible but desirable. Nor would these necessarily militate against the child attaining a long survival with no or relatively slight complications.

Weil[24] recognizes some of these aspects in his 1968 paper on current concepts in juvenile diabetes, which contains specific treatment recommendations, including the use of properly supervised self-selected diet by the child.

From the G.R.S. experience, it appears that one of the major problems is that after the child has been repeatedly overprotected, cautioned, and forbidden ardently desired activities which are normal ones for nondiabetic children, he reacts by taking advantage of his situation in the only way he can find. If he cannot, then he makes himself believe that he does not want to. So what had initially been externally imposed protective restrictions become unconscious internally imposed and often excessive restrictions. These can result in self-withdrawal and self-isolation.

Symptoms of these responses by G.R.S. as a child and adolescent diabetic included the following: chronic use of vague somatic complaints to avoid social involvements and responsibilities that became available (after he had lagged sufficiently behind peer development to make such involvements stressful or mutually hostile), mention of diabetic restrictions as global excuses against group playing and even school attendance, and exclusive pursuit of solitary hobbies or those which involved the child only with (nonthreatening) adults.

Summary

To my knowledge, this is the first case report in the English literature and the third in the world literature of a 40 year juvenile onset diabetic survival with no clinically demonstrable physical damage. Physical damage is used in a restricted sense. It is an in-depth study of and by a 50-year-old male physician, diabetic since the age of 5½ years. Only unmodified insulin has been used. This is suggested as a possible factor, with generally good metabolic control, in preventing damage. It is the common denominator with the two cases reported previously. Unmodified insulin has had a previously unreported prolongation of action during the past 18 years. Hyperlabile or "brittle" diabetes has occurred in the past ten years. Unusual psychological, emotional, and social problems may arise in a child diabetic due to overprotection by concerned parents. The parents must serve as a guide in overcoming some of these, while the child, himself, should be given some of the responsibility for directing his own care.

References

1. Blöch J, Korp W: Report of ten patients with a 40 year history of diabetes. *Wien Klin Wschr* **75**:378-380, 1963.
2. von Csapo G, Hobi M: Over 40 years existence of diabetes mellitus without specific complications. *Med Klin* **62**:871-872, 1967.
3. White P: Childhood diabetes. *Diabetes* **9**:345-355, 1960.
4. Belmonte MM: The future of the diabetic child. *Canad Med Assoc J* **88**:1112-1116, 1963.
5. Hirohata T: The natural history of diabetes (mortality). *Diabetes* **16**:875-881, 1967.
6. Davidson ET: Juvenile diabetes mellitus. *J Florida Med Assoc* **55**:209-211, 1968.
7. Chung Hsueh-Li, et al: Diabetes mellitus: A clinical analysis of 922 cases. *Chinese Med J* **81**:511-525, 1962.
8. Smith JL: Asteroid hyelitis and diabetes mellitus. *Trans Amer Acad Ophthal Otolaryng* **69**:269-278, 1965.
9. Luxenberg M, Sime D: Relationship of asteroid hyelosis to diabetes mellitus and plasma lipid levels. *Amer J Ophthal* **67**:406-413, 1969.
10. Treuting TF: Role of emotional factors in the etiology and course of diabetes mellitus: A review of recent literature. *Amer J Med Sci* **244**:93-109, 1962.
11. Swift CR: Adjustment problems in juvenile diabetes. *Psychosom Med* **29**:555-571, 1967.
12. Birkbeck JA, Klonoff H, McTaggart AH: Emotional disturbance in juvenile diabetics. *Diabetes* **17**:317-318, 1968.
13. MacLean N, Ogilvie RF: Observations on the pancreatic islet tissue of young diabetic subjects. *Diabetes* **8**:83-91, 1959.
14. John HJ: Diabetes mellitus in children: A review of 500 cases. *J Pediat* **35**:723-744, 1949.
15. Baumslag H, Yodaiken, RE: New perspectives in the family histories of juvenile diabetics. *Diabetes* **17**(suppl 1):316, 1968.
16. Cahill GF Jr: Some thoughts concerning the treatment of diabetes mellitus, in Ingelfinger FJ et al (eds): *Controversy in Internal Medicine*. Philadelphia, WB Saunders Co, 1966, pp 503-511.
17. Ashton N: Retinal microaneurysm in the non-diabetic subject. *Brit J Ophthal* **35**:189-211, 1951.
18. Wise GN: Retinal microaneurysms. *Arch Ophthal* **57**:151-156, 1957.
19. Chester EN, Banker BQ: Role of lipid thrombi in the pathogenesis of diabetic retinopathy. *Arch Intern Med* **120**:397-407, 1967.
20. Lacey AH: International insulin standards. *Diabetes* **17**:705-707, 1968.
21. Molnar GD: Observations on the etiology and therapy of "brittle" diabetes. *Canad Med Assoc J* **90**:953-959, 1964.
22. Gastineau CF: The care of unstable diabetes. *Maryland Med J* **17**:68-70, 1968.
23. Pond H: Special problems of diabetic child. *Practitioner* **200**:527-532, 1968.
24. Weil WB: Juvenile diabetes mellitus. *New Eng J Med* **278**:829-831, 1968.

Superinfection of an Amoebic Abscess by *Salmonella enteritidis*

J. Joseph Marr, MD, and MAJ Roderick C. Haff, MC, USAF, St. Louis

Hepatic abscess can be a difficult diagnosis in the evaluation of a fever of unknown origin. Recently an unusual example of superinfection of an amoebic abscess by *Salmonella enteritidis* was admitted to this hospital. This existence of concurrent infection by two such unusual and unrelated organisms provides another example of the enigma of *Salmonella* infections in general and demonstrates the ability of this organism to appear unexpectedly in areas of decreased host resistance in an otherwise healthy individual.

Patient Summary

The patient was a 20-year-old Negro man, admitted to the medical service, with fever of three weeks' duration.

Three weeks prior to admission to Barnes Hospital, he attempted to prevent a friend from falling down some stairs by leaning over a bannister and taking hold of his leg. The bannister pressed against the epigastrium and right upper quadrant of the patient's body, and for several moments he sustained the full weight of the other's 68 kg (150 lb). He felt well thereafter and thought no more of the incident until the following morning when he began to have some pain in the right upper chest and right shoulder. He was seen in the emergency room for this complaint and was told that he had "probably strained a muscle" and that the pain would resolve itself in several days. Approximately ten days later he began to have fever with increasing pain in the same area and an associated dry cough. He returned to the emergency room where a chest roentgenogram and complete blood cell count were unremarkable; he was thought to have a viral respiratory illness.

Two days later the fever became more severe, primarily at night; it was accompanied by a chilly sensation and sweating. These symptoms continued for approximately eight days. During this time the pain in his right chest and shoulder persisted and now had a distinctly pleuritic quality. He returned to the emergency room and was admitted.

His blood pressure was 110/70 mm Hg; pulse rate, 110 beats per minute and regular; respirations of 24 per minute were accompanied by splinting of the right chest. The physical examination was unremarkable except for his appearance, which was that of a severely ill Negro man and the findings of tenderness over the right shoulder, liver, and right flank areas. Diaphragmatic excursion was limited on that side, and the liver was diffusely enlarged to 3 fingerbreadths below the costal margin in the midclavicular line.

Laboratory values and hospital course are recorded in Fig 1. The urine was normal. The chemical profile was within normal limits, with the exception of an alkaline phosphatase value of 20 King-Armstrong units and a serum glutamic oxaloacetic transaminase (SGOT) value of 70 units. The bilirubin and blood urea nitrogen values were normal.

Fluoroscopy of the chest showed the diaphragm to be elevated and restricted in movement. A large filling defect in the right posterolateral portion of the liver was observed on the scan obtained after injection of 2 millicuries of colloidal form of indium ^{113m}In (Fig 2, *left* and *center*).

Because of the possibility of an amoebic abscess, the patient was treated with chloroquine phosphate for 24 hours prior to aspiration of the liver; the following day 150 cc of red-brown purulent material were removed (Fig 2, *right*). A microscopic examination of this material showed only necrotic tissue and gram-negative bacilli in clumps. After the institution of broad-spectrum antibiotic therapy, open drainage was undertaken through the bed of the 11th rib in the posterior axillary line, with the use of a large rubber tube. A biopsy of the wall of the abscess was performed and cultures were obtained for bacteria and amebae. During the procedure there was bleeding from the hepatic parenchyma which required replacement with 4 units of whole blood during the next 24-hour period.

Thereafter, he improved steadily with a slow resolution of the fever over a period of several days and a decrease in liver size and tenderness. Culture and sugar fermentation tests made on the organism indicated that it was a *Salmonella*, group-D. When these results were obtained, administration of cephalothin sodium (Keflin) and gentamicin sulfate was discontinued and ampicillin sodium, 1 gm, four times a day, was begun. Subsequent serotyping confirmed the organism as *S enteritidis* (Table 1). Because smear and

Received for publication July 9, 1970; accepted Dec 15.

From the departments of medicine and surgery, Washington University School of Medicine and the Barnes Hospital, St. Louis.

The views expressed herein are those of the authors and do not reflect the views of the Air University, the US Air Force, or the Department of Defense.

Reprint requests to Department of Internal Medicine, Washington University School of Medicine, Barnes and Wohl hospitals, 4550 Scott Ave, St. Louis 63110 (Dr. Marr).

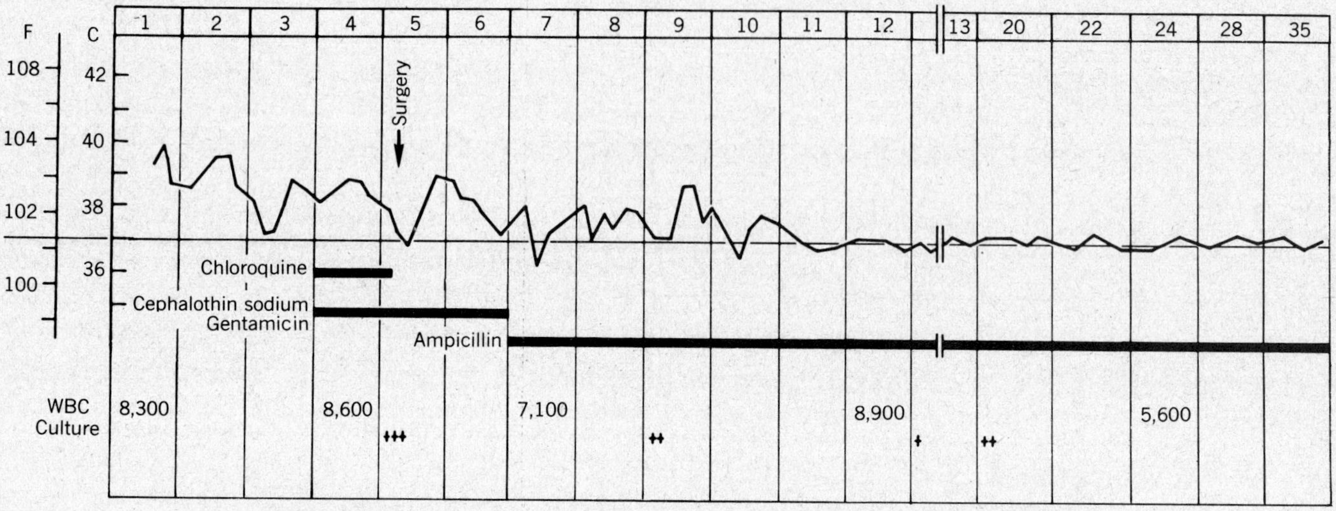

Fig 1.—Hospital course. Arrow indicates time of surgical drainage of abscess; white blood cell counts and duration of positive cultures from the abscess drainage are indicated.

Table 1.—Phase 1 Antigenic Type of the Patient's Organism

Somatic Studies	
Polyvalent	Positive
Polyvalent	Positive
Group D	Positive
All others	Negative

Flagellar Studies

Phase 1		Phase 2
Polyvalent	Positive	None present
Polyvalent B	Positive	
G complex	Positive	
Group g	Positive	
Group m	Positive	
All other groups	Negative	

Table 2.—Composite of Serologic Studies During Hospital Course*

	S typhi		*S enteritidis*		*E histolytica*	
Hospital Day	Somatic	Flagellar	Somatic	Flagellar	HA	CF
1	80	0	20	20	4,096	8
3	640	0	160	20		
7	640	0	160	80		
14	1,280	0	320	160		
22	1,280	0	320	160		
28	640	0	320	160	4,096	
31	640	0	320	160		

* Titers are expressed as the reciprocal of the serum dilution.

Fig 2.—Hepatic scan, posterior (left) *and lateral* (center) *view, done prior to aspiration of the abscess.* Right, *Upright abdominal roentgenogram taken after aspiration of the abscess.*

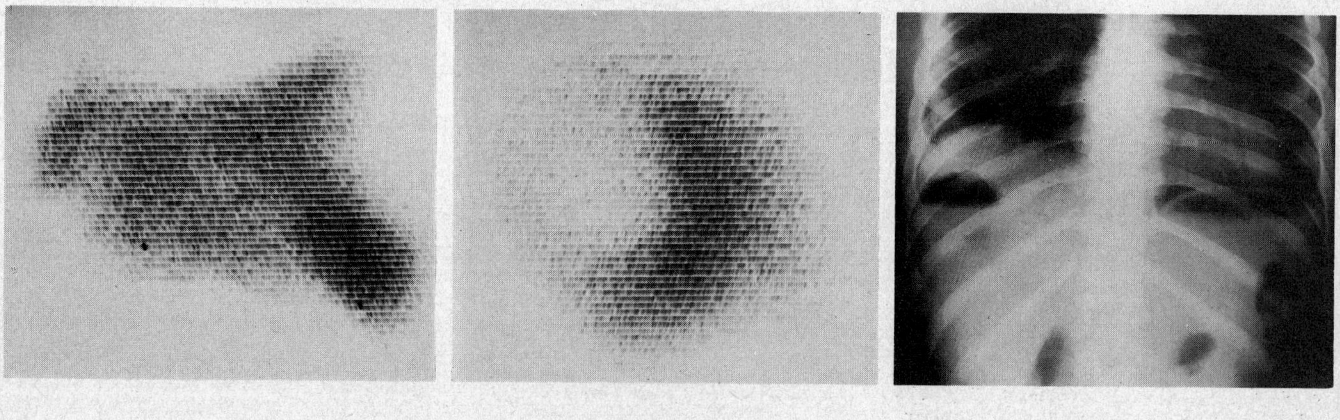

culture of the abscess material revealed only bacteria, it was believed that the lesion was a pyogenic abscess. Chloroquine therapy was therefore discontinued.

Six days following the drainage of the abscess, the patient was afebrile and remained clinically well, although organisms were recovered from the wound for the next three weeks. Serologic studies drawn on admission and at several points during his convalescence are indicated in Table 2. Neither *Entameba histolytica* nor *S enteritidis* was cultured from the stool. A second liver scan on the tenth hospital day showed a marked decrease in the cavity. Serial upright roentgenograms of the abdomen demonstrated almost complete disappearance of air in the liver when the drainage tube was removed on the 31st hospital day.

On the 21st hospital day the report of the elevated amebic antibody titer (Table 2) was received. At that time, despite his improving clinical status, he was treated for amebiasis with chloroquine phosphate, 250 mg, three times a day, with a total of 11 gm, and tetracycline hydrochloride, 500 mg, four times a day, for two weeks.

Comment

Upon review of the patient's history and serologic data, we believe that the probable sequence of events was inapparent infection with *E histolytica,* hemorrhage into the abscess following trauma, and then secondary bacterial infection. The sudden appearance of pain in a previously asymptomatic hepatic abscess subsequent to trauma is a phenomenon well recognized in the tropical medicine literature.[1]

The markedly elevated amebic hemagglutination titer (HA) and the presence of a complement-fixation (CF) titer of 1:8 lend support to the diagnosis of extraintestinal amebiasis.[2,3] Extensive evaluation of the serologic tests for diagnosis of amebiasis have shown that HA titers of this magnitude, in the absence of gastrointestinal symptoms, are obtained only in extraintestinal amebiasis.[2] Apparently false-positive HA titers occur but are rare and not of this magnitude.[4] The presence of an elevated CF titer establishes that the infection was probably less than a year or two in duration.[2] The inability to culture the protozoan (Tsuchiya's egg medium) and the failure to find the organism in the abscess wall with PAS stains do not militate against amoebae being the factor in its inception. The absence of culture or biopsy evidence for amoebic infection is most likely the result of the bacterial superinfection. Amoebic abscesses will at times become sterile in the absence of superinfection, presumably due to the presence of the amoebic histiolytic enzymes and the acid pH. However, when superinfection by bacteria occurs, the amoebae are almost invariably destroyed and evidence of their former presence is lost.[1]

The source for the amoebic infection is unknown: neither the patient's wife nor child had serologic or cultural evidence of infection by *Salmonella* or *Entameba.* He has not been out of the country, nor even out of the St. Louis area. The last reported recovery of *E histolytica* in this area was in April 1969, the only case of symptomatic amebiasis in the last five years.

The nature of the secondary bacterial invader is of some interest. *Salmonella* are not usually present in hepatic abscess and a review of the English literature yields only four other documented cases. The first was in a 29-year-old Chinese man in 1934[5] and the second in a 24-year-old African man in 1952.[6] In both of these instances the infecting organism was *S enteritidis.* A third report by Joseph et al[7] mentioned an hepatic abscess due to *S arizona,* and Essien et al[8] described the superinfection of an hepatic amoebic abscess by a *Salmonella.*

Identification of the organism as a Salmonellae, group-D, was made by the appropriate fermentation tests. The demonstration that it was *S enteritidis* was made possible by the presence of phase 1 specific antigens (Table 1). Because *S enteritidis* and *S typhi* have mutual somatic antigens, the serum titer against the latter organism was determined concurrently with that against the patient's organism (Table 2). The expected concomitant rise in antibody titer against the somatic antigens of *S typhi* was observed, although the rise was significantly less than that to the somatic antigens of *S enteritidis.* However, the rise in antibody titer to the H antigen of the patient's organism with a persistently negative titer to the flagellar antigen of *S typhi* eliminates the possibility of an acute infection by the latter.

Salmonella have been found to cause localized infections in virtually every part of the body, although in review of 7,779 cases of infections with these organisms only 572, or 7%, were focal.[9] Abscesses were found in one-fourth of these, and most were directly or indirectly connected to the gastrointestinal tract as perirectal, perineal, subphrenic, or periappendical abscesses. Others were found in the brain, lungs, skin, spleen, and middle ear. The development of secondary infection in retention cysts of the kidney, corpus luteum cysts, ovarian cysts, uterine myomata and carcinomas, and pheochromocytomas has also been described.[10] However, a review of the mentioned literature and several other series of *Salmonella* infections[9,11-14] has failed to reveal any mention of liver abscess.

It is of interest that the leukocyte

count in this patient did not vary and was never out of the normal range. This is, of course, characteristic for *Salmonella* infection but clearly unusual for primary amoebic abscess. The average white blood cell count for amoebic abscess is in the range of 15,000/cu mm in several series.[15,16]

The propensity of *Salmonella* organisms to localize in areas of decreased resistance is generally appreciated; however, none of the reviews already mentioned describes this organism in the liver parenchyma. Furthermore, it is rather remarkable that *S enteritidis* and *S arizona* should be found, since they are relatively uncommon pathogens for man although prevalent in poultry and rodents. The vast majority of gastrointestinal *Salmonella* infections of man in the United States are due to *S typhimurium*[17] and *S enteritidis* in second or third place in order of frequency. However, extraintestinal focal infections or septicemias only rarely involve organisms other than *S typhimurium* or the *S paratyphi* group.[9,14] Thus it would be presumed, based on prevalence of *Salmonella*, that *S enteritidis* would not be a likely secondary invader of man in three of these instances.

The only other series of *Salmonella* infections with any liver parenchymal involvement is that of Osler.[18] In his personal experience of 1,500 infections, three had hepatic abscesses. He described them as due to *S typhosa*. However, in view of the cross-reaction of *S enteritidis* with *S typhosa* one might speculate that these also may have been due to *S enteritidis*, since serologic typing at that time was not developed enough to allow one to make the distinction.

The treatment employed in this instance was that of broad spectrum antibiotic therapy prior to drainage, and specific therapy after cultures were obtained. The drainage procedure was extraserosal; we believe it to be the method of choice. The emphasis in the surgical literature has been toward transperitoneal drainage,[7] but because of the possibility of amoebic abscess the extraserosal method was employed.

Finally, it was of interest that the wound continued to yield *S enteritidis* for 3½ weeks despite adequate amounts of ampicillin. This persistence is in keeping with the well-known ability of members of the *Salmonella* genus to persevere despite specific antimicrobial therapy. Although the drug may have curtailed the dissemination of these organisms it would appear that it had no influence on the rate at which they were eradicated from the abscess.

Summary

A young man suffered trauma to an asymptomatic hepatic amoebic abscess. This abscess subsequently became superinfected with *S enteritidis.*

Localized infections by *Salmonella* are somewhat unusual, and documented instances of liver infection are rare. Moreover, those organisms which have been described in hepatic abscesses have been relatively uncommon pathogens for man. The possible significance of this is unknown.

Salmonella enteritidis persisted in the drainage tract for 3½ weeks despite adequate chemotherapy. The drug had apparently little influence on the rate at which the organisms were eradicated from the abscess.

References

1. Manson-Bahr P: Amoebic abscess of the liver: Its diagnosis and treatment. *Proc Roy Soc Med* **25**:1-10, 1931.
2. Kessell JF, Lewis WP, Pasquel CM, et al: Indirect hemagglutination and complement fixation tests in amebiasis. *Amer J Trop Med Hyg* **14**:540-549, 1965.
3. Milgram EA, Healy GR, Kagan IG: Studies on the use of the indirect hemagglutination test in the diagnosis of amebiasis. *Gastroenterology* **50**:645-649, 1966.
4. Healy GR: The specificity of the indirect hemagglutination test in the immunodiagnosis of amebiasis in temperate North America. *J Parasit* **56**:427, 1970.
5. Hah-Liong L: *Salmonella enteritidis* in liver abscess. *Chinese Med J* **49**:577-580, 1935.
6. Hirschowitz BI: Pyogenic liver abscess: A review with a case report of a solitary abscess caused by *Salmonella enteritidis. Gastroenterology* **21**:291-299, 1952.
7. Joseph WC, Kahn AM, Longmire WP: Pyogenic liver abscess. *Amer J Surg* **115**:63-68, 1968.
8. Essien EM, Ahimic HS, Laja AO: *Salmonella typhi* in amoebic liver abscess. *W Afr Med J* **14**:121-124, 1965.
9. Saphra I, Winter JW: An evaluation of 7,779 human infections at the New York Salmonella Center. *New Eng J Med* **236**:1128-1134, 1957.
10. Bennett IL, Hook EW: Infectious disease: Some aspects of salmonellosis. *Ann Rev Med* **10**:1-20, 1959.
11. Han T, Sokal JE, Neter E: Salmonellosis in disseminated malignant diseases. *New Eng J Med* **276**:1045-1052, 1967.
12. MacReady RA, Reardon JR, Saphra I: Salmonellosis in Massachusetts. *New Eng J Med* **256**:1121-1128, 1957.
13. Black PH, Kunz LV, Swartz MN: Salmonellosis: A review of some unusual aspects. *New Eng J Med* **262**:811, 864, 921, 1960.
14. Baker MP, Bragdon JH: Septicemia due to *Salmonella enteritidis. New Eng J Med* **237**:175-179, 1947.
15. Manson-Bahr P, Willoughby H: On the leucocyte count in liver abscess. *Trans Roy Soc Trop Med Hyg* **22**:465-467, 1929.
16. Ochsner A, DeBakey M, Murray S: Pyogenic abscess of the liver. *Amer J Surg* **40**:292-319, 1938.
17. *Salmonella Surveillance.* National Communicable Disease Center, 1965-1969.
18. Osler WO: *The Principles and Practice of Medicine*, ed 7. New York, D Appleton & Co, 1909, pp 57-105.

Retroperitoneal Fibrosis

Response to Corticosteroid Therapy

Luigi P. Morandi, MD, and Peter J. Grob, MD, Zurich, Switzerland

Retroperitoneal fibrosis was first described by Albarran[1] in 1905 and defined as a disease entity by Ormond[2] in 1948. Despite the fact that many cases have since been observed and reviewed,[3-7] the etiology, pathogenesis, and natural history of this disorder remain obscure and therapy is still the subject of discussion.

We report on two patients with retroperitoneal fibrosis presenting as outstanding features prompt regression of symptoms after treatment with corticosteroids. In one patient this effect was observed repeatedly during a relapsing course of the disease during a period of 11 years with involvement of both ureters and an iliac vein.

Patient Summaries

PATIENT 1.—An office employee had a *first episode* of right flank pain in December 1958 at the age of 52 years. Past history disclosed rheumatic fever at the age of 28 years, with resulting stenosis of the aortic valve. Thyroidectomy was performed because of toxic goiter at the age of 47 years. An excretory urogram showed slight medial deviation of the right ureter. Treatment with 30 mg of prednisone daily led to the disappearance of pain within days. Prednisone administration was slowly reduced and discontinued four weeks after initiation of therapy.

A *second episode* of pain in the right flank began in April 1959. The intravenous urogram of June 24, 1959, disclosed a medial deviation and constriction of the upper part of both ureters with a bilateral hydronephrosis which was more pronounced on the right side. Exploratory laparotomy revealed a dense fibrotic mass anterior to the lumbar spine, which enclosed the great vessels and the ureters. Histological examination of this material showed a nonspecific, chronic, slightly fibrosing inflammation with lymphadenitis and perilymphadenitis (Fig 1), which established the diagnosis of retroperitoneal fibrosis. The patient was then given daily doses of 3 mg of dexamethasone. Again, the pain disappeared within days. One month later the intravenous urogram was nearly normal. The drug regimen was maintained for 17 months, the dosage was slowly reduced to 0.5 mg/day, and finally discontinued. No signs of disease could be detected in the following years; the repeatedly performed urograms and results of urinalyses were normal.

A *third episode* occurred in May 1966 (5½ years after cessation of dexamethasone therapy) the patient became aware of an increasing swelling of the left leg. His general condition deteriorated and pain occurred in the left lumbar region and left hypogastrium. The excretory urogram (July 1966) disclosed a slight hydronephrosis on the left side and a dilatation of the proximal part of the left ureter. A narrowing of the left external iliac vein with reflux could be detected by phlebography (Fig 2). As seen by lymphography, the lymph nodes of the pelvic and left inguinal region were slightly enlarged. In July 1966, dexamethasone therapy was resumed with a dosage of 3 mg/day. Pain, swelling of the left leg, and the palpable mass in the hypogastrium disappeared within days. The excretory urogram performed 51 days later revealed normal findings. Similarly, the phlebogram done six months later presented almost normal aspects of the formerly affected external iliac vein. However, in October 1967, while treated with dexamethasone at a maintenance dosage of 0.5 mg/day, pain reappeared, but this time on the right flank. An excretory urogram showed a poor concentration of dye in the right kidney. A constriction of the right ureter of 1 cm length, at the upper border of the second sacral vertebra was demonstrated by a retrograde pyelogram. The dosage of dexamethasone was raised from 0.5 to 3 mg daily, whereupon the pain subsided. A pyelogram performed six weeks after readjustment of therapy was normal. Therefore, dexamethasone was slowly reduced, then maintained at a dose of 1 mg and withdrawn in August 1968, 25 months after initiation of therapy. The patient has since been free from fibrosis-related symptoms.

Concomitant Diseases.—Since 1959 the patient suffered from anginal pain of varying intensity and since 1968 he showed signs of left ventricular failure. In November 1969, a severe postrheumatic aortic stenosis was successfully corrected by insertion of a Starr-Edwards prosthesis and obstruction of the left anterior descending coronary branch was relieved by a bypass procedure. Biopsy material of heart muscle, pericardium, and epicardium taken at this occasion showed no fibrosis.

PATIENT 2.—A business man was first hospitalized in February 1970 at the age of 65 years with the chief complaint of bilateral flank pain. The pain had become increasingly severe since October 1969. The intravenous urogram disclosed a nonfunctioning right kidney and a slight hydronephrosis on the left side due to a compression in the upper third part of the ureter. A surgical exploration of the right ureter revealed a dense, fibrotic mass enclosing the ureter, the iliac vein, and all of the neighboring structures. Histological examination of biopsy material showed a nonspecific slightly fibrosing inflammation with abundant lymphocytes and plasma cells predominantly around blood vessels. Treatment with 60 mg of prednisone was followed by disappearance of pain within days. An intravenous urogram performed five weeks after initiation of therapy was almost normal, except for a moderate hydronephrosis of the formerly nonfunctioning right kidney. Since March 1970 the patient has been maintained on a

Received for publication July 29, 1970; accepted Nov 25.
From the Department of Internal Medicine, University Hospital, Zurich, Switzerland.
Reprint requests to Department of Medicine, University Hospital, 8006 Zurich, Switzerland (Dr. Grob).

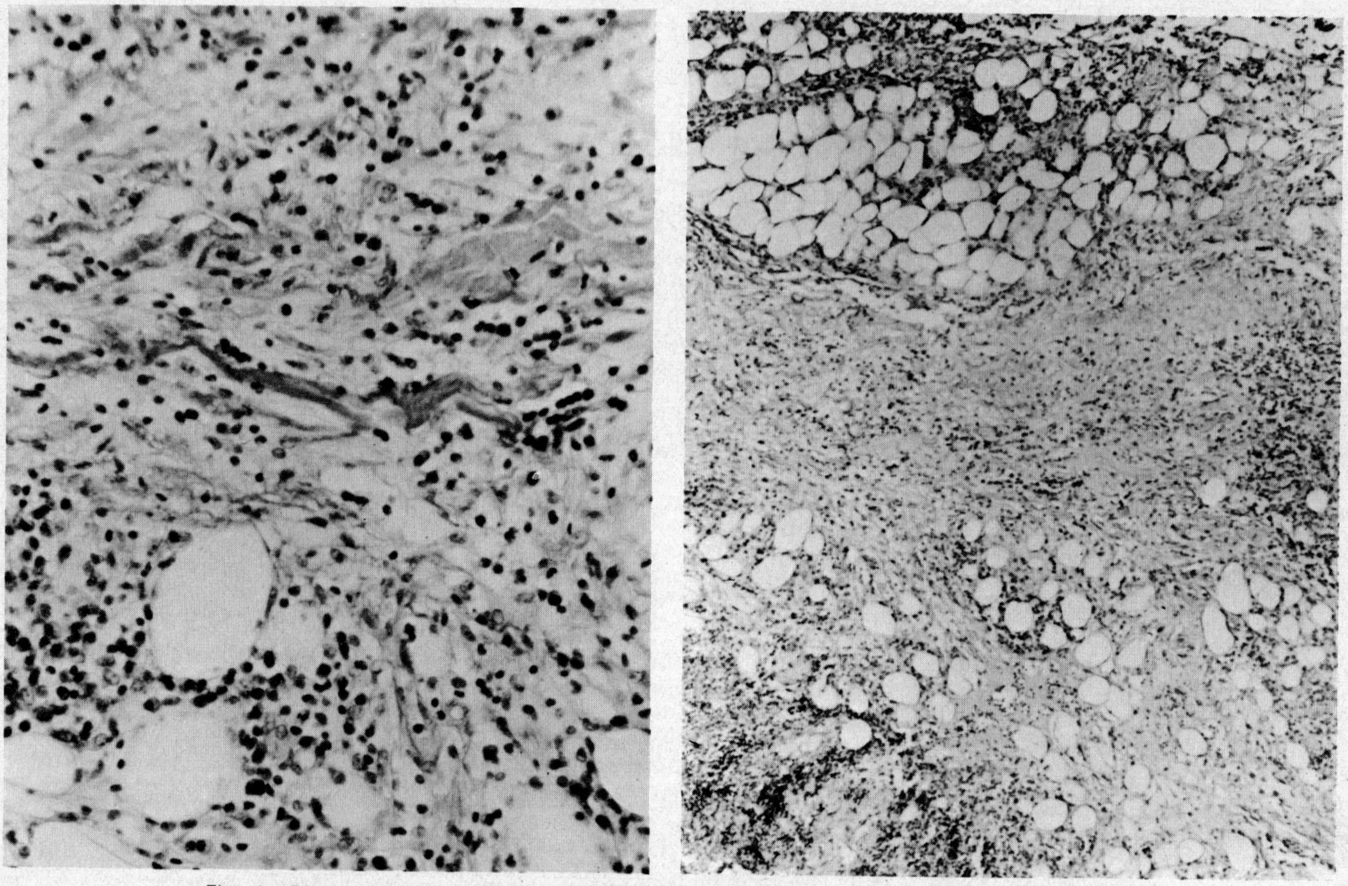

Fig 1.—Biopsy specimen (July 1959). Right, *Fine-fibrillar fibrosis and lymphoplasmacellular infiltration between two lobules of fatty tissue (Van Gieson, ×100).* Left, *Fibrosis and lymphoplasma cellular infiltration between bands of connective tissue (hematoxylin-eosin, ×360).*

regimen of 30 mg of prednisone and is without symptoms.

Further Examinations.—The sedimentation rate was elevated in both cases during the acute stages of the disease and remained so for months even after symptoms subsided. Immunoelectrophoreses of serum proteins gave normal findings. The serum immunoglobulins and β_1C levels were within normal limits when assayed by radioimmune diffusion technique. Repeated latex fixation tests for rheumatoid factor and passive hemagglutination tests for antithyroglobulin were negative, as were indirect immunofluorescence tests for the detection of antinuclear antibodies and of antibodies against parietal gastric cells, thyroideal tissue, and fibrous material.

The immunofluorescence test for the detection of tissue-bound γ-globulin and complement on biopsy material obtained during surgical intervention on the heart in patient 1 (November 1969) revealed no pathological findings. Similar tests on biopsy material of diseased tissue in patient 2 were difficult to interpret since nonspecific fluorescence was very strong due to abundant elastic and fibrous material.

Comment

In the first patient an *intermittent course* of the disease is presented with subsequent involvement of both ureters at different sites and of the left external iliac vein. Similar observations have been described by Raper[3] in a case with subsequent involvement of the ureters, the common bile duct, and the aorta within an 11-year period and by Kay[8] in a case with subsequent involvement of the ureters, the iliac vein, and the vena cava within a 7-year period. These observations are contradictory to the view[9] that retroperitoneal fibrosis is a self-limiting disease. Involvement of various organs such as arteries,[5,10-14] veins,[12,14-16] duodenum,[16] mesocolon, and colon[17] is not unusual and depends on the extent of the fibrotic process.

Retroperitoneal fibrosis is commonly treated by surgery or by surgery combined with corticosteroids.[7] Therefore, relatively little is known about the efficacy of corticosteroids alone, and respective data are contradictory. Some authors described positive effects[18-23] while others could see none.[24-27] In our patients, the effectiveness of *corticosteroid* seemed to be confirmed by the repeatedly observed normalization of the pyelograms and the rapid disappearance of clinical symptoms. A relapse occurring during treatment of patient 1 could be controlled by increasing the dosage. Disagreeing views on the effectiveness of corticosteroids may be due to the fact that therapy was initiated at varying stages of the disease. Buckberg and co-workers[28] described a prompt response to corticosteroids in a case presenting abundant cellular infiltration of involved tissue, but found no beneficial effect in those cases where hyaline fibrosis was predominant. In our patients, the histological picture was characterized by abundant cellular elements. This suggested an early stage of the disease. Varying therapeutic effects could also be due to different schedules of treatment. As demonstrated by the history of the first patient, acute attacks may occur if medication is not continued long enough.

An evaluation of the effectiveness of any kind of treatment for retroperitoneal fibrosis is also hampered by the fact that spontaneous regression of symptoms has been described.[18,29-32] For this reason, it is difficult to evaluate the significance of apparent steroid-induced remission with certainty.

Etiology and pathogenesis of idiopathic retroperitoneal fibrosis are still obscure. Its concomitant occurrence with sclerosing cholangitis,[33-35] in combination with sclerosing mediastinitis,[28,36-38] and with Riedel's struma,[33,35,39,40] has led to the assumption that retroperitoneal fibrosis might represent a manifestation of a systemic disease of connective tissues. Comings and co-workers[35] described the occurrence of these manifestations in two brothers from a first-cousin marriage. They used the term "multifocal fibrosclerosis" and suggested a genetic etiology.

Retroperitoneal fibrosis has also been described with a concomitant, massive perivascular fibrosis in the region of the aorta and the coronary arteries[41,42] and with generalized arteritis including a marked involvement of the coronary arteries.[43] In our first patient, coronary arteries were also affected but there is no evidence as to a relationship with the fibrotic process.

Some observations point to possible connections of retroperitoneal fibrosis and autoimmune diseases. Thus, in isolated cases the following diseases have been observed in association with retroperitoneal fibrosis: lupus erythematosus,[44] periarteritis nodosa,[9] disseminated vasculitis and membranoproliferative glomerulonephritis,[45] intrahepatic sclerosing cholangitis,[46] and a case of Raynaud's disease and pulmonary fibrosis in the presence of antinuclear factors in the bood.[47]

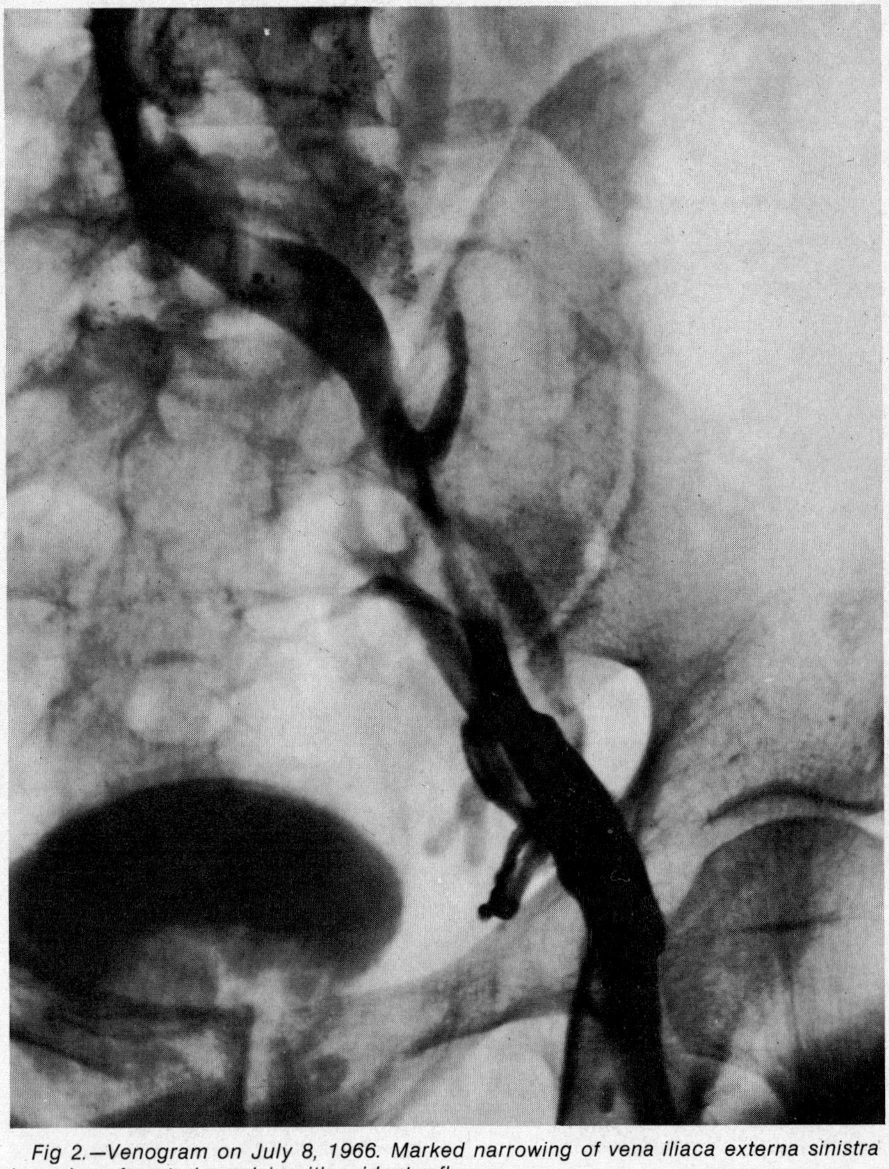

Fig 2.—Venogram on July 8, 1966. Marked narrowing of vena iliaca externa sinistra in region of posterior pelvis with evident reflux.

In this respect it is of interest that hydralazine may induce syndromes resembling lupus erythematosus, periarteritis nodosa, as well as retroperitoneal fibrosis. This suggests a common pathogenic mechanism.[48,49] Also methysergide (Sansert) is known to induce retroperitoneal fibrosis.[49] Our patients have, however, not been treated with one of these drugs and routine immunological tests revealed no abnormalities. Thus, evidence for the immunopathogenic mechanism is still lacking for this mysterious disease.

Summary

Two patients with retroperitoneal fibrosis are described who showed prompt regression of symptoms after treatment with corticosteroids. In one of these patients this effect was observed repeatedly during a relapsing course of the disease during a period of 11 years with subsequent involvement of both ureters at different sites and an iliac vein. Cellular elements were abundant in the affected tissue of both patients, which suggested an early stage of the disease. Routine immunologic examinations gave no evidence for an immunopathogenic basis of this disease.

References

1. Albarran J: Rétention rénale par périuréterite: Libération externe de l'uretère. *Assoc Franc d'Urol* p 511-517, 1905.
2. Ormond JK: Bilateral ureteral obstruction due to envelopment and compression by inflammatory retroperitoneal process. *J Urol* **59**:1072-1079, 1948.
3. Raper FP: Idiopathic retroperitoneal fibrosis involving the ureters. *Brit J Urol* **28**:436-446, 1956.
4. Dineen JP, Asch T, Pearce JM: Retroperitoneal fibrosis: An anatomic and radiologic review with a report of four new cases and an explanation of pathogenesis. *Radiology* **75**:380-390, 1960.
5. Ormond JK: Idiopathic retroperitoneal fibrosis: An established clinical entity. *JAMA* **174**:1561-1568, 1960.
6. Utz DC, Henry JD: Retroperitoneal fibrosis. *Med Clin N Amer* **50**:1091-1099, 1966.
7. Jones JN, Ross EJ, Matz LR, et al: Retroperitoneal fibrosis. *Amer J Med* **48**:203-208, 1970.
8. Kay RG: Retroperitoneal vasculitis with perivascular fibrosis. *Brit J Urol* **35**:284-291, 1963.
9. Ormond JK: Idiopathic retroperitoneal fibrosis: A discussion of the etiology. *J Urol* **94**:385-390, 1965.
10. Furlong JH, Connerty HV: Compression of the aorta and ureters by a retroperitoneal inflammatory mass. *Delaware Med J* **30**:63-67, 1958.
11. Larson RE, Ross JV: Intermittent claudication secondary to idiopathic fibrous retroperitonitis: Report of an unusual case. *Circulation* **28**:1145-1148, 1963.
12. Hackett E: Idiopathic retroperitoneal fibrosis: A condition involving the ureters, the aorta, and the inferior vena cava. *Brit J Surg* **46**:3-9, 1958.
13. Perlow S: Obstruction of the iliac artery caused by retroperitoneal fibrosis. *Amer J Serg* **105**:285-287, 1963.
14. Schaefer HC, Varughese G, Klein E, et al: Vascular manifestations of idiopathic retroperitoneal fibrosis. *Amer J Surg* **111**:257-261, 1966.
15. Hinshaw HC, Rutledge DI: Lesions in superior mediastinum which interfere with venous circulation. *J Lab Clin Med* **27**:905-916, 1942.
16. Schneider CF: Idiopathic retroperitoneal fibrosis producing venacaval, biliary, ureteral and duodenal obstructions. *Ann Surg* **159**:316-320, 1964.
17. Leffall LD, White JE, Mann M: Retroperitoneal fibrosis: Two unusual cases. *Arch Surg* **89**:1070-1076, 1964.
18. Hawk WS, Hazard JB: Sclerosing retroperitonitis and sclerosing mediastinitis. *Amer J Clin Path* **32**:321-334, 1959.
19. Raper FP: Idiopathic retroperitoneal fibrosis involving the ureters. *Proc Roy Soc Med* **53**:690-691, 1960.
20. O'Regan R, Treahy PA, Prior IAM: Idiopathic retroperitoneal fibrosis: A case presenting with renal failure, treated effectively with adrenal steroids. *New Zeal Med J* **60**:518-554, 1961.
21. Morandi L, Camponovo F, Siebenmann R: Corticosteroid-therapie bei der chronischen fibrosierenden Retroperitonitis (sogenannte retroperitoneale Fibrose). *Schweiz Med Wschr* **93**:1409-1414, 1963.
22. Shaheen DJ, Johnston A: Bilateral ureteral obstruction due to envelopment and compression by an inflammatory retroperitoneal process: Report of two cases. *J Urol* **82**:51-57, 1959.
23. Stueber PJ: Primary retroperitoneal inflammatory process with ureteral obstruction. *J Urol* **82**:41-50, 1959.
24. Harrow BR, Sloane JA: Idiopathic retroperitoneal fibrosis. *JAMA* **182**:38-43, 1962.
25. Patoir G, Spy E, Proye C: Fibrose rétropéritonéale. *J Chir* **85**:23-37, 1963.
26. Eiseman B, Yech KS: Portal hypertension with idiopathic retroperitoneal fibrosis. *Brit J Surg* **50**:225-227, 1962-1963.
27. Cibert J, Durand L, Riviere C: Les compressions uretérales par sclérose du tissue cellulo-adipeux péri-uretéral "périuretérites primitives." *J Urol Med Chir* **62**:705-733, 1956.
28. Buckberg GD, Dilley RB, Longmire WP: The protean manifestations of sclerosing fibrosis. *Surg Gynec Obstet* **123**:729-736, 1966.
29. Benfield JR, Harrison RW, Moulder PV, et al: Bilateral nodular pulmonary granulomas and retroperitoneal fibrosis: Simulated metastatic malignant neoplasm and spontaneous remission of ureteral obstruction. *JAMA* **182**:579-581, 1962.
30. Mahoney EM, Edwards EA: Spontaneous regression of leg edema and hydronephrosis following idiopathic retroperitoneal fibrosis. *Amer J Surg* **103**:514-517, 1962.
31. Lund F, Pedersen J: Periureteritis fibrosa (Gerota's fascitis). *Acta Med Scand* **167**:105-109, 1960.
32. Thompson RJ, Carter R, Gibson LD, et al: Acute idiopathic retroperitoneal fibrosis. *Ann Surg* **153**:399-406, 1961.
33. Haché L, Utz DC, Woolner LB: Idiopathic fibrous retroperitonitis. *Surg Gynec Obstet* **115**:737-744, 1962.
34. Bartholomew LG, Cain JC, Woolner LB, et al: Sclerosing cholangitis: Its possible association with Riedel's struma and fibrous retroperitonitis: Report of two cases. *New Eng J Med* **269**:8-12, 1963.
35. Comings DE, Skubi KB, Van Eyes J, et al: Familial multifocal fibrosclerosis. *Ann Intern Med* **66**:884-892, 1967.
36. Hawk WA, Hazard JB: Sclerosing retroperitonitis and sclerosing mediastinitis. *Amer J Clin Path* **32**:321-334, 1959.
37. Cameron DG, Ing ST, Boyle M, et al: Idiopathic mediastinal and retroperitoneal fibrosis. *Canad Med Assoc J* **85**:227-323, 1961.
38. Morgan AD, Loughridge LW, Calne RY: Combined mediastinal and retroperitoneal fibrosis. *Lancet* **1**:67-70, 1966.
39. Pesch KJ, Kracht J: Retroperitoneale Fibrose bei Myxöden. *Frankfurt Z Path* **73**:97-99, 1963.
40. Turner-Warwick R, Nabarro JDN, Doniach D: Riedel's thyroiditis and retroperitoneal fibrosis. *Proc Roy Soc Med* **59**:12-14, 1966.
41. Reed WG, Stinely RW: Massive periaortic and periarterial fibrosis: Report of a case. *New Eng J Med* **261**:320-323, 1959.
42. Hardmeier T, Hedinger C: Beziehungen zwischen der retroperitonäalen Fibrose und der sogenannten Takayasuschen Arteriitis. *Schweiz Med Wschr* **94**:1669-1676, 1964.
43. Jones EA, Alexander MK: Idiopathic retroperitoneal fibrosis associated with an arteritis. *Ann Rheum Dis* **25**:356-359, 1966.
44. Lipman RL, Johnson B, Berg G, et al: Idiopathic retroperitoneal fibrosis and probable systemic lupus erythematosus. *JAMA* **196**:1022-1023, 1966.
45. Reidbord HE, Hawk WA: Idiopathic retroperitoneal fibrosis and necrotizing vasculitis: Report of a case, with autopsy findings and etiologic consideration. *Cleveland Clin Quart* **32**:19-27, 1965.
46. Hellstrom HR, Perez-Stable EC: Retroperitoneal fibrosis with desseminated vasculitis and intrahepatic sclerosing cholangitis. *Amer J Med* **40**:184-187, 1966.
47. Que GS, Mandema E: A case of idiopathic retroperitoneal fibrosis presenting as a systemic collagen disease. *Amer J Med* **36**:320-329, 1964.
48. Graham JR, Suby HI, LeCompte PR, et al: Fibrotic disorders associated with methysergide therapy for headache. *New Eng J Med* **274**:359-368, 1966.
49. Graham JF, Suby HI, LeCompte PM, et al: Inflammatory fibrosis associated with methysergide therapy. *Res Clin Stud Headache* **1**:123-164, 1967.

Special Commentaries

The Care and Management of the Dying

Russell Noyes, Jr., MD, Iowa City

If the medical profession seeks to preserve the sanctity of human life, then we, its members, must cherish that life in all of its forms and care for it even in its declining, final stages. When we fail to do so, we undermine society's sense of social responsibility and diminish the worth of every human being. Dying persons, then, are eminently deserving of our attention and concern. If this concern is strengthened by a dim awareness of our own mortality, so much the better. Perhaps a compassionate response will thereby be enhanced. But in addition we have need for some understanding of the emotional aspects of the dying process to guide our treatment efforts. This article will review the meaning attached to dying, examine the psychological reaction to it, and offer principles for the care and management of dying persons.

Meaning

Dying, the last stage of life, though it may arouse fear may also have profound significance for the life that experiences it. It is potentially a climactic moment when an individual may confront his mortality. At this moment a man may view his life in perspective and achieve previously unattained humility. He may increase his maturity or strengthen his faith. Dying provides a true test of beliefs, and a man's courage in facing death may bear witness to their strength. The person who maintains his dignity and courage while dying in effect preserves it for a lifetime and for the memory of his surviving family.

The attitudes of earlier periods present a striking contrast to our own. The nobility of the ancients found its most exalted expression in dying. Followers of the Stoic philosophy, for example, while not believing in immortal life, saw in death a gateway to freedom. He who found his life abhorrent was at liberty to end it. Man remained unconquerable as long as the door was open and his most faithful ally, death, did not desert him. The Stoics taught men to hope for little in the next world but to fear nothing in this one. Seneca, their foremost spokesman, said, "Slavery loses its bitterness when by a step I can pass to liberty. Against all the injuries of life, I have the refuge of death."[1] Consistent with their view of life, they considered learning how to die to be a matter of utmost importance.

During the Middle Ages emphasis shifted from dying nobly at the end of life to preparing the soul throughout life for its journey into the next world. This life was despised as being filled with misery and tainted with sin. Men were urged to prepare for death, which would unalterably fix their existence in eternity. The deathbed was seen as a great battlefield where the devil unleashed a final bitter assault upon the soul. Learning to die properly, therefore, became of the highest importance. Rules for holy dying were detailed and explicit. A man was to die gladly and willingly, and having confessed his sins and fixed his mind upon examples of unwavering faith such as that of Job, he was to emulate Christ in his own dying.

With the Renaissance, emphasis shifted from the next world back to this one. In life's last act was its climax. The magnified individualism of the period was reflected in the manner of dying. In Shakespeare's tragedies, for example, his protagonists continued to express their characters when passing through the gates of death. Though fatally stabbed, Mercutio ironically continued to jest. Romeo was amorous: "Thus with a kiss I die!" Hamlet called upon Horatio "To report my cause aright." Death was accepted and confronted in the same way that other aspects of life were faced. The standards of behavior for dying were also those for living.

Traditional concepts of appropriate dying such as the ones described provided individuals during certain historical periods, with patterns to follow in dying. Today the situation is quite different. Death and life no longer have continuity, and those who confront it feel at a loss in dealing with it. Terminally ill patients tend to deny and avoid death. Physicians tend to share the attitudes of their patients and cannot entirely be criticized for joining society in this tendency. Yet, as they collaborate with patients to evade the reality before them, they often erect a barrier to communication and understanding. The dying person

Received for publication May 5, 1970; accepted Aug 26.

From Iowa State Psychopathic Hospital, Iowa City.

Reprint requests to Iowa State Psychopathic Hospital, 500 Newton Rd, Iowa City 52240 (Dr Noyes).

may become isolated as a consequence. In addition to this sharing of denial physicians are threatened professionally by death. In their struggle to save lives—a struggle which they ultimately lose—they discover, when facing fatal illness, that their scientific skills no longer avail them. Instead they find that they must function almost entirely as comforters. In this often less well developed role, their personalities and humanity must serve them.

Not only physicians but most persons harbor fear of death in some degree. This stems from a variety of sources. It will aid the examination of these sources if death is divided into three distinct, though interrelated, aspects: dying, end of life, and afterlife. The first is dying. The pain and suffering that may accompany dying arouses apprehension, but the frequency of this complication is probably exaggerated in the public mind. The great clinician and teacher, Sir William Osler, who called himself a "student for many years of the art and act of dying" reported on a series of 500 deathbed cases.[2] He studied them with respect to modes of death and sensations accompanying each. Of the total, 90 patients, or 18%, suffered bodily pain and only 11 patients, or 2%, suffered mental apprehension. He concluded:

> We speak of death as the king of terrors and yet how rarely the act of dying appears to be painful. How rarely do we witness agony in the last hours. Strict, indeed, is the fell sergeant in his arrest but few feel the iron grip. The hard process of nature's law is for most of us, mercifully effected and death, like birth, is but a sleep and a forgetting.[3]

Among the disturbing prospects for some dying individuals are altered consciousness, disfigurement, and loss of control of bodily functions. Some fear becoming abhorrent and burdensome to loved ones. Others fear particularly the thought of regression, a return to childlike thinking and behavior which accompanies the dying process. Having suffered in childhood when dependence on other human beings was a necessity, they seek to avoid a return to that state. In dying they fear becoming helpless and vulnerable.

Perhaps for some, the most fearful anticipation of all is awakened by imagining the social demands of dying. Not only is courage and dignity demanded but one must cope with grieving relatives. According to Montaigne, the queer and dreadful faces and trappings with which we surround death are more frightening than death itself:

> An entirely new way of living; the cries of mothers, wives, children; the visits of people dazed and benumbed by grief; the presence of a number of pale and weeping servants; a darkened room; lighted candles; our bedside besieged by doctors and preachers; in short, everything horror and fright around us.[4]

A second aspect contributing to fear is the end of life. Some anticipate leaving unrealized goals as they depart from this life. Others sense the emptiness of wealth and status, values that formerly gave rise to striving. Above all, dying individuals dread leaving loved ones. Most of our experiences with bereavement involve the loss of a single family member, but the dying person foresees losing all members and himself as well. Faced with this outlook, and realizing his utter helplessness, he may become acutely aware of his need for transcendent beliefs.

A final aspect of death contributing to fear is afterlife. Death is an unknown; we are like children stumbling into the dark as we approach it. Where feelings of guilt or sinfulness are present, as they frequently are, some, according to their beliefs, grow apprehensive of possible punishment. Since Old Testament times death has symbolized punishment. During the Middle Ages a man's suffering, even while dying, was regarded as punishment and it was said ". . . that sickness before a man's death is a purgatory to him when it is suffered patiently, gladly, and with a free and kind will of heart."[5] As a part of our judicial system we punish serious crimes by the death penalty. Not unnaturally, some dying persons ask themselves why such a fate has befallen them. Unfortunately, they commonly conclude that their suffering and death represents punishment.

Psychological Reaction

It is useful, though artificial, to think of the psychological reaction to dying as occurring in stages. Each is typically characterized by certain adaptive mechanisms and emotional reactions. Given sufficient time and the proper circumstances, a dying individual may arrive at a final stage of acceptance. The first stage, however, is usually one of denial. As messages begin to reach the terminally ill person, his initial reaction is usually one of stunned disbelief. These messages arrive from various sources, and it is a mistaken notion that only patients who are told that they are dying know this. Drawn facial expressions and a variety of somatic sensations tell the truth just as plainly. Of course, those who are directly informed may not believe that they are dying, and those who do may never speak of it. Their silence may be an expression of kindly consideration towards their families as they seek to spare loved ones the increased distress of an emotional confrontation. Dying persons may not wish to point up their helplessness or seem to demand rescue.

The realization of death shocks a man's former denial and affronts his sense of omnipotence. Thus an appreciation of the fact that one is dying must be gained gradually. As denial gives way to acceptance, the strength of either may vary from one day to the next. The man who one day speaks of the approaching end of his life might the next day speak in quite an opposite fashion.

With partial acceptance a second stage appears. The dying patient, anticipating bereavement, begins to grieve. Lindemann, in his classical study of grief, noted that this reaction may appear in anticipation of the loss about to be experienced.[6] The syndrome in the dying closely resembles the grief of surviving relatives. It includes sadness, preoccupation with anticipated losses, physical distress, feelings of anger, feelings of guilt, and a paralysis of activity. The physical distress, including nervousness, insomnia, weakness, poor appetite, and weight loss, may be falsely ascribed to the coexisting terminal illness. Preoccupation with anticipated losses naturally bring a flood of memories which, though often cherished, may also arouse painful associations.

Feelings of bitterness and resentment often grow intense and may take the form of blaming an unjust fate. Overflowing hostility at times spreads over all relationships but occasionally may be focused in all its fury upon a single person—the doctor. Kübler-Ross observes that nurses are likewise quite often the target of displaced anger.[7] Diffused hostility may result in unresponsiveness to human relationships to which family and professionals may react negatively.

Feelings of guilt and regretful ruminations occur as dying individuals turn blame upon themselves and search their memory for events which might account for their fate. A portion of their sense of guilt may stem from hostility experienced towards their families. Doubting that their love has been wholehearted, they sense that their leave-taking is not entirely out of harmony with their wishes. If we accept Freud's notion that even loving relationships contain an element of hostility, then we can imagine that few people die while being totally free of feelings of guilt.[8]

A final stage of acceptance may be achieved by terminally ill individuals. In arriving at this stage they are assisted by a number of mechanisms both adaptive and defensive. One of these is regression, which, when it becomes profound, may include a desire for immediate gratification, emphasis upon the present moment, and extreme dependence upon the physician. With this latter development the doctor is viewed as god-like and is imbued with magical powers. Such a relationship is crucial where hope is to be maintained.

As the patient's strength wanes, his interest diminishes, and he may develop an attitude of quiet expectation. In these last hours of life, according to Sir Henry Holland:

> No previous reason or feeling can afford a right estimate of the relation the mind assumes to death . . . even where no impairment of its faculties has occurred. This is especially true when long painful sickness has been the prelude to the event. But the exhaustion also from acute pain of short continuance alters this relation; and even without sickness or suffering of any kind, the mere diminution of vital power by general decay produces the same effect. The earnestness to live abates, as the possession of life is gradually withdrawn.[9]

Dying persons do not regularly agonize over their departure. The misconception that they do results, perhaps, from the wish among those of us living vigorously that the dying should suffer, lest in not doing so they should seem to show a disdain for the life which we cherish, or should seem happy to leave us behind.

The stage of acceptance is possible where hope is maintained. Some intermix a measure of hope for miraculous cure with their acceptance. And, as already noted, the physician may become an object of tremendous faith. But as the end draws near and as emotional investment in life is withdrawn some will show, according to their faith, a growing religious concern. Faith in God may at this time develop to a high point. Hallucinations of departed loved ones, frequently reported a century ago and regarded then as portents of impending death, suggest, when they occur, the strong influence of expectations of a life after death. Clarke expressed the interpretation of many of his period regarding a terminal alteration of consciousness observed in some patients.[10] He said that just as they were freed from the flesh they might catch sight of the "glory beyond":

> Entranced by a glimpse of what the eye hath not seen, nor ear heard, and of which man has formed no conception, his gaze would be riveted upon a glory, invisible to his earthly companions. His features would be transfigured, and those around would be amazed, perhaps appalled at the sight, as some fishermen were, two thousand years ago, upon a mountain in Galilee by the transcendent glory of a familiar face . . . such must be the ineffable expression of transfigured humanity upon the features of whoever gets a sight of heaven, before he has left the earth.[10]

Treatment

Our objective in the treatment of dying persons is euthanasia. This term refers, in its original meaning used here, to a painless and peaceful death. Included in the concept is the medical art of accomplishing easy dying. Rohlfs, writing in 1880, regarded euthanasia as so important that he called the art "obstetrics of the soul" and gave to it the rank of an independent medical discipline.[11] Marx, whose thesis was published in Latin in 1826, left the medical profession with a classic.[12] His treatment of the subject is worthy of review. He recommended that patients be cared for in an atmosphere of quiet, cleanliness, and affectionate attention. The entire plan of treatment, he advised, should be confined within the symptomatic and palliative indication. Marx urged physicians beyond the dispensing of medicines to the "administering of some kind of higher comfort." "Whoever refuses his part in his duty," he said, "and assigns it solely to priests, deprives himself of the most noble and rewarding aspect of his work." He urged that the doctor offer an attitude of quiet confidence and optimism rather than any distortion of fact or promise of cure. To the last, Marx attended his patients. Having observed that the final sense to abandon the dying was that of hearing, he felt that it should not be "blotted out with noise nor with lamentation nor with mournful sound of funeral song."

In addition to alleviating pain and emotional suffering, physicians should strive to spare their patients indignity and isolation. Much isolation occurs in the strange, impersonal surroundings of hospitals and is increased by the intrusion of life-maintaining apparatus. A major indignity is that of treating patients as though they were diseases. As we move away from the organic orientation in medicine, death will increasingly be recognized as a psychological and social, as well as, organic event. The demeaning practice of maintaining physical life after an individual has departed psychologically will be seen in new perspective. However, a physician's most demeaning practice is that of robbing his patient of his death by not allowing him to talk about it or share in decisions regarding the length and quality of his last days. Decisions regarding life-prolonging procedures should, whenever possible, be placed in the hands of patients themselves and, when this is not reasonable, in the hands of the family.

The physician should not only foster a continuing atmosphere of dignity and social belonging, but should also strive to preserve his patient's sense of individuality and style of life. He should strive to assist his patient to achieve a death which is fitting and appropriate according to his character. An independent, hard-working, family head might be sorely threatened by fatal illness. Yet he might be given a large measure of responsibility for his own care and allowed a certain freedom of activity where these factors were seen as important.

Communication with the fatally ill is a delicate art the principles of which have been set down by Verwoerdt.[13] The approach to a patient regarding his prognosis depends to an extent upon the style and comfort of the physician in such matters. Armed with the realization that patients are not usually devastated by knowing that they are dying, he may make ambiguous though truthful prognostic statements. These should not be formal or final statements, for such would have the effect of blocking further communication. They might rather be viewed as invitations. Having opened the door, he will carefully assess the response and at that moment, or, more probably at some later time, be prepared to talk to his patient about what dying means to him.

It is natural to ask what to do when, as one leaves the room, a patient inquires, "Doctor, am I dying?" Is this a request for information, a demand for reassurance, or an expression of hostility? Only a further exchange can answer this question. Thus, from the beginning there can be no advance mapping of the course; there are no stock responses that can be recommended. Rather, the physician must rely upon his experience, his human desire to aid his dying patients, and his belief that his object is not so much one of saying the right thing in an anxiety evoking situation as it is revealing compassionate understanding which he feels.

Patients often find it easier to share their feelings about death with their physicians because they realize that their doctor does not have the same personal stake in their dying that family members have. The family is intimately involved, however, and the patients' dying is indeed a family affair. The doctor not only must share prognostic information and report progress but he will wish the family to know in a general way about communications with the patient regarding his final illness. He must involve them in decision making and occasionally provide them with emotional support to assist them in expressing their own grief.

The physician's task is one of providing or arranging for emotional, physical, and spiritual support. Emotional support can be offered when anxiety and uncertainty regarding distressing symptoms and disfigurements are encountered in the course of dying. These may be alleviated by honest reassurance. Patients often need encouragement to express fears of this type. The physician must be unhurried and open. He must put a premium upon maintaining rapport through a difficult period. On occasion he will become aware of a nurse who has developed a close emotional bond with a terminally ill person arising out of her intimate contact with him. He may then support and praise her efforts.

The grief of the dying cannot truly be shared. Neither can it be assuaged by false reassurance. It may be recognized and understood, however, and its expression encouraged. The most appropriate response to an expression of grief may be thoughtful silence. A response to guilt, and especially to anger, is difficult to avoid, and nurses especially must be supported and encouraged not to interpret these emotions personally. Regressive behavior is likewise trying but more tolerable when one realizes that it represents a dying patient's effort to cope with his last hours.

Adequate control of the pain associated with terminal malignancy is extremely important. It is tremendously reassuring to patients when they feel that the doctor intends to control distressing symptoms as they arise. One can scarcely disagree with Jaffe when he says, ". . . no patient should ever wish for death because of his physician's reluctance to use adequate amounts of potent narcotics."[14] There is little reason for withholding even substantial doses of narcotics, especially longer acting preparations such as methadone hydrochloride, from dying patients. These drugs should be available to patients in pain whose death can be predicted with certainty and from whom the drug need never be withdrawn.

The experience of pain is profoundly influenced by a patient's interpretation of its meaning and by anxiety. In addition to recognizing the source of anxiety and providing appropriate reassurance, it may be controlled by the use of the minor tranquilizing medications such as chlordiazepoxide hydrochloride (Librium) or diazepam (Valium). These agents are also effective in reducing the symptoms of grief and are free of many of the troublesome side effects of the phenothiazines and tricyclic antidepressants.

The physician must also help to restore, maintain, or enhance his patient's faith in a universal order. The roles of priest and physician were once indistinguishable, and clearly patients attribute priestly functions to their physicians. They should, therefore, be aware of patients' needs for transcendental beliefs and should be prepared to collaborate with clergymen in responding to these needs. But at the same time they should view it as their duty to continue their personalized care of their patients throughout the dying process without delegating it wholly to others. The task is a difficult one, but the aim is both worthy and noble. As Montaigne said, "He who would teach men to die would teach them to live."[4]

Summary

If physicians are to assume their role of primary importance in the care of dying patients, they need an awareness of the meaning such patients attach to dying and the psychological reaction they experience. Fear of death may derive from a variety of sources and be expressive of concern associated with dying, the end of life, and afterlife. Many of these fears are exaggerated and some are shared by physicians. The psychological reaction to dying occurs in stages. Initial denial is followed by anticipatory grief and finally acceptance. The objective in the treatment of dying persons is one of aiding them to achieve a painless and peaceful death, a concept well-developed historically. The physician needs a technique for communicating with dying patients and needs to provide emotional, physical, and spiritual support.

References

1. Seneca: *Oh Consolation of Marcia,* 6. 21.
2. Osler W: Science and immortality, in *The Student Life and Other Essays.* Boston, Houghton Mifflin Co, 1931, p 117.
3. Osler W: Thoughts on dying. *Canad Med Surg* **16**:511, 1888.
4. Montaigne M: That to philosophize is to learn to die, in Frame D (trans): *The Complete Works of Montaigne.* Stanford, Calif, Stanford University Press, 1948, vol 1, p 68.
5. Camper FMM (ed): *Ars Moriendi, The Book of the Craft of Dying.* New York, Longmans Green & Co Inc, 1917, chap 2.
6. Lindemann E: Symptomatology and management of acute grief. *Amer J Psychiat* **101**:141-148, 1944.
7. Kübler-Ross E: *On Death and Dying.* New York, Macmillan Co, 1969, p 45.
8. Freud S: Thoughts for the times on war and death, in *Collected Papers of Sigmund Freud.* New York, Basic Books Inc, 1959, vol 4.
9. Holland H: *Medical Notes and Reflections,* ed 2. London, Longman Green & Co Inc, 1840, p 289.
10. Clarke EH: *Visions, A Study of False Sight.* Cambridge, Houghton Osgood and Co, The Riverside Press, 1878, p 278.
11. Rohlfs: *Geschichte der deutschen Medizin,* Stuttgart, 1880.
12. Marx CFH: *Medical Euthanasia,* thesis. Göttingen, Germany, 1826. W Cane (trans), published in *J Hist Med* **7**:401-416, 1952.
13. Verwoerdt A: *Communication With The Fatally Ill.* Springfield, Ill, Charles C Thomas, Publisher, 1966.
14. Jaffe JH: Narcotic analgesics, in Goodman LS, Gilman A (eds): *Pharmacologic Basis of Therapeutics.* New York, Macmillan Co, 1965, p 264.

Criteria for the Evaluation of the Severity

Use of These Criteria

Patients should be placed in *one* class from *each* of three major categories: (I) Severity of Signs and Symptoms; (II) Severity of Renal Functional Impairment; and (III) Level of Performance. In each major category, the user should select the highest class whose criteria are fulfilled.

For example, a patient would be graded as II-C-1 if signs and symptoms fit class II under Severity of Signs and Symptoms, if the creatinine clearance is 30% of predicted normal, and if all usual types of physical activity can be carried out. If the patient is unable to carry out his or her usual types of most strenuous physical activity, the classification would be II-C-2. If the patient develops only one class III criterion under Severity of Signs and Symptoms (eg, nausea and vomiting), then he or she would be left in class II. Six months later, as osteodystrophy appears, the criteria for inclusion in class III would be fulfilled. If, at the same time, the creatinine clearance is 4% of predicted normal and physical activities are limited severely, the patient would be classified as grade III-F-4.

Prepared by the Council on the Kidney in Cardiovascular Disease of the American Heart Association.

(I) Classification of Signs and Symptoms by Severity

This classification is designed to describe the severity of the clinical manifestations of renal disease which are displayed by the patient. The patient should be placed in the highest class whose criteria are fulfilled.

Class I.—Requires (a) plus one or more of (b) through (f):

(a) No symptoms directly referable to renal disease

(b) Fixed proteinuria (> 200 mg/24 hours)

(c) Repeatedly abnormal urine sediment or bacteriuria in properly obtained urine specimens

(d) Demonstrable radiographic abnormality of the upper genitourinary tract

(e) Hypertension attributable to past or active renal disease

(f) Biopsy-proven parenchymal renal disease

Class II.—Any two or more of the following:

(a) Symptomatic because of symptoms **directly** referable to the kidney (eg, hypoproteinemic edema, dysuria, flank pain, renal colic, nocturia)

(b) Radiographic evidence of osteodystrophy

(c) Stable anemia attributable to renal disease

(d) Metabolic acidosis attributable to renal disease

(e) Severe hypertension (diastolic blood pressure > 110 mm Hg)

Class III.—Any two or more of the following:

(a) Symptomatic osteodystrophy

(b) Symptomatic peripheral neuropathy

(c) Nausea and vomiting without primary gastrointestinal cause

(d) Limited ability to conserve or excrete usual dietary load of sodium and water; tending to sodium depletion, dehydration, or congestive heart failure

(e) Impaired mentation attributable to renal disease.

Class IV: Any two or more of the following:

(a) Uremic pericarditis

(b) Uremic bleeding diathesis

(c) Asterixis and severely impaired mentation, with or without convulsion

(d) Hypocalcemic tetany

Class V:

(a) Coma

(II) Classification of Renal Functional Impairment

Exact classification (primary criterion) should be based on measurement of the glomerular filtration rate (GFR) (commonly approximated by the creatinine clearance) when possible, since the plasma creatinine concentration may vary in the presence

Established Renal Disease

of muscular wasting and decreased creatinine production. When clearance values are unavailable, the plasma creatinine concentration (secondary criterion) may be used but the subscript "c" should be added to the classification, eg, Class D_c.

Class	Primary	Secondary
A	GFR normal	Serum creatinine normal
B	GFR reduced > 50%	Serum creatinine normal to 2.4 mg/100 ml
C	GFR 20%-50% of predicted normal	Serum creatinine 2.5-4.9 mg/100 ml
D	GFR 10%-20% of predicted normal	Serum creatinine 5.0-7.9 mg/100 ml
E	GFR < 10% of predicted normal	Serum creatinine 8-12 mg/100 ml
F	GFR < 5% of predicted normal	Serum creatinine >12 mg/100 ml

(III) Performance Classification

A description of what the patient thinks he is able to do and not what the physician thinks he should be able to do.

Class 1.–Capable of performing all his **usual** types of physical activity.

Class 2.–Unable to perform the most strenuous of **usual** types of physical activity for that particular patient, eg, sports activity, fast walking, running, shoveling, lawn mowing.

Class 3.–Unable to perform all his usual **daily** physical activities on more than a part-time basis, eg, household duties, employment, driving an automobile, playing with children.

Class 4.–Severe limitation of usual physical activity. May need assistance for some facets of self-care, ie, shaving. Mentation may or may not be impaired. May be confined to bed.

Class 5.–Semi-coma or coma.

In the absence of uniform criteria for the description of patients with chronic renal disease, it is difficult to assess the severity of a patient's illness, to determine his need for a specific therapy, and to evaluate therapeutic effectiveness unless a detailed clinical resume is available. The Renal Section of the Council on Circulation of the American Heart Association has attempted to develop criteria to assist in the more uniform description of the patient with chronic renal disease. It is hoped that these criteria, besides serving as a short-hand index of severity of disease in individual patients, will be of particular value in series of cases appearing in the medical literature. Instead of such gradings as "severe renal impairment," "moderate uremia," "partially rehabilitated," "mildly symptomatic," which are frequently used for reasons of space, a more precise and meaningful description can be given using the indexes outlined here.

In full realization that a lengthy tabulation may not be used by the busy clinician, we have kept the criteria as simple and brief as possible. Nonetheless, because of the frequent disparity between a patient's clinical manifestations of disease, the absolute reduction in his renal function, and his performance capabilities, it has been felt necessary to include all three of these categories to describe more accurately the severity of disease and its effect upon the patient.

Editor's Note

A special set of criteria for the diagnosis of kidney disease and related disorders has been drawn up by the Council on the Kidney in Cardiovascular Disease of the American Heart Association and is being printed here simultaneously with its appearance in Circulation *and* Annals of Internal Medicine. *An editorial comment upon these criteria will appear in a subsequent issue of* THE ARCHIVES. *It was felt important to have this appear as soon as it was available, and it is therefore published in this issue prior to receipt of the editorial commentary.*

Clinical Commentary

The Goldblatt Kidney

Leonard B. Berman, MD, Cleveland

The clinical concept of the Goldblatt kidney began as an unplanned child, went through a stormy adolescence, and has now emerged, in its 35th year, as a serious and interesting adult. It is the purpose of this paper to provide brief sketches of those periods, to characterize the present situation, and finally to speculate about the future.

Goldblatt was a properly brought up young man, which is to say he had been taught that hypertension *produced* sclerosis of the large and small branches of the arterial system, including those of the kidneys, and that the cause of the hypertension was unknown. His experience as a pathologist, however, repeatedly confronted him with the fact that the hypertensive patient at necropsy showed vascular sclerosis in the kidney which was more frequent and severe than that seen in any other organ. It was possible that the renal vessels were more vulnerable to damage by pressure than vessels elsewhere. But it was also possible that arteriolosclerosis of the kidney came first and was, somehow, the cause of the hypertension. This latter concept attracted several investigators and experimental attempts to produce hypertension by interfering with the renal circulation were a popular scientific pastime in the first third of this century. The experimenters failed either because there was no elevation of blood pressure or renal function was destroyed in the experiment. It was this latter point that precluded any analogy with human essential hypertension wherein renal function was preserved.

For Goldblatt to experimentally pursue his concept of renal arteriolosclerosis and renal ischemia preceding and causing hypertension, a means was required of inducing such vessel changes in the experimental animal. There was, and still is, no known way to induce arteriolosclerosis in a normotensive animal's kidneys. Yet the analogy that persistently presented itself to Goldblatt's mind was that arteriolosclerosis behaved as if each afferent arteriole leading to its glomerulus were partially occluded by a tiny clamp (one million clamps in each human kidney). Could he, therefore, simulate the million clamps with one large clamp, ie, a clamp on each main renal artery? And so, he set out to produce hypertension with preservation of renal function by partially constricting both renal arteries. The arterial constriction was intended to represent the arteriolosclerotic process. Success would demonstrate that his concept of human essential hypertension was possible, although it would not prove it. His first achievement was the clamp. Its virtues were chronicity and adjustability, ie, the clamp could be left on the renal artery indefinitely and the degree of constriction could be increased or lessened at will. Since each renal artery was constricted separately, with an interval of several weeks between operations, Goldblatt had the opportunity to observe the effects of unilateral constriction and here is where the turn of events surprised him. The blood pressure in the animal with *unilateral* constriction of the main renal artery rose and remained elevated for weeks or, occasionally months. Permanent hypertension, on the other hand, was accomplished by constriction of both renal arteries, or by constriction of one renal artery and removal of the contralateral kidney. As for the hypertension in the dog with unilateral constriction, prompt cure could be obtained by removing either the clamp or the clamped kidney. Thus,

Received for publication Dec 21, 1970; accepted Feb 8, 1971.

From the Department of Nephrology, Mt. Sinai Hospital of Cleveland.

Reprint requests to Department of Nephrology, Mt. Sinai Hospital of Cleveland, University Circle, Cleveland 44106 (Dr. Berman).

two distinct and historic experimental results were achieved, one of them entirely accidental, and the other a stated goal of the experiments; one of them destined to occupy the clinicians' attention for the next quarter of a century; the other to be repeatedly confirmed but not yet related to human disease. A word of explanation is in order. The hypertension which followed unilateral constriction came as a surprise to Goldblatt. It was an unplanned event presenting itself to a prepared mind. The demonstration of cure by removing the clamp or the kidney made it a matter of intense clinical interest. This result, published in 1934,[1] is directly responsible for the clinical concept of a Goldblatt kidney. The other experimental result, possibly of far greater importance, had no immediate therapeutic implication and is, by now, in some danger of being forgotten. Let us restate the point here. Goldblatt produced persistent hypertension with preservation of renal function by constricting both renal arteries. This was precisely his original intention. His success, which was the first of its kind, provided an experimental analogue of essential hypertension and supported his original hypothesis that a million tiny clamps in each kidney (arteriolosclerosis) comes first and results, in some undefined manner, in hypertension.

The practical world of clinical medicine, and indeed the inhabitants of the sister planet of experimental medicine (including Goldblatt) became completely taken up with the mechanism of the curable hypertension related to unilateral constriction and its application to patients. The mechanisms first considered by Goldblatt included endocrinologic, neurogenic, and humoral. The first two were quickly ruled out by ablation experiments and attention finally came to rest on a humoral pathway.

Goldblatt himself provided some of the earliest evidence in favor of a humoral mechanism. He demonstrated that occlusion of the renal vein prevented the hypertension which otherwise followed constriction of the corresponding main renal artery. Other investigators made the case conclusive by various means such as grafting an ischemic kidney into a normotensive dog and observing elevation of the blood pressure when the circulation was restored to the transplanted kidney. The assumption was made that renal ischemia had resulted in the accumulation of a pressor substance which was released into the general circulation. But which substance? A logical candidate was renin, the substance isolated from normal animal kidneys in 1898, by Tigerstedt and Bergmann.[2] Goldblatt's experiments led to the rediscovery of renin and the now familiar story of the humoral mechanism of experimental renal hypertension. Many investigators played an important part in these investigations, among whom were Pickering, Printzmetal, Page, Helmer, Houssay, Braun-Menendz, Skeggs, Kahn, and many others. One of the first steps was the accidental discovery by Friedman et al[3] that renin itself is not a pressor substance. Later work by Page and others showed that renin acts instead upon renin substrate to form a new substance, (angiotensin) which is vasoconstrictor and pressor.

Meanwhile, the clinical hunt for human counterparts to the Goldblatt kidney had been going on (1940 to 1960) with a large amount of enthusiasm and a very small amount of restraint. It was not possible during most of that period to measure renin clinically. Identification of the patient who could be cured by surgery rested, therefore, on indirect and treacherous grounds. Aortographic demonstration of renal arterial stenosis, for example, was not correctly understood but was taken to be a sufficient criterion for surgery. A high failure rate was inevitable. Separate measurements of each kidney's function, looking for a specific pattern of increased sodium reabsorption on the affected side, was an improvement. But false positives could easily be produced by bilateral, asymmetric intrarenal arteriosclerosis, not amenable to surgery. In more recent times, the identification of curable renovascular hypertension rests on a more rational base, ie, the measurement of renin activity in renal vein blood. Thus, Goldblatt's happy accident of 26 years ago is a working concept in clinical medicine today and continues to provide a basis for newer work in hypertension. For example, in patients with end-stage renal failure and hypertension, about 15% can be shown to have renin dependent hypertension curable by bilateral nephrectomy.[4]

But what of Goldblatt's original hypothesis? What of his demonstration that bilateral constriction of the renal arteries mimics human essential hypertension in several important respects? What of the vast majority of hypertensive patients who have no demonstrable interference with either renal artery (and therefore no surgical approach to treatment)? Do these people have a million Goldblatt clamps in each kidney? The major problem, by far, has been a failure to demonstrate any increased renin secretion in essential hypertension. Kaneko's work[5] with the renin response to acutely lowered blood pressure in essential hypertension is a promising exception to this general statement. It might be argued that the kidneys in this situation are acting through a different, nonrenin mechanism, but there is as yet no way of directly proving a renal origin in human essential hypertension. The question of a renal origin remains open, but that is not to say inactive Goldblatt, himself, continues to seek the missing proof. Two of his present approaches are of interest. First, the long-term infusion of very low, perhaps unmeasurable amounts of renin may produce hypertension over long periods of time. By analogy, essential hypertension may represent the slow, prolonged release of small amounts of renin. Goldblatt and Haas have shown that kidney tissue from such patients contains more renin than normal, but further proof is lacking. A second line of approach has been that of renin immunization, which follows the lead of Wakerlin[6] and others. Renin is a protein, albeit an impure one, and can be used as an antigen in heterologous species to create antirenin antibodies. Such antibodies neutralize the enzymatic (angiotensin producing) properties of renin, thus preventing a hypertensive response to renin. Dogs, and other species, made hypertensive with bilateral Goldblatt clamps have been rendered normotensive by injections of heterologous (eg, hog) renin, in association with the development of an antirenin titer. In extending this work to humans, formidable problems have quickly become apparent. For example, human renin is not antigenic in humans. Nonhuman renin creates antibodies which are ineffective against human renin. Therefore, how may we immunize humans? Deodhar and Goldblatt showed that homologous renin could be rendered antigenic by changing the molecule slightly. They showed that homologous renin (dog) could be rendered antigenic for the dog by acetylation. In one striking case, they cured a dog who had been hypertensive for six years, with injections of acetylated dog renin and the development of a high antirenin titer to dog renin.[7] Acetylated human renin injected into hypertensive humans was the next step and is currently being investigated, but a high titer of antirenin to human renin has not yet been achieved.

In recent years, Goldblatt and Haas have turned their attention to angiotensin, and in particular, its curious behavior when injected intraarterially. Investigation of the lack of pressor response to intraarterial injections led them to the discovery of angiotensin cofactor (1968),[8,9] a substance present in blood which, when mixed with angiotensin and injected intraarterially, restores the pressor response. An explanation of the behavior of cofactor may possibly be found in its newly recognized vasodilating properties. Thus, intraarterial angiotensin by itself produces prompt vasospasm in the injected artery and traps the pressor agent. Cofactor acts presumably by preventing the vasospasm and permitting the entrance of angiotensin into the general circulation.[10]

Future

What lies ahead? Perhaps we can someday evaluate a hypertensive patient by measuring each link in the renin chain, eg, substrate, converting enzyme angiotensin 1 and 2, and the final link, ie, vascular reactivity; and perhaps, indeed, we shall immunize the hypertensive patient against renin in the practice of "nephrallergy." Ultimately, we may return to and illuminate the dark corner in which Goldblatt's original question still sits—the question that asks whether the kidney in essential hypertension is victim or culprit.

References

1. Goldblatt H, Lynch J, Hanzal RF, et al: Studies on experimental hypertension: I. The production of persistent elevation of systolic blood-pressure by means of renal ischemia. *J Exp Med* **59**:347-380, 1934.
2. Tigerstedt R, Bergmann PG: Niere and Kreislauf, Skandinav. *Arch Physiol* **8**:223-271, 1898.
3. Friedman B, Abramson PI, Marx W: Pressor substance in the cortex of the kidney. *Amer J Physiol* **124**:285-294, 1938.
4. Vertes V, Cangiano JL, Berman LB, et al: Hypertension in end-stage renal disease. *New Eng J Med* **280**:978-981, 1969.
5. Kaneko Y, Ikeda T, Takeda T, et al: Renin release in patients with benign essential hypertension. *Circulation* **38**:353-362, 1968.
6. Wakerlin GD: Antibodies to renin as proof of the pathogenesis of sustained renal hypertension. *Circulation* **17**:653-657, 1958.
7. Deodhar SD, Haas E, Goldblatt H: Production of antirenin to homologous renin and its effect on experimental renal hypertension. *J Exp Med* **119**:425-432, 1964b.
8. Haas E, Goldblatt H, Lewis L, et al: Inhibition of angiotensin and its protection by a cofactor in blood. *Amer J Physiol* **215**:1420-1428, 1968.
9. Haas E, Goldblatt H, Lewis L, et al: Angiotensin-protective cofactor. *Amer J Physiol* **217**:981-987, 1969.
10. Berman LB, Roza O, Mitra S, et al: *The Mechanism of Action of Angiotensin Cofactor*, abstracted, American Society of Nephrology, 1970, p 8.

Review

Infectious Disease Problems of Narcotic Addicts

Charles E. Cherubin, MD, New York

With the recent widespread increase in narcotic addiction, we as physicians are professionally responsible for the medical care of the increasing number of addicts whom we see in hospitals or in private practice; no one can now justifiably feel himself isolated from treating such patients. Further, they suffer from a high incidence of infrequent or rare infectious diseases and offer the researcher an unusual opportunity to study the disease mechanisms and therapy.

There is a decidedly increased mortality among addicts.[1] In New York the principal cause of death appears to be a syndrome of sudden collapse accompanied by pulmonary edema subsequent to an intravenous injection.[2]

Other conditions associated with narcotic usage are such infectious disease as tetanus, septicemia, hepatitis, an unknown type of chronic liver disease, endocarditis, and superficial abscesses.[1,3,4] We no longer see in this city the malaria which was at one time the most widely recognized addiction associated disease state.[5] However, because of the frequency of malaria and of addiction, in servicemen in Southeast Asia, we might be seeing needle-transmitted malaria again. Indeed, in the past few months several cases of *Plasmodium vivax* malaria in addicts have been seen in California, Illinois, and North Carolina (Communicable Disease Center, *Morbidity and Mortality Weekly Reports,* March 27, 1971, and May 8, 1971).

Received for publication Jan 7, 1971; accepted April 27.
From the Department of Medicine, New York Medical College and the Office of the Hospital Epidemiologist, Harlem Hospital Center, New York.
Reprint requests to Department of Medicine, Metropolitan Hospital, 97th St & 1st Ave, New York 10029 (Dr. Cherubin).

Tetanus

Tetanus and narcotic addiction form the most unusual and dramatic association of drug abuse with any infectious disease. This association is over 90 years old.[6] Until 15 years ago, case reports and hospital reviews made drug addiction a notable but infrequent cause of tetanus. Then in 1955, reports from Chicago's Cook County Hospital[6] and New York City's Harlem Hospital[7] indicated that the majority of tetanus cases they had treated recently were those of drug addicts.

As early as 1942, in the city of New York, there was an unusual point source epidemic of tetanus which involved addicts who had shared the same adulterated drug.[8] In 1959, Greenberg made the observation in an unpublished report that the disease in narcotic addicts was markedly different from that in nonaddicts.[9]

During the period 1950 to 1961, tetanus contributed 8.3% of the deaths of addicts seen by the Office of the Chief Medical Examiner.[10] For the past 15 years we have had an average about nine cases a year in this city.

The author has investigated tetanus in the city of New York during the period 1950 to 1970.[9,11] The majority of cases diagnosed in New York since 1955 have been drug addicts. These were mainly the Negro women and men in their 20's and 30's who lived in central or east Harlem and who had been using subcutaneous injections—"skin popping."

The age distribution was that of addicts in general. There was an overly high proportion of women. This was thought to be due to the combined effects of their lesser protection by circulating antibody and their greater use of "skin popping."[12] The Harlem concentration of cases was felt to be a result of the very much greater—though unexplained—use of subcutaneous injections in that area.

The increased mortality rate among addicts with the disease seems to be related to the nature of the initial tissue injury, that is, to a puncture wound and possibly to the inclusion of quinine in the injected material.[11]

Few hospitals are equipped, or prepared, to provide care for the more severe cases of tetanus. These require intensive 24-hour anesthesia, nursing, and medical care for periods of three weeks or more. Consequently, the mortality rate has remained high despite our efforts.

English workers have demonstrated extremely high levels of catecholamines[13,14] in patients with tetanus. They have attributed the alternating periods of hypertension and hypotension, the hyperpyrexia, the cardiac arrhythmias, and the sudden deaths seen in severe cases to this cause.

Fluctuating unstable blood pressures have been seen in all patients with severe tetanus, but the author's own experience is that the hyperpyrexia seems nearly always due to infection (usually pulmonary), the arrhythmias are often related to hypoxia and reversible with improved ventilation, and the deaths are due to diffuse confluent and sometimes necrotizing bronchopneumonia if they are not directly traceable to respiratory equipment failure.

During the first few days of intensive therapy, there is what appears to be a marked positive fluid balance in cases of severe tetanus. This has not been previously men-

Serologic Reactivity of Addict Sera Compared With Controls (%)

Group	No.	VDRL	Fluorescent Treponemal Antibody-Absorptin Test (FTA-ABS)	C-Reactive Protein 1-2+	C-Reactive Protein 3-4+	Latex Fixation	Monotest	γ-Globulin 15% to 20%	γ-Globulin >20%	SH Antigen
Male addicts	100	6	4	26	4	...	9	38	40	4
Female addicts	100	12	6	30	4	8	12	26	43	2
Male controls	100	...	...	21	...	...	3	18	6	1
Female controls	100	...	...	12	...	1	2	24	11	...

Febrile Agglutinins (% to Nearest Whole Number)*

Group	No.	Typhoid O			Typhoid H			Paratyphoid A			Paratyphoid B			*Brucella abortus*			*Proteus* OX_{19}		
		80	160	320+	80	160	320+	80	160	320+	80	160	320+	80	160	320+	80	160	320+
Male addicts	95	26	11	10	7	1	1	12	1	...	8	5	...	11	2	1	24	6	1
Female addicts	80	29	25	6	10	13	8	5	6	...	31	9	1	19	8	...	11	3	3
Male controls	95	16	3	...	7	1	...	5	...	...	2	...	...	...	1	...	3	1	...
Female controls	80	16	3	...	10	5	3	3	...	...	4	4	...	...	...	...	3	1	...

* Reciprocal of antibody titers.

tioned or investigated. At this time, when generalized seizures are poorly controlled, there is an extraordinary diaphoresis. The serum sodium is usually relatively low (125 to 135 mEq/liter), while the urine specific gravity is uniformly high (>1.020). This, and a single personal observation of a lower than normal serum osmolality, concomitant with a high urine osmolality, suggests inappropriate antidiuretic hormone release rather than fluid and electrolytic loss through sweat. On the third to fifth day these findings disappear.

In the second or third week there is again evidence of fluid retention with dependent and, occasionally, pulmonary edema. However, this has been described in patients on positive-pressure respirators for prolonged periods of time.[15] The edema does appear to respond to diuretics. This fluid retention has also been attributed to inappropriate antidiuretic hormone (ADH) secretion.[15] As yet there is no direct evidence for it during either period of therapy.

In contrast to the elaborate preparations that must be made for the treatment of addicts with tetanus, the prevention of the disease is simple. It involves immunization with tetanus toxoid of all addicts seen in medical facilities and public institutions. Only a few of the city's hospitals or agencies have such a program at the present time.

Pneumonia

One would anticipate from the description of addicts with tetanus that they would also suffer from unusual and severe pneumonias. Indeed, a report concerning English drug addicts describes a predominance of staphylococcal and gram-negative pneumonias.[16] We, in this city, see far more in the way of pneumococcal bronchopneumonia in addicts.[17] At Harlem Hospital, indeed, the majority of male patients below the age of 40 who are hospitalized for pneumonia are drug users. The disease is usually uncomplicated and responds satisfactorily to penicillin. The only unusual clinical feature of these pneumonias in addicts, besides their apparent increased incidence, is that about half are bilateral basilar bronchopneumonias, a distribution not as frequent in nonaddicts of that age with pneumonia. Between July 1969 and June 1970, 75 addicts with pneumonia were seen on the medical wards at Harlem Hospital. Forty-one percent had bilateral infiltrates. In nearly all of these cases a pneumococcal etiology was confirmed or strongly implicated. In an age-matched group of nonaddicts with pneumonia, seen during the same period, only 24% had similar bilateral basilar pneumonitis. Indeed, some of them may have also been addicts.

On questioning, a substantial proportion of addicts with this variety of pneumonia gave a history of an "overdose" (really a period of unconsciousness which follows an intravenous injection) occurring about a day prior to the onset of pulmonary symptoms. This suggests that perhaps the pneumonias arise as secondary infections following mild episodes of "heroin pulmonary edema." Such a sequence is supported by clinical experience with addicts with acute pulmonary edema as described by a report from the Bronx Municipal

Hospital Center.[18] In contrast, at Metropolitan Hospital this sequence of events and bilateral pneumonitis are encountered infrequently among the large number of addicts seen with pneumonia.

Several authors have attributed the fever and leukocytosis seen in half to two thirds of patients with heroin pulmonary edema to the pyrogenic properties of the drug mixtures injected,[3,19] while others have seen them as evidence of pneumonia.[1,18] This last view seems to be simpler and more logical. If the injected material had such pyrogenic properties, addicts would have fever and a leukocytosis much of the time. Clinical experience also supports the view that these febrile episodes are superimposed bacterial pneumonias. Of 28 heroin pulmonary edema cases seen as inpatients at Harlem Hospital over a year's time, 13 had an admission temperature of 100 F (37.8 C) or more. Eleven of the 13 had a leukocytosis (white blood cell count [WBC] >10,000). Of the remaining 15 who had a temperature of less than 100 F on admission, only nine had a leukocytosis. Furthermore, six of the 15 (including most of those with a leukocytosis) became febrile within a day after their admission. This would suggest a bacterial pneumonitis in an altered lung parenchyma far more than a direct effect of the drug itself.

There have been anecdotal reports of platelike aletectasis[20] and diverse pulmonary diseases[21] in drug users. Lung abscesses and necrotizing pneumonias also are seen in addicts; there were three cases of each among the 75 addicts with pneumonia seen in the 12-month period mentioned. During this time, in comparison there were 27 cases of lung abscess seen in nonaddicts.

Infective Endocarditis

Our knowledge of endocarditis in addicts has been almost entirely dependent upon reports of unusual cases. The result has been that, at three different times, three different conclusions about the nature of the disease have been drawn: initially, it was a candidiasis; then, nonhemolytic streptococcal infections of the aortic and mitral valves; and most recently, staphylococcal endocarditis. Louria summarized our knowledge of endocarditis in addicts up to this point.[3]

What was then wanted was a broad review of the city's experience with endocarditis in addicts, rather than the unusual case. In New York a different method of sampling than had been previously attempted was possible. All addicts who die and are identified as such are autopsied by the Office of the Medical Examiner. Thus, a definite pathologic diagnosis of infective endocarditis could be made on those patients who would ordinarily be lost to study. All identifiable cases of endocarditis which occurred in New York in the eight-year period, 1960 to 1967, were investigated. Twenty-nine hospitalized and seven nonhospitalized cases were identified and studied. Sole tricuspid valve involvement was found in only 9%; a bilateral endocarditis involving the tricuspid valve was noted in another 9%. The most commonly affected valves were, in order of frequency, the aortic and the mitral. Staphylococci were the causative organism in 48% of the hospitalized patients; unusual streptococci were found in 14%; and candida were found in three patients. Gram-negative rods or no organisms at all were isolated in the remaining patients.[22] Major embolic episodes were common in these patients; seven died suddenly outside of the hospital from cerebral or myocardial emboli.

Although there does appear to be an increased frequency of tricuspid and candida endocarditis in the addicts as compared with nonaddicts, the literature is probably biased toward the overreporting of these unusual cases of endocarditis in addicts.

In contrast to these findings has been a recent report from Cook County Hospital,[23] in which half of the addicts with endocarditis had *Streptococcus viridans* as the infecting organism. This must be a most unusual situation. A survey of the infectious disease consultants in New York city does not support similar conclusions. The experience with addict endocarditis at Lexington Kentucky Hospital as reported by Sapira[4] is similar to that in New York. In a three-year period at Harlem Hospital, 1968 to 1970, 12 addicts with endocarditis have been diagnosed: six were infected with *Staphylococcus aureus;* two, *Candida;* one, *Strep viridans;* one, *Klebsiella;* and one with no identified organism. There were three patients with tricuspid valve involvement; the remainder had aortic or mitral valve infections. During the same period, only four nonaddicts with endocarditis were diagnosed, two of whom had a *Staph aureus* and two, a *Strep viridans.*

The frequency of staphylococcal, gram-negative, and *Candida* valve infections is probably related to the addict's multiple, daily, unsterile injections and to superficial infections. The selection of the aortic valve as the predominant site of endocarditis in addicts is probably the result of their having a relatively low frequency of preexisting rheumatic and, therefore, of mitral valvular heart disease. The large pressure gradient across the aortic valve apparently makes it more susceptible to bacterial endocarditis, even in the absence of visible malformation.

Hepatitis and Liver Disease

Acute hepatitis transmitted by the communal use of contaminated needles has been the subject of many reports.[24-26] It is the foremost cause of addict admissions to the medical services at municipal hospitals. The occurrence of separate, multiple recurrent episodes of jaundice in addicts has been noted; such a history is found in about one in 20 cases of hepatitis in addicts seen in the hospital.

The presence of persistent abnormal liver function tests in three fourths of one series of heroin addicts after a minimum of seven months imprisonment and in another series autopsy evidence of chronic hepatic inflammation have been used to argue that chronic viral hepatitis is a common sequel to narcotic injections.[27] Liver biopsies in these studies have shown small foci of intense round cell infiltration, particularly in the periportal areas.[28,29]

To investigate this problem a study was recently undertaken which had some unexpected results.

Sera taken from patients with hepatitis who denied drug usage, and from users of intravenous heroin and methamphetamine, with and without clinical evidence of hepatitis, were tested for the presence of the serum hepatitis (SH) related antigen by the Ouchterlony technique of Prince.[30] This antigen appears to be specific for long-incubation-period hepatitis[31] and is identical with the Australia antigen of Blumberg et al.[32]

It was found that 50% of sera from adolescents and young adults with hepatitis, at Harlem Hospital and New York Hospital, whether they admitted to or denied drug usage, were positive for SH antigen.[33] Considering the relative insensitivity of the test and the duration of symptoms prior to hospitalization (two weeks on average), it was concluded that the majority of adult cases of hepatitis included in this study were caused by the agent of long incubation period hepatitis.

Two and two tenths percent of drug users without icteric hepatitis also had detectable quantities of this antigen.[33] By comparison, the frequency of antigen detection in volunteer blood donors was 0.1%. This estimate of chronic SH carriers in addicts may be an overestimate since the people tested were on a detoxification ward and some of those with antigen may have had anicteric hepatitis of recent onset. I have observed that the SH rate among former addicts in Daytop Village who had not used drugs for some time seems somewhat lower, about 1.2%.

To examine the problems of chronic liver disease in narcotics users, liver sections of consecutive addicts autopsied at the Medical Examiner's Office (none of whom died of liver disease) were compared with age-matched controls. In addition, 300 former drug users in a rehabilitation program, Daytop Village, were followed (unpublished data). The autopsy liver sections were read by two pathologists without knowledge of the subjects' histories. Of the 44 readable liver sections from addicts, 11 were interpreted as chronic aggressive hepatitis, 1 as chronic aggressive hepatitis with granulomata (this case was SH positive), 10 as chronic persisting hepatitis, 14 as nonspecific reactive hepatitis, 5 as normal, and 3 as fatty infiltration. Of the 56 controls, none had chronic persisting or chronic aggressive hepatitis; they had either normal livers, nonspecific reactive hepatitis, fatty infiltration, or Laennec's cirrhosis.

Among the living former drug users, 50% gave a history of hepatitis. Among whites the frequency was 58%, while among nonwhites it was 27%. This is a unique finding and as yet unconfirmed and unexplained. There was a notable decline in serum glutamic pyruvic transaminase (SGPT) values, but not in serum glutamic oxaloacetic transaminase (SGOT) values, parallel with the duration of time off of drugs. On entry 50% had SGPT values of over 50 units/ml; after eight months 20% still had SGPT values of over 50 units/ml and in half of these the values were greater than 100 units/ml. Liver biopsy of three chronic antigenemic patients demonstrated chronic aggressive hepatitis. Biopsy of those with persistent transaminase elevations showed mainly chronic persistent hepatitis. The combined data suggest that a substantial minority of drug users develop a self-perpetuating chronic liver disease, probably viral in etiology. The majority, however, have a self-limited disease—possibly—perpetuated by repeated exposures to the virus or to other components in illicit intravenous drug injections (Cherubin CE, et al, unpublished data).

False Positive Serologic Tests

Finally, we come to the area of false-positive diagnoses. In narcotic addicts all serologic tests for syphilis are to be regarded with caution.[34-36] In a study of the serologic reactivity of sera from narcotic addicts admitted for detoxification, nearly a quarter were found to react to the unheated serum reagin test or the Venereal Disease Research Laboratory (VDRL) test. Confirmatory tests were positive in only 12% of the men and 15% of the women. There was no observed effect of age or sex on the 6% to 13% of the sera that gave biologic false-positive reactions.[37]

Nearly 20% of the sera gave low-titer reactions (1/8 to 1/16) on lymphogranuloma venereum complement fixation (CF), and 6% to 16% reacted on Q fever CF testing.[37]

Sera were also tested with the standard battery of febrile agglutinins (typhoid O and H, paratyphoid A and B, *Brucella*, and *Proteus* OX_{19}). The addicts possessed higher titers than did an age- and sex-matched group of controls taken from specimens submitted to the department of health for syphilis serology. Indeed, the titers in addicts were higher than those found in the select group of sera submitted to the health department specifically for febrile agglutinins. Addicts' sera appears to have a broad and nonspecific reactivity to the standard febrile agglutinins, and the interpretation of these tests in such patients is correspondingly difficult if not impossible.[38]

A change in admissions policy in the addict treatment center, previously studied, then occurred with the preferential admission of younger drug users, not previously treated, and multiple substance users. This resulted in a fall in the syphilis serology rate by one half (20% to 10%). There was no change in the reaction rate of addict sera with the C-reactive protein tests or the test for mononucleosis (Monotest), but there was a decline in the rate of reactions in the latex fixation. The reaction rates of addict sera in these tests was, however, much greater than that of the controls. These nonspecific reactions did not correlate with each other, nor did they appear related to serum hypergammaglobulinemia which was seen in more than 20% of addicts or with the presence of SH antigen.[39]

In the Table, the serologic reactivity of addict sera is demonstrated. The febrile agglutinin titers were performed on a separate sample of addict sera. The controls were sera submitted for syphilis serology.

A recent investigation of opsonins and immunoglobulins in addicts showed that higher levels did occur in addicts than in controls.[40] However, it is not clear that cases and controls were adequately matched for race and background. Thus, the study might have demonstrated the hyperglobulinemia of blacks or of the poor, and not that of addicts.

Thus, although we know that nonspecific serologic reactions occur with addict sera, we do not know, as yet, why (along with much else in addicts) they do occur.

Summary

Addicts frequently suffer from a variety of uncommon infectious diseases: tetanus, staphylococcal and mycotic endocarditis, chronic hepatitis, etc. They, therefore, present an unusual opportunity for the physician or clinical investigator to pursue therapeutic or etiologic investigations in these diseases. The gaps in our knowledge are numerous and wide. Addicts with tetanus are difficult to control and appear to have an undefined water retention syndrome. Those with pneumonia have an unusually high frequency of bilateral basilar infiltrates. The incidence of endocarditis in addicts is inordinately high and the etiologic organism is frequently of unusual nature. Addicts appear to suffer from a relatively high frequency of chronic hepatitis even after they stop drug usage. In addiction, the biologic false-positive serologic reactions, infrequent in the general population, are common among drug users and represent a clinical diagnostic problem and a unique circumstance for the study of these phenomena.

Joelene Noel and Audrey Adams, nurse epidemiologists, assisted with the case-finding, follow-up, and compilation of data on patients in Harlem Hospital. The chiefs of service and the housestaffs of medicine, pediatrics, obstetrics and gynecology, and pathology of Harlem Hospital provided assistance.

References

1. Cherubin CE: The medical sequelae of narcotic addiction. *Ann Intern Med* **67**:23-33, 1967.
2. Siegel H: Helpern M, Ehrenreich T: The diagnosis of death from intravenous narcotics. *J Forensic Sci* **11**:1-16, 1966.
3. Louria D, Hensle BS, Rose J: The major medical complications of heroin addiction. *Ann Intern Med* **67**:1-22, 1967.
4. Sapira JD: The narcotic addict as a medical patient. *Amer J Med* **45**:555-588, 1968.
5. Most H: Falciparum malaria among drug addicts: Epidemiologic studies. *Amer J Pub Health* **30**:403-410, 1940.
6. Levinson AK, Marske RL, Shein MD: Tetanus in heroin addicts. *JAMA* **157**:658-660, 1955.
7. Bedel MD, Paley SS: Introduction of human tetanus through minor wounds. *New York J Med* **55**:1186-1188, 1955.
8. Rouche B: A pinch of dust, in *Eleven Blue Men*. Boston, Little Brown & Co, 1953.
9. Cherubin CE: Urban tetanus. *Arch Environ Health* **14**:802-808, 1967.
10. Helpern M, Rho YM: Deaths from narcotism in New York city. *New York J Med* **66**:2391-2408, 1966.
11. Cherubin CE: Epidemiology of tetanus in narcotic addicts. *New York J Med* **70**:267-277, 1970.
12. Cherubin CE, Millian SL, Palusci E, et al: Investigations in tetanus in narcotic addicts in New York city. *Amer J Epid* **88**:215-223, 1968.
13. Keilty SR, Gray RC, Dundee VW, et al: Catecholamine levels in severe tetanus. *Lancet* **2**:195, 1968.
14. Prys-Roberts C, Kerr JH, Corbett JL, et al: Treatment of sympathetic overactivity in tetanus. *Lancet* **1**:542-546, 1969.
15. Sladen A, Laver MB, Pontoppidan H: Pulmonary complications and water retention in prolonged mechanical ventilation. *New Eng J Med* **279**:448-453, 1968.
16. Briggs JH, McKerron CG, Souhami RL, et al: Severe systemic infections complicating mainline heroin addiction. *Lancet* **2**:1227-1231, 1967.
17. Cherubin CE, Brown J: Systemic infections in heroin addicts. *Lancet* **1**:298, 1968.
18. Steinberg AD, Karliner JS: The clinical spectrum of heroin pulmonary edema. *Arch Intern Med* **122**:122-127, 1968.
19. Sapira JD, McDonald RD: Drug abuse–1970. *DM* November 1970.
20. Gelfand ML, Hammer H, Hevizy T: Asymptomatic pulmonary atelectases in drug addicts. *Dis Chest* **52**:782-787, 1967.
21. Stern WZ, Spear PW, Jacobson HE: Roentgen finding in acute heroin intoxication. *Amer J Roentgen* **102**:522-532, 1968.
22. Cherubin CE, Baden M, Kavaler F, et al: Infective endocarditis in narcotic addicts. **69**:1091-1098, 1968.
23. Ramsey RG, Gunnar RM, Talein JR: Endocarditis in the drug addict. *Amer J Card* **25**:608-618, 1970.
24. Steigman F, Hyman S, Goldbloom R: Infectious hepatitis (homologous serum type) in drug addicts. *Gastroenterology* **15**:642-646, 1950.
25. Alter AA, Michael M Jr: Serum hepatitis in a group of addicts. *New Eng J Med* **259**:387-389, 1958.
26. Levine RA, Payne MA: Homologous serum hepatitis: In youthful heroin users. *Ann Intern Med* **53**:164-178, 1960.
27. Potter HP, Cohen NN, Norris RR: Chronic hepatic dysfunction in heroin addicts. *JAMA* **174**:2049-2051, 1960.
28. Kaplan N: Chronic liver disease in narcotic addicts. *Amer J Dig Dis* **8**:402-410, 1963.
29. Norris RF, Potter HP Jr: Hepatic inflammation in narcotic addicts. *Arch Environ Health* **11**:662-668, 1965.
30. Prince AM: An antigen detected in the blood during the incubation period of serum hepatitis. *Proc Nat Acad Sci* **60**:814-821, 1968.
31. Prince AM, Hargrove RL, Szmuness W, et al: Immunologic distinction between infectious and serum hepatitis. *New Eng J Med* **282**:987-991, 1970.
32. Blumberg BS, Sutnick AI, London WT: Australia antigen and hepatitis. *JAMA* **207**:1895-1896, 1969.
33. Cherubin CE, Hargrove RL, Prince AM: Serum hepatitis (SH) related antigen in illicit drug users. *Amer J Epidem* **91**:510-517, 1970.
34. Boak RA, Carpenter CM, Miller JN: Biologic false positive reactions for syphilis among narcotic addicts. *JAMA* **175**:326, 1961.
35. Harris A, Brown L, Portnovy J, et al: Narcotic addiction and BFP reactions in tests for syphilis. *Public Health Rep* **77**:537-543, 1962.
36. Harris WD, Andrei J: Serologic test for syphilis among narcotic addicts. *New York J Med* **67**:2967-2974, 1967.
37. Cherubin CE, Millian SJ: Serologic investigation in narcotic addicts: I. VDRL, LGV, H simplex and Q fever. *Ann Intern Med* **69**:739-742, 1968.
38. Vogel H, Millian SJ, Cherubin CE: Febrile agglutinins in narcotic addicts. *Amer J Clin Path* **3**:932-935, 1970.
39. Millian SJ, Cherubin CE: Serologic investigations in narcotic addicts: III. *Amer J Clin Path*, to be published.
40. Nickerson DS, Williams RC, Boxmeyerm, et al: Increased opsonic capacity of serum in chronic heroin addiction. *Ann Intern Med* **72**:671-677, 1970.

Books

The Heart, Arteries, and Veins, ed 2. Edited by J Wills Hurst, MD, R Bruce Logue, MD. Price, not given. Pp 1,615, with many photographs, pictures, and diagrams. Blakiston Co, 330 W 42nd St, New York, 1970.

Out of the plethora of medical books that materialize each year, perhaps a dozen or so emerge as "best sellers." Some are original texts which present the essence of information about a new disease or discipline or techniques, material that has appeared in the journals during the preceding years. Some are fresh editions of classic tomes, old familiar friends, updated. Alas, the majority are poor to mediocre and should never have been written, much less honored by publication between hard covers.

But the task of sifting and scanning and separating wheat from chaff is amply rewarded by the occasional discovery of that superb text that somehow you had missed previously. Such a book is *The Heart* edited by Hurst and Logue. This is the second edition of this multiauthored (82) text, and it must be ranked with the modern classics of medicine. One cannot devour a book of 1,615 pages; it must be nibbled and chewed and savored. This one has occupied a significant portion of my reading time, in a most pleasurable fashion, during the past month.

The editors have been very circumspect in selection of team members; they hand-picked their experts to write about what they know best. For example, P. D. White on evolution of knowledge of the heart and its diseases; Gorlin on physiology of the coronary circulation; editor Hurst on physical examination; P. Harvey on heart sounds; Sones on cinecoronary anteriography; Marriott on arrythmias and conduction disturbances; Kirklin and Wallace on surgery of congenital heart disease; Edwards on various aspects of cardiac pathology; Brest and Moyer on hypertension; Blount and Grover on pulmonary hypertension; Dexter on pulmonary embolism and acute cor pulmonale; Braunwald on idiopathic hypertrophic subaortic stenosis; Parmley and Mattingly on traumatic heart disease; Lamb on the effects of air travel and altitude; and Goldberg on pharmacology of cardiovascular drugs. Of course, there are dozens of others, ideally matched author to subject.

It makes for a most authoritative text. Variations in style between chapters is subtle, more organizational than syntactic. In sharp-shooting the excellent index I could detect no significant flaws or hiatuses; current concepts of therapy, precoronary care, and new surgical techniques reside quite comfortably beside discussions of cardiac embryology, basic electrocardiography, physical examination, and a detailed discussion of the vast area of diseases of the heart and vessels. There are even chapters on insurance and medical-legal aspects of heart disease. Nowhere could I detect any excess verbiage—in fact for a fat book the text is remarkably lean. References follow every chapter, many as current as 1969.

Of course, one must have a favorite chapter—my vote must go to Harvey and his clicks, hisses, and rumbles. As I read I could almost hear him reproducing with phenomenal fidelity the loud M1—opening snap—middiastolic rumble climaxing in a crescendo, all reproduced from his own hi-fi voice box.

It is a thoroughly laudable book. The editors are to be congratulated once again. It should reside proudly beside Friedberg and Woods on just about everybody's medical book shelf.

ROBERT H. MOSER, MD
Haiku, Hawaii

Communications to this Department may be sent directly to Robert H. Moser, MD, the Maui Medical Group, Maui Professional Center, Wailuku, Maui, Hawaii 96793, or to the Chief Editor for transmittal to him.

Pathogenesis of Diabetes Mellitus. By E Cerasi, R Luft. Price, $31.50. Pp 354. John Wiley & Sons Inc, 605 Third Ave, New York 10016, 1970.

This volume is based on the Nobel Symposium held in Stockholm from Sept 3 to 6, 1969. The four introductory lectures have all been published elsewhere either in whole or in part. This is also true for most of the special lectures. However, there might be an advantage in having them assembled in one compact volume, especially to readers other than the small band of diabetologists who are actively engaged in diabetes research.

On the bright jacket it was stated that "the Symposium was aimed at indicating the route that research in the field of diabetes sooner or later would have to follow." The symposium falls somewhat short of this aim. The predominant theme is that disturbances of the dynamics of insulin secretion are the cause of diabetes mellitus. The sluggish response of beta cells to a glycemic stimulus is considered to be the initial, genetically brought-about expression of an abnormally reacting beta cell, a view championed by Cerasi and Luft. Undoubtedly the secretory capacity of the beta cells is defective so that a higher glycemic stimulus is necessary to produce insulin release at rates approximately normal. However, this by no means explains the decreased effectiveness of insulin in lowering the hyperglycemia in maturity onset diabetics. Furthermore, disturbed glucose metabolism resulting in hyperglycemia should not be equated with diabetes mellitus. It was formerly believed that virtually all the specific complications of diabetes mellitus were sequelae dependent on poor or inadequate glucose metabolism. It has now been recognized that diabetes mellitus is a disease with protean manifestations, ie, vascular and biochemical as well as those directly attributable to abnormal glucose metabolism. Only the article by M.D. Siperstein in Introductory Lecture No. 4, "The Relationship of Carbohydrate Derangements to the Microangiopathy of Diabetes" represents these new concepts. In view of these considerations, perhaps the title of this volume should be changed from "Pathogenesis of Diabetes Mellitus" to "Insulin Biosynthesis and Secretion."

This handsome volume will be a nice addition to the private library of research fellows and internists, if they are willing to invest $31.50.

SHIAO-WEN SHEN, MD
Tucson, Ariz

Antibiotics in Clinical Practice. Edited By Hillas Smith, MD. Price, $11.75. Pp 346, with nine illustrations. Williams & Wilkins Co, 428 E Preston St, Baltimore, 1969.

Antibotics in Clinical Practice, by Hillas Smith, was first published in Great Britain in 1969, and this same edition is now distributed in North America. The author emphasizes in the preface that the majority of books dealing with antibiotics give little emphasis to the clinical aspects of their use. The present book is meant to be primarily clinical. It has been written mainly for physicians practicing inside or outside the hospital and for senior students. It is not intended for microbiologists, nor for specialists in the antibiotic field. Due to the solitary authorship of the book there is uniformity of style and approach to the various problems, but there is also a disparity between the quality of the various chapters. The author states that special attention has been accorded septicemia endocarditis, chemoprophylaxis, the difficulties encountered in antibiotic control of patients with liver and kidney disorders, and patients with altered immunity states.

There is a great deal of useful information in this book concerning individual antimicrobial agents which are discussed in Part 1 and the application of these antibiotics in a number of important commonly encountered infections. It is unfortunate that it has a number of inconsistencies and omissions. In a classification of the antibiotics as being either bactericidal or bacteriostatic, kanamycin sulfate and gentamicin have been omitted from the list of bactericidal agents. One inconsistency of the book is that for various penicillins and cephalosporin antibiotics chemical structural formulas are given, but they are not available for any of the other antimicrobial agents.

Cephaloridine is discussed much more extensively than cephalothin sodium because it is in more popular Great Britain. It is my feeling that the potential toxicity of cephaloridine should be taken more seriously; it has resulted in the United States to limiting on the allowed dose for the average adult to 4 gm/24 hr. The author states on page 48 that cephalothin seems more toxic than cepahloridine, but the opposite statement seems correct.

Since this book is intended for senior students and nonexperts in infectious diseases, certain statements are vague. For example, on page 71 it is stated that in treatment of peritonitis, when perforation of the bowel occurs, the tetracyclines have a definite place in therapy. This statement is true but it should have been stated that tetracyclines represented insufficient treatment for this infection. Additional antimicrobial agents are required for proper coverage of the intestinal flora which has leaked into the peritoneal cavity.

In the chapter on chloramphenicol the author discusses the use of this antibiotic in meningitis, in Klebsiella pneumonia, and in some other infection. However, it is quite doubtful whether chloramphenicol is the antibiotic of choice in any other infection besides typhoid fever. It may be considered as second line antibiotic after appropriate cultures and sensitivity studies have indicated that chloramphenicol is the agent which would be useful if an adequate substitute agent is not available. On page 95 it is stated that neomycin sulfate may be given parenterally in serious systemic infections where other antibiotics have failed. It would be hard to construct any clinical situation in 1970 in which this statement is applicable. In a brief discussion on the applicability of gentamicin in gram-negative septicemias, various portals of entry are listed, but the most frequent portal of entry for such infections, the urinary tract, is not listed (this omission is corrected elsewhere in the book). In the dose requirement for gentamicin the author states that 0.8 to 1.2 mg/kg/day given in three equal doses is adequate. It was also stated that a total daily dose of 2 mg/kg should not be exceeded. It is of importance to emphasize that for infections of average seriousness 3 mg/kg/day of gentamicin can be given. In connection with the administration of the antifungal agent amphotericin B intravenously, it is not stated that side effects are minimized by administering the intravenous infusion during a period of at least six hours. Although it is correct to state that the dose is gradually increased during a period of days until 1 mg/kg is given each day, it should be clear that often this is not possible due to side effects. Yet many patients have been cured of serious systemic fungal infections such as histoplasmosis, blastomycosis, and candidiasis with daily doses of amphotericin B well below the 1 mg/kg.

It should also be pointed out in connection with the treatment of endocarditis due to *Streptococcus viridans* that practically all patients suffering from this infection can be cured with penicillin G, 20 million units, and streptomycin, 0.5 gm every 12 hours intramuscularly in two to three weeks provided that no hemodynamic complications occur. This is certainly much shorter than the four to six weeks treatment suggested by the author with pencillin G alone. The chapter on treatment of staphylococcal infections is rather vague and sometimes confusing. It is true that penicillin G (providing the organism is sensitive) is the most effective single antibiotic and certainly should be the antibiotic of choice. However, often in the early phase of the diagnosis the microorganism has been identified but its sensitivities are unknown. It would have been well to point out that in all serious staphylococcal infections a drug like methicillin sodium or oxacillin should be given in high doses or that either one of these may be combined with penicillin G until sensitivity studies have been reported. The treatment of a staphylococcal pneumonia and of staphylococcal septicemia may very well require four weeks, and it is probably safer to treat most serious staphylococcal pneumonias and staphylococcal septicemias for that period of time. Therefore, the statement that therapy must be continued for a minimum of two weeks is vague. Staphylococcal enterocolitis probably is best treated with vancomycin hydrochloride 0.5 to 1 gm every six hours orally. It certainly has not been demonstrated that cloxacillin is more effective than vancomycin as may be inferred from the statement on page 183.

When the author lists alternative possibilities for the treatment of serious staphylococcal infections (when penicillin resistance is demonstrated), the order of listing indicated is cephaloridine, lincomycin, erythromycin, fucidic acid, and vancomycin. It would have been advisable to list cephalothin as the antibiotic of choice in such instances and lincomycin and erythromycin should only be chosen in low grade and chronic infections, such as osteomyelitis. On the other hand, vancomycin should be high on the list of substituting agents since practically all *Staphylococcus aureus* strains are sensitive to it and this drug appears to be the drug of choice when penicillin G, methicillin, or cephalothin cannot be used in a serious staphylococcal infection.

On page 195 it is stated that Diphtheroids and *Staphalbus* are common contaminants (in a discussion of false-positive cultures). This is certainly correct, but it should also be pointed out in the same paragraph that *Staphalbus* may cause endocarditis and, therefore, should always be taken seriously when recovered from the blood stream. A statement to this effect, however, can be found elsewhere in the book. It is somewhat unfortunate that in the discussion of the clinical diagnosis of endocarditis due to *Strep viridans* a statement is made that there is fever, malaise, anemia, cardiac murmurs, and splenomegaly. Especially for medical students and for physicians who do not see many patients with endocarditis, a statement would have been helpful indicating that any patient who has a heart murmur and an unexplained fever even in the absence of anemia and splenomegaly as well as minor or major embolic phenomena should be suspected of having endocarditis.

On page 198 it is mentioned that *Staph albus* is frequently responsible for a low grade infection such prosthetic devices (in the more immediate postoperative period) cannot be found in the text. On page 200 it is stated that patients with myelomatosis are unusually susceptible to infections with gram-negative organisms. It would be well to point out that in myelomatosis it is pyogenic cocci, especially the pneumococcus which causes pulmonary and blood stream infections. On page 203 it is stated that for staphylococcal infection a combination of penicillin G and cloxacillin is recommended. This statement appears to be only correct in the initial phase of treatment, but one of the two agents can be omitted after antimicrobial sensitivity data are available to the physician. The statement on the same page that "Methicillin can be used instead of Cloxacillin but, as it is rather more toxic and probably less active, it is not recommended" has no sound basis. It would have been more correct to state that enterococcal septicemia can usually be treated with penicillin G alone and that enterococcal endocarditis should be treated with a combination of penicillin G and streptomycin. Nothing is said about the duration of treatment of this serious illness and it is hoped that in a next edition a period of treatment of four weeks will be recommended. Little is said also about the possibilities of combining ampicillin with kanamycin and penicillin G with kanamycin in patients who have organisms which do not seem to be killed by standard combinations of penicillin and streptomycin.

There are many useful tables in this book. It would gain considerably in usefulness by the addition of more specific information with regard to the period of time required for the treatment of certain infections and by correction of some inaccuracies and incomplete statements.

PAUL E. HERMANS, MD
Rochester, Minn

A Short Textbook of Haematology. By RB Thompson, MD. Price, $8. Pp 384. JB Lippincott Co, E Washington Sq, Philadelphia 19105, 1970.

This is a short textbook of "haematology" designed to fill the gap between major textbooks and chapters in more comprehensive texts. By and large, the author succeeds in his purpose. Its 384 pages are about 30% the number of Wintrobe's 1,287, and 56% of de Gruchy's 681; but since the latter costs only a few dollars more, is better illustrated and written somewhat more felicitously, many readers will prefer it.

The book is well organized, with chapters on red and white blood cells, blood groups, iron metabolism, anemias, the spleen, proliferative disorders, paraproteinemias, and hemorrhagic disorders. References are current (through 1968) and emphasize the British literature. Emphasis is on pathophysiology and clinical description, and in some cases rather specific therapeutic measures are spelled out.

Errors are few and insignificant. The author finds room for speculation. This keeps the book from being dull, but renders it subject to challenge. Examples include the comments on hormonal activity of the spleen, and on the absence of splenomegaly in cases of metastasis to bone marrow. The author relates hypochromia in polycythemia vera to venesections, which would not explain the phenomenon in untreated cases. In the therapy of incompatible blood transfusion reactions, most authorities would have reservations about the author's suggestion of transfusion of compatible blood, and many would advocate intravenous administration of mannitol.

The term "anemia of infection" is used rather loosely to include the anemias seen with neoplasia and burns, as well as infections; a less confusing term would probably be "anemia of chronic disease." Similarly the term "aplastic anemia" is used loosely to encompass also refractory anemias with normal or increased cellularity; this seems to introduce unnecessary confusion.

Of significance for practitioners is the statement that the most common etiologic agent for aplastic anemia (other than cytotoxic agents) is no longer chloramphenicol but phenylbutazone (Butazolidin).

The sections on leukemia and lymphomas have been rewritten extensively and are quite up to date. The statement that there is no place for surgery in the therapy of Hodgkin's disease seems true for lymph nodes but may need revision with respect to the spleen. Most American physicians will take exception to the old-fashioned notion that the patient with Hodgkin's disease should not be told his diagnosis.

The two chapters on megaloblastic anemias are particularly good, reflecting the author's special interest in this subject. The section on hemorrhagic disorders also serves to clarify a complex subject.

In summary, this is an interestingly written short textbook of hematology which should be helpful both to practicing physicians and to medical students.

HARVEY ROTHBERG, MD
Princeton, NJ

A Primer on Immunologic Disorders. By Heniz J Wittig, MD; William A Welton, MD; Robert Burrell, PhD. Price $6.75. Pp 123. Charles C Thomas Publisher, 301-327 E Lawrence Ave, Springfield, Ill, 1970.

The authors of this monograph, pediatric allergist, dermatologist, and immunologist, propose to present "basic information on immunologic mechanisms and their application to diagnosis and treatment of human disease" as well as "condensing the high points of current literature." Basically, the problem is whether any of these broad topics which include basic immunology, clinical aspects of atopic diseases, autoimmune systemic connective-tissue disorders, transplantation immunology, and disorders with excess or deficiencies with immunoglobulins, can be adequately covered to provide sufficient practical knowledge for any level of interest in a book of less than 100 pages. Many sections are most brief and sketchy. For example, primary acquired agammaglobulinemia, is dispensed with in two sentences! Immunoglobulin E receives only brief comment and serum levels are not mentioned, although they have been done for years. Therapy for severe status asthmaticus is outlined in less than one page, in a manner totally inadequate to make this presentation of any practical value. Thus, in most cases, this book will serve little purpose; other sources of reference will have to be consulted.

ROBERT E. REISMAN, MD
Buffalo

Allergy of the Nervous System. Edited by Frederic Speer, MD. Price, $13.50. Pp 259. Charles C Thomas Publisher, 301-327 E Lawrence Ave, Springfield, Ill 62703, 1970.

Much of this volume is devoted to an evangelistic hard sell for an allergic etiology for a raft of neurologic and psychiatric conditions such as headache, epilepsy, tension-fatigue syndrome, behavior disorder, neuroses, and psychoses. The evidence presented for such a conclusion is almost completely anecdotal. The sweeping generalizations made from observation of individual cases are unlikely to impress even the least critical of physician readers. The chapter on "Allergic Neuropathies and Demyelinating Diseases" by Philip M. Gottlieb stands out as an exception, being well written and a much better balanced presentation of available data relating experimental allergic encephalomyelitis and experimental allergic neuritis to naturally occurring disease. It would be unfortunate if this chapter were to bestow credibility on many of the concepts presented elsewhere in the book.

The concept that allergic reactions can produce a tremendous variety of clinical syndromes involving the nervous system seems likely to be valid even though definitive proof is often lacking. To reverse this and propose that, therefore, most neurologic or psychiatric syndromes of poorly documented pathophysiology are due to allergy does not seem reasonable to me.

LTC DARRELL S. BUCHANAN, MC, USA
San Francisco

Scientific Foundation of Obstetrics and Gynecology. Edited by Elliot E Philipp, MA, MB, BCh, FRCS, FRCOG, Josephine Barnes, MA, DM, FRCP, FRCS, FRCOG; Micheal Newton, MA MB, BCh, MD, FACS, FACOG. Price, $30. Pp 750, with 488 illustrations. FA Davis Co, 1915 Arch St, Philadelphia 19103, 1970.

Do you owe a Christmas gift to your wife's OB-GYN man? Give him this handsome volume, which, opened on his library table at page 240, plates 2 and 3, will add a dash of color, encourage comment, and reduce at least some of his guests to nonconversing, compulsive readers. For between these covers is very rich fare indeed. God knows the American OB-GYN man needs intellectual stimulation, and *refreshing* intellectual stimulation, and it's here (proof: about 60 of the 80 contributors are from the United Kingdom). The book is catholic and comprehensive: it starts with a model introduction to DNA, and all that, by a Belgian (P. Malpoix-Higgins), and ends with an interesting discussion on the topic of radioactive isotopes by a Japanese (H. Fujimori), who describes some unusual clinical applications.

As with any compendious volume of multiple authorship there are marked differences among the chapters. Some are virtual monographs, ripened out of many prior publications and heavy with references; others are brief essays. The book is divided into 13 sections. The general introduction includes an essay on tumors by R.J.B. King which is short but full of interesting insights. The next section is entitled "Female Genital Tract," and covers the anatomy and physiology of the uterus and adnexa, their innervation and lymphatic drainage. Section 3, "Ovum and Fetus," includes the longest of the monographs, a restatement of classical work on the development of the placenta by W. J. Hamilton and J. D. Boyd. Section 4 is on circulation and hemodynamics in mother and fetus. Section 5 (chapters on carbohydrates, lipid, protein, calcium, and folate metabolism), section 8 (chapters on liver, kidney, and fluid and electrolyte balance) and the chapters in section 10 on thyroid, adrenal and pancreas, are probably not superior to similar material in the best of current textbooks of internal medicine. They do contain aspects which relate to pregnancy, however, and these justify their presence in this volume. The three chapters on the newborn (section 6) deal with the first breath, the development of lung tissue, the respiratory distress syndrome, and brown adipose tissue. Three of the six chapters in the section on the central nervous system (section 9) are concerned with that ever-flowing source of complaint (and customers), the female bladder. The urinary tract also bulks large in the section on bacteriology (section 11). Section 10 is entitled "Endocrinology," a subject which, quite naturally, pervades the book. This section includes chapters by A. C. Crooke, M. F. Jayle and E. C. Amoroso on gonadotropins, tests of gonadal function, and the placenta, respectively.

The subjects of menstruation and ovulation are discussed in other sections by S. L. Israel and C. A. Gemzell, respectively. The topic of lactation has a section to itself (section 8) by (of course) A. T. Cowie and S. J. Folley.

There is a section on drugs, cytotoxic and teratogenic (section 12) and the concluding section (section 13) concerns genetics, geographics, statistics, mathematics, ultrasonics, electronics, and nucleonics. Genetics tends to be reintroduced at too elementary a level in too many places in the book: it deserves a full section to itself.

A good index is provided. The illustrations are large and attractive, but they also reveal to what an extent reproductive physiology is arrested at the morphological and descriptive level. There is something permanent about anatomy, however, and the reader can rest assured that the information contained in the many handsome photomicrographs will be valid for a long time to come.

This book is interesting and valuable, and is recommended to all who wish to advance their knowledge of human reproduction.

GEORGE S. RICHARDSON, MD
Boston

BOOKS RECEIVED

Ultrasound in Clinical Obstetrics. By William J Garett, MD, David E Robinson, ME. Price, $11.75. Pp 116, Charles C Thomas Publisher, 301-327 E Lawrence Ave, Springfield, Ill 62703, 1970.

Chemical Control of Fibrinolysis-Thrombolysis. Edited by Joseph M Schor, PhD. Price, $17.95. Pp 328. John Wiley & Sons Inc, 605 Third Ave, New York 10016, 1970.

Introduction to Steroid Biochemistry and Its Clinical Application. By Murray A Freedman, MD, Sandra N Freedman, MD. Price, $10.75. Pp 201 with 5 illustrations. Harper & Row Publishers Inc, 49 East 33rd St, New York 10016, 1970.

Involuntary Movement Disorders. By Irving Spencer Cooper, MD. Price, $29.50. Pp 432, with 521 illustrations. Hoeber Medical Division, Harper & Row Publisher Inc, 49 E 33rd St, New York 10016, 1969.

Membrane Proteins. By New York Heart Association. Price, $8.50. Pp 360, with many figures. Little Brown & Co, 34 Beacon St, Boston 02106, 1969.

Clues to Diagnosis in Congenital Heart Disease. By Alden S Gooch, MD; Vladir Maranho, MD; Harry Goldberg, MD. Price, $15. Pp 336, with 512 illustrations. FA Davis Co, 1915 Arch St, Philadelphia 19103, 1969.

A History of Preventive Medicine. By Harry Wain, MD. Price, $14.75. Pp 407, with no illustrations. Charles C Thomas Publisher, 301-327 E Lawrence Ave, Springfield, Ill 62703, 1970.

Synopsis of Anatomy. By Liberato JA Didio, MD. PhD. Price, $17.75. Pp 530, with 388 illustrations. CV Mosby Co, 3207 Washington Blvd, St. Louis 63103, 1970.

Modern Treatment: Treatment of Pyelonephritis: Diuretics in the Management of Fluid Retention. By John H Moyer, MD; Charles D Swartz, MD; Henry O Heinemann, MD. Price, $20. Pp 496. Harper & Row Publishers Inc, 49 East 33rd St, New York 10016, 1970.

Coronary Heart Disease (Cardiovascular Clinics), vol 1 No. 2. By AN Brest, MD. Price, $8. Pp 325, with 98 illustrations. FA Davis Co, 1915 Arch St, Philadelphia 19193, 1969.

Handbuch der Speziellen Pathologischen Anatomie und Histologie. H Fek, MD; R Haapl, MD; G Rothe, MD. Price, $46.20. Pp 401, with 181 illustrations. Springer-Verlag, 175 Fifth Ave, New York 10010, 1969.

Internal medicine at large

Response to chemotherapy

In vitro studies of a cancer patient's immune response before and after chemotherapy may give some indication of his chances of survival and the effects of the treatment on his tumor.

In addition, according to Jules Harris, MD, of the University of Ottawa, there appears to be a "vulnerable period" six to nine days after the completion of a course of chemotherapy during which stimulation of the immune response might prolong the interval between courses of chemotherapy, perhaps even leading to prolonged remission.

Dr. Harris, who is an assistant professor of medicine and director of the laboratory of immunology at the University of Ottawa, and A.R. Cheema, MD, of the Department of Developmental Therapeutics, M.D. Anderson Hospital and Tumor Institute, Houston, reported some of their results at the Chicago meeting of the Society for Clinical Oncology. Dr. Cheema's co-worker is E.R. Hersh, MD.

Dr. Cheema's study involved 40 patients whose metastatic solid tumors were treated by chemotherapy. The regimen consisted of five-day courses of single drugs or combinations of drugs repeated every two to four weeks. Each patient's immune responses were studied before, one day after, and ten days after therapy by assessing his lymphocytes' and "blastogenic responses" to phytohemagglutinin and a streptococcal antigen. These blastogenic response tests are indices of the functional integrity of the lymphocytes.

One day after the chemotherapy course ended, the blastogenic response (i.e., immunological reactivity) was suppressed in all 40 patients. Significant differences appeared ten days later. The blastogenic response exceeded the pretreatment level in 23 patients who survived from 5 to more than 13 months (mean 11 months) and whose tumors regressed. In the other 17, who survived a mean of 2.1 months and whose tumors continued to progress, the blastogenic response remained suppressed or did not exceed pretreatment levels.

Dr. Harris and colleagues studied 12 patients with solid, non-lymphomatous tumors who were treated with a 5-day course of a combination of cyclophosphamide, vincristine, methotrexate, and 5-fluorouracil.

The protocol called for giving the patients a second course of the drugs after a nine-day interval. One of the indicators measured in the study was the lymphocyte response to phytohemagglutinin; the investigators found that the blastogenic response after chemotherapy was 3 to 12 times greater than before in the patients whose immune functioning had been near normal levels prior to therapy.

"These were the patients who showed a favorable response to chemotherapy," Dr. Harris said. "We believe there is a synergism between the drugs and the patient's immune response."

The investigators found also that the period in which lymphocyte function recovered and exceeded pretreatment values was from six to nine days after completion of chemotherapy. "We believe that if, during this three-day period, the patient's

continued

Highlights This Month

A Houston physician reports that the type as well as the incidence of breast cancer correlate with family history of the disease . . . page 334.

Nitroso compounds are studied for their carcinogenic potential . . . page 335.

A proflavine dye seems to prevent recurrence of Types I and II herpesvirus infections . . . page 336.

Internists in the news . . . pages 341, 344.

Chemotherapy continued

immune response is stimulated by some other method, such as administering BCG, or an extract of the patient's own tumor cells or even passive immunotherapy (from another patient) the 'overshoot' phenomenon may go even higher. Thus, it may be possible to wait much longer before the next course of drugs is used," added the investigator.

Before attempting this, the investigators will test other measures of the immune response, such as whether the patient's lymphocytes will react against his tumor cells or other in vitro correlates of delayed hypersensitivity.

Heredity and breast cancer

A study of 6,550 breast cancer patients hospitalized between 1944 and 1969 suggests a correlation between a patient's family history of the disease and differences in disease type and frequency.

David E. Anderson, PhD, professor of biology in the Section of Medical Genetics at the University of Texas M.D. Anderson Hospital and Tumor Institute, Houston, said that the risk of breast cancer "developing in daughters and sisters of families already containing two affected sisters is three to eight times higher than that of women of similar age belonging to families with other hereditary neoplasms."

He added, however, that "whether or not these latter families are representative of the general population with regard to breast cancer occurrence is not known at present."

The study showed a 9.6% rate of bilateral breast cancer in patients with a family history of the disease. The frequency of bilateral disease in the breast cancer patients without any family history of breast cancer was 2.8%—close to the 3.0% found in other studies of cancer patients.

This difference in frequency of bilateral disease was the most noticeable distinction between the "familial" (500) and "nonfamilial" (6,050) patients, but the distinction became even more striking when the patients' ages were studied. Bilateral disease occurred in 15.5% of younger "familial" patients (those diagnosed between 20 and 44 years of age). Among "nonfamilial" patients in the same age group, the rate was 3.4%. The rate of bilateral disease remained higher (9.8%) in "familial" patients diagnosed between the ages of 45 and 54, compared to 2.4% in patients in the same age group without a family history of the disease. (Dr. Anderson does not consider the differences between the two groups significant after the age of 55.)

In addition to having more bilateral disease, "familial" patients also seem to develop the disease at an earlier age than "nonfamilial" patients. Even so, the survival time of both groups was statistically the same. Half of the patients in the "familial" group lived at least 32 months after initial diagnosis, while half the "nonfamilial" patients survived 33 months.

Comparison of the early and late "familial" patients also suggests that

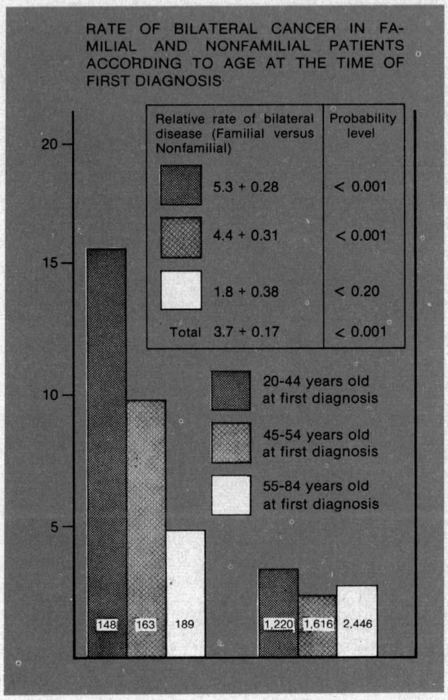

benign uterine tumors occur more often in the late onset group, while ovarian cysts and tumors and benign breast disease are more frequent in the early onset group. Dr. Anderson said, however, that age alone may explain some of these differences, and that the findings in the early onset group should not be considered significant.

Blood type O was generally correlated with early familial breast cancer, while type A was generally associated with late breast cancer. Other genetic markers were not found to have a significant relationship to the occurrence of the disease.

Dr. Anderson spoke at the second National Conference on Breast Cancer in Los Angeles.

Environmental carcinogens

Nitrosamines and nitrosamides, compounds which are known to cause cancer in animals, may be synthesized in the body from chemicals commonly found in the human environment. A West German investigator recently described experiments aimed at determining the possible risk these chemicals pose to man.

Johannes Sander, MD, of the Hygiene-Institut of Tubingen University, told a symposium on "Cancer and the Environment" in Houston that the nitroso compounds are formed by the reaction of nitrites with secondary amines and alkylamides. Nitrites and some nitrite-yielding substances are used as drugs and as food additives in meat, fish, and flour. Nitrogen oxides are also inhaled, and nitrite can be formed by nitrate-reducing bacteria.

The secondary amines and alkylamides necessary for the formation of the carcinogenic nitroso compounds are also abundant. They are found in drugs, plants, and foods, in tobacco, detergents, and pesticides, and several of these compounds are used in industry.

Although the necessary ingredients are present in the environment, obviously not everyone who is exposed to them develops cancer. Dr. Sander's group has conducted five groups of experiments to find out why. Their preliminary results:

• Studies of *in vitro* nitrosation of secondary amines and alkylamides showed that the reaction will occur in a neutral or slightly acidic environment if there is a high concentration of nitrite or a long enough reaction period. But "very potent carcinogens which are derived from strongly basic amines of low molecular weight . . . are not easily formed in biological materials," while relatively non-carcinogenic aromatic nitrosamines develop easily in nitrate-containing media.

• Under the right conditions—such as ultraviolet light—nitrites are liberated by cultures of nitrate-reducing bacteria (enterbacteria). If amines are present, nitrosamine formation "corresponds to a chemical synthesis in all respects." Maximal yields occur between pH4 and 5. The mouth is a good site for such a reaction, especially among smokers, because "several secondary amines which are constituents of tobacco smoke are dissolved in the saliva."

• In man, nitrate can be reduced to nitrite by bacteria in the stomach, especially under the neutral or weakly acid conditions that prevail after a meal.

• No nitrosamine compounds were found in the stomachs of rats and mice after the administration of strongly basic secondary amines and nitrite, but such compounds were found after the ingestion of weakly basic compounds. Some of the nitroso derivatives were carcinogenic, and the dosages were low. "There is no big difference between the amount of nitrite which is allowed to be present in nitrite-treated food—this is 0.02% of nitrite in several countries including the US—and the dosage which was necessary to produce tumors in this animal experiment," said Dr. Sander.

• The increased use of fertilizers and other agricultural chemicals leads to the formation of more nitrite in the soil as an intermediate product of nitrifying and denitrifying bacteria. Further, several secondary amines occur either as metabolites of plants or bacteria in the soil or are added to it as chemicals.

Dr. Sander pointed out that his work is far from conclusive, and that further studies are needed on minimum dose levels for carcinogenesis, the role of cocarcinogenic substances, and the epidemiology of cancer.

Drugs and lab tests

A Missouri physician reports that the results of most laboratory tests are not affected by any drugs that a patient might be taking.

Hubert J. Van Peenen III, MD, came to this conclusion after computer analysis of test results in 4,727 patients.

"In the vast majority of patients," he said, "grossly abnormal values cannot be properly ascribed to medication but to the patients' underlying disease." When, for example, the clinician blames hyperuricemia on diuretics, he is going along with "a medical myth, exactly similar to the myth that infectious mononucleosis commonly causes a biologic false positive test for syphilis."

Dr. Van Peenen reported his study to the Section on Pathology at the Annual Convention of the American Medical Association meeting in Atlantic City.

Internal medicine at large

Herpesvirus therapy

A dramatic new therapy for both acute and recurrent herpes virus infection was reported at the Second International Congress of Virology in Budapest.

According to a team from Baylor College of Medicine topical use of a proflavine dye has prevented recurrence of chronic herpes infection in over 100 patients with lesions at various sites, including the lips and the genitalia. The particular agent used was proflavine hemisulphate 3, 6-diaminoacridine sulphate dihydrate. The agent has been effective against both Types I and II herpesviruses. Even after initial treatment, there were very few recurrences in the course of the two-year study, especially with respect to Type II herpes, the investigators said.

The crux of the unusual treatment, Conrad D. Moore, MD, explained, lies in the combined effect of the dye substance and white light applied to the affected areas. The interaction of these agents with virus is so rapid and so pronounced that "in a matter of seconds a virus concentration of 8 logs can be completely inactivated."

Dr. Moore reported that proflavin in concentration as low as 1/4000 has proved effective against conjunctivitis and gonorrhea ophthalmia. Furthermore a controlled study of over 100 animals in whom the corneas had been scratched and infected with herpesvirus showed that the drug-light treatment had produced a cure or a significant improvement in all instances. The dye had been applied to the involved cornea three times daily and the beam from an ordinary 150-watt bulb had been directed at the eye for up to 5 minutes two or three times a day.

After the 6th day, the cornea began to clear and treatment was stopped at the end of two weeks. The animals were kept under observation for 27 to 37 days and no recurrent herpetic lesions were detected, Dr. Moore declared.

Although the virus remains antigenic, after exposure to this combined treatment, the viral DNA appears to be altered in such a way that it can no longer initiate viral replication, noted Joseph L. Melnick, PhD, head of Baylor's Department of Virology and one of the collaborators in the proflavin study. The remaining members of the team are virologist Craig Wallis, MS, research investigator Michael D. Kuns and two dermatologists, Troy D. Felber, MD, and John Knox, MD. Dr. Felber presented a similar report at the 120th annual convention of the American Medical Association.

Dr. Melnick also emphasized that the novel treatment immediately destroys extracellular herpesvirus, a finding that has not been an attribute of previous anti-herpes agents. Such extracellular herpesvirus generally persists and becomes a source of recurrent infection with the same viral agent.

The dye-light technique, the Baylor virologist added, "should provide an ideal means of making inactivated vaccines since the method does not seem to diminish or alter the antigenicity of the virus." He pointed out that an inactivated vaccine for pseudorabies, also a herpes agent, has already been used to confer passive immunity to piglets.

Gonorrhea

Women with gonorrhea secrete IgA antibody in the genital tract in response to the gonococci, reports Richard J. O'Reilly, MD, of the Venereal Disease Research Laboratory of the Center for Disease Control in Atlanta. He represented the CDC research team, which was following up the work of other groups who found stimuli such as viral infections cause mucous membranes to secrete IgA antibody. He said the finding may eventually lead to a vaccine against gonorrhea, but that many technical problems must be overcome before a clinical antibody test is feasible.

Dr. O'Reilly presented a paper to the Section on Dermatology at the Annual Convention of the American Medical Association meeting in Atlantic City. He said that the fluorescent staining technique distinguishes locally secreted IgA antibody in vaginal washings from serum antibody that may have "leaked" into the vagina.

Leslie C. Norins, MD, PhD, director of the VDRL, said that "these genital tract antibodies demonstrated by Dr. O'Reilly may represent the female body's first line of defense against gonorrhea, and they may be a mechanism whereby infected women hold their gonorrhea in check and remain carriers, rather than developing fulminating infections."

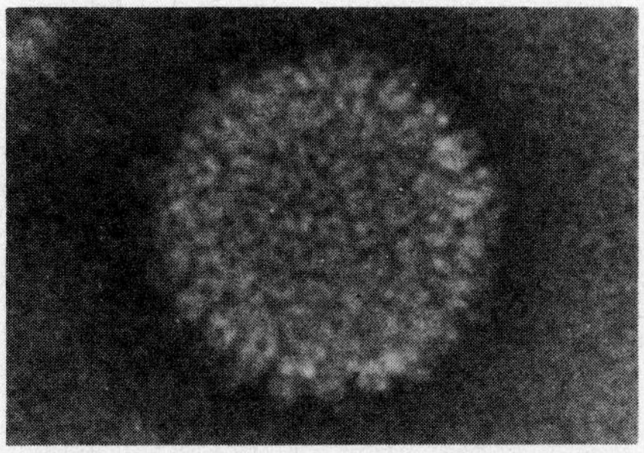

Crystal-like capsomeres on the protein coating of a herpes simplex virus are visible in the electron microphotograph above.

Manipulating genes

Researchers in Buffalo have shown that human herpesvirus cells added to mouse cells in vitro pass genetic material into the mouse cells.

The transferred genes enable the mouse cells to produce thymidine kinase, an enzyme that these cells had been incapable of synthesizing before being infected with the virus. The transformation seemed to be permanent and stable.

The study, using human herpes simplex virus type I cells, was conducted by William F. Munyon, MD, and co-workers at Roswell Park Memorial Institute, and reported at the Chicago meeting of the American Association for Cancer Research.

The research indicates that, in transforming cells, herpes simplex virus can produce new inheritable properties in these cells. Other research has shown that such properties may be oncongenic if infection occurs under certain conditions. Finally, the findings may be applied to studies in genetic engineering.

"The most satisfactory treatment for hereditary diseases which are due to the lack of a particular gene would be the replacement of the missing gene in a particular tissue of the body. Viruses, because of their tissue specificity and their ability to donate genetic material to cells, may in the future be therapeutic agents and not disease-producing agents," Dr. Munyon said.

In order to prevent the viruses from killing the mouse cells, the investigators used ultraviolet light to damage most of the viral DNA. They found that the number of colonies of cells that were transformed was related to: how much virus had been added to the culture, how much ultraviolet irradiation the viruses had received, cell density, and the period of incubation in the growth medium.

The investigators also found that no genes were passed to the mouse cells if the virus was first exposed to rabbit serum that contained antibodies to the virus.

Ultrasound technique

Ultrasound has been found to be a rapid, noninvasive technique for diagnosing ascites according to Philadelphia investigators.

The procedure can detect small quantities of fluid—as little as 100 cc—according to Barry B. Goldberg, MD, of the Episcopal Hospital in Philadelphia. He presented a paper on the procedure to the Section on Radiology at the Annual Convention of the American Medical Association meeting in Atlantic City.

Dr. Goldberg said there was a good correlation between the ultrasonic readings and results of isotope-dilution studies conducted in ascites patients. However, if the amount of fluid exceeds 10 liters, there is a tendency to underestimate the volume, he said.

The investigator and his co-workers found ascites in 51 of 85 patients. Paracentesis, surgery, or autopsy confirmed a positive result in 24 cases. In six cases, the negative results were confirmed either by autopsy or by surgery.

Dr. Goldberg said that the sensitivity of the technique should be useful for diagnosing patients with abdominal trauma, cirrhosis, intra-abdominal malignant neoplasm or inflammatory processes.

Sour news for sweeteners

The Food and Drug Administration has set limits on the saccharin content in certain foods and beverages and has endorsed a recommendation made last year by the National Academy of Sciences on daily individual intake.

Adult consumption of the artificial sweetener (the only noncaloric one now generally available) should not exceed 1 gm/day, or somewhat more than the amount contained in 25 cups of saccharin-sweetened soft drinks. (The average individual daily consumption of saccharin is 3 grains, or 0.2 gm.)

The regulation would limit saccharin content of beverages and fruit juices to 12 mg/fluid ounce (or 7 mg if sugar is also added); in processed

continued

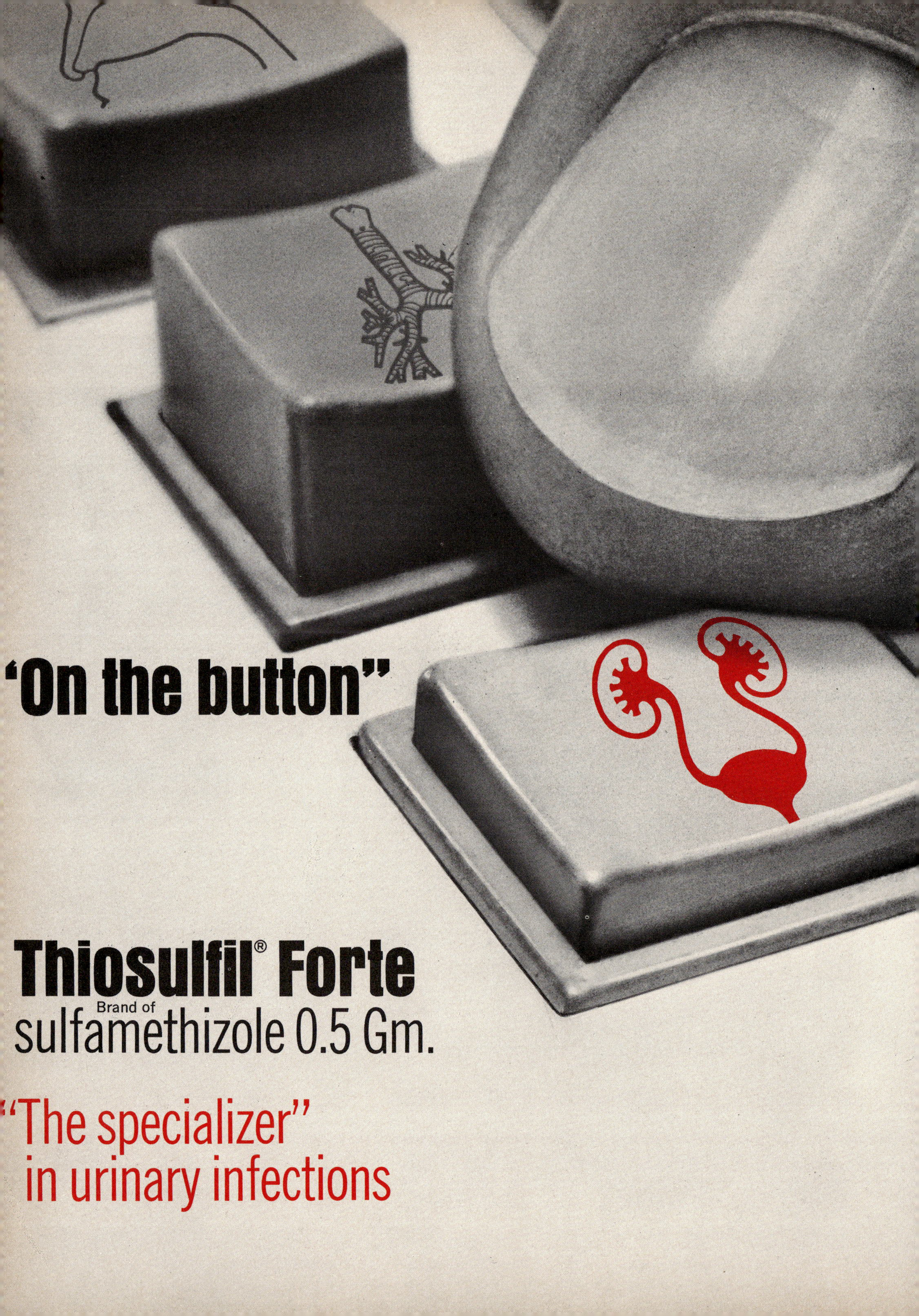
'On the button"
Thiosulfil® Forte
Brand of
sulfamethizole 0.5 Gm.
"The specializer"
in urinary infections

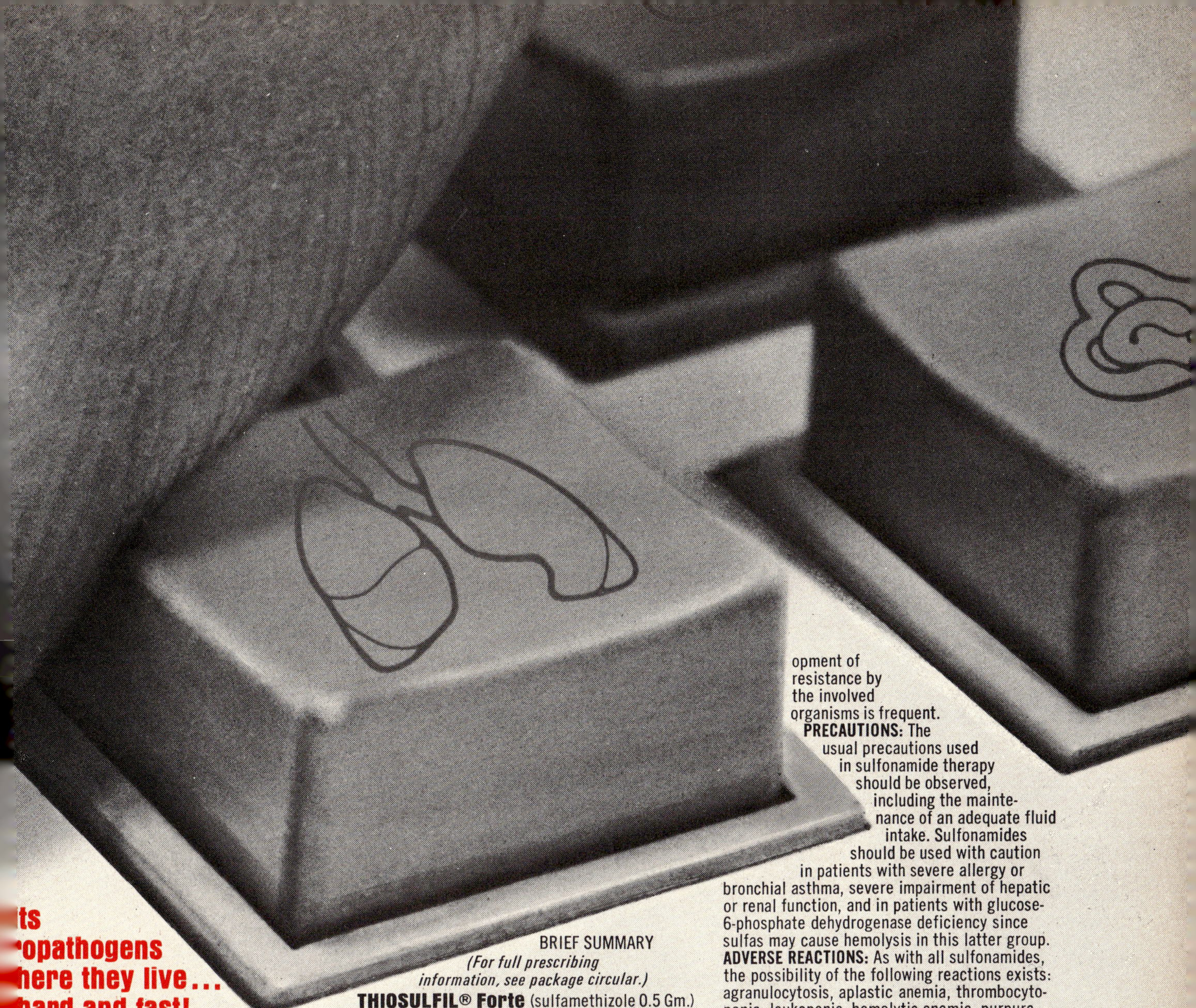

ts
opathogens
here they live...
hard and fast!

A *true specific* in cystitis...
a *true specific* in pyelitis.
In fact, THIOSULFIL Forte
ulfamethizole 0.5 Gm.) accumu-
es so *little* in the respiratory
ct and other tissues that it has
y *one* indication—urinary
ct infections due to susceptible
ganisms.
Rapidly absorbed and excreted,
IOSULFIL Forte delivers its
cent antibacterial action *locally*.
thin eight hours, about 80
cent of the drug is in the
nary tract in free, active form—
fight the infection where it is.
The patient on THIOSULFIL
rte uses less sulfonamide...
s more action for his money.
d there's no need for excessive
ding or priming doses.

BRIEF SUMMARY
(For full prescribing information, see package circular.)

THIOSULFIL® Forte (sulfamethizole 0.5 Gm.)
Bacteriostatic agent for use in Urinary Tract Infection (due to susceptible organisms)

INDICATIONS: THIOSULFIL is indicated in the treatment of acute and chronic urinary tract infections—cystitis, urethritis, prostatitis, pyelonephritis, and pyelitis—caused by susceptible bacteria, normally *Escherichia coli, Klebsiella aerobacter, Staphylococcus aureus, Proteus mirabilis,* and less frequently, *Proteus vulgaris.* As with most antibiotics and all antimicrobials, THIOSULFIL is most effective in acute, uncomplicated urinary tract infections. **CONTRAINDICATIONS:** Sulfonamides should not be used in patients hypersensitive to sulfa drugs. They should not be used in infants less than two months of age, in pregnancy at term, and during the nursing period because sulfonamides pass the placenta and are excreted in the milk and may cause kernicterus. **WARNINGS:** Sulfonamides should not be used to treat group A streptococci infections or their sequelae. The occurrence of sore throat, fever, pallor, purpura, or jaundice during sulfonamide administration may be an early indication of serious blood dyscrasias. Frequent blood counts and renal function tests should be carried out during sulfonamide treatment, especially during prolonged administration. Microscopic urinalyses should be done once a week when a patient is treated for longer than two weeks. Urine cultures should be made to confirm eradication of bacteriuria. (Para-aminobenzoic acid must be added to the culture media while the patient is on sulfonamide.) Because sulfonamides are bacteriostatic, development of resistance by the involved organisms is frequent. **PRECAUTIONS:** The usual precautions used in sulfonamide therapy should be observed, including the maintenance of an adequate fluid intake. Sulfonamides should be used with caution in patients with severe allergy or bronchial asthma, severe impairment of hepatic or renal function, and in patients with glucose-6-phosphate dehydrogenase deficiency since sulfas may cause hemolysis in this latter group. **ADVERSE REACTIONS:** As with all sulfonamides, the possibility of the following reactions exists: agranulocytosis, aplastic anemia, thrombocytopenia, leukopenia, hemolytic anemia, purpura, hypoprothrombinemia, methemoglobinemia, erythema multiforme (Stevens-Johnson Syndrome), generalized skin eruptions, exfoliative dermatitis, anaphylactoid reactions, periorbital edema, conjunctival and scleral injection, photosensitization, arthralgia, allergic myocarditis, drug fever, chills, toxic nephrosis with oliguria and anuria, periarteritis nodosum, L. E. phenomenon, hepatitis, pancreatitis, stomatitis, nausea, emesis, abdominal pains, diarrhea, anorexia, headache, peripheral neuritis, mental depression, convulsions, ataxia, hallucinations, tinnitus, vertigo, and insomnia. The sulfonamides bear certain chemical similarities to some goitrogens, diuretics (acetazolamide and the thiazides), and oral hypoglycemic agents. Goiter production, diuresis, and hypoglycemia have occurred rarely in patients receiving sulfonamides and cross-sensitivity may exist with these agents. However, the incidence of severe reactions following the use of THIOSULFIL (sulfamethizole) has been very low. **HOW SUPPLIED:** THIOSULFIL Forte—No. 786—Each tablet contains sulfamethizole 0.5 Gm. (scored), in bottles of 100 and 1,000. Also in unit dose package of 100. THIOSULFIL—No. 785—*Tablets*—Each tablet contains sulfamethizole 0.25 Gm. (scored), in bottles of 100 and 1,000. No. 914—*Suspension*—Each 5 cc. (teaspoonful) contains sulfamethizole 0.25 Gm., in bottles of 16 fluidounces.

Ayerst. AYERST LABORATORIES
New York, N.Y. 10017

7128

FDA continued

foods to 30 mg per serving; and in sweeteners for the table, to 40 mg per serving.

The FDA will also be reviewing many of the 600 food substances on the GRAS (generally recognized as safe) list. Saccharin and other food additives will receive a new classification apart from the list, and the sweetener will have a provisional status while testing continues.

Charles Edwards, MD, FDA Commissioner, said that "the action does not require a change in the diet of most Americans and will not affect any of the current uses of saccharin." He added that the regulations have been instituted, in part, to prevent an increase in saccharin levels in foods and beverages while testing continues.

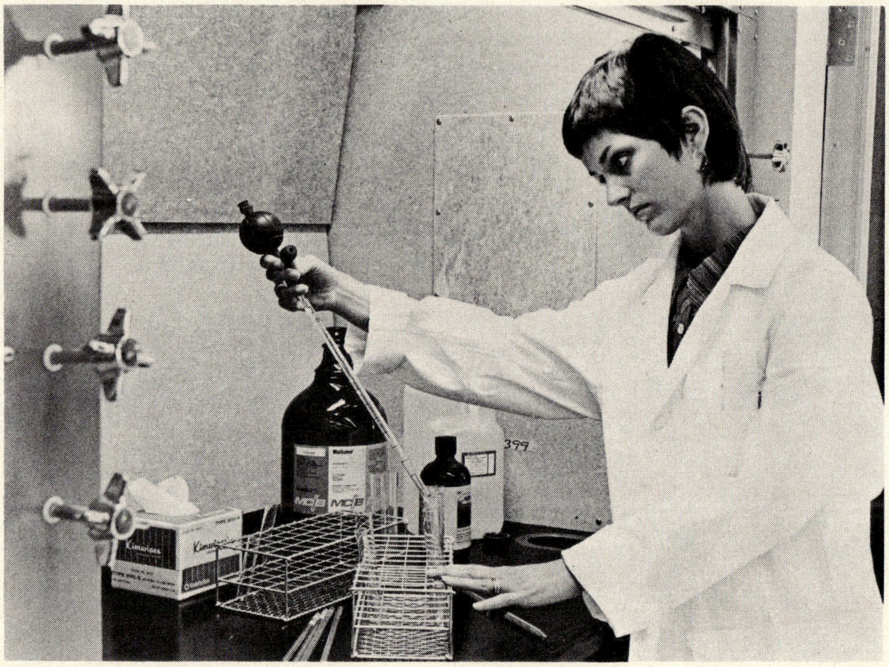

Staff medical technologist Cynthia Johnson draws off a noxious chemical within a blower-equipped hood in the new Educational Center.

Pathology center

"A national organization of the physicians engaged in our specialty is of prime importance. The scientific programs of this organization will take up subjects particularly suited to our specialty and of value to our everyday work."

The speaker was Philip Hillkowitz, MD, who was to become the first president of the American Society of Clinical Pathologists. The year was 1922. The place was Missouri Baptist Hospital, St. Louis. Two-score physicians, listed as clinical pathologists in the Directory of the American Medical Association, were in a discussion which would result in organization of the ASCP.

As the 50th anniversary of that May 22-23 meeting approaches, the ASCP announced—at the dedication of its new Educational Center—that it is observing a golden anniversary "Year of Pathology." For most of the golden anniversary year the association will be headed by William D. Dolan, MD, Arlington, Va, who headed the building fund committee for the new center before becoming president of the organization.

The new center, for which Dr. Dolan's committee raised more than $2 million, will concentrate under one roof many of the programs ASCP has developed over the years. Among other things, the center:

- acts as the national source for creation and distribution of ASCP educational materials,
- accommodates seminars, lectures, demonstrations, and laboratory workshops for up to 120 participants,
- uses modern means of communication (including a television studio which now is being equipped) for education,
- allows for expansion (up to 100%) over the next decade as technology dictates, and
- provides facilities for ASCP staff.

From the 145 charter members a half-century ago, the ASCP has grown to today's record high of more than 16,000, of whom 6,000 are physicians and 10,000 are medical technologists.

Alex F. Robertson, MD, has been named chairman of the Department of Pediatrics at the Medical College of Georgia. Dr. Robertson will leave his positions as professor of pediatrics and head of the Division of Neonatology at the Ohio State University College of Medicine to assume his new post.

Robert E. Hodges, MD, will become professor of medicine at the University of California Davis School of Medicine. He leaves his position as professor of internal medicine at the University of Iowa College of medicine to assume his new duties.

George Meiklejohn, MD, will serve as acting dean of the University of Colorado School of Medicine. Dr. Meiklejohn, professor and chairman of the Department of Medicine at the medical school, will be replacing **David W. Talmage,** MD, until a successor is appointed.

Monroe D. Eaton, MD, will become senior scientist in medical microbiology at Stanford University School of Medicine. He is retiring from the position of professor of bacteriology and immunology, emeritus, at Harvard Medical School.

George L. Wied, MD, has been named the 1971 recipient of the **Esther Langer Memorial Award** of the Ann Langer Cancer Research Foundation. Dr. Wied is the Blum-Riese Professor of Obstetrics and Gynecology and Pathology in the University of Chicago Division of the Biological Sciences and Pritzker School of Medicine.

Stanley Deutsch, MD, PhD, will become professor and head of the Department of Anesthesiology at the University of Oklahoma Medical Center. Formerly, he was chairman of the Department of Anesthesiology at Michael Reese Hospital and Medical Center and professor of anesthesiology at the University of Chicago Pritzker School of Medicine. Dr. Deutsch succeeds **R. Gibson Parrish,** MD, professor and vice chairman at the Oklahoma medical center, who has been department head temporarily since last summer.

Arthur Ebbert, Jr., MD, has been appointed professor of clinical medicine at Yale Medical School. Also promoted at the medical school, **Sherman M. Weissman,** MD, was named professor of medicine and molecular biophysics and biochemistry.

Saul Zwi, MD, has been named visiting professor in the Department of Medicine of the University of Chicago Division of Biological Sciences and the Pritzker School of Medicine. He is chief of the Respiratory Unit in the Johannesburg Hospital, South Africa.

The alumni association of the College of Physicians and Surgeons of Columbia University has presented awards to: **John K. Lattimer,** MD, (Gold Medal), professor and chairman of the Department of Urology; **Lowyd Ballantyne,** MD, (Silver Medal), assistant to the chief of surgery and associate attending at Roosevelt Hospital; and **Jeffrey M. Brensilver,** MD, (Bronze Medal), a 1971 graduate of the medical school who plans to continue his studies in internal medicine.

Stuart H. Q. Quan, MD, is the new president of the James Ewing Society. **Arthur I. Holleb,** MD, will be president-elect of the organization.

Richard E. Behrman, MD, has assumed the positions of professor and chairman of the Department of Pediatrics at the College of Physicians and Surgeons of Columbia University, and director of pediatric services at Babies Hospital and the Pediatric Clinics. Previously, he was professor of pediatrics and director of the Division of Prenatal Medicine at the University of Illinois Medical School, Chicago.

Robert R. Cadmus, MD, has been chosen the new executive director of the Medical Center for Southeastern Wisconsin. Dr. Cadmus is leaving his position as president of the College of Medicine and Dentistry of New Jersey at Newark to undertake his new duties at the Wisconsin medical center. Facilities associated with the center include Milwaukee Children's Hospital; Froedtert Memorial Lutheran Hospital; Milwaukee Psychiatric Hospital; the Milwaukee County institutions; Veterans' Administration Hospital at Wood, Wisc; Curative Workshop, and the Milwaukee Blood Center.

Marcus M. Reidenberg, MD, assistant professor of pharmacology and medicine at Temple University School of Medicine, will become part of the seven-member consultant group on the Use and Testing of Antiobesity Drugs. The group will report its findings to the Food and Drug Administration.

Volume 128, Number 3, September 1971

Archives of Internal Medicine

Original Articles

Conventional Radiation Therapy in Acromegaly

A Review and Reassessment

Ann M. Lawrence, MD, PhD; Steven M. Pinsky, MD; and Ira D. Goldfine, MD, Chicago

External pituitary radiotherapy is sufficiently free of serious side effects to argue for it being a first choice of treatment in acromegaly provided it is therapeutically effective. Of 28 acromegalic patients who had received external radiotherapy to the pituitary gland, 22 or 78% had normal or very near normal basal serum growth hormone levels. This experience compares with a recent report of favorable results with conventional radiation therapy but contrasts with experience from some centers. Disparate results between centers argue for analysis of factors which may contribute to varying therapy results. Some of these factors, as well as the comparative morbidity associated with external radiotherapy and other forms of treatment in acromegaly, are reviewed and considered. External radiation therapy of the pituitary in acromegaly continues to represent appropriate therapy in this disease.

Many years passed from the late 1800's when some of the first presumptions were made that the pituitary gland probably played an essential role in causing acromegaly[1-3] to when Harvey Cushing's neurosurgical intervention in this disease marked a first attempt at definitive treatment.[4,5] Transfrontal and transphenoidal hypophysectomy are associated with considerable morbidity, however, and mortality resulting from an intracranial approach to therapy in acromegaly is higher than by other modes of treatment. At the turn of the century, x-irradiation of the pituitary as treatment for acromegaly was first reported[6-7] thus offering what appeared to be a simpler and safer approach to management of acromegaly. Morbidity being less than that associated with a neurosurgical approach, roentgen therapy to pituitary tumors quickly became a popular form of treatment. In the five decades or more since Belclere's report[7] of the first successful treatment by external radiation, modifications of high energy radiation therapy have been introduced with what was believed by many to represent improved clinical benefits to acromegalic patients so treated.[8-15]

Prior to 1965, almost without exception, reports in the surgical, medical, and radiologic literature attested to the clinical benefits of radiation therapy for approximately 70% of patients with acromegaly.[8-12,14,15] Nevertheless, difficulties in the judging of "clinical activity" were acknowledged and a reliable assay for growth hormone was heralded as a tool needed to add objectivity to clinical assessment in this disease.[14] When the radioimmunoassay of growth hormone became available,[16] conventional radiation therapy was disparaged by several groups as less successful therapeutically than formerly believed due to the finding of high serum growth hormone levels in patients with previous radiotherapy to the pituitary gland.[17-19] Considerable impetus was given to the development of alternative therapeutic approaches because of these reports.[20-27] Where once the choice of therapy for a given acromegalic patient was fairly simple, an array of procedures are now available with choices largely being made on the basis of local expertise and interest.

Since ideal treatment still is to render the acromegalic process quiescent without disturbing normal pi-

Received for publication Nov 18, 1970; accepted Jan 25, 1971.

From the departments of medicine and radiology, the University of Chicago Pritzker School of Medicine.

Reprint requests to Department of Medicine, University of Chicago Pritzker School of Medicine, Chicago 60637 (Dr. Lawrence).

tuitary function, if at all possible, we have continued to use radiotherapy of the pituitary as a first approach to treatment in acromegalic patients without threat to vision. Patients judged unresponsive to an initial high dose of radiation (4,000 to 6,000 roentgens) were to be considered candidates for a subsequent implantation procedure using strontium 90-yttrium 90 probe insertion.[28] Since 1964, in the course of evaluating growth hormone levels in 34 acromegalic patients, it has become apparent that radiation therapy in acromegaly is, in reality, an effective means of treatment in this disease[29] and clearly approximates or exceeds the clinical success rate of 70% when clinical criteria alone were used to judge therapeutic success.[10-15] Although it can be argued that normal basal growth hormone levels are not, in and of themselves, a full basis for assigning inactivity to the acromegalic process, consecutive measurements of growth hormone levels at spaced intervals following treatment do complement usual clinical and laboratory assessment. As such, growth hormone levels clearly serve as a comparative basis for judging relative change in growth hormone production and release in any given acromegalic patient.

Further, other groups have recently compiled their experience with radiation therapy for acromegaly and report a success rate which is essentially similar to that which we have observed.[30,31] It seems appropriate that additional experience be delineated in order to give a basis for recommending that radiation therapy continue to hold a prominent place in the therapeutic armamentarium for acromegaly. It is the purpose of this report to review the experience at the University of Chicago with pituitary radiotherapy in acromegaly since the 1940's. Since 1964, clinical assessment of acromegalic activity has been coupled with measurements of basal serum immunoreactive growth hormone titers. This report includes many patients currently being followed up who received pituitary radiation prior to 1964 as well as a group of patients who were studied prior to treatment and have been followed up for at least twelve months since completing a single course.

Table 1.—Basal GH Levels and Clinical State of Disease in Acromegalic Patients Irradiated Prior to 1965

Subject No.	Sex	Course	Dose (R)	Human Growth Hormone (mμg/ml)	Activity
1	M	Cobalt 60	3,382	23	Active
2	F	Cobalt 60	6,600*	30	Active
3	M	Cobalt 60	3,000	22	Active
4	M	Cobalt 60	3,000	5	Inactive
5	M	Cobalt 60†	4,500	3	Inactive
6	M	Cobalt 60	3,060	5	Inactive
7	F	Cobalt 60	4,000*	7	Inactive
8	F	Cobalt 60	4,046	6	Inactive
9	F	Cobalt 60	3,100	10	Inactive
10	F	Cobalt 60	4,485	7	Inactive
11	F	Cobalt 60	5,420	5	Inactive
12	M	Cobalt 60	3,428	8	Inactive
13	F	Cobalt 60	5,400*	8	Inactive
14	F	VDG‡	3,206	6	Inactive
15	F	VDG	2,950	5	Inactive
16	M	VDG	1,680	2	Inactive

* Two courses.
† Subtotal hypophysectomy with irradiation two years later when still active.
‡ VDG = Van de Graff.

Table 2.—Change in Basal Growth Hormone Levels and Clinical Status of Disease in Acromegalic Patients Irradiated Since 1965

Subject No.	Sex	Dose (R)	Date	Human Growth Hormone (mμg/ml) Before	After		Activity	% Decrease
17	M	5,500	1965	50	25	(1969)	Active	50
18*	F	6,500	1966	55	65	(1969)	Active	gain 87
19†	F	5,500	1965	332	185	(1967)	Active	44
20‡	M	5,400	1968	35	1	(1969)	Hypopituitary	97
21	M	6,500	1966	27	1	(1970)	Inactive	96
22	F	5,000	1970	20	4	(1970)	Inactive	80
23	M	5,446	1964	55	5	(1965)	Inactive	93
23	M	3,500	1964	35	3	(1966)	Inactive	91
24	F	3,500	1965	28	8	(1966)	Inactive	71
25	M	6,000	1965	30	1	(1966)	Inactive	97
26§	M	6,000	1965	300	10	(1966)	±Inactive	97
27	M	6,000	1965	50	5	(1966)	Inactive	90
			Totals	1,017	313		Average % Decrease	74
			Averages	84.75	26		% Decrease	69

* Only patient with pneumoencephalographic demonstration of supracellular extension.
† Pneumoencephalogram showed air in sella—? cyst with rupture.
‡ Eleven opposing fields; other cobalt 60 used rotational fields.
§ Van de Graff; all others treated with cobalt 60.

Patients and Methods

Twenty-eight patients with acromegaly, followed up since 1964 with serial basal and ambulatory immunoreactive growth hormone measurements added to the usual clinical and laboratory methods of evaluating activity in this disease, make up the material for this report. Eight additional patients have been treated by other means or were treated too recently to be included in this review. In addition to periodic outpatient department checks, all patients have been admitted to the University of Chicago Clinical Research Center for more detailed investigations, designed principally to assess anterior pituitary function before and after therapy.

Of this group of 28, 16 had received radiation therapy 4 to 27 years before their first measurement of growth hormone was obtained (Table 1). One patient (13) received two courses of radiation therapy elsewhere, in 1966 and 1968, before being seen by us in 1970. The other 12 patients were diagnosed from 1964 on (Table 2), underwent study beforehand, and were then treated with the use of a rotational field technique with 360° rotation centered on the pituitary gland. For this rotational therapy pneumoencephalograms have been performed routinely since 1964 because of the importance of definite localization of tumor extent. Using pneumoencephalogram films, port roentgenograms are taken in three positions to assure that the radiation beam passes through the pituitary from each port. The size of the portal is determined by the size of the tumor. In most cases 4 × 4cm or 5 × 5cm ports were used. Most of the patients were treated on a cobalt 60 rotational unit; three patients were treated with x-rays from a 2 mev Van de Graaff generator which utilizes a rotating chair. One patient had undergone a partial surgical hypophysectomy two years before radiation; therapy was given because of continued clinical activity of his disease. Calculated tumor doses were 3,500 R to 6,500 R in patients treated since 1964. In the 15 patients treated before then, tumor doses ranged from 1,800 to 6,600 R. Three patients treated prior to 1965 received two interrupted courses. All others received fractionated therapy starting with small doses of between 50 to 100 R, ultimately achieving a dose of 1,000 R a week with the use of five daily fractions.

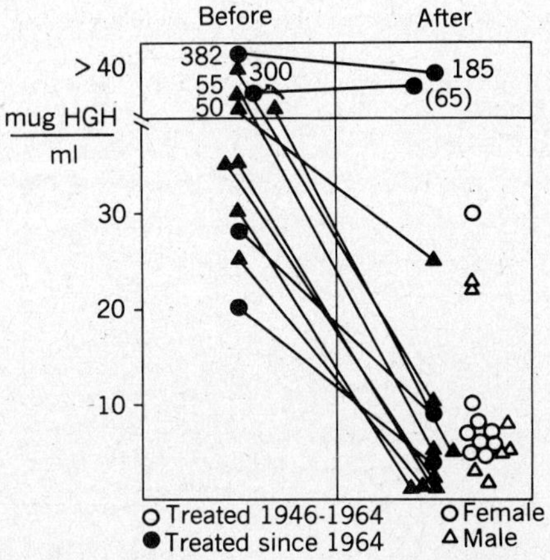

Serum human growth hormone (HGH) levels in 28 acromegalic patients before and after external radiotherapy to the pituitary gland.

Basal overnight fasting sera for growth hormone measurements were obtained upon awakening at approximately 7 AM and after three days in the hospital during which time patients consumed a constant calorie weight maintenance diet. Serum growth hormone was measured using very minor modifications of the method described by Catt et al.[32] Normal early morning basal values at this center using this method are 4 ± 4 mμg/ml for adult men, 6 ± 4 mμg/ml for women.

Results

Basal growth hormone levels obtained in the fashion described above were not noted to fluctuate greatly in our active and inactive acromegalic patients. Although random specimens obtained during the day and night did vary greatly, it was possible to obtain stable values in all patients who underwent control saline infusions provided they were allowed to rest for approximately 30 minutes prior to starting the infusion. Basal sera drawn in the manner described did not vary by greater than 20% on consecutive morning samples and seldom showed even this great a range of variation.

In the 16 previously treated patients, 13 or 81% had basal growth hormone levels in the normal or very near normal range (Table 1, Fig 1); each of these had been judged clinically inactive for at least one year prior to the first measurement of serum growth hormone. Of the 12 patients treated since 1965, nine or 75% have demonstrated lowering of basal serum growth hormone levels into the normal range (Table 2, Fig 1) six months to four years after treatment. Lowering of growth hormone levels in these patients has also been associated with disappearance of clinical and other laboratory findings of this disease. Although three patients in this group are unequivocally active two to four years after radiotherapy, substantial lowering of basal growth hormone values has occurred in two of these. The only patient in whom growth hormone levels have not changed following therapy is the one patient in whom suprasellar extension of the pituitary tumor was demonstrated by pneumoencephalography. Combining the two groups yielded 21 treated patients (77%) with normal or nearly normal basal growth hormone levels and six with values clearly in the active acromegalic range (Fig 1). In all instances where basal growth hormone levels were within the normal range the physician caring for a given patient believed the individual to have clinically quiescent disease.

Six patients remain active with elevated growth hormone levels 2 to 9 years after radiotherapy. By relying on examination of sequential snapshots and history of signs and symptoms it seems that the time lapse between clinically manifest disease and pituitary radiotherapy was greater than 12 years in all but one of these patients. Of the 21 inactive patients, only one had an estimated delay between symptoms and therapy of greater than ten years. Thirteen of this group had had evidence of acromegaly for less than five years before receiving pituitary radiotherapy. Of the three patients treated since 1965 who are still active, one (patient 18) demonstrated pneumoencephalographic evidence of suprasellar extension; 12 other patients had pneumoencephalograms and none showed extension above the confines of the sella turcica. Patient 19, still active three years after receiving 5,500 R, demonstrated air within the sella which suggests the possibility of cystic rupture into the subarachnoid space. Because of patient refusal, pneumoencephalogram was not performed in patient 17, who also has continued active acromegaly.

Comment

Active acromegaly requires treatment. In addition to cosmetic disfiguration and protean but disturbing symptomatology which includes fatigue, depression, diaphoresis, and headaches; disability due to unopposed hypersecretion of growth hormone also results. Diabetes mellitus, crippling osteoarthritis, entrapment syndromes, heightened risk of neoplasia, hypopituitarism, and threat to vision are among the morbid consequences of untreated disease. Moreover, acromegaly may seriously pose a threat to longevity by intracranial extension of the tumor or by myocardial decompensation due to acromegalic heart disease.[33] Reduced life expectancy because of increased risk of cerebral-vascular and respiratory disease has been documented.[34] Treatment, however, should ideally remove the hypersomatrophism without producing hypopituitarism, a serious and disabling substitute, which some would argue is a high price to pay for rendering acromegaly inactive.

Conventional external pituitary radiotherapy is sufficiently free of serious side effects as to argue for it being the obvious first choice of treatment in this disease if it is therapeutically effective. Since the initial reports of 1965 to 1967[17-19] which question the effectiveness of radiotherapy, other groups have reviewed their experience and, with us,[29] have concluded that this therapeutic method clearly should not be abandoned.[30,31] The wider experience utilizing basal growth hormone values to complement clinical evaluation in acromegaly argues for a success rate with radiation therapy which is comparable to that obtained with implantation of sources of ionizing radiation, freezing with cryoprobe implantation, and heavy-particle bombardment.[31] Indeed it has been suggested that some of the success of surgical hypophysectomy should be attributed to radiation therapy which is received by most pituitary tumor patients either before or after operation.

The discrepancy with regard to treatment success in acromegaly between different centers which offer radiation therapy does, however, require analysis. Many factors may significantly contribute to apparent differences in success rate. Technical features would appear to be an obvious source of variation, barring reports of growth hormone levels in biased series which reflect primarily patients referred because of failure to respond to irradiation. Energy source, total dose delivered, number of courses, treatment period, portal size, and location are but some of the technical features of radiotherapy which have undergone modification since the turn of the century. High energy radiation therapy with cobalt 60, 2 mev x-ray equipment (Van de Graaff generator), or 4 to 8 mev linear accelerator has generally replaced use of orthovoltage therapy. Single courses have replaced multiple interval courses at most centers since there are data suggesting that this schedule results in a higher success rate and may also bring about beneficial results more quickly.[9,11,12,14,15] Protracted fractional techniques starting with 50 to 100 R and building to higher daily doses have generally been adopted. Multiple opposing stationary or rotational fields have replaced single or dual portals and the volume of the irradiated field has been further cut by the use of small 4 × 4cm or 5 × 5cm ports.[13,35] Whether rotational field therapy offers a greater incidence of success over the use of multiple opposing stationary ports is not clear from the available literature. Although as many as 40% of patients treated with doses as low as 2,000 to 2,500 R have experienced clinical remission,[11] better results have been reported with high energy radiation using cobalt 60 in patients receiving 3,500 R or greater.[12-15] Sheline and co-workers[14] found only 26% clinical remission in patients receiving tumor doses below 3,500 R with an improved success rate of 78% in those receiving in excess of this dose. At present, calculated tumor doses at most centers approximate 4,500 to 6,500 R using cobalt 60 or similar sources. Although an appreciable increase in success rate may acrue from doses in excess of 3,500 R, there is little support for believing that doses in excess of 5,000 R achieve improved results. Further there are unquestionably factors other than strictly technical ones which influence a given acromegalic patient's response to pituitary irradiation. Cystic tumors, it has been suggested, represent a variety much more resistant to the effects of radiation therapy[9-12] and although this cannot be accurately forecast before therapy, it is estimated from neurosurgical and autopsy observations that 15% to 20% of pituitary adenomata are cystic.[10,36] Pneumoencephalograms in two of our six patients still active years following therapy, demonstrated air within a sella mass which suggests the possibility of cystic rupture into the subarachnoid space. Since pituitary radiotherapy has on rare occasion contributed to radiation-induced vasculitis and glial necrosis in portions of the temporal lobe exposed to high dose levels in the path of the beam,[37-39] it may be argued that compromise of the hypothalamopituitary portal vasculature due to variable vascular suseptibility to radiation damage may play an additional determining role in whether therapy will succeed or not. It would seem that a more serious analysis of these many factors including sex, age, ethnic characteristics, size of tumor, duration of disease, and other variables should be carried out on a broader scale than has been done to date.

Thus it would appear from our observations and additional recent reports that properly administered external radiation therapy can achieve quite acceptable therapeutic results in more than 70% of acromegalic patients so treated. Early diagnosis and treatment, and absence of cystic degeneration or supracellular extension, may significantly contribute to the therapeutic success rate. These results with high energy radiation therapy thus compare favorably with reports of success rates using yttrium 90, strontium 90, gold Au 198, and cryoprobe implantations and transphenoidal surgical hypophysectomy.[31] Heavy particle therapy has also been associated with lowering of growth hormone levels into the normal range in 70% of acromegalic patients when levels were reevaluated two years after treatment. Evaluation five to nine years after this form of therapy suggests that an even higher success rate may be achieved over this longer period.[40] By the same token, however, 81% of all patients in our series who were studied 4 to 27 years after completing conventional therapy had normal basal values and clinically inactive disease. Whether this represents delayed effects of radiation therapy or the natural course of the disease process is of course open to question.

In addition to comparing the success rate of pituitary irradiation, consideration must be given also to the comparative morbidity of x-ray treatment and other therapeutic approaches, namely surgical hypophysectomy, destructive implantations, and proton beam bombardment. Brain damage has been reported in three acromegalic patients who had previously received high dose super voltage x-ray or high energy γ-radiation to the pituitary.[39] Cumulative doses were 9,775 R, 10,126 R, and 8,150 R. Symptoms and signs of progressive brain damage and findings of intense gliosis and vasculitis at craniotomy were seen six months, one, and three years after completion of treatment. Consensus is lacking as to the exact cause of radionecrosis of brain tissue although the unusually high absolute doses and multiple treatment periods may have been largely responsible in these particular patients. Some believe that gliosis and necrosis are secondary to neuronal damage. Many investigators, however, feel that the vasculoglial architecture of the brain is the more radiovulnerable. Because of the lack of anastomatic channels in the brain, damage to the supporting vasculature is especially detrimental to critical blood supply in brain areas so affected. The latent period which has been associated with radionecrosis in portions of the brain consequent to pituitary radiation seems to fit more with the expected outcome of damage to vasculo-connective tissue and local ischemia, than with radiation induced damage to nervous tissue per se.[37-39]

Further, it appears that the degree of radiation associated brain damage is proportional to the absolute dose, the volume of the brain included in the field, the initial starting dose, and the time course over which the radiation therapy is fractionated. Repeated radiation exposures in the form of spaced series may result in greater damage, often after a delay of many years, than that of a single consecutive series of treatments calculated to deliver the same dose. By the same token, radiation delivered in too concentrated a period, although fractionated, may operate to significantly damage vascular substratum, whereas larger doses may cause no damage if protracted over a longer period starting with small daily doses which are gradually built up. Modern techniques cognizant of these and other factors, which utilize multiple stationary or rotational fields, small ports, low starting doses, and a single fractionated course over 4 to 6 weeks have virtually eliminated radiation induced brain necrosis from patients receiving irradiation to pituitary tumors. Nevertheless, consensus is still lacking as to the absolute tolerable dose, with estimates ranging between 4,500 and 6,500 R. Such estimates have been largely based on animal models studied over short intervals, and rare reports of the tragic development of radionecrosis in man have been noted not to occur until many years after therapy has been completed.

Transient temporal area epilation and extraocular muscle palsies due to injury of cranial nerves 3, 4, and 6 have been reported with pituitary radiotherapy. Spontaneous pituitary hemorrhage has occurred in patients with pituitary adenomas but rare cases have been reported where tumor hemorrhage or so-called "pituitary apoplexy" developed soon after initiation of radiation therapy.[41] There may be reason for believing that tumor doses should not exceed 50 to 100 R daily at the outset; this admonition would seem a more serious one in patients presenting with bulky, large tumor masses, in those with compromise to visual fields, or where there is pneumoencephalographic demonstration of suprasellar extension of the tumor.

Rarely sarcomatous degeneration has occurred in pituitaries of patients previously treated with external radiation. This complication is rare, however, with only four cases reported in irradiated acromegalics.[42,44] In each case multiple courses of relatively low-dose radiation was given. There has been a tendency to ascribe cause to radiation received and these reports have, in turn, been the cause of considerable concern. That radiation may not be the culprit should be considered as seriously. No instance of pituitary carcinoma or sarcoma has been reported in any patient who has received radiation to a presumed normal pituitary for a variety of disorders including breast cancer, hypertension, thyrotoxicosis, menstrual irregularities, etc.[9,11,44,45] Atkinson, in his monograph on acromegaly, believed he had found 43 pituitary sarcomas in a review of 248 autopsied cases of acromegaly who had never received irradiation.[46] This report from 1930 and others before it,[3,47] which note a fairly frequent occurrence of sarcomatous degeneration in pituitary tumors, have been largely disparaged by subsequent reports[48] as probably representing erroneous histopathologic interpretations. Nevertheless, we have available for review slides taken from the autopsy of an acromegalic-giant where a fibrosarcoma of the pituitary gland is clearly evident in a patient who had never received radiation therapy. Furthermore, it is possible to cause pituitary tumors in certain strains of animals by removing one or another target gland.[49] Here it is believed that a break in the pituitary-target gland axis leads to excessive stimulation of the pituitary by specific hypothalamic releasing factors. Clinical examples of this development in man are also recognized.[50-54] Since there is some reason for believing the hypothalamus may excessively stimulate pituitary somatotrophs in acromegaly,[55,56] it could be argued that sarcomatous degeneration in four patients who had previously been irradiated is coincidental in a disease process with a heightened risk for neoplastic degeneration with or without therapy. Indeed it may be that this complication was more frequent prior to effective therapy with high energy radiotherapy when the basic disease process was allowed to persist for a longer time. In each of the previously reported cases of sarcomas developing in pituitaries of irradiated acromegalic patients, more than one course of irradiation had been administered with relatively low-dose therapy. If supervoltage x-ray or gamma teletherapy should be held responsible for the development of these malignancies, it may be that the initial lower doses, given to patients who were treated by the space-interval technique, played a decisive role. The carcinogenic role of radiation in doses of 1,200 to 3,000 R to connective tissue is well recognized. Indeed, no instance of pituitary sarcoma has been reported in any pituitary tumor patient who received a dose in excess of 3,500 R in a single treatment course.

Finally, the amount of time required for radiation therapy to the pituitary to be effective in acromegaly varies greatly. Occasional patients have demonstrated improvement in weeks, and three out of our eight patients demonstrated lowering of elevated growth hormone levels into the normal range by 2½ and 3 months after therapy had been completed. All of the eight patients treated since 1964 who became clinically inactive demonstrated decrease in serum growth hormone levels to normal within 2½ years. Sheline and co-workers[14] noted that 70% of their patients who responded beneficially to pituitary radiation were clinically well in from six months to one year. However, since greater time for complete remission may be required in certain individuals, extended follow-up may be more appropriate than subjecting the patient to alternative therapies too early.

Thus, the somewhat longer time required for therapeutic results and the extremely rare occurrence of radiation induced brain damage or pituitary hemorrhage must be weighed against the frequency and kinds of morbidity which may accrue from other forms of therapy in acromegaly. The risks of anesthesia and the development of meningitis, pituitary or sphenoid sinus hemorrhage, cerebrospinal fluid rhinorrhea, inadvertent injury to structures within and without the cavernous sinus, and improper localization of the radiation source or cryoprobe within the pituitary tumor are among the potential hazards or difficulties associated with the implantation procedures. There may also be a greater risk to anterior-pituitary function with these techniques. Local total destruction of the tumor, as well as some normal pituitary tissue, accompanies implantation procedures and it is believed, by its advocates, that given the remarkable reserve of pituitary cells, this kind of partial hypophysectomy will not adversely affect function. Proton beam α-particle bombardment, because of lessened radiation exposure to adjacent structures, can deliver doses in excess of 6,000 R to the pituitary for treatment of acromegaly. Whether local destruction or greater exposure of normal pituitary tissue to ionizing radiation will result in too great an incidence of hypopituitarism must await long-term study. There is as yet insufficient composite data to make any accurate judgment in this regard. It is entirely uncertain whether any therapeutic advantage accrues from doses much in excess of 4,500 R. Success, as measured both clinically and by lowering of circulating growth hormone titers, using doses of 3,500 to 4,500 R already appears to approximate the success rate experienced by groups using other forms of therapy including pituitary implants and modifications of proton bombardment.

Finally, how does radiation therapy produce its therapeutic effect? It is generally taken for granted that this is due to greater radiosensitivity of the more actively metabolizing tumor cells compared to the remarkable radio-resistance of normal pituicytes. It needs to be emphasized, however, that there is very little support in the literature for this contention. Short-term observations support the presumption that normal pituitary tissue is radio-resistant. Two terminal breast cancer patients received 8,100 and 10,000 R to the pituitary gland and failed to show any histologically verifiable changes when these glands were examined 2½ to 3 months later.[45] Some workers have described early vascular degeneration in the presence of edema in some patients dying soon after irradiation but point out that this appeared to occur in particularly vascular adenomata.[9] Other reports, however, attest to the complete absence of any visible radiation changes in pituitaries of acromegalic patients who sustained clinical benefit but died of unrelated problems months or years later.[11,57] Bachman[11] was impressed with the observation that glands from clinically inactive, treated patients exhibited the same picture of adenomatous hyperplasia or adenoma formation as did pituitaries taken from clinically active, untreated acromegalics.

Many earilier reports have pointed to the prevalence of adenomatous hyperplasia of chromophobic or eosinophilic cells in the pituitary glands of acromegalic patients[2-4,11] which suggests the possibility that hyperplasia may frequently precede true adenoma formation. These observations may importantly bear on other abnormalities in acromegaly which have raised the possibility that acromegaly may be caused in some cases by inappropriate and excessive release of hypothalamic growth hormone releasing substance,[55,56] perhaps analogous to the current conceptualization of the pathogenesis of Cushing's disease.[58] If confirmatory evidence for this intriguing hypothesis should be forthcoming, then our traditional preoccupation with techniques designed to injure the pituitary will require some reconsideration. It is tempting in this regard to wonder whether conventional radiation therapy, when it is effective, is so because of significant radiation delivered to the hypothalamus. Further, it is possible that there are also deleterious effects of radiation to the vasculo-glial tissue of the hypothalamic-pituitary portal system. Since available biopsy and autopsy materials have tended to show lack of radiation necrosis in irradiated pituitaries, it may be that subtle damage to the vascular support may account for the observed therapeutic effects of pituitary irradiation in acromegaly by reducing the flow of releasing factors to the pituitary gland from the hypothalamus. This might explain apparent radiation effectiveness in acromegalics with as little as 2,000 R despite good evidence that pituicytes are far more radio-resistant and could help to explain clinical benefit in treated patients whose pituitary glands histologically demonstrate hyperplastic or adenomatous changes but no real evidence of radionecrosis when examined at postmortem.[11]

Thus, a reassessment of the results of irradiation in the treatment of active acromegaly opens several areas for question and may challenge long held assumptions as to the etiology of acromegaly, its natural course, and the appropriateness of radiation therapy as a favored form of treatment. It appears that properly performed modern radiation therapy techniques effect an equal cure rate in acromegaly when compared to implantation techniques and proton beam therapy.[31] The threat of brain damage from radiation therapy seems now to be a very remote one when modern techniques are used which substantially minimize the volume of central nervous system exposed to radiation. Pituitary hemorrhage, although occurring spontaneously, may be initiated by improper technique if large doses over a short period of time are used at the onset of a therapy course. A review of the older literature, which took note of frequent spontaneous pituitary sarcomas and of the case reports of carcinomatous degeneration in irradiated tumors in acromegaly, suggests that in the latter instance this may have been either circumstantial or associated with multiple course therapy utilizing low doses of radiation during the first treatment period.

Nevertheless, because of the apparent discrepancy in results on basal growth hormone levels in radiation treated acromegalic patients between various centers, there is still a clear need to collate as many identifiable variables of currently employed techniques against clinical and laboratory success so that the optimum radiation therapy program for treatment of acromegaly can be established. There are serious questions raised by the available literature as to whether there is any advantage to attempting to increase dosage above 5,000 R with available high energy sources. Additional consideration to whether or not this disease originates in the pituitary or in the hypothalamus will probably be forthcoming. If evidence for the latter should mount, then examination of alternative techniques designed to effect hypothalamic activity must be sought as well.[29] However, until there is a clear understanding of the pathogenesis of acromegaly, it would appear that external radiation therapy continues to offer an exceptionally innocuous route of therapy as a first recourse. Other more aggressive and seemingly more noxious therapeutic methods should be reserved as secondary approaches to radiation treatment failures. Quite obviously, neurosurgical intervention must be resorted to in those patients in whom either pneumoencephalographic evidence of extracellular extension or serious compromise of visual fields or both is obtained since rapid neurosurgical decompression in these instances represents the only possible chance of preserving vision and may, when accompanied by postoperative radiation therapy, actually preserve adequate pituitary function as well. Nevertheless, since it is rare that all of the pituitary tumor can be removed at surgery, it seems appropriate that radiation therapy be coupled to operative intervention when this approach is undertaken.

Thus this study adds further support to the contention that radiation therapy of the pituitary in acromegaly is an appropriate and effective form of treatment. Better than 70% of patients so treated appeared to sustain clinical and laboratory remission, many within one year of completion of therapy. The causes for treatment failures are not clear although suprasellar extension, and cystic degeneration may play a role. Pneumoencephalographic study will aid in identifying those patients with extrasellar extension. Possibly too, autonomous adenomas, no longer responsive to hypothalamic control, may represent tumors particularly resistant to the effects of radiation therapy. It is of interest that the duration of disease prior to treatment in our group of six therapy failures was greater than 12 years in all but one patient, an interval considerably longer than that which was estimated for the inactive group. Whether earlier diagnosis and prompt treatment will improve the success rate remains to be seen. Finally, in addition to substantiating the role of radiation therapy in the treatment of acromegaly, serial growth hormone measurements in these patients will clearly aid in determining proper dosage and treatment planning.

This investigation was supported in part by Public Health Service research grants T01-AM-05170 and RR-55 and the Fisher Endocrine Research Fund.

Nonproprietary and Trade Names of Drug

Gold Au 198—*Aureoloid-198, Auroscan-198, Aureotope.*

References

1. Minkowski O: Über einem Fall von Akromegalie berliner. *Klin Wschr* **24**:371-374, 1887.
2. Fränkel SA, Benda C: Klinische und anatomische Beiträge zur Lehre von der Akromegalie. *Deutsch Med Wschr* **23**:513-515, 1901.
3. Lewis D: Hyperplasia of the chromophile cells of hypophysis as the cause of acromegaly. *Johns Hopkins Hosp Bull* **16**:157, 1905.
4. Cushing H: The hypophysis cerebri: Clinical aspects of hyperpituitarism and hypopituitarism. *JAMA* **53**:249-255, 1909.
5. Cushing H: *The Pituitary Body and Its Disorders.*

Philadelphia, JB Lippincott Co, 1912.
6. Gramegna A: Un cas d' acromégalie traitè par la radiotherapie. *Rev Neurol* **17**:15-17, 1909.
7. Béclère A: The radio-therapeutic treatment of tumours of the hypophysis, gigantism and acromegaly. *Arch Roentgen Radiol* **14**:147-150, 1909.
8. Dyke CG, Davidoff LM: *Roentgen Treatment of Diseases of the Nervous System.* Philadelphia, Lea & Febiger Publishers, 1942.
9. Kerr HD: Irradiation of pituitary tumors. *Amer J Roentgen* **60**:348-359, 1948.
10. Davidoff LM, Feiring EH: Surgical treatment of tumors of the pituitary. *Amer J Surg* **75**:99-136, 1948.
11. Bachman AL, Hariss W: Roentgen therapy for pituitary adenoma: Correlation of tumor dose with response in 64 cases. *Radiology* **53**:331-341, 1949.
12. Buschke F: Radiotherapy of pituitary adenomas. *Western J Surg* **58**:271-278, 1950.
13. Buschke F: *Progress in Radiation Therapy.* New York, Grune & Stratton Inc, 1958.
14. Sheline GE, Goldberg MB, Feldman R: Pituitary irradiation for acromegaly. *Radiology* **76**:70-75, 1961.
15. Correa JN, Lampe I: Radiation treatment of pituitary adenomas. *J Neurosurg* **19**:626-631, 1962.
16. Glick SM, Roth J, Yalow RS, et al: Immunoassay of human growth hormone in plasma. *Nature* **199**:784-787, 1963.
17. Glick SM, Roth J, Yalow RS, et al: The regulation of growth hormone secretion. *Recent Progr Hormone Res* **21**:241-283, 1965.
18. Beck P, Schalch PS, Parker ML, et al: Correlative studies of growth hormone and insulin plasma concentrations with metabolic abnormalities in acromegaly. *J Lab Clin Med* **66**:366-379, 1965.
19. Roth J, Glick SM, Hollander CS: Acromegaly and other disorders of growth hormone secretion. *Ann Intern Med* **66**:760-788, 1967.
20. Joplin GF, Frazer R, Steiner R, et al: Partial pituitary ablation by needle implantation of gold-198 seeds for acromegaly and Cushing's disease. *Lancet* **2**:1277-1280, 1961.
21. Molinatti GM, Camanni F, Massara F, et al: Implantation of yttrium-90 in sella turcica in 16 cases of acromegaly. *J Clin Endocr* **22**:599-611, 1963.
22. Linfoot JA, Greenwood FC: Growth hormone in acromegaly: Effect of heavy particle pituitary irradiation. *J Clin Endocr* **25**:1515-1518, 1965.
23. Forrest APM, Greenwood FC, Stewart HJ, et al: Pituitary implantation for pituitary tumors. *Proc Roy Soc Med* **58**:475-480, 1965.
24. Kaufman B, Pearson OH, Shealy CN, et al: Transnasal-transphenoidal yttrium-90 pituitary implantation in therapy of acromegaly. *Radiology* **86**:915-920, 1966.
25. Dashe AM, Solomon DH, Rand RW, et al: Stereotaxic hypophyseal cryosurgery in acromegaly and other disorders. *JAMA* **198**:591-596, 1966.
26. Adams JE, Seymour RJ, Earll JM, et al: Transphenoidal cryohypophysectomy in acromegaly. *J Neurosurg* **28**:100-104, 1968.
27. Kjellberg RN, Shintani A, Frantz AG, et al: Protonbeam therapy in acromegaly. *New Eng J Med* **278**:689-695, 1968.
28. Harper PV, Strandford N, Paloyan E, et al: Destruction of the hypophyses with an Sr^{90}-Y^{90} needle. *Ann Surg* **160**:743-754, 1964.
29. Lawrence AM, Kirsteins L: Progestins in the medical management of acromegaly. *J Clin Endocr* **30**:646-652, 1970.
30. Sahnd GR, Nadeau A: Late effects of cobalt therapy on growth hormone secretion, in *Third International Congress of Endocrinology,* abstracted. *Excerpta Medica* **157**:46, 1968.
31. Roth J, Gorden P, Brace K: The efficacy of conventional pituitary irradiation in acromegaly. *New Eng J Med* **282**:1385-1391, 1970.
32. Catt K, Tregear GW: Solid-phase radioimmunoassay in antibody-coated tubes. *Science* **158**:1570-1571, 1968.
33. Pepire CJ, Aloia J: Heart muscle disease in acromegaly. *Amer J Med* **48**:530-534, 1970.
34. Wright AD, Hill DM, Lowy C, et al: Mortality in acromegaly. *Quart J Med* **39**:1-16, 1970.
35. Bouchard J: *Radiation Therapy of Tumors and Diseases of the Nervous System.* Philadelphia, Lea & Febiger Publishers, 1966, p 244.
36. Dott NM, Bailey P, Cushing H: A consideration of hypophysial adenomata. *Brit J Surg* **13**:314-366, 1925.
37. Lampe I: Radiation tolerance of the central nervous system, Buschke F (ed): in *Progress in Radiation Therapy.* New York, Grune & Stratton Inc, 1958, pp 224-236.
38. Raskin R: Central nervous system damage after radiation therapy. *Int Surg* **48**:430-441, 1967.
39. Peck FC, McGovern ER: Radiation necrosis in acromegaly. *J Neurosurg* **25**:536-542, 1966.
40. Lawrence JH, Tobias CA, Linfoot JA, et al: Successful treatment of acromegaly: Metabolic and clinical studies in 145 patients. *J Clin Endocr* **31**:180-198, 1970.
41. Hamwi GJ, Skillman TG, Tufts KC: Acromegaly. *Amer J Med* **29**:690-699, 1960.
42. Wheelock MC, del Regato JA: Eosinophilic adenoma of pituitary with sarcomatous changes. *Cancer Seminar* **3**:77-79, 1962.
43. Goldberg MB, Sheline GE, Malamud N: Malignant intracranial neoplasms, following radiation therapy for acromegaly. *Radiology* **80**:465-470, 1963.
44. Greenhouse AH: Pituitary sarcoma: Possible consequences of radiation. *JAMA* **190**:269-273, 1964.
45. Kelly KH, Feldsted ET, Brown PO, et al: Irradiation of the normal human hypophysis in malignancy: Report of three cases receiving 8100-10,000r tissue dose to the pituitary gland. *J Nat Cancer Inst* **11**:967-983, 1951.
46. Atkinson FRB: *Acromegaly.* London, John Bale Sons & Danielsson Ltd, 1932.
47. Revaut P: Acromégalie avec diabète sucré tumeur du corps pituitaire et gigantisme viscéral. *Soc Med Hop Paris* **17**:352-360, 1900.
48. Kraus JE: Neoplastic disease of the human hypophysis. *Arch Path* **39**:343-349, 1945.
49. Furth J, Dent JN, Burnett WT, et al: The mechanism of induction and the characteristics of pituitary tumors induced by thyroidectomy. *J Clin Endocr* **15**:81-97, 1955.
50. Nelson DH, Meakin JW, Dealy JB, et al: ACTH producing tumor of the pituitary gland. *New Eng J Med* **259**:161-164, 1958.
51. Van Wyk JJ, Guembach MM: Syndrome of precocious menstruation and galactorrhea: An example of hormonal overlap in pituitary feedback. *J Pediat* **57**:416-435, 1960.
52. Gordon SJ, Moses AM: Multiple endocrine organ refractoriness to trophic hormone stimulation: A patient with an enlarged sella turcica and increased FSH secretion. *Ann Intern Med* **63**:313-316, 1965.
53. Melnyk Clifford, Greer M: Functional pituitary tumor in an adult possibly 20 to long-standing myxedema. *J Clin Endocr* **25**:761-766, 1965.
54. Leiba S, Landau B, Ber A: Target gland insufficiency and pituitary tumors. *Acta Endocr* **60**:112-120, 1969.
55. Cryer PE, Daughaday WH: Regulation of growth hormone secretion in acromegaly. *J Clin Endocr* **29**:386-393, 1969.
56. Lawrence AM, Goldfine ID, Kirsteins L: Growth hormone dynamics in acromegaly. *J Clin Endocr* **31**:239-247, 1970.
57. Goldberg MB, Lisser H: Acromegaly: Consideration of its course and treatment. *J Clin Endocr* **2**:477-501, 1942.
58. Rovit RL, Duane TD: Cushing's syndrome and pituitary tumors. *Amer J Med* **46**:416-427, 1969.

The response to upright posture, measured by changes in renin activity in renal (RVR) and peripheral (PVR) veins was studied in eight normotensive, healthy adults on a normal sodium intake. Measurements were made while the subjects were supine and after 15 and 30 minutes upright. The RVR increased from a mean of 236 ± 82 ng/100 ml to 530 ± 170 ng/100 ml and 655 ± 217 ng/100 ml, 15 and 30 minutes after the subjects assumed the upright posture ($P < 0.05$). During the same interval, PVR increased in proportion to the renal venous changes. These data provide control values in healthy human adults for simultaneous RVR and PVR measured by the Boucher method.

Peripheral and Renal Vei

Effect of Postural Stimulatio

Tatiana A. Assaykeen, PhD; Ronald A. Castellino, MD; Thomas A. Love, MD; and Thomas A. Stamey, MD, Stanford, Calif

Each living renal transplant donor at Stanford Medical Center is routinely investigated by renal arteriography and selective renal venography. This provided a unique opportunity to study simultaneous renal (RVR) and peripheral (PVR) vein renin activity in healthy, normotensive patients. Two females and six males, from 23 to 52 years of age, were studied while on a regular diet and without premedication. The right renal vein was catheterized[1] via a right femoral vein. While the individuals were supine, 20-ml samples of blood were obtained simultaneously from the renal vein and an antecubital vein. The patient was then placed upright (80° to 90°) on the fluoroscopic tilt table, and after 15 minutes a second renal vein sample was drawn. Repeat samples from renal and antecubital veins were taken after an additional 15 minutes upright. The catheter position was monitored by intermittent fluoroscopy and was kept patent with heparinized 5% dextrose in water. Following completion of the sampling, contrast media was injected to confirm the position of the catheter in the renal vein. No contrast media was used prior to this injection. The blood samples were collected on ice in a solution of 3.8% ethylenediamine tetra acetic acid (EDTA) and the plasma was assayed for renin activity (nanograms of angiotensin generated per 100 ml of plasma per three-hour incubation) according to a slight modification[2] of the method of Boucher et al.[3]

When normotensive, healthy patients were stimulated by upright posturing, there was a significant increase ($P < 0.05$) in RVR when compared to RVR while supine (236 ± 82 ng/100 ml, to 530 ± 170 ng/100 ml, and 655 ± 217 ng/100 ml; 15 and 30 minutes upright). There was no significant difference in RVR when the 15 and 30 minute upright samples were compared. The PVR also increased with postural stimulation in the four of five patients in whom this comparison could be made. The mean rise for this group, however, was not significant. Utilizing data from patients 1, 3, 4, 5, and 8, the PVR rose from a mean of 222±89 ng/100 ml to

Received for publication Nov 16, 1970; accepted Feb 25, 1971.

From Stanford University School of Medicine, Stanford, Calif. Dr. Love is now with Chelsea Naval Hospital, Boston.

Reprint requests to Department of Surgery, Division of Urology, Stanford University School of Medicine, Stanford, Calif 94305 (Dr. Assaykeen).

Renin Activity

n Normotensive Healthy Adults

Normotensive Donors—Venous Renin Activity*

Patient No.	Age (yr)	Sex	Supine Renal	Supine Antecubital	Upright 15 Minutes Renal	Upright 30 Minutes Renal	Upright 30 Minutes Antecubital
1	28	F	100	120	180	490	210
2	25	M	140	50	620	350	...
3	52	M	560	250	920	1,870	1,270
4	47	F	80	40	280	300	180
5	23	M	160	150	270	220	170
6	27	M	160	...†	400	740	390
7	50	M	40	...	60	40	40
8	31	M	650	550	1,510	1,230	1,180
			236±82‡	193±78	530±170 ($P<0.05$)§	655±217 ($P<0.05$)	491±190 ($P>0.05$)

* In nanograms per 100 ml per three hours.
† Laboratory accident.
‡ Mean ± 1 standard error of the mean.
§ Level of significance when compared to the respective supine value.

602 ± 255 ng/100 ml, a 2.7-fold rise; and the RVR rose from 310 ± 122 ng/100 ml to 822 ± 317 ng/100 ml, also a 2.7-fold increase. In both the supine and 30 minute upright positions, the RVR was 1.4-fold higher than the corresponding PVR.

The values in the Table represent levels for RVR and PVR in normotensive and otherwise healthy patients and indicate the normal response to postural stimulation in both renal and peripheral venous blood. Our values for PVR before and after postural stimulation compare with those of Cohen et al.[4] They, however, did not report values for RVR. Kaneko et al[5] reported simultaneous values for PVR and RVR in normotensive patients, utilizing another method for measuring renin and employing a different stimulus, acute reduction of arterial pressure with sodium nitroprusside infusions. During control periods their RVR was 1.3-fold greater than simultaneous PVR. This figure compares well with our value of a 1.4-fold difference.

The data presented confirm the reported effects of postural stimulation on renin secretion,[4] indicate the relationship between RVR and PVR during stimulation of renin secretion, and provide baseline values for comparison of data from hypertensive patients when the Boucher method is utilized.

This investigation was supported in part by Public Health Service training grant 5 TOI AM 05513.

References

1. Seldinger SI: Catheter replacement of the needle in percutaneous arteriography: A new technique. *Acta Radiol* **39**:368-376, 1953.

2. Assaykeen TA, Otsuka K, Ganong WF: Rate of disappearance of exogenous dog renin from the plasma of nephrectomized dogs. *Proc Soc Exp Biol Med* **127**:306-310, 1968.

3. Boucher R, Veyrat R, de Champlain J, et al: New procedures for measurement of human plasma angiotensin and renin activity levels. *Canad Med Assoc J* **90**:194-201, 1964.

4. Cohen EL, Conn JW, Rovner DR: Postural augmentation of plasma renin activity and aldosterone excretion in normal people. *J Clin Invest* **46**:418-428, 1967.

5. Kaneko Y, Ikeda T, Takeda T, et al: Renin release during acute reduction of arterial pressure in normotensive subjects and patients with renovascular hypertension. *J Clin Invest* **46**:705-716, 1967.

Saline Suppression of Plasma Aldosterone in Hypertension

MAJ David C. Kem, MC, USA, Honolulu; Myron H. Weinberger, MD, Indianapolis; Darrel M. Mayes, Honolulu; and Charles A. Nugent, MD, Tucson, Ariz

Nine normal subjects and 18 patients with essential hypertension had similar suppression of plasma aldosterone concentration to 5 ng/100 ml or less after intravenous infusion of 2 liters of isotonic saline during four hours of recumbency. Six patients with aldosteronism and adrenal adenomas or glucocorticoid suppressible hyperplasia failed to suppress normally. One hypertensive hypokalemic patient with low plasma renin activity had elevated plasma deoxycorticosterone and failed to suppress his plasma aldosterone concentration below 5 ng/100 ml. Three of four patients with renovascular stenosis and hypertension suppressed normally. The fourth patient with a postinfusion plasma aldosterone concentration of 7 ng/100 ml was found to suppress normally when this value was expressed as percent of the two-hour upright value. This saline infusion, recumbency test is rapid and requires minimal patient preparation.

Expansion of the extracellular and intravascular volumes by oral administration of sodium chloride with[1,2] and without mineralocorticoids[3] and by intravenous infusion of saline[4] and albumin[5] has been used to investigate abnormalities in the control of aldosterone secretion in hypertensive patients. Presumably, suppression of renin by these stimuli in responsive individuals leads to decreased angiotensin generation and aldosterone production. These stimuli are expected to suppress aldosterone production and excretion in patients with essential and renovascular hypertension, but not in those with primary aldosteronism.[6] (For brevity, "primary aldosteronism" is used in this article to refer to patients with excessive aldosterone production and suppressed renin activity. Adenomas, idiopathic hyperplasia, and glucococorticoid suppressible hyperplasia all show these characteristics[7] although each has different morphologic and therapeutic features.) Patients with primary aldosteronism are expected to have greater than normal autonomy of aldosterone production. A number of problems characterize the use of these tests in identifying patients with primary aldosteronism and in distinguishing these patients from individuals with secondary aldosteronism. The tests take several days to perform, all require collection of 24-hour urine specimens, and some do not allow confident separation of patients with primary from those with secondary hyperaldosteronism.[5]

Measurement of plasma aldosterone has been used to document hyperaldosteronemia.[2,8-12] Plasma aldosterone concentration may be within normal limits in patients with primary aldosteronism in spite of obtaining the samples from subjects who were either sodium-replete or taking a diet in which sodium was unrestricted.[11] Even if plasma aldosterone con-

Received for publication Jan 11, 1971; accepted May 17.

From the departments of internal medicine, Tripler Army Hospital, Honolulu (Dr. Kem); the Indiana University Medical Center, Indianapolis (Dr. Weinberger); the University of Hawaii School of Medicine, Honolulu (Mr. Mayes); and the University of Arizona College of Medicine, Tucson (Dr. Nugent). Dr. Kem is now with the University of Texas Southwestern Medical School, Dallas. Mr. Mayes is now with the Inter-Science Institute, Los Angeles.

Read in part before the 52nd Annual Meeting of the Endocrine Society, St. Louis, June 10, 1970.

Reprint requests to Department of Internal Medicine, University of Arizona College of Medicine, Tucson, Ariz 85724 (Dr. Nugent).

centration were elevated, its determination would not be expected to separate primary and secondary forms of hyperaldosteronism except possibly when done as part of a test of the mechanisms controlling aldosterone production.

This study was undertaken to determine whether acute suppression of plasma aldosterone by a single intravenous infusion of 2 liters of isotonic saline in recumbent patients might provide an effective tool for the diagnosis of hyperaldosteronism and differentiate between those of primary and secondary origin.

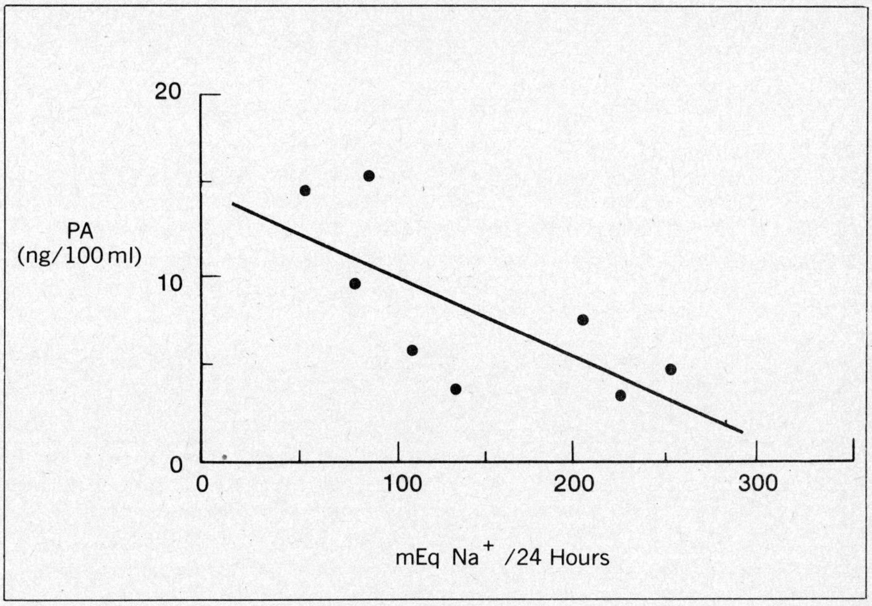

Fig 1.—Relation between sodium excretion on the day prior to infusion and the eight-hour recumbent plasma aldosterone (PA) concentration in eight normal subjects.

Fig 2.—Plasma aldosterone (PA) after eight hours recumbency (→), after two hours upright (↑), and after four hours recumbency and infusion (→ after infusion). The dotted line indicates the highest value after infusion in groups 1, 2a, and 2b.

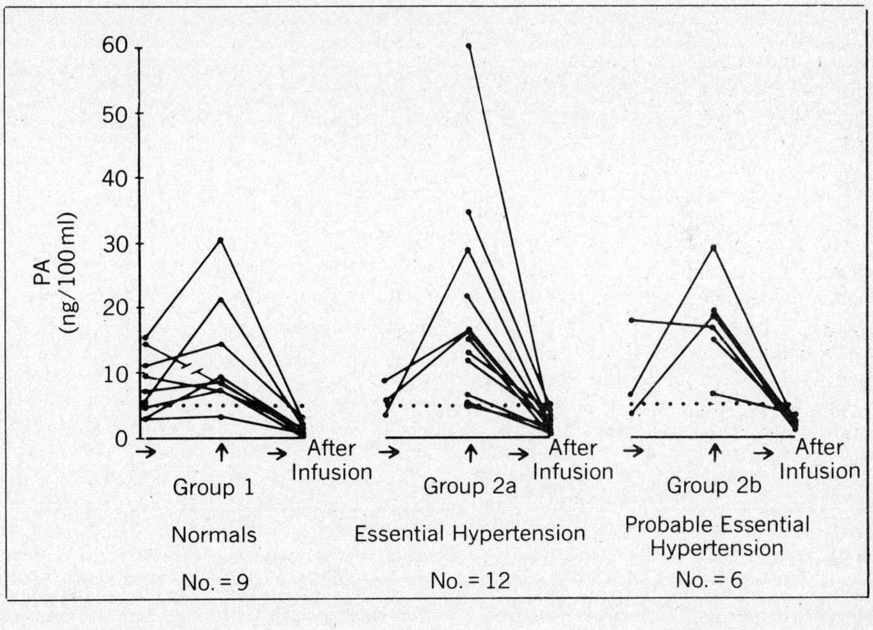

Materials and Methods

Plasma aldosterone was measured by radioimmunoassay.[13] Urine aldosterone was measured using either a double isotope derivative method[14] or radioimmunoassay of aldosterone released from urine by hydrolysis at pH 1 for 16 hours and processed in the same manner as plasma aldosterone. Plasma renin activity (PRA) in most patients was measured by the method of Gunnells et al.[15] Results of PRA analysis obtained by radioimmunoassay of generated angiotensin I[16] are specifically designated. Blood for PRA was chilled immediately after venipuncture and the plasma was separated at 2 C and frozen until it was analyzed. Evaluation of all patients included a hostory; physical examination; urinalysis; determination of serum electrolytes, urinary catecholamines, and 17-ketogenic steroids[17]; and either para-aminohippuric acid (PAH) renograms[18] or rapid sequence intravenous pyelograms.[19] Aortography and differential renal vein PRA were obtained in patients thought to have renovascular disease because of abnormal screening tests.[20] Adrenal venography was performed in patients with aldosteronism for localization of tumors and for determination of hyperplasia.[21]

Drugs containing estrogens were discontinued for at least one month and diuretics for at least one week before the study. Dietary sodium was not controlled prior to the saline infusion. Patients collected a 24-hour urine specimen the day prior to the saline infusion for determination of sodium and potassium excretion. Prior to the infusion patients were recumbent overnight for eight hours until 6 AM. At this time, blood for aldosterone and PRA determinations was obtained from recumbent inpatients and both inpatients and outpatients were asked to remain upright for two hours. Breakfast was withheld and at 8 AM blood was obtained for aldosterone, PRA, and serum electrolyte determinations. The patients were then placed in the supine position, and 2 liters of isotonic saline were infused evenly over a four-hour period. Blood for aldosterone and PRA determinations was obtained after two and four hours of saline infusion and recumbency. Blood pressure and pulse rate were monitored during the infusions.

Informed consent to perform the study was given by all volunteer subjects and patients before the saline infusion.

Nine normal volunteers (group 1) were

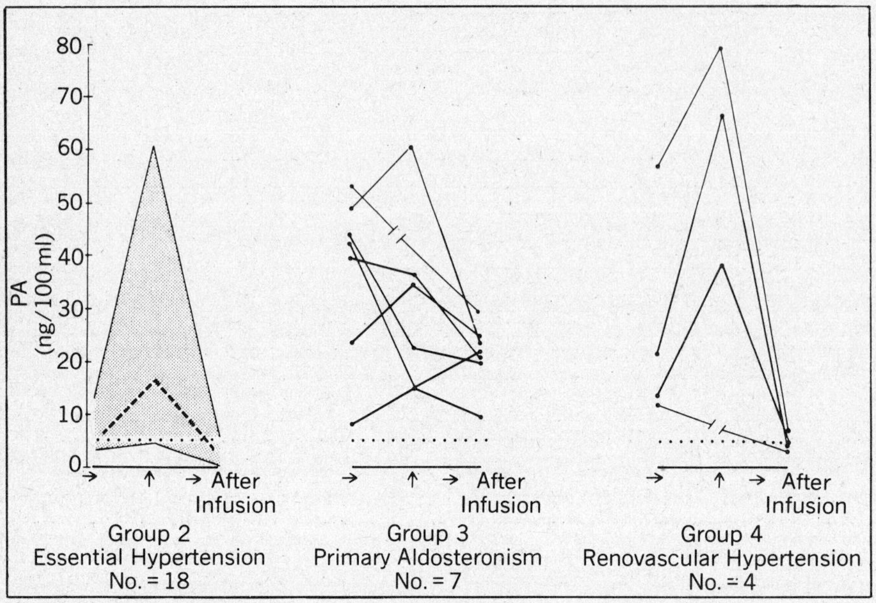

Fig 3.—Plasma aldosterone in groups 2, 3, and 4. The solid lines for ggroup 2 encompass the range of individual values and the dashed lines represent the median values. The horizontal dotted line is the same as in Fig 2. y = 14.4 -0.046x, r = -0.71.

Fig 4.—The percent suppression of plasma aldosterone is plotted as a function of the plasma aldosterone concentration after infusion. Data enclosed in boxes represent suppression as percent of eight-hour recumbent values.

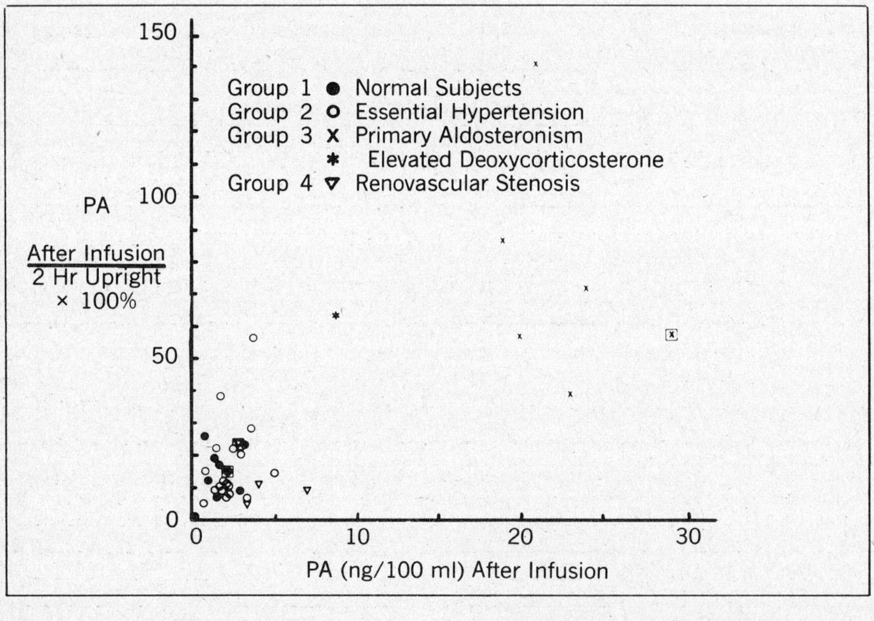

studied. All were healthy men with no history of hypertension or renal disease.

Ten men and eight women with a diagnosis of essential hypertension were studied. Patients with malignant hypertension or diastolic blood pressure greater than 140 mm Hg were excluded from the study. In 12, the diagnosis was based on normal results of screening tests (group 2a). Six patients with probable essential hypertension had unilateral abnormalities on renograms or rapid-sequence pyelography but had normal aortography or renal vein PRA determinations or both (group 2b).

Six hypertensive, hypokalemic patients with elevated urinary aldosterone excretion before and after potassium supplementation and with suppressed PRA were studied (group 3). Adrenal adenomas have been removed from five with resolution of hypokalemia and amelioration of hypertension. Three patients (28, 29, and 30) although improved, have not become normotensive since surgery. One patient (31) has glucocorticoid-suppressible aldosteronism and a hyperplastic left adrenal demonstrated by venography. The right adrenal vein was not catheterized. After 1 mg per day of dexamethasone (Decadron), plasma aldosterone concentration decreased to less than 1 ng/100 ml within two days. Hypokalemia was corrected within two weeks and the serum potassium concentration has remained normal for ten months. Hypertension of greater than 20 years' duration has markedly diminished but not disappeared during this time. One additional patient (34) with hypokalemia, hypertension, low PRA, and elevated plasma deoxycorticosterone concentration has been included in group 3. Urinary aldosterone excretion was 3μg per day. Pending results of studies for other mineralocorticoids which may be contributing to his hypokalemia and hypertension, surgery has been deferred. All seven patients in group 3 became normokalemic after treatment with spironolactone.

Four hypertensive patients with renovascular stenosis (group 4) were studied. All had unilateral abnormalities on intravenous pyelography and renal arteriography and a twofold or greater difference in renal vein PRA. Three patients had an elevated two-hour upright PRA. Patients 35 and 38 had normal blood pressures following unilateral nephrectomy and vascular repair. Patient 36 was excluded from surgical therapy because of advanced age. Patient 37 had severe renovascular stenosis and a small kidney but there was no improvement in hypertension following unilateral nephrectomy.

The Wilcoxon Signed-Ranks test and Mann Whitney two-sample rank test were used to examine data.[22] The null hypothesis was rejected when P was < 0.05 (one-tailed).

Results

Sodium excretion on the day prior to the study (Table) was similar in all patient groups except for three of four patients with renovascular stenosis and hypertension (group 4) who excreted large amounts of sodium.

The concentration of plasma aldosterone determined in recumbent normal subjects correlates with the 24-hour urine sodium excretion ($r = -0.71$, $P = 0.05$, Fig 1). Normal subjects (group 1) had significantly higher plasma aldosterone concentrations ($P < 0.025$) after they had been upright for two hours than after being recumbent overnight (Table and Fig 2). After saline infusion and four hours of recumbency plasma aldosterone decreased to a median of 1.5 ng/100 ml. This is significantly lower than the values of samples collected after eight hours of recumbency and after two hours in the upright position ($P < 0.005$). In order to examine whether this suppression might be due to posture alone, three subjects were similarly studied, but the saline infusion was omitted. Plasma aldosterone values for these subjects are as follows: 11, 7, and 6 ng/100 ml after eight hours of recumbency; 36, 10, and 8 ng/100 ml after standing for two hours; and 14, 5.2, and 4.6 ng/100 ml after lying down for four hours.

Plasma aldosterone concentrations in samples from patients with probable essential hypertension (group 2b) were similar to those in patients with essential hypertension (2a) both before and after saline infusion. There was no additional evidence that the renographic or pyelographic abnormalities identified in group 2b were associated with any other cause of hypertension nor did they demonstrate any resistance to suppression of plasma aldosterone concentration. We have therefore combined groups 2a and 2b as group 2 (essential hypertension) in Table 1 and in Fig 3. The median plasma aldosterone concentrations in samples obtained from patients in group 2 at all times were similar to those found in normal subjects. All patients with essential hypertension suppressed plasma aldosterone to 5 ng/100 ml or less after

Effect of Saline Infusion on PA and PRA

Patient No.	Sodium (mEq) 24-hr Excretion	PA (ng/100 ml) 8-hr Recumbency	PA (ng/100 ml) 2-hr Upright	PA (ng/100 ml) After Infusion	PA Suppression % 2-hr Upright	PRA (ng/100 ml/hr) 2-hr Upright	PRA (ng/100 ml/hr) After Infusion
Group 1							
1	51	15		2.2			
2	79	9.4	7.4	0.0	0		
3		11	14	3.2	23		
4	89	15	31	2.9	9		
5	109	5.3	21	1.5	7		
6	134	3.2	9.3	1.6	17		
7	204	7.1	8.5	1.0	12		
8	226	2.9	3.1	0.8	26		
9	252	4.5	7.3	1.4	19		
Median	122	7.1	8.9	1.5	15		
Range	(51-252)	(2.9-15)	(3.1-31)	(0.0-3.2)	(0-26)		
No.	8	9	8	9	8		
Group 2a							
10	13		22	2.2	10	555	266
11	32		61	3.4	5	327	106
12	60	5.9	16	1.9	12		
13	90		4.8	1.8	38	92	25
14	93		13	3.6	28	174	96
15	106		35	5.0	14	317	75
16	119	8.7	17	1.7	10	102	40
17	136		6.7	1.5	22	123	45
18	153		12	2.6	22	150	46
19	154	3.4	29	2.3	8	567	75
20	163		15	0.7	5	133	63
21	199		5.2	0.8	15	102	77
Median	113	5.9	15.5	2.1	13	150	75
Range	(13-199)	(3.4-8.7)	(4.8-61)	(0.7-5.0)	(5-38)	(92-567)	(25-266)
No.	12	3	12	12	12	11	11
Group 2b							
22	99	6.7	29	2.1	7		
23	112	18	16	1.4	9	112	71
24	151	3.7	19	1.8	9	171	77
25	247		6.8	3.8	56	100	25
26	338		15	3.0	20	152	92
27			19	2.1	11	217	124
Median	151	6.7	18	2.1	10	152	77
Range	(99-338)	(3.7-18)	(6.8-29)	(1.4-3.8)	(7-56)	(100-217)	(25-124)
No.	5	3	6	6	6	5	5
Group 2 (comb)							
Median	116	6.3	16	2.1	11	151	75
Range	(13-338)	(3.4-18)	(4.8-61)	(0.7-5.0)	(5-56)	(92-567)	(25-266)
No.	17	6	18	18	18	16	16
Group 3							
28	13*	39	36	20	56	102	67
29	13*	42	15	21	140	7	10
30	185	48	61	23	38	5	<5
31	460	23	34	24	71	88†	<50†
32	76	43	22	19	86	4	4
33	nl diet*	51		29		22‡	20
34	nl diet*	7.5	14	8.8	63	63	29
Median		41	28	21	67	36	10
Range		(7.5-51)	(14-61)	(8.8-29)	(38-140)	(4-102)	(0-67)
No.		7	6	7	6	6	7
Group 4							
35	414	21	67	3.3	5	500†	114†
36	314	13	38	4.1	11	292†	106†
37	50	12		2.8		119‡	61
38	196	57	80	7.0	9	2,747	101
Median		17	67	3.7	9	500	104
Range		(12-57)	(38-80)	(2.8-7.0)	(5-11)	(292-2,747)	(61-114)
No.		4	3	4	3	3	4

* Dietary intake excretion not measured.
† Bioassay.
‡ Eight-hour recumbent.

saline infusion and recumbency. The median plasma aldosterone concentration of group 2 after infusion was similar to that of group 1.

Six patients with documented primary aldosteronism had concentrations of plasma aldosterone after eight hours of recumbency which were near or above the highest found under similar circumstances in groups 1 and 2 (Fig 2 and 3). After two hours of upright posture, all five patients studied had plasma aldosterone concentrations which were within the range found in groups 1 and 2. All seven group-3 patients failed to suppress normally after saline infusion (Fig 3 and 4). The lowest plasma aldosterone concentration after saline infusion in the six patients with documented primary aldosteronism was 19 ng/100 ml and the median of 21 ng/100 ml for the same patients was significantly higher than that of groups 1 and 2 ($P < 0.005$). Patient 34 does not have typical primary aldosteronism since he has low urinary aldosterone excretion and a markedly elevated plasma deoxycorticosterone concentration. While he had the lowest plasma aldosterone concentrations of any patient in group 3, he also failed to suppress below 5 ng/100 ml.

Four patients with documented unilateral renovascular stenosis and hypertension (group 4) were studied. Three had elevated plasma aldosterone concentrations after being recumbent overnight and after two hours in the upright position. Three patients' plasma aldosterone decreased normally to less than 5 ng/100 ml following the saline infusion. The fourth patient (38) suppressed her plasma aldosterone concentration to 7 ng/100 ml which is slightly above the highest value found in the patients with essential hypertension. She had the highest 8-hour recumbent and two-hour upright values. The median suppression for group 4 was 9% (range 5 to 11) of the two-hour upright value. The response to saline infusion in these patients was similar to that in groups 1 and 2 and clearly different from that of group 3 (Fig 2, 3, and 4).

The effect of saline infusion on PRA was examined in groups 2a, 2b, 3, and 4 (Table). The PRA was similar in groups 2a and 2b, both in the two-hour upright posture and after suppression by saline infusion. The median PRA after saline infusion was 50% of the two-hour upright value. The PRA values in all patients in group 3 after overnight recumbency or after being upright for two hours were low relative to sodium excretion. Five of the seven patients had further suppression following infusion. The three patients with renovascular stenosis and elevated plasma aldosterone concentrations also had elevated PRA after two hours of upright posture. These values were in the highest range seen in the patients with essential hypertension in spite of the fact that all three patients were excreting large amounts of sodium. It is of interest that after saline infusion all four had PRA values similar to those in group 2.

The possibility that variations in prior salt intake might effect the saline infusion test was investigated in patients with essential hypertension by separating the patients into those excreting more and less than 100 mEq of sodium per day prior to the saline infusion. Both groups suppressed plasma aldosterone equally after saline infusion.

Initially, blood samples for aldosterone were drawn two and four hours after starting the saline infusion. In group-2 patients, the median plasma aldosterone concentration after two hours of saline infusion was 3.4 ng/100 ml (range 2.2 to 8.5 ng/100 ml). Because of the limited effectiveness of a two-hour saline infusion in suppressing plasma aldosterone in patients with essential hypertension, only four-hour plasma aldosterone values have been used subsequently.

There was no significant difference between mean serum potassium concentrations before and after infusion in patients with essential hypertension. In patients with primary aldosteronism, the greatest decrease after infusion was 0.5 mEq/liter and this was not accompanied by any change in symptoms.

Over 50 infusions have been performed. Two hypertensive patients had transient elevations of diastolic blood pressure (15 mm of Hg over baseline) which returned to normal before the infusion was finished.

Comment

George et al[5] used intravenous infusions of albumin to examine the effect of volume expansion on aldosterone production in normal subjects and in patients with primary and secondary aldosteronism. Patients were given a diet low in sodium, and aldosterone excretion and secretion were measured before and after infusion of 50 or 100 gm of albumin per day for three to eight days. The test showed elevated values for aldosterone secretory rates in all six patients with primary aldosteronism after infusion. However, on the basis of this test, six of 11 patients with secondary aldosteronism could not be differentiated from patients with primary aldosteronism.

Espiner et al[4] used intravenous saline infusions to expand plasma volume in normal individuals and patients with aldosterone-producing adenomas maintained on diets containing 10 mEq of sodium per day. They infused their patients with 2 liters of isotonic saline for four hours on two consecutive days. Aldosterone secretion values obtained on the second day allowed clear separation of the two groups. Patients with secondary aldosteronism were not included in their study. A drop in serum potassium ranging from 0.2 to 1.2 mEq/liter was noted in all of their patients with adenomas. This was attributed in part to urinary potassium loss through increased exchange of potassium for sodium in the distal tubule during the two-day period.

Slaton et al[6] infused patients with primary aldosteronism with isotonic solutions containing either dextran or plasma proteins and sodium chloride over two to four hours and measured 24-hour urinary aldosterone excretion after starting the infusion. Seven of ten patients with an aldosterone-producing adenoma failed to suppress aldosterone excretion significantly below baseline. Results in normal subjects were not included for comparison with three patients whose values were suppressed.

These studies indicate that patients with an aldosterone-producing adenoma of hyperplasia can, with only a few exceptions, be separated from normal subjects by measurement of aldosterone secretion of excretion before and after direct volume expansion. Nevertheless, the relative difficulty and expense of performing such tests and their reported inability to differentiate primary from secondary forms of aldosteronism have discouraged their utilization in clinical medicine. Thus, George et al[5] could find no advantage of acute volume expansion over that of determining the serum potassium response to oral administration of sodium chloride.

Failure to control posture and dietary sodium intake would decrease the value of determination of plasma aldosterone concentration in the diagnosis of primary aldosteronism. Plasma aldosterone is increased by upright posture (Fig 2) and by decreased sodium intake (Fig 1). Plasma aldosterone also follows a circadian pattern in normal individuals with peak values in the morning and lowest values at 6 PM and midnight.[23] Patients with primary and idiopathic aldosteronism have a similar pattern and occasionally have values within the normal range.[24,25]

Our study shows that in response to recumbency and the infusion of 2 liters of isotonic saline over a four-hour period, normal subjects (group 1) and patients with essential hypertension (group 2) have easily suppressed plasma aldosterone levels in spite of widely varying sodium excretion. Luetscher et al[12] gave 18 gm or more of sodium chloride orally to normal subjects and patients with essential hypertension. They reported impaired suppression of plasma aldosterone concentration in their hypertensive patients. In our study, we found both groups suppressed similarly. This difference might be attributable to patient selection, relative strength of stimulus, or, possibly, different mechanisms by which suppression occurs when rapid intravenous salt loading in recumbent patients is used rather than prolonged oral loading in ambulant patients.

Hypertensive patients, including those with primary aldosteronism, have been reported to have an accelerated excretion rate of infused sodium when compared with normal subjects.[26,27] The similarity of plasma aldosterone concentration after infusion in groups 1 and 2 in our study suggests that differences in the rate of sodium excretion do not alter the response of this hormone to rapid volume expansion. There was no significant difference in suppression of plasma aldosterone in patients excreting small or large amounts of sodium in our study. While severe sodium restriction should be avoided, no other dietary measures seem indicated prior to the procedure.

All seven patients with hypermineralocorticoidism due either to an adenoma or to hyperplasia (group 3) had impaired suppression of plasma aldosterone concentration. These patients also have either a blunted or a paradoxical response of plasma aldosterone concentration to changes of posture.

We have used the highest plasma aldosterone concentration found after infusion in normal subjects and patients with hypertension (5 ng/100 ml) as one criterion to separate individuals with normal and impaired suppressibility. However, for classification of some patients, it may be more helpful to examine the percent suppression of plasma aldosterone concentration plotted as a function of the plasma aldosterone concentration after infusion (Fig 4). Our six patients with documented primary aldosteronism in group 3 have impaired suppressibility and high plasma aldosterone concentrations after infusion. The data on these patients are well separated from those of normal subjects and patients with essential and renovascular hypertension Patient 34 (group 3) occupies an intermediate position. In using this saline infusion test for the diagnosis of primary aldosteronism, even if a patient (such as patient 38 in group 4) has a slightly elevated postinfusion plasma aldosterone concentration, a marked percentage decrease in aldosterone concentration following saline infusion would place the patient with groups 1, 2, and 4 in the lower left-hand corner of Fig 4.

The secondary aldosteronism in three of our four patients with renovascular hypertension was unexpected. Hypokalemia was absent though none were taking diets very low in sodium content. Our studies, utilizing direct measurement of plasma aldosterone, confirm those of Vecsei et al[28] who used secretory and metabolic clearance data to calculate mean plasma aldosterone concentration. In their study 14 of 18 patients with renovascular disease had elevated plasma aldosterone concentrations. Kotchen et al[29] reported that the best therapeutic responses to surgery in patients with renovascular stenosis were in those having secondary aldosteronism. Our experience has been similar with good therapeutic responses to surgery in two patients with secondary aldosteronism. The third patient has responded well to appropriate medical therapy. The patient with a normal plasma aldosterone concentration relative to sodium intake had no decrease of hypertension after unilateral nephrectomy.

It has been helpful to obtain two-hour upright PRA determinations in investigating patients for primary aldosteronism. When the values are interpreted relative to the 24-hour urinary sodium excretion preceding the test, markedly suppressed levels support excluding renovascular hypertension. The finding of a high PRA and plasma aldosterone concentration relative to sodium excretion followed by normal suppression of plasma aldosterone after infusion is consistent with a renovascular basis for hypertension. The PRA determination after infusion has not been of diagnostic value and might be omitted. Patients with questionably abnormal suppressibility and mildly elevated plasma aldosterone concentrations after infusion should be studied by alternative techniques for investigating primary and secondary aldosteronism[1-7,10,11,21] or they could be restudied by saline infusion after six months.

This investigation was supported in part by Public Health Service research grants HE-06308, FR-00057, and AM-11455 and by a research and development grant from the US Army awarded to Tripler General Hospital.

MAJ Carroll Martin, MC, USA; MAJ Darrel Combs, MC, USA; MAJ George Dewey, MC, USA; MAJ Frederick Stoddard, MC, USA; MAJ Richard Merrill, MC, USA; and CAPT LeeRoy Joyner, MC, USA, assisted in studying the patients. LTC Jorges Gutierrez, MC, USA, and Joseph Bookstein, MD, performed and interpreted the renal venography studies. John Ladd, MD, referred and followed-up one of the patients in group 3.

References

1. Biglieri EG, Slaton PE, Kronfield SJ, et al: Diagnosis of an aldosterone-producing adenoma in primary aldosteronism. *JAMA* **201**:510-514, 1967.

2. Horton R: Stimulation and suppression of aldosterone in plasma of normal men and in primary aldosteronism. *J Clin Invest* **48**:1230-1236, 1969.

3. Weinberger MH, Dowdy AJ, Nokes GW, et al: Plasma renin activity and aldosterone secretion in hypertensive patients during high and low sodium intake and administration of diuretic. *J Clin Endocr* **28**:359-371, 1968.

4. Espiner EA, Tucci JR, Jagger PI, et al: Effect of saline infusions on aldosterone secretion and electrolyte excretion in normal subjects and patients with primary aldosteronism. *New Eng J Med* **277**:1-7, 1967.

5. George JM, Wright L, Bell NH, et al: The syndrome of primary aldosteronism. *Amer J Med* **48**:343-356, 1970.

6. Slaton PE, Schambelan M, Biglieri EG: Stimulation and suppression of aldosterone secretion in patients with an aldosterone-producing adenoma. *J Clin Endocr* **29**:239-250, 1969.

7. Salti IS, Stiefel M, Ruse JL, et al: Non-tumorous "primary" aldosteronism. *Canad Med Assoc J* **101**:1-16, 1969.

8. Peterson RE: Determination of peripheral plasma aldosterone, in Baulieu EE, Robel P (eds): *Aldosterone*. Oxford, England, Blackwell Scientific Publications, 1964, pp 145-161.

9. Balikian HM, Brodie AH, Dale SL, et al: Effect of posture on the metabolic clearance rate, plasma concentration and blood production rate of aldosterone in man. *J Clin Endocr* **28**:1630-1640, 1968.

10. Fraser R, Brown JJ, Chinn R, et al: The control of aldosterone secretion and its relationship to the diagnosis of hyperaldosteronism. *Scot Med J* **14**:420-440, 1969.

11. Brown JJ, Davies DL, Fraser R, et al: Plasma electrolytes, renin and aldosterone in the diagnosis of primary hyperaldosteronism. *Lancet* **2**:55-59, 1968.

12. Luetscher JA, Weinberger MH, Dowdy AJ, et al: Effects of sodium loading, sodium depletion and posture on plasma aldosterone concentration and renin activity in hypertensive patients. *J Clin Endocr* **29**:1310-1318, 1969.

13. Mayes D, Furuyama S, Kem DC, et al: A radioimmunoasay for plasma aldosterone. *J Clin Endocr* **30**:682-685, 1970.

14. Kliman B, Peterson RE: Double isotope derivative assay of aldosterone in biological extracts. *J Biol Chem* **235**:1639-1648, 1960.

15. Gunnells JC, Grim CE, Robinson RR, et al: Plasma renin activity in healthy subjects and patients with hypertension. *Arch Intern Med* **119**:232-240, 1967.

16. Haber E, Koerner T, Page LB, et al: Application of a radioimmunoassay for angiotensin I to the physiologic measurements of plasma renin activity in normal human subjects. *J Clin Endocr* **29**:1349-1355, 1969.

17. Metcalf MG: A rapid method for measuring 17-hydroxy-corticosteroids in urine. *J Endocr* **26**:415-423, 1963.

18. Nordyke RA, Tonchen A: The radiohippuran renogram. *JAMA* **183**:440-443, 1963.

19. Maxwell MH, Gonick HC, Wiita R, et al: Use of the rapid-sequence intravenous pyelogram in the diagnosis of renovascular hypertension. *New Eng J Med* **270**:213-220, 1964.

20. Mannick JA, Huvos A, Hollander WE: Post-hydralazine renin release in the diagnosis of renovascular hypertension. *Ann Surg* **170**:409-415, 1969.

21. Conn JW, Rovner DR, Cohen EL, et al: Preoperative diagnosis of primary aldosteronism. *Arch Intern Med* **123**:113-123, 1969.

22. Goldstein A: *Biostatistics*. New York, Macmillan Co, 1964, pp 15-63.

23. Michelakis AM, Horton R: The relationship between plasma renin and aldosterone in normal man. *Circ Res* **27**:185-194, 1970.

24. Kem DC, Mayes D, Nugent CA: Saline suppression of plasma aldosteronism and renin in hypertension, abstracted, in *Program of the 52nd Annual Meeting of the Endocrine Society*, 1970, p 64.

25. Kem DC, Weinberger MH, Mayes D, et al: ACTH and renin in the circadian rhythm of plasma aldosterone. *Clin Res* **18**:603, 1970.

26. Baldwin DS, Biggs AW, Goldring W, et al: Exaggerated natriuresis in essential hypertension. *Amer J Med* **24**:893-902, 1958.

27. Rovner DR, Conn JW, Knopf RF, et al: Nature of renal escape from the sodium-retaining effect of aldosterone in primary aldosteronism in normal subjects. *J Clin Endocr* **25**:53-64, 1965.

28. Vecsei P, Dusterdieck G, Jahnecke J, et al: Secretion and turnover of aldosterone in various pathological states. *Clin Sci* **36**:241-256, 1969.

29. Kotchen TA, Lytton B, Morrow LB, et al: Angiotensin and aldosterone in renovascular hypertension. *Arch Intern Med* **125**:265-272, 1970.

Macular Cherry-Red Spot, Corneal Clouding, and β-Galactosidase Deficiency

A new syndrome which combines clinical features of several storage diseases (mucopolysaccharidoses, sphingolipidoses, and mucolipidoses), but which is nonetheless unique, is characterized by autosomal recessive inheritance and the *presence* of dwarfism, gargoyle facies, mental retardation, seizures, corneal clouding, macular cherry-red spot, β-galactosidase deficiency, dysostosis multiplex, and hearing deficit. It is also characterized by the *absence* of clinically enlarged organs, vacuolated blood cells, and mucopolysacchariduria.

Clinical, Biochemical, and Electron Microscopic Study of a New Autosomal Recessive Storage Disease

Morton F. Goldberg, MD; Edward Cotlier, MD;
Larry G. Fichenscher, MD; Kenneth Kenyon, MD;
Rafael Enat, MD; and Stephen A. Borowsky, MD, Chicago

The cherry red spot in the macular area of the retina has been clinically useful in detecting disorders of sphingolipid storage, such as Tay-Sachs' disease (familial amaurotic idiocy).[1,2] Observation of corneal clouding has similarly been helpful in characterizing several types of mucopolysaccharide storage, such as Hurler's disease (gargoylism).[3-6] Within both groups of disorders, several entities have been characterized by deficiency of β-galactosidase or other lysosomal acid hydrolases.[7-23]

Within the last few years, a variety of patients with rare, metabolic storage diseases has been reported which cannot, by clinical criteria, be fitted precisely into the known sphingolipidoses (SLSs) or mucopolysaccharidoses (MPSs). These patients have had features of both types of storage diseases. In an attempt to bring order out of an otherwise nosologic chaos, a new category of storage diseases, the mucolipidoses (MLSs), has therefore been promulgated recently.[23] Nonetheless, certain unusual cases still defy classification.[24-41]

The purpose of this report is to describe a family with characteristics of a storage disease that resembles the MPSs, SLSs, and MLSs in certain respects (corneal clouding, macular cherry-red spot, and β-galactosidase deficiency), but that seemingly is unique.

Report of Family

SUBJECT IV-4.—The proband is a 12-year-old boy of Mexican ancestry (Fig 1). His parents' marriage was consanguineous: the subject's paternal grandfather and his maternal great-grandmother were siblings.

The patient's neonatal history was unremarkable. He sat at 6 months, walked at 16 months, and talked at 2 years of age. By the age of 2 to 3 years, he was thought to be a slow learner. His facial appearance was moderately coarse (Fig 2) and was considered by his parents to be similar to two of his nine siblings (subjects IV-5 and IV-9), who appeared to have suffered from a similar systemic disease (Fig 1).

At the age of 3 years, he was toilet trained. At this time physical examination revealed only a "functional" heart murmur. A pediatrician found no indication of brain damage.

Abnormally slow learning was first documented at the age of 6 years, when he was unable to perform satisfactorily in nursery school. A Stanford-Binet test revealed an intelligence quotient of 50. He subsequently attended a special school for retarded children.

At the age of 8 years, an illiterate test of vision revealed acuities of 20/70 oculus dexter and 20/60-1 oculus sinister. A cherry-red spot in each macula was noted (Fig 3).

At the age of 10, he developed frequent generalized seizures. The patient was pleasant and cooperative and weighed 25.9 kg (57 lb [< 25th percentile]). He was 133.35 cm (4 ft 4½ in) tall (~ tenth percentile) and had a head circumference of 53 cm (~ 20th percentile). Corrected vision was 20/40 OD and 20/60 OS. He had vertical nystagmus and horizontal end-point nystagmus. An audiogram revealed a bilateral sensorineural hearing loss. Findings of neurologic examination were otherwise unremarkable except for occasional extensor plantar reflexes. Electroencephalography showed a mildly abnormal record, with many spike and wave complexes consistent with a seizure disorder. His seizures were moderately well controlled with *N*-methyl phenobarbital, but he had intermittent twitching and occasional episodes of sudden falling to the floor without loss of consciousness. A Wechsler intelligence test for children revealed an IQ of 58.

Skull roentgenograms showed a J-shaped sella (Fig 4), similar to that seen in several MPSs,[5] but were otherwise normal. X-ray films of the mouth showed unusually thin tooth enamel, multiple impacted teeth, and surrounding eruption cysts (Fig 5). These findings resembled dental anomalies of the Hurler syndrome (MPS type I) and the Morquio syndrome (MPS type IV).[43] Roentgenograms of the dorsolumbar spine showed a hypoplastic L-2 vertebral body

Received for publication April 16, 1971; accepted May 14.

From the Department of Ophthalmology, University of Illinois Eye and Ear Infirmary, Chicago. Dr. Fichenscher is now with Presbyterian-St. Luke's Medical Center, Chicago. Dr. Kenyon is now with the Wilmer Institute, Johns Hopkins Hospital, Baltimore. Drs. Enat and Borowsky are now with the West Side Veterans Administration Hospital, Chicago.

Read in part before the meeting of the Association for Research in Vision and Ophthalmology, Sarasota, Fla, April 27, 1971.

Reprint requests to 1855 W Taylor, Chicago 60612 (Dr. Goldberg).

and universal vertebra plana with central beaking (Fig 6) resembling, therefore, the vertebral anomalies of the MPSs.[43,44]

Bone marrow showed an active erythroid series consistent with iron deficiency anemia. Vacuolated or abnormally granulated cells were not seen either in the marrow or in the peripheral blood.

A skin biopsy from the deltoid area showed no abnormal fibroblasts on tissue culture nor abnormal connective tissue elements on electron microscopy.

At the age of 12 years, his height was 133.35 cm (< 3rd percentile) and his weight was 38.8 kg (82.5 lb) (< 50th percentile). He stood erect and had no visible bodily, articular, or cartilaginous abnormalities except for moderate sternal protrusion and thin extremities. Multiple, slightly raised, thickened, cutaneous patches, which measured approximately 5 × 10 mm, were present over the thorax and abdomen. Vision was 10/70 OD and 10/50 OS. Gross inspection showed clear corneas, but slit lamp examination revealed ground glass stromal translucency, which was most marked posteriorly and peripherally, and which resembled that described in the MPSs.[3-5] Both optic disks appeared slightly pale, and there was a definite cherry-red fovea oculus uterque caused by perifoveal grayness of the retina.

A repeat examination of his peripheral blood and bone marrow cells revealed no abnormal vacuolation or granulation. Serum enzyme values (serum glutamic oxaloacetic transaminase [SGOT], serum glutamic pyruvic transaminase [SGPT], lactic dehydrogenase [LDH], alkaline phosphatase, and isocitric dehydrogenase) and bilirubin were all within normal limits. His partial thromboplastin time was slightly prolonged (51.6 seconds; normal = 30 to 45 seconds). An Ivy bleeding time was at the upper limit of normal. His prothrombin time was 79.2% of normal.

Urinalysis for mucopolysaccharides was qualitatively and quantitatively normal (8.4 mg of total mucopolysaccharides per liter of urine). A repeat study by another laboratory showed 4.6 mg of hexuronic acid per liter of urine. No metachromatic granules could be found in a highly concentrated urine specimen.

A lumbar puncture showed an opening pressure of 180 mm H_2O and a closing pressure of 170 mm H_2O. The clear cerebrospinal fluid contained 106 mg/100 ml protein and 70 mg/100 ml glucose. No white blood cells were visible microscopically.

Several biopsies were performed without complication under local anesthesia. Two specimens of liver were obtained with a Menghini needle. One was used for biochemical investigations, and one was divided in half for light microscopic, histochemical, and electron microscopic studies. A biopsy specimen of fornix conjunctiva was utilized for biochemical and for electron microscopic studies. Biopsy specimens of both normal and abnormal appearing skin were utilized for biochemical, light microscopic, electron microscopic, histochemical, and tissue culture studies (see the following for details). Biochemical studies of cultured skin fibroblasts showed the total mucopolysaccharide content to be $5 \mu g/10^6$ cells (within normal limits).

Subject IV-5.—The proband's older brother died at the age of 3 years after being struck by a car. Little is known of him except that he resembled the proband (subject IV-4) and subject IV-9 in facial appearance and was thought to be retarded by his parents.

Subject IV-9.—The proband's older sister was apparently well until the age of 13 years, when she had the onset of frequent, generalized seizures. She had a gargoyle facies, kyphoscoliosis, keel chest, and thin extremities (Fig 7).

Like her brother, subject IV-4, she suffered from continuous facial twitches and purposeless movements of her extremities. By the age of 22 she was unable to walk or to control her bladder or bowel functions. She could not swallow and required a gastrostomy. Neurologic examination revealed brisk, equal deep tendon reflexes, normal plantar reflexes, and good muscle tone. Her eyes were never examined by an ophthalmologist.

A chest roentgenogram revealed broadened ribs and kyphoscoliosis.

Urine was negative for mucopolysaccharides and amino acids.

At the age of 22 she developed status epilepticus and died shortly thereafter of inanition and left ventricular heart failure.

Autopsy Findings in Subject IV-9

At autopsy, the liver weighed 1,100 gm and showed only congested vessels histologically. The spleen weighed 160 gm but was normal histologically. The heart weighed 135 gm and had markedly thickened mitral and aortic valves. Freeze-dried specimens of the aortic and mitral valves, the liver, spleen, and skin were stained with hematoxylin-eosin and with PAS and were histologically unremarkable. Alcian blue staining of the freeze-dried heart valves was similarly negative.

Microscopic examination of bone showed abnormal endochondrial ossification with irregular proliferation of vessels and accumulations of histiocytic-like cells with foamy cytoplasm. These cells appeared restricted to the nonmarrow-containing portions of the bone.

The brain weighed 910 gm but had no gross abnormalities. Microscopically, the leptomeninges were normal. There was a significant but nonspecific loss of neurons in the cerebral cortex and in the dentate and inferior olivary nuclei. The number of Purkinje cells was also diminished. No vacuolation or other morphologic evidence of lipid storage was seen. Freeze-dried specimens of brain were stained with PAS and were normal. The optic nerves and tracts were well myelinated.

Methods

Histologic and Electron Microscopic Methods in Subject IV-4.—*Liver.*—Half of the liver biopsy specimen was immediately frozen in isopentane chilled to -160 C in liquid nitrogen, and cut in the cryostat at -30 C. Some sections were placed on slides, but the majority were dried in vacuo from the frozen state, which yielded essentially frozen-dried sections which were processed histochemically after affixing on slides with a small amount of egg albumin. Stains employed were the following: periodic acid leuchofuchsin (with and without counterstaining with light green; with and without prior treatment with α-amylase

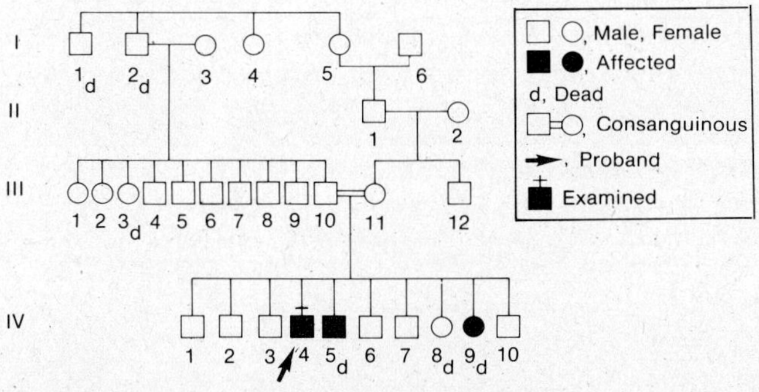

Fig 1.—Pedigree of family. Note consanguinity.

and β-amylase), alcian blue (with and without nuclear fast red), colloidal iron (with and without prior treatment with α-amylase and β-amylase), Luxol fast blue (with and without neutral red), and Sudan black (with and without nuclear fast red). The remaining half of the liver biopsy was immediately fixed in phosphate-buffered glutaraldehyde and postfixed in osmium tetroxide. It was embedded in epoxy resin, and thick sections were stained with toluidine blue. Thin sections were stained with uranyl acetate and lead citrate and were examined on an electron microscope (RCA EMV 4).

Skin and Conjunctiva.—Normal and abnormal skin biopsy specimens were frozen, sectioned, and stained by techniques identical to those employed for the liver specimen. Skin and conjunctival biopsies were also fixed in barbital (Veronal) acetate-buffered 2% osmium tetroxide at 0 C for 45 minutes. They were then dehydrated in increasing concentrations of ethanol and embedded in epoxy resin (Araldite). Thin sections were stained with uranyl acetate and lead citrate and were examined with the electron microscope (JEM 100-B).

Biochemical Methods in Subject IV-4 and in Controls.—Biopsy specimens of the sub-

Table 1.—Acid Hydrolases* in Liver Biopsy Specimens of Proband and Normal Subjects

	Normal	Proband
β-Glucosaminidase	158-342	141
β-Galactosidase	26-42	30.1
β-Glucosidase	1.5-3.8	6.8
α-Mannosidase	6.3	9.5
Sulfatase	8.5-24.0	11.2

* In μmols per gram of wet weight per hour.

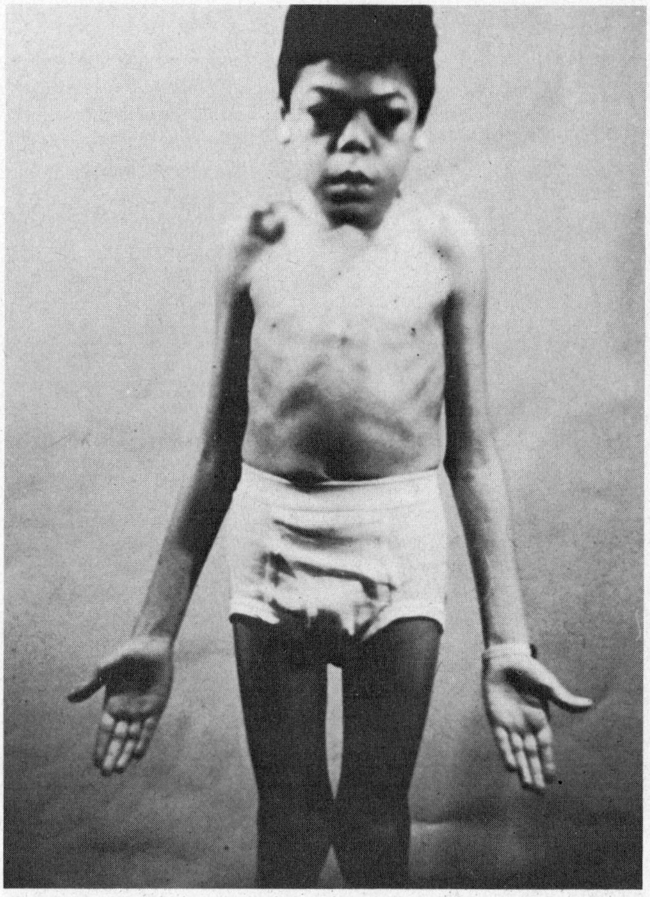

Fig 2.—Subject IV-4. Note moderately coarse facies, slender habitus, and erect posture.

Table 2.—Acid Hydrolases in Two Skin Biopsy Specimens From Proband and in Two Normal Subjects

	A*		B†		Proband's % of Normal	
	Normal	Proband	Normal	Proband	A*	B†
β-Glucosaminidase	2.20-2.39	1.67-2.67	0.870-0.947			
Mean	2.29	2.17	0.908	0.964	95	106
β-Galactosidase	1.07-1.80	0.07-0.21	0.424-0.713			
Mean	1.36	0.19	0.539	0.084	14	15
β-Glucosidase	0.29-0.33	0.08-0.10	0.115-0.130			
Mean	0.31	0.09	0.122	0.039	29	32
α-Mannosidase	1.31-1.98	1.11-1.60	0.519-0.785			
Mean	1.64	1.41	0.650	0.626	85	96
β-Glucuronidase	0.95-1.43	1.86-1.90	0.376-0.567			
Mean	1.11	1.88	0.440	0.835	169	189
α-Fucosidase	2.80-2.95	2.30-3.20	1.110-1.169			
Mean	2.87	2.70	1.138	1.199	96	105
Sulfatase	0.07-0.09	0.09-0.11	0.027-0.035			
Mean	0.08	0.10	0.031	0.044	125	133

* In μmols per gram of wet weight per hour.

† In μmols per gram of protein per minute (average of reactions of two normal subjects: 4.2% protein; average of biopsies 1 and 2 from the proband: 3.75% protein).

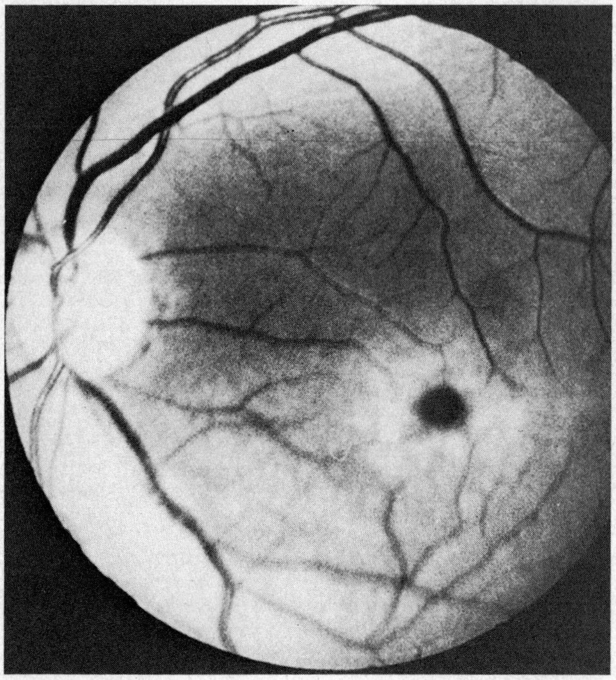

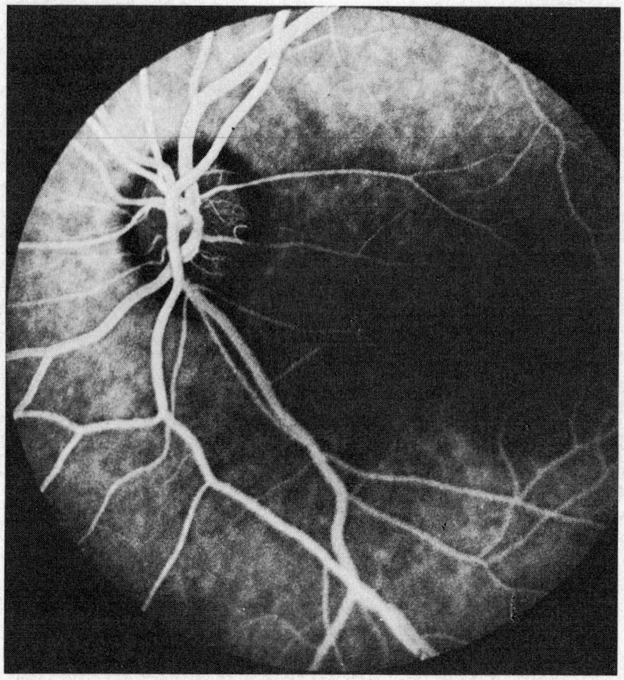

Fig 3.—Fundus of left eye. Left, *Black and white print obtained from kodachrome fundus photograph. Note cherry-red spot in center of macula, caused by perifoveal grayness.* Right, *Arteriovenous phase of fluorescein angiogram is normal in appearance.*

Fig 4.—Lateral view of skull roentgenogram of subject IV-4. Note J-shaped sella, similar to that seen in mucopolysaccharidoses.[5]

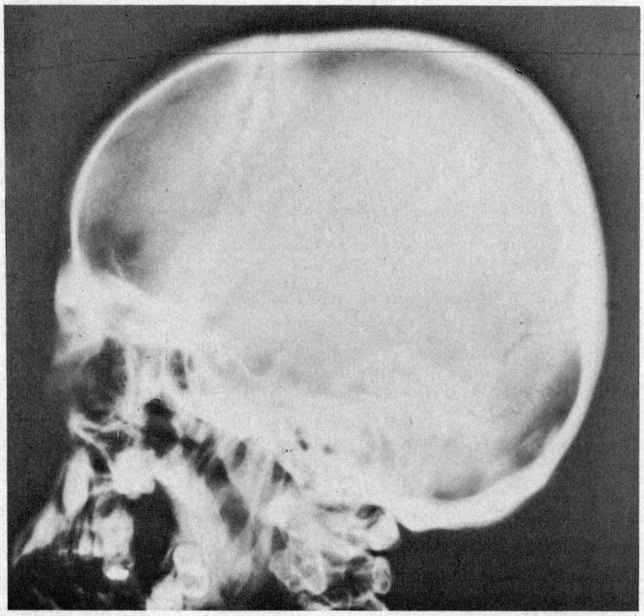

Fig 5.—X-ray film of teeth, which shows unusually thin tooth enamel, multiple impactions, and eruption cysts. These abnormalities have also been described in the mucopolysaccharidoses.[42]

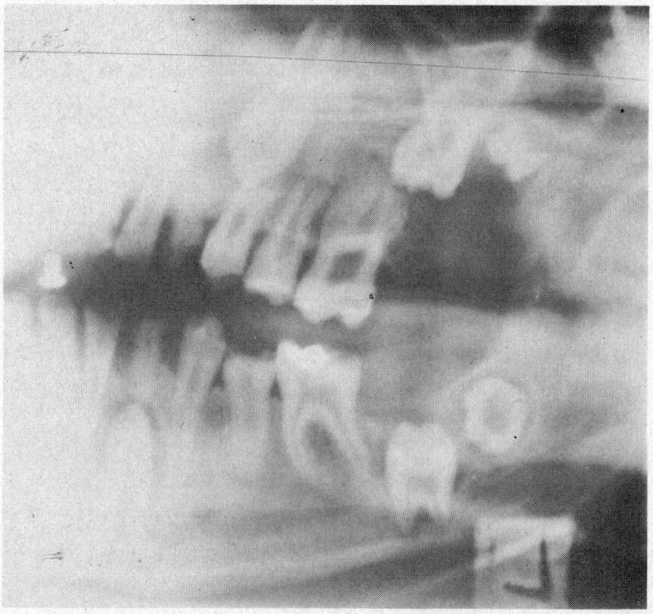

ject's skin, conjunctiva, and liver; two biopsy specimens of skin and conjunctiva from normal patients; and liver material obtained at autopsy from patients without neurological disease were homogenized in 1 to 2 ml of distilled water and stored at -20 C until processed. Pieces of skin were cut into smaller fragments with scissors. Shreds of skin fragments incompletely homogenized were removed. Serum was stored at -20 C until processed.

Hexosaminidase, Galactosidase, Mannosidase and Glucosidase in Tissues.—The 4-methylumberylferryl derivatives of β-D-N acetyl glucosaminide, β-D-galactopyranoside, β-D-glucopyranoside and α-D-mannoside were used as substrates at a concentration of 1 millimol/liter. The buffer was 0.1M citrate buffer at pH 3.5 to 5.0. The reaction mixtures of 100μl 0.1M buffer, 100μl substrate, and 5μl to 10μl of homogenate were incubated at 37 C in stoppered test tubes placed in a shaking water bath for 60 minutes. All samples were run in duplicates. The samples were transferred to ice, and 1 ml of 0.4M glycine-NaOH buffer at pH 10.4 was added. The samples were read in a fluorometer (Turner) adapted to 1-ml test tubes with a primary filter (760) and secondary filters (48 and 2A). 4-Methylumbelliferone was used as the standard. The assay was based on a fluorometric assay for glycosidases.[45]

Glucuronidase, Fucosidase and Sulfatase in Tissues.—The *p*-nitrophenol derivatives of β-D-glucuronic acid, α-D-fucoside and sulfate were used as substrates at a concentration of 2 millimols/liter. The buffer was 0.1M acetate buffer at pH 4.5. The reaction mixtures of 80μl of substrate in buffer and 20μl of tissue homogenate were incubated at 37 C for one hour in stoppered microtubes and placed in a shaking water bath for 60 minutes. The samples were then cooled in ice, and 100μl of 0.4M glycine-NaOH buffer were added. The samples were centrifuged for 5 minutes at 2,000 rpm, and the supernatants were read at 420 mμ in the 50μl micro-cells of the spectrophotometer (Beckman DU). *p*-Nitrophenol standards were used.

Hexosaminidase A and B and β-Galactosidase in Serum.—Ten microliters of serum was used for hexosaminidase assay with 1 millimolar β-D-acetyl glucosaminide. The buffer and the inactivation at 50 C were as described by O'Brien et al[20] with our modification of the method for microsamples (E. Cotlier, MD, unpublished data). β-Galactosidase in serum was determined according to the technique of Ockerman.[46]

Proteins.—In liver and skin samples, proteins were determined according to the technique of Lowry et al.[47]

Results

Histologic and Electron Microscopic Methods in Subject IV-4.—*Liver.*—Contrary to findings in the classic MPSs,[48] hepatic parenchymal cells of the subject were normal with both light and electron microscopic examination (Fig 8). Abnormalities were not observed with hematoxylin-eosin or with the histochemical stains. With the electron microscope, numerous vacuoles were seen in the cytoplasm of sinusoidal lining cells (Fig 9). The vacuoles were 1μ to 5μ in diameter and were surrounded by a single membrane. They gave the cells a bubbly appearance. Most often their contents were clear. However, a few vacuoles contained granular material which was of moderate electron density. The vacuolization of the reticuloendothelial cells in the presence of intact hepatocytes appeared similar to that observed in I-cell mucolipidosis. However, membranous lamellar vacuoles were not seen in subject IV-4, unlike the situation in I-cell disease

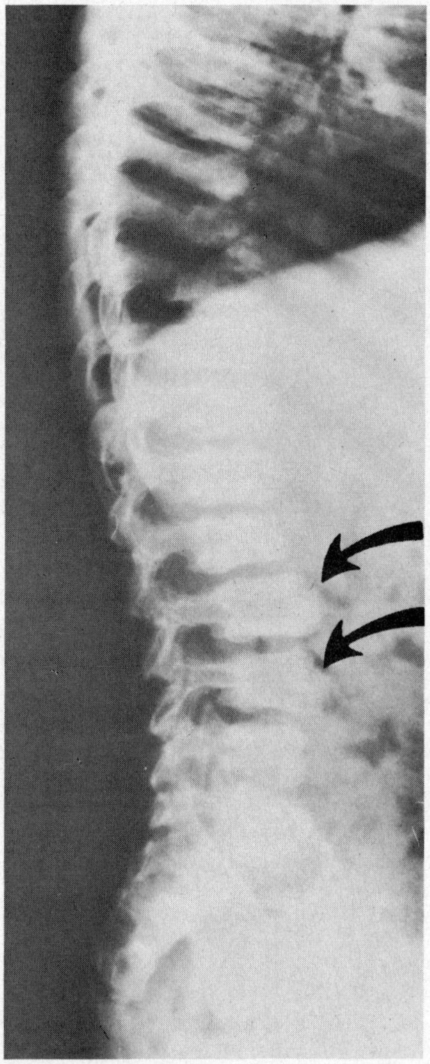

Fig 6.—Roentgenogram of dorsolumbar spine. Note anterior beaking of vertebral bodies (arrows).

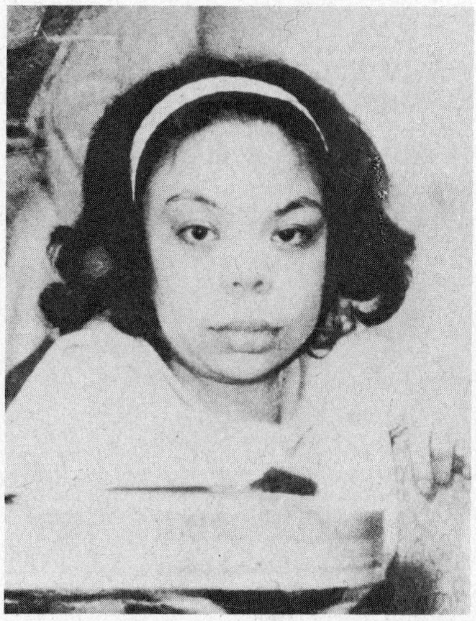

Fig 7.—Subject IV-9. Note gargoyle type of facies. (Photograph reproduced posthumously from polaroid print).

Table 3.—Acid Hydrolases in Conjunctival Biopsy Specimens of Proband and Normal Subjects

	Conjunctiva*		Proband's % of Normal
	Normal	Proband	
β-Glucosaminidase	7.2-8.1	13.0	168
Mean	7.7		
β-Galactosidase	3.0-3.6	1.8	55
Mean	3.3		
β-Glucosidase	2.1-3.2	2.6	100
Mean	2.6		
α-Mannosidase	2.7-3.9	1.9	58
Mean	3.3		
β-Glucuronidase	1.8-2.1	3.1	158
Mean	1.95		
α-Fucosidase	0.7-1.6	0.9	78
Mean	1.16		
Sulfatase	1.5-1.8	1.3	76
Mean	1.71		

* In μmols per gram of wet weight per hour.

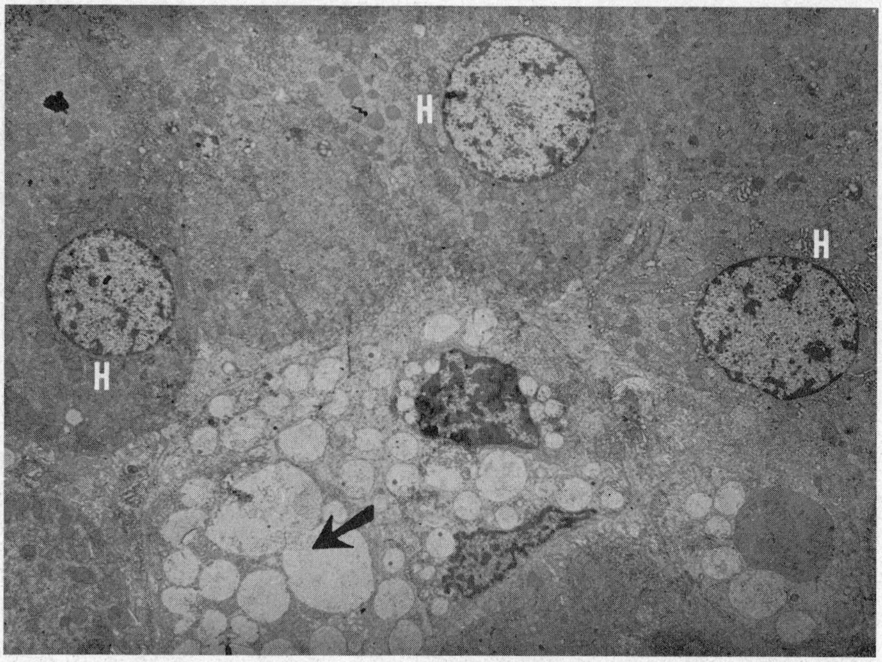

Fig 8.—Electron micrograph (× 2,160) of liver biopsy from subject IV-4. Three normal hepatocytes (H) *are seen at top. A vacuolated sinusoidal lining (Kupffer) cell is seen at bottom* (arrow).

Fig 9.—Electron micrograph (× 3,310) of liver biopsy from subject IV-4. The cytoplasm of a sinusoidal lining cell contains numerous vacuoles.

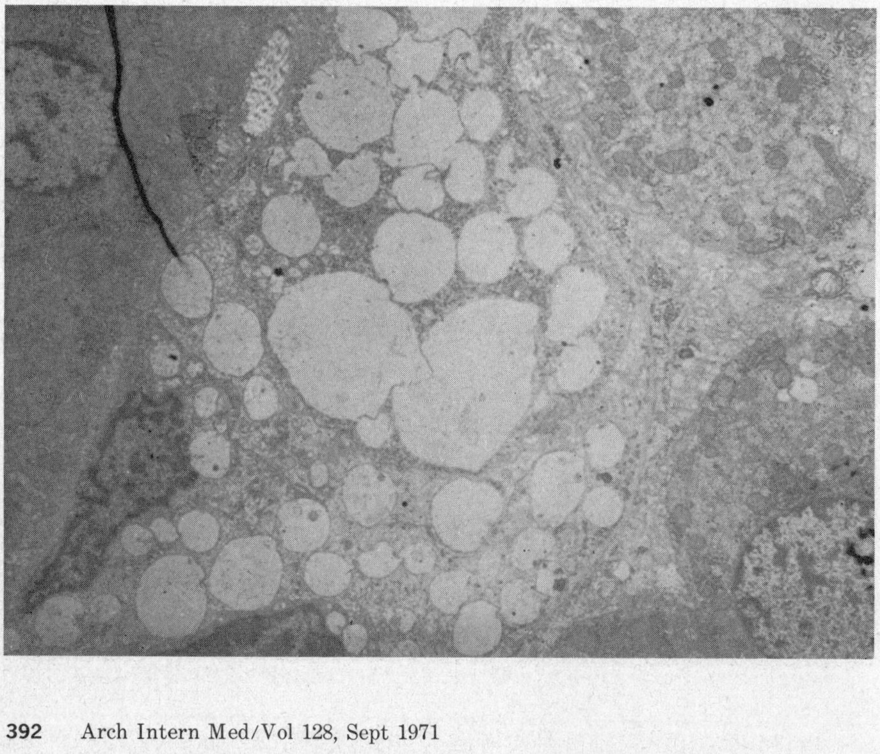

(K.R. Kenyon, MD, et al, unpublished data).

Skin and Conjunctiva.—Light microscopy revealed no cutaneous abnormalities in subject IV-4 with hematoxylin-eosin or with the histochemical stains. Similarly, electron microscopy revealed no abnormalities in the normal skin, abnormal skin, or conjunctiva. The basal epithelial cells of all three tissues did not contain abnormal inclusions. In the subepithelial region of these tissues, vacuole-distended histiocytes (prominent in the MPSs and in I-cell mucolipidosis[49]) were not apparent (Fig 10). The fibroblasts did not demonstrate excessive cytoplasmic vacuolization, and there were no collections of abnormal extracellular material.

Biochemical Results in Subject IV-4.—*Liver.*—Activities of acid hydrolases in liver from the subject did not differ significantly from those of control livers (Table 1).

Skin.—In Table 2 the activities of acid hydrolases in skin of two normal patients and subject IV-4 are shown. The average of acid hydrolases in normal skin was in close agreement with those values reported by Ockerman.[46] Average values for acid hydrolases (in μmols per gram per hour) in skin from the subject indicated normal values of β-hexosaminidase (2.17), α-mannosidase (1.41), α-fucosidase (2.70), β-glucuronidase (1.88), and sulfatase (0.10). The skin of the subject, however, was markedly deficient in β-galactosidase; biopsy 1 (clinically normal) with values of 9% of the controls, biopsy 2 (clinically abnormal) with values of 18.5% of the controls. The mixture of equal volumes of normal skin and the subject's skin (biopsy 1) homogenates resulted in β-galactosidase values insignificantly different from those expected (Fig 11), indicating that inhibitors of the enzyme reaction were not present in the subject's skin. A moderate deficiency of β-glucosidase was also found: the average of the two skin biopsies from the subject was 29% of the enzyme activity of controls. The pH distribution curves of β-galactosidase, β-glucosidase and β-glucosaminidase in skin of controls and the subject are shown in Fig 12.

Conjunctiva.—A conjunctival biopsy specimen from the subject was deficient in β-galactosidase with values 55% those of controls (Table 3).

Serum.—Hexosaminidase values (in μmols/liter/hour) were normal (total, 523; A, 405; B, 118). β-Galactosidase was also within normal limits in the subject's serum (0.275μmols/liter/min).

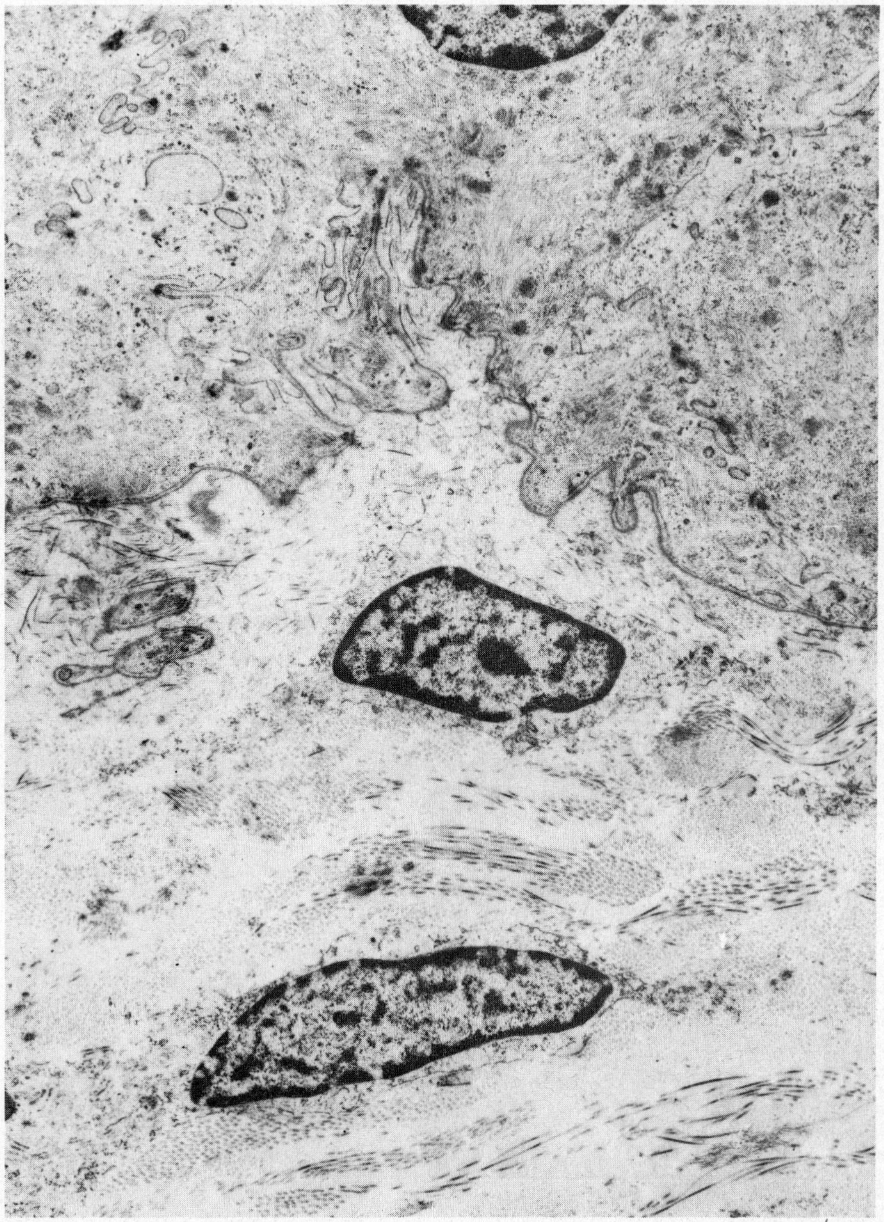

Fig 10.—Electron micrograph (×10,000) of biopsy from fornix conjunctiva of subject IV-4. Basal epithelial cells (at top) *and two subepithelial fibroblasts* (bottom) *are unremarkable. Unlike mucopolysaccharidoses and mucolipidoses,[49] abnormal vacuoles are not seen.*

Comment

Nosology.—Precise diagnostic separation of inherited storage diseases is complicated by the overlapping of clinical syndromes, by the frequent simultaneous storage of more than one major class of compounds (eg, the Gm_1 gangliosidosis syndromes[50] and metachromatic leukodystrophy[51,52]), by the fact that an enzyme deficiency may not be specific to one disease only,[6,13,14,20,23] and by the sophistication of many of the laboratory techniques that are required for complete description of a disease. Nonetheless, precise diagnosis remains a worthy objective for accurate genetic counseling to affected or potentially affected families and for treatment of diseased individuals if, at any time in the future, new pharmacologic agents or genetic engineering techniques become applicable.[53]

The mucopolysaccharidoses are defined as primary, gene-determined disorders of mucopolysaccharide metabolism[54,55] and are characterized by the presence of abnormal types and amounts of mucopolysaccharides in the urine. At least six types have been delineated.[54] Of these, types I (Hurler syndrome), IV (Morquio syndrome), V (Scheie syndrome), and VI (Maroteaux-Lamy syndrome) have grossly visible corneal clouding (Table 4). Type II (Hunter syndrome) is characterized by clinically clear corneas, but biomicroscopic clouding has been observed in older patients.[3,4] In addition to the effect of clouding in

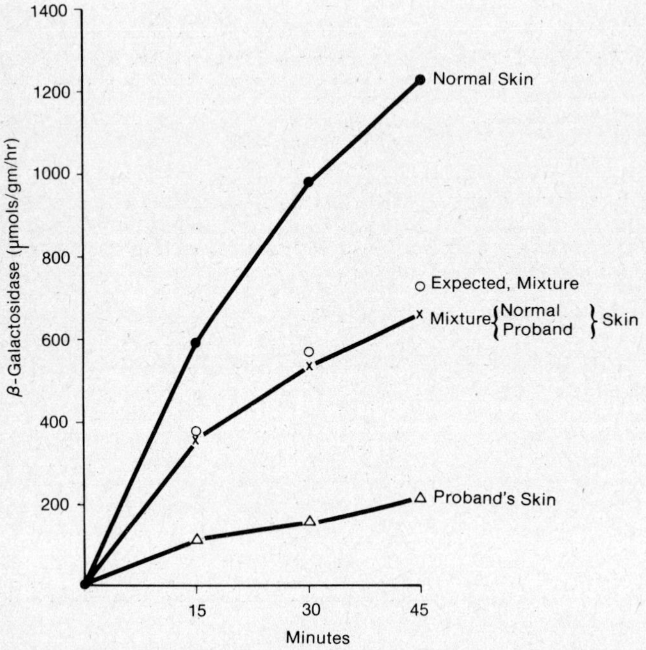

Fig 11.—Marked deficiency of β-galactosidase is found in skin of subject IV-4. A mixture of equal volumes of normal skin and the subject's skin homogenates resulted in β-galactosidase values insignificantly different from those expected, which indicates that inhibitors of the enzyme were not present in the subject's skin.

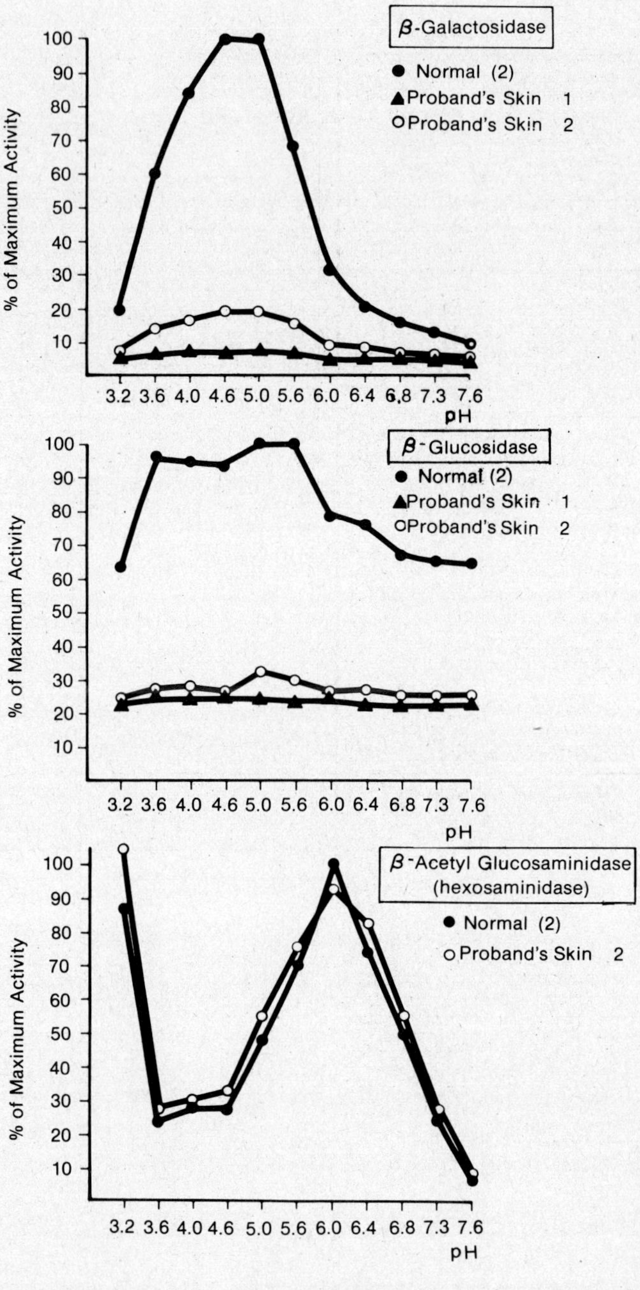

Fig 12.—pH distribution curves of β-galactosidase, β-glucosidase, and β-acetylglucosaminidase in skin. Marked deficiency of β-galactosidase, moderate deficiency of β-glucosidase, and no deficiency of β-acetyl glucosaminidase are seen in skin of subject IV-4 when compared to normal.

the MPSs, vision may also be adversely affected by optic atrophy and by pigmentary degeneration of the retina,[4,5] but macular cherry-red spots have not been described (Table 4).

Subject IV-4 resembles the MPSs in his facial appearance, skin plaques, reduced intellect, cloudy corneas, J-shaped sella, lumbar vertebral beaking, dental defect, dwarfism, hearing deficit, and deficiency of skin β-galactosidase (Table 5). The pedigree also strongly suggests an autosomal recessive type of inheritance, due to consanguinity and the ratio of affected to nonaffected individuals in generation IV (Fig 1). The absence of abnormal mucopolysaccharides in the tissues and in the urine and the presence of a macular cherry-red spot in the proband, however, indicate a disease with characteristics different from the classic MPSs.

The sphingolipidoses are primary,

Table 4.—Storage Diseases With Cloudy Cornea but Normal Macula

Mucopolysaccharidoses[3–5]	
	MPS type I
	MPS type II (in older cases, with slit lamp only)
	MPS type IV
	MPS type V
	MPS type VI
Sphingolipidosis[61,62]	
	Fabry's disease (biomicroscopically visible whorl-like dystrophy in corneal epithelium)
Mucolipidosis[23]	
	MLS type III (pseudo-Hurler polydystrophy)
Primary corneal dystrophies[62]	
	Groenouw's type II (macular corneal dystrophy)
	Schnyder's crystalline corneal dystrophy
Unclassified cases[25–27]	

Table 5.—Similarities of Proband to Known Storage Diseases

Mucopolysaccharidoses	
	Coarse facies
	Thick skin plaques
	Reduced intellect
	Deficient β-galactosidase
	Cloudy cornea
	J-shaped sella
	Lumbar vertebral beaking
	Enamel tooth defect
	Dwarfism
	Hearing loss
Sphingolipidoses	
	Macular cherry-red spot
	No mucopolysacchariduria
	Reduced intellect
	Deficient β-galactosidase
	Abnormal cerebrospinal fluid
Mucolipidoses	
	Coarse facies
	Reduced intellect
	Deficient β-galactosidase
	Dysostosis multiplex
	Cloudy cornea plus macular cherry-red spot

Table 6.—Storage Diseases With Macular Grayness or Cherry-Red Spot Without Corneal Clouding*

Sphingolipidoses	
	Tay-Sachs' disease (Gm_2 gangliosidosis type I)[2,50]
	Sandhoff's disease (Gm_2 gangliosidosis type II)[50]
	Niemann-Pick disease[2]
	Lactosyl ceramidosis[59]
Mucolipidoses	
	Farber's disease[63]
	Sea-blue histiocyte syndrome or chronic Niemann-Pick disease† (yellow perifoveal granules)[2,64,65]
	Mucolipidosis I (lipomucopolysaccharidosis) (Spranger, J.W.)
Unclassified cases[24,33,36,38,39,41]	

* Not all of these patients had slit lamp examination to exclude biomicroscopic corneal clouding.

† Proper nosologic characterization of this disease has not yet been accomplished.

Table 7.—Storage Diseases With Macular Cherry-Red Spot Plus Corneal Clouding

Sphingolipidosis	
	Childhood metachromatic leukodystrophy[60]
Mucolipidoses	
	Gm_1 type I (generalized gangliosidosis)[13,50]
	MLS type I (lipomucopolysaccharidosis)[23]
Unclassified cases[31,33,34,40]	
Proband (this report)	

Table 8.—Storage Diseases With Deficient β-Galactosidase

Mucopolysaccharidoses[6,7,21,43]	
	MPS I
	MPS II
	MPS III
Sphingolipidoses	
	Krabbes' disease[15,16]
	Lactosyl ceramidosis[59]
	Fabry's disease is characterized by deficiency of α-galactosidase[9,12]
Mucolipidoses[23]	
	Gm_1 type I
	Gm_1 type II
Proband (this report)	

gene-determined disorders, in which tissue storage of sphingosine-containing lipids is the biochemical hallmark. At least eight distinct types have been described.[2,50,56-58] Of these, macular cherry-red spot or macular grayness without corneal clouding has been described in Tay-Sachs' disease, Sandhoff's disease,[50] Niemann-Pick disease, and in lactosyl ceramidosis[59] (Table 6). One form of metachromatic leukodystrophy, a sphingolipidosis, has had both macular cherry-red spot plus corneal clouding (Table 7).[60]

Subject IV-4 resembles the SLSs because of reduced intellect, abnormal cerebrospinal fluid, autosomal recessive inheritance, deficient β-galactosidase, absence of mucopolysacchariduria, and presence of macular cherry-red spot (Table 5). However, his longevity (and that of his sister, subject IV-9), normal-sized liver and spleen, serum and tissue enzyme concentrations, and MPS-like features (and those of his sister) preclude a diagnosis of one of the classic SLSs.[2,14,50,56-58,61,62]

Mucolipidoses, like the MPSs and SLSs, are inherited metabolic diseases. They are characterized by the combined storage of mucopolysaccharides, sphingolipids, and glycolipids.[23] Five types have been described in which the pathogeneses are as yet undefined: MLS type I (lipomucopolysaccharidosis), MLS type II (I-cell disease), MLS type III (pseudo-Hurler polydystrophy), Farber's disease,[63] and the sea-blue histiocyte syndrome (or chronic form of Niemann-Pick disease).[64,65] Five other types (Gm_1 generalized gangliosidosis, types I and II, fucosidosis, mannosidosis, and infantile sulfatidosis with mucopolysacchariduria) have enzyme defects which have been identified.[23] Of the MLSs, macular grayness or cherry-red spot without corneal clouding has been described, thus far, only in Farber's disease.[2] In addition, Spranger (unpublished data, 1971) has noted two patients with MLS type I with cherry-red maculas, in whom slit lamp examination failed to show corneal clouding (Table 6). Also, yellow perifoveal granules have been noted in the chronic form of Niemann-Pick disease or the sea-blue histiocyte syndrome[64,65] (Table 6). The combination of macular cherry-red spot plus corneal clouding has been noted in Gm_1 generalized gangliosidosis type I[13] and in MLS type I[23] (Table 7). Corneal clouding in the absence of retinal abnormalities has been considered to be characteristic of MLS type III (Table 4).[23,54]

Subject IV-4 resembles certain of the MLSs because of the combined corneal and retinal abnormalities, the coarse facial features, the dysostosis multiplex, and the absence of abnormal urinary mucopolysaccharides (Table 5). He differs from the MLSs because of the absence of vacuolated cells in the hepatic parenchyma, marrow, and peripheral blood; the presence of normal levels of fucosidase, mannosidase, and sulfatase; the absence of histochemical evidence suggesting mucopolysaccharide or lipid storage; and the absence of metachromatic material in the urine. Despite these exclusionary characteristics, subject IV-4 most resembles certain cases thought by Spranger and Wiedemann to be examples of MLS type I,[23] and it is possible that further heterogeneity exists within this group. As yet, biochemical identification of an abnormally stored substance has not been possible, because the subject is alive and appropriate tissue is unavailable. However, on clinical grounds, abnormal storage is presumed to be the cause of the macular cherry-red spot, corneal clouding, reduced intellect, etc.

Biochemistry.—At least eight clinical syndromes associated with galactosidase deficiency are known* (Table 8). The storage of both gangliosides and mucopolysaccharides in several of the MPS syndromes can result from the absence of a ubiquitous heat-labile fraction of β-galactosidase.[6] More profound clinical signs and early metabolite accumulation and death result from a total β-galactosidase deficiency, as in the generalized gangliosidoses.[8] Galactocerebroside β-galactosidase deficiency has been found in Krabbe's disease (globoid cell leukodystrophy)[15,16] and may well be responsible for loss of myelin and globoid cell infiltration. In Fabry's disease a mild deficiency of α-galactosidase results in accumulation of ceramide trihexoside, a glycoprotein with galactose in the terminal group.[9-11] A new clinical syndrome, lactosyl ceramidosis resulting from a β-galactosidase (galactosyl hydrolase) deficiency has also been described recently.[59]

The deficiency of β-galactosidase in skin of subject IV-4 was very marked. The values were even lower than those in skin of the MPS syndromes. In addition, skin from subject IV-4 showed moderate deficiencies of β-glucosidase, an enzyme not previously tested in the skin of subjects with mucopolysaccharidoses. It is likely that a β-hexosidase in skin may break down both *d*-galactose and *d*-glucose. The velocities indicate a preferential treatment towards *d*-galactose. Gatt attempted separation and purification of β-galactosidase and β-glucosidase from brain β-hexosidase.[66] However, the final yield and minimal Michaelis constant (K_m) differences between the two brain fractions indicated that a single enzyme may be present. A similar lack of specificity has been demonstrated for brain and spleen acetyl-B-*N*-hexosaminidase. This enzyme lacks a selective specificity towards glucosaminide and galactosaminide substrates.

Due to the scarcity of the biopsy material, no attempts could be made to identify the metabolite(s) that probably accumulate(s) in various tissues of subject IV-4. It is likely that such a metabolite might have a galactose or a lactose group in a terminal position. Among glycolipids, GM_1-monosialoganglioside

NANA
|
(Cer-Glc-Gal-GalNAc-Gal), disialoganglioside and trisialoganglioside

(NANA)
|
NANA
|
NANA
|
(Cer-Glc-Gal-NAcGal-Gal), GM_3-

NANA
|
hematoside (Cer-Glc-Gal), GL-3 (Cer-Glc-Gal-Gal), Lactosyl ceramide (Cer-Glc-Gal), and Krabbe's gan-

*References 6,7,9-11,15,16,21,23,43,57

glioside (Gal-Cer), could be substrates for β-galactosidase. Among mucopolysaccharides, keratan sulfate (GlcNAc-Gal) requires a β-galactosidase for its breakdown.

It must be emphasized, however, that chondroitin sulfate B and heparitin sulfate (two mucopolysaccharides that are abnormally present in MPS syndromes I, II and III, all of which are characterized by deficient β-galactosidase), do not contain β-D-galactoside residues in their structure. This clinico-chemical discrepancy casts doubts on whether β-galactosidase is the primary enzyme deficiency in these MPSs or simply an ancillary finding. Fluharty and coworkers[67] failed to demonstrate β-galactosidase deficiency in fibroblast cultures of heterozygous carriers of MPS types I, II, and III. Furthermore, all electrophoretic fractions of β-galactosidase were present in skin fibroblast cultures of homozygous individuals with MPS types I and III.[68]

In the conjunctiva of subject IV-4, only a moderate β-galactosidase deficiency (55% of controls) and normal β-glucosidase values were found. Thus this subject can be classified as deficient, though not totally lacking in β-galactosidase. However, repeated electron microscopic examination of the subject's skin and conjunctiva failed to reveal any abnormal storage material. This disparity between the biochemical and ultrastructural findings casts further doubt on the possible primary role of β-galactosidase deficiency in the pathogenesis of this—and possibly other—storage diseases.

In addition, deficiency of total β-hexosidase was not found in the liver of subject IV-4 despite evidence of vacuolated reticuloendothelial cells. The fact that an enzyme deficiency was not found in the liver biopsy specimen of this subject is in contrast with decreased levels of β-galactosidase in liver of the MPS syndromes[21] and GM_1 gangliosidosis type I.[69] This subject may represent a milder and tissue-specific β-galactosidase deficiency. This could account for his longer life span (and that of his sister, subject IV-9); his lack of obvious visceral involvement; and the localization of lesions to organs such as retina, skin, bone, and brain, where the combined glycolipid-mucopolysaccharide breakdown may be slower than in other tissues.

David Kaplan, MD, performed the qualitative and quantitative studies on urinary mucopolysaccharides; S.T. Nerenberg, MD, PhD, performed the studies on urinary metachromasia and mucopolysacchariduria; Reuben Matalon, MD, performed the anatomic and biochemical studies of cultured skin fibroblasts; Samuel Pruzansky, DDS, interpretated the dental x-ray films; H.R. Catchpole, PhD, assisted with the histochemical studies; and R. Herbst, Jr., MD, cared for the proband.

References

1. Tay W: Symmetrical changes in the region of the yellow spot in each eye of an infant. *Trans Ophth Soc UK* **1**:55-57, 1881.
2. Cogan DG, Kuwabara, T: The sphingolipidoses and the eye. *Arch Ophthal* **79**:437-452, 1968.
3. Goldberg MF, Maumenee AE, McKusick VA: Corneal dystrophies associated with abnormalities of mucopolysaccharide metabolism. *Arch Ophthal* **74**:516-520, 1965.
4. Goldberg MF, Duke JR: Ocular histopathology in Hunter's syndrome: Systemic mucopolysaccharidosis type II. *Arch Ophthal* **77**:503-512, 1967.
5. Goldberg MF, Scott CI, McKusick VA: Hydrocephalus and papilledema in the Maroteaux-Lamy syndrome (mucopolysaccharidosis type VI). *Amer J Ophthal* **69**:969-975, 1970.
6. Ho MW, O'Brien JS: Hurler's syndrome: Deficiency of a specific beta galactosidase isoenzyme. *Science* **165**:611-613, 1969.
7. Ockerman PA, Kohlen P: Glycosidases in skin and plasma in Hunter's syndrome. *Acta Paediat Scand* **57**:281-289, 1968.
8. Singer HS, Schaffer IA: White-cell beta-galactosidase activity. *New Eng J Med* **282**:571, 1970.
9. Kint JA: Fabry's disease: Alpha-galactosidase deficiency. *Science* **167**:1268-1269, 1970.
10. Mapes CA, Anderson RL, Sweeley CC: Enzyme replacement in Fabry's disease, an inborn error of metabolism. *Science* **169**:987-989, 1970.
11. Romeo G, Migeon BR: Genetic inactivation of the alpha-galactosidase locus in carriers of Fabry's disease. *Science* **170**:180-181, 1970.
12. Clarke JTR, Knaack J, Crawhill JC, et al: Ceramide trihexosidosis (Fabry's disease) without skin lesions. *New Eng J Med* **284**:233-235, 1971.
13. Emery JM, Green WR, Wyllie RG, et al: Gm_1-gangliosidosis: Ocular and pathological manifestations. *Arch Ophthal* **85**:177-187, 1971.
14. Okada S. Veath ML, O'Brien JS: Juvenile GM_2 gangliosidosis: Partial deficiency of hexosaminidase A. *J Pediat* **77**:1063-1065, 1970.
15. Suzuki K, Suzuki Y: Globoid cell leucodystrophy (Krabbe's disease): Deficiency of galactocerebroside beta-galactosidase. *Proc Nat Acad Sci* **66**:302-309, 1970.
16. Malone MJ: Deficiency in a degradative enzyme system in globoid leukodystrophy. *Amer Soc Neurochem Trans* **1**:56, 1970.
17. Kaback MM, Howell RR: Infantile metachromatic leukodystrophy: Heterozygote detection in skin fibroblasts and possible applications to intrauterine diagnosis. *New Eng J Med* **282**:1335-1340, 1970.
18. Julius R, Buehler B, Aylworth A, et al: Diagnostic techniques in metachromatic leukodystrophy. *Neurology* **21**:15-18, 1971.
19. Stumpf D, Austin J: Metachromatic leukodystrophy (MLD): IX. Qualitative and quantitative differences in urinary arylsulfatase A in different forms of MLD. *Arch Neurol* **24**:117-124, 1971.
20. O'Brien JS, Okada S, Chen A, et al: Tay-Sachs disease: Detection of heterozygotes and homozygotes by serum hexosaminidase assay. *New Eng J Med* **283**:15-20, 1970.
21. MacBrinn M, Okada S, Woollacott M, et al: Beta-galactosidase deficiency in the Hurler syndrome. *New Eng J Med* **281**:338-342, 1969.
22. Wiesmann VN, Lightbody J, Vassella F, et al:

Multiple lysosomal enzyme deficiency due to enzyme leakage? *New Eng J Med* **284**:109-110, 1971.

23. Spranger JW, Wiedemann HR: The genetic mucolipidoses: Diagnosis and differential diagnosis. *Humangenetik* **9**:113-139, 1970.

24. Pesme P, Verger P: Forme juvenile de l'idiotie amaurotique familiale avec degenerescence maculaire du type Tay-Sachs. *Bull Soc Franc Ophtal* **59**:56-67, 1946.

25. Horton WA, Schimke RN: A new mucopolysaccharidosis. *J Pediat* **77**:252-258, 1970.

26. Brown SI, Kuwabara T: Peripheral corneal opacification and skeletal deformities: A newly recognized acid mucopolysaccharidosis simulating rheumatoid arthritis. *Arch Ophthal* **83**:667-677, 1970.

27. Philippart M, Sugarman GI: Chondroitin-4-sulphate mucopolysaccharidosis: A new variant of Hurler's syndrome. *Lancet* **2**:854, 1969.

28. Clausen J, Dyggve HV, Melchior JC: Mucopolysaccharidosis: Paper electrophoretic and infrared analysis of the urine in gargolylism and Morquio-Ullrich's disease. *Arch Dis Child* **38**:364-374, 1963.

29. Clausen J, Dyggve HV, Melchior JC: Chemical and enzymic studies of a family with skeletal abnormalities associated with mental retardation. *Clin Chem Acta* **29**:197-207, 1970.

30. Dyggve HV, Melchior JC, Clausen J: Morquio-Ullrich's disease: An inborn error of metabolism? *Arch Dis Child* **37**:525-534, 1962.

31. Jervis GA: Hallervorden-Spatz disease associated with atypical amaurotic idiocy. *J Neuropath Exp Neurol* **11**:4-18, 1952.

32. Favarger P, Wildi E: Chemical analysis and histochemical examination of an atypical case of Tay-Sachs' disease, in Cumings JN (ed): *Cerebral Lipidoses, A Symposium.* Springfield, Ill, Charles C Thomas, Publisher, 1957, pp 146-158.

33. Villani G: Su un particolare reperto degenerativo della cornea in tre casi atypici di idiozia amaurotica familiare. *Boll Oculist* **12**:1328-1338, 1933.

34. Cacchione A: Su tre casi atypici d-idiozia amaurotic familiare con particolare reperto degenerativo della cornea. *Note Rev Psychiat* **64**:149-164, 1935.

35. Franceschetti A, Francois J, Babel J: Les heredo-degenerescences chorio-retiniennes (degenerescences tapetoretiniennes). *Rap Soc Franc Masson* **2**:915-916, 1963.

36. Tittarelli R, Giagheddu M, Spadetta V: Typical ophthalmoscopic picture of "cherry-red spot" in an adult with the myoclonic syndrome. *Brit J Ophthal* **50**:414-420, 1966.

37. de Leon GA, Kaback MM, Elfenbein IB, et al: Juvenile dystonic lipidosis. *Johns Hopkins Med J* **125**:62-77, 1969.

38. Anderson B, Margolis G, Lynn WS: Ocular lesions related to disturbances in fat metabolism. *Amer J Ophthal* **45**:23-41, 1958.

39. Wyburn-Mason R: On some anomalous forms of amaurotic idiocy and their bearing on the relationship of the various types. *Brit J Ophthal* **27**:145-173, 193-307, 1943.

40. Berard-Badier M, Paillas JE, Gastaut H, et al: Essai sur la signification des demyelinisations dans l'idiote amaurotique infantile. *Psychiat Neurol* **132**:50-93, 1958.

41. Szabo L, Polgar J, Vass Z, et al: A Hurler's syndrome variant. *Lancet* **2**:1314, 1967.

42. Gorlin RJ, Pindborg JJ: *Syndromes of the Head and Neck.* New York, McGraw-Hill Book Co Inc, 1964, pp 378-383.

43. Spranger JW, Koch F, McKusick VA, et al: Mucopolysaccharidosis VI (Maroteaux-Lamy's disease). *Helv Paediat Acta* **25**:337-362, 1970.

44. Linker A, Evans LR, Langer LO: Morquio's disease and mucopolysaccharide excretion. *J Pediat* **77**:1039-1047, 1970.

45. Leaback DH, Walker PG: Studies on glucosaminidase 4: The fluorometric assay of N-acetyl-B-glucosaminidase. *Biochem J* **78**:151, 1961.

46. Ockerman PA: Acid hydrolases in skin and plasma in gargoylism: Deficiency of β-galactosidase in skin. *Clin Chem Acta* **20**:1-6, 1968.

47. Lowry OH, Rosenbrough NJ, Furr AL, et al: Protein measurement with the folin phenol reagent. *J Biol Chem* **193**:265-275, 1951.

48. Callahan WP, Lorincz AE: Hepatic ultrastructure in the Hurler syndrome. *Amer J Path* **48**:277-298, 1966.

49. Quigley H, Goldberg FM: Scheie syndrome and macular corneal dystrophy: An ultrastructural comparison of conjunctiva and skin. *Arch Ophthal* **85**:553-564, 1971.

50. O'Brien JS: Ganglioside storage diseases, in Hirschhorn K, Harris H (eds): *Advances in Human Genetics*, to be published.

51. Rampini S, Isler W, Baerlocher K, et al: Die Kombination von metachromatischer Leukodystrophie und Mukopolysaccharidose als selbständiges Krankheitsbild (Mukosulfatidose). *Helv Paediat Acta* **25**:436-461, 1970.

52. Bischel M, Austin J, Kemeng M: Metachromatic leukodystrophy (MLD): VII. Elevated sulfated acid polysaccharide levels in urine and postmortem tissues. *Arch Neurol* **15**:13-28, 1966.

53. DiFerrante N, Nichols BL, Donnelly PV, et al: Induced degradation of glycosaminoglycans in Hurler's and Hunter's syndromes by plasma infusion. *Proc Nat Acad Sci* **68**:303-307, 1971.

54. McKusick VA: The nosology of the mucopolysaccharidoses. *Amer J Med* **47**:730-747, 1969.

55. McKusick VA, Kaplan D, Wise D, et al: The genetic mucopolysaccharidoses. *Medicine* **44**:445-483, 1965.

56. Brady RO: Prenatal diagnosis of lipid storage diseases. *Clin Chem* **16**:811-815, 1970.

57. Brady RO: Metabolic disorders of sphingolipid metabolism in man. *Chem Phys Lipids* **5**:261-269, 1970.

58. Brady RO: The genetic mismanagement of complex lipid metabolism. *Bull NY Acad Med* **47**:173-182, 1971.

59. Dawson G, Stein AO: Lactosyl ceramidosis: Catabolic enzyme defect of glycosphingolipid metabolism. *Science* **170**:556-558, 1970.

60. Cogan DG, Kuwabara T, Moser H: Metachromatic leukodystrophy. *Ophthalmologica* **160**:2-17, 1970.

61. Weingeist TA, Blodi FC: Fabry's disease: Ocular findings in a female carrier: A light and electron microscopic study. *Arch Ophthal* **85**:169-176, 1971.

62. Goldberg MF: A review of selected corneal dystrophies associated with systemic diseases, in Bergsma D (ed): *The Second Conference on the Clinical Delineation of Birth Defects.* National Foundation March of Dimes, March 1971, vol 3, No. 3.

63. Moser HW, Prensky AL, Wolfe HJ, et al: Farber's lipogranulomatosis: Report of a case and demonstration of an excess of free ceramide and ganglioside. *Amer J Med* **47**:869-890, 1969.

64. Silverstein MN, Ellefson RD, Ahern EJ: The syndrome of the sea-blue histiocyte. *New Eng J Med* **282**:1-4, 1970.

65. Sebestyen J, Galfi I: Retinal functions in Niemann-Pick lipidosis. *Ophthalmologica* **157**:349-356, 1969.

66. Gatt S, Rapport MM: Isolation of β-galactosidase and β-glucosidase from brain. *Biochem Biophys Acta* **113**:567-576, 1966.

67. Fluharty AL, Porter MT, Lassila EL, et al: Acid glycosidases in mucopolysaccharidoses' fibroblasts. *Biochem Med* **4**:110-120, 1970.

68. Benson PF, Bowser-Riley F, Giannelli F: Beta-galactosidases in fibroblasts: Hurler and Sanfilippo syndromes. *New Eng J Med* **283**:999-1000, 1970.

69. Callahan JW, Wolfe LS: Isolation and characterization of keratan sulfates from the liver of a patient with GM_1 gangliosidosis type I. *Biochem Biophys Acta* **215**:527-543, 1970.

Adverse Reactions to Sulfisoxazole, Sulfamethoxazole, and Nitrofurantoin

Manifestations and Specific Reaction Rates During 2,118 Courses of Therapy

Jan Koch-Weser, MD; Victor W. Sidel, MD; Marion Dexter, RN; Catherine Parish, RN; Diana C. Finer; and Paula Kanarek, MA, Boston

Hospitalized patients were monitored during 2,118 courses of therapy with sulfisoxazole, sulfamethoxazole, or nitrofurantoin. Overall frequency of adverse reactions severe enough to require discontinuation of the responsible drug was 3.1% for sulfisoxazole, 3.3% for sulfamethoxazole, and 9.2% for nitrofurantoin. Reaction rates were highly dependent on the duration of therapy. Toxic reactions were far more common to nitrofurantoin (5.1%) than to the sulfonamides (0.3%). They consisted mainly of gastrointestinal disturbances, were more common in women, and their frequency increased sharply with daily dose per patient weight. Sulfisoxazole was associated with allergic reactions in 2.8% of patients, sulfamethoxazole in 3.0%, and nitrofurantoin in 4.1%. Skin rashes, eosinophilia, and drug fever were the common manifestations. Serious reactions to all three drugs were rare (0.14%) and renal toxicity or immediate-type hypersensitivity reactions were not observed.

The therapeutic usefulness of drugs depends both on their effectiveness and on their potential for adverse reactions. When two drugs with similar therapeutic indications are available, informed choice requires accurate knowledge of the benefit-to-risk ratio of both. Therapeutic effectiveness can usually be determined by well-designed studies on relatively few patients. In contrast, significant adverse reactions occur in a small percentage of patients and their quantitation requires careful observation of a large number of patients exposed to the drug.

Accurate knowledge of adverse reaction rates is available for very few drugs. It is rarely developed during studies of therapeutic efficacy prior to the general clinical use of the drug. It cannot be derived from analyses of spontaneous reports of drug-related adverse events to drug companies, medical journals, or government regulatory agencies. Such reports represent only a small and unknown fraction of the adverse reactions actually occurring.[1,2] Furthermore, the number of patients exposed to the drug is generally not known. In the absence of accurate numerator and denominator information, statements concerning reaction rates to individual drugs represent only guesses. The most practical and reliable method for determining the risk of adverse drug reactions under clinical conditions is prospective surveillance of hospitalized patients and evaluation at the time and place of occurrence of all untoward events that might be drug-related.[2,3]

This paper reports the results of such a prospective study on adverse effects of sulfisoxazole, sulfamethoxazole, and nitrofurantoin, three drugs which often represent therapeutic alternatives in the treatment of urinary tract infections. The study was designed to determine the overall reaction rate to these drugs, the risks of specific manifestations, and the influence of patient characteristics and of drug dosage on the reaction rate. The findings indicate that administration of nitrofurantoin carries a higher risk of adverse effects than therapy with the two sulfonamides and that the rate of serious reactions to all three drugs is quite low.

Methods

Between April 1967 and July 1968 all patients hospitalized at the Massachusetts General Hospital for whom treatment with sulfisoxazole, sulfamethoxazole, or nitrofurantoin was initiated were immediately identified through daily examination of order and medication sheets by study clerks. Forty percent of patients treated with sulfisoxazole (randomly selected by the terminal digit of their hospital number) and all patients receiving the other drugs were then observed daily for adverse drug reactions. Each patient's course was monitored by a specially trained surveillance nurse throughout his therapy with one of the three drugs and thereafter for three days or until discharge or death. In addition, all patients who suffered adverse effects from these drugs were followed in the hospital after therapy until the reaction had completely cleared.

Initially, each patient's history was reviewed and his personal characteristics recorded together with all pertinent diagnoses, clinical data, and results of laboratory examinations. Thereafter, standardized records were kept of the patient's clinical course, laboratory data, and dosage schedules of all drugs administered. Untoward changes in a patient's clinical course or laboratory findings during therapy with sulfisoxazole, sulfamethoxazole, or nitrofurantoin were evaluated by a clinical pharmacologist at the time of their occurrence and after discharge. Those unto-

Received for publication Aug 12, 1970; accepted Oct 27.

From the Clinical Pharmacology Unit, departments of pharmacology and medicine, and the Community Medicine Unit, Department of Medicine, Harvard Medical School and Massachusetts General Hospital, Boston.

Reprint requests to Clinical Pharmacology Unit, Department of Medicine, Massachusetts General Hospital, Fruit St, Boston 02114 (Dr. Koch-Weser).

Table 1.—Reaction Rates to Individual Drugs

	Total Utilizations	Total Reactions		Toxic Reactions		Allergic Reactions	
	No.	No.	Reaction Rate (%)	No.	Reaction Rate (%)	No.	Reaction Rate (%)
Sulfisoxazole	1,002	30	3.1	3	0.3	28	2.8
Sulfamethoxazole	359	12	3.3	1	0.3	11	3.0
Nitrofurantoin	757	70	9.2	39	5.1	31	4.1

Table 2.—Manifestations of Reactions

	Sulfisoxazole and Sulfamethoxazole		Nitrofurantoin	
Dermatologic reactions	29		15	
Macular eruption		7		3
Maculopapular eruption		6		4
Urticarial eruption		5		3
Angioneurotic edema		2		1
Erythema multiforme		2		1
Pruritus only		2		0
Other eruptions (Purpuric, petechial, vesicular erythema nodosum, exfoliative dermatitis)		5		3
Gastrointestinal reactions	8		75	
Anorexia, nausea		3		38
Vomiting		3		28
Abdominal pain		1		4
Gastrointestinal bleeding		1		2
Diarrhea		0		3
Hematologic reactions	20		13	
Eosinophilia		16		10
Hemolytic anemia		1		1
Megaloblastic anemia		0		1
Leukopenia		1		1
Thrombocytopenia		1		0
Hypoprothrombinemia		1		0
Drug Fever	16		15	
Serum sickness	1		2	
Vasculitis	1		1	
Cholestatic jaundice	1		0	
Pulmonary infiltration	0		2	
Polyserositis	0		1	
Polyneuropathy	0		1	

Table 3.—Reaction Morbidity

	Sulfisoxazole and Sulfamethoxazole				Nitrofurantoin			
	Toxic Reactions		Allergic Reactions		Toxic Reactions		Allergic Reactions	
	No.	%	No.	%	No.	%	No.	%
None	0	0.0	9	23.1	0	0.0	4	12.9
Mild	3	75.0	22	56.4	33	84.6	11	35.5
Moderate	1	25.0	6	15.4	6	15.4	15	48.4
Severe	0	0.0	2	5.1	0	0.0	1	3.2
Total	4	100.0	39	100.0	39	100.0	31	100.0

ward events which after careful analysis of all available information could not be attributed to the patient's underlying disease or to other therapy and which cleared upon cessation of therapy with sulfisoxazole, sulfamethoxazole, or nitrofurantoin were considered to represent adverse reactions to one of these drugs. In approximately nine out of ten cases this judgement coincided with that of the physicians responsible for the patient's care. For the purpose of this study only those adverse effects severe enough to require specific treatment, reduction, or cessation of therapy with the offending drug, or its future avoidance were considered adverse drug reactions.[1,4]

Detailed data concerning all patients monitored, their drug therapy, and any adverse reactions were coded and entered on punch cards. Adverse reactions were classified as toxic or allergic according to their generally accepted mechanisms. Specific reaction rates and the effects of patient and therapy characteristics on reaction rates were determined using appropriate computer programs. To compare the allergic and toxic reaction rates to nitrofurantoin and to sulfonamides the almost identical results for sulfisoxazole and sulfamethoxazole were pooled. All statistical analyses were performed by chi-square tests including, where appropriate, consideration of linear trends.

Results

The numbers of patients monitored throughout their treatment with sulfisoxazole, sulfamethoxazole, or nitrofurantoin are shown in Table 1. With the exception of two patients treated with sulfisoxazole intravenously, all patients received these drugs by mouth. Sulfisoxazole and nitrofurantoin were almost always administered four times per day, sulfamethoxazole twice daily. Prophylaxis of urinary infection was the therapeutic aim in 34.3% of the courses of sulfonamides and in 19.1% of nitrofurantoin utilizations. All other patients received the drugs for treatment of urinary infections and there were no major differences among the three drugs in the infecting organisms treated.

Table 1 shows the number and type of adverse reactions to the three drugs studied. Both toxic and allergic reaction rates to sulfisoxazole

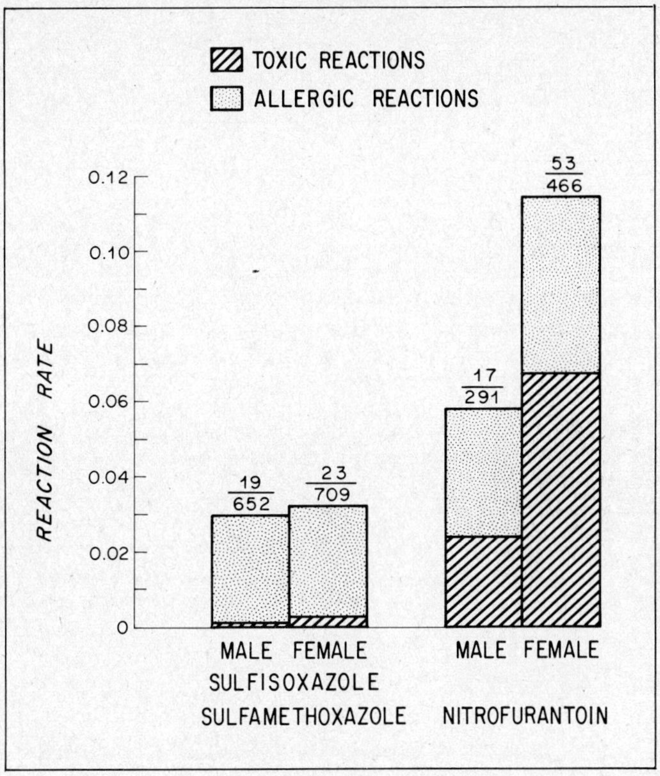

Fig 1.—Sex-specific reaction rates to sulfonamides and nitrofurantoin.

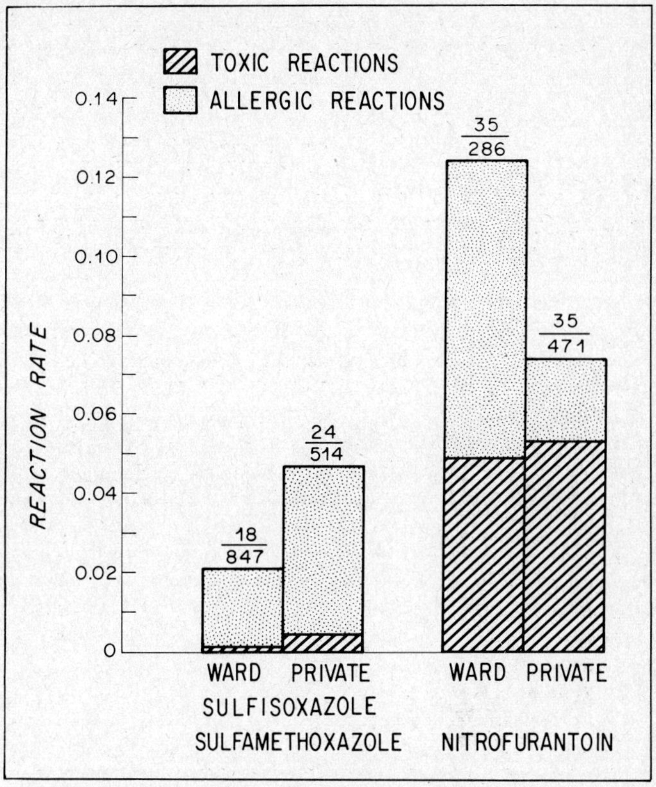

Fig 2.—Reaction rates on ward and private services.

and sulfamethoxazole were almost identical. Specific reaction rates to the two drugs also did not differ significantly. Accordingly, the results for the two sulfonamides were pooled and compared with those for nitrofurantoin. The overall incidence of adverse reactions to nitrofurantoin was significantly higher than that to the sulfonamides ($P < 0.001$). This difference was primarily due to the much more common occurrence of toxic reactions to nitrofurantoin ($P < 0.001$). Allergic reactions also appeared more frequently during nitrofurantoin than during sulfonamide therapy, but the difference did not reach the 95% confidence level.

Table 4.—Age-Specific Reaction Rates

Age	Total Utilizations	Toxic Reactions		Allergic Reactions	
	No.	No.	Reaction Rate (%)	No.	Reaction Rate (%)
	Sulfisoxazole and Sulfamethoxazole				
<15	120	0	0.0	1	0.8
15 to 44	284	1	0.4	10	3,5
45 to 64	379	1	0.3	14	3.7
65 to 74	292	1	0.3	8	2.7
>74	286	1	0.3	6	2.1
Total	1,361	4	0.3	39	2.9
	Nitrofurantoin				
<15	95	1	1.1	3	3.2
15 to 44	122	9	7.4	6	4.9
45 to 64	229	11	4.8	16	7.0
65 to 74	168	8	4.7	5	3.0
>74	143	10	7.0	1	0.7
Total	757	39	5.1	31	4.1

Manifestations of the 42 adverse reactions to sulfisoxazole and sulfamethoxazole and of the 70 to nitrofurantoin are listed in Table 2. Gastrointestinal disturbances constituted the great majority of toxic reactions and were far more common during therapy with nitrofurantoin than with the sulfonamides ($P < 0.001$). Drug fever occurred during 2.0% of nitrofurantoin utilizations but in only 1.2% of patients treated with the two sulfonamides. The incidence of adverse reactions with dermatologic or hematologic manifestations to the sulfonamides and to nitrofurantoin was similar. Hypersensitivity reactions of the immediate type were not observed in any patient.

Table 3 shows the morbidity resulting from toxic and allergic reactions to the sulfonamides and nitrofurantoin. Most of the toxic gastrointestinal reactions to nitrofurantoin resulted in only mild morbidity. On the other hand, allergic reactions to nitrofurantoin tended to be associated with greater morbidity than al-

Table 5.—Effect of Mean Daily Dose on Reaction Rate

	Total Utilizations	Toxic Reactions		Allergic Reactions	
	No.	No.	Reaction Rate (%)	No.	Reaction Rate (%)
Sulfisoxazole					
2.00 or less	330	1	0.3	7	2.1
2.01 to 3.50	341	1	0.3	8	2.3
3.51 or more	331	1	0.3	13	3.9
Total	1,002	3	0.3	28	2.8
Sulfamethoxazole					
1.80 or less	191	0	0.0	5	2.6
1.81 or more	168	1	0.6	6	3.6
Total	359	1	0.3	11	3.1
Nitrofurantoin					
199 or less	258	9	3.5	10	3.9
200 to 299	242	12	5.0	10	4.1
300 or more	257	18	7.0	11	4.3
Total	757	39	5.1	31	4.1

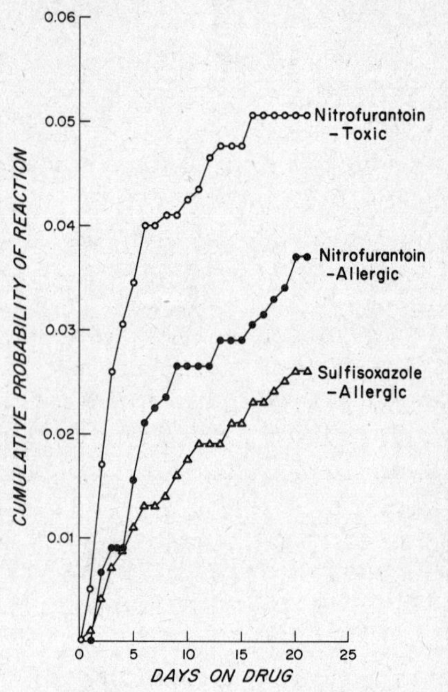

Fig 3.—Cumulative probability of adverse reactions by days on nitrofurantoin or sulfisoxazole.

lergic reactions to sulfisoxazole and sulfamethoxazole. This reflects the fact that fewer allergic reactions to nitrofurantoin than to the sulfonamides manifested themselves only in the skin.

Sex-specific reaction rates to the two sulfonamides and to nitrofurantoin are given in Fig 1. During therapy with sulfisoxazole and sulfamethoxazole the sexes showed a similar incidence of both toxic and allergic reactions. Nitrofurantoin treatment was also associated with an almost identical incidence of allergic reactions in males and females, but toxic reactions to nitrofurantoin were significantly more common in females ($P<0.01$).

Age-specific adverse reaction rates to the three drugs are shown in Table 4. Among adults patient age was not a factor in the rate of toxic reactions, but only one such reaction occurred in children. The incidence of allergic reactions to the two sulfonamides and to nitrofurantoin increased up to the age of 45 to 64 years and fell thereafter.

The toxic reaction rate to nitrofurantoin was strikingly dependent on patient weight: 14.5% for adult patients weighing less than 120 pounds, 9.5% for patients between 120 and 150 pounds, and 2.6% for patients over 150 pounds. This linear trend was highly significant ($P<0.001$) and obtained in both men and women. Patient weight did not influence the incidence of allergic reactions to any of the three drugs.

Toxic reactions to the sulfonamides and to nitrofurantoin were equally common on ward and private services (Fig 2). The incidence of allergic reactions to the sulfonamides was significantly higher on the private service ($P<0.01$), but the reverse was true for nitrofurantoin ($P<0.01$). Reliable histories of previous exposure to these drugs which might account for the differences could not be obtained from most patients. Reaction rates in medical and surgical patients were almost identical.

Table 5 shows the distribution of mean daily dosages received by the monitored patients and the effect of dose on reaction rate. In no patient did the mean daily dosage of sulfisoxazole, sulfamethoxazole, or nitrofurantoin exceed 5.0, 3.0, and 0.4 gm, respectively. No statistically significant effect of the mean daily dose on the incidence of allergic reactions was demonstrated for any of the three drugs, but the reaction rates tended to increase with the amount of drug administered. Toxic reactions to nitrofurantoin increased significantly with the mean daily dose ($P<0.001$). The frequency of these reactions was even more strikingly dependent on mean daily dose per pound of body weight. Only 1.6% of patients receiving less than 4 mg/kg, but 23.6% of those given more than 7 mg/kg suffered toxic effects.

The cumulative probability of the occurrence of allergic reactions to sulfisoxazole or of allergic or toxic reaction to nitrofurantoin is illustrated in Fig 3. The data were obtained using the multiple decrement life table method by adding the daily probabilities of reaction on all days preceding and including the one under consideration. These curves characterize a patient's cumulative risk of suffering a reaction of the specified type to the two drugs in terms of the duration of his therapy with the drug. This method of presentation of risk data clearly demonstrates the marked dependence of reaction risk on duration of exposure. The cumulative probability of both toxic and allergic reactions increased progressively with days on therapy.

Eighty percent of the observed toxic reactions to nitrofurantoin appeared during the first six days, and no further reactions occurred after the 16th day of treatment. The daily probabilities of allergic reactions to nitrofurantoin or sulfisoxazole were also highest during the first week but declined only slightly thereafter, and allergic reactions continued to occur during the third and fourth week of treatment. Allergic reactions during the first week must have represented previous sensitization to these commonly used drugs, but therapeutic histories were too unreliable to verify this.

Comment

The specific purpose of this study was to determine the incidence of the common adverse reactions to three drugs used to treat urinary tract infection and to evaluate patient and dosage factors which influence reaction rates. Previous knowledge concerning the adverse effects of these drugs has been a byproduct of efficacy studies in small groups of patients or has come from sporadic spontaneous reports of clinical observations. Such information is of little value for the calculation of reaction rates.[1,2]

Estimates of the incidence of adverse reactions to these three drugs have varied enormously. Yow suggested that serious reactions occur in fewer than 0.1% of patients treated with sulfisoxazole.[5] Kutscher et al analyzed the published experience during the first seven years of clinical use of sulfisoxazole and found tenfold variations in the reported incidence of many adverse manifestations.[6] Lehr estimated the overall reaction rate to sulfisoxazole as 0.028 to 0.088.[7] Adverse reactions to nitrofurantoin have been observed in 3.5% to 40% of patients, but many of these were trivial and dosages were often higher than now generally used.[8-10] No comparisons of reaction rates to sulfisoxazole and nitrofurantoin during their therapeutic use in similar populations have been attempted.

A major difficulty in comparing adverse reaction rates is the failure of most reports to state their definition of such events. In our studies only those undesirable effects of drugs severe enough to require withdrawal or reduction of dosage, treatment, or future avoidance of the drug have been considered adverse drug reactions.[1,4] This operational definition is readily understood and accepted by physicians and encompasses the significant risks of drug therapy.[2] It excludes many expected and minor symptoms which are common in hospitalized patients and can rarely be attributed to a specific drug.

Our findings suggest a higher incidence of significant untoward events associated with the use of sulfisoxazole or nitrofurantoin than suggested by previous reports. Prospective surveillance predictably gives a far more complete picture of the adverse potential of drugs than occasional reports of such events.[1,2] The causal role of one of the three drugs could not always be established with certainty. The clinical situation was often complex and some adverse events attributed to these drugs may have been due to other factors. The reverse may also have occurred. Almost certainly, however, careful monitoring and evaluation of untoward changes in a patient's course on the basis of all available evidence at the time and place of the occurrence yields more reliable information than the generally incomplete data in spontaneous reports to manufacturers, regulatory agencies, or medical journals.

Adverse drug reaction rates are far more meaningful if duration of therapy, dosage, and patient characteristics are specified.[11,12] The crucial dependence of reaction risks on duration of exposure has been previously stressed[12] and was confirmed in this study. The increased rate of toxic reactions to nitrofurantoin with daily dose and even more strikingly with daily dose per body weight is expected since such reactions are related to drug concentration in the body. A sharply progressive increase in the frequency of gastrointestinal reactions with increasing dosage of nitrofurantoin has been observed by others and daily doses over 7 mg/kg are intolerable to a high percentage of patients.[8,9] The marked increase in the frequency of nausea and vomiting with increasing daily dosage per body weight suggests that they result from an action of nitrofurantoin on the central nervous system rather than on the gastrointestinal tract. This is further supported by the rare evidence of local irritation such as heartburn, abdominal pain, or gastrointestinal bleeding and by the occurrence of nausea and vomiting after intravenous injection.[13] In our experience, the slowing of absorption of nitrofurantoin by its ingestion with food or by administration in macrocrystalline form[14] does not prevent the occurrence of severe nausea and vomiting. It seems likely that these symptoms are related more closely to the average concentration of the drug in body fluids than to the rate of absorption. This concentration would be reduced by the above maneuvers only if absorption became incomplete and then drug concentration in the urine would also be lowered.

Allergic reaction rates to all three drugs studied also increased with mean daily dose although the trend did not reach statistical significance. A relationship between dosage of sulfonamides and sensitization has been suggested by Lehr.[7] We have previously observed an increase in frequency of allergic reactions with dosage during prolonged treatment with semisynthetic penicillins. These relationships are not apparent if the course of therapy is short, since then only previously sensitized individuals will suffer allergic reactions and any dose can elicit an allergic reaction in a sensitized patient.

Patient characteristics other than weight and previous exposure clearly influence the rate of reactions to these drugs. The frequency of allergic reactions is lowest in children, reaches a peak in the group 45 to 64 years of age, and declines thereafter. The lower allergic reaction rate in children probably results from their lesser previous exposure. No ready explanation offers itself for the decreasing frequency in the aged; it was not due to short courses of therapy. We have found the same relatively low allergic reaction rate in old age during therapy with semisynthetic penicillins. The rarity of toxic reactions in children likely reflects low drug concentrations in their bodies due to the common reduction of dosage in proportion to body weight rather than surface area. Women had far higher toxic reaction rates to nitrofurantoin than men. Higher frequency of drug-induced nausea and vomiting in women has been a consistent finding in our studies on adverse drug reactions and has been reported by others.[10,15] It is only partly explained by the failure to adjust drug dosage to the lesser weight of women.

No new types of adverse reactions to the three drugs studied were detected. Generation of such information is not the main purpose of studies of this type which are primarily intended to define the quantitative importance of the more common adverse reactions.[2] Intensive, prospective studies can uncover previously unrecognized adverse drug reactions and interactions,[16,17] but short-term surveillance of 1,000 or fewer patients receiving drugs which have been used in millions of patients for many years is not likely to reveal those very rare or delayed adverse reactions which have escaped detection. However, some serious adverse reactions to the sulfonamides (hepatitis, serum sickness, hypoprothrombinemia, thrombocytopenia) and to nitrofurantoin (pulmonary infiltration, polyserositis, serum sickness, polyneuropathy) which are considered quite rare were encountered once or more during this study. Surveillance of a five to ten times larger group of patients treated with these drugs might well allow the badly needed estimate of the frequency of such serious reactions which represent the crucial risks of drug therapy.

The rate of untoward effects severe enough to require discontinuation of therapy is significantly higher for nitrofurantoin than for sulfisoxazole or sulfamethoxazole. While the great majority of these reactions cause only mild or moderate morbidity and clear promptly when therapy is stopped, a patient given nitrofurantoin is three times more likely not to tolerate this therapy than a patient treated with sulfisoxazole or sulfamethoxazole. For all three drugs the risks of serious reactions of renal toxicity, and of immediate-type hypersensitivity reactions appears quite low.

This study was supported in part by contracts FDA 67-24, FDA 68-11, and FDA 69-10 with the Food and Drug Administration. Dr. Koch-Weser is a Burroughs Wellcome Scholar in Clinical Pharmacology. Dr. Sidel is a Faculty Fellow of the Milbank Memorial Fund.

John Webb, director of pharmacy, Susan Baker, Joanne Byrnes, Ann E. Eaton, Elizabeth Federman, Lois Henderson, Patricia Simmons, Naidene Waller, and Janet Wittes participated in the Massachusetts General Hospital Adverse Drug Reaction Study.

Nonproprietary and Trade Names of Drugs

Sulfisoxazole—*Entusil, Gantrisin.*
Sulfamethoxazole—*Gantanol.*
Nitrofurantoin—*Furadantin, Macrodantin, Nitrex, Steri-med, Trantoin.*

References

1. Koch-Weser J, Sidel VW, Sweet RH, et al: Factors determining physician reporting of adverse drug reactions: Comparison of 2,000 spontaneous reports with surveillance studies at the Massachusetts General Hospital. *New Eng J Med* **280**:20-26, 1969.

2. Gardner P, Cluff LE: The epidemiology of adverse drug reactions: A review and perspective. *Johns Hopkins Med J* **126**:77-87, 1970.

3. International drug monitoring: The role of the hospital. *WHO Techn Rep Ser*, No. 425, pp 1-24, 1969.

4. Koch-Weser J: Definition and classification of adverse drug reactions. *Drug Inform Bull* **2**:72-78, 1968.

5. Yow EM: Observations on the use of sulfisoxazole (Gantrisin) in 1,000 consecutive patients, with particular reference to the frequency of undesirable side effects. *Amer Prac* **4**:521-525, 1953.

6. Kutscher AH, Lane SL, Segall R: The clinical toxicity of antibiotics and sulfonamides: A comparative review based on 104,672 cases treated systemically. *J Allerg* **25**:135-150, 1954.

7. Lehr D: Clinical toxicity of sulfonamides. *Ann NY Acad Sci* **69**:417-447, 1957.

8. Mintzer S, Kadison ER, Shlaes WH, et al: Treatment of urinary tract infections with a new antibacterial nitrofuran. *Antibiot Chemother* **3**:151-157, 1953.

9. Trafton HM, Beutner EH, Petronio JJ, et al: Furadantin in urinary-tract infections: Clinical and laboratory studies. *New Eng J Med* **252**:383-387, 1955.

10. Dumittan SH: Enquête sur 100 cas d'infection urinaire chronique traités par la nitrofurantoine. *Schweiz Med Wschr* **11**:296-302, 1960.

11. Jick H, Slone D, Borda IT, et al: Efficacy and toxicity of heparin in relation to age and sex. *New Eng J Med* **279**:284-286, 1968.

12. Koch-Weser J, Sidel VW, Federman EB, et al: Adverse effects of sodium colistimethate: Manifestations and specific reaction rates during 317 courses of therapy. *Ann Intern Med* **72**:857-868, 1970.

13. Halliday A, Jawetz E: Sodium nitrofurantoin administered intravenously: A limited study to define its clinical indication. *New Eng J Med* **266**:427-432, 1962.

14. Hailey FJ, Glascock HW Jr: Gastrointestinal tolerance to a new macrocrystalline form of nitrofurantoin: A collaborative study. *Curr Ther Res* **9**:600-605, 1967.

15. Seidl LG, Thornton GF, Smith JW, et al: Studies on the epidemiology of adverse drug reactions. *Bull Hopkins Hosp* **119**:299-315, 1966.

16. Slone D, Jick H, Lewis GP, et al: Intravenously given ethacrynic acid and gastrointestinal bleeding: A finding resulting from comprehensive drug surveillance. *JAMA* **209**:1668-1671, 1969.

17. Koch-Weser J: Potentiation by glucagon of the hypoprothrombinemic action of warfarin. *Ann Intern Med* **72**:331-335, 1970.

Pyogenic Vertebral Osteomyelitis

Treatment With Antimicrobial Agents and Bed Rest

M. Colin Jordan, MD, and William M. M. Kirby, MD, Seattle

Four patients were treated with antibiotics and simple bed rest for pyogenic vertebral osteomyelitis. The initial clinical response to therapy was good in all patients, with a rapid fall in temperature and a marked decrease in back pain within two or three days. The duration of hospitalization averaged 42 days and all four patients were ambulatory when discharged. Spontaneous intervertebral fusion occurred in three patients and all have returned to work. The duration of follow-up has ranged from 17 to 30 months and no relapses or complications have occurred. The fourth patient died of a myocardial infarction ten days after discharge. At autopsy, the vertebral bodies and disk space were sterile and reparative bony sclerosis had begun. In these four cases, the clinical response to bed rest and antibiotics was equivalent to that obtained with rigid immobilization. This regimen avoids the inconvenience and hazards of body casts and the duration of hospitalization may be shortened.

Pyogenic infections of the vertebral bodies and their intervening disk spaces are relatively uncommon. For this reason, and also because these infections tend to manifest themselves in a bizarre fashion, correct diagnosis is often delayed. Attention is frequently directed away from the spine by abdominal pain, neuromuscular disturbances, or genitourinary symptoms. While these diagnostic difficulties have been repeatedly described,[1-4] there has been a paucity of objective therapeutic information since the advent of antibiotics.

Orthopedic surgeons consider effective treatment to consist primarily of immobilization, usually in a body cast, and assign antimicrobial therapy an adjunctive or supportive role.[4-8] This approach stems largely from the preantibiotic era when surgical debridement and immobilization were the only therapy available. The extent to which antimicrobial agents have modified the need for immobilization is not known and no controlled series are available.

During the past three years we have had an opportunity to treat four patients with pyogenic disk space and vertebral infections with antimicrobial agents and simple bed rest. The immediate clinical response, as well as the long-term results, suggest that rigid immobilization of the vertebral column is not necessary in uncomplicated cases of spinal osteomyelitis.

Received for publication Oct 21, 1970; accepted Nov 9.

From the Department of Medicine, University of Washington School of Medicine, Seattle.

Reprint requests to Department of Medicine, University of Washington School of Medicine, Seattle 98105 (Dr. Kirby).

Methods

Four patients with bacterial infections of the disk space and adjacent vertebral bodies were seen by us between January 1967 and December 1968. Clinical data are summarized in Table 1. None of them was immobilized in a body cast. Treatment consisted of bed rest for three or four weeks in the hospital in conjunction with the parenteral administration of antimicrobial agents. Two patients (patients 2 and 4) were allowed the early use of a bedside commode while patients 1 and 3 remained in bed for two or three weeks. After treatment with antibiotics given parenterally was discontinued, the appropriate chemotherapeutic was then administered orally for several weeks and the patients were seen at frequent intervals as outpatients.

Table 1.—Summary of Clinical Data in Four Patients With Pyogenic Vertebral Osteomyelitis

Patient No.	Age, yr	Infection Site	Causative Organism	Source of Culture	Antimicrobial Therapy	No. Days in Hospital	No. Days of Therapy*	Current Status of Patient
1	57	T10-11	*Staph aureus*	Needle aspiration	Methicillin, penicillin	39	125	Working as typist (30 mo)†
2	66	L4-5	*Sal san diego*	Blood, stool	Chloramphenicol ampicillin	35	91	Asymptomatic, housewife (24 mo)
3	63	L2-3	*Staph aureus*	Knee joint, urine	Methicillin, cephalothin, erythromycin	40	49	Died of myocardial infarction
4	56	L2-3	*P mirabilis*	Blood, needle aspiration	Ampicillin	56	117	Working as bus driver (17 mo)

* Total duration of inpatient and outpatient antibiotic therapy.
† Parentheses indicate duration of follow-up from initiation of therapy.

Patient Summaries

PATIENT 1.—A 57-year-old typist had a tooth extraction and received antibiotics for a dental abscess in April 1966. Subsequently she noted weight loss, malaise, fatigue, and anorexia and diffuse back pain developed in May 1966, followed by intermittent abdominal pain. A barium meal demonstrated a small duodenal ulcer. In September 1966 a laparotomy was performed because of persistent abdominal pain and revealed only a few adhesions. By November 1966 the patient was bedfast with severe pain in the back and abdomen and there was no improvement with ten days of tetracycline hydrochloride therapy. On admission to University Hospital, Jan 3, 1967, she was lethargic and appeared chronically ill. Her temperature was 101.3 F (38.6 C). The back was rigid with marked tenderness over the lower thoracic vertebrae but no abnormalities were found on neurologic examination. Roentgenograms of the dorsal spine (Fig 1, *top*) showed loss of the disk space between the 10th and 11th vertebrae with bony destruction and sclerotic reactions involving both vertebral bodies. There was widening of the paravertebral shadows at the same level, which suggested abscess formation. Needle aspiration of the disk space was performed and culture of the purulent material obtained grew large numbers of coagulase-positive *Staphylococcus aureus*, sensitive to penicillin G. Blood cultures were sterile. Treatment was initiated with parenteral administration of methicillin sodium but was changed to intravenous administration of penicillin G (20,000,000 units daily) when antibiotic sensitivities were reported. The patient was at complete bed rest with an underlying bed board for 21 days while receiving penicillin parenterally, and there was marked improvement in her back pain and mental status during this time. Fever subsided within a few days and the erythrocyte sedimentation rate (ESR) gradually fell to normal (Table 2). On the 27th hospital day she was allowed to sit on the edge of her bed and she was ambulatory on the 30th day. On the 39th day the patient was discharged and phenoxymethyl penicillin potassium was administered orally for an additional three months. Roentgenograms showed progressive reossification and fusion of the vertebral bodies during the ensuing months, as shown on follow-up films made in March 1968 (Fig 1, *bottom*). The patient returned to work in August 1967.

Table 2.—Changes in Erythrocyte Sedimentation Rate During Therapy of Four Patients With Spinal Osteomyelitis

Patient	Erythrocyte Sedimentation Rate*: Admission	Discharge	Follow-up
1	94	47	15 (19 mo)
2	65	22	11 (13 mo)
3	74	44†	Died
4	89	30	6 (10 mo)

* Computed in milimeters per hour.
† Myocardial infarction and hypersensitivity reaction to methicillin during hospitalization.

Comment.—The indolent nature of pyogenic vertebral osteomyelitis, particularly when brief courses of antimicrobial therapy have masked many of the symptoms and signs, has been noted by several authors.[1,2,7,9] This patient complained of back pain for seven months before the correct diagnosis was established and an unnecessary laparotomy was performed because of abdominal pain. The association of abdominal pain and vertebral osteomyelitis, especially when the thoracic spine is involved, has been stressed by Sullivan.[4,6] Although the osteomyelitis had been present for several months, there was an excellent response both symptomatically and objectively to antibiotic therapy and rest without immobilization.

PATIENT 2.—A 66-year-old housewife became ill on March 7, 1968, with fever, nausea, vomiting, and diarrhea and she was admitted to a community hospital with a temperature of 104 F (40 C). Blood cultures contained *Salmonella san diego.* She was treated with parenterally and orally administered chloramphenicol sodium succinate (6.0 gm/day) for ten days with a rapid fall in her temperature. Lower lumbar pain developed on March 12, 1968, but roentgenograms revealed only minimal osteoarthritis. After discharge the back pain increased and was not relieved by indomethacin. X-ray films of the lumbar spine were again normal but the pain became steadily worse and nocturnal fever developed. On May 4, 1968, the patient was admitted to University Hospital where she was found to have low grade fever and mild tenderness over the lumbar spine. Roentgenograms demonstrated partial destruction of the fifth lumbar vertebra with collapse of the disk space between the fourth and fifth vertebral bodies (Fig 2, *left*). Stool cultures contained *Sal san diego* but the blood was sterile. Hemoglobin electrophoresis was normal. Contrast studies of the gallbladder, upper-gastrointestinal tract, and colon were normal. Therapy was begun with a continuous intravenous infusion of ampicillin sodium (9.0 gm/day). Supportive therapy consisted of bed rest with a bed board and commode privileges. The patient gradually became afebrile during the next several days and her back pain disappeared. The ESR mirrored the clinical response (Table 2). On the 24th hospital day she began sitting on the side of her bed and oral administration of ampicillin (6.0 gm/day) was begun on the 30th day. After 35 days of hospitalization she was discharged with full ambulation and instructed to continue antibiotic therapy for ten more weeks. Roentgenograms taken during the next 14 months showed gradual reossification of the opposed vertebral bodies and complete fusion (Fig 2, *right*). The patient had resumed her household duties and was totally asymptomatic.

Comment.—Despite the development of back pain following an episode of bacteremia, the diagnosis of spinal osteomyelitis was not made in this case for eight weeks. X-ray film abnormalities, which may lag behind the clinical signs for as long as two months,[1] were absent on two occasions and this contributed to the delay in diagnosis. Even a retrospective examination of the previous films failed to show evidence of the abnormality. As stressed by Clawson and Dunn,[10] laminagraphy may be of value in detecting early lesions. Although there have been reports describing an association between salmonella osteomyelitis and sickle cell disease[11] and between salmonellosis and various malignancies,[12] neither was found in this patient.

PATIENT 3.—A 63-year-old salesman had a long history of degenerative joint disease involving the cervical and lumbar spine and both knees. Prednisone, 10 to 20 mg daily, was given for several months with minimal improvement. During the summer of 1967 he received several injections of cortisone acetate into the left knee, which later became red and swollen. On Aug 25, 1967, he was admitted to University Hospital complaining of chills, fever, and pain in the lower back. His temperature was 101.3 F (38.5 C) and there was tenderness and swelling over the third and fourth lumbar vertebrae. *Staphylococcus aureus* was cultured from the inflamed left knee joint and from the urine; blood cultures were negative.

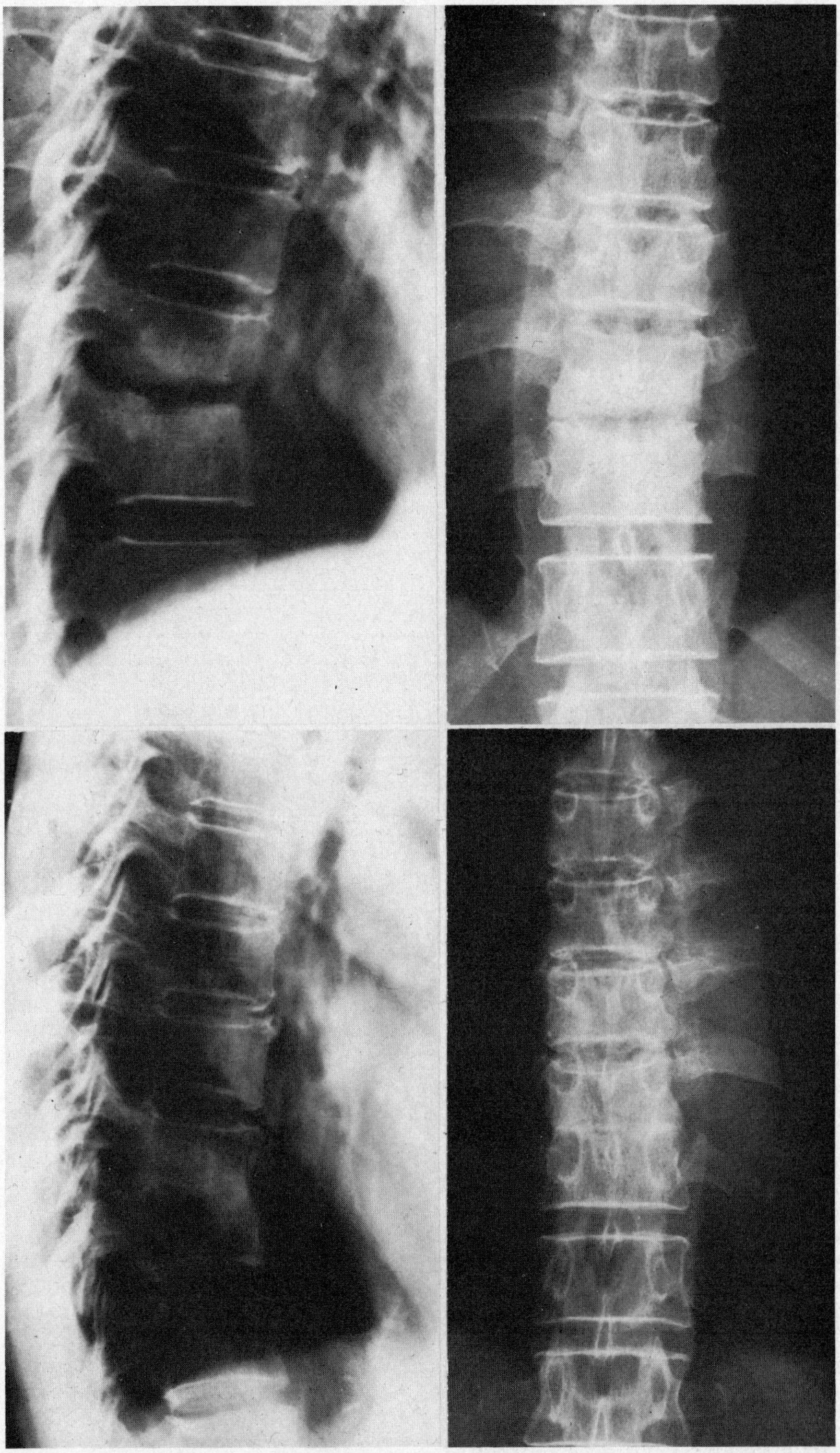

Fig 1.—Top, Osteomyelitis of 10th and 11th thoracic vertebrae, with paravertebral swellings suggesting abscess formation, at onset of antibiotic therapy (patient 1). Bottom, *Roentgenogram 14 months later. Bony fusion and regression of paravertebral swellings.*

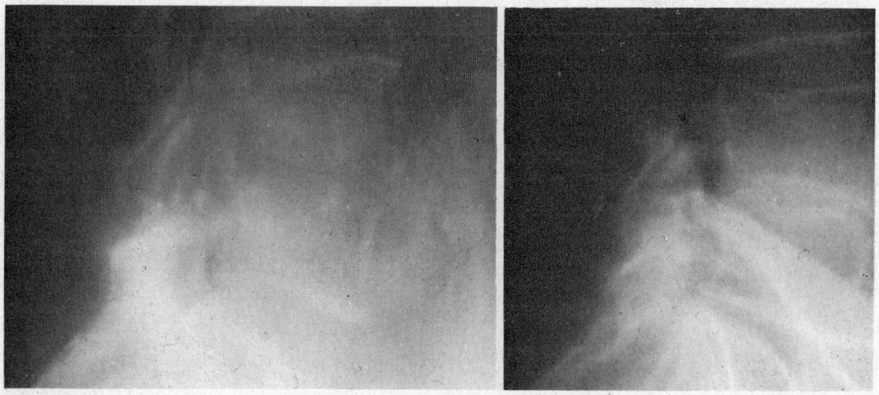

Fig 2.—Left, *Extensive involvement of fourth and fifth lumbar vertebrae and adjoining interspace prior to therapy.* Right, *Excellent reossification and fusion 13 months later (patient 2).*

Roentgenograms of the lumbar spine revealed osteomyelitis of the third lumbar vertebra with collapse of the subjacent disk space. Treatment was begun with methicillin 12 gm/day intravenously and the left knee bursa was irrigated locally with methicillin until pus could no longer be drained. A plaster splint was applied to the leg and the patient was placed on a Foster frame which he found confining and uncomfortable. Progressive improvement was noted but on the tenth day he developed high fever, hematuria, and mild eosinophilia and the blood urea nitrogen level rose to 35 mg/100 ml. Methicillin therapy was stopped and he was given cephalothin sodium (6 gm/day) with an abrupt fall in temperature within 24 hours. On the 15th day a regular hospital bed with a board under the mattress was substituted for the Foster frame and he found this comfortable with minimal pain in the back and knee. After 24 days of antibiotics given parenterally he was given erythromycin estolate orally (2 gm/day). A myocardial infarction occurred at this time and necessitated postponement of attempts at mobilization. On Oct 2, 1967, (38th hospital day) the patient was ambulatory for brief periods and was discharged on the following day. X-ray films at that time revealed early signs of bony reaction around the affected disk space. The ESR had fallen to 33 mm/hr prior to the myocardial infarction but was 44 mm/hr at the time of discharge. When seen in the outpatient clinic one week later, he was ambulatory and complained only of occasional pain in both knees. Erythromycin therapy was continued. Several days later the patient suddenly collapsed and died at home. Autopsy revealed a healed and an acute myocardial infarction with rupture of the interventricular septum. Microscopic examination of the kidneys showed diffuse interstitial nephritis with tubular damage. The major portion of the affected lumbar disk had been replaced with fibrous tissue and chronic inflammation was found in both vertebral bodies. Cultures of these tissues were negative.

Comment.—This patient's excellent clinical response to antibiotics and bed rest, as well as the negative cultures and signs of healing at autopsy, indicate that the spinal osteomyelitis would have gradually progressed to a complete cure if the second myocardial infarction had not occurred. Interstitial nephritis during methicillin therapy has been observed by several authors and probably represents a true hypersensitivity reaction to the drug.[13,14] Cephalothin was substituted with no difficulty in this patient.

Fig 3.—Left, *Lytic defect in lower part of second lumbar vertebrae, with narrowing of disk space, at time of admission.* Middle, *Loss of the disk space and signs of bony healing following laminectomy and several weeks of antibiotic therapy.* Right, *Fusion of involved vertebrae 17 months after treatment was started (patient 4).*

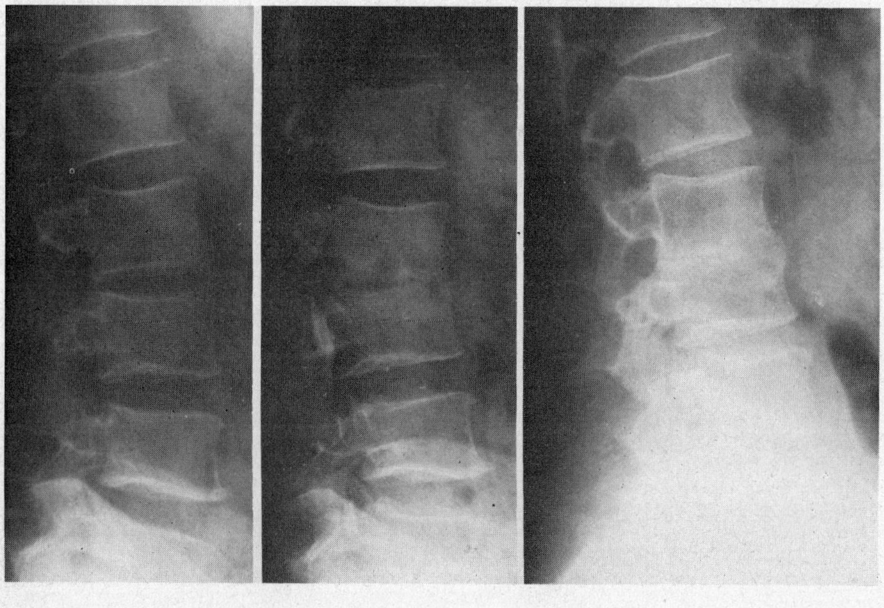

Patient 4.—A 56-year-old bus driver developed back pain in November 1968 not relieved by analgesics. In early December he noted chills and fever, urinary hesitancy, and dysuria. A blood culture was positive for *Proteus mirabilis* at a community hospital but back pain and fever continued despite treatment with various antimicrobial agents. Upon transfer to University Hospital, Dec 28, his temperature was 104 F (40 C), there was tenderness over the lumbar spine, and hyperactive reflexes and unsustained clonus were noted in the right leg. Roentgenograms showed narrowing of the second lumbar disk space with lytic defect involving the inferior aspect of the second lumbar vertebra (Fig 3, *left*). A cisternal myelogram was normal. Several blood cultures and material obtained from the disk

space by needle aspiration were positive for *P mirabilis*. The patient was at bed rest with a bed board and received ampicillin 12 gm/day intravenously. The back pain subsided promptly and the temperature and ESR declined progressively. Two weeks after antibiotic therapy was initiated a second myelogram, performed because of persistent neurologic signs involving the right leg, was interpreted as showing an epidural defect on the right side. Surgical exploration of the area was performed with laminectomy and removal of granulation tissue. No epidural abscess was present. Cultures of the excised tissue revealed a light growth of *P mirabilis*. Following surgery, antibiotics and bed rest were continued and he wore a back brace intermittently (Fig 3, *middle*). After 33 days of parenteral therapy, ampicillin sodium was given orally, 4.0 gm/day. On the 56th hospital day the patient was discharged ambulatory, although mild clonus and hyperreflexia of the right leg were still present. Ampicillin trihydrate therapy was discontinued after 117 days and the patient returned to work. When seen in June 1970 he had gained 20 kg (44 lb) and roentgenograms showed fusion of the involved vertebrae (Fig 3, *right*).

Comment.—Because of persisting neurologic signs, this patient underwent a surgical exploration and his hospital stay was prolonged. Nevertheless, he was eventually cured with bed rest and antimicrobial therapy. Vertebral infections caused by gram-negative bacilli are usually related to urinary infections or surgical manipulation of the urinary tract[2,3,7] and organisms are thought to reach the vertebrae via the pelvic lymphatics and general circulation.[15,16]

Comment

The objective of therapy in spinal osteomyelitis is the elimination of infection followed by fusion of the affected vertebral bodies.[3-7] During the past three decades there has been a gradual evolution to more conservative methods of treatment. Operative vertebral fusion was often used in the preantibiotic era but has been performed less frequently in recent years.[1,4-6] At present, some surgeons favor early exploration of these lesions in order to obtain diagnostic material and to remove infected tissue.[17,18] Others prefer needle aspiration for diagnosis and reserve operative intervention for the drainage of paraspinous abscesses or for emergency decompression of the spinal cord.[1,7]

Aside from surgery, immobilization has been the cornerstone of orthopedic management of spinal osteomyelitis,[4-8] and antimicrobial agents have been considered an important adjunctive form of therapy. However, Sullivan[4-6] has stated that antibiotics should not be used in disk space infections unless there is evidence of spread of the suppurative process to the adjacent soft tissues. Prolonged immobilization (usually from two to four months) in a plaster cast extending from breast to knee is recommended by him as the sole mode of therapy in uncomplicated cases. Antibiotics are withheld on the theory that continued intervertebral inflammation might be more likely to result in spontaneous fusion with obliteration of the infected disk space.[4,6,19] However, antibiotics have been used in addition to immobilization in most reported series with excellent results.[1-3,7,16] Spontaneous intervertebral fusion has usually occurred within 6 to 24 months.

Although spontaneous arthrodesis is a valuable indicator of successful therapy, many patients have been cured without roentgenographic evidence of fusion. Ambrose et al[1] noted spontaneous fusion in only seven of their 19 patients, most of whom were treated with antimicrobial agents and immobilized in plaster casts. Relapses did not occur in any of these patients. Apparently patients who fail to achieve complete arthrodesis reach a state of fibrous stabilization which functions just as effectively as when there is bony fusion.[1,20]

While some degree of rest is desirable during the initial phase of therapy when symptoms may be severe, the degree of limitation necessary in conjunction with antimicrobial therapy is not known. In spinal tuberculosis, where the reparative bony reaction occurs much more slowly than in pyogenic infections,[17,21] chemotherapy and simple bed rest have resulted in rates of vertebral fusion similar to those obtained with prolonged immobilization.[22,23] Bed rest was sufficient immobilization for the four patients with pyogenic infections described in this report. Spontaneous intervertebral fusion occurred in three instances and bony reaction was progressing in the fourth patient when he died of a myocardial infarction. The clinical responses and the rate of fall of the erythrocyte sedimentation rate were similar to those described for patients treated with rigid immobilization.[4-8] Each patient was ambulatory at the time of discharge and received oral antimicrobial therapy as an outpatient for several weeks without relapse of the infection. Undoubtedly the excellent results are partly attributable to the fact that all four patients had primary infections of relatively recent onset caused by readily identified organisms susceptible to bactericidal antibiotics. In addition, paraspinous abscesses, draining sinuses, and other complications were not encountered.

There have been several reports of complications associated with the use of hip spica and body casts. Kaminsky[24] recently described the development of gynecomastia in five young men immobilized for several weeks in hip spicas. All four patients in whom steroid excretion was measured had elevated urinary 17-hydroxycorticosteroid levels and three had increased urinary pituitary gonadotropins (follicle-stimulating hormone). Persistent irritation of the breasts by the plaster cast, resulting in a pituitary response, was felt to be the most likely cause of the gynecomastia. An apparently rare complication of plaster immobilization is the "body cast syndrome."[25,26] Five of the 12 reported cases have been fatal. Marked gastric atony and distention occur and are followed by copious vomiting, aspiration, electrolyte disturbances, and, in some instances, cardiac arrest. In addition to these complications, the likelihood of pulmonary thromboembolism and "hypostatic" pneumonia is increased by prolonged immobilization and restriction of ventilation. Furthermore, a cast discourages or precludes adequate physical examination which must be performed repeatedly in many cases because of underlying disorders. Aside from these medical factors, the inconvenience and discomfort of the body cast are a constant source of irritation to patients.

Although hematogenous pyogenic osteomyelitis is characterized by a marked tendency to recur and become chronic,[16,24] sequestrum formation is minimal in vertebral osteomyelitis and antimicrobial therapy without sequestrectomy is much more likely to be successful than in long-bone infections.[27,28] Our results indicate that a conservative therapeutic approach, consisting of simple bed rest and the administration of appropriate bactericidal antibiotics, is safe and effective in selected cases.

Nonproprietary and Trade Names of Drugs

Cephalothin sodium—*Keflin*.
Ampicillin—*Alpen, Amcill, Polycillin, Principen*.

References

1. Ambrose GB, Alpert M, Meer CS: Vertebral osteomyelitis: A diagnostic problem. *JAMA* **197**:619-622, 1966.
2. Stone DB, Bonfiglio M: Pyogenic vertebral osteomyelitis. *Arch Intern Med* **112**:491-500, 1963.
3. Bruno MS, Silverberg TN, Goldstein DH: Embolic osteomyelitis of the spine as a complication of infection of the urinary tract. *Amer J Med* **29**:865-878, 1960.
4. Sullivan CR, Symmonds RE: Disk infections and abdominal pain. *JAMA* **188**:655-658, 1964.
5. Sullivan CR, Bichel WH, Svien HJ: Infections of vertebral interspaces after operations on intervertebral discs. *JAMA* **166**:1973-1977, 1958.
6. Sullivan CR: Diagnosis and treatment of pyogenic infections of the intervertebral disc. *Surg Clin N Amer* **41**:1077-1086, 1961.
7. Garcia A Jr, Crantham SA: Hematogenous pyogenic vertebral osteomyelitis. *J Bone Joint Surg* **42**:429-436, 1960.
8. Chapnis R: Staphylococcal spondylitis. *Rheumatism* **21**:39-44, 1965.
9. Changed character of osteomyelitis, editorial. *Brit Med J* **3**:255-256, 1967.
10. Clawson DK, Dunn AW: Management of common bacterial infections of bones and joints. *J Bone Joint Surg* **49**:164-182, 1967.
11. Hook EW, Campbell CG, Weens HS: Salmonella osteomyelitis in patients with sickle cell anemia. *New Eng J Med* **257**:403-407, 1957.
12. Han T, Sokal JE, Neter E: Salmonellosis in disseminated malignant diseases. A seven-year review (1959-1965). *New Eng J Med* **276**:1045-1052, 1967.
13. Baldwin DS, Levine BB, McCluskey RT: Renal failure and interstitial nephritis due to penicillin and methicillin. *New Eng J Med* **279**:1245-1252, 1968.
14. Simenhoff ML, Guild WR, Dammin GJ: Acute diffuse interstitial nephritis. Review of the literature and case report. *Amer J Med* **44**:618-625, 1968.
15. Coman DR, de Long RP: The role of the vertebral venous system in the metastasis of cancer to the spinal column: Experiments with tumor-cell suspensions in rats and rabbits. *Cancer* **4**:610-618, 1951.
16. Wiley AM, Trueta J: The vascular anatomy of the spine and its relationship to pyogenic vertebral osteomyelitis, *J Bone Joint Surg* **41**:796-809, 1959.
17. Pritchard AE, Robinson MP: Staphylococcal infection of the spine. *Lancet* **2**:1165-1166, 1961.
18. Johnson RW Jr: In discussion of Garcia and Crantham.[7] *J Bone Joint Surg* **42**:436, 452, 1960.
19. Sullivan CR, McCaslin FE: Further studies on experimental spondylitis and intercorporeal fusion of the spine. *J Bone Joint Surg* **42**:1339-1348, 1960.
20. Stern WE, Balch RE: Surgical aspects of nonspecific inflammatory and suppurative disease of the vertebral column. *Amer J Surg* **112**:314-325, 1966.
21. Kulowski J: Pyogenic osteomyelitis of the spine: An analysis and discussion of 102 cases. *J Bone Joint Surg* **18**:343-364, 1936.
22. Falk A: Results of long-term chemotherapy in spinal tuberculosis: XVII. A follow-up study of 235 patients. *Amer Rev Resp Dis* **95**:1-5, 1967.
23. Konstam PG, Blesovsky A: The ambulant treatment of spinal tuberculosis. *Brit J Surg* **50**:26-38, 1962.
24. Kaminsky HH: Gynecomastia in patients immobilized in spica casts. *JAMA* **210**:2395-2396, 1969.
25. Schwartz DR, Wirka HW: The cast syndrome: A case report and discussion of the literature. *J Bone Joint Surg* **46**:1549-1552, 1964.
26. Berk RN, Coulson DB: The body cast syndrome. *Radiology* **94**:303-305, 1970.
27. Waldvogel FA, Medoff G, Swartz MN: Osteomyelitis. A review of clinical features and therapeutic considerations and unusual aspects. *New Eng J Med* **282**:316-322, 1970.
28. Trueta J: The three types of acute hematogenous osteomyelitis: A clinical and vascular study. *J Bone Joint Surg* **41**:671-680, 1959.

Vitamin E and Porphyrin Metabolism in Man

Padmanabhan P. Nair, PhD; Esteban Mezey, MD; Hari S. Murty, PhD;
Jeffrey Quartner; and Albert I. Mendeloff, MD, Baltimore

Four patients with symptoms of porphyria were treated with water soluble vitamin E. In all four patients, urinary excretion of δ-aminolevulinic acid, porphobilinogen, coproporphyrins, and uroporphyrins, which were initially elevated, decreased to normal levels following therapy. The initial vitamin E levels in whole blood which were lower than normal responded to treatment with the vitamin and paralleled clinical improvement. The effects of vitamin E on porphyrin metabolism were examined in a group of six male chronic alcoholic patients without clinical evidence of chronic liver disease. The coproporphyrinuria associated with alcoholism was found to be nonresponsive to vitamin E. Our observations indicate that the action of vitamin E in porphyria is probably not mediated through a reversal of the effects of any concurrent alcoholism.

Vitamine E, or α-tocopherol, the principal member of the group of methyl substituted tocols, has remained an enigma ever since its discovery five decades ago. A deficiency of this vitamin in experimental animals is characterizaed by species- and tissue-specific manifestations which affect one or more organ systems.[1-3] In primates and in man recent studies have shown the existence of an anemia associated with a lack of this vitamin, the abnormality being traceable to a defect in heme synthesis.[4-7]

The administration of vitamin E has been shown to depress the urinary excretion of porphyrins and porphyrin precursors in lead poisoning in rabbits,[8] in allylisopropylacetamide (AIA) induced porphyria in rats,[9] and in human porphyria cutanea tarda.[10] These observations led us to postulate that vitamin E could function in the regulation of the rate-determining enzymatic steps in the biosynthesis of porphyrins[11,12] and heme.[13] In this study we have compared the effects of vitamin E (Aquasol E) administration on porphyrin metabolism in human porphyria with those in alcoholics on a controlled regimen. The results show that vitamin E induces a significant depression in the urinary excretion of porphyrins and their precursors in porphyria, whereas the vitamin has no effect on similar changes in chronic alcoholism.

Received for publication Nov 25, 1970; accepted Feb 8, 1971.

From the Biochemistry Research Division, Department of Medicine, Sinai Hospital of Baltimore, Inc.; the Department of Medicine and the Alcoholism Research Unit, Baltimore City Hospitals; and the Johns Hopkins University School of Medicine, Baltimore.

Reprint requests to Sinai Hospital of Baltimore, Inc, Greenspring and Belvedere Ave, Baltimore 21215 (Dr. Mendeloff).

Materials and Methods

Subjects.—Patient 1.—A 58-year-old white man was first seen in consultation by the chief of dermatology of this hospital on June 22, 1963, for complaints of recurrent blisters on the dorsal surface of the hands, face, and neck. Physical examination showed a well-nourished man in his middle fifties. Vesicular eruptions with erosions which formed crusts and scars were seen on the dorsal surface of the hands, fingers, cheeks, and external auricles, and on the sides and the back of the neck. In addition, his face, which appeared plethoric, had a number of milia and some suffusion of both conjuctivae.

Family history was unremarkable, except for an aunt who had diabetes. The patient himself had had a laryngeal polypectomy in December 1962 and was being treated with thyroid tablets by his family physician. He admitted to drinking at least a fifth of a gallon of alcoholic beverages socially every week and was frequently exposed to the sun while golfing. A reddish discoloration of the urine was noted by his family physician about a month prior to his first visit to the dermatologist. Physical examination was entirely negative except for the skin lesions.

Routine laboratory studies showed a moderate polycythemia, and skin biopsy revealed a subepidermal bulla. Liver function test values were generally normal, except for sodium sulfobromsulphthalein (BSP) retention of 25% and serum globulin of 3.7 gm/100 ml. Wood's light examination on five different occasions showed reddish fluorescence of the urine, which upon extraction and spectroscopic analysis, contained elevated levels of uroporphyrins. A diagnosis of porphyria cutanea tarda was made, and the only suggested treatment at that time was the avoidance of alcohol, which was, however, not adhered to by the subject.

In November 1968, on the basis of our earlier findings on the role of vitamin E in the regulation of heme metabolism in experimental porphyria, this patient was referred to us for special studies on the action of vitamin E in this condition. During the five years intervening between the time of the original diagnosis and his entry into our study, there were no reported periods of remission. Determinations of total blood vitamin E, urinary excretion of creatinine, aminolevulinic acid (ALA), porphobilinogen (PBG), and uroporphyrins, and coproporphyrins, were made on four separate occasions during a ten-day period to establish the variations in these constituents. The subject was then placed on vitamin E (Aquasol E) therapy administered orally (100 mg/day) for a period of four weeks while all the special studies were repeated at weekly intervals. Towards the end of the second week of therapy, the patient showed a dramatic improvement in his cutaneous lesions, which paralleled a return to normal of his urinary porphyrin excretions. At the end of the fourth week, since the patient was in complete remission, the level of vitamin E administered was reduced to a single dose of 100 mg/week. During the entire period of the study, no attempt was made to alter his dietary habits or his usual intake of alcoholic beverages. He was followed at monthly intervals for about a year. He has remained free of symptoms during this period and there was no recurrence of the cutaneous lesions following periods of exposure to sunlight during outdoor activities.

PATIENT 2.—This 27-year-old white woman had had frequent episodes of abdominal pain for three years before several PBG tests in the urine were positive. A negative laparotomy one year after onset of symptoms, a negative smoking and drinking history, and normal findings on physical examination and liver function tests on several occasions lent added support for the diagnosis of acute intermittent porphyria. She had a bizarre personality and a host of associated symptoms which included obstinate constipation and visual disturbance.

She was admitted to the hospital for observation and collection of urine for determination of PBG and ALA. She was then placed on a regimen of vitamin E, 100 mg per day, and readmitted to the hospital for four subsequent two-day periods to permit accurate urine collections. During this entire treatment period of four weeks no change in symptoms occurred.

PATIENT 3.—This 59-year-old man gave a history of intermittent epigastric pain for two years until in mid-1969 he had more severe pain with radiation to the back, accompanied by nausea and vomiting, and a weight loss of 7.3 kg (16 lb). Despite negative results on gastrointestinal radiologic studies, a normal hematocrit value and amylase concentrations, and normal urine, a slightly diabetic glucose tolerance test gave reason for exploratory laparotomy, carried out for suspected pancreatic disease. The pancreas was normal at operation, but there were some isolated areas of fat necrosis on the mesentery of the small bowel. A month after operation he had recurrence of his former pain, but now much more severe, and he was unable to gain weight. He required senna therapy to move his bowels. Findings of physical examination and routine laboratory studies were again normal. Several urine samples were strongly positive for porphobilinogen.

During the next several weeks quantitative studies of his excretion of PBG and ALA were carried out. Excretion of both substances was markedly increased. His serum tocopherol level was low. He was then given vitamin E therapy at 100 mg per day and has been observed for over a year. His pain slowly disappeared and did not recur until he had not taken vitamin E for three months. Urinary excretion of porphyrins, ALA, and PBG returned to normal values following therapy with vitamin E.

PATIENT 4.—This 45-year-old Negro woman came to the outpatient department complaining of increasing pigmentation over both malar eminences and forehead. Findings of general physical examination were remarkable only for a moderately enlarged firm liver. She gave a history of intermittent consumption of 6 ounces of scotch whiskey mixed with milk for a period of several years. Laboratory studies were normal except for BSP retention of 13% at 45 minutes. Urinary excretion of PBG and ALA were abnormally high, and she was treated with vitamin E, 100 mg per day. No advice was given regarding her alcohol intake. Approximately four weeks after beginning her therapy with vitamin E she first noted lessening of the hyperpigmentation of the face, which went on to complete disappearance in eight weeks. Urinary excretion values of ALA, PBG, and porphyrins paralleled the clinical return to normal.

Patient Studies.—Six male chronic alcoholic patients without clinical evidence of chronic liver disease were studied. The duration of their alcohol intake varied from 28 to 48 years (mean, 38 years). All had been drinking in excess of 200 gm of alcohol daily up to at least 24 hours prior to admission. Four gave a history of prior hospital admissions for alcoholism, and two had a history of one or more episodes of delirium tremens. Dietary intake had been poor (less than 20 gm of protein a day) in three of the patients. Pertinent clinical and laboratory findings are summarized in Table 1. Upon admission the patients were placed on a normal protein diet and a regimen of alcohol. This diet consisted of 3,200 calories of which protein made up 14.9% (120 gm); fat, 17.5% (80 gm); carbohydrate, 18.7% (150 gm); and alcohol 48.9% (280 gm). Ninety-five percent alcohol was diluted in noncaloric juice and administered in eight daily doses at two-hour intervals from 8 AM to 10 PM. Eight days after admission, a twenty-four-hour urine collection was obtained, following which the patients were started on a regimen of vitamin E, 100 mg, orally, daily for five days. Urine was collected again for 24 hours immediately following the fifth dose of vitamin E, and it was assayed for porphyrins and porphyrin precursors. Creatinine determinations were made on the urine samples to ensure completeness of the twenty-four hour collections.

Laboratory Procedures.—Vitamin E was determined in whole blood by gas-liquid chromatographic procedures developed in this laboratory.[14-16] In this method vitamin E was isolated from whole blood after mild saponification, converted to its trifluoroacetate derivative, and chromatographed on a mixed phase column.

Urinary δ-aminolevulinic acid and porphobilinogen were determined by the method of Marver et al.[17] Urinary coproporphyrins and uroporphyrins were measured spectrophotometrically by standard laboratory procedures.[18,19]

Results

Blood Levels of Vitamin E in Porphyria.—Initially, vitamin E concentrations in whole blood were lower than the normal values for our laboratory (Table 2). However, the blood levels of the vitamin rose steadily following vitamin E therapy.

Effect of Vitamin E in Porphyria.—It can be seen from Table 3 that upon

Table. 1.—Clinical and Laboratory Findings in Six Male Chronic Alcoholic Patients

Patient No.	Age (yr)	Duration of Alcohol Intake	Liver Size (cm)*	Hemoglobin (gm/100 ml)	Serum Enzymes GOT/GPT† (IU/Liter)	Serum Bilirubin Total (mg/100 ml)	Serum Alkaline Phosphatase (KA Units)	Serum Albumen (gm/100 ml)	Prothrombin Concentration (%)	BSP Retention (%, 45 min)†	Liver Fat	Biopsy Necrosis
1	63	48	12	17.6	94/51	1.0	12.8	3.9	72	22	not done	
2	47	28	2	15.0	123/86	1.3	10.3	3.1	50	24	marked	focal
3	44	28	4	12.5	147/62	1.0	10.5	3.0	100	15	mild	focal
4	52	37	2	14.3	29/31	0.8	10.2	4.4	100	3	mild	none
5	52	36	0	14.8	27/17	0.8	9.8	4.5	69	3	mild	none
6	57	43	1	14.4	86/62	1.0	14.6	3.3	100	9	moderate	focal
Range of normal laboratory values				14.0-17.0	<40/35	<1.0	<14	3.5-5.7	80-100	<7		

† GOT = glutamic oxacetic transaminase; GPT = glutamic pyruvic transaminase.
* Centimeters below the right costal margin at the mid-clavicular line at which the liver edge was palpable.
‡ Percent retention of sulfobromphtalein sodium after 45 minutes.

Table 2.—Blood Levels of Vitamin E Before and After Therapy*

	Patient 1	Patient 2	Patient 3
Before therapy	0.52	0.16	0.17
After therapy†	2.46	0.37	0.46

* Values are given in mg/100 ml; normal values = 1.0 to 1.3 mg/100 ml whole blood.
† Four to six weeks after therapy with 100 mg vitamin E daily.

Table 3.—Urinary Excretion of δ-Aminolevulinic Acid and Porphobilinogen Before and After Vitamin E Therapy

	δ-Aminolevulinic Acid (μmol/24 hr)				Porphobilinogen (μmol/24 hr)			
	Patient 1	Patient 2	Patient 3	Patient 4	Patient 1	Patient 2	Patient 3	Patient 4
Before therapy*	698	582	25.9	57	572	34.6	24.1	23.9
After therapy†	22	5.2	2.3	1.5	5.5	0.17	1.8	0.53

* Mean of three to four individual 24 hour determinations.
† Approximately four to six weeks after starting therapy.

Table 4.—Urinary Excretion of Porphyrins Before and After Vitamin E Therapy

	Coproporphyrins (mg/24 hr)				Uroporphyrins (mg/24 hr)			
	Patient 1	Patient 2	Patient 3	Patient 4	Patient 1	Patient 2	Patient 3	Patient 4
Before therapy*	8.5	0.82	9.1	7.8	10.5	0.16	2.5	58.9
After therapy†	3.1	0.76	1.9	0.52	2.79	0.25	ND‡	2.3

* Mean of three to four individual 24-hour determinations.
† Approximately four to six weeks after starting therapy.
‡ ND = not detectable.

Table 5.—Effect of Vitamin E Administration on the Urinary Excretion of Porphyrin Precursors and Porphyrins

Patient No.	δ-Aminolevulinic Acid (μmol/24 hr) Control	Vitamin E	Porphobilinogen (μmol/24 hr) Control	Vitamin E	Coproporphyrins (μg/24 hr) Control	Vitamin E	Uroporphyrins (μg/24 hr) Control	Vitamin E
1	3.45	4.96	0.88	0.41	519	439	351	382
2	3.28	2.18	0.24	1.10	145	711	136	48
3	6.47	4.86	1.12	0.69	579	2045	0	0
4	2.66	1.11	0.97	0.57	317	1245	514	24
5	9.23	3.91	1.59	0.98	264	466	43	86
6	3.66	1.58	0.41	1.22	253	274	124	83
Normal values	11.4 ± 3.8		3.7 ± 2.1		120-300		5-30	

administration of vitamin E, ALA and PBG values, which were initially elevated, were significantly reduced to levels generally considered normal. Similarly, Table 4 presents data showing a significant decrease in urinary excretion of coproporphyrins and uroporphyrins. The urinary excretion of creatinine was not affected by vitamin E therapy.

Effect of Vitamin E in Chronic Alcoholism.—Table 5 shows the laboratory findings in the six male chronic alcoholic subjects placed on this study. The urinary excretion of ALA and PBG was within normal limits in all six subjects before and after administration of vitamin E. Urinary coproporphyrins were elevated in three of the patients before and in five after the administration of vitamin E. In only one of five patients with elevated urinary uroporphyrin excretion, did the level return to normal following therapy with vitamin E.

Comment

Porphyrias are characterized by the overproduction of heme precursors such as δ-aminolevulinic acid, porphobilinogen, and porphyrins. Since these compounds are either intermediates in the early stages of the biosynthetic (Figure) pathway to heme and heme proteins or end products in a branched pathway, the regulatory mechanisms controlling their formation play an important role in the pathogenesis of both genetic and acquired porphyrias.

According to current concepts, control of the biosynthesis of heme could be exercised (*a*) at the step involving the formation of the rate-limiting enzyme, ALA synthetase,[20] (*b*) by a negative feedback inhibition by free heme of its own synthesis[21] or by heme as a corepressor in the formation of ALA synthetase,[20,22] or (*c*) indirectly, by the regulation of the synthesis of globin which functions

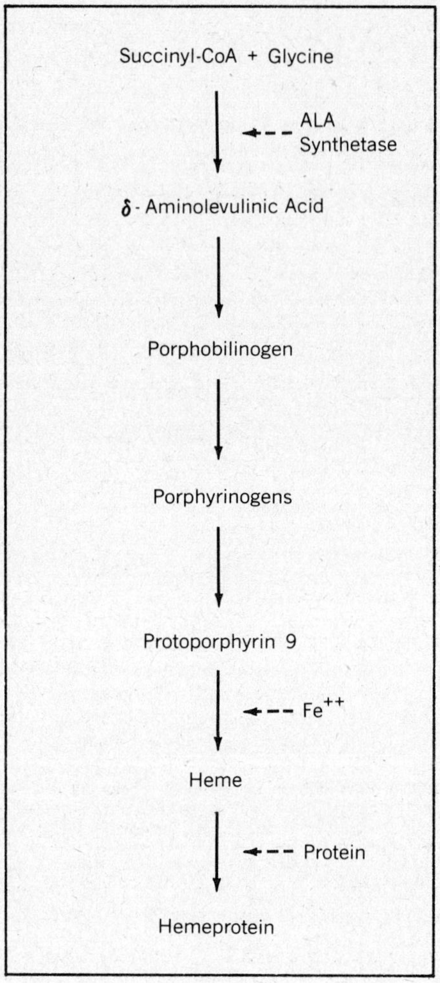

Outline of the biosynthesis of hemeproteins.

as a scavenger of free heme.[23] While an uncoupling of any of these regulatory mechanisms could lead to the development of the manifestations of porphyria, any attempt to postulate a specific aberration at this stage would be premature. The issue is further complicated by the fact that in porphyria other acquired contributory factors, such as alcoholism in two of the cases, superimpose their effects upon any inherited metabolic predisposition to the development of the condition. Thus, the action of vitamin E in effecting a remission will have to be viewed cautiously, although from kinetic studies we have obtained evidence indicating that vitamin E acts by blocking or reversing the induction of hepatic ALA synthetase.[11,12] Since porphyrin excretion in our chronic alcoholic subjects remained unaltered after therapy with vitamin E, the action of the vitamin in porphyria is not mediated through a reversal of the effects of alcoholism.

The initial pretreatment values for blood vitamin E illustrate the existence of a deficiency associated with this clinical condition. However, among the three subjects studied, only in one did we notice a prompt and sustained rise in blood levels of this vitamin following oral therapy. It is also interesting to point out that in this same patient, clinical improvement paralleled the rise in blood vitamin E. Since, in the other two patients, blood levels did not approach values we consider as normal, and since in these patients relief from the symptoms of the disease were delayed, the observations are suggestive of a positive correlation between the two factors. This raises the question whether some porphyrics might have a concurrent defect in the absorption and transport of this fat-soluble vitamin. Further studies will be necessary to elucidate this aspect of our findings.

In chronic alcoholics and in normal healthy volunteers, an increase in the urinary excretion of coproporphyrins has been reported.[24-28] However, in contrast, enhanced excretion of the porphyrin precursors, ALA and PBG, has been described in subjects in Africa with cutaneous porphyria in whom there was no evidence of a hereditary factor and the ingestion of adulterated alcoholic beverages was a likely cause.[29,30] In the present study, chronic alcoholics receiving alcohol while on an adequate diet had significant increases in the urinary excretion of both uroporphyrins and coproporphyrins, while the urinary excretion of ALA and PBG remained within normal limits. While all six patients had biochemical or histological evidence or both of liver-cell damage, cirrhosis of the liver, which has been shown to be associated with porphyrinuria, was not found in the five patients that had liver biopsies. The porphyrinuria induced by alcohol is usually asymptomatic and reversible, and only a small proportion of alcoholics develop symptoms of cutaneous porphyria. Alcohol, however, is a precipitating factor in the hereditary form of cutaneous porphyria.

The administration of vitamin E to our alcoholic subjects for a period of five days had no significant effect on the urinary excretion of coproporphyrins and resulted only in the depression of uroporphyrin excretion in one of the patients. In this case, the failure to demonstrate decreases in the urinary excretion of porphyrins following vitamin E therapy may be due to a different mechanism by which alcohol induces porphyrinuria.

This investigation was supported in part by Public Health Service research grants AM-02131, RO1, MH 14251, and general research support grant 5SO-1FR-05478 from the National Institutes of Health.

Israel Zeligman, MD, and Charles E. Carr, MD, referred patients for the study and made the follow-up studies possible.

References

1. Mason KE: The tocopherols: VII. Effects of deficiency, in Sebrell WH Jr, Harris RS (eds): *The Vitamins: Chemistry, Physiology and Pathology.* New York, Academic Press Inc, 1954, vol 3, pp 514-562.

2. Dinning JS: Vitamin E responsive anemia in monkeys and man. *Nutr Rev* **21**:289-291, 1963.

3. Roels OA: Present knowledge of vitamin E. *Nutr Rev* **25**:33-37, 1967.

4. Majaj AS, Dinning JS, Azzam SA, et al: Vitamin E responsive megaloblastic anemia in infants with protein-calorie malnutrition. *Amer J Clin Nutr* **12**:374-379, 1963.

5. Porter RS, Fitch CD: Vitamin E deficiency in the monkey: X. Protoporphyrin and heme synthesis by peripheral blood and bone marrow. *Scand J Hemat* **3**:175-185, 1966.

6. Whitaker JA, Fort EG, Vimokesant S, et al: Hematologic responses to vitamin E in anemia associated with protein calorie malnutrition. *Amer J Clin Nutr* **20**:783-789, 1967.

7. Darby WJ: Tocopherol-responsive anemias in man. *Vitamins Hormones* **26**:685-699, 1968.

8. DeRosa R: The effect of δ-tocopherol on experimental lead poisoning: Behaviour of urinary coproporphyrin and of the blood picture. *Acta Vitamin* **8**:167-172, 1954.

9. Murty HS, Nair PP: Prevention of allylisopropylacetamide induced experimental porphyria in the rat by vitamin E. *Nature* **223**:200, 1969.

10. Murty HS, Pinelli A, Nair PP, et al: Porphyria cutanea tarda: Therapeutic response to vitamin E, abstracted. *Clin Res* **173**:474, 1969.

11. Murty HS, Medina EV, Brooks SK, et al: Vitamin E and regulation of heme synthesis, abstracted. *Fed Proc* **29**:694, 1970.

12. Nair PP, Murty HS, Grossman N: The in vivo effect of vitamin E in experimental porphyria. *Biochem Biophys Acta* **215**:112, 1970.

13. Murty HS, Caasi PI, Brooks SK, et al: Biosynthesis of heme in the vitamin E deficient rat. *J Biol Chem* **245**:5498-5504, 1970.

14. Nair PP, Sarlos I, Machiz J: Microquantitative separation of isomeric dimethyltocols by gas-liquid chromatography. *Arch Biochem Biophys* **114**:488-493, 1966.

15. Nair PP, Machiz J: Gas-liquid chromatography of isomeric methyltocols and their derivatives. *Biochem Biophys Acta* **144**:446-451, 1967.

16. Nair PP, Luna Z: Identification of δ-tocopherol from tissues by combined gas-liquid chromatography, mass spectrometry, and infrared spectroscopy. *Arch Biochem Biophys* **127**:413-418, 1968.

17. Marver HS, Tschudy DP, Perlroth MG, et al: The determination of aminoketones in biological fluids. *Anal Biochem* **14**:53-60, 1966.

18. Schwartz S, Berg MH, Bossenmaier I, et al: Determination of porphyrins in biological materials, in Glick D (ed): *Methods of Biochemical Analysis.* New York, Interscience Publishers Inc, 1960, vol 8, pp 221,293.

19. Bauer JD, Ackermann PG, Toro G: Urinalysis, in Bray G (ed): *Clinical Laboratory Methods,* St. Louis, CV Mosby Co, 1968, p 43.

20. Granick S: The induction in vitro of the synthesis of δ-aminolevulinic acid synthetase in chemical porphyria. A response to certain drugs, sex hormones and foreign chemicals. *J Biol Chem* **241**:1359-1375, 1966.

21. Karibian D, London IM: Control of heme synthesis by feedback inhibition. *Biochem Biophys Res Commun* **18**:243-249, 1965.

22. Waxman AD, Collins A, Tschudy DP: Oscillations of hepatic δ-aminolevulinic acid synthetase produced in vivo by heme. *Biochem Biophys Res Commun* **24**:675-683, 1966.

23. Grayzel AI, Fuhr JE, London IM: Effects of inhibitors of protein synthesis on the synthesis of heme in rabbit reticulocytes. *Biochem Biophys Res Commun* **28**:705-710, 1967.

24. Franke K, Fikentscher R: Die Bedeutung der quantitativen Porphyrin bestimmung mit der Lumineszenzmessung fur die Prufung der Leberfunkcion and fur Ernahrungs Fragen. *Munch Med Wschr* **82**:171-172, 1935.

25. Brugsch JT: Toxic porphyrinuria following chronic alcoholism. *Proc Staff Meet Mayo Clin* **39**:609-613, 1937.

26. Sutherland DA, Watson CJ: Studies of coproporphyrins: VI. The effect of alcohol on the per diem excretion and isomer distribution of the urinary coproporphyrins. *J Lab Clin Med* **37**:29-39, 1951.

27. Zieve L, Hill E, Schwartz S, et al: Normal limits of urinary coproporphyrin excretion determined by an improved method. *J Lab Clin Med* **41**:663-669, 1953.

28. Orten JM, Doehr SA, Bond C, et al: Urinary excretion of porphyrins and porphyrin intermediates in human alcoholics. *Quart J Stud Alcohol* **24**:598-609, 1963.

29. Gelfand M, Mitchell JD: Bantu porphyria: A clinical study of 16 cases. *Trans Roy Soc Trop Med Hyg* **51**:62-68, 1957.

30. Lamont N McE, Hathorn M, Joubert SM: Porphyria in the Africans: A study of 100 cases. *Quart J Med* **30**:373-392, 1961.

Lidocaine Infusion in Acute Myocardial Infarction

Effects on Left Ventricular Function

Shahbudin H. Rahimtoola, MB, MRCPE; M. Ziad Sinno, MD; Henry S. Loeb, MD; Ruben Chuquimia, MD; Kenneth M. Rosen, MD; and Rolf M. Gunnar, MS, MD, Chicago

The effects of lidocaine hydrochloride infusion (1 and 3 mg/min) on left ventricular (LV) function were assessed in 23 patients with acute myocardial infarction (AMI). There were no significant changes in heart rate, systemic arterial pressure, central venous pressure, cardiac output, preejection period (PEP), left ventricular ejection time (LVET), the PEP/LVET ratio, or calculated systemic vascular resistance. Left ventricular pressures were obtained in six patients. There was no change in calculated LV stroke work. The LV end-diastolic pressure (LVEDP) was unchanged in five patients, but one patient had an increase of LVEDP and of mean aortic pressure that was not associated with changes in other recorded parameters. Lidocaine hydrochloride infusion at 1 and 3 mg/min in patients with AMI does not result in a measurable alteration of cardiac performance.

Lidocaine hydrochloride is a useful antiarrhythmic agent[1] and is frequently used for treatment of ventricular dysrhythmias that arise after an acute myocardial infarction (AMI).[2,3]

Lidocaine has a dose-dependent negative inotropic effect in the isolated canine and human cardiac muscle.[4] In intact dogs, lidocaine administration in the usual therapeutic amounts does not significantly change left ventricular (LV) function[4]; but in higher dosages there is a decrease of myocardial contractile force[5] and depression of LV function.[4,6]

Lidocaine administered to patients during cardiac surgery and during cardiac catheterization does not produce significant circulatory depression[7] and does not result in any significant change in LV function.[8] After AMI lidocaine has been shown to produce no significant change in cardiac output, arterial pressure, or heart rate,[3] but knowledge of its effects on LV function is lacking.

This study assesses the effects of lidocaine administration on LV function after AMI in man. We could not demonstrate a significant change in ventricular performance at dosage levels of 1 and 3 mg/min.

Materials and Methods

Lidocaine studies were carried out in 23 patients admitted to the coronary care unit of Cook County Hospital. There were 18 men and five women; their ages ranged from 37 to 73 years (mean, 57 years).

The diagnosis of AMI was based on the history, enzyme (serum glutamic oxaloacetic transaminase [SGOT], lactic dehydrogenase [LDH], and creatine phosphokinase [CPK]) changes,[9] and characteristic alteration of the electrocardiogram.[10,11] Eighteen patients were judged to have a transmural myocardial infarct on the basis of pathological Q waves on the ECG, and five patients were judged to have a nontransmural myocardial infarction. Nine of the lidocaine studies were carried out within 24 hours of the onset of the symptoms, an additional ten in the second 24 hours, and the remainder of the studies were carried out within four days of the onset.

Intravascular pressures were recorded via a No. 5 nylon catheter and using strain gauges (Statham P23db). Catheters were introduced percutaneously into the brachial artery and antecubital vein. The brachial artery catheter was advanced to the central aorta and in six patients the catheter was passed across the aortic valve into the left ventricle, under fluoroscopic and manometric pressure monitoring. The venous catheter was advanced to the central venous system. Cardiac output was determined by the indicator dilution technique with the use of indocyanine green and a densitometer (Waters). Heart sounds were recorded by using a contact crystal microphone (Hewlett-Packard). The carotid tracing was obtained with the use of a pulse wave attachment (Hewlett-Packard). All the variables were recorded on a photographic recording system (Hewlett-Packard). Cardiac output, cardiac index (CI), and left ventricular stroke work (LVSW) were calculated in the standard manner.

Systolic time intervals were derived from the ECG, aortic pressure pulse, and phonocardiogram, as described by Weissler et al.[12] The QS_2 is the time from the Q wave of the ECG to the first high frequency vibration of the second heart sound, LVET is the left ventricular ejection time derived from the aortic pressure pulse or from the carotid pulse tracing, and, preejection period (PEP) is the time from the Q wave of the ECG to the onset of ventricular ejection and is derived by subtracting LVET from QS_2. The PEP/LVET ratio was calculated. The values of PEP and LVET were corrected (c) for heart rate as described by Weissler et al.[12] Systolic time intervals are parameters of ventricular function.[13] The PEP/LVET ratio has been related to the ejection fraction[14] and by implication to myocardial perform-

Received for publication Nov 11, 1970; accepted Feb 10, 1971.

From the Department of Adult Cardiology, Division of Medicine and the Hektoen Institute for Medical Research, Cook County Hospital and the Department of Medicine, Abraham Lincoln School of Medicine, University of Illinois College of Medicine, Chicago.

Reprint requests to Department of Adult Cardiology, Division of Medicine, Cook County Hospital, 1825 W Harrison St, Chicago 60612 (Dr. Rahimtoola).

Changes in Pressure, Blood Flow, and Systolic Time Intervals During Lidocaine Infusion

Indexes*	Control Mean	Control Range	Control-Lidocaine (1mg/min) Patient No.	Control-Lidocaine (1mg/min) Mean Difference	Control-Lidocaine (1mg/min) SEM	Control-Lidocaine (3 mg/min) Patient No.	Control-Lidocaine (3 mg/min) Mean Difference	Control-Lidocaine (3 mg/min) SEM
Heart rate (beats per min)	80.0	61-109	22	3.6	3.9	23	2.6	1.5
Ao$\bar{P}$ (mm Hg)	104.7	72-129	20	6.3	5.1	21	—0.9	1.9
CVP (mm Hg)	5.6	1-15	22	0.0	0.3	23	1.1	0.5
CI (liters/min/sq m)	2.4	1.7-4.8	22	0.2	0.1	23	—0.0	0.1
SV (ml/beat)	59.9	31-102	22	4.3	3.0	23	—2.1	1.8
SVR (units)	23.9	12.3-33.4	20	0.5	1.4	21	2.7	3.0
LVEDP (mm Hg)	29	13-36	5	—2.4	1.8	6	+0.7	1.9
LVSW (gm-meter)	83	18-189	5	—7.2	7.0	6	—2.8	6.1
PEP_c (msec)	141.6	96-187	19	6.3	7.5	18	0.9	1.7
$LVET_c$ (msec)	372.2	333-419	19	24.2	18.3	18	—3.7	2.3
PEP/LVET Ratio	0.481	.260-0.756	19	0.008	0.028	18	0.014	0.008

* *P* value for all indexes was >0.05. Ao$\bar{P}$ = mean aortic pressure, CVP = central venous pressure, CI = cardiac index, SV = stroke volume, SVR = systemic vascular resistance, LVEDP = left ventricular end-diastolic pressure, LVSW = left ventricular stroke work, PEP_c = preejection period corrected for heart rate, $LVET_c$ = left ventricular ejection time corrected for heart rate, SEM = standard error of mean.

ance, since myocardial performance is an important determinant of the ejection fraction.[15,16]

Procedure

Informed consent for the studies was obtained. After the catheters were in position and the patient was in a clinically steady state for about one half hour, pressures, indicator dilution curves (IDC), and phonocardiograms were recorded. Lidocaine hydrochloride was administered by continuous intravenous infusion in a dose of 1 mg/min and pressures, IDC, and phonocardiograms were again recorded. Lidocaine hydrochloride infusion was increased to 3 mg/min and the recordings were repeated. Each dose of lidocaine was given for 30 to 60 minutes. Throughout the study the patient received oxygen at 6 liters/min by nasal cannula.

Results

The mean difference, standard error of the mean, and the *P* value for the paired determinations before and after lidocaine administration are shown in the Table. In Fig 1 are depicted the mean values (± SD) for heart rate, mean aortic pressure (Ao$\bar{P}$), CI, systemic vascular resistance (SVR), left ventricular end-diastolic pressure (LVEDP), PEP_c, $LVET_c$, and the PEP/LVET ratio prior to, and during, lidocaine infusion (1 and 3 mg/min).

There was no significant change ($P > 0.05$) in any of the variables that were recorded and in those that were calculated. In spite of abnormal LV function in most of these patients, there was no demonstrable deterioration of LV function during lidocaine infusion. This is illustrated graphically in Fig 2 in one patient who initially had a cardiac index of 1.1, stroke volume of 19 ml, LVEDP of 36 mm Hg, PEP_c of 164 msec, and PEP/LVET ratio of 0.610.

In one patient the LVEDP increased from 14 to 23 mm Hg during

Fig 1.—Mean value (± SD) of the various variables during the control period (c), and during lidocaine hydrochloride infusion, 1 and 3 mg/min (L_1 and L_3). There is no significant change in any of the measurements ($P > 0.05$).

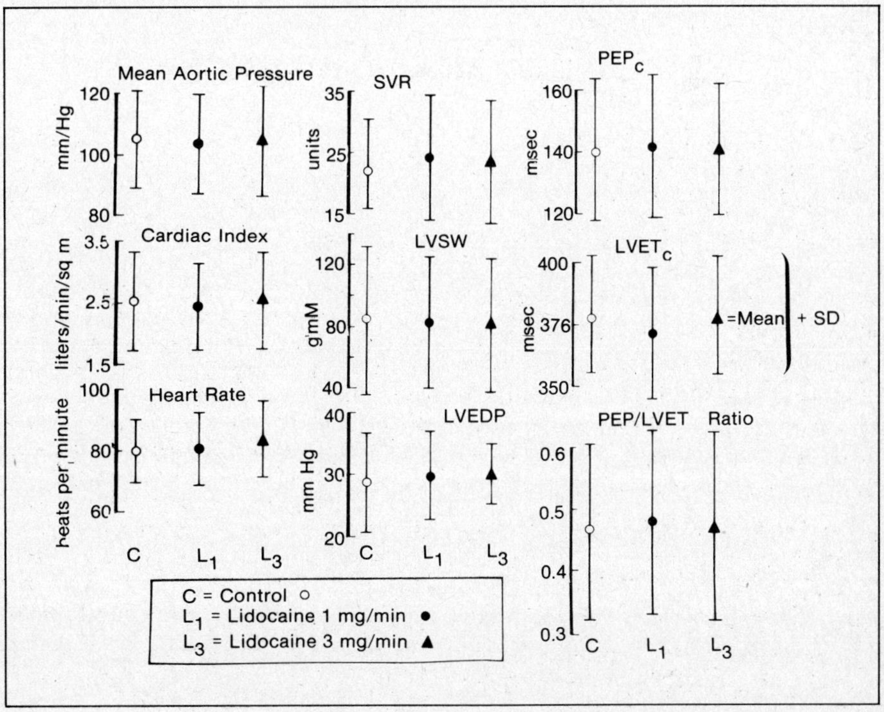

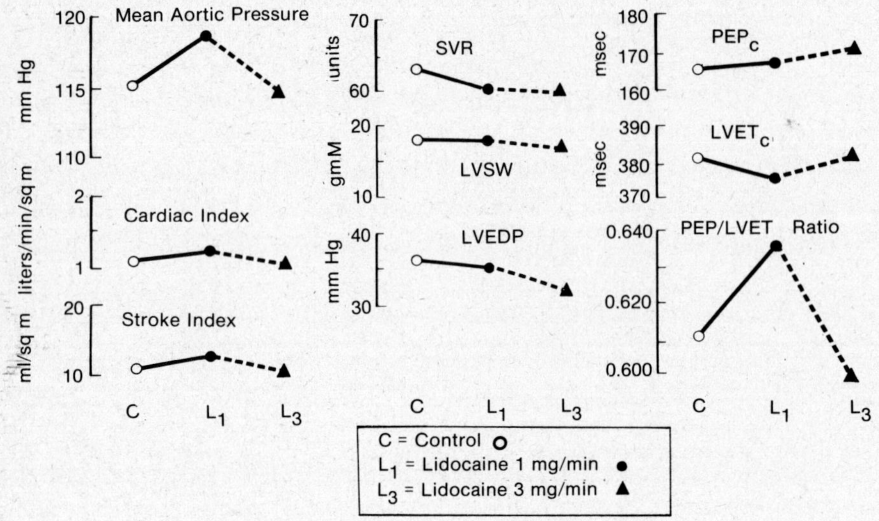

Fig 2.—The effects of lidocaine hydrochloride infusion, 1 and 3 mg/min (L_1 and L_3), in one patient with AMI who had considerable impairment of LV function. There was no real change in any of the variables even though the values were abnormal during the control period (c).

lidocaine administration but the mean arterial pressure had simultaneously increased from 102 to 115 mm Hg while the other variables showed no change.

Comment

Left ventricular function was impaired in most of our patients following AMI.[17] This study has shown that in patients with AMI, lidocaine hydrochloride infusion in doses of 1 and 3 mg/min had no demonstrable effect on cardiac performance. In one patient there was an increase of LVEDP and arterial pressure with no change in any of the other variables. It is possible that in this one patient the increase in LVEDP was the result of the increased aortic pressure during lidocaine infusion and not the result of a progressive deterioration in cardiac performance.

Robinson et al[18] have shown that lidocaine, in a dose of 5 mg/kg, produced significant depression of ventricular function after experimental myocardial infarction. The dosage of lidocaine that was used in the study just cited was very much in excess of that used clinically in AMI.

Lidocaine produced no significant delay in atrioventricular or intraventricular conduction.[19] Lidocaine infusion in doses of 1 to 2 mg/min is frequently used in AMI for suppression of ventricular dysrhythmias.[3,20,21] The results reported in this study demonstrate that lidocaine hydrochloride in doses of 1 and 3 mg/min can be infused in patients with AMI without causing depression of LV function.

This investigation was supported in part by Public Health Service grant HE-08834-07 from the National Heart and Lung Institute.

Minu K. Patel, MSc, performed the statistical analysis of the data.

References

1. Frieden J: Antiarrhythmic drugs: VII. Lidocaine as an antiarrhythmic agent. *Amer Heart J* **70**:713-715, 1965.

2. Lown B, Fakhro AM, Hood WB Jr, et al: The coronary care unit. *JAMA* **199**:188-198, 1967.

3. Jewitt DE, Kishou Y, Thomas M: Lignocaine in the management of arrhythmias after acute myocardial infarction. *Lancet* **1**:266-270, 1968.

4. Nayler WG, Molunes I, Carson V, et al: The effect of lignocaine on myocardial function high energy phosphate stores, and oxygen consumption: A comparison with propanolol. *Amer Heart J* **78**:338-345, 1969.

5. Austen WG, Moran JM: Cardiac and peripheral vascular effects of lidocaine and procaineamide. *Amer J Cardiol* **16**:701-707, 1965.

6. Asokan SK, Frank MJ, Regan TJ: Assessment of myocardial depression with therapeutic doses of lidocaine and procaineamide. *Amer J Cardiol* **21**:91, 1968.

7. Harrison DC, Sprouse JH, Morrow AG: The antiarrhythmic properties of lidocaine and procaineamide: Clinical and physiologic studies of their cardiovascular effects in man. *Circulation* **28**:486-491, 1963.

8. Schumacher RR, Lieberson AD, Childress RH, et al: Hemodynamic effects of lidocaine in patients with heart disease. *Circulation* **37**:965-972, 1968.

9. Cohen L: Contributions of serum enzymes and isozymes to the diagnosis of myocardial injury. *Mod Conc Cardiovasc Dis* **36**:43-54, 1967.

10. Massie E, Walsh TJ: *Clinical Vectorcardiography and Electrocardiography.* Chicago, Year Book Publishers Inc, 1960, pp 592.

11. Gunnar RM, Pietras RJ, Blackaller J, et al: Correlation of vectorcardiographic criteria for myocardial infarction with autopsy findings. *Circulation* **35**:158-171, 1967.

12. Weissler AM, Harris WS, Schoenfeld CD: Systolic time intervals in heart failure in man. *Circulation* **37**:149-159, 1968.

13. Weissler AM, Harris WS, Schoenfeld CD: Bedside technics for the evaluation of ventricular function in man. *Amer J Cardiol* **23**:577-583, 1969.

14. Gerrard CJ Jr, Weissler AM, Dodge HT: The relationship of alterations in systolic time intervals to ejection fraction in patients with cardiac disease. *Circulation* **42**:455-462, 1970.

15. Miller GAH, Kirklin JW, Swan HJC: Myocardial function and left ventricular volumes in acquired valvular insufficiency. *Circulation* **31**:374-384, 1965.

16. Dodge HT, Baxley WA: Hemodynamic aspects of heart failure. *Amer J Cardiol* **22**:24-34, 1968.

17. Gunnar RM, Sinno MZ, Loeb HS, et al: Left ventricular preformance during first two days after acute myocardial infarction. *Circulation* **62**:111-162, 1970.

18. Robinson SL, Schroll M, Harrison DC: The circulatory response to lidocaine in experimental myocardial infarction. *Amer J Med Sci* **258**:260-269, 1969.

19. Rosen KM, Lau SH, Weiss MB, et al: The effect of lidocaine on atrioventricular and intraventricular conduction in man. *Amer J Cardiol* **25**:1-5, 1970.

20. Lown B, Vassaux C: Lidocaine in acute myocardial infarction. *Amer Heart J* **76**:586-587, 1968.

21. Gianelly R, Von der Groeben JO, Spivack AP, et al: Effect of lidocaine on ventricular arrhythmias in coronary heart disease. *New Eng J Med* **277**:1215-1219, 1967.

Clinical Notes

Progressive Multifocal Leukoencephalopathy

Lynn W. Lyon, MD;
William F. McCormick, MD; and
Sydney S. Schochet, Jr., MD,
Iowa City

In 1958, Åström et al[1] described three cases of a clinically progressive, asymmetric disorder of the central nervous system (CNS) which they named "progressive multifocal leukoencephalopathy" (PML). This disorder was associated with Hodgkin's disease and chronic lymphocytic leukemia in their patients. In reviewing the literature at that time, they found five additional cases which fulfilled their criteria for PML.[2-5]

Since 1958, many additional cases of PML associated with a variety of underlying disease processes have been described.[6-56] The purpose of the present report is to describe a new case of PML occurring in a patient with macroglobulinemia, an association not previously reported. Clinical, pathological, and virologic findings are described.

Received for publication June 10, 1970; accepted Sept 10.

From the departments of neurology and pathology (Neuropathology), University of Iowa College of Medicine, Iowa City.

Reprint requests to Room 28, Medical Laboratories, Iowa City 52240 (Dr. McCormick).

Patient Summary

A 61-year-old white man was first seen in a local hospital in December 1958 complaining of shortness of breath and abdominal distension. Physical examination revealed a right upper quadrant abdominal mass and a right pleural effusion. He was described as "grossly intact" on neurologic examination. His hemoglobin level was 11.1 gm/100 ml, and white blood cell count (WBC) was 6,000/cu mm. Roentgenograms of his chest revealed the presence of a right pleural effusion and left lower lobe "metastatic lesions." Thoracentesis with cytological examination failed to show evidence of malignancy. An exploratory laparotomy revealed a large mass arising from the liver. Biopsy material from this mass was interpreted as "malignant lymphoma of the liver." Treatment with mechlorethamine hydrochloride and cobalt 60 irradiation was instituted, with clinical resolution of the abdominal mass and pleural effusion. The patient was then lost to follow-up, but apparently did well for approximately the next nine years.

In June 1968 the patient was first admitted to the University of Iowa Hospitals with 20% second and third degree burns from a gasoline explosion. A left pleural effusion and left supraclavicular mass were found. His hemoglobin value was 12 mg/100 ml, and WBC was 8,900/cu mm. An x-ray film of the chest showed left lower lobe and superior mediastinal lesions. Multiple thoracenteses with cytologic examination failed to demonstrate atypical cells. The patient's burns healed without grafting, and he was discharged "against medical advice" in August 1968 before further evaluation of his systemic illness could be accomplished.

The patient was readmitted to University Hospital on Nov 19, 1968, with severe, recurring epistaxis, which required left internal maxillary artery ligation for control. During a three-month hospitalization (November 1968 through January 1969), the patient's underlying disease was evaluated. Physical examination revealed a large left supraclavicular mass, several enlarged supraclavicular and infraclavicular lymph nodes, and pleural effusion. The liver and spleen were not palpable, and there were no abdominal masses. The neurological examination was described as "intact." Laboratory values included hemoglobin, 12.3 gm/100 ml; WBC, 8,000/cu mm; platelets, 230,000/cu mm; normal urine, and sulfobromophthalein hydrochloride BSP, 13% retention at 45 minutes. Serum protein electrophoresis showed increased γ-globulin level (5.5 gm/100 ml) with a marked increase in the IgM fraction on immunoelectrophoresis. Ultracentrifugation studies demonstrated increased IgM. Tests for cryoglobulin and cryofibrinogen were negative, as was the Coombs' test. Bence Jones protein was absent from the urine. A bone marrow aspiration from the sternum showed normal maturation of the myeloid and erythroid elements and a mild increase in eosinophils and monocytes. Review of the 1959 liver biopsy failed to confirm the previous diagnosis of malignant lymphoma and was interpreted as "polymorphous cellular infiltration of the liver—malignant vs inflammatory." A lymph node biopsy was interpreted as "most compatible with macroglobulinemia." Serum immunoelectrophoresis was interpreted as "Waldenström's macroglobulinemia." Treatment with cyclophosphamide (Cytoxan) was initiated in January 1969. The patient was discharged to be followed on an outpatient basis.

Readmission was necessary in late February because of hoarseness and diminishing vision. Laryngoscopic examination disclosed a submucosal tumor encroaching on the larynx from the left. The biopsy specimen was inadequate for diagnosis. Neurological examination revealed the patient to be lethargic but rational and oriented. There was mild dysarthria and diminished visual acuity. Diffuse weakness was noted, but no focal motor signs were illicitable. Over the next two months, however, the patient followed a progressive deteriorating course with decreasing mental capability, diminishing visual acuity, increasing dysarthria, and a progressive left spastic hemiparesis. X-ray films of the skull were normal. An EEG was abnormal, with focal right posterior delta activity. A brain scan made after administration of sodium pertechnetate Tc 99m was normal. A lumbar puncture showed an opening pressure of 190 mm H_2O and clear cerebrospinal fluid (CSF) with seven mononuclear cells and a protein level of 76 mg/100 ml. The patient was treated with cyclophosphamide, and cobalt 60 therapy directed at the brain. His deteriorating course continued, and he died on April 20, 1969.

Autopsy Findings.—At the time of autopsy the patient was poorly nourished and moderately emaciated. The lungs were heavy, weighing 640 and 610 gm, right and left, respectively. A 9 cm fresh infarct was present in the right lower lobe and an ill-defined area of consolidation, largely nonhemorrhagic and measuring some 8 cm, was present in the left lower lobe. Thromboemboli were demonstrated in the vessels leading to the infarcted area on the right. Scattered consolidated foci of bronchopneumonia were present bilaterally. A 75 gm, grayish-tan, moderately firm and fleshy, dumbbell-shaped mass was present in the left supraclavicular fossa and extended into the anterior superior mediastinum. A 12 cm, roughly spherical mass was present in the left hemithorax immediately behind the sternum and attached to the left leaf of the diaphragm. The spleen was not enlarged, weighing 110 gm. The liver was likewise not enlarged and was normal. There was an area of thickening and induration in the greater curvature of the stomach, 20 cm from the gastroesophageal junction. In the center of this 12-cm area of induration was a 4 cm area of ulceration. No other gross abnormalities were found in the thoracicoabdominal viscera.

Microscopic examination confirmed the presence of the pulmonary infarct and of bilateral areas of acute bronchopneumonia. The ill-defined area of induration in the left lower lobes contained large numbers of plasma cells, lymphocytes, and macrophages, with a plasma cell predominance. Some of the plasma cells contained PAS-positive material in their cytoplasm. The area of induration and ulceration of the stomach was found to show full thickness infiltration by large numbers of similar-appearing plasma cells. Multiple sections through the large thoracic mass attached to the left hemidiaphragm and of the dumbbell-shaped lesion involving the supraclavicular and superior mediastinal area also revealed homogeneous fields of plasma cells with PAS-positive material in their cytoplasm. Sections of multiple lymph nodes in the abdomen, mediastinal, and inguinal areas revealed scattered small collection of plasma cells throughout. Examination of the bone marrow from sternum, vertebra, and iliac crests revealed a relatively mild increase in the numbers of plasma cells in all locations with several larger collections near the periostium of the vertebrae.

Gross examination of the brain revealed slight increase in weight (1,422 gm) and asymmetrical cerebral hemispheres with the right larger than the left. A portion of the right frontal lobe was rapidly frozen at −74 C and stored in a dry ice chest for virologic isolation. The remainder of the brain and the spinal cord were fixed in formaldehyde solution for gross and microscopic examination. There was severe, diffuse congestion of the superficial cortical vessels. No transtentorial hernias were present. Frontal atrophy of moderate severity was present bilaterally. There was a discrete, 8 cm area of general expansion and partial obliteration of the sulci in the posterior aspect of the right frontal lobe and in the superior parietal lobule. The brain was quite soft—almost fluctuant—deep to this area of gyral expansion. On sectioning, a relatively large, indistinctly demarcated, destructive lesion was present in the right cerebral hemisphere subjacent to the area of cortical expansion and softening noted on the uncut specimen. The lesion maximally involved the central and convolutional white matter (Fig 1), but in some areas completely transected the cortex. The more central portions of this lesion were granular and finely fenestrated, with mi-

Fig 1.—Massive destructive lesion in right cerebral hemisphere involving maximally the central and convolutional white matter.

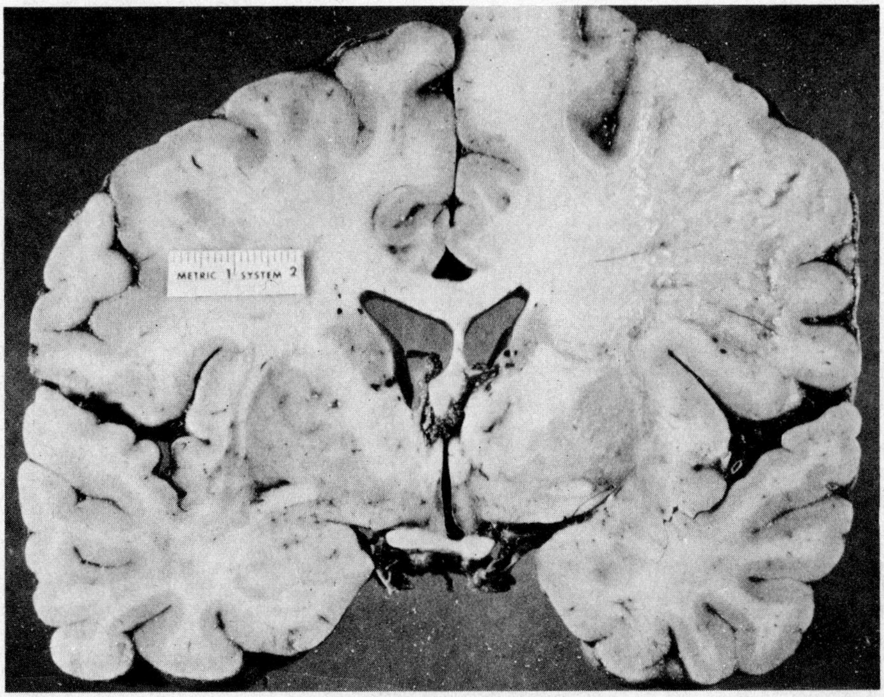

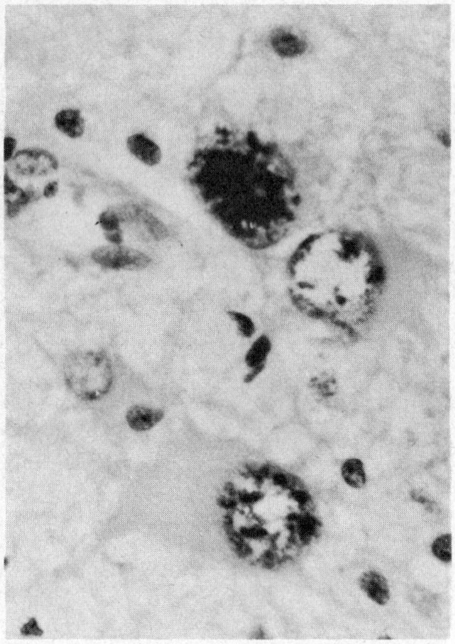

Fig 2.—Numerous bizarre giant astrocytes present in the destructive lesions (hematoxylin-eosin stain, ×600).

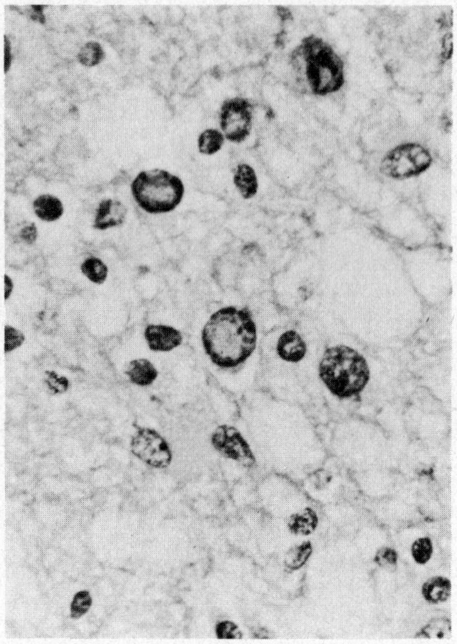

Fig 3.—Oligodendroglial cells contain ill-defined, eosinophilic, type-A intranuclear inclusions (hematoxylin-eosin stain, ×480).

Fig 4.—A nucleus containing paracrystalline arrays of virus particles resembling papova-virus (uranyl acetate-lead citrate stain, ×22,500).

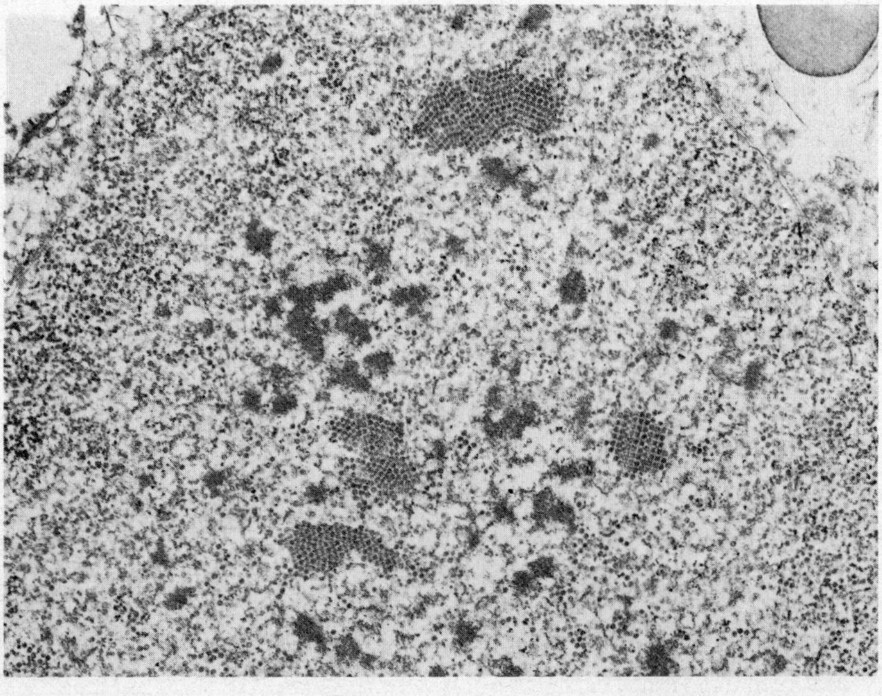

nute cysts. The tissues were minimally discolored yellow to gray. There was moderate expansion of the convolutional white matter surrounding the areas of overt involvement with resulting deformation of the right lateral ventricle. There was gross sparing of the nuclear components of the striatum. A 1.5 cm area of softening and slight yellowish discoloration was present in the left thalamus and several small (1-2 mm) discrete, gray, softened foci were present in the central white matter of the left parietal lobe. Grossly, the brain stem, cerebellum, and the spinal cord were not remarkable.

Microscopically, the large lesion in the right cerebral hemisphere and the multiple smaller lesions in the left cerebral hemisphere were similar in appearance, consisting of rarified and gliotic areas containing vessels cuffed by lymphocytes, occasional plasma cells, and lipid-laden macrophages. There was prominent glial proliferation with numerous bizarre, giant astrocytes (Fig 2), binucleated astrocytes, gemistocytes, and enlarged astrocytes with abnormal mitotic figures. Numerous oligodendroglial cells contained ill-defined, eosinophilic, type-A intranuclear inclusions (Fig 3).

For electron microscopic studies, blocks of formaldehyde solution-fixed brain from areas of maximal gross alteration were postfixed in 1% phosphate buffered osmium tetroxide.

After dehydration in a graded series of alcohols, the tissue was embedded in an epoxy resin. Sections 2μ thick, stained with toluidine blue were screened in order to select blocks suitable for further sectioning. The thin sections were stained with uranyl acetate and lead citrate prior to examination in an electron microscope.

Although the tissue showed extensive fixation artifacts, distinctive nuclei corresponding to the inclusion-bearing glial cells were readily identified. These nuclei were characterized by a thin peripheral band of clumped chromatin surrounding a central zone filled with osmophilic spheroids and filaments (Fig 4 and 5). The spherical particles had an average diameter of 40 mμ and were occasionally grouped in paracrystalline arrays. No further details could be resolved. The filaments averaged 35 mμ in diameter and were of indeterminant length (Fig 6).

Other glial cells recognizable as astrocytes contained large bizarre nuclei and skeins of intracytoplasmic glial filaments. No virus-like particles could be identified

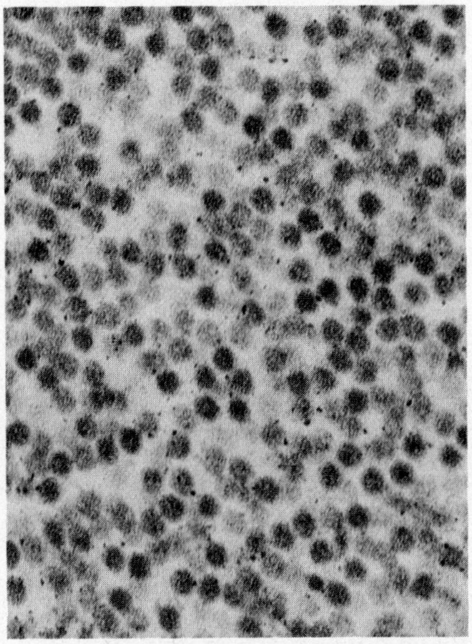

Fig 5.—Individual virions, averaging 40 mμ in diameter, in an oligodendroglial nucleus (uranyl acetate-lead citrate stain, × 75,000).

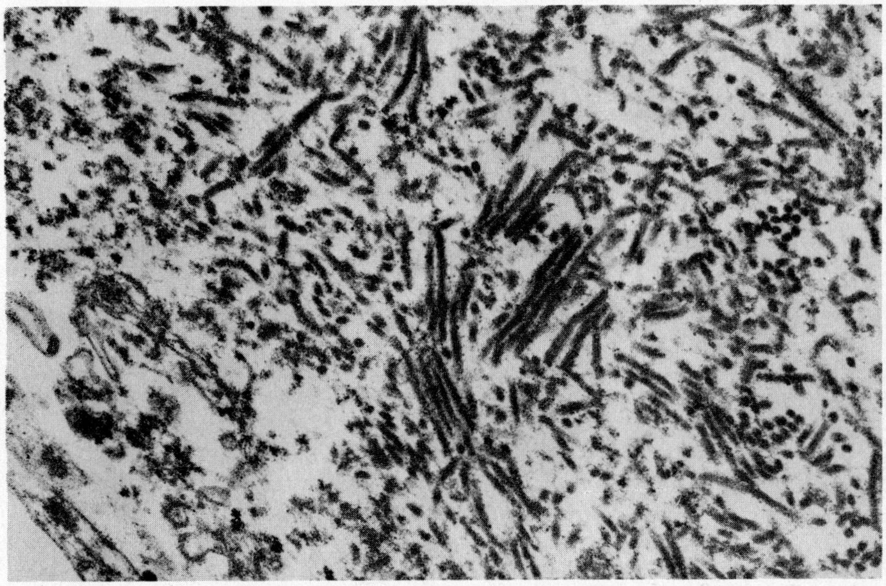

Fig 6.—Filamentous forms averaging 35 mμ in diameter were present in many oligodendroglial nuclei (uranyl acetate-lead citrate stain, × 44,000).

in these cells.

Virologic Studies.—Portions of the frozen brain were thawed and ground to a 10% suspension using sterile powdered glass in mortar and pestle. Following slow speed centrifugation the supernatant was cultured on appropriate media to establish that the sample was free of mycoplasma, bacteria, and fungi. Intracranial inoculation of the supernatant fluid in day-old white Swiss mice was carried out with no observed morbidity or mortality in 28 days.

Cultures of human fetal liver (HFL) grown on Earles' minimum essential medium with 5% sterile fetal calf serum were inoculated with the supernatant fluid from the original 10% brain suspension. Tissue culture fluid was harvested after the cell sheet was destroyed. The fluid was inoculated into BHK-21 (clone 15) cultures and appeared to cause generalized cytopathic effect without focal lesions. Cells from the BHK-21 cultures were centrifuged in order to form compact pellets. These were fixed with 1% osmium tetroxide and processed for electron microscopy, but no virus particles could be recognized.

Comment

Classically, PML is a focal or asymmetric disorder that develops in adult life usually superimposed on a background of chronic illness. A total of 73 cases[1-56] have been described in the literature and are summarized in the Table with regard to the underlying disease process. The present case describes the association of PML and Waldenström's macroglobulinemia. Men are affected almost twice as frequently as women. The onset of neurological symptoms attributed to PML has no apparent relation to either the severity or duration of the underlying disease process. Once neurological involvement becomes evident, the illness usually pursues a rapidly progressive course leading to death within one to several months. However, Hedley-Whyte et al[6] and Stam[7] have each described single cases with 5 and 19 year survivals, respectively. Age at death has varied from 17 to 82 years with the median age being 57 years.

The symptoms and signs in PML are referable to the involved areas of the nervous system. Pyramidal tract involvement is the most frequently encountered neurological deficit being present in 76% of described cases. Intellectual impairment (74%), visual deficit (37%), language disorders (24%), and cerebellar signs (24%) are also common. Brain stem signs (20%), sensory deficits (16%), and seizures (11%) have been reported less constantly. Diminution of vision was the initial neurological symptom in the present case, followed shortly by progressive intellectual deterioration, hemiparesis, and dysarthria. Death occurred three months after the onset of neurological involvement.

The clinical laboratory has been of little aid in establishing the diagnosis of PML. Hematologic studies usually reflect the underlying disease process. Serum proteins have been investigated in several cases,[32,33,35,38,40,44,55] but we know of no previous descriptions of macroglobulinemia. In the present case macroglobulins have been demonstrated by immunoelectrophoresis and by ultracentrifugation techniques. Skull x-rays have always been interpreted

Primary Disease Processes Associated with Progressive Multifocal Leukoencephalopathy

Associated Disease	Reference	No. of Cases
Hodgkin's disease	1, 2, 5, 8, 15, 16, 22 (2 cases), 28, 34 35 (2 cases), 38, 39 (3 cases), 43	17
Leukemia		15
Acute lymphocytic leukemia	32	1
Chronic lymphocytic leukemia	1 (2 cases), 10, 21, 23, 35, 36, 50, 53	9
Acute myelogenous leukemia	36	1
Chronic myelogenous leukemia	8 (2 cases), 20, 52	4
Malignant lymphoma (excluding Hodgkin's disease)	6, 8 (2 cases), 9, 10, 14, 22, 27, 29, 30, 42, 46, 48, 56	14
Carcinoma, metastatic	8, 38 (2 cases), 42	4
Sarcoidosis	3, 44, 49	3
Tuberculosis	4, 13, 51	3
Multiple myeloma	33, 40	2
Collagen vascular disease		2
Systemic lupus erythematosus	31	
Rheumatoid arthritis	52	
Miscellaneous		
Whipple's disease	45	1
Polycythemia vera	37	1
Malignant thymic teratoma	39	1
Primary hypersplenism	55	1
Macroglobulinemia	Present case	1
No associated disease process known	4, 7, 8, 11, 19, 21, 24, 25, 54	9
		74

as normal. Cerebrospinal fluid findings are normal in most cases* although mild elevations of protein and mononuclear pleocytoses have been reported.[1-3,39,41,54] Electroencephalograms commonly show both diffuse and focal abnormalities, but are in no way characteristic.† The use of brain scans has been infrequently reported. Three cases[6,11,25] with normal scans and one with an abnormal scan[54] have been reported. Angiograms have been negative.[6,11,19,25,33,35,44,53,55,56] Air contrast studies are unrevealing,[19,25,52] except in those patients with cortical atrophy and ventricular enlargement.[3,7,8,35,44] A focally abnormal EEG and mild CSF abnormalities were the only laboratory findings suggestive of neurologic abnormality in the present case.

Pathologically, PML is characterized by multiple lesions of variable size and cytological characteristics suggesting progressive stages in the development of the destructive process. Initially, these lesions consist of widely disseminated foci of demyelination with relative sparing of the axis cylinders. Later these foci tend to become confluent producing large, plaque-like areas of demyelination with varying degrees of axonal loss. Progressive multifocal leukoencephalopathy is a multifocal process that can involve all areas of the CNS and, at least on some occasions, the peripheral nervous system (PNS). Involvement of the cerebral hemispheres has been described in all reported cases. Cerebellar and brain stem involvement are reported in approximately 50% of cases. Spinal cord involvement has been noted in six cases,[6,29,31,35,41,44] while peripheral nerve involvement has been reported in two cases.[28,41] There are striking alterations in the glia within the areas of demyelination. The oligodendroglial nuclei are enlarged and many contain ill-defined acidophilic inclusions. The astrocytes display a variety of configurations. Many are only slightly enlarged, stellate, and have intensely acidophilic cytoplasm. Other astrocytes are markedly enlarged and have very large ovoid nuclei, multiple nuclei, or nuclei that are grotesquely multilobed. Atypical mitotic figures are occasionally encountered.

In 1961, Richardson[8] first suggested immunologic hyporeactivity with subsequent viral invasion of the nervous system as the pathogenetic mechanism in PML. The immunologic status of many of the patients with PML is incompletely established. More recently, Ellison[9] studied a case of PML diagnosed antemortem in a patient with lymphosarcoma and found severe impairment of delayed hypersensitivity and of antibody formation. Numerous investigators[10-25] have demonstrated virus-like particles that closely resemble members of the Papova group of viruses. This group, first described by Melnick[26] in 1962, now includes the papilloma viruses, the polyoma, SV40 and K viruses. The identity of the group is based largely on morphologic similarities of the virions. All display an icosahedral capsid; however, the exact number of capsomeres is uncertain. Two subgroups can be defined on the basis of the diameter of the virions. The members of the papilloma subgroup have a diameter of about 55 mμ. The other subgroup which includes the polyoma, SV40 and K virus have smaller diameters, ranging from 45 to 50 mμ. The virus-like particles observed in this case, as in previously reported cases, have a diameter more consistent with the polyoma, SV40, K virus subgroup. Although the virions in this case were 40 mμ, slightly smaller dimensions would be expected in thin sections of formalde-

*References 1,6,8,10,14,19,20,22,23,25,28,33,35, 36,38-40,44,45.

†References 1,3,6-8,11,14,19,20,22,25,27,32,33,35, 36,39,40,41,44,52,54-56.

hyde solution fixed tissue than in negatively stained unfixed material.

Filamentous forms have been observed in homogenates of tissue infected with polyoma, SV40, human wart, and rabbit papilloma virus. In intact tissue, filaments like those in PML have been observed only following infection with the polyoma agent. Such forms have been variously regarded as a virion precursor or as the result of aberrant capsomere assembly. Although attempts to culture a virus from cases of PML have been unsuccessful,[10,18,28] a viral etiology still seems most probable. It has been suggested that "papova-like virus particles are present as unobtrusive symbionts" in human brain tissue.[57] During the course of a clinically unrecognized infection by a syncytiogenic agent (eg, one of the paramyxoviruses) the papova-like agent may be activated resulting in its replication and disease.

The cells harboring these virus-like particles in the brain tissue have usually been regarded as the inclusion-bearing oligodendrocytes. Ultrastructurally, the astrocytes often appear unusually large and bizarre in configuration but contain no virus particles. It seems probable that the virus initially attacks the oligodendrocytes resulting in the demyelination. The unusual astrocytic response may be secondary to the demyelination and resulting breakdown products. Unusual forms of astrocytes have been observed in and around demyelinated foci in multiple sclerosis and postinfectious encephalomyelitis. On the other hand, it is tempting to speculate whether the bizarre astrocytes might result from transformation by one of the oncogenic papova viruses. With SV40 virus it has been shown that transformation can only occur during the S-period.[58] The proliferation of astrocytes in response to the infection or demyelination or both would provide a large population of susceptible cells in close proximity to the oligodendrocytes harboring recognizable vegetative virions. Furthermore, if these astrocytes behaved similar to cultures of fetal hamster brain cells, the transformation would produce initially unstable, predominantly lethal nuclear alterations.[59] True neoplasms might develop but only after many cell generations and from a small number of these cells.

It has been suggested by Koprowski et al,[57] that a biologically active papova-like agent might be isolated from patients with PML if the patients' brain tissue is cultured in the presence of a syncytiogenic agent. It is unfortunate that this was not done in this case.

We did not inoculate brain material from this case into primates or into a large variety of nonprimate mammals due to the limitations of our laboratory facilities. A portion of the frozen brain from this patient was sent to another laboratory in an attempt to isolate the virus with negative results at this time, nine months later.

Summary

Progressive multifocal leukoencephalopathy (PML) is an uncommon infection of the nervous system, generally found in patients with decreased host immunity. Morphologically, the lesions are characterized by inclusion bearing oligodendrocytes, bizarre astrocytes, and papova-like virus particles in the glial cells. It is suggested that the oligodendroglial changes reflect infection while the astroglial changes represent transformation by the papova-like virus, an agent known to be oncogenic in nonhuman species. All attempts to isolate the virus by conventional virologic procedures have thus far been unsuccessful.

Serum immunoelectrophoresis was performed by the Immunoglobin Reference Center, Springfield, Va.

References

1. Åström K-E, Mancall EL, Richardson EP Jr: Progressive multifocal leukoencephalopathy: A hitherto unrecognized complication of chronic lymphatic leukemia and Hodgkin's disease. *Brain* **81**:93-111, 1958.

2. Bateman OJ Jr, Squires G, Thannhauser SJ: Hodgkin's disease associated with Schilder's disease. *Ann Intern Med* **22**:426-431, 1945.

3. Christensen E, Fog M: A case of Schilder's disease in an adult with remarks to the etiology and pathogenesis. *Acta Psych Neurol* **30**:141-154, 1955.

4. Hallevorden J: Eigenartige und nicht rubizierbare prozesse, in Bumke: *Handbuch der Geisteskrankheiten.* Berlin, Springer-Verlag, 1930, vol 11, pp 1063-1107.

5. Winkelman NW, Moore MT: Lymphogranulomatosis (Hodgkin's disease) of the nervous system. *Arch Neurol Psychiat* **45**:304-318, 1941.

6. Hedley-Whyte ET, Smith BP, Tyler HR, et al: Multifocal leukoencephalopathy with remission and five year survival. *J Neuropath Exp Neurol* **25**:107-116, 1966.

7. Stam FC: Multifocal leukoencephalopathy with slow progression and very long survival. *Psychiat Neurol Neurochir* **69**:453-459, 1966.

8. Richardson EP Jr: Progressive multifocal leukoencephalopathy. *New Eng J Med* **265**:815-823, 1961.

9. Ellison GW: Progressive multifocal leukoencephalopathy. *J Neuropath Exp Neurol* **28**:501-506, 1969.

10. Dolman CL, Furesz J, Mackay B: Progressive multifocal leukoencephalopathy. *Canad Med Assoc J* **97**:8-12, 1967.

11. Fermaglich J, Hardman JM, Earle KM: Spontaneous progressive multifocal leukoencephalopathy. *Neurology* **20**:479-484, 1970.

12. Howatson AF, Nagai M, ZuRhein G: Polyoma-like vi-

rions in human demyelinating brain disease. *Canad Med Assoc J* **93**:379-386, 1965.

13. Ikuta F: Particles of Papova virus group associated with progressive multifocal leukoencephalopathy. *Clin Neurol* **6**:671-674, 1967.

14. Martin JB, Banker BQ: Subacute multifocal leukoencephalopathy. *Arch Neurol* **21**:590-602, 1969.

15. Morecki R, Porro RS: Progressive multifocal leukoencephalopathy. *Arch Neurol* **22**:253-258, 1970.

16. Muller J, Watanabe I: Progressive multifocal leukoencephalopathy. *Amer J Clin Path* **47**:114-123, 1967.

17. Papadimitriou JM, Kakulas BA, Sadka M: Virus-like particles in proximity to myelin in a case of progressive multifocal leukoencephalopathy. *Proc Aust Assoc Neurol* **4**:133-140, 1966.

18. Schwerdt PR, Schwerdt CE, Silverman LS, et al: Virions association with progressive multifocal leukoencephalopathy. *Virology* **29**:511-514, 1966.

19. Silverman L, Rubinstein LJ: Electron microscopic observations on a case of progressive multifocal leukoencephalopathy. *Acta Neuropath* **5**:215-224, 1965.

20. Tomiyasu U, Baker RN, Wollman J: Progressive multifocal leukoencephalopathy and the "slow viruses." *Bull Los Angeles Neurol Soc* **33**:59-69, 1968.

21. Vanderhaeghen JJ, Perier O: Leucoencéphalite multifocale progressive. *Acta Neurol Belg* **65**:816-837, 1965.

22. Woodhouse MA, Dayan AD, Burston J, et al: Progressive multifocal leukoencephalopathy: Electron microscope study of four cases. *Brain* **90**:863-870, 1967.

23. ZuRhein GM: Polyoma-like virions in a human demyelinating disease. *Acta Neuropath* **8**:57-68, 1967.

24. Zuphein GM, Chou SM: Papova virus in progressive multifocal leukoencephalopathy, in *Infections of the Nervous System, Association for Research of Nervous and Mental Diseases.* Baltimore, Williams & Wilkins Co, 1968, vol 44, pp 307-362.

25. ZuRhein GM, Chou SM: Particles resembling papova viruses in human cerebral demyelinating disease. *Science* **148**:1477-1479, 1965.

26. Melnick JL: Papova virus group. *Science* **135**:1128-1130, 1962.

27. Adams JH, Short IA: Progressive multifocal leucoencephalopathy: A neurological complication of diseases involving the reticuloendothelial system. *Scot Med J* **10**:195-202, 1965.

28. Dolman CL, Cairns ARM: Leukoencephalopathy associated with Hodgkin's disease. *Neurology* **11**:349-353, 1961.

29. Sadka M: Progressive multifocal leukoencephalopathy. *Proc Aust Assoc Neurol* **1**:13-17, 1963.

30. Adlersberg L: Sur un case de leuco-encéphalopathie plurifocale progressive. *Presse Med* **72**:3337-3340, 1964.

31. Bauer W, Chamberlin W, Horenstein S: Spinal demyelination in progressive multifocal leukoencephalopathy. *Neurology* **19**:287, 1969.

32. Behar A: Progressive multifocal leukoencephalopathy in a case of acute lymphatic leukemia. *Israel J Med Sci* **1**:650-654, 1965.

33. Bethlem J, Van Gool J, Den Hartog Jager WA: Progressive multifocal leukoencephalopathy associated with multiple myeloma. *Acta Neuropath* **3**:525-528, 1964.

34. Castaigne P, Buge A, Escourolle R, et al: La leucoencéphalopathie multifocal progressive. *Presse Med* **73**:1167-1170, 1965.

35. Cavanagh JB, Greenbaum D, Marshall AHE, et al: Cerebral demyelination associated with disorders of the reticuloendothelial system. *Lancet* **2**:524-529, 1959.

36. Chandor SB, Forno LS, Wivel NA: Progressive multifocal leukoencephalopathy. *J Neurol Neurosurg Psychiat* **28**:260-271, 1965.

37. D'Agostino AN, Pease GL, Kernohan JW: Cerebral demyelination associated with polycythemia vera. *J Neuropath Exp Neurol* **22**:138-147, 1963.

38. Deep WD, Fraumeni JF, Tashima CK, et al: Leukoencephalopathy and dermatomyositis in Hodgkin's disease. *Arch Intern Med* **113**:635-640, 1964.

39. De la Pava S, Pickren JW: Progressive multifocal leukoencephalopathy. *New York J Med* **65**:795-799, 1965.

40. Del Duca V Jr, Morningstar WA: Multiple myeloma associated with progressive multifocal leucoencephalopathy. *JAMA* **199**:671-673, 1967.

41. Fisher CM, Williams HW, Wing ES Jr: Combined encephalopathy and neuropathy with carcinoma. *J Neuropath Exp Neurol* **20**:535-547, 1961.

42. Flament-Durand J, Waelbroeck C: Leucoencéphalopathie multifocal progressive á expression neurologique primaire, au cours d'un réticulosarcome rénal. *Acta Neurol Belg* **66**:41-52, 1966.

43. Gallai M, Eckhardt A, Ambrózy G: Über einen Fall von sich zu Hodgkinscher Krankheit hinzugesellender progressiver multifokaler leukoencephalopathie. *Psychiat Neurol* **145**:356-368, 1963.

44. Headington JT, Umiker WO: Progressive multifocal leukoencephalopathy. *Neurology* **12**:434-439, 1962.

45. Hecker R, Reid RTW: Cerebral demyelination in Whipple's disease. *Med J Aust* **49**:211-212, 1962.

46. Jellinger K, Seitelberger F: Beitrag zur "progressiven multifokalen Leukoencephalopathie." *Deutsch Z Nervenheilk* **187**:749-769, 1965.

47. Johnstone RF, Green RA, Headington JT: Progressive multifocal leucoencephalopathy. *Arch Intern Med* **111**:353-362, 1963.

48. Lloyd OC, Urich H: Acute disseminated demyelination of the brain associated with lymphosarcoma. *Lancet* **2**:529-530, 1959.

49. Loken AC, Refsum S, Jacobsen W: Progressive multifocal leukoencephalopathy in a case of sarcoidosis. *Acta Med Belg* (special issue), 1962, pp 494-500.

50. Mancall EL: Progressive multifocal leukoencephalopathy. *Neurology* **15**:693-699, 1965.

51. Namiki H, Matsuyama H: A case of progressive multifocal leukoencephalopathy. *Acta Path Jap* **15**:1-10, 1965.

52. Slooff JL: Two cases of progressive multifocal leucoencephalopathy with unusual aspects. *Psychiat Neurol Neurochir* **69**:461-474, 1966.

53. Sibley WA, Weisberger AS: Demyelinating disease of the brain in chronic lymphatic leukemia. *Arch Neurol* **5**:300-307, 1961.

54. Smith JL: Progressive multifocal leukoencephalopathy. *Arch Ophthal* **62**:828-832, 1959.

55. Weinstein VF, Woolf AL, Meynell MJ: Progressive multifocal leukoencephalopathy and primary hypersplenism. *J Clin Path* **16**:405-418, 1963.

56. Woolsey RM, Nelson JS: Progressive multifocal leukoencephalopathy. *Neurology* **15**:662-666, 1965.

57. Koprowski H, Barbanti-Brodano G, Kalg M: Interaction between papova-like virus and paramyxovirus in human brain cells: A hypothesis. *Nature* **225**:1045-1047, 1970.

58. Roe FJC, Rowson KEK: The induction of cancer by combinations of viruses and other agents, in Richter GW, Epstein MA (eds): *Review of Experimental Pathology.* New York, Academic Press Inc, 1968, vol 6, p 181.

59. Shein HM: Neoplastic transformation of hamster astrocytes and choroid plexus cells in culture by polyoma virus. *J Neuropath Exp Neuol* **29**:70-88, 1970.

Familial Paraproteinemia

J. Andrew Grant, MD, Bethesda, Md; and George R. Blumenschein, MD, and Charles E. Buckley, III, MD, Durham, NC

Waldenström[1] described three patients with excess homogeneous serum immunoglobulins but no evidence of malignancy and subsequently named the syndrome "benign monoclonal gammopathy."[2] Larsson[3] identified the first familial occurrence of benign monoclonal gammopathy and multiple myeloma in siblings. Subsequently, a number of reports of familial paraproteinemia have appeared.[4-13] The incidence of familial paraproteinemia is higher than can be accounted for by chance alone.[4,7,8] The cause of this familial association remains obscure. The present report of a mother with multiple myeloma and a son with benign monoclonal gammopathy illustrates an experimental approach toward evaluation of a possible genetic defect by examining the immunoglobulin products of these aberrant plasma cell clones from two related individuals.

The basic immunoglobulin molecule consists of two heavy and two light chains. There are five immunoglobulin classes based on the five types of heavy chains. Light chains also can be divided into two types, κ and λ. Bence Jones proteins are homogeneous light chains which are thought to be produced by a single plasma cell clone. On the basis of amino acid sequence analyses of Bence Jones proteins, it has been shown that a light chain can be divided into (1) an amino-terminal half (variable region) which is unique to each light chain and (2) a carboxy-terminal half (common region) which is nearly identical for all light chains of a given type.[14] Considerable evidence supports the conclusion that the amino acid sequences of the common and variable regions from a light chain are determined by two separate genes.[15] A single amino acid variation in the common region of λ-light chains occurs at position 190 (an arginine-lysine interchange), which correlates with the two forms of the serological Oz groups (+ or −).[16] The Oz (+) and Oz (−) peptides can be separated on peptide maps.

Williams et al,[4] Berlin et al,[5] and Seligmann et al[12] have demonstrated by immunological and physico-

Received for publication Aug 28, 1970; accepted Feb 2, 1971.

From the Immunology Branch, National Cancer Institute, Bethesda, Md, and the Department of Medicine, Duke University Medical Center, Durham, NC. Dr. Blumenschein is now with the Department of Medicine, Passavant Hospital, Chicago. Dr. Grant is now with the Johns Hopkins University School of Medicine.

Reprint requests to Division of Clinical Immunology, Good Samaritan Hospital, O'Neill Research Laboratories, 3 North, 5601 Loch Raven Blvd, Baltimore 21212 (Dr. Grant).

chemical means that the paraproteins produced within families have no consistent correlation. Peptide mapping was used to compare the primary amino acid sequences of serologically similar light chains (both λ) from the paraproteins of this mother and son. Extensive differences are demonstrated between these light chains. Thus the paraproteins in these relatives are the products of two different plasma cell clones, which express distinctly different light chain structural genes.

Patient Summaries

PATIENT 1.—The patient, a 57-year-old woman, was first seen at Duke University Medical Center in October 1967, because of a rapidly enlarging mass on her forehead of several weeks duration. She had experienced increasing fatigue and exertional dyspnea for over a year and had recently been told by her personal physician that she was anemic. High thoracic spine pain and left chest wall tenderness had been present for over six months. The patient appeared as a pale, elderly white woman with normal vital signs except for blood pressure of 165/85 mm Hg. A firm 4 × 4 cm mass extruded from the center of her forehead and 2 × 2 cm nodules were palpable in the right parietal bone and the left occipital bone. Her fifth thoracic spine was tender and slightly prominent. The left lateral rib cage from the 5th to 11th ribs was tender to palpation. There were no palpable lymph nodes and the liver and spleen were not enlarged.

Hemoglobin and hematocrit values were 12.2 gm/100 ml and 37%, respectively. White blood cell count was 4,547/cu mm with a normal differential cell count. Urine contained a monoclonal γ-migrating protein, later shown to be of the λ-type with a sedimentation coefficient ($S_{20,w}$) of 4.5. Initially, the patient excreted 4.7 gm of Bence Jones protein per 24 hours. Roentgenograms showed multiple small circumscribed lesions in the table of the skull, collapse of T-5 multiple small punched out areas in other thoracic vertebra, and multiple circumscribed lesions in all ribs. A sternal bone marrow aspirate contained greater than 80% plasma cells. The blood urea nitrogen (BUN) value was 8 mg/100 ml. Cellulose acetate serum electrophoresis and immunoelectrophoresis suggested moderate reduction of all immunoglobulins but no anomalous immunoglobulins.

The patient responded to biweekly intravenous infusions of cyclophosphamide (500 mg/sq m). This dosage was adjusted to maintain an absolute granulocyte count of 1,000/cu mm. Improvement was reflected in a disappearance of the skull nodules, reduced bone pain, a decrease in the 24-hour excretion of Bence Jones protein, and a slight rise in hemoglobin value.

PATIENT 2.—The patient, a 39-year-old, career, noncommissioned military officer, was in good health until the age of 36 when (in the spring of 1966) he developed the abrupt onset of asthma. Throughout the remainder of that year he had recurring severe asthmatic episodes lasting from one to two weeks, often necessitating emergency hospitalization. It was not until the spring of 1967 when daily oral prednisone therapy was begun that he noted a lessening of his symptoms. In March 1967 he was found to have an elevated diastolic blood pressure and was treated with triamterene, methyldopa, and hydrochlorthiazide.

During a thorough medical evaluation for his respiratory illness in July 1967, he was found to have a homogeneous γ-globulin spike on serum electrophoresis. Bone marrow examination showed normal maturation of myeloid and erythroid elements and between 5% to 10% plasma cells. Urine contained no protein and a metastatic series failed to show bony lesions.

Following the diagnosis of myeloma in his mother, the patient first came to the Duke University Medical Center for evaluation in January 1968. He was an obese, cooperative white man whose blood pressure was 110/90 mm Hg; pulse rate, 86 beats per minute and regular; and respirations, 16/min following slight exertion. He had no palpable lymph nodes. Inspiratory and expiratory wheezes were heard. Findings of abdominal examination were normal. His hemoglobin level was 17.0 gm/100 ml and white blood cell count, 11,000/cu mm with a differential cell count of 52% neutrophils, 7% eosinophils, 3% basophils, 34% lymphocytes, and 4% monocytes. The urine contained no protein. The following values were within normal ranges: BUN, calcium, phosphorus, and alkaline phosphatase. Bone marrow aspiration from his sternum showed a myeloid/erythroid ratio of 2:1, slight erythroid hyperplasia, and 5% plasma cells. Roentgenograms of the skull and chest were normal. Cellulose acetate electrophoresis of his serum showed a 27 mg/ml monoclonal γ-globulin spike and normal albumin. Immunoelectrophoresis revealed a typical homogeneous arc of the IgG-λ type. Sedimentation coefficient of the homogeneous immunoglobulin was 7.5 $S_{20,w}$. Quantitative immunoglobulin determinations by radial diffusion[17] showed IgG, 31.0 mg/ml; IgA, 0.7 mg/ml; IgM, 1.3 mg/ml; κ-determinants as IgG, 3.5 mg/ml; and λ-determinants as IgG, 20.5 mg/ml. (Normal values are IgG, 12.4 ± 2.2 mg/ml; IgA, 2.8 ± 0.7 mg/ml; IgM, 1.2 ± 0.35 mg/ml; κ, 8.0 ± 2.0 mg/ml; and λ, 4.5 ± 1.2 mg/ml.) He was last evaluated in June of 1967, at which time his respiratory symptoms were stable. Serum electrophoresis showed that the paraprotein had declined in concentration to 18 mg/ml. Subsequently, the patient was lost to follow-up.

A sister and brother of patient 2 were examined for evidence of paraproteins in their sera by serum electrophoresis. The sister had a heterogeneous increase in γ-globulin. The brother had no abnormalities. There were no other siblings or any offspring of this generation.

Methods and Materials

Bence Jones protein was purified from urine of patient 1 by diethyl amino ethyl (DEAE) cellulose (Whatman DE-52) chromatography using a pH 8.0 tris (hydroxy methyl) amino methane hydrochloride (tris HCl) linear gradient from 0.01M to 0.40M.

Serum from patient 2 was fractionated by gel exclusion chromatography (using Sephadex G-200) and eluted with normal saline buffered at pH 7.4. The 7S peak was further fractionated by DEAE-cellulose gradient chromatography already described. A sharp fraction was obtained which contained only a homogeneous IgG-λ by immunoelectrophoresis. Reduction and alkylation of this protein was performed according to Fleischman et al[18] with the use of 0.15M β-mercaptoethanol and 0.175M iodoacetamide. Heavy and

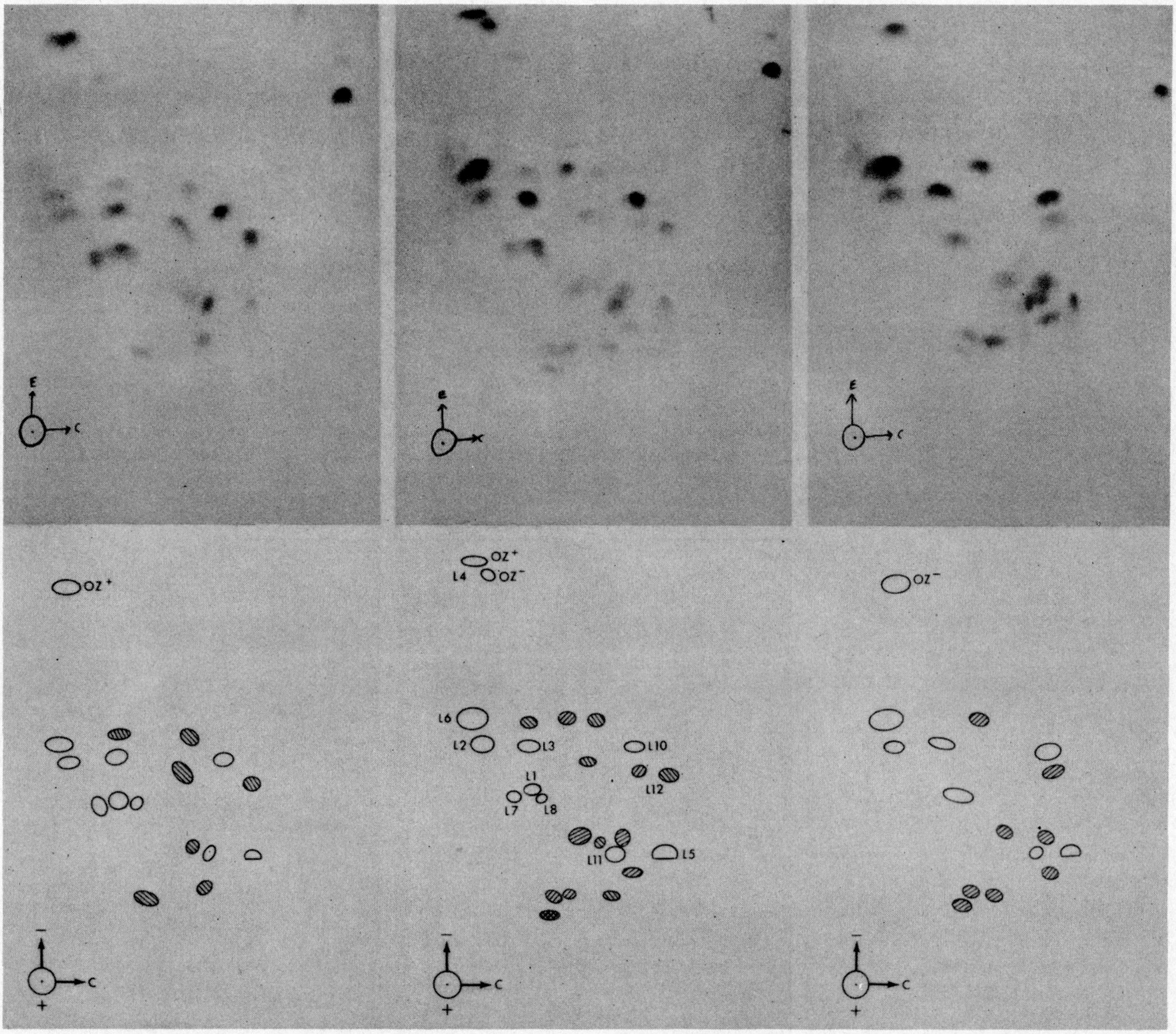

Fingerprint maps of immunoglobulin light chains. Maps were prepared according to method of Katz et al.[20] Top left, *Map was obtained from a trypsin digest of 2 mg of aminoethylated light chains (Bence Jones protein) from patient 1.* Top right, *Map is a similar preparation using 2 mg of light chains from patient 2.* Top center, *Map is a mixture of 1 mg from both patient 1 and patient 2. Interpretative drawings are below each map. In directions of chromatography and electrophoresis are indicated. Common region peptides are indicated by unshaded areas and are labeled beginning from the C-terminal according to Hood and Ein.*[22] *The Oz peptide (L4) appears in two forms, ie, the Arg-containing Oz (—) and Lys-containing Oz (+) peptide. The protein of patient 1 is Oz (+) and the protein of patient 2, Oz (—). Variable peptides are cross-hatched differently for each protein. The switch peptide between the common and variable regions (amino acids 104-111) is L12 and migrates differently for each protein.*

light chains were separated using Sephadex G-100 chromatography in 1N acetic acid.

Light chains from both patients 1 and 2 were aminoethylated[19] to convert cystine to the tryptic substrate aminoethylcysteine. The protein dissolved in 0.1M NH_4HCO_3 was digested with 2% 1-(1-tosylamido-2-phenol) ethylchloromethyl ketone-trypsin for three hours at 37 C. Peptide maps were prepared according to the method of Katz et al.[20]

Two peptides, the Oz peptide (L4) and the "switch" peptide L12 in the Figure, were eluted with water from peptide maps of light chains from patients 1 and 2. Peptides were hydrolyzed in 6N HCl for 20 hours at 37 C and amino acid composition determined on an amino acid analyzer (Beckman 120C). The N-terminal amino acid of the switch peptides was identified by dansylation.[21]

Results

Tryptic peptide maps of light chains from patients 1 and 2 are shown in the Figure. A map containing a mixture of each protein is in the center and is useful in demonstrating similarities and differences in migration properties of peptides from the two proteins. In the interpretative drawings below, open circles represent λ-common region peptides and are numbered from the C-terminal according to Hood and Ein.[22] Identity of common region peptides from each protein is shown by similar migration in the mixed map as well as by comparison with peptide maps from other λ-chains.[22] One exception is the Oz peptides (L4) which were isolated and shown to have a composition identical to Oz (+) for patient 1 and Oz (−) for patient 2.

The so-called switch peptide L12, lying at the junction of the common and variable region, is often cleaved by trypsin in λ-chains to give an octapeptide (104-111). It was noted on a mixed map that this peptide from

Switch Peptide of λ-Chains*

Protein	Position 105 ... 110
Sh	Leu Thr Val Leu Gly Gln Pro Lys
Patient 1	Leu(Thr,Val,Leu,Gly,Glx,Pro)Lys
Patient 2	Val(Thr,Val,Leu,Gly,Glx,Pro)Lys
New	Val Thr Val Leu Gly Gln Pro Lys

*The tryptic switch peptides from paraprotein light chains of patients 1 and 2 were eluted from peptide maps (Figure). Parentheses indicate the composition determined on the amino acid analyzer and amino acids are aligned by homology. The N-terminal amino acids were identified by the dansyl technique.[21] The C-terminal lysine, is assumed since this is the only trypsin substrate in the peptides. The sequences of Sh and New are obtained from Putnam et al[23] and Langer et al,[24] respectively. Numbering is that of protein Sh.[23]

paraprotein light chains of patients 1 and 2 had different migration properties (see L12, Figure). Composition and N-terminal identification showed that the peptides probably differed only at position 104 (Table), and each resembles previously sequenced Bence Jones proteins.

Shaded peptides (Figure) represent probable variable region peptides and are shaded in different directions for each protein. In the mixed map it is shown that most of the peptides appear to be unique for each light chain. This demonstrates extensive differences between the two light chain variable regions from paraproteins of this mother and son.

Comment

The diagnosis of multiple myeloma is unequivocal in the mother, patient 1, who has neoplastic plasma cells and Bence Jones proteinuria. The appearance of a homogeneous immunoglobulin spike in a person without a demonstrable plasmacytoma, as in the case of the son, patient 2, has been termed benign monoclonal gammopathy by Waldenström.[2] However, follow-up of the latter patient was unfortunately limited.

Axelsson and Hällen[8] and Axelsson et al[9] surveyed 6,995 persons in Scandinavia and found that three families had seven individuals (2, 2, and 3 in each family) with monoclonal immunoglobulin spikes. Williams et al[4] examined the kindred of 33 patients with paraproteins and 24 control families. Five of the paraprotein families had other members with coincidental paraproteins; only one family in the control group had a member with paraproteinemia. Spengler et al[7] found four families out of 22 with a paraprotein proband to have two members with paraproteins. These reports support the conclusion that familial paraproteinemia occurs more frequently than can be explained by chance. Certainly environmental or genetic factors or both may be involved but, presently, no identification is possible.

One possible genetic mechanism for familial paraproteinemia is that the same plasma cell clone escapes control of cell division in relatives and proliferates. This model predicts that paraproteins from two related individuals would be identical. While earlier reports suggested that this was not true,[4,5,12] a more rigorous examination of the primary amino acid sequence of both the common and variable regions of paraprotein λ-light chains from a mother and son was in order.

Peptide mapping showed that the common regions of the two light chains differed in the Oz peptide L4 (Figure), the only common region peptide where normal variation of sequence has been previously reported. One of the possible causes for the two (Oz [+] and OZ [−]) forms of the common region seen in normal individuals is two separate common region structural genes.[15,22] Thus, the common regions of the paraprotein light chains of patients 1 and 2 may be encoded by separate genes. The only other peptide with an easily characterized sequence and with different migration properties in peptide maps was the switch peptide L12. A leucine-valine interchange was observed at position 104 (Table and Figure). Almost all variable region peptides from light chains of patients 1 and 2 are different, which shows that these polypeptides are also encoded by different variable region structural genes.

Sequence differences have been demonstrated by peptide mapping in both the common and variable regions of these two paraprotein light chains. This must correlate with different common and variable region structural genes in the plasma cell clones synthesizing these proteins. Thus we have clearly eliminated one possible genetic mechanism for abnormal monoclonal plasma cell proliferation in familial paraproteinemia.

Summary

Certain families have a higher incidence of paraproteins in two or more members than would be expected on the basis of coincidence. One possible explanation would be that plasma cell clones, with similar structural genes for the paraprotein synthesized by these cells, proliferate in related individuals. This hypothesis predicts that paraproteins from two members of the same family would be identical. The paraproteins of a mother with multiple myeloma and a son with probable benign monoclonal gammopathy were isolated. Light chains were both of the λ-type but had differences on peptide maps in both the common and variable regions of the proteins. These data demonstrate that the structural genes operative in paraprotein light chain production in these first-degree relatives are clearly different. Each paraprotein is produced by a distinct plasma cell clone.

This investigation was supported in part by US Public Health Service training grant AL00031. Dr. Buckley is a research career development awardee, US Public Health Service grant AI14,797.

Roy Woods, PhD, assisted with the determination of quantitative immunoglobulin concentrations.

Nonproprietary and Trade Names of Drug

Methyldopa—*Aldomet.*

References

1. Waldenström J: Incipient myelomatosis or "essential" hyperglobulinemia with fibrinogenopenia: A new syndrome? *Acta Med Scand* **117**:216-247, 1944.

2. Waldenström J: Studies on conditions associated with disturbed gamma globulin function (gammopathies). *Harvey Lect* **56**:211-231, 1961.

3. Larsson SO: Myeloma and pernicious anemia. *Acta Med Scand* **172**:195-205, 1962.

4. Williams RC, Erickson JL, Polesky HF, et al: Studies of monoclonal immunoglobulins (M-components) in various kindreds. *Ann Intern Med* **67**:309-327, 1967.

5. Berlin SO, Odeberg H, Weingart L: Familial occurrence of M-components. *Acta Med Scand* **183**:347-350, 1968.

6. Wysocki K, Mackiewicz S: Familial anomalous β_{2A}-globulin. *Arch Intern Med* **116**:351-356, 1965.

7. Spengler GA, Bütler R, Fischer C, et al: On the question of familial occurrence of paraproteinemia. *Helv Med Acta* **33**:208-219, 1966.

8. Axelsson U, Hällen J: Familial occurrence of pathological serum proteins of different gamma globulin groups. *Lancet* **2**:369-370, 1965.

9. Axelsson U, Bachmann R, Hällen J: Frequency of pathological proteins (M-components) in 6,995 sera from an adult population. *Acta Med Scand* **179**:235-247, 1966.

10. Alexander LL, Benninghoff DL: Familial multiple myeloma. *J Nat Med Assoc* **57**:471-475, 1965.

11. Alexander LL, Benninghoff DL: Familial multiple myeloma. *J Nat Med Assoc* **59**:278-281, 1967.

12. Seligmann M, Danon F, Mihaesco C, et al: Immunoglobulin abnormalities in families of patients with Waldenström's macroglobulinemia. *Amer J Med* **43**:66-83, 1967.

13. Danon F, Clauvel JP, Seligmann M: Les "paraproteines" de type IgG et IgA en dehors de la maladie de Kahler. *Rev Franc Etudes Clin Biol* **12**:681-701, 1967.

14. Asofski R, Binaghi RA, Edelman GM, et al: An extension of the nomenclature for immunoglobulins. *Bull WHO* **41**:975-978, 1969.

15. Hood L, Talmage DW: Mechanism of antibody diversity: A germ line basis for variability. *Science* **168**:325-334, 1970.

16. Ein D: Nonallelic behavior of the Oz groups in human lambda immunoglobulin chains. *Proc Nat Acad Sci USA* **60**:982-985, 1968.

17. Fahey JL, McKelvey EM: Quantitative determination of serum immunoglobulins in antibody-agar plates. *J Immun* **94**:84-90, 1965.

18. Fleischman JB, Pain RH, Porter RR: Reduction of γ-globulins. *Arch Biochem Biophys* **1**(suppl):174-180, 1962.

19. Raftery MA, Cole RD: On the aminoethylation of proteins. *J Biol Chem* **241**:3457-3461, 1966.

20. Katz AM, Dreyer WJ, Anfinson CB: Peptide separation by two-dimensional chromatography and electrophoresis. *J Biol Chem* **234**:2897-2900, 1959.

21. Gray WR: Dansyl chloride procedure. *Meth Enzym* **11**:139-151, 1967.

22. Hood L, Ein D: Genetic implications of common region sequence comparison of lambda immunoglobulin chains differing at position 190. *Science* **162**:679-681, 1968.

23. Putnam FW, Titani K, Wikler M, et al: Structure and evolution of kappa and lambda light chains. *Cold Spr Harb Symp Quant Biol* **32**:9-29, 1967.

24. Langer B, Steinmetz-Kayne M, Hilschmann N: The complete amino acid sequence of Bence Jones protein, new λ-type. *Hoppe-Seyler's Z Physiol Chem* **349**:945-951, 1968.

α Heavy Chain Disease

A Variant of Mediterranean Lymphoma

Avinoam Zlotnick, MD,
and Micha Levy, MD,
Jerusalem, Israel

The Mediterranean type of abdominal lymphoma has recently been described as a separate disease entity by Ramot et al,[1] Eidelman et al,[2] and Seijffers et al.[3] The disease affects mainly young people of Mediterranean origin and is characterized by severe diarrhea accompanied by abdominal pain, hypocalcemia, and malabsorption. Proteinuria is present in some cases. Analysis of the proteins in the serum and the urine in one of these cases led Seligmann et al[4,5] to the discovery of α heavy chain disease. To the best of our knowledge, only seven patients with this disease have been reported up to 1969.[4-9] This is a report of an additional case in which the abnormal protein disappeared from the serum during a remission induced by cyclophosphamide and prednisone.

Received for publication Aug 28, 1970; accepted Sept 24.

From Department of Medicine "A" and the Research Laboratory for Autoimmune Diseases, Hadassah University Hospital and Medical School, Jerusalem, Israel.

Reprint requests to Department of Medicine "A," Hadassah University Hospital, PO Box 499, Jerusalem, Israel (Dr. Zlotnick).

Patient Summary

A 20-year-old Jewish man, born in Iraq but living in Israel since the age of 2 years, was admitted to our department in August 1966.

At the age of 15 he started to suffer from watery diarrhea with up to ten bowel movements daily and occasional pain in the umbilical region. He did not notice blood in the stool and had no fever. Antiamebic treatment and a cellulose-free diet were of no avail.

His condition gradually worsened, and he lost 5 kg of body weight in a few months. At the age of 20 he was admitted to another hospital where physical examination revealed a poor nutritional state, distended abdomen, and increased peri-

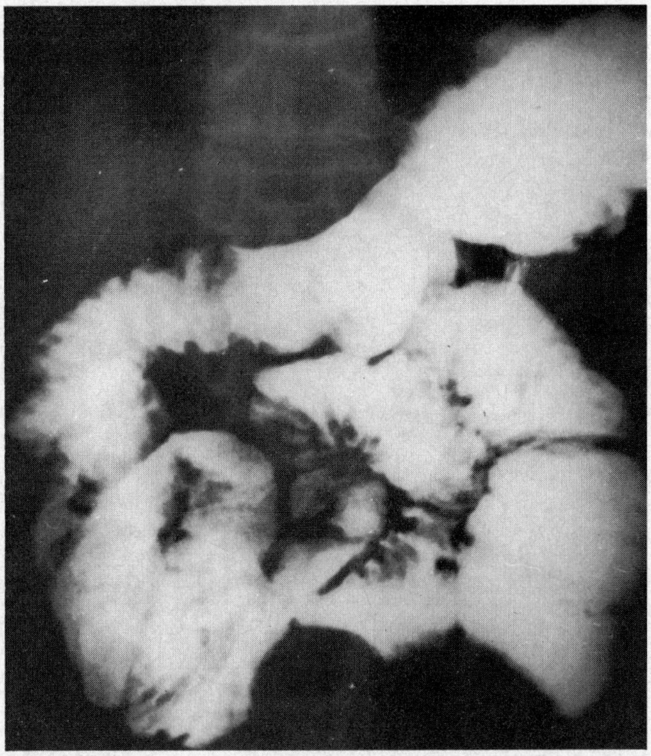

Fig 1.—Barium swallow. Note dilatation of first to third parts of duodenum with absence of normal mucosal pattern.

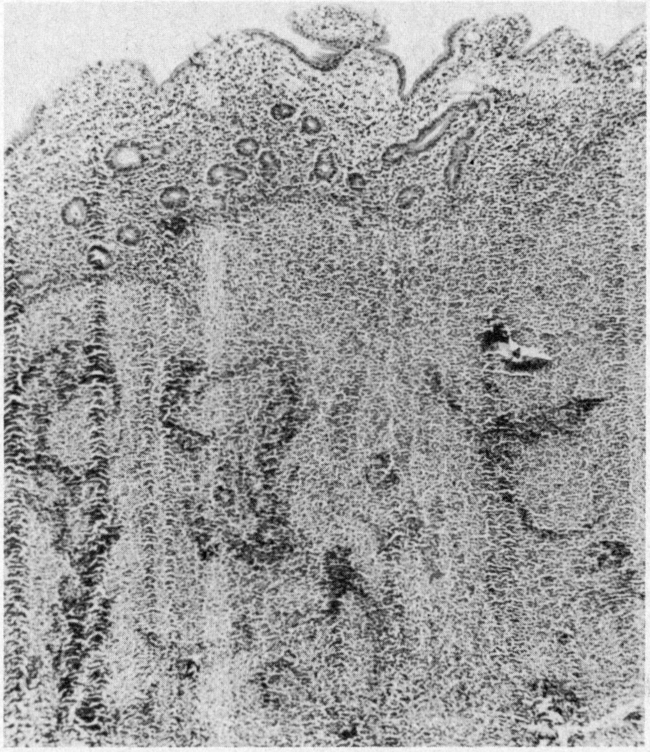

Fig 2.—Small intestinal biopsy showing the flattening of villi. Infiltrate extends from mucosa through muscles (hematoxylin-eosin stain, ×54).

stalsis. The liver and the spleen were not palpable and no lymphadenopathy was detected. Clubbing of the fingers and toes was noted. A xylose absorption test and the carotene content of the serum were compatible with malabsorption, and sprue was diagnosed. Treatment with prednisone and a gluten-free diet did not improve his condition. The patient was then admitted to our department. On admission he weighed 41 kg (90 lb), and his height was 170 cm (67 in); the temperature was 37 C (98.6 F). Muscle wasting and weakness were pronounced. There were no other abnormal findings.

Laboratory examination revealed the following values: urinalysis, normal; erythrocyte sedimentation rate, 10 mm after one hour, 20 mm after two hours (Westergren); hemoglobin, 13 gm/100 ml; white blood cell count (WBC), 7,850/cu mm; with a differential count of 53% lymphocytes, 40% neutrophils, and 7% monocytes. Serum urea, glucose, sodium, potassium, chloride, amylase, bilirubin, and liver flocculation test values were normal. The serum alkaline phosphatase value was 4.4 units/100 ml (Bodansky), uric acid level, 6.1 mg/100 ml; serum calcium level, 9.9 mg/100 ml; serum phosphorus level, 3.1 mg/100 ml; serum iron value, 43μg/100 ml; iron binding capacity, 240μg/100 ml; and vitamin B_{12}, 200μg/ml. The serum albumin level was 3.6 gm/100 ml; globulin, 3.7%. Serum electrophoresis revealed the following values: albumin, 51.0%; α_1-globulin, 5.2%; α_2-globulin, 16.6%; β-globulin, 11%; and γ-globulin, 28.2%. No paraprotein was detected. Serum carotene level was 40 units/ml. The oral glucose tolerance curve was flat (fasting, 110, 106, 124, 122, 130, and 104 mg/100 ml at half hour intervals). The five-hour urinary excretion of D-xylose after a 5 gm oral load was 1.0 gm (normal > 1.2 gm).

The stool was watery, yellowish, and, on microscopy, was found to contain multiple fat droplets, muscle fibers, and starch granules. Parasites were not found and cultures for pathogenic bacteria were negative.

Findings of x-ray examination of the

Fig 3.—Higher magnification of Fig 2. Infiltrate consists of small lymphocytes with hyperchromatic nucleus and few plasma cells in between them (hematoxylin-eosin stain, ×540).

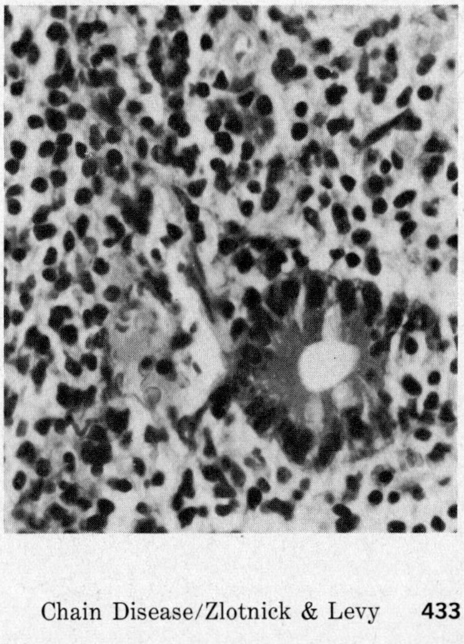

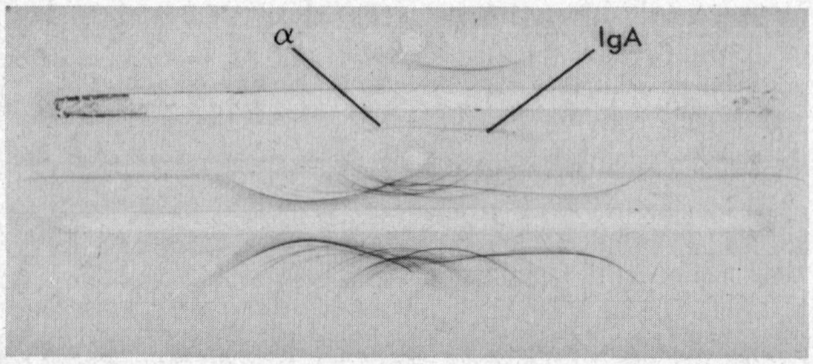

Fig 4.—Immunoelectrophoresis of patient's serum (center well) and a normal control serum (outer wells). Lower trough contains anti-whole human serum and upper trough, anti-IgA serum. Note increased mobility towards the anode of the α heavy chain (α) and formation of a spur with the normal IgA globulin (IgA).

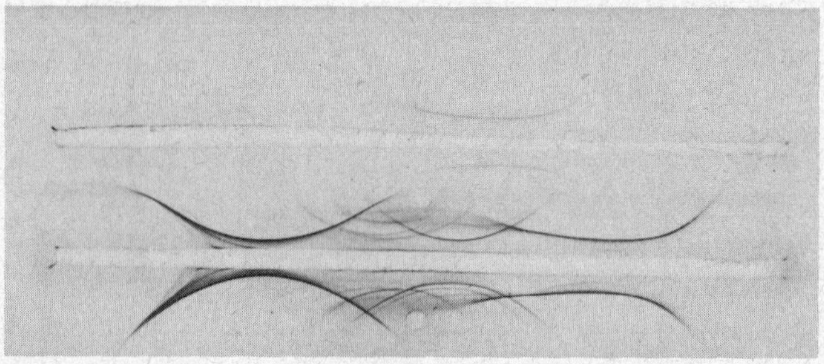

Fig 5.—Same arrangements as in Fig 4. Note disappearance of the α heavy chain.

chest, esophagus, and stomach were normal. The small intestine showed an irregular and thickened wall, with multiple filling defects; there was narrowing and dilatation of loops throughout the whole length of the small intestine. Only after three hours did the contrast material reach the distal part of the ileum (Fig 1).

A peroral small bowel biopsy obtained from an area just beyound the ligament of Treitz, revealed flattening of the villi, sparsity of crypts, and a heavy cellular infiltration of the mucous membrane with lymphocytes and a few plasma cells (Fig 2 and 3). This finding was compatible with a diagnosis of lymphosarcoma of the small bowel. A bone marrow aspirate was interpreted as normal. The diagnosis of Mediterranean type of abdominal lymphoma with malabsorption was established.

Course.—The patient was seen regularly in the outpatient department and readmitted to our department on several occasions during the following three years. Since his first hospitalization he has constantly taken prednisone, 20 to 40 mg daily; or corticotropin, 15 to 25 units daily.

Ten intravenous injections, each of 1 mg vincristine sulfate, were given at weekly intervals between October 1966 and March 1967. This treatment was stopped, however, because of lack of effect on his symptoms, the appearance of parasthesiae in the fingers and disappearance of the deep tendon reflexes. The patient continued to have five to ten watery bowel movements daily, felt extremely weak, and was unable to work.

In June 1967 he was admitted once more, this time because of marked edema of the legs. Laboratory studies revealed the following values: proteinuria, 1 to 2 gm/24 hr, total serum protein, 4.4 gm/100 ml; serum albumin, 2.1 gm/100 ml; serum cholesterol, 68 to 89 mg/100 ml; serum potassium, 2.3 mEq/liter; and prothrombin time, 12% of normal. The patient was treated with steroids, blood, plasma, vitamins, and potassium chloride. His condition improved, the edema disappeared, and the number of bowel movements decreased. Immunoelectrophoresis of the serum revealed the presence of an α heavy chain.

In January 1968 a mass could be felt in the lower abdomen, and the hemoglobin value dropped to 10.6 gm/100 ml. Following the administration of 900 mg of cyclophosphamide intravenously, the mass disappeared and the hemoglobin level went up to 11.5 gm/100 ml. Since then, he has received 100 to 350 mg of cyclophosphamide weekly. His general condition improved, the number of bowel movements decreased to three to four per day, he put on weight, and the edema disappeared. The total serum protein level rose to 7.3 gm/100 ml.

Two episodes of high fever (December 1968 and April 1969) responded well to cyclophosphamide, 900 mg intravenously.

Osteoporosis, probably due to continuous treatment with steroids and malabsorption, was detected in 1969 when the patient complained of pain in his back.

During the last six months, in the eighth year of his illness, his bowel movements have been almost normal. The main complaints are low back pain and occasional twitching in his hands and feet. The abdomen is rarely swollen. There is no detectable lymphadenopathy or abdominal mass. Blood chemistry is normal, the erythrocyte sedimentation rates are 15 mm after one hour, 55 mm after two hours; urine, normal; hemoglobin value, 13.8%; WBC, 7,800 with a normal differential count; serum albumin level, 2.9 gm/100 ml; and globulin value, 3.4 gm/100 ml.

Special Studies

Cellulose Acetate Electrophoresis.—This procedure was performed with a microzone cell electrophoresis apparatus using barbital (Veronal) buffer pH 8.6, ionic strength 0.1. The strips were stained with Ponceau S and scanned in a recording densimeter-integrator.

Immunoelectrophoresis.—This procedure was performed with the microapparatus of Scheidegger[10] using the following antisera: (1) horse antihuman serum (Hyland, lot 38303), (2) goat anti IgA human globulin (lot 71-212), and (3) rabbit antihuman κ and λ sera, prepared in our laboratory and rendered monospecific by absorption with serum from a patient with agammaglobulinemia and with κ and λ proteins.

Results

Cellulose acetate electrophoresis of the patient's serum and concentrated urine revealed slightly increased α_2

globulin (16.6%) but no abnormal band. However, immunoelectrophoresis of the patient's serum with a polyvalent antiserum showed an abnormal IgA globulin. When the serum was analyzed with a specific IgA antiserum, a precipitin line extending toward the anode and cross-reacting with the normal IgA precipitin line was noted (Fig 4). The normal IgA precipitin line showed a spur with the abnormal IgA line, indicating that the latter lacked some antigenic determinants present in the normal IgA. The abnormal line did not react with either anti-κ or anti-λ sera. M. Seligmann, MD, who examined this serum, could further confirm our findings by showing that it failed to inhibit the reaction between κ and λ light chains and anti-κ and anti-λ antisera. Using special antisera he was able to show that the fast moving protein in the patient's serum was an α heavy chain, containing antigenic determinants identical to those of the purified α heavy chains isolated from his patients previously diagnosed as suffering from α heavy chain disease.

Immunoelectrophoresis of the patient's serum during a clinical remission after treatment with prednisone (Meticorten) and cyclophosphamide showed that the pathologic fast-moving α heavy chain had disappeared (Fig 5). The latter, however, reappeared during an exacerbation of the disease and disappeared again after an additional course of cyclophosphamide.

Comment

Brandstaetter (in an oral communication, 1964) first drew attention to the fact that malabsorption in young Arabs and Oriental Jews living in Israel is most frequently associated with the occurrence of lymphoma of the small intestine. Later Ramot et al[1] and Eidelman et al[2] described in detail the clinical and pathologic findings in 13 and 9 patients, respectively, with this disease. Seijffers et al[3] described another case and coined the name Mediterranean lymphoma. The possibility was raised that an environmental factor or a genetic predisposition might play a role in the etiology of the disease. The incidence of Mediterranean lymphoma in Israel was found to be 8/100,000 in Arabs between the ages of 15 to 30 years and 3/100,000 among Oriental Jews (who immigrated from Africa or Asia). No Ashkenazy Jews were found among those affected by the disease.[7]

Crabbé et al[11] have shown that about 85% of the antibody producing cells, found in the lamina propria of the gastrointestinal tract contain IgA globulin. Two molecules of IgA globulin, released by these cells, attach themselves to the transport piece protein produced by the epithelial cells and form an IgA antibody dimer which can pass the epithelial barrier and be excreted into the gastrointestinal tract. It has been shown that the IgA antibody dimer has the capacity to fix complement and to lyse different bacteria[12] which the IgA monomer is unable to do. Thus a new defence mechanism has been established for the gastrointestinal tract. It is therefore not surprising that many cases of malabsorption may be associated with an IgA globulin deficiency due to suppression of production of the whole IgA molecule.[8] A new disease entity, the α chain disease, in which there is a suppression of light chain production and an overproduction of α heavy chains has recently been described by Seligmann et al[4] and Rambaud et al[5] in a Syrian patient suffering from Mediterranean lymphoma. They subsequently added three additional cases, all of which were Arabs with Mediterranean lymphoma.[6] Since Seligmann et al's first description several other patients with α heavy chain disease have been reported by Ramot and Hulu[7]; Jones, cited by Hobbs[8]; and Laroche et al.[9]

The characteristic features of Mediterranean lymphoma are that it is prevalent in patients 15 to 30 years of age and that all patients so far have been Jews or Arabs from the Mediterranean basin. The only Mexican patient, whose case was described by Jinich et al,[13] was of Jewish-Syrian extraction. The disease is characterized by severe diarrhea, abdominal pain, and malnutrition. The diarrhea is profuse and the discharge may reach 14 liters daily. There is usually an extensive loss of fluid and electrolytes, leading to severe hypokalemia and hypocalcemia.[3] Abdominal pain may be mild or severe, appearing in bouts and sometimes terminating in subileus or ileus. Steatorrhea is always present. The glucose tolerance curve is flat and xylose absorption is impaired. Total serum protein content is normal or low. Serum alkaline phosphatase is increased in the absence of abnormal liver function tests or bone destruction.

Findings of x-ray examination of the gastrointestinal tract are characterized by dilatation of the second and third parts of the duodenum and less frequently of the jejunum and ileum. The small intestinal wall is thickened, simulating the presence of polyps.

Electrophoresis of the serum in the patients with α heavy chain disease may be normal or may show a broad band extending from the α_2 to β_2 region. The urine may show the same finding or may be normal in spite of the presence of the pathologic protein in the serum.[4,5] Immunoelectrophoresis of the serum, however, invariably shows an IgA band extending towards the anode and sometimes crossing the albumin precipitation line. The pathologic line may also be present in the urine. Since in previous work on Mediterranean lymphoma, protein studies were not performed regularly, it is impossible to determine the prevalence of α heavy chain disease in this entity.

In all previously reported cases of α heavy chain disease, the abnormal protein persisted in the serum during the period that the patient was under observation. Our case is apparently unique in that the abnormal protein disappeared after treatment with prednisone and cyclophosphamide. Decrease in the amount of paraprotein as a result of treatment with cytotoxic agents has been reported in multiple myeloma.[14] The disappearance of the protein in our case is most probably due to the fact that it was not present in large quantities in the serum. The absence of α heavy chain in the urine of our patient may be explained, as in other cases, by the tendency of the α chains to form polymers with high molecular weights, which can, therefore, not pass through the glomerular filter.

The histologic finding of the intestinal mucosa in α heavy chain disease is very characteristic. There is a flattening or complete absence of the intestinal villi and a predominantly plasma cell infiltration. Some of these cells give a positive reaction with PAS stain.[7] The histologic finding in the intestinal biopsy in our case was characterized by the sparsity of plasma cells, which might explain the small quantity of α chains in the serum and its rapid disappearance following treatment.

The increasing number of reported cases with α heavy chain disease may indicate that the Mediterranean lymphoma is a rather heterogenous entity, and the α heavy chain disease should be singled out as a separate entity.

Summary

A form of lymphoma of the small intestine, causing malabsorption in young Arabs and oriental Jews, has recently been described and named Mediterranean lymphoma. An overproduction of the α heavy chain has been found in seven such cases reported during the last two years. An additional case of α heavy chain disease in a 20-year-old man suffering from Mediterranean lymphoma is reported here. This is apparently the first reported case in which the pathological immunoglobulin disappeared after treatment with prednisone and cyclophosphamide.

This investigation was supported in part by the Israel Cancer Foundation.

I. S. Levij, MD, Department of Pathology, Hadassah University Hospital interpreted the biopsy specimen and prepared the photomicrographs. E. Schwartz, MD, Department of Radiology interpreted the x-ray pictures.

Nonproprietary and Trade Names of Drugs

Corticotropin—*Actest, Acthar, Actrope, Cortigel, Cortrophin, Depo Acth, Duracton.*

Vincristine sulfate—*Oncovin.*

References

1. Ramot B, Shahin N, Bubis JJ: Malabsorption syndrome in lymphoma of the small intestine. *Israel J Med Sci* **1**:221-226, 1965.
2. Eidelman S, Parkins RA, Rubin CE: Abdominal lymphoma presenting as malabsorption. *Medicine* **45**:111-137, 1966.
3. Seijffers MJ, Levy M, Hermann G: Intractable watery diarrhea, hypokalemia and malabsorption in a patient with Mediterranean type of abdominal lymphoma. *Gastroenterology* **55**:118-124, 1968.
4. Seligmann M, Danon F, Hurez D, et al: Alpha chain disease: A new immunoglobulin abnormality. *Science* **162**:1396-1397, 1968.
5. Rambaud JC, Bognel C, Prost A, et al: Clinico-pathological study of a patient with "Mediterranean" type of abdominal lymphoma and a new type of IgA abnormality ("alpha chain disease"). *Digestion* **1**:321-324, 1968.
6. Seligmann M, Rambaud JC: IgA abnormalities in abdominal lymphoma (α-chain disease). *Israel J Med Sci* **5**:151-157, 1969.
7. Ramot B, Hulu N: Clinical and pathological aspects of intestinal lymphoma and the relation to paraproteinemia of alpha chain. *Harefuah* **76**:396-398, 1969.
8. Jones A, cited by Hobbs JR: Immunoglobulins and malabsorption. *Proc Roy Soc Med* **62**:982, 1969.
9. Laroche C, Seligmann M, Meyillon H, et al: Nouvelle observation d'une maladie des chaînes lourdes alpha. *Presse Med* **78**:55-59, 1970.
10. Scheidegger JJ: Une micro-méthode de l'immuno-électrophorèse. *Int Arch Allerg* **7**:103-110, 1955.
11. Crabbé PA, Carbonara AD, Heremans JF: The normal human intestinal mucosa as a major source of plasma cell containing IgA immunoglobulin. *Lab Invest* **14**:235-248, 1965.
12. Adinolfi M, Glynn AA, Lindsay M, et al: Serological properties of γA antibodies to *Escherichia coli* present in human colostrum. *Immunology* **10**:517-526, 1966.
13. Jinich H, Rojas E, Webb JA, et al: Lymphoma presenting as malabsorption. *Gastroenterology* **54**:421-425, 1968.
14. Waldenström J: Treatment of multiple myeloma. *Brit J Haemat* **5**:217-220, 1968.

IgM Heavy Chain Fragments in Waldenström's Macroglobulinemia

Nirmala Bhoopalam, MD, Chicago; Bak Moo Lee, MD, Berwyn, Ill; and
Vincent J. Yakulis, and Paul Heller, MD, Chicago

Waldenström's macroglobulinemia is an immunoproliferative disorder characterized by the presence of large amounts of monoclonal macroglobulin (IgM) in the serum, apparently produced by abnormally proliferating lymphocytes.[1] While in the original description of Waldenström the number of lymphocytes was not increased in the peripheral blood, the bone marrow showed characteristic lymphocytic infiltrations and in later reports on macroglobulinemia the disease was associated with peripheral lymphocytosis.[2] Thus, macroglobulinemia has variable morphologic manifestations.

IgM consists of five subunits which have the general structure of all immunoglobulins, namely a pair of type specific heavy chains and a pair of light chains of either the κ type or the λ type. Five such subunits combine to form an IgM molecule $(\mu_2\ \kappa_2)_5$ or $(\mu_2\ \lambda_2)_5$. In 20% to 30% of the patients Bence Jones protein is also present.[3] Most patients also have traces of uncombined subunits (IgMs), but free μ chains in this disease have not yet been described. There have been recent reports[4-6] of a patient with chronic lymphocytic leukemia in whose serum an immunoglobulin fraction was detected with μ-chain specificity which migrated electrophoretically with the α_2-globulin fraction and was devoid of light chains. The total α_2 fraction was approximately 1.4% as calculated from the electrophoregram depicted in the publication.[5] Neither IgM molecules nor IgM subunits were demonstrable, but free light chains of the κ type were found in the serum and urine.

The present report deals with a patient who had in the serum in addition to monoclonal IgM (19S) two fractions with μ specificity of lower molecular weight, one of which was identified as consisting of heavy-chain determinants only. Free light chains (Bence Jones protein) of the λ type were also present. The patient had a blood picture of chronic lymphocytic leukemia.

Received for publication Dec 14, 1970; accepted Jan 7, 1971.

From the Department of Medicine, University of Illinois Abraham Lincoln School of Medicine and Veterans Administration West Side Hospital, Chicago (Drs. Bhoopalam and Heller and Mr. Yakulis), and the Laboratory Service, MacNeal Memorial Hospital, Berwyn, Ill (Dr. Lee). Dr. Lee is now with the Jacksonville State Hospital, Jacksonville, Ill.

Reprint requests to PO Box 8195, Chicago 60680 (Dr. Heller).

Patient Summary

A 75-year-old white woman was admitted to the hospital on April 4, 1970, because of shortness of breath, ankle edema, and ascites. She had been receiving digitalis and diuretics for several years because of congestive heart failure attributed to arteriosclerotic heart disease. A few weeks prior to admission, her physician detected enlarged cervical lymph nodes and hepatosplenomegaly. The patient was emaciated, lethargic, pale, and severely dyspneic. The temperature was 100.8 F (38.2 C); the pulse rate, 100 beats per minute and regular; and the blood pressure, 135/60 mm Hg. The anterior and posterior cervical lymph nodes were enlarged, the largest measuring approximately 3 cm in diameter. Most of them were discrete. The apical impulse was in the left sixth intercostal space and forcible. A grade 3 ejection murmur was noted over the apical area. The base of the right hemithorax was dull to percussion and breath sounds were absent. The abdomen was markedly distended; shifting dullness was demonstrable. Because of the ascites, hepatomegaly and splenomegaly were not detectable. There was 3+ edema of the lower extremities. Ophthalmoscopy revealed distended veins with periodic constrictions ("box-car phenomenon") and several fresh hemorrhages. The hematocrit value was 28%; hemoglobin value, 8.5 gm/100 ml; and the leukocyte count was 45,000/cu mm with 78% mature lymphocytes. There was marked rouleux formation. The specific gravity of the urine was 1.010 and there was a trace of protein. A mucoid sputum sample showed pneumococci on direct examination and culture. The values of some of the tests on the blood serum were as follows: glutamic oxaloacetic transminase, 65 units/ml (normal 50); lactic acid dehydrogenase, 360 units/ml (normal 200); uric acid, 14 mg/100 ml; serum urea, 58 mg/100 ml; serum calcium, 8.8 mg/100 ml; serum phosphorus, 4 mg/100 ml; serum albumin, 1.9 gm/100 ml; and globulins, 6.5 gm/100 ml. The chest roentgenogram showed right pleural effusion and mild cardiac enlargement. The electro-

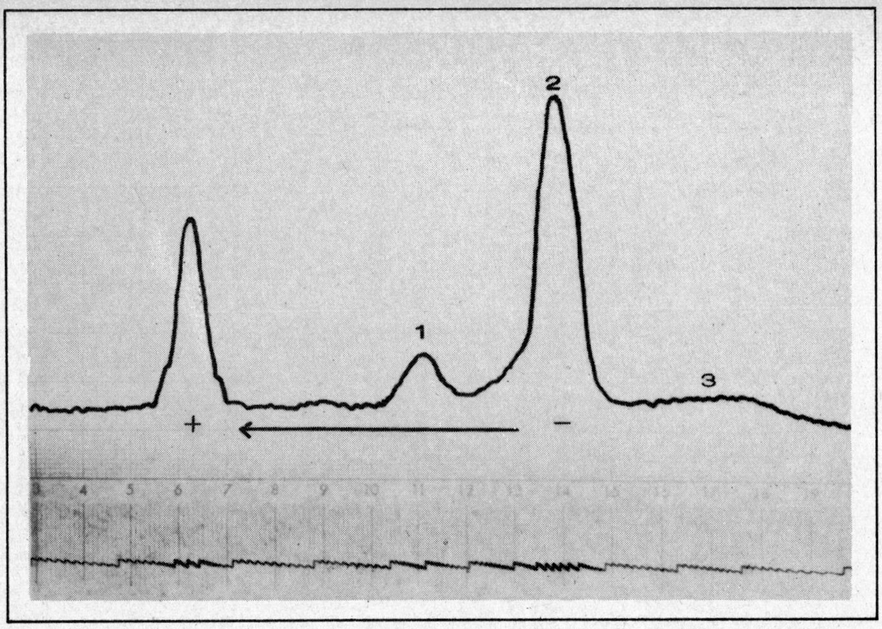

Fig 1.—Tracing of electrophoregram (cellulose acetate, pH 8.6) of serum. (1) α_2-region containing the IgM heavy chain fragment (see immunoelectrophoregram) Fig 2. (2) β-region containing IgM. (3) γ-region (note decrease of normal γ-globulin fraction).

cardiogram showed sinus tachycardia with depressed ST segments and inverted T waves in lead I, II, V_5, and aV_L. The bone marrow was hypercellular with predominance of small lymphocytes. A lymph-node biopsy showed complete distortion of normal architecture and diffuse infiltrations with large immature and plasmacytoid lymphocytes. There also was proliferation of histiocytes, and the capsule and the perinodal adipose tissue were infiltrated with lymphocytes. The patient was given digoxin, furosemide, and penicillin G potassium, but her course was relentlessly downhill, the temperature rose to 104 F (40 C), and she died three days after admission. Full autopsy was not permitted, but samples of liver and spleen were obtained by Vim-Silverman needle. The splenic tissue was diffusely infiltrated with the same kind of cells as were seen in the lymph node, and the hepatic architecture was preserved with many lymphocytes in the dilated sinusoids.

Fig 2.—Immunoelectrophoresis of normal (NS) and patient's serum developed with antiserum to total immunoglobulin fraction, IgM, κ and λ chains. Note three prepitin arcs in reaction of patients serum with anti IgM and only two arcs in reaction of patients serum with anit-λ, indicating the presence of μ chain fraction devoid of light chain in patients serum. The most cathodic arc is formed by IgM and the second arc by IgM subunits.

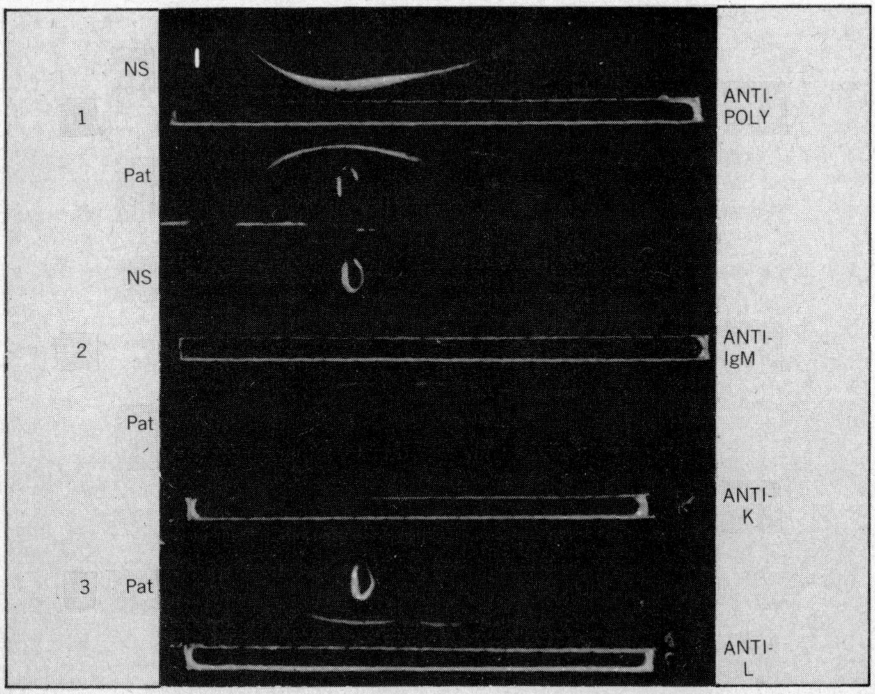

Special Studies of the Immunoglobulins

Immunoelectrophoresis (IEP) was performed in barbital-buffered agarose, pH 8.2, 0.03M. Rabbit antisera to human serum, μ, κ, λ, chains and to the total immunoglobulin fraction were used.[7] The serum of the patient was subjected to gel filtration (in Sephadex G-200) equilibrated with 0.15M sodium chloride and the resulting fractions concentrated by vacuum dialysis. Electrophoresis of the serum and of the isolated filtration fractions was done on cellulose acetate or agarose gel. For the demonstration of free light chains (Bence Jones protein) in serum the antisera to κ and λ light chains were absorbed with pooled normal IgG (human γ-globulins, fraction II).[8] Light chain typing of immunoglobulins was performed according to the method of Radl.[9] This technique consists of immunoelectrophoresis in agar gel into which either κ or λ light chains had been incorporated prior to electrophoresis. During electrophoresis all immunoglobulins containing the light chain corresponding to the incorporated antiserum are precipitated and those containing the other light chains escape precipitation and can then be identified by appropriate antisera.

The electrophoregram of the patient's serum showed in addition to the monoclonal peak near the cathode a more anodically moving fraction (Fig 1). Quantitative immunoglobulin determinations by radial immunodiffusion yielded the following values: IgG, 320 mg/100 ml (normal 900 to 1,200 mg/100 ml); IgA, 18 mg/100 ml (normal 150 to 295 mg/100 ml); IgM, 7,000 mg/100 ml (normal 95 to 145 mg/100 ml). Immunoelectrophoresis of the patient's serum developed with an antiserum to μ chains showed three precipitin arcs in a pattern of complete identity, while the immunoelectrophoregram of normal serum had a single arc near the point of application of the serum (Fig 2). When antiserum to light chains was used, a single arc with antiserum to κ was demonstrated near the point of application and a double arc with antiserum to λ light chains. Thus, the most anodic precipitin arc demonstrated by antiserum to μ chains failed to react with antisera to the light chains, and, therefore, further studies were performed to corroborate this evidence for the presence of a fraction consisting of heavy chain fragments only. Sephadex G-200 filtration of the patient's serum yielded three peaks corresponding to three different populations of molecules all of which reacted with antiserum to IgM (Fig 3). In normal serum only the first peak (exclusion peak) contains IgM. The third filtration fraction also contained serum albumin as shown by immunoelectrophoresis, and, therefore, the anti-IgM reactive fraction in this peak can be assumed to have a molecular weight of approximately 68,000, which corresponds to that of the heavy chain fragment. In addition, this fraction also reacted with antisera to free λ light chains presumably due to the presence of polymerized light chains. The second peak contained IgG, and, therefore, the fraction in this peak reacting with anti-IgM had to be assumed to consist of IgM subunits. When antisera to light chains were incorporated into the agar gel prior to electrophoresis, some of the molecules reacting with anti-IgM escaped precipitation and, therefore, were devoid of light chains.

The quantification of IgM by radial immunodiffusion resulted in a value of 7,000 gm/100 ml. Because of the above evidence of molecules of smaller size in the patient's serum and the increased diffusion rate of smaller molecules in the agar gel, this figure is slightly too high, but the correction factor could not be calculated.

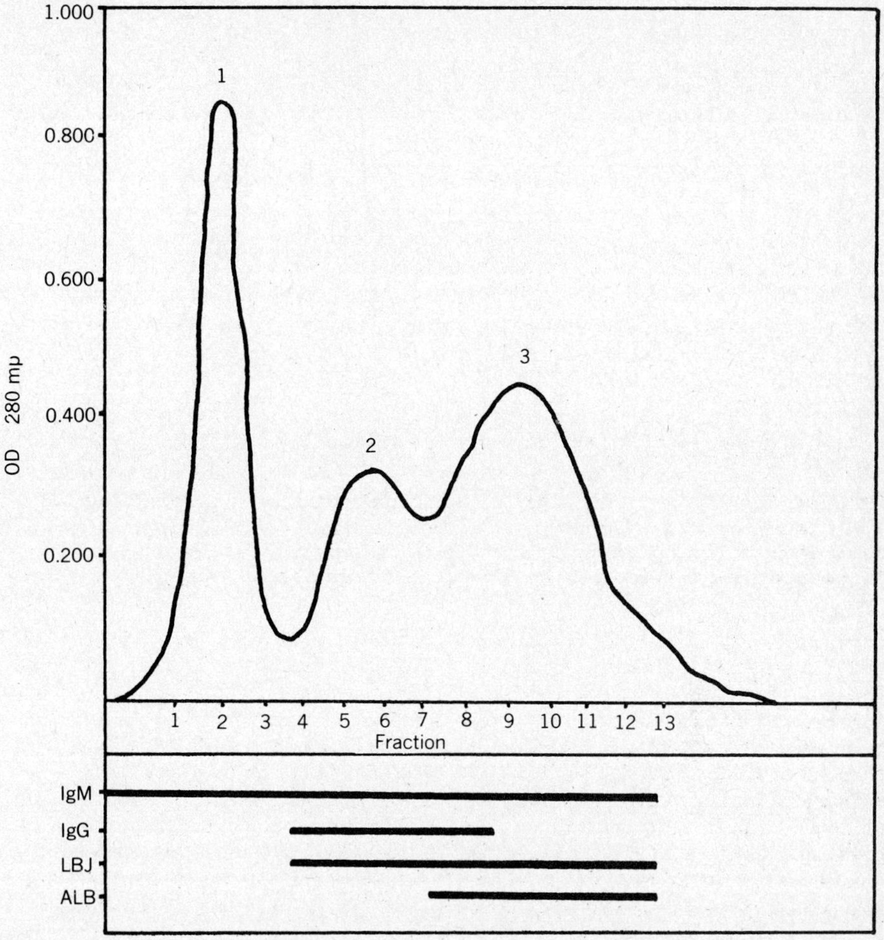

Fig 3.—Sephadex G-200 filtration of the patients serum. (1) Exclusion peak (19S). (2) ∽7S fractions. (3) ∽4.5S fractions. Fractions with μ specificity were present in all three peaks. LBJ signifies Bence Jones protein of the λ type; ALB signifies serum albumin.

Fig 4.—Immunoelectrophoresis of normal and patient's serum with anti IgM (upper pattern) *and of IgM and of $NaBH_4$ treated IgM* (lower pattern). *Note similarity of the pattern of the patients IgM with those of $NaBH_4$ treated IgM.*

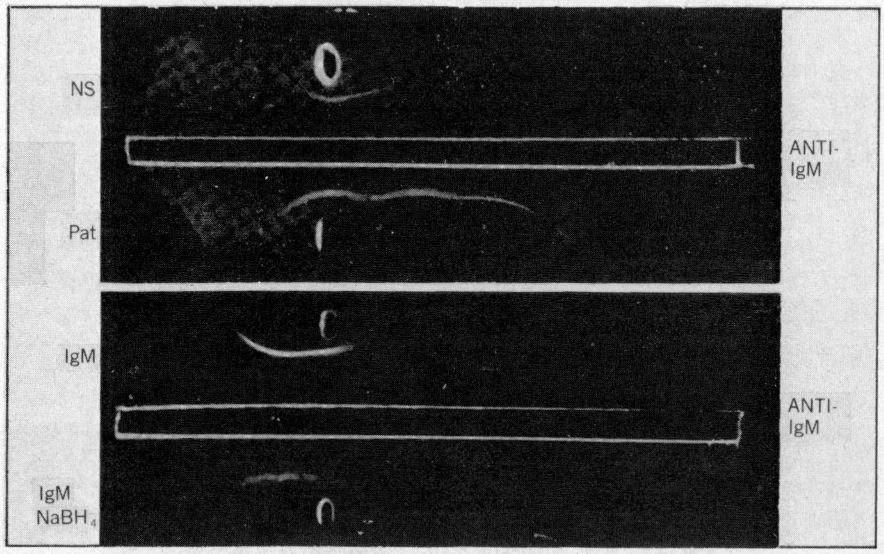

Comment

The immunochemical findings in this patient are of interest because they reflect the mechanism of immunoglobulin synthesis by malignant lymphocytes in a unique manner. Normal immunoglobulin synthesis usually is balanced and leads to the assembly of whole molecules without significant overproduction of light or heavy chains. Most of the patients with macroglobulinemia[10] have, in addition to the fully assembled IgM molecule, trace amounts of IgM subunits. Overproduction of IgM subunits alone cannot be solely responsible for the appearance of subunits in the serum; there also must be an abnormality of assembly due to structural alterations in these subunits, perhaps caused by mutational amino acid substitutions which might have deprived the subunit molecules of chemical groups capable of reacting with the neighboring subunits to form polymers. As mentioned in the introduction, immunoglobulin fractions with the immunochemical characteristics of μ chains, devoid of light chains, were demonstrable in the serum of a patient with chronic lymphocytic leukemia in sufficient quantity to result in a small homogeneous peak in the α_2 region of the cellulose acetate electrophoregram,[4-6] similar to the second peak in our patient. Further studies performed by Forte et al[5] have led these investigators to conclude that this protein represented heavy chain or a fragment thereof. The lack of assembly of this fraction into complete immunoglobulin molecules could not be attributed to overproduction alone because free light chains of the κ type were also found which suggests the inability of the μ chains to form the normal covalent bond with light chains.[5,6] The findings in the patient of this report differ from those described by Forte et al in their patient with lymphocytic leukemia in the following way: Our patient had the clinical picture of Waldenström's macroglobulinemia (7 gm/100 ml; IgM) and the immunochemical studies revealed as the predominant abnormality the presence of an IgM peak in addition to the peak in the α_2 region. By immunoelectrophoresis this latter peak did not react with anti-κ or anti-λ serum and, therefore, must be assumed to be due to free heavy chains or heavy chain fragments. The estimation of the molecular weight was in agreement with this assumption. Moreover, the immunoelectrophoretic pattern of the patient's serum developed with anti-IgM also resembled that of IgM subjected to reductive cleavage by sodium borohydride which, as shown previously,[11] results in the cleavage of IgM into heavy chain fragments of IgM devoid of light chains (Fig 4). Thus, in our patient three protein fractions with μ reactivity were detected: complete molecules, IgM subunits, and heavy chain fragments. In addition, free light chains were also present in the serum. The combination of these abnormalities raises the possibility of unbalanced synthesis of the polypeptide chains of the IgM molecules, some of which have lost the capacity for combining with each other prior to their secretion from the cell. It is likely that this defect in the assembly of subunits and of heavy and light chains was due to peculiarities in the amino acid sequence of the μ chains synthesized by the abnormal clone of lymphocytes. Unfortunately the early death of this patient precluded the collection of more material for more detailed studies.

Summary

The serum of a patient with Waldenström's macroglobulinemia was found to contain heavy chain fragments of IgM, free λ-type light chains, and IgM subunits, in addition to large amounts of monoclonal IgM.

The combination of these abnormalities indicates unbalanced synthesis of the heavy chains of IgM, some of which have lost the capacity for combining with light chains prior to their secretion from the cell, probably because of abnormalities in their primary structure. The latter also appear to be responsible for the presence of a large number of IgM subunits in the serum.

This investigation was supported in part by Veterans Administration research funds.

Nonproprietary and Trade Names of Drug

Furosemide—*Lasix.*

References

1. Waldenström JC: Incipient myelomatosis or essential hyperglobulinemia with fibrinogenopenia: New syndrome? *Acta Med Scand* **117**:216-247, 1944.
2. Mackay IR, Taft LI, Woods EF: Clinical features and pathogenesis of macroglobulinemia. *Brit Med J* **1**:561-563, 1957.
3. Waldenström JG: *Monoclonal and Polyclonal Hypergammaglobulinemia.* Nashville, Tenn, Vanderbilt University Press, 1968, p 53.
4. Ballard HS, Hamilton LM, Marcus AJ, et al: A new variant of heavy-chain disease (γ M chain disease). *New Eng J Med* **282**:1060-1063, 1970.
5. Forte FA, Prelli F, Yount WJ, et al: Heavy chain disease of the U (γ M) type: Report of the first case. *Blood* **36**:137-144, 1970.
6. Buxbaum J, Franklin EC, Scharff MD: Immunoglobulin M heavy chain disease: Intracellular origin of the Mu chain fragment. *Science* **169**:770-772, 1970.
7. Costea N, Yakulis V, Heller P: The dependence of cold agglutinin activity on K chains. *J Immun* **99**:558-563, 1967.
8. Zelkowitz L, Yakulis V: Immunologic methods for detection and quantification of Bence Jones proteins. *J Lab Clin Med* **76**:973-980, 1970.
9. Radl J: Light chain typing of immunoglobulins in small samples of biological material. *Immunology* **19**:137, 1970.
10. Solomon A, McLaughlin CL: Biosynthesis of low molecular weight (7S) and high molecular weight (19S) immunoglobulin M. *J Clin Invest* **49**:150-160, 1970.
11. Yakulis V, Schmale J, Costea N, et al: Production of Fc fragments of IgM. *J Immun* **100**:525-529, 1967.

Chromosome Aberrations in the Child of a Kidney Transplant Recipient

Daniel E. Leb, MD, Pittsburgh; and Bernard Weisskopf, MD, and Bob S. Kanovitz, MD, Louisville

Successful kidney transplantation in young women results in the resumption of normal ovulatory menstrual cycles, so it is not surprising that pregnancies in renal transplant recipients have been reported.[1-4] Since azathioprine is known to produce fetal death and stunt fetal growth and is a teratogenic agent in animals,[5-8] there is valid concern for the human fetus. So far no abnormalities of infants born to women taking azathioprine have been described.[1-4,9,10]

This report documents the occurrence of chromosomal abnormalities in the child of a cadaver kidney transplant recipient.

Materials and Methods

Chromosome analysis was performed on peripheral blood leukocytes cultured in the presence of phytohemagglutinin with the use of a slight modification of the technique described by Moorhead et al.[11] The slides were stained with Giemsa stain. Chromosomes in 100 metaphases were studied under light microscopy with an oil immersion objective. Karyotypes were prepared by photographic enlargement and photographs mounted according to the Chicago Conference of Standardization of Human Cytogenetics.

Patient Summary

A 26-year-old white woman developed renal failure secondary to chronic glomerulonephritis in September 1966. Bilateral nephrectomy and splenectomy were done in March 1967, preparatory to cadaver transplantation. The patient was maintained on periodic hemodialysis until Jan 22, 1968, when she received a cadaver renal allograft. Matching was restricted to major blood group. Diuresis occurred after 15 days of tubular necrosis and by the 35th day after transplant the creatinine clearance was 63 ml/min. Initial immunosuppression consisted of large doses of azathioprine and prednisone, 400 mg of cactinomycin, and 450 roentgens local irradiation to the graft. Maintenance immunosuppression which continued throughout her pregnancy consisted of azathioprine, 75 to 100 mg, and prednisone, 20 mg (Fig 1).

Her last normal menstrual period was Nov 4, 1968, and she had a positive pregnancy test by the end of December. Hypertension, edema, and albuminuria developed in the third trimester and a diagnosis of preeclampsia was made. She was treated with bed rest and thiazides with a good response. On July 26, 1969, she was delivered of a healthy viable, female infant weighing 4.1 kg (5 lb 9 oz) after 8½ hours of labor.

Results of physical examination and laboratory studies of the child at birth were normal except for the chromosome studies. Findings of physical examination, psychologic testing, and radiographic and chemical studies of the infant were also normal at 7 months of age.

Results

Figure 2 illustrates some of the abnormalities found in the chromosome study done on the baby one day after birth.

Some of the chromosomes cannot be identified with certainty. Portions of the missing chromosomes are obviously those mounted to the side of the karyotypes; however, the extensive fusion, translocation of fragments, and bridging makes it impossible to identify the fragments with any assurance. For example, in Fig 2, *right,* a portion of the overlap bridge may consist of at least one identifiable, large, metacentric chromosome of the A group, however, we believe that this is not superimposition but true bridging.

One week later a second study of the infant's chromosomes failed to reveal the bridging seen in the previous study; however, breaks, translocations, and deleted chromosomes persisted as illustrated in Fig 3. The persistence of chromosomal damage may have been dependent on the excretion rate of azathioprine and the time needed for generation of leukocytes not affected by the drug.

The Table summarizes the serial studies of chromosomes in this infant. By November the findings were within normal limits and no sig-

Received for publication Nov 16, 1970; accepted Jan 21, 1971.

From the Renal Division, Department of Medicine, University of Pittsburgh School of Medicine, Pittsburgh; and the departments of medicine and pediatrics, University of Louisville School of Medicine and Child Evaluation Center, Louisville.

Read in part before the 50th annual meeting of the American College of Physicians, April 14, 1970.

Reprint requests to Department of Medicine, Presbyterian-University Hospital, Room 11430, 230 Lothrop St, Pittsburgh 15213 (Dr. Leb).

nificant increase in chromosomal abnormalities was noted three months later.

Careful questioning of the mother failed to reveal evidence of ingestion of other potentially mutagenic drugs. She had received thiazides and steroids which have not been reported to produce the abnormalities seen here. Study of the mother's chromosomes was done 3½ months after delivery, at which time 12% of metaphases obtained from her lymphocytes were abnormal. Figure 4 illustrates abnormalities typical of those found. Gaps, breaks, and extra fragments were seen; however, the bridging which characterized the initial study of the infant was not found. A subsequent study 3½ months later (7 months postpartum) was within normal limits; however, only 28 metaphases suitable for study were obtained. Failure to obtain ideal growth of lymphocytes in other patients on azathioprine has been noted, but the significance of this phenomenon is unclear at present.

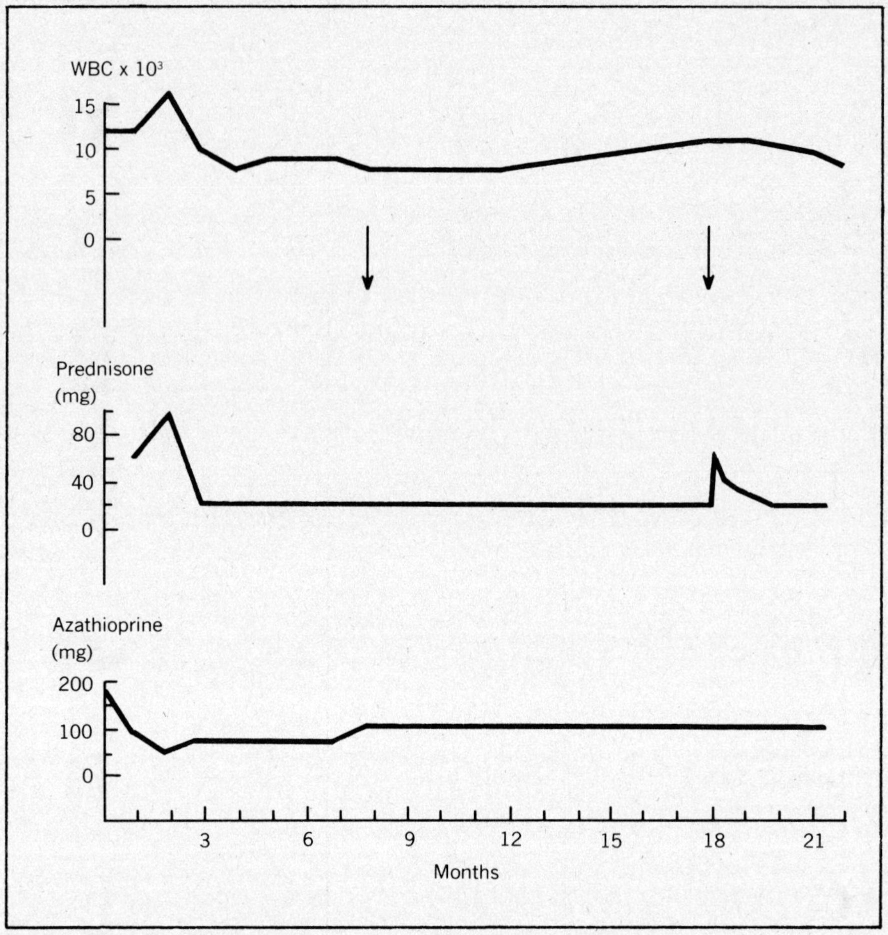

Fig 1.—White blood cell count and immonosuppression in the kidney transplant patient. Arrows *indicate the last normal menstrual period and the date of delivery. The cactinomycin and radiation administered during the first week are not shown.*

Comment

Conflicting data in the literature yield an unclear picture regarding the effects of azathioprine on chromosomes. Jensen[12-14] studied chromosomes obtained from bone marrow of patients before, during, and after azathioprine therapy. He found 11 of 15 patients developed structural changes or deviation in the normal diploid number of chromosomes while on a regimen of azathioprine. The changes subsided after cessation of treatment. The patient population he studied consisted of patients with collagen diseases, cirrhosis of the liver, and chronic glomerulonephritis, but not transplant patients. Eberle et al[15] studied a similar group of adults who were given 1.5 to 2.5 mg/kg of azathioprine per day. In contrast to Jensen, they noted significant abnormalities prior to administration of azathioprine and found no significant difference in chromosome abnormalities between treated and untreated patients. The studies are not strictly comparable since Eberle et al obtained cells from peripheral blood and, as Jensen points out, there may be a discrepancy between bone marrow and peripheral blood studies due to the origin of the cells, bone marrow perhaps being a more sensitive index.

Animal studies of teratogenic activity, fetal stunting, and death indicate that the latter effect may be a dose-related phenomenon while the former does not appear to be.[5-8] Azathioprine is metabolized to 6-mercaptopurine. Biesele[16] has demonstrated that 6-mercaptopurine produces increased chromosome breaks in mouse fibroblast tissue culture; thus, teratogenicity[7] and chromosome damage have been demonstrated in the same species, albeit, in separate studies and under totally different experimental conditions.

Abnormal Metaphases in the Child of a Kidney Transplant Patient

	Metaphases	
Date	Examined	% Abnormal
7/28/69	100	11
8/04/69	100	19
11/10/69	100	3
2/24/70	100	5

Tallent et al[17] recently reported the occurrence of myelomeningocele and rib abnormalities in the child of a male transplant recipient. The father received 1,350 rads of local irradiation to the graft five years previously and was apparently taking 125 mg azathioprine daily when the

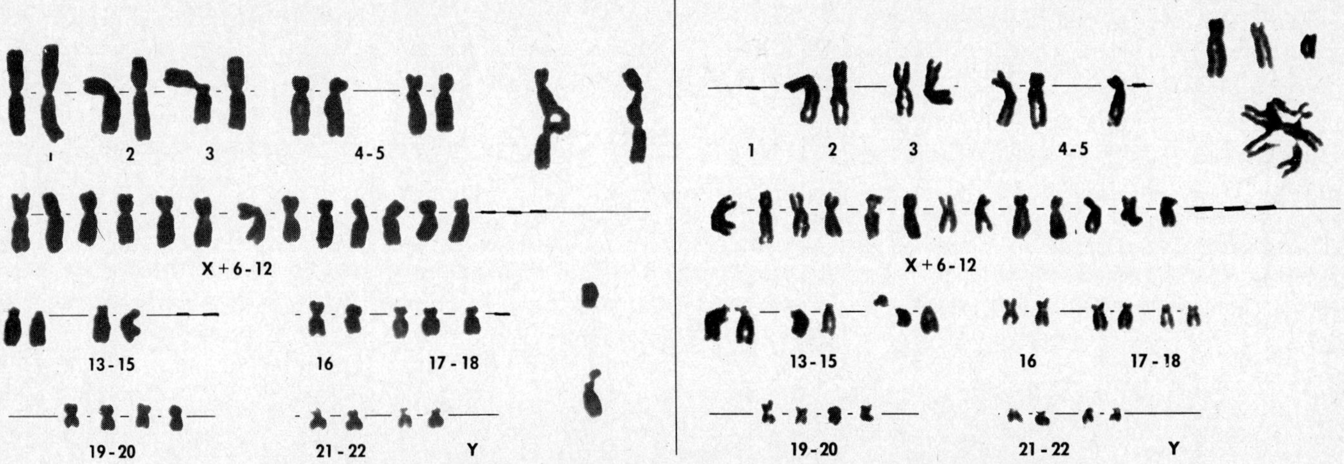

Fig 2.—Left and right, *Selected karyotypes from the original study of the child, one day after birth. Note the breaks, extensive bridging, and missing chromosomes.*

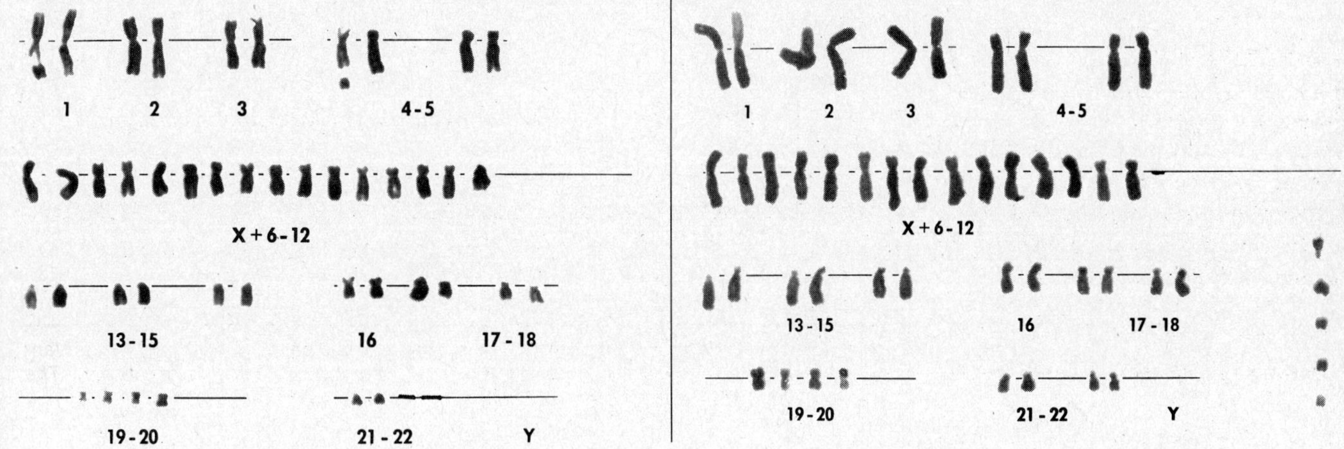

Fig 3.—Left and right, *Selected karyotypes from the study of the child, one week after birth. The damage may be less extensive. No bridging is seen. Note the breaks, unidentifiable fragments, and missing chromosomes.*

Fig 4.—Left and right, *Selected karyotypes obtained from the study of the mother, 3½ months postpartum. Note the breaks and extra fragments.*

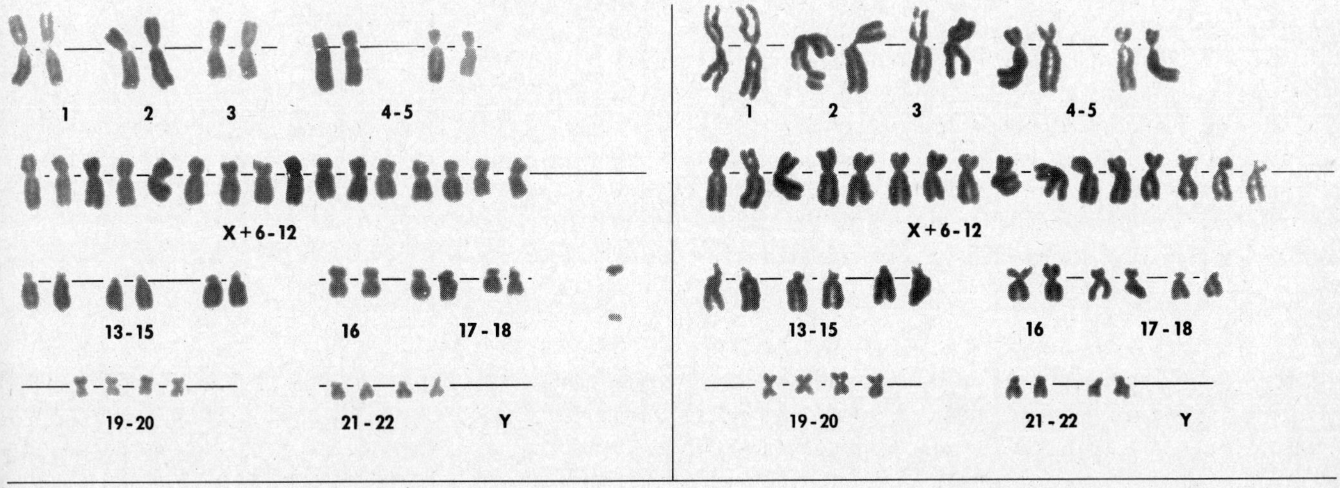

child was conceived. Although the child's congenital defects cannot definitely be attributed to the father's immunosuppression, the defects are similar to those reported by Githens et al in mice.[7] Chromosome studies were not reported.

The findings in the present case are consistent with much of the available data. The appearance of chromosome damage in the infant may indicate that azathioprine crosses the placental barrier in man since no other potential mutagen could be found. The disappearance of the abnormalities seen in the later studies, consistent with Jensen's findings,[12-14] supports this hypothesis. The only other suggestion of toxicity of azathioprine to the human fetus is her birth weight. Although the number of patients is far too small for statistical analysis, this infant and those reported in the literature have tended to weigh less than average for newborns.

We cannot explain the disappearance of chromosome abnormalities in the mother on the second study. Our preliminary studies of chromosomes from peripheral blood of other kidney transplant patients on a regimen of azathioprine indicate that abnormalities occur but may disappear in subsequent studies. The failure to obtain satisfactory growth in the second study on the mother may be an effect of azathioprine, but no conclusion is possible at this time.

Two problems are raised by this case. First, although the chromosome abnormalities found in peripheral blood subsides with time, such abnormalities may persist in tissues not studied. In particular, the primordial ova which have undergone haploid division by birth are of interest. If chromosome damage has occurred here, it might well be responsible for the occurrence of abnormalities in the next generation.

Second, the question of the possible subsequent development of cancer both in the transplant recipient and her child must be raised. Recent reports[18] and our own experience indicate that there may be increased incidence of neoplasm in transplant patients. Boveri, in 1914, postulated that chromosome abnormalities were important in the etiology of malignancies[19] and there are many subsequent reports of chromosome abnormalities related to many types of tumors.[20] Azathioprine, 100 mg/kg, administered three times a week for four weeks to NZB mice, resulted in the development of malignant lymphomas.[21] The chromosome damage reported here, which appears to result from azathioprine administration, might provide a clue to the mechanism of the occurrence of neoplasms in transplant patients. The relationship of mutagens, such as azathioprine, to carcinogenesis must be further explored.

Summary

Chromosomal damage was found in peripheral blood lymphocyte cultures obtained at birth from the child of a kidney transplant recipient on a regimen of azathioprine. Subsequently the changes disappeared. Chromosome abnormalities were also found in the transplant recipient. The findings are consistent with the available reports of the effects of azathioprine and bring to light the problem of persistent damage to the infants' chromosomes and the relationship of chromosome damage to cancer.

This investigation was supported in part by Public Health Service Chronic Dialysis Center grant 39466-03-68, training grant 5T1 HE 5619-04, and special project grant from the Maternal and Child Health Service; and by a Birth Defect Center grant from the National Foundation of the March of Dimes.

Nonproprietary and Trade Names of Drugs

Azathioprine—*Imuran.*
Cactinomycin—*Sanamycin.*

References

1. Murray JE, Reid DE, Harrison JH, et al: Successful pregnancies after human renal transplantation. *New Eng J Med* **269**:341-343, 1963.
2. Board JA, Lee HM, Draper DA, et al: Pregnancy following kidney transplantation from a non-twin. *Obstet Gynec* **29**:318-323, 1967.
3. Kaufman JJ, Dignam W, Goodwin WE, et al: Successful, normal childbirth after kidney homotransplantation. *JAMA* **200**:338-341, 1967.
4. Whitsell JC, Merkatz IR, Tunner WS, et al: Growth, development and fertility following kidney transplantation, in *Abstracts of the American Society of Nephrology*, 1969, p 74.
5. Thiersch JB: Effect of 6-(1'-methyl-4' nitro-5' imidazolyl)-mercaptopurine on the rat litter in utero. *J Reprod Fertil* **4**:297-312, 1962.
6. Murray JE, Sheil AG, Moseley R, et al: Analysis of mechanism of immunosuppressive drugs in renal homotransplantation. *Ann Surg* **160**:449-470, 1964.
7. Githens JH, Rosenkrantz JG, Tunnock SM: Teratogenic effects of azathioprine (Imuran). *J Pediat* **66**:959-961, 1965.
8. Tuchmann-Duplessis H, Mercier-Parot L: Reactions prouoquees chez l'embryon par deux antimetabolites chimiquement voisins. *Bull Schweiz Akad Med Wiss* **22**:153-165, 1966.
9. Gillibrand PN: Systemic lupus erythematosus in pregnancy treated with azathioprine. *Proc Roy Soc Med* **59**:834, 1966.
10. Powell D: Pregnancy in active chronic hepatitis on immunosuppressive therapy. *Postgrad Med J* **45**:292-295, 1969.
11. Moorhead PS, Nowell PG, Mellman WJ, et al: Chromosome preparations of leukocytes cultured from human peripheral blood. *Exp Cell Res* **20**:613-616, 1960.
12. Jensen MK, Soborg M: Chromosome aberrations in human cells following treatment with Imuran. *Acta Med Scand* **179**:249-250, 1966.
13. Jensen MK: Chromosome studies in patients treated with azathioprine and amethipterin. *Acta Med Scand* **182**:445-455, 1967.
14. Jensen MK: Effect of azathioprine on the chromosome complement of human bone marrow cells. *Intern J Cancer* **5**:147-151, 1970.
15. Eberle P, Honstein W, Perings E: Chromosomes in patients treated with Imuran. *Humangenetik* **6**:69-73, 1968.
16. Biesele JJ: Chemically induced imitations of mitotic anomalies common to cancer cells. *Ann NY Acad Sci* **71**:1054, 1958.
17. Tallent MD, Simmonds RI, Nojarian JS: Birth defects in child of male recipient of kidney transplant. *JAMA* **211**:1854-1855, 1970.
18. Penn I: Malignant lymphomas in transplantation patients: A review of the world experience. *Int J Clin Pharmacol* **3**:49-54, 1970.
19. Boveri TH: *Zur Frage der Erstehung Maligner Tumoren*. Jena, Gustave Fischer, 1914.
20. Miles CP: Chromosomal alterations in cancer. *Med Clin N Amer* **50**:875-885, 1966.
21. Casey TP: Azathioprine (Imuran) administration and the development of malignant lymphomas in NZB mice. *Clin Exp Immun* **3**:305, 1968.

Bradycardic Rhythms During Peritoneal Dialysis

LCDR Edwin A. Rutsky, MC, USNR, Portsmouth, Va

Peritoneal dialysis has been utilized extensively in the management of patients with acute and chronic renal failure and in acute drug intoxication. Although many of the hazards of this procedure have been discussed in detail,[1-6] the occurrence of vagal-induced bradycardia and hypotension have been mentioned only briefly.[2,7,8] That serious and life-threatening arrhythmias may be produced by peritoneal dialysis-induced vagotonia has not been emphasized. This report stresses the potentially serious nature of such arrhythmias observed during the performance of peritoneal dialysis in three patients.

Patient Summaries

PATIENT 1.—A 54-year-old woman was admitted to the Portsmouth Naval Hospital in December 1969 following the onset of pericarditis associated with chronic renal failure. Physical examination showed the blood pressure to be 136/92 mm Hg and the pulse rate, 94 beats per minute. Moderate cardiomegaly and a typical three-component pericardial friction rub were present. Pitting edema was present in the lower extremities. The blood urea nitrogen (BUN) value was 58 mg/100 ml and the serum creatinine value, 8.0 mg/100 ml. An electrocardiogram demonstrated increased left ventricular voltage and nonspecific ST-segment changes. The chest roentgenogram showed generalized cardiomegaly.

Peritoneal dialysis was performed via a stylet catheter. The procedure, which was uneventful, was repeated ten days later. The serum electrolyte level was normal at that time. Incomplete drainage of dialysate from the abdomen led to progressive abdominal distention during the second dialysis. While the dialysis catheter was being repositioned, the patient complained of abdominal pain and became cyanotic and acutely short of breath. Concomitantly, the radial pulse decreased from 80 to 15 beats per minute and became irregular. Intravenous administration of 0.5 mg of atropine sulfate accelerated the pulse rate to 100 beats per minute within 30 seconds. An electrocardiogram subsequently demonstrated a sinus tachycardia. The results of physical examination and the chest roentgenogram were unchanged. The dialysis was continued, after replacement of the catheter, without any immediate cardiac arrhythmia. The patient suffered a cardiac arrest later that day and died. No evidence of a myocardial infarction or pulmonary embolus was found at postmortem examination. The heart was enlarged and revealed fibrinous pericarditis and moderate focal coronary arteriosclerosis.

PATIENT 2.—A 19-year-old woman was admitted to the Portsmouth Naval Hospital in February 1970 because of abdominal pain and intractable vomiting. Physical examination showed the blood pressure to be 142/92 mm Hg and the pulse rate, 94 beats per minute. Extensive exudates were present in the optic fundi. The results of the remainder of the examination were unremarkable. At the time of admission the BUN value was 107 mg/100 ml and the serum creatinine level was 16 mg/100 ml.

Peritoneal dialysis was performed twice using a stylet catheter. Following the second dialysis, bilateral pulmonary infiltrates and arterial hypoxemia necessitated endotracheal intubation and mechanical ventilatory assistance. The arterial oxygen tension ranged between 40 and 50 mm Hg while the patient received 100% oxygen. In order to facilitate mechanical ventilation, she received 16 mg of morphine sulfate intravenously during a four-hour period. Thirty minutes after the last dose of morphine was given, her blood pressure fell to 72/42 mm Hg and an idioventricular rhythm developed (heart rate, 40 beats per minute). Intravenous administration of nalorphine hydrochloride (3.0 mg), epinephrine (1.0 ml of 1:10,000 epinephrine), and atropine sulfate (1.0 mg) restored the blood pressure to 100/60 mm Hg and reestablished a normal sinus rhythm (heart rate, 70 beats per minute). A third peritoneal dialysis was begun shortly thereafter. With infusion of 1,500 ml of dialysis fluid, bradycardia again occurred and progressed to complete cardiac standstill. Resuscitative efforts restored a normal sinus rhythm but the patient later developed diffuse intravascular coagulation and died. Autopsy disclosed focal myocarditis with necrosis in an otherwise normal heart.

PATIENT 3.—A 27-year-old woman was admitted to the Portsmouth Naval Hospital in March 1960 after apparently having ingested 25 acetaminophen tablets. Physical examination showed a confused, agitated woman with a blood pressure of 120/86 mm Hg, a pulse rate of 120 beats per minute, and a respiratory rate of 36 per minute. Laboratory studies included determination of serum electrolytes which showed a sodium value of 137 mEq/liter; potassium value, 4.5 mEq/liter; and chloride value, 110 mEq/liter. The carbon dioxide content was undetectable. The arterial pH was 6.92 and the arterial CO_2 tension was 0 mm Hg. The BUN value was 8 mg/100 ml, the blood glucose level was 350 mg/100 ml, and the undiluted serum was trace-positive for acetone.

The serum potassium level fell to 1.4 mEq/liter after initial parenteral therapy with insulin, sodium bicarbonate, and potassium chloride. The patient required resuscitation on two occasions because of cardiac asystole and ventricular fibrillation. Endotracheal intubation was performed and mechanical ventilatory assistance was utilized thereafter. Morphine sulfate was given intravenously (total dose, 14 mg in 24 hours) to improve mechanical ventilation. Potassium chloride was given parenterally until the serum potassium level rose to 3.9 mEq/liter. However, the serum potassium progressively increased to a peak level of 9.6 mEq/liter and the blood glucose rose to 1,600 mg/100 ml. The cardiac rhythm changed from a sinus tachycardia to an atrioventricular (A-V) junctional (or sinoventricular) rhythm. Peritoneal dialysis was begun in an effort to control the hy-

Received for publication July 29, 1970; accepted Feb 8, 1971.

From the Department of Medicine, Naval Hospital, Portsmouth, Va.

The opinions or assertions contained herein are those of the author and are not to be construed as official or reflecting the views of the Navy Department or the Naval Service at large.

Reprint requests to Department of Medicine, Division of Nephrology, University of Alabama Medical Center, Birmingham, Ala 35233 (Dr. Rutsky).

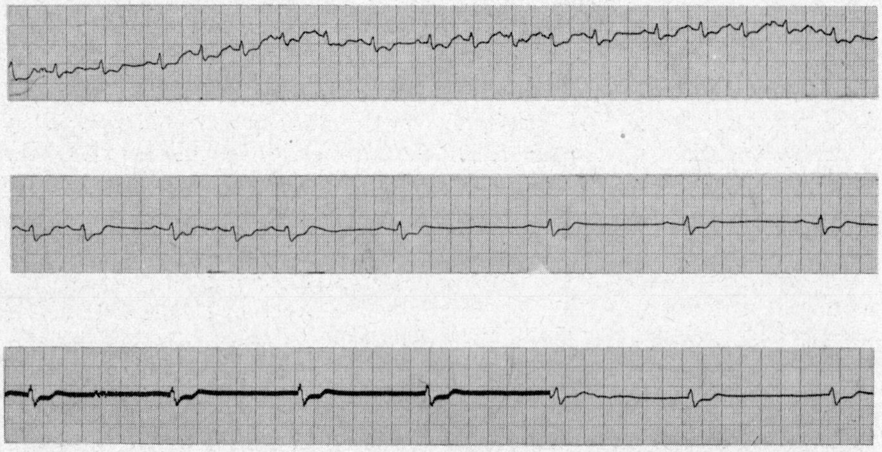

Patient 3. Top, *Rhythm strip showing an irregular sinus tachycardia just prior to infusion of dialysis fluid into the abdomen.* Middle, *Rhythm strip several minutes after* top. *Dialysis fluid infusing into the abdominal cavity was accompanied by the development of sinus bradycardia.* Bottom, *Rhythm strip just after* middle. *Development of an A-V junctional rhythm during the infusion of dialysis fluid into the abdomen.*

perkalemia. Atropine sulfate (0.2 mg) was given intravenously before the dialysis catheter was inserted. An idioventricular rhythm developed five minutes after infusion of the first 2 liters of dialysis fluid. A second intravenous dose of 1.0 mg of atropine sulfate did not affect the heart rate and cardiac asystole ensued. The abdomen was drained of dialysate during resuscitation and a cardiac rhythm was reestablished (sinus tachycardia). When dialysis fluid was again infused into the abdomen, a slow A-V junctional rhythm was produced (Figure) in spite of another intravenous dose of 1.0 mg atropine sulfate. Dialysis was discontinued because of the unstable cardiac rhythm. The patient died several hours later after still another episode of cardiac asystole. The heart was normal at postmortem examination.

Comment

Vasovagal phenomena have been observed previously during the performance of peritoneal dialysis. Hager and Merrill described a patient in whom bradycardia and hypotension developed each time dialysis fluid was infused into the abdomen, and they suggested that this might be prevented by the administration of atropine.[8] Similarly, Miller and Tassistro stated that vagal-induced bradycardia or hypotension may complicate peritoneal dialysis.[2]

The physiological control of cardiac rhythmicity and the results of vagal nerve stimulation upon cardiac conduction have been reviewed extensively.[9] Vagal-induced bradyarrhythmias may be of serious consequence. Bradycardia per se may cause a significant reduction in the cardiac output[10] and there is evidence that vagal nerve stimulation may depress ventricular function in the dog, even when the fall in heart rate is prevented by atropine.[11,12] When conduction and hemodynamic changes are extreme, the result may be syncope of either the Stokes-Adams[13] or vasodepressor[14-17] variety.

There is ample evidence that reflex bradycardia, other cardiac arrhythmias, and hypotension may result from manipulation of the gastrointestinal tract,[18-23] distention of the abdominal cavity,[23] or irritation of the peritoneum.[24] Increased vagal tone at least is a contributing factor in the production of such arrhythmias since they frequently may be abolished or prevented by atropine.[21,23,24]

Peritoneal dialysis may activate the vagus nerve by similar mechanisms. Abdominal distention is an obvious occurrence. Peritoneal irritation may result immediately from the direct trauma of inserting the peritoneal stylet catheter and subsequently from either chemical[6] or bacterial peritonitis.[2,6] In addition, the emotional reaction of the patient, by itself, may trigger a vasodepressor response.[14]

The effects of vagal stimulation upon the heart may be influenced by a number of other factors encountered frequently in patients who require peritoneal dialysis. Underlying heart disease, as in patient 1, may accentuate the hemodynamic changes of bradycardia. Stokes-Adams attacks are more apt to result from increased vagal tone when anatomic abnormalities of the conduction system are present.[13]

Morphine may contribute to the development of vagal-induced bradyarrhythmias (patients 2 and 3). The vagomimetic action of morphine has been observed especially in the setting of acute myocardial infarction[10] but also in the experimental animal.[25,26] While similar effects have not been found in normal individuals or in patients with aortic valve disease,[27,28] it is possible that morphine has a significant vagomimetic action only in a setting conducive to vagotonia, such as peritoneal dialysis.

Hyperkalemia is a well-known depressant of cardiac pacemaker tissue.[9,29] Hyperkalemia also has been shown to potentiate the depressor effects of experimental vagal stimulation upon sinoatrial (S-A)[25,26] and A-V conduction.[26] Thus, it is possible that hyperkalemia and the vagomimetic action of morphine had impaired S-A and A-V automaticity when dialysis was initiated in patient 3. The initial small does of atropine may have accentuated the conduction abnormality even further.[30] The sequence of events suggests that additional vagotonia induced by peritoneal dialysis on two occasions produced progressive bradycardia and cardiac asystole which could not be prevented by large amounts of atropine.

Peritoneal dialysis is used often in the management of patients similar to those described in this report. Such patients frequently have myocardial disease and severe electrolyte and acid-base imbalance, and they often receive morphine. All of these factors may heighten cardiac responsiveness to reflex vagal stimulation. Many of these patients may receive digitalis which, by its vagal stimulatory effects[31] and direct actions upon the heart, may worsen the results of reflex vagotonia.

The bradyarrhythmias which may occur are potentially lethal and do not always respond to usual doses of atropine. The physician and paramedical personnel in attendance should be aware of this complication of peritoneal dialysis and appropriate resuscitative equipment should be readily available. Constant monitoring of the cardiac rhythm may be advisable in selected patients. Occasionally, hemodialysis may be preferable when unstable bradyarrhythmias occur with peritoneal dialysis.

Summary

Serious bradyarrhythmias were observed during the course of peritoneal dialysis in three patients. In each patient, the arrhythmia appeared in conjunction with abdominal distention by dialysis fluid or during the course of manipulation of the dialysis catheter. The arrhythmias were due in part to reflex-vagotonia since the bradycardia was rapidly abolished in one patient by atropine. The evidence that the vagus nerves play an important role in the genesis of such arrhythmias is discussed. Additional factors such as underlying myocardial disease, administration or morphine sulfate, and hyperkalemia may increase the susceptibility of the heart to the effects of reflex vagal stimulation. Vagal-induced bradyarrhythmias probably occur more frequently during peritoneal dialysis than has previously been recognized.

References

1. Barry KG, Schwartz FD, Hano JE, et al: Peritoneal dialysis: Current applications and recent developments, in Schreiner GE (co-ordinating ed), Becker EL (ed): *Proceedings of the Third International Congress of Nephrology, Washington, DC, 1966: Clinical Nephrology.* Basel, S Karger AG, 1967, vol 3, pp 288-304.

2. Miller RB, Tassistro CR: Peritoneal dialysis. *New Eng J Med* **281**:945-949, 1969.

3. Levin S, Winkelstein JA: Diet and infrequent peritoneal dialysis in chronic anuric uremia. *New Eng J Med* **277**:619-624, 1967.

4. Lasker N, Shalhoub R, Habibe O, et al: Management of end-stage kidney disease with intermittent peritoneal dialysis. *Ann Intern Med* **62**:1147-1169, 1965.

5. Palmer RA, Newell JE, Gray EJ, et al: Treatment of chronic renal failure by prolonged peritoneal dialysis. *New Eng J Med* **274**:248-254, 1966.

6. Maher JF, Schreiner GE: Hazards and complications of dialysis. *New Eng J Med* **273**:370-377, 1965.

7. Ribot S, Jacobs MG, Frankel HJ, et al: Complications of peritoneal dialysis. *Amer J Med Sci* **252**:505-517, 1966.

8. Hager EB, Merrill JP: Peritoneal dialysis and acute renal failure. *Surg Clin N Amer* **43**:883-896, 1963.

9. Hoffman BF, Cranefield PF: The physiological basis of cardiac arrhythmias. *Amer J Med* **37**:670-684, 1964.

10. Zipes DP: The clinical significance of bradycardic rhythms in acute myocardial infarction. *Amer J Cardiol* **24**:814-825, 1969.

11. Sarnoff SJ, Brockman SK, Gilmore JP, et al: Regulation of ventricular contraction: Influence of cardiac sympathetic and vagal nerve stimulation on atrial and ventricular dynamics. *Circ Res* **8**:1108-1122, 1960.

12. Daggett WM, Nugent GC, Carr PW, et al: Influence of vagal stimulation on ventricular contractility, O_2 consumption and coronary flow. *Amer J Physiol* **212**:8-18, 1967.

13. Pomerantz B, O'Rourke RA: The Stokes-Adams syndrome. *Amer J Med* **46**:941-960, 1969.

14. Stead EA Jr: Fainting. *Amer J Med* **13**:387-388, 1952.

15. Weissler AM, Warren JV, Estes EH Jr, et al: Vasodepressor syncope, factors influencing cardiac output. *Circulation* **15**:875-882, 1957.

16. Greene MA, Boltax AJ, Ulberg RJ: Cardiovascular dynamics of vasovagal reactions in man. *Circ Res* **9**:12-17, 1961.

17. Glick G, Yu PN: Hemodynamic changes during spontaneous vasovagal reactions. *Amer J Med* **34**:42-51, 1963.

18. Maher CC, Crittenden PJ, Shapiro PF: An electrocardiographic study of viscerocardiac reflexes during major operations. *Amer Heart J* **9**:664-676, 1934.

19. Reid LC, Stephenson HE Jr, Hinton JW: Cardiac arrest. *Arch Surg* **64**:409-420, 1952.

20. Stephenson HE Jr, Reid LC, Hinton JW: Some common denominators in 1,200 cases of cardiac arrest. *Ann Surg* **137**:731-744, 1953.

21. Smith BH: The nature and treatment of the coeliac plexus reflex in man. *Lancet* **2**:223-227, 1953.

22. Mendelsohn D Jr, Monheit R: Electrocardiographic and blood pressure changes during and after biliary-tract surgery. *New Eng J Med* **254**:307-313, 1956.

23. Gilbert NC, Fenn GK, LeRoy GV: The effect of distention of abdominal viscera on the coronary blood flow and on angina pectoris. *JAMA* **115**:1962-1967, 1940.

24. Weissler AM, Warren JV: Syncope and shock, in Hurst JW, Logue RB (eds): *The Heart.* New York, McGraw-Hill Book Co Inc, 1970, p 542.

25. Feigenbaum H, Wunsch CM, Fisch C: Interrelationship of potassium and vagal action on the sinoatrial pacemaker and on atrioventricular conduction. *J Clin Invest* **44**:399-405, 1965.

26. Fisch C, Knoebel SB, Feigenbaum H, et al: Potassium and the monophasic action potential, electrocardiogram, conduction and arrhythmias. *Progr Cardiovasc Dis* **8**:387-418, 1966.

27. Jaffe JH: Narcotic analgesics, in Goodman LS, Gilman A (eds): *The Pharmacological Basis of Therapeutics.* New York, Macmillan Co, 1965, pp 255-256.

28. Lowenstein E, Hallowell P, Levine FH, et al: Cardiovascular response to large doses of intravenous morphine in man. *New Eng J Med* **281**:1389-1393, 1969.

29. Surawicz B: Relationship between electrocardiogram and electrolytes. *Amer Heart J* **73**:814-834, 1967.

30. Innes IR, Nickerson M: Drugs inhibiting the action of acetylcholine on structures innervated by postganglionic parasympathetic nerves (antimuscarinic or atropinic drugs), in Goodman LS, Gilman A (eds): *The Pharmacological Basis of Therapeutics.* New York, Macmillan Co, 1965, p 527.

31. Moe GK, Farah AE: Digitalis and allied cardiac glycosides, in Goodman LS, Gilman A (eds): *The Pharmacological Basis of Therapeutics.* New York, Macmillan Co, 1965, pp 673-683.

Effect of Bilateral Nephrectomy in Postpartum Nephrosclerosis

Charlotte C. Erickson, MD;
Michael D. Lagios, MD;
Patricia Schoenfeld, MD;
and Richard J. Cohen, MD,
San Francisco

Several recent reports have called attention to a newly recognized syndrome of irreversible postpartum renal failure and microangiopathic hemolytic anemia that develops following normal pregnancy.[1-6] The cause of renal failure and its relationship to the accompanying hemolysis remain unknown. A patient with this syndrome eventually required bilateral nephrectomy for control of malignant hypertension. The pathologic findings and postoperative course in this case suggest that the renal abnormalities may play a prominent role in the production of the fragmented red blood cells and hemolysis observed in this syndrome.

Received for publication Aug 12, 1970; accepted Oct 28.

From the medical, the clinical pathology, and laboratory medicine services, San Francisco General Hospital and the departments of medicine and clinical pathology and laboratory medicine, University of California School of Medicine, San Francisco.

Reprint requests to Editorial Office, San Francisco General Hospital, 1001 Potrero Ave, San Francisco 94110.

Patient Summary

A 20-year-old woman in the eighth month of her first pregnancy was hospitalized in December 1968, for evaluation of proteinuria. Mild proteinuria, ankle edema, and a hematocrit value of 30% were first noted in August 1968, during her first trimester of pregnancy. Blood pressure at that time was 110/70 mm Hg. Treatment with a low sodium diet, vitamins, oral diuretics, folic acid, and parenteral iron failed to produce significant improvement. The patient had no previous history of renal disease or anemia. Physical examination on admission revealed a moderately obese female in the 35th week of pregnancy. Blood pressure was 130/80 mm Hg. A trace of pedal edema was present bilaterally; no other abnormalities were noted. Laboratory tests yielded the following values: hemoglobin, 9.2 gm/100 ml; hematocrit, 26%; white blood cell count (WBC), 12,300/cu mm with normal differential count; reticulocytes, 0.05%; serum iron, 95μg/100 ml; iron binding capacity, 360μg/100 ml. A fluorescent spot test

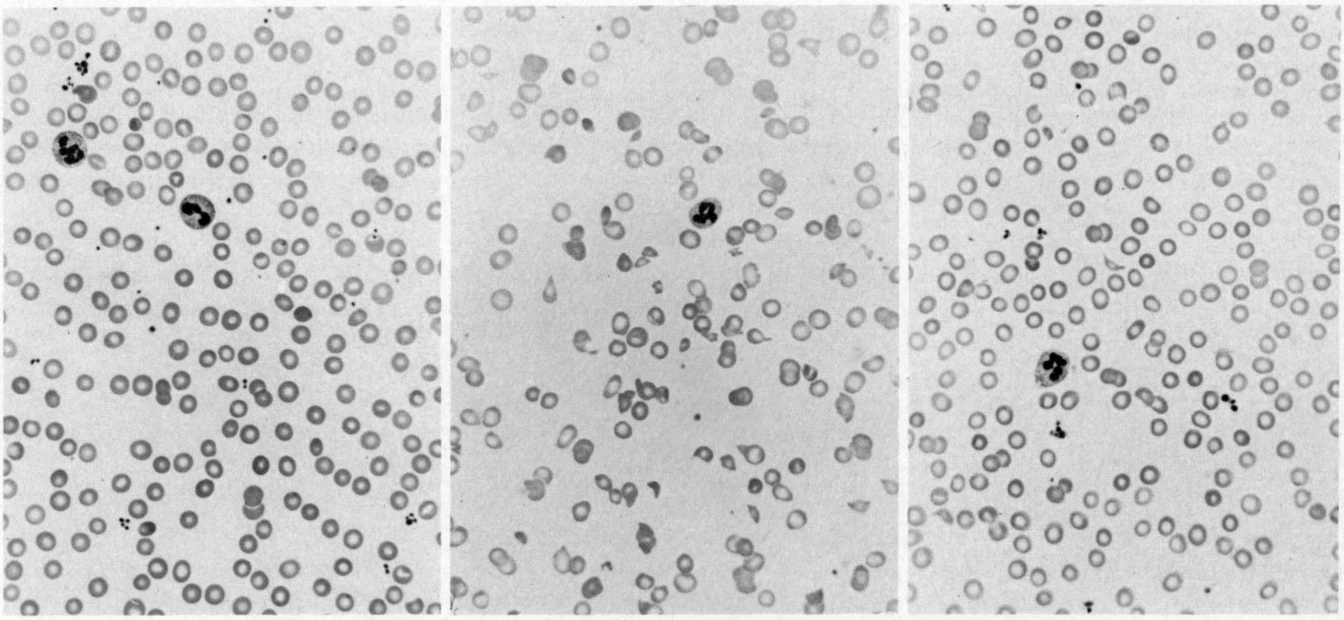

Fig 1.—Peripheral blood smears. Left, *Eighth month of pregnancy.* Center, *Six weeks postpartum.* Right, *Five days following bilateral nephrectomy (Wright's stain, ×400).*

for glucose-6-phosphate dehydrogenase activity yielded normal values and sickle cell preparations were negative.

Peripheral blood smears showed normal red blood cell morphology (Fig 1, *left*). Sternal bone marrow aspirate showed mild erythroid hypoplasia. Iron stores were slightly reduced. Urinalysis revealed a specific gravity of 1.020, proteinuria (2+), and two to three red and white blood cells per high-power field. Blood urea nitrogen (BUN) level was 6 mg/100 ml; serum creatinine value, 0.6 mg/100 ml; and creatinine clearance, 157 ml/min; 24-hour urinary protein excretion was 920 mg. Urine cultures repeatedly showed no growth.

The patient was discharged and followed in the clinic during the remainder of her pregnancy; no change in anemia or proteinuria occurred. Neither hypertension nor clinical evidence of toxemia were noted. On Jan 26, 1969, a normal female infant was delivered without complication and the patient was discharged on the fourth postpartum day at which time the hematocrit level was 32%.

The patient was rehospitalized on Feb 21, because of nausea, vomiting, generalized edema, and oliguria. The patient was notably pale and lethargic. Blood pressure was 156/108 mm Hg and pulse rate 108 beats/min. Advanced periorbital and pretibial edema were present. Funduscopic examination showed arteriolar narrowing without exudate or hemorrhage. Laboratory values were as follows: hemoglobin, 5.4 gm/100 ml; hematocrit, 18%; red blood cell count, 2×10^6/cu mm; reticulocytes, 18%; platelets, 192,000/cu mm; and WBC, 11,500/cu mm with a differential count of 89% mature neutrophils, 1% band neutrophils, 3% eosinophils, and 7% lymphocytes. The peripheral blood smear (Fig 1, *center*) showed marked anisocytosis and poikilocytosis with numerous schistocytes, burr cells, and spherocytes. Urinalysis demonstrated a specific gravity of 1.007; pH, 5.0; and proteinuria (3+). There were 75 to 100 white blood cells per high-power field with numerous granular and hyaline casts. Urine output averaged less than 250 ml per day. Direct and indirect Coombs' tests were negative. Serum analysis showed a lactic dehydrogenase level of 616 international units (IU) (upper normal limit, 116 IU) with marked elevation of fraction 1. Blood urea nitrogen level was 181 mg/100 ml and creatinine level was 43.6 mg/100 ml. Serum glutamic oxaloacetic transaminase, total proteins and albumin/globulin ratio, sodium, potassium, chloride, carbon dioxide combining power, and calcium values were within normal limits as were the prothrombin time and partial thromboplastin time. Antinuclear antibody tests and lupus erythematosus (LE) cell preparations were negative. Latex-bound antifibrinogen test (Fi Test) for serum fibrin degradation products (FDP) was negative. Assay[7] of FDP by the tanned red blood cell hemagglutination immunoinhibition technique[8] was less than 8μg/ml on repeated occasions (normal = less than 8μg/ml). Reexamination of the bone marrow demonstrated marked erythroid hyperplasia with normal activity of other marrow elements.

Retrograde pyelograms obtained soon after admission showed no evidence of ureteral obstruction and tomograms revealed normal-sized kidneys. Anuria and hemolytic anemia with severe red blood cell fragmentation continued despite numerous transfusions and full supportive measures. On Feb 28, a Scribner shunt was inserted and hemodialysis was begun and repeated three times a week. Blood pressure was controlled at normotensive levels with methyldopa (250 mg, three times daily) and phenobarbital (32 mg, four times daily). Open renal biopsy was performed on March 13, without complication. On March 21, repeated grand mal convulsions and mental stupor developed. Blood pressure was 190/130 mm Hg

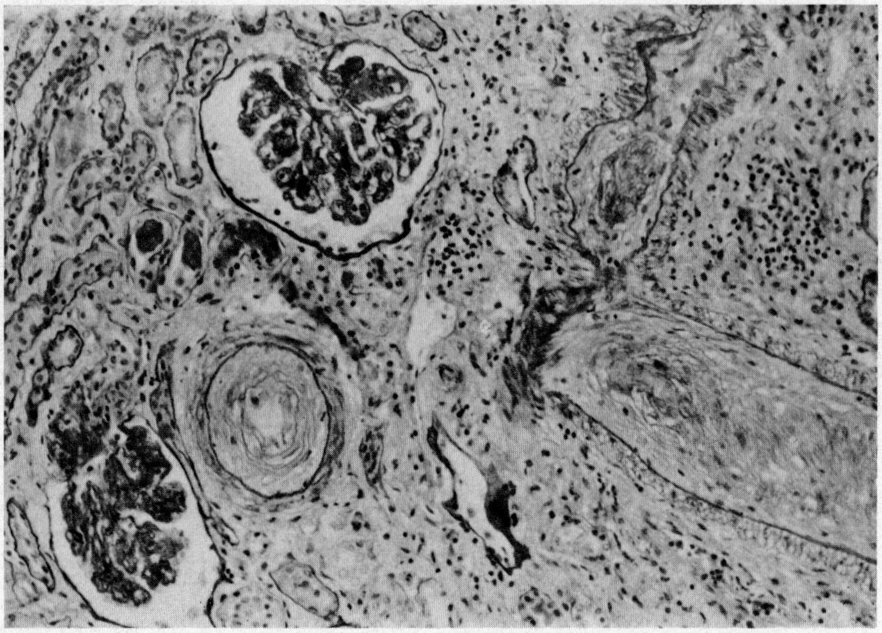

Fig 2.—Nephrectomy specimen demonstrating two obsolescent glomeruli with ischemic collapsed capillary loops. Intralobular arteries show marked distension of the media by intimal proliferation (performic acid-Schiff stain, ×280).

and could not be controlled with increasing doses of methyldopa (up to 3 gm/day), reserpine parenterally, magnesium sulfate, and more frequent hemodialysis. Funduscopic examination revealed the appearance of bilateral retinal hemorrhage. On March 29, almost two months following delivery, bilateral nephrectomy was performed. Six hours following surgery blood pressure dropped to 110/70 mm Hg and has remained within the normal range without antihypertensive medication since that time. Signs of hemolysis and red blood cell fragmentation disappeared progressively during the first five days after nephrectomy (Fig 1, *right*) and have not recurred. The postoperative hematocrit value remained stable at 34% without any further transfusion requirement. Within two months after surgery, retinal hemorrhage was no longer seen on the dunduscopic examination. Hemodialysis has been performed regularly for 18 months postoperatively on an outpatient basis.

Special Studies

The specimen obtained by open renal biopsy was processed for light and electron microscopy and immunofluorescent antihuman globulin studies immediately after surgical removal. Tissues for electron microscopy were fixed in glutaraldehyde, postfixed in osmium, and embedded in Araldite.

The biopsy specimen contained 26 glomeruli, characterized by collapsed glomerular tufts with shrunken capillary lumens and marked convolutions of the basement membranes. Moderate hilar mesangial proliferation and occasional hyalinization were present. None of the glomeruli was normal and several showed complete hemorrhagic necrosis. No fibrin thrombi were seen. Acute malignant arteriolar nephrosclerosis of arcuate and intralobular vessels was present (Fig 2). These vessels were nearly occluded by edematous concentrically laminated endothelial proliferation. Appropriate histochemical methods revealed considerable acid mucopolysaccharide ground substance but no mature collagen or reduplication of elastic lamella as might be seen in a chronic process and no fibrin was demonstrated. Juxtaglomerular granulation was prominent in nearly every glomerulus where the hilum was visualized. Fibrinogen, IgA, IgG, IgM, and complement component C′3 could not be demonstrated with the appropriate fluorescein-labeled antisera, all of which gave positive reactions in suitable controls.

Electron microscopy of glomeruli demonstrated irregular convoluted basement membranes, mesangial proliferation, and focal endothelial slough. There were no electron-dense deposits or lucencies in the basement membrane. Blood vessels showed endothelial and subendothelial necrosis in many areas. Morphologically identifiable polymerized fibrin was not demonstrable in blood vessels or glomeruli. Specimens from the excised kidneys showed more advanced malignant arteriolar nephrosclerosis with necrosis of afferent arterioles and juxtaglomerular hyperplasia.

Comment

This patient manifests the clinical findings of the newly recognized syndrome described as "irreversible postpartum renal failure,"[2,4,6] "postpartum hemolytic uremic syndrome,"[9] "postpartum malignant nephrosclerosis,"[1,3] and "postpartum malignant hypertension."[9] The syndrome is characterized by a normal pregnancy and delivery followed in a few days to a few weeks by the rapid onset of acute renal failure, hemolytic anemia, and severe hypertension. Ten of 13 reported cases have ended in death. In three of the 13 cases reported previously, proteinuria was noted late in the third trimester but was not accompanied by hypertension, toxemia, or abnormalities of renal function which could suggest the eventual seriousness of the problem. The proteinuria discovered during our patient's eighth month of pregnancy was extensively evaluated, short of renal biopsy, but no other abnormalities of renal function were found. Proteinuria may thus represent an early but nonspecific manifestation of the syndrome.

Hemolytic anemia, characterized by large numbers of severely fragmented red blood cells, microspherocytes, and reticulocytosis (Fig 1, *center*), was an especially prominent clinical feature in our patient. These morphologic abnormalities were noted in all of the reported cases of this syndrome and are identical to the red blood cell changes observed in hemolytic anemia accompanying thrombotic thrombocytopenia purpura, malignant hypertension, acute renocortical necrosis, and acute necrotizing glomerulonephritis. Brain et al[10] suggested that the abnormal red blood cell morphology in this group of disorders might be the result of traumatic contact between red blood cells and the pathologically altered intima of small blood vessels, leading to the general acceptance of the term "microangiopathic hemolytic anemia." The small intralobular arteries and afferent arterioles in the biopsy and nephrectomy specimens from the present case were almost totally occluded by endothelial proliferation (Fig 2). Electron microscope studies showed distorted red blood cells that had dissected beneath denuded endothelial membranes into the perivascular space (Fig 3). Red blood cells being forced through such altered vessels under a sustained elevated blood pressure might well be subjected to the stresses and damage necessary to produce the observed fragmentation and hemolysis.

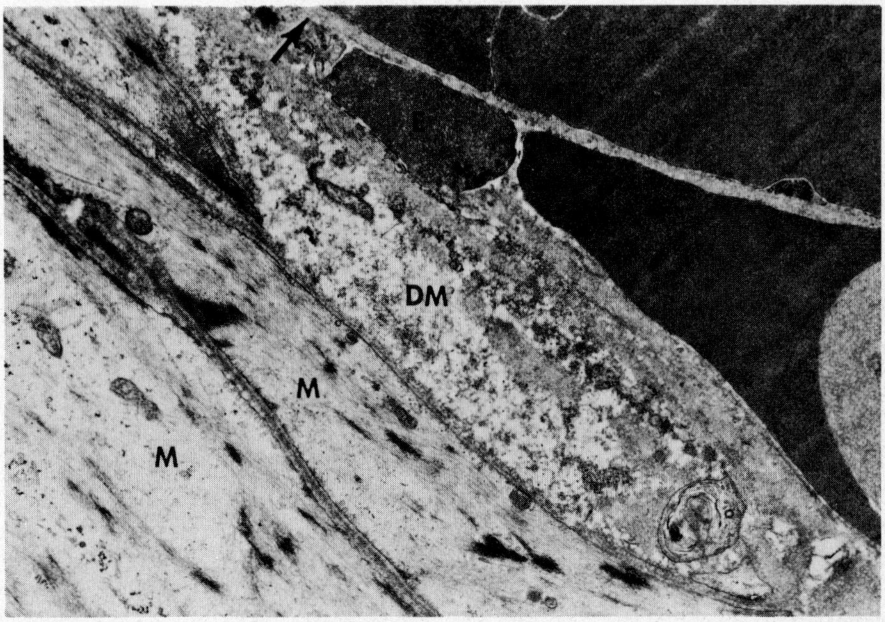

Fig 3.—Electron photomicrograph of degenerating intralobular artery from biopsy specimen showing denuded endothelial basement membranes (arrow), *with two erythrocytes dissecting into perivascular space. Smooth muscle cells immediately adjacent to the vascular surface show degenerative changes (DM), while deeper in the media only compression is evident, (M). Morphologically identifiable fibrin is not evident (scale = 1μ).*

The results of bilateral nephrectomy in our patient suggest that the vascular abnormalities responsible for the erythrocyte deformities and hemolysis are localized to the kidneys. All microangiopathic red blood cell changes disappeared rapidly following the removal of both kidneys and have not recurred in the 16 months since surgery. Similar results were noted by Giromini and Laperrouza[11] in an adult with hemolytic uremic syndrome who underwent bilateral nephrectomy plus splenectomy.

Pathologic examination of the kidneys in previously reported cases of postpartum nephrosclerosis frequently revealed circumferential intimal proliferation in arcuate and intralobular vessels similar to that seen in patients with malignant hypertension, systemic sclerosis, and homograft rejection with no evidence of a primary glomerular lesion. Many specimens from patients in the late phases of postpartum nephrosclerosis showed fibrin thrombi and fibrinoid necrosis of afferent arterioles and the glomerular stalk. This has led to the speculation that fibrin deposition may underlie the fulminant nephrosclerosis, occurring as part of a localized or disseminated intravascular coagulation. Bull and Kuhn[12] suggested that red blood cells passing through small blood vessels to which fibrin strands have become attached are obstructed and torn up by these intravascular strands and thus produced hemolysis and striking morphologic abnormalities. In vitro experiments have demonstrated prominent erythrocyte fragmentation following forced passage of red blood cells through a polymerizing fibrin clot or through special nonfibrin strands.[13] Several investigators have attempted to use heparin in the treatment of this syndrome but have found no obvious beneficial clinical effect.[2,4,6]

Our patient had no evidence of enhanced intravascular coagulation. At no time did the platelet count fall to below 192,000/cu mm. Results of routine coagulation studies were normal throughout the entire course of the disease and quantitative assays for the presence of FDP were repeatedly normal. All surgical specimens, processed with maximal care, showed no fibrin under light and electron microscopy or with fluorescein-labeled antisera to fibrinogen. The repeated failure to demonstrate fibrin thrombosis or fibrinoid material makes it dubious that intravascular coagulation contributed significantly either to the severe microangiopathic hemolytic anemia or to the hypertension and renal failure.

The pathogenesis of the progressive refractory renal failure in this syndrome remains unknown. Rosenmann et al[5] postulated that an autoimmune mechanism might be responsible for the development of this feature and demonstrated the localization of IgG, IgM, and complement component C′3 in the glomeruli of one patient. Immunofluorescent studies of the biopsy specimen in our case failed to demonstrate IgG, IgA, IgM, or C′3 proteins in the glomeruli or vessels.

Since prolonged survival of patients with the postpartum nephrosclerotic syndrome is possible after bilateral nephrectomy the procedure should be considered in those patients whose clinical course is rapidly deteriorating despite vigorous therapy with hemodialysis, antihypertensive drugs, corticosteroids, and heparin. The results of bilateral nephrectomy were dramatic in our patient: fragmented red blood cells almost totally disappeared five days after surgery and the severe hypertension was completely corrected in the immediate postoperative period. Such results implicate the kidneys not only in the pathogenesis of the microangiopathic hemolytic anemia, but also in the pathogenesis of the refractory and malignant hypertension.

Summary

Irreversible acute renal failure, microangiopathic hemolytic anemia, and malignant hypertension developed one month postpartum in a 20-year-old woman. Despite hemodialysis and vigorous attempts to control the hypertension, convulsions and progressive stupor developed necessitating bilateral nephrectomy. Hypertension and microangiopathic hemolytic anemia rapidly disappeared thereafter, suggesting that the abnormalities localized within the kidneys were responsible for these clinical features. The pathogenesis of this fulminant postpartum syndrome is unknown, but enhanced intravascular coagulation with fibrin deposition could not be demonstrated as a significant factor in the production of this patient's renal or hematologic disease. Prolonged survival (18 months to date in the present case) is possible following the performance of bilateral nephrectomy and such action should be considered in those patients showing progressive clinical deterioration.

Nonproprietary and Trade Names of Drug

Methyldopa–*Aldomet.*

References

1. Scheer RL, Jones DB: Malignant nephrosclerosis in women post partum: A not on microangiopathic hemolytic anemia. *JAMA* **201**:600-608, 1967.
2. Robson JS, Martin AM, Ruckley VA, et al: Irreversible post-partum renal failure. *Quart J Med* **37**:423-435, 1968.
3. Wagoner RD, Holley KE, Johnson WJ: Accelerated nephrosclerosis and postpartum acute renal failure in normotensive patients. *Ann Intern Med* **69**:237-248, 1968.
4. Ogg CS, Cameron JS: Post-partum renal failure. *Lancet* **1**:1317, 1969.
5. Rosenmann E, Kanter A, Bacani RA, et al: Fatal late postpartum intravascular coagulation with acute renal failure. *Amer J Med Sci* **257**:259-273, 1969.
6. Clarkson AR, Meadows R, Lawrence JR: Post-partum renal failure: The generalized Shwartzman reaction. *Aust Ann Med* **18**:209-216, 1969.
7. Castelan DJ, Hirsh J, Martin M: Latex-bound antifibrinogen test for plasma fibrinogen assay. *J Clin Path* **21**:638-642, 1968.
8. Merskey C, Lalezari P, Johnson AJ: A rapid, simple, sensitive method for measuring fibrinolytic split products in human serum. *Proc Soc Exp Biol Med* **131**:871-875, 1969.
9. McKay DG: Progress in disseminated intravascular coagulation, pt II. *Calif Med* **111**:279-290, 1969.
10. Brain MC, Dacie JV, Hourihane DO: Microangiopathic haemolytic anaemia: The possible role of vascular lesions in pathogenesis. *Brit J Haemat* **8**:358-374, 1962.
11. Giromini M, Laperrouza AC: Prolonged survival after bilateral nephrectomy in an adult with haemolytic-uraemic syndrome. *Lancet* **2**:169-170, 1969.
12. Bull BS, Kuhn IN: The production of schistocytes by fibrin strands (a scanning electron microscope study). *Blood* **35**:104-111, 1970.
13. Bull BS, Rubenberg ML, Dacie JV, Brain MC: Microangiopathic haemolytic anaemia: Mechanisms of red-cell fragmentation: In vitro studies. *Brit J Haemat* **14**:643-652, 1968.

ECG Analysis No. 2

Premature Atrial Contraction

Douglas P. Zipes, MD, and Charles Fisch, MD, Indianapolis

As was described last month for premature ventricular beats, the interaction of the basic heart rate, the degree of prematurity, and electrophysiologic properties of refractoriness and conduction determine what follows in the wake of any premature impulse. The fact that discharge of a premature atrial contraction (PAC) originates in the atrium affords the impulse greater opportunity to reach the sinus node before the latter can fire. Therefore, a PAC most often disturbs the timing of the sinus node by discharging it and causing the next impulse to begin from that point. One would surmise that this would make the interval between the PAC (P′) and the next normal P wave (P′-P) exactly the same as a normal P-P interval. However, two factors prevent this from occurring. First, the P′-P interval may be lengthened by the time it takes the impulse to discharge the atrium and then travel to, and discharge the pacemaker cells within the sinus node, and reemerge to the atrium (Fig 1). Second, premature discharge of a pacemaker such as the sinus node may depress its rhythmicity and delay its return.[1,2] In general, the earlier this occurs after recovery of excitability the greater the amount of depression produced. The contour of the P wave following a PAC may differ from normal because premature discharge of the sinus node may cause a shift in the pacemaker locus, to another site still within the sinus node itself, or to an ectopic locus, or result in alteration of intra-atrial conduction. In Fig 2, the P′-P interval following the first PAC exceeds the P-P interval by 130 msec, probably owing to depression of the sinus pacemaker by the PAC. Note also the slightly different contour of the two P waves following the PAC. Most likely this indicates a change in intra-atrial conduction because the rate remains the same as the original sinus rate and the pacemaker is thus still within the sinus node. The next PAC occurs later in diastole, does not depress sinus node return, and the P′-P interval is only 10 to 20 msec longer than the P-P interval. Conduction from atrium to sinus node may account for this difference. The third PAC is again early and creates changes similar to the first PAC.

Since the refractory period of the atrioventricular (A-V) node exceeds that of the atria, conduction of a very early PAC may be slowed across the A-V node causing P-R prolongation, or even be completely blocked (Fig 3). In general, a long P′-R interval (indicating retarded A-V conduction) follows a short R-P′ interval (indicating an early PAC, occurring close to the preceding QRS) since A-V conduction proceeds over pathways not yet fully repolarized. It is possible that sinus node-to-atrium conduction (S-A) also lengthens, but the standard ECG does not register sinoatrial conduction. Sometimes an early PAC may not be slowed sufficiently in the A-V node to allow complete ventricular repolarization; the impulse may then be conducted aberrantly over partially repolarized tissue in the ventricles to produce functional bundle branch delays or block (Fig 4). This subject and the effects of cycle length on refractory period will be explored further in later sessions.

Premature systoles may affect conduction of subsequent beats. For example, when multiple PACs occur in succession, an early PAC which discharges the A-V junction but fails to reach the ventricles may slow conduction of the following P wave by leaving a trail of partially repolarized A-V junctional fibers.

An early PAC may conduct slowly through the A-V junction to the ventricles and then return over an alternate pathway to the atria, and produce an atrial "echo" (reciprocal or return extrasystole). In Fig 5, the third P wave is premature and conducts with a long P-R interval. A negative P wave, indicating retrograde atrial activation, follows the QRS (atrial echo) and delays the next sinus node discharge. The second to last P wave in the top ECG conducts with less A-V slowing and does not return to the atria. Sustained reentry of an impulse between atria and A-V nodal region may cause some types of supraventricular tachycardia. Slow conduction through the sinus node also may produce echoes.

Vagal discharge prolongs the refractory period of the sinus node, while shortening that of the atria. Under these circumstances, a PAC may engage the atria but not the sinus node to produce a rather infrequent event, an interpolated PAC.

Received for publication April 20, 1971; accepted April 28.

From the Indiana University Medical Center, Krannert Institute of Cardiology, Indianapolis.

Reprint requests to 1100 W Michigan St, Indianapolis 46202 (Dr. Zipes).

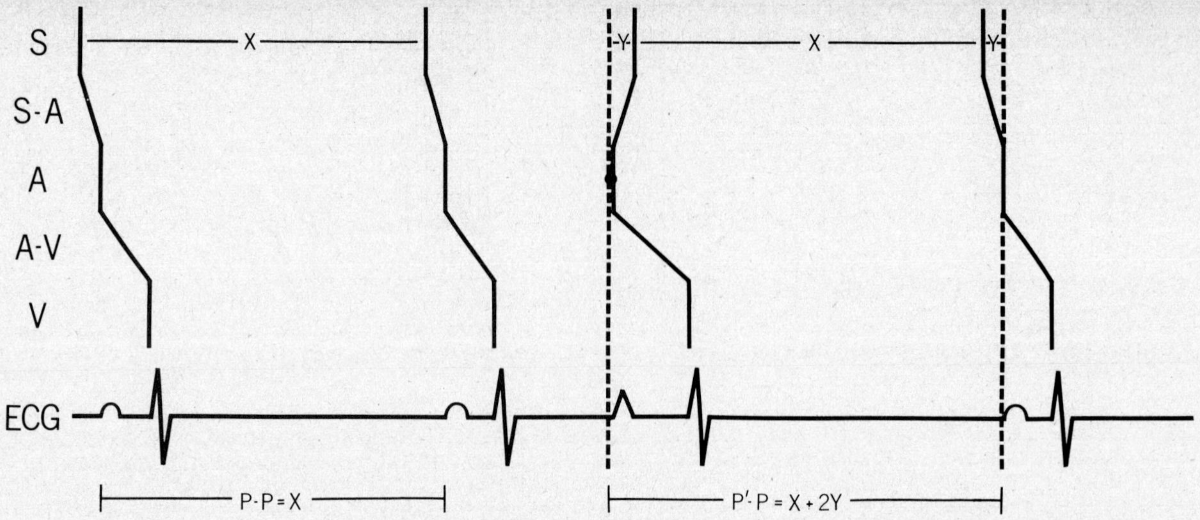

Fig 1.—Diagramatic example of a PAC. Sinus interval equals X msec. Third P wave represents PAC which reaches S-A node Y msec after onset of P wave, discharging sinus node and causing next sinus cycle to begin at that time. Therefore, P'-P interval equals X + 2Y msec. A noncompensatory pause is present.

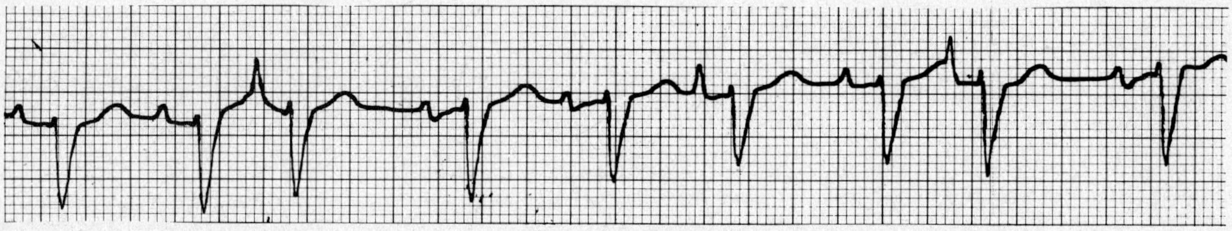

Fig 2.—PAC depressing sinus node discharge. Monitor lead. Sharply pointed P waves represent PACs which, when they occur early, delay return of sinus node. The P'-P interval is much longer than P-P interval. Contour of P waves following early PACs differs from normal P wave, indicating a shift in pacemaker locus or a change in intra-atrial conduction.

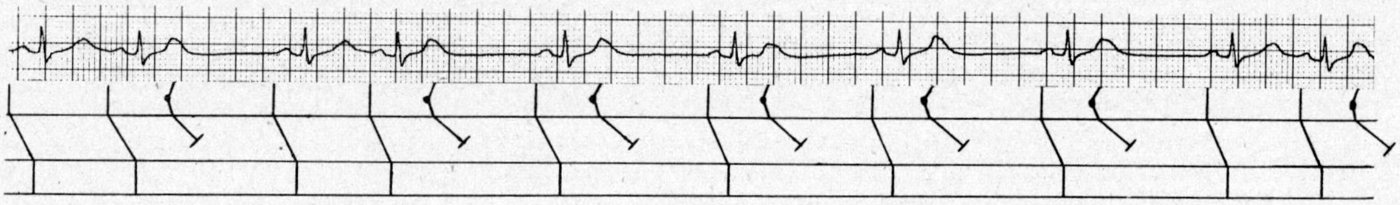

Fig 3.—Nonconducted PACs. Ladder diagram indicates atrial activity, A-V conduction, and ventricular activity. The P wave of a nonconducted PAC lies buried within the T wave of the QRS complexes which precede the pauses. Note difference between normal T waves and those in which a P' hides. When analyzing an arrhythmia displaying an unexpected pause in sinus beating, always search for a PAC buried in the preceding T wave.

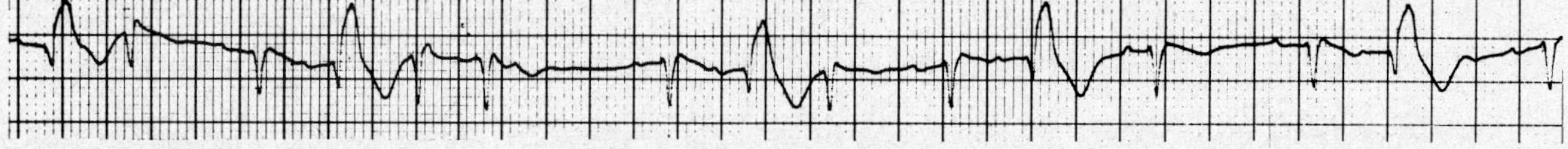

Fig 4.—Aberrantly conducted PACs, lead VI. Multiple PACs occur; those which terminate a short cycle that follows a long cycle have an rsR' configuration because of functional right bundle branch block.

In the top tracing of Fig 6, a sinus P wave follows the PAC at the proper time making the interval between the normal P waves flanking the PAC equal to a normal sinus interval. In the lower tracing, the PAC occurs slightly later and invades the sinus node.

A compensatory pause after a PAC occurs less commonly than a noncompensatory pause, but since either may happen, the length of the pause after a premature systole may not be used conclusively to differentiate a PAC from a premature ventricular beat (Fig 7).

When sinus arrhythmia alters the rhythm or when an escape beat terminates the pause following a PAC, precise interpretation of the electrophysiologic events becomes difficult.

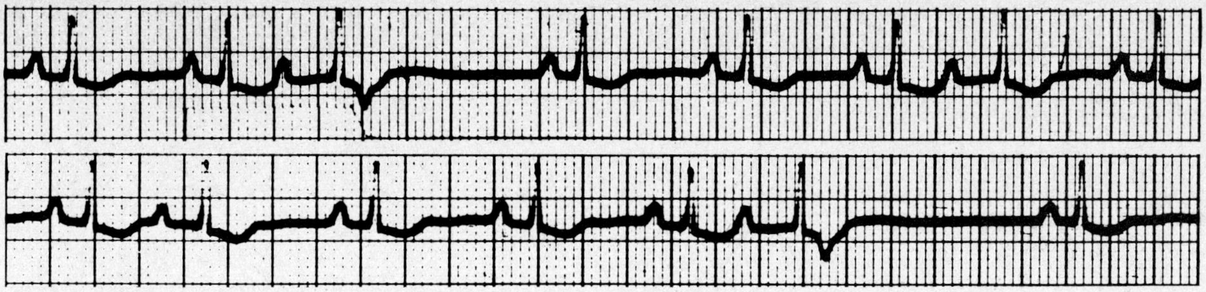

Fig 5.—PAC producing atrial echo beats, lead II. First PAC (top) and last (lower tracing) occur sufficiently close to preceding beat (short R-P′) to conduct with delay across A-V junction (long P′-R). During this slowed conduction, impulse returns to chamber of origin, reexcites atria and produces atrial echo. Other two PACs have slightly longer R-P′ intervals, shorter P′-R intervals, and do not return to atria.

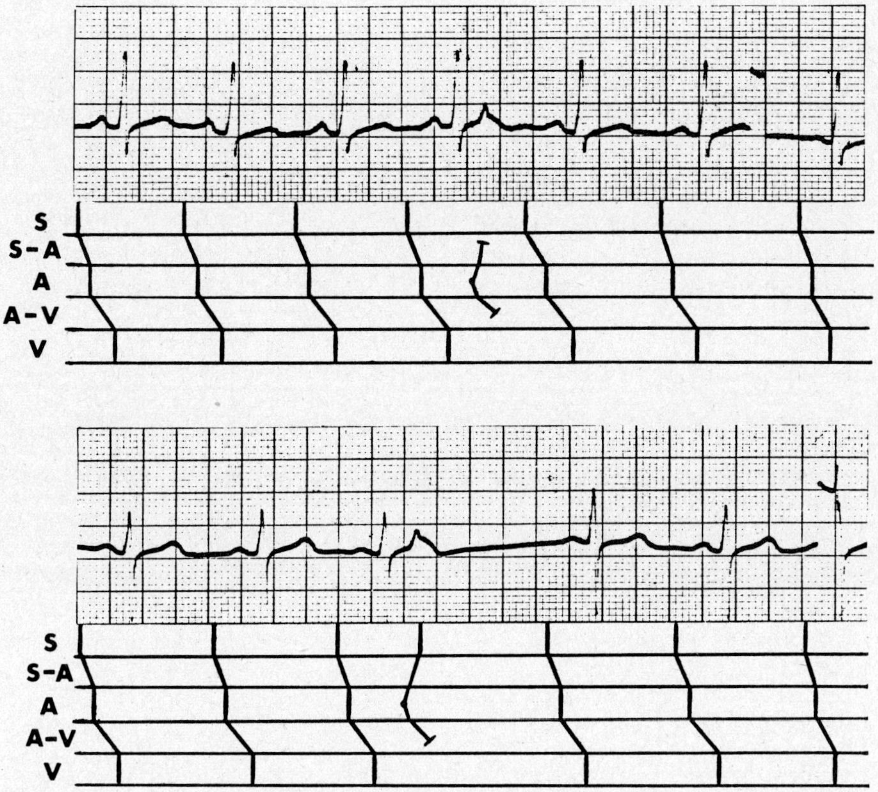

Fig 6.—Interpolated PAC. Top tracing (lead II), PAC does not penetrate sinus node, nor does it reach ventricles. Sinus discharge continues uninterrupted. The S-A conduction of sinus impulse following PAC may be slowed. Slight sinus irregularity is present. Lower tracing (lead III), PAC occurs minimally later and reaches the sinus node to produce a noncompensatory pause.

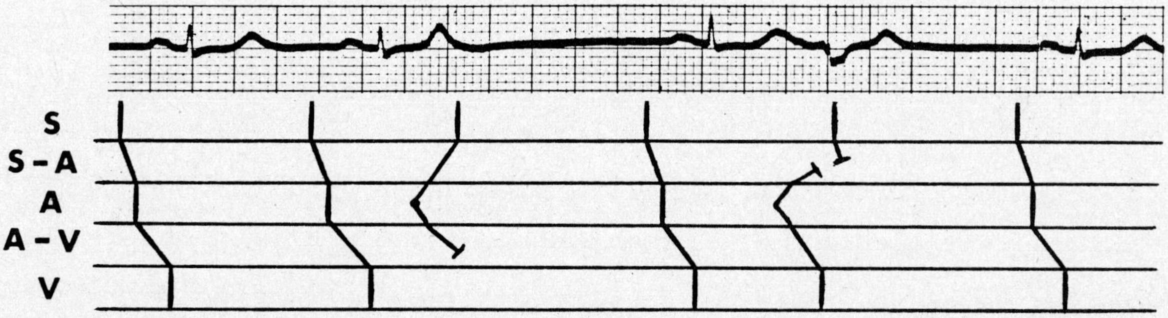

Fig 7.—PAC producing compensatory pause, lead II. First PAC discharges sinus node and initiates noncompensatory pause. Longer coupling interval of second PAC allows sinus node discharge which prevents invasion by PAC. Second PAC conducts aberrantly through ventricles.

References

1. Pick A. Langendorf R, Katz LN: Depression of cardiac pacemakers by premature impulses. *Amer Heart J* **41**:49-57, 1951.

2. Lange G: Action of driving stimuli from intrinsic and extrinsic sources on in situ cardiac pacemaker tissue. *Circ Res* **17**:449-459, 1965.

How to Implement the Weed System

(In Order to Improve Patient Care, Education, and Research by Improving Medical Records)

J. Willis Hurst, MD, Atlanta

Obstacles to implementing the Weed system for improving medical records so as to improve patient care, medical education, and research relate to the acceptance of an innovative system, to the mechanics of the system, and to the creation of an excellent problem list. Obstacles to acceptance and mechanics can be overcome by a small group of interested people who make a sincere effort to influence those around them but the creation of an excellent problem list requires intense work and a thought process that is the essence of a medical education. The method of creating an excellent problem list is discussed.

Lawrence Weed is correct in his views regarding the improvement of patient care, education, and research by improving medical records.[1] He has highlighted the medical record as a document which should enable one to learn while he cares for the patient. He has suggested the following system[2] (Fig 1). By enumerating a patient's *problems* it becomes possible to develop *plans*, to write *orders*, to compose *progress notes*, and to write a *discharge summary* which are identified by the same number. The *problem list*, which serves as an index to the chart, should be placed at the front of the record so it can be found quickly. The objective of the system is to produce a document to improve patient care that can be used as easily as a dictionary.

To date the author has identified three kinds of obstacles associated with the execution of the Weed system on the medical services of the Department of Medicine of Emory University School of Medicine (Grady Memorial Hospital, Emory University Hospital and the Veterans Administration Hospital) in Atlanta. They are as follows: (1) *obstacles related to the acceptance of an innovative development*, (2) obstacles related to the mechanics of the system, and (3) *obstacles related to the creation of an excellent problem list.*

Obstacles Related to the Acceptance of an Innovative Development.—Many blockades are encountered because all of the individuals concerned do not—in the beginning—share the same degree of interest in the system. Some will see no need for such a system and a few will consider it a punitive exercise. Others will find it difficult to execute the plan on a consistent basis. They may even understand the value of such a display system, but their old habits prevent them from executing it in a reliable way. Senior staff have more difficulties in this regard than do junior students. These obstacles must be expected by anyone who inaugurates the system. The obstacles that occur are *no* different to those found when *any* new system or change is initiated.

Obstacles Related to the Mechanics of the System.—Some individuals may honestly believe that they are executing the Weed system, but a scrutiny of their charts will reveal that they are not. For example, the numbered problem list may be in its proper place—the first sheet on the chart—but the orders may be written using numbers that are unrelated to the problem list. This, of course, will cause great difficulties since the nurse would be taught incorrectly. She could not learn from such a record because her signals would be wrong. In fact, such a record teaches her improperly. The point is that the display and mechanical aspects of the system must be understood and then employed with devoted reproducibility. This set of difficulties should be expected by anyone who elects to begin the system. Such difficulties can be eliminated by appropriate meetings with students, house staff, senior staff, paramedical personnel, nurses, medical librarians, and administrators. The number of meetings required

Received for publication Feb 11, 1971; accepted April 14.
From the Department of Medicine, Emory University School of Medicine, Atlanta. Dr. Hurst is professor and chairman of the Department of Medicine.
Reprint requests to 69 Butler St SE, Atlanta 30303 (Dr. Hurst).

must be determined by "sensing" the need for them. One can be sure, however, that *many* discussions will be required to develop the system. Whoever is responsible for the development of this system must be willing to spend some time each day working with this set of obstacles, and a large number of people must see that the "nitty gritty" details of the mechanical aspects of the system are in fact being accomplished. No errors can be accepted. The solution to this set of problems is not intellectually taxing. To do something "by the numbers" does not require much brain power. It does, however, require an understanding as to why it is useful and why it must be done with great precision on every occasion. The most defeating opinion, however, is the assumption that doing it by the numbers is all there is to the Weed system. The real value of the system only emerges after the concept has been accepted and the mechanics of the method have become second nature to those who use it.

Obstacles Related to the Creation of an Excellent Problem List.—Let us assume that the idea of the Weed system has been accepted by the students, house officers, fellows, senior staff, nurses, paramedical personnel, medical librarians, and administrators. Let us also assume that medical data are appreciated, stored, and accounted for with as much dependability as money is stored and accounted for in a bank. The intellectual aspect of the system can then reach its full flower. The *problem list* is not simply the identification of the data base by numbers but rather must emerge out of the data base. Accordingly, the problem list may be incorrect if (1) *the data base is wrong or inadequate or* (2) *if a correct data base is interpreted improperly.* These errors will now be discussed in more detail.

Incorrect Problem List as the Result of an Inadequate Data Base.—An excellent problem list cannot be created unless the data base is adequate. If an asymptomatic patient with a completely negative past history is being examined and the physician does not hear the faint murmur of aortic valve regurgitation, he cannot create an accurate problem list for his patient. If a physician does not examine—or have someone examine—the cells of the cervix, then he cannot detect early cancer by that technique and it will not be possible to have a meaningful problem list when that anatomic area of the body has been ignored.

Data collecting requires skill and that skill requires practice. It is like playing the piano. To appreciate the skill, to understand the way a piano works, and to understand music and the system by which it is communicated (by notes on a sheet of paper) are not enough to make a superb musician. To be a superb musician it is necessary to sit down to the piano and practice—and practice—and practice—until it is right.

In the future data collection may not be done solely by the physician. Even now a reliable nurse can be taught to record the blood pressure in all four extremities with great accuracy. Too often the doctor may not do it because he knows it takes too long, even though he knows it should be done. We are now entering a new era when the data base on patients will beenlarged by nonphysician assistants and by computer techniques. The physician must begin to view the procurement of a data base (history, physical examination, and laboratory data) on his patients in a different way. He should have complete data when it is possible, and he must develop reliable ways of making it complete. Obviously, a more useful *problem list* can be synthesized from an accurate, complete data base than can emerge out of a data base that was acquired in a "hit and miss" fashion.

Incorrect Problem List as a Result of Improper Interpretation of the Data Base.—If the data base is accurate and complete, the physician has the opportunity of making a good problem list for his patient. Such will not happen automatically since it requires disciplined thought to make a meaningful problem list from raw data. The physician must manipulate and interpret the facts accumulated in the data base in such a way as to synthesize a meaningful *problem list.* As a matter of fact, the ability to manipulate and interpret data in a logical manner is a major objective of an educational system. This is why the physician spends at least 12 years after high school in an educational system. Allied health personnel who assist in data gathering may not have the educational background required to arrange the facts into a meaningful problem list. To rephrase, it is the physician's responsibility to manipulate and interpret the data base in a logical way since that is what his educational system is all about.

The thought process employed by a physician which involves the manipulation and interpretation of data is a lesson in self-discipline. This is a separate kind of discipline from data collection, for which the physician is responsible but which he may or may not collect himself. (See previous discussion.) John Gardner's views on self-discipline are pertinent to this discussion. He wrote:

> Not only the claims of civility but the realities of individual development call for some measure of self-discipline. Every great artistic performance is a consequence of self-discipline long and faithfully applied. So is every great athletic or intellectual performance. Disciplined in that sense—schooling, a consciousness adherence to standards, an effort to bring performance into line with an admired ideal—is the essence of craftsmanship.[3]

It is easy to identify a superficial problem list. The hallmark of a superficial problem list is the mere listing of a few symptoms, physical findings, and laboratory abnormalities. Such a list indicates that the individual who prepared it does not yet know that signs, symptoms, and laboratory abnormalities are not the ideal end for which plans can be written. The beginning student will have this difficulty because he has not learned the discipline of synthesizing data into meaningful ends (diagnoses) and he must work on the matter until he can do so. For example, suppose the laboratory reports that the hematocrit value is 28%. The beginner writes the problem as "anemia." He then may prescribe a therapeutic plan without establishing the cause of the anemia. He should have written the problem as "hematocrit of 28%." He then should write a plan that would establish the cause of the abnormality. Should he discover from the result of his plans that the problem is depleted iron stores, he then has a new problem to explain, ie, *why* does the patient have depleted iron stores. A new plan may be needed to answer that question. In another patient the beginner may decide that a set of data add up to heart failure. He writes down heart failure as a problem but does not realize he must establish an etiology for it. The data which might enable him to make an etiologic diagnosis may even be available but he has not disciplined his mind to try to do so. The seasoned physician knows that the identification of a physiologic abnormality—heart failure—may be the beginning but it is not the end of his problem solving. He tries to establish the etiology of the heart disease that has caused the heart failure. When he cannot, he knows that his data base is either inadequate or he is unable to interpret it. A consultant may be needed to solve such a problem.

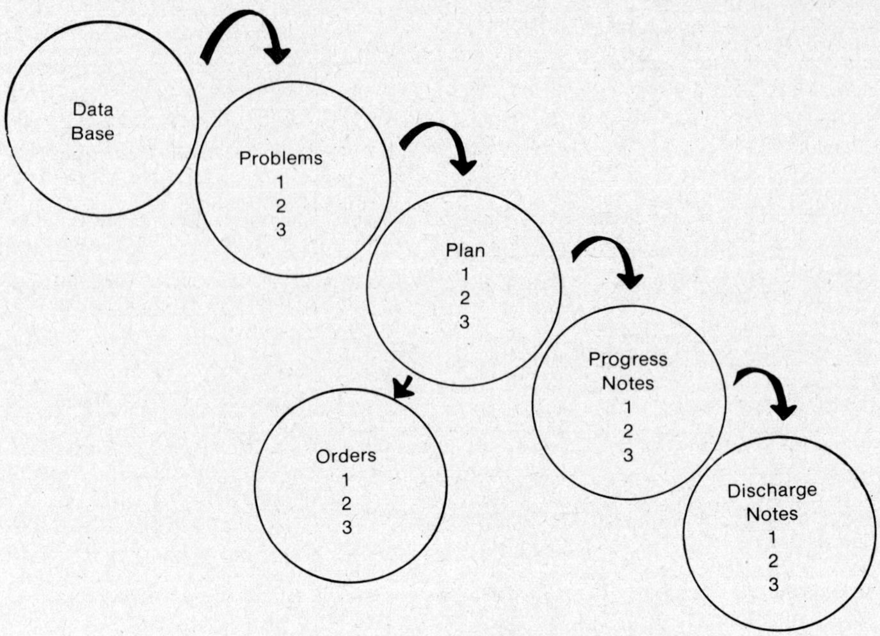

Fig 1.—Diagram illustrating Weed's display system.

The highly disciplined thought process that moves the observer from raw data to a problem list must be practiced—and practiced—and practiced until it is executed routinely with as little struggle as one has in putting on one's shoes.

The *problem list* must be ~~acute~~ accurate since the *initial plan, orders, progress notes,* and *discharge notes* are predetermined by the *problem list.* The creation of an excellent problem list can be abetted by the following suggestion.

What is a Problem?—A beginner quickly turns his thoughts toward such a question. This is appropriate. He soon realizes that a problem may be defined as something that "concerns the patient." It may or may not concern the physician. He also soon realizes that a problem may be something that concerns the physician but does not "concern" the patient. After considering both of these definitions he realizes that he must combine them. A problem can be defined as something that concerns the patient, or the physician, or both. The physician must learn to survey the data base and to organize and condense his views into a problem list. He should remember that for each problem he writes he must consider executing an initial plan. Accordingly, if he is to write an *initial plan* for a problem then the problem must be found in the problem list. It should also be remembered that the problem should be listed even when he plans to do nothing since such a decision requires a note of explanation in many instances. No *orders* can be written, except under emergency circumstances, unless they are a part of an *initial plan* which is written after the *problem list* has been created.

Who Determines if a Problem List is Correct?—This is a common question when the environment includes students, house officers, fellows, and senior staff. The problem list created by one person must not be judged as "right" or "wrong" by some other person. The other person can only say that he would have made a different list but he cannot say the first person's list is incorrect. It must be remembered that all students and all physicians do not have the same degree of knowledge at any point in time. If such were true it would be reasonable to expect that all persons would write the same problem list when they saw the same patient. To expect such would defeat an important aspect of Weed's system. It must be constantly recalled that each individual must collect data and then manipulate and interpret the data. The individual who writes a problem list must do so honestly and he can only draw upon his own brain to do so. Therefore the list he creates is an

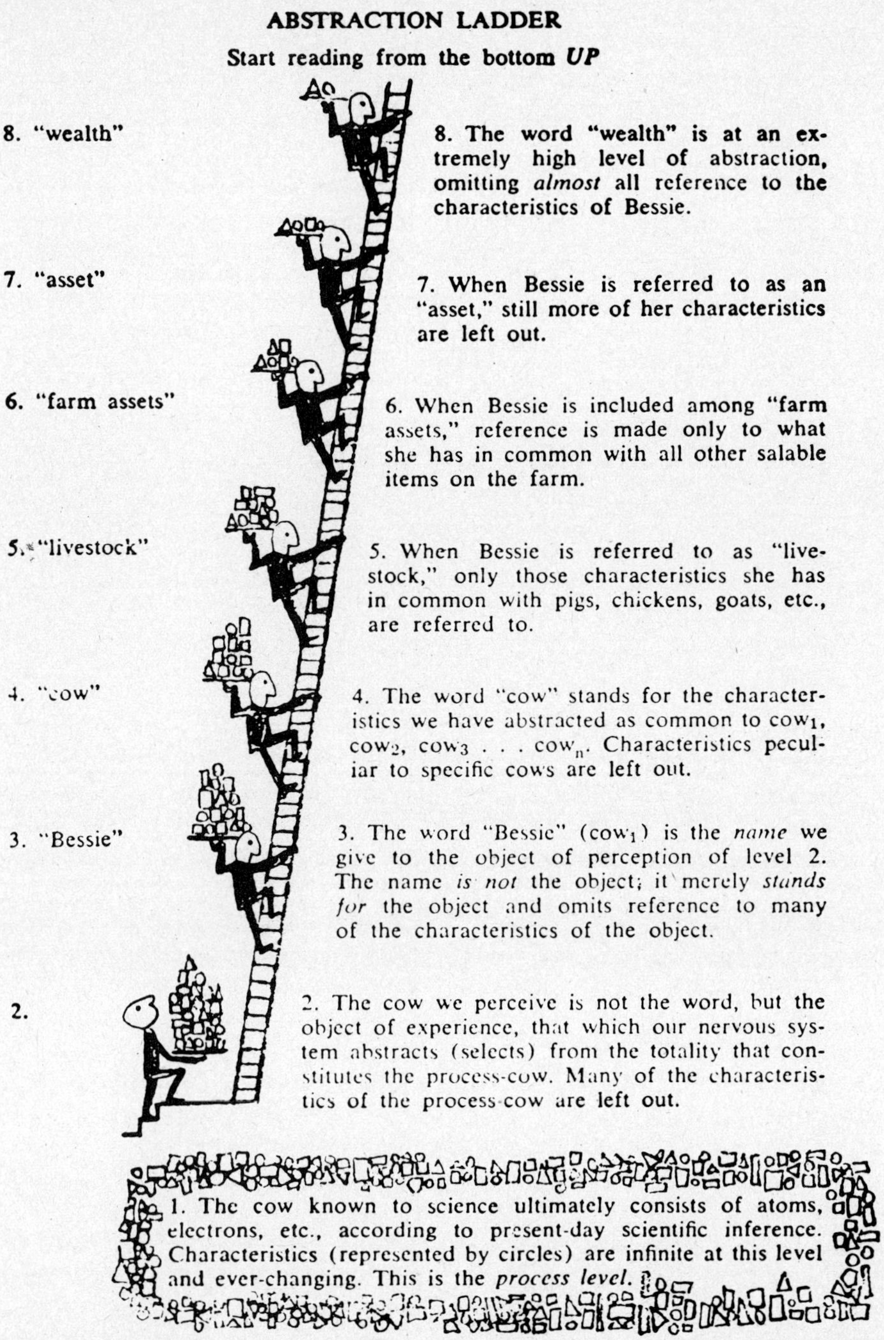

Fig 2.—The abstraction ladder. Bessie the Cow *is used in this illustration (from Hayakawa).*[4]

honest and useful one *for him.* He cannot be expected to do more than that. Another individual who has more skill in collecting and interpreting data may study the patient and create a more meaningful problem list. The *explanation* given for the difference between the first problem list and the second problem list is known as *teaching.* The individual who wrote the first list was not wrong—he was an honest learner. It must be remembered that the Weed system is a problem-solving system. An appropriate test would be whether or not the patient's problems were solved and not whether two people wrote identical records.

It is Essential to List in the Problem List Exactly What One Knows—No More and No Less.—The author has been surprised to learn that many individuals have not schooled themselves to do this. One factor responsible for the difficulty is a lack of understanding of language. Hayakawa's book *Language in Thought and Action* is especially useful in correcting this fault.[4]

Hayakawa wrote:

> To think more clearly, to speak and write more effectively, and to listen and read with greater understanding—these have been the goals of the study of language from the days of the medieval trivium to present-day high school and college English.[4]
>
> Perhaps an illustration will clarify the writer's position. What is the teacher's duty when a child says in class, "Taters ain't doin' good this year?" Traditionally, teachers of English and speech have seen their first duty as that of correcting the child's grammar, pronunciation, and diction in order to bring these up to literate standards. The teacher with a semantic orientation will give priority to a different task. He will ask the student such questions as "What potatoes do you mean? Those on your father's farm, or those throughout the country? How do you know? From personal observation? From reports from credible sources?" In short, the teacher of semantics will concern himself, and teach his student to concern themselves, first of all with the truth, the adequacy, and the degree of trustworthiness of statements. Often when students who are bored with studying grammar and diagraming sentences become interested in the content and purposes of communication, their hostility to linguistic instruction vanishes, and problems of grammatical and syntactical propriety are solved in passing.[4]

Hayakawa's definition of semantics is important to know. He writes, "Semantics is the study of human interaction through communication."[4] Hayakawa's chapter "How We Know What We Know" should be read by all medical students—again and again. In this chapter he introduces the reader to the *Abstraction Ladder,* which is based on "The Structural Differential," a diagram originated by Alfred Korzybski to explain the

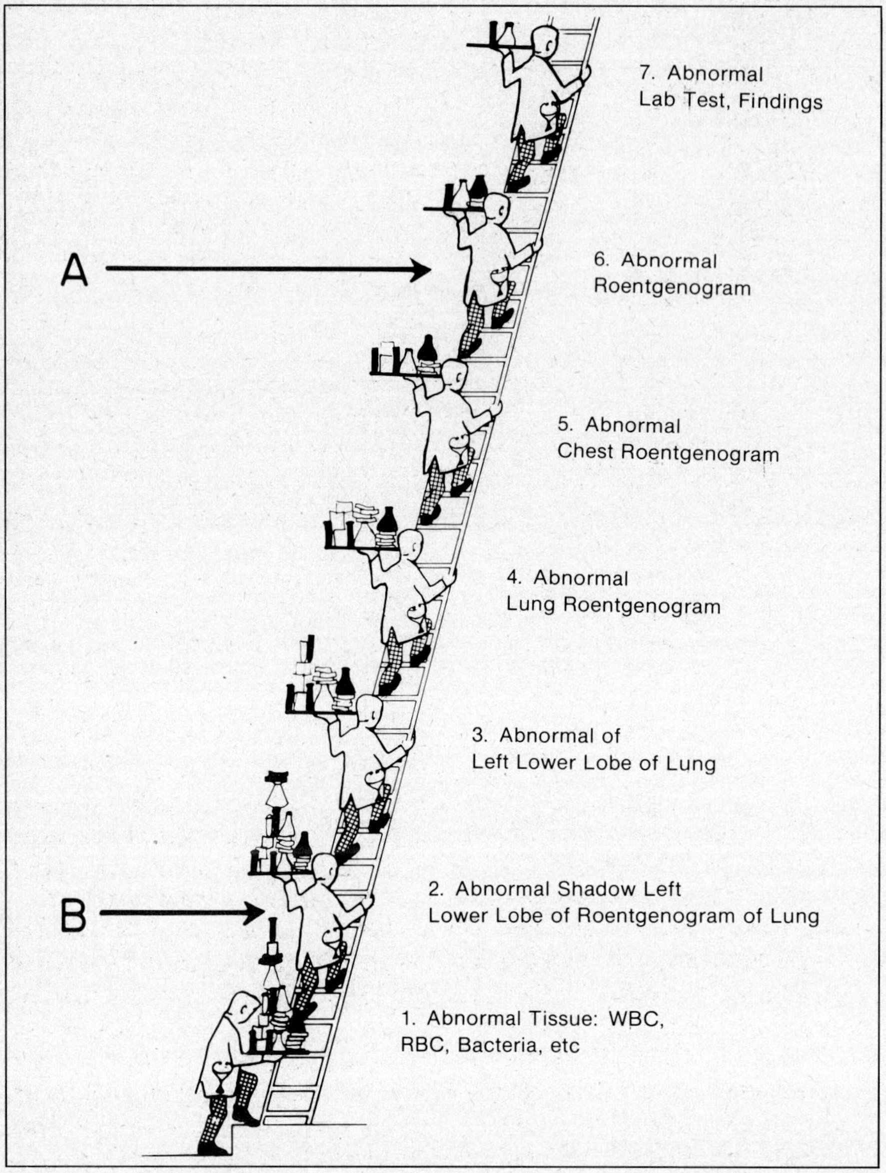

Fig 3.—An abstraction ladder associated with an abnormal finding on the chest roentgenogram. Start reading from the bottom up. A *would be identified by a high level abstracter. The low level abstracter would diagnose pneumonia.* B *illustrates the proper level of abstraction based on the data available.*

process of abstracting. He uses "Bessie" the cow to illustrate the process of abstracting (Fig 2).[4]

A ladder of abstraction can be constructed for every word or concept. An example of medical problem is shown in Fig 3. The top rung of the ladder signifies a low level of abstraction. Suppose the data base reveals that there is an abnormal roentgenogram. A high-level abstracter would simply write down abnormal roentgenogram. Put to a challenge, however, the observer would probably realize that he really knows more than that about the problem. He will usually know that it is an abnormal roentgenogram of the *chest*. Pressed further he will realize that is is an abormal roentgenogram of the *lungs*. Pressed even further he will realize that it is an abnormal roentgenogram of the *left lower lobe* of the lung. He may even recognize that there is an abnormal *shadow* in the left lower lobe of the lung. The observer knows that much. He does not know enough to go lower on the ladder of abstraction. To do so would force him to be too specific with the data available. The *shadow* could be due to a pulmonary infarction or pneumonia but he cannot say which from the roentgenogram alone. The low-level abstracter would glance at the film and say that the patient had pneumonia. He would be more specific than the data allows. When one identifies an abnormality it is wise to consider all of the rungs on the appropriate ladder of abstraction. Having "seen" the full ladder the objective is to select the rung of the ladder that indicates what one *knows*—no more and no less. This approach is of enormous value in identifying a problem since it prevents one from being too general when the data would allow him to be more specific or too specific when the data does not allow it. This approach is of enormous assistance in creating a meaningful problem list.

The words we use to represent thoughts we wish to communicate are located on a rung of some ladder of abstraction. In order to learn how to communicate properly we must know the ladder we are using and must also know where on the ladder a given symbol or word is located. Some individuals are persistently high-level abstracters. One could say that they have their feet firmly planted in the clouds. Other individuals are persistently low-level abstracters. They are the individuals who cannot see the forest for the trees. Hayakawa writes,

> The interesting writer, the informative speaker, the accurate thinker, and the sane individual, operate on all levels of the abstraction ladder, moving quickly and gracefully and in orderly fashion from higher to lower, from lower to higher—with minds as lithe and deft and beautiful as monkeys in a tree.[4]

Since words are abstract symbols, used to communicate what we think, it is obvious that one cannot create an excellent problem list without consid-

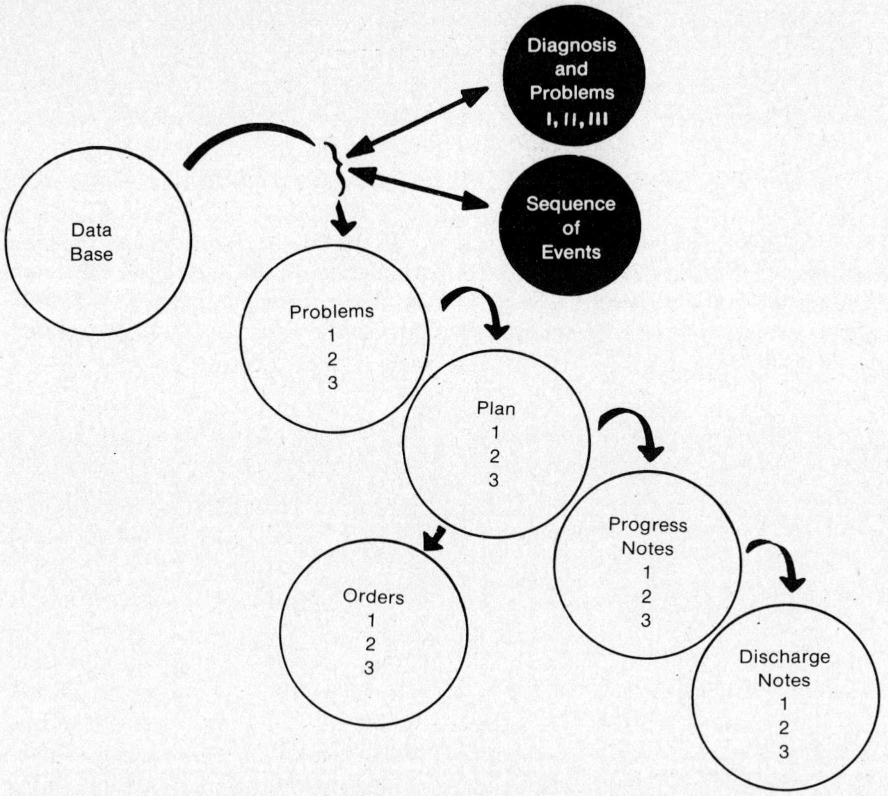

Fig 4.—Diagram illustrating addition of Diagnoses and Problems *and* Sequence of Events *to the Weed system. The discipline of establishing* Diagnoses and Problems *and the* Sequence of Events *assists the physician in creating the proper problem list from the data base.*

ering the level of abstraction or classification of the words we used. Accordingly, semantics becomes one of the more important disciplines to be considered by a physician.

Alvan Feinstein has written a classic book, *Clinical Judgment.*[5] The entire book is relevant to the problem of creating an excellent problem list. He, too, points out the problems associated with the language we use. He wrote,

> Human taxonomy provides a classification for designating a host who has a disease. Pathologic taxonomy provides a classification for designating (or diagnosing) the host's disease. There is no organized medical system, however, for classifying the illness that is the clinical interaction of host and disease. The illness of patients—an entity of nature constantly observed by clinicians, constantly analyzed by clinicians, and constantly treated by clinicians—has no taxonomy.

Since the illness of patients has no accepted taxonomy, we must expect difficulty in the creation of a problem list. Whereas Feinstein makes no claims that he has developed appropriate and final clinical taxonomy, it is clear to those who study his works that he has aimed a beacon light at the problem so that we can all examine it more thoroughly. His book should be read by all students and physicians since it deals with the collection of clinical data, the manipulation of data, and the interpretation of data. Problem lists improve after reading Feinstein.

The facts accumulated in the data base must be examined from different vantage points. The facts remain the same but the purpose of the observations may vary. Whereas there may be many ways to manipulate and interpret the facts in the data base, I will discuss only two of them.

The Establishment of Diagnoses and Problems.—The data acquired by the data-gathering methods of the history, physical examination, and laboratory may consist of a hodgepodge of facts. The physician who is surveying the data may be able to "order" a portion of the data into a more meaningful word symbol known as *diagnoses.* For example, he may be able to make a diagnosis of "coronary atherosclerotic heart disease with recent angina pectoris" without collecting additional data. On the other hand, he may discover on physical examination that the patient has a large liver but he may have no idea why the liver is large. He cannot and must not jump to a diagnosis without adequate data. Since no diagnosis can be made, then this is termed a *problem* rather than a diagnosis. I believe that it is wise to maintain a difference between a problem that can be ordered into a diagnosis and that which is a mere problem. At least this should be done as one first views a mass of facts. Some facts can be ordered into more meaningful symbols and other facts must be left as isolated findings.

Those facts that can be ordered into a diagnostic set should be manipulated in a special way. One method of manipulation was introduced to the profession in 1928 by the New York Heart Association publication *Criteria for the Classification and Diagnosis of Heart Disease.* The name was changed in 1939 to *Nomenclature and Criteria for Diagnosis of Diseases of the Heart.* The name was changed again in 1953 to *Nomenclature and Criteria for the Diagnosis of Diseases of the Heart and Blood Vessels.* The sixth edition, published in 1964 has been titled *Diseases of the Heart and Blood Vessels-Nomenclature and Criteria for Diagnosis.* The experts who wrote the first edition were obviously concerned that physicians were not using proper nomenclature or adequate criteria for the diagnosis of cardiovascular disease. All subsequent editions have continued to clarify the nomenclature and the criteria that should be used to establish a diagnosis. These books have had profound influence on the profession. They point out the necessity of arriving at a system diagnosis such as *heart disease*. They further expect the *etiology* to be sought and listed in acceptable terms. The *anatomy* must be *highlighted* as must the altered *physiology* and *function*. The concepts set forth in the book are applicable to all medical disciplines and not just cardiology.

In summary, it is wise to try to establish a system diagnosis which includes four subdiagnoses. The subdiagnoses include the following: an etiologic diagnosis, anatomic diagnosis, physiologic diagnosis, and functional diagnosis. The *problem list* should emerge from the diagnosis and subdiagnoses but will not be identical with them. Whenever such a diagnosis, including the appropriate etiologic, anatomic, physiologic, and functional subdiagnosis cannot be made, the appropriate taxonomy is used. For example, should a large liver be found on physical examination but the etiology and the degree of physiologic derangement are not known and there is no interference with total body function, one can only use anatomic taxonomy. The problem is a *large liver*. The effort to establish *diagnoses and problems* serve as a stimulus for the physician to try to establish etiologic, anatomic, physiologic, and functional diagnosis when he can. This separates the data base into those findings that can be ordered so that they are understood and those findings that cannot be ordered and are, in fact, simply findings. One may ask why not use the list created under the heading of *diagnoses and problems* as the *problem list*. A little experience with the system will soon show that a problem list should not include all of the items shown under the heading and that some problems not listed under the *diagnoses and problems* list should be included in the problem list.

I recommend the use of a separate heading of *diagnoses and problems* and that *roman numerals* be used to enumerate the list of items listed under the heading (Fig 4). *Arabic numbers* should be used in the problem list that is placed at the front of the chart.

The Establishment of the Sequence of Events.[6]—It is strange but true that a long list of problems can be created and the physician may not understand the interrelationships of the problems. A diagram made up of arrows and lines which interconnect the problems is an excellent way to stimulate such thought processes (Fig 4). In some situations a diagram showing the sequence of events that lead to the final illness may even teach the difficulties of *not* instituting preventive measures! In other situations such a diagram highlights the precipitating factors and aggravating factors. Such a diagram may teach that a certain illness may have resulted from a cluster of many problems.

Note that the addition of the *diagnoses and problems* and the *sequence of events* do not in any way alter the Weed concept or the features of its display. The reason these two items are added to the system is to insure the physician that he does not jump too quickly or without much thought from the raw *data base* to the formation of a *problem list*. In effect, these two features are added as stoplights in the hope of encouraging the physician to manipulate and interpret the data base with great care. These two features—or stoplights—are shown in Fig 4. Note that they are shown as side reactions to the flow of the Weed system.

Is the System Solving Problems?—Remember the Weed system is not merely a problem identifying system; it is a *problem-solving* system. Many individuals believe they are executing the Weed system even when the problem list on the patient is not being continually updated. The very minute a problem is solved it should be indicated on the problem sheet. One can see the tracks of the problem identifiers going down the problem sheet. One can see the tracks made by problem solvers going across the problem sheet (from left to right).

Any efforts to improve medical care and education by improving medical records will create new problems. Piet Hein's grook is pertinent to this point. He wrote:

We shall have to evolve
problem-solvers galore-
since each problem they solve
creates ten problems more.[7]

The Weed system will not solve all the problems but it does move us to a new set of problems. In doing I believe it improves the care of the patient and assists in the educational process of those involved. Piet Hein also wrote:

Problems worthy of attack
prove their worth by hitting back.[8]

Portions of *The Recovery of Confidence* are reproduced with permission from the author, J.W. Gardner, and the publisher, W.W. Norton & Company, Inc., Publishers.

Portions of *Language in Thought and Action* and Fig 2 are reproduced with permission from the author, S.I. Hayakawa, and the publisher, Harcourt, Brace & World, Inc.

References

1. Hurst JW: Ten reasons why Lawrence Weed is right. *New Eng J Med* **284**:51-52, 1971.
2. Weed LL: Medical records that guide and teach. *New Eng J Med* **278**:593-599, 652-657, 1968.
3. Gardner JW: *The Recovery of Confidence*. New York, WW Norton & Company Inc Publishers, 1970, p 81.
4. Hayakawa SI: *Language In Thought and Action*, ed 2. New York, Harcourt Brace & World Inc, 1939, VII-IX (preface).
5. Feinstein AR: *Clinical Judgment*. Baltimore, Wilkins & Wilkins Company, 1967, p 127.
6. Hurst JW: *Four Hats*. Chicago, Year Book Medical Publishers Inc, 1970, p 82.
7. Hein P: *More Grooks*. London, Hodder Paperbacks Ltd, 1968, p 32.
8. Hein P: *Grooks*. Cambridge, Mass, MIT Press, 1966, p 2.

The Art and Science of Presenting a Patient's Problems

(As an Extension of the Weed System)

J. Willis Hurst, MD, Atlanta

The proper presenation of a patient's medical problems by an expert is an artistic and scientific achievement that stimulates and teaches those who hear him. Since experts are rare, it is not uncommon for the one who presents a patient's medical problems to achieve a negative result. Some years ago, in an effort to improve the art, I wrote a short satire entitled "The Art of Poor Case Presentation" hoping to highlight—and thereby eradicate—the destructive aspects of the act of presenting.[1,2] Unfortunately, the satire did not produce any visible evidence of benefit even though it was widely read. Now, some years later, another approach is needed in order to improve the art of presenting a patient's problem. Accordingly, the objective of this discussion is to describe a method of "patient presentation" which recognizes the changes which are occurring in our medical education and patient care systems. The changes that are occurring may even eliminate the need for patient presentations, but, until that day comes, the current techniques of patient presentation should be changed considerably.

Received for publication May 20, 1971; accepted June 25.

From the Department of Medicine, Emory University School of Medicine, Atlanta. Dr. Hurst is professor and chairman of the Department of Medicine.

Reprint requests to Department of Medicine, Emory University School of Medicine, 69 Butler St SE, Atlanta 30303 (Dr. Hurst).

How to Present a Patient's Problems

The best presentation emerges from the knowledge attained by executing the Weed system.[3,4] The Weed system is a logic and display system which consists of five steps. The physician collects biologic data from the patient by taking a history, performing a physical examination, and obtaining appropriate laboratory tests. These efforts create the *data base*. The data base is then considered in such a way as to allow the physician to develop a *complete problem list* which denotes all of the patient's problems. Each problem is assigned an arabic number and the list is placed on a special sheet at the front of the chart. A separate *plan* is written for each problem and is identified by the same number and title that was assigned to the problem. The orders for each problem are assigned the same number as the problem for which the orders were written. *Progress notes* are written for each problem and are assigned a similar number and title. The *discharge note* displays the problems identified by numbers and titles and summarizes the data base which enabled the physician to arrive at his final conclusions regarding the patient. The discharge note should also reveal the exact treatment that was prescribed for each problem, the condition of the patient at the time of discharge, and the disposition of the patient. The system described by Weed is a problem-solving system. The initial problem list may reveal problems that are in various stages of resolution. The plans created for the problems should help resolve those problems that are identified as being at a high level of abstraction. When a problem is solved, an arrow is drawn to the right of the problem and the newly discovered solution is listed along with the date. In this way the complete problem list becomes an accurate, up-to-date summary of the patient's medical status. The author has emphasized two additional side steps of the Weed system in order to insure the development of an excellent problem list.[5] The two side steps are really steps in self-discipline and include manipulating the raw data into etiological, anatomical, physiological, and functional diagnoses (which are shown in Roman numerals) and the establishment of a *sequence of events* which is designed to show the temporal relationships of all of the patient's illnesses. When raw data are looked at in this way, an excellent problem list will be created.

When a patient's problems are presented to some other person (or persons), it follows that he should deviate from the traditional method of presentation when he has organized his thinking according to Weed's plan. The following principles should be considered when one presents a patient's problems:

1. Certain preliminary plans should be executed by the presenter before the presentation actually begins. The presenter must assess the situation in which the patient's problems are to be presented and determine the exact objectives of the exercise. The presenter must have all of the necessary items to present the patient's problems. He must have the chart, the appropriate roentgenograms, electrocardiograms, etc. The types of teaching aids that will be needed must be determined before the presentation begins and they must be checked out to make certain that they are in working order. The chart itself—with the problem list clearly displayed—may be the teaching aid on ward rounds when the group is small. On the other hand, it may be proper to use a blackboard, an overhead projector that projects written material onto the screen, or prepared slides when the group is large.

The presenter should make the decision regarding the wisdom of presenting the patient's problems in front of the patient. As a general rule, the presentation should not be made in front of the patient. *The time physicians and students spend with patients should be devoted entirely to the patient. Each patient is unique and what each says and reveals must be listened to and studied carefully.* Physicians and students should not—as a general rule—discuss *their* problems associated with data collection and interpretation at the bedside even though they are specifically related to the patient under consideration. The details of the presentation should be presented elsewhere and specific points are clarified when the patient is confronted. Stated another way, the patient must always be the center of the discussion when the group-patient encounter occurs. The individual responsible for the presentation should discuss the plans with the patient. The presenter should explain that the group of physicians intend to review the patient's problems and that they will come by to see the patient in the room or have the patient come to a conference room.

The leader of the group must be highly skilled. He must make the patient emotionally and physically comfortable. He must show appropriate concern for the patient's wellbeing. He must indicate to the patient that he and the group are reviewing every detail of all of the patient's problems and that the exercise they are engaged in is designed to contribute to his comfort and treatment. As Osler emphasized, it is usually appropriate to leave the bedside with an optimistic statement of some sort even if it is no more than stating that the physicians caring for the patients are working diligently on the patient's problems.

2. The presenter must remember when he presents to a group that verbal sounds cannot be heard when he mumbles. He must be aware of the location of each member of the group and speak where every individual can hear him. He must determine how formal he should be before he presents. Should he present the material to a large group ("grand rounds") he should stand erect and present in a formal manner. On the other hand, if he is presenting to a small group in a small workroom he might not stand and the presentation should be less formal.

3. The style and form of the presentation should be as follows:

A. The presentation should begin with the following type of statement: Mrs. Brown is 40 years old. It is improper to say that Mrs. Brown is a female. It is not necessary to refer to the race of the patient unless it is scientifically important to do so.

B. Following the introductory statement that Mrs. Brown is 40 years old, the presenter should say, "She has the following problems." He then presents the complete problem list which he has developed utilizing the Weed system. The problem list located at the front of the chart may be viewed by all when the group is small. When the group is large the presenter must display the complete problem list on the blackboard, project it on the screen using an overhead projector, or use a slide. The presenter then states each problem by the number and indicates the problem or problems which precipitated the reason or reasons for the patient seeking medical care at that particular time. The group listening should then have an overview of the patient's illness. Each single problem can then be viewed in the context of all of the other problems.

C. The presenter then states that he wishes to give the *data base* on one or more of the problems. The number of problems he discusses depends upon his understanding of the objectives of the exercise. He should then indicate the reasons why he has chosen the problems he wishes to discuss. If the presenter does not know why he is presenting, the effort is doomed to failure. The presenter should then give the data base, including the historical points; the abnormal physical findings; and the available laboratory data that is related to that *particular problem.* The presenter should not relate the entire history, give the results of the total physical examination, or give all of the laboratory data. He should, in essence, select that portion of the data base he believes fulfills the acceptable criteria that allowed him to establish the name given to the problem he is discussing. The presenter will find it useful to actually highlight the information related to the history, physical examination, and laboratory by identifying the data as (*a*) data obtained by history, (*b*) data obtained from the physical examination, and (*c*) data obtained in the laboratory. The points made under each heading should be given in the order of their diagnostic specificity. The diagnostic clue that is thought to be of the greatest value should be enumerated first. This will teach the presenter that diagnostic clues do not all have the same diagnostic value. During this phase of the presentation, the presenter displays the appropriate roentgenograms, ECGs, etc.

D. Following the preceding the presenter again states the purpose of the presentation and thereby reminds the group that the emphasis will be placed on certain problems and not others or that there is equal emphasis on all problems. At times the presenter will indicate that the purpose of the presentation is to demonstrate certain abnormalities in the patient and discuss them later or the presenter may have specific questions to ask the attending man who is the "leader" of the group.

E. The presenter then asks the group if they have any questions regarding the presentation. The presenter should hope that the members of the group do ask questions. This gives him a chance to clarify or to extend his remarks in a very specific way.

4. The patient is seen after the presentation has been completed. The leader of the exercise then asks the patient appropriate questions and checks and demonstrates a few of the important physical findings. Every individual in attendance must focus his entire attention on the patient. Members of the group must not talk to each other while the patient is talking or when the physical findings are being demonstrated. The group encounter with the patient can be helpful, reassuring, and humane from the patient's point of view or can be the reverse unless every member of the group, especially the leader, is sensitive to the potential good or harm of such an activity.

5. The discussion is completed after the physicians have left the bedside or the patient has left the teaching room. The type of discussion is, of course, determined by having a clear view of the objectives of the activity.

6. When possible the presenter—who should have a good relationship with the patient—should see the patient after the session is over in order to assess whether the patient misinterpreted the encounter with the group or if the patient was made anxious by the group.

Summary

The "presentation of a patient's problems" is used as a teaching technique for and by students, house officers, and seasoned physicians. As long as this technique is used—and it may not be used in the future—it is proper to scrutinize the activity carefully. When it is done poorly, medical education suffers. When it is done well, medical education improves. Since medical education determines the quality of patient care, it follows that we must demand excellence in all aspects of the educational system if we expect to have excellent patient care. The time has come when we must emphasize a different type of "patient presentation." The method of patient presentation should be patterned after the concepts promulgated by Weed in his efforts to improve education and patient care by developing the problem-solving record system. It makes no sense to develop a problem-oriented record and to give a source-oriented presentation.

This document highlights many of the problems associated with the presentation of a patient to a group of students and physicians. Many teaching failures will be eliminated if the method of patient presentation follows the Weed principles.

References

1. Hurst JW: The art of poor case presentation. *Harvard Med Alum Bull* October, 1957.
2. Hurst JW: The art of poor case presentation, in *Four Hats.* Year Book Medical Publishers Inc, 1970, pp 132-136.
3. Weed LL: *Medical Records, Medical Education, and Patient Care.* Cleveland, Case Western Reserve University Press, 1969, pp 1-273.
4. Hurst JW: Ten reasons why Lawrence Weed is right. *New Eng J Med* **284**:51-52, 1971.
5. Hurst JW: How to implement the Weed system: (In order to improve patient care, education, and research by improving medical records). *Arch Intern Med* **128**:456-462, 1971.

The Psychology of Physical Illness as Portrayed in Thomas Mann's *The Magic Mountain*

Harry S. Abram, MD, Nashville, Tenn

Although several of Thomas Mann's works deal with physical illness (carcinoma of the uterus in *The Black Swan*, cholera in *Death in Venice*, and even organ transplantation in *The Transposed Heads*), none do so as intimately and intricately as his monumental novel *The Magic Mountain*[1] written in 1924. In this novel Mann uses the vehicle of a young man's reaction to tuberculosis and sanatorium life (prior to antituberculosis medication) for his profound exposition of life, death, and the meaning of man's existence. As it would be presumptuous to cover any or all of these areas, I have limited this essay to the psychology of physical illness as portrayed in the hero's adaptation to tuberculosis, and its application to our understanding of patient response to chronic illness. The commentary, along with my review of Solzhenitzyn's *The Cancer Ward*,[2] substantiates my conviction that great novelists have made significant but unrecognized contributions to the literature of medical psychology.

Received for publication Jan 13, 1971; accepted April 5, 1971.

From the Department of Psychiatry, Vanderbilt University Medical Center, Nashville, Tenn.

Reprint requests to Department of Psychiatry, Vanderbilt University Medical Center, Nashville, Tenn 37203 (Dr. Abram).

The Novel

The story of *The Magic Mountain* is a simple one. The hero, Hans Castorp, is a 23-year-old man from Hamburg who visits his cousin, Joachim Ziemssen, a patient at the International Sanatorium Berghof in Davos-Platz in the Canton of the Grisons, Switzerland. The visit, intended originally for three weeks, begins in August 1907 before Castorp begins his job with the ship-building firm of Tunder and Wilm's. The novel ends seven years later when Castorp is last seen on a battlefield in World War I. In the interim, he is diagnosed as having tuberculosis prior to his leaving his cousin after the three-week visit; the following seven-year period becomes, in Erikson's terminology a "psychosocial moratorium"[3] during which Castorp works out his conflicts involving life, death, and disease in a maturing and at times traumatic fashion.

Autobiographical Aspects.—As in *The Cancer Ward*, there is an autobiographical element in the creating of the novel. In 1953 Mann noted in his postscript "The Making of *The Magic Mountain*"

> In the year 1912—over a generation ago now—my wife was suffering from a lung complaint, fortunately not a very serious one; yet it was necessary for her to spend six months at a high altitude in a sanatorium at Davos, Switzerland. . . . I visited my wife some weeks at Davos. There is a chapter in *The Magic Mountain* entitled "Arrival" where Hans Castorp dines with his cousin Joachim in the sanatorium restaurant, and tastes not only the excellent Berghof cuisine but also the atmosphere of

the place and the life "bei uns hier oben." If you read that chapter, you will have a fairly accurate picture of our meeting in this sphere and my own strange impressions of it.

The impressions grew stronger and stronger during the three weeks I spent at Davos visiting my wife while she was a patient. They are the same three weeks Hans Castorp originally meant to spend at Davos—though for him they turned into seven fairytale years of his enchanted stay. At least *one* of his experiences is a pretty exact transference to my hero of things that happened to me. I mean the examination of the carefree visitor from the "flatland," and the resulting discovery that he himself is to become a patient too. . . .

If I had been Hans Castorp, the discovery might have changed the whole course of my life. The physician assured me that I should be acting wisely to remain there for six months and take the cure. If I had followed his advice, who knows, I might still be there! I wrote *The Magic Mountain* instead.

I have chosen the themes of dependency, regression, and neurotic attitudes toward illness to exemplify Mann's handling of patient's reactions to physical disease in the novel.

Dependency and Regression.—Mann, in his autobiographical comments, hints at neurotic dependency and regression in illness in his statement that he may never have left the sanatorium if he had agreed to stay for the "cure." In the novel, Settembrini, a tuberculous philosopher at the sanatorium, warns Castorp of the excessive dependency which can develop with illness. One senses throughout the novel that he is speaking for Mann. (In fact, Mann in his 1953 postscript writes that Settembrini is "sometimes a mouthpiece for the author, but by no means the author himself.")

There was Fräulein Kneifer, Ottilie Kneifer, last year. She came of a good family—the daughter of an important government official. She was here some year and a half and had grown to feel so much at home that when her health was quite restored—it does happen up here; people do sometimes get well—she couldn't bear to leave. She implored the Hofrat to let her stop; she could not and would not go; this was her home, she was happy here. But the place was full, they wanted her room, and so all her prayers were in vain; they stood out for discharging her cured. Ottilie was taken with high fever, her curve went well up. But they found her out by exchanging her regular thermometer for a "silent sister." You aren't acquainted as yet with the term, it is a thermometer without figures, which the physician measures with a little rule, and plots the curve himself. Ottilie, my dear sir, had 98.4°; she was normal. Then she went bathing in the lake—it was the beginning of May; we were having frost at night; the water was not precisely ice-cold, say a few degrees above. She remained sometime in the water, trying to contract some illness or other—alas, she was, and remained, quite sound. She departed in anguish and despair, deaf to all the consolations her parents could give. "What shall I do down there?" She kept crying. "This is my home!" I never heard what became of her.

Settembrini's warning (to avoid the dependency and regression of illness) comes frequently and in various forms. He observes that the patients "imagine themselves entitled to pity, and justified of their bitterness, irony, and cynicism" and admonishes Castorp, "guard yourself altogether from taking their mental attitude! . . . The atmosphere in which we live is obviously very favorable to such miasmic growths, I may hope, or rather, I must fear, that you understand my meaning."

Associated with such dependency are the regressive responses to illness. With illness, the patient regresses to earlier types of behavior in response to the stress of the disease and being placed in an environment (hospital or sanatorium) in which he is cared for and protected. He must relinquish temporarily his independence and responsibility to place himself in the hands of others, as he had as a child and infant. Such a response is a natural one and essential at the time of illness. But as Settembrini (speaking for Mann) remarks, the dependency for some patients proves too pleasurable and is difficult to renounce after the illness for more mature styles of living. Regarding regression Settembrini tells young Castorp:

I would urge it upon you: hold yourself upright, preserve your self-respect, do not give ground to the unknown. Flee from this sink of iniquity, this island of Circe, whereon you are not Odysseus enough to dwell in safety. You will be going on all fours—already you are inclining toward your forward extremities, and possibly you will begin to grunt—have a care!

Neurotic Attitudes Toward Illness.—In these areas Mann is concerned with the patient's preoccupation and fascination with his illness. As Herr Settembrini expressed it, "people [the patients] were possessed of two ideas, and only two: temperature—and then again temperature" and spoke of "the disease which was the business of life up here." For example, at one of Castorp's first meals at the sanatorium he overhears a typical conversation.

Frau Stöhr, sitting there in her woolen blouse, gave the table to know she had been examined that forenoon; she went into particulars, affectedly drawing back her upper lip from the rodent-like teeth. There were rhonchi to be heard in the upper right side, and under the left shoulder-blade the breathing was still very limited; the "old man" said she would have to stop another five months.

In the third week when Castorp tells his table-mates that he has tuberculosis, "they shook their fingers at him, they winked maliciously, they put their heads on one side, crooked their forefingers beside their ears and waggled them in a pantomime suggestive of their delight at having found him out, who had played the innocent so long." Indeed, after the diagnosis is made, one of the physicians congratulates Castorp, "with his head tipped back sideways, and one hand on the young man's shoulder, smiling so heartily that the yellowish teeth showed in his beard, he shook him warmly by the hand."

In such instances Mann believes that illness is given a dignity which it does not deserve and which leads to neuroticism. Settembrini, in another of his dialogues with Castorp, remarks:

But I take issue where you regard the combination of disease with dullness as a sort of aesthetic inconsistency, an error in taste on the part of nature, a "dilemma for the human feelings," as you were pleased to express yourself. When you professed to regard disease as something so refined, so—what did you call it?—possessing a "certain dignity"—that it doesn't "go with" stupidity. That was the expression you used. Well, I say no! Disease has nothing refined about it, nothing dignified. Such a conception is in itself pathological, or at least tends in that direction. Perhaps I may best arouse your mistrust of it if I tell you how ancient and ugly this conception is. It comes down to us from a past seething with superstition, in which the idea of humanity has degenerated and deteriorated into sheer caricature; a past full of fears, in which well-being and harmony were regarded as suspect and emanating from the devil, whereas infirmity was equivalent to a free pass to heaven. . . .

The dilemma, my dear sir, the tragedy, begins where nature has been cruel enough to split the personality, to shatter its harmony by imprisoning a noble and ardent spirit within a body not fit for the stresses of life.

Resolution of Neurotic Attitudes.—As noted earlier, in the course of the novel Castorp works through many conflicts related to his illness. He finds meaning in life and yet is able to accept the inevitability of death. The latter comes when he looks at his own hand through a fluoroscope.

He [the physician] was so kind as to permit the patient, at his request, to look at his own hand through the screen. And Hans Castorp saw, precisely what he must have expected, but what it is hardly permitted man to see, and what he had never thought it would be vouchsafed him to see: he looked into his own grave. The process of decay was forestalled by the powers of the light-ray, the flesh in which he walked disintegrated, annihilated, dissolved in vacant mist, and there within it was the turned skeleton of his own hand, the seal ring he had inherited from his grandfather, hanging loose and black on the joint of his ringfinger—a hard, material object, with which man adorns the body that is fated to melt away beneath it, when it passes on to another flesh that can wear it for yet a little while. With the eyes of his Tienappel ancestress, penetrating, prophetic eyes, he gazed at this familiar part of his own body, and for the first time in his life he understood that he would die.

Castorp subsequently becomes involved with the "suffering and dying in the establishment," remarking "Well, I have made up my mind to concern myself a bit in future with the severe cases of the moribund." He visits them at the bedside, talks with them about their sickness and fear of death, and related to them in a beneficial and positive manner. He even sends them gifts, such as flowers, and thus antedates Eissler who in his excellent book *The Psychiatrist and the Dying Patient*[4] stresses the importance of the gift to the dying patient. Castorp's final realization of the meaning of life, disease, and death comes in the amazing chapter entitled "Snow" in which he is lost in a violent blizzard.

For all interest in disease and death is only another expression of interest in life, as is proven by the humanistic faculty of medicine, that addresses life and its ails always so politely in Latin, and is only a division of the great and pressing concern which, in all sympathy, I now name by its name: the human being, the delicate child of life, man, his state and standing in the universe. . . . I will keep faith with death in my heart, yet will remember that faith with death and the dead is evil, is hostile to humankind, so soon as we give it power over thought and action. *For the sake of goodness and love, man shall let death have no sovereignty over his thoughts.*

Comment

As in my review of *The Cancer Ward,* I cannot cover all aspects of *The Magic Mountain* related to the psychology of illness but merely hope that isolated vignettes stir the reader back to read the original works. Indeed, I wonder if these and similar books should not be required reading for all medical students. Mann, in the novel, also discusses other problems such as suicide in the physically ill, the physician with physical illness, and the relationship of psychoanalysis to organic disease. Yet in this presentation I wished to emphasize the concepts of regression, dependency, and the neurotic aspects of chronic illness. One may correctly say that we no longer have sanatorium life and that anti-tuberculosis medication and advanced thoracic surgical techniques have replaced such institutions as the Berghof. Yet we see similar reactions in other chronic illnesses, particularly heart disease, diabetes, and patients requiring long-term hemodialysis. In such patients neurotic attitudes, particularly excessive dependency and overconcern with bodily functions, can lead to crippling and incapacitating states. Hope and active involvement in life are essential ingredients to successful rehabilitation. Or, as Mann ends this remarkable novel:

Out of this universal feast of death, out of this extremity of fever, kindling the rain-washed evening sky to a fiery glow, may it be that Love one day shall mount?

References

1. Mann T: *The Magic Mountain.* HT Lowe-Porter (trans), London, Secker & Warburg, 1961.
2. Abram HS: The psychology of terminal illness as portrayed in Solzhenitzyn's *The Cancer Ward. Arch Intern Med* **124**:758-760, 1969.
3. Erickson EH: Problem of ego identity. *J Amer Psychoanal Assoc* **4**:56-121, 1956.
4. Eissler KR: *The Psychiatrist and the Dying Patient.* New York, International Universities Press Inc, 1956.

Editorial

Consumerism in Medicine

As part of the revolutionary zeal that has flourished during the past ten years, consumer advocacy has developed as a significant force in the community. Best exemplified by Ralph Nader and his staff of associates and volunteers, the sequence of study, analysis, and demand for change on behalf of the consumers' interest has become known as the process of consumerism. The major element in all of this activity has been the unyielding insistence that the people who are to use the product or who are to be recipients of a service are entitled to an important voice in how that product is produced or how that service is dispensed. As far as the profession of medicine is concerned, consumer participation has existed for many years in the form of boards of advisors or of trustees for community hospitals. But such consumer activity—in light of present day ventures—would be considered to be perfunctory. Such hospital boards have not had representation from all of the various types of consumers that use the constituent institutions. Consumerism calls for a style of militant advocacy which is more than advisory or consultative.

The process of consumerism—wherever it has been successfully launched—has built into it either the implied, or even the explicit, notion that there is an inherent anatagonism between the producer and the supplier. Consumer advocates, when asked to speak to this element in their philosophy, quickly indicate that such adversary posturing need not always be the case. "If the shoe fits . . ." is the closing rejoinder. The point, however, is that the consumer is saying that even if he doesn't know best, he at least expects the producer to hear him out—and usually more than just a hearing—before important decisions are made about the product or service being provided. In medicine, this is a particularly difficult issue, because for generations it has been an accepted truism that the complex professional elements that determine the decisions of the physician can only be completely handled by individuals who have been trained as physicians. Thus for years hospital directors have been actually "directed" by the senior physicians of their staff, and various health care programs for communities have been designed and managed almost solely by physicians. Clearly, this insularity of decision-making is no longer held to be tenable.

All three areas of medicine—provision of care, education, and research—are now being similarly influenced by consumer participation. The care sector is the most visible because it affects directly the most people. Thus the establishment of the free clinics in many urban areas has been accomplished with the appointment of governing boards consisting of community representatives who very directly guide the day to day management of these clinics. In some units, the recruitment of professional staff is also decided by the consumer-run governing committee, and, in these instances the advice and counsel of other staff physicians may or may not be persuasive. In several urban hospitals, the community representatives have also requested direct participation in the management of these facilities. Last year, the "revolt" that took place at a hospital in New York City was remarkable for, among many features, the fact that consumer representatives were stationed in the clinic corridors so as to provide continuous surveillance of the type of service being offered to the patients and their families. The observations of these advocates were then submitted to the governing board so that the board could be properly advised as to the performance of the professionals.

Less invasive in nature, but equally important in terms of potential influence, has been the quite open change in hospital boards so as now to include a wide base of representation from the community. This has occurred both in the urban ghettos and in the rural areas. Men and women now serve as advisors and trustees to major health care institutions—witness the community-run board of the Johns Hopkins affiliated East Baltimore program—where previously only affluence and social status determined such appointments. The system is changing and, though it may not be yet quite as "democratic" as some consumer advocates would wish, there is a very definite modification in old styles.

As far as medical education is concerned, it depends upon who is to be considered the "consumer"—the medical student himself or the public who is financing the educational venture. In terms of the student, he now has quite a strong voice in the educational process. At many medical schools there is now voting student participation on almost all standing committees. Active contributions towards curriculum modification and program design are being conducted. Here at the University of Illinois, students aid in the design of appraisal examinations, help in the planning of new courses, and have an important voice in such key functions as chairman recruitment committees. The students are now being looked to as "young faculty" and this has been a very salutary development.

In terms of the underwriting public, less specific major change has occurred for medical schools although if one is willing to view Congress and the various state legislatures as representing the public interest, then the role of the consumer in higher education is more powerful and more articulate than ever before. No new medical school or no new significant expansion of an already existing school can possibly take place without confirmation and sanction by the legislatures. And this includes the so-called private schools whose budgets are almost completely dependent upon federal and/or state funding.

Last, there is consumer participation in research programs, an area which at first glance would seem to be the least likely to warrant or require public participation. Scientific investigations depend first and foremost upon the interest and competence of the scientific scholar. What to study and how to study it are matters that depend upon the entire body of information that now exists and then upon the methods and talents of the investigators who are disciplined in specific fields. But the matter does not rest there. The funds for most scientific research derive from the public—either government grants or tax-deductible "private" philanthropies—and thus those who give the money intend to have a significant voice in how it is spent.

In effect this is really not a new turn of affairs, for in the past when the scientists wanted more support they have turned to the public for help: the American Heart Association, the American Cancer Society, the National Foundation-March of Dimes, and the National Kidney Foundation are but a few examples. In these organizations the scientists have asked the laymen to go out and raise money for their programs, and then they have used these funds for the studies which the various scientific review boards have considered to be worthy of support. For the most part, this has all worked out quite well. As long as the scientists are relatively comfortable with the arrangement, the public's efforts toward raising monies are usually encouraged with no crosscurrents. In fact, those laymen who work hardest at being "producer" advocates—by being extraordinarily effective with other consumers—are held in high regard by the scientific community. There has been a very happy marriage between the scientists and their public protagonists. What happens when not all the scientists agree on how to run their scientific affairs? A good deal of distress ensues. The recent Cancer Authority legislation is a prime case in point.

In this latter situation, a panel of scientific advisors recommended the establishment of a Cancer Authority separate from the jurisdiction of the National Institutes of Health. Many scientists disagreed. The Congress held hearings. The differing scientific views were presented. But the public support for one view far outweighed the public support for the other. The "separatists" were joined by several public relation experts and national columnists. The mail response to one columnist's specific appeal for a show of support was so remarkable as to make clear to Congress that a political issue was at stake that could not be denied. Thus the administration of scientific research became politicized: the vote in the Senate for the separate Cancer Authority was 79 to 1!

What is the medical profession to do with all this "consumer" advocacy? Obviously it must live with it. Can it go about the task of effectively exercising its professional skills—clinical, educational, and investigative—in the presence of powerful public influence? Clearly it will have to. But it does mean that planning for the future will now demand an active partnership with public representatives. When the American Medical Association—through its Committee for Political Action—pursued legislative support for its causes, many scientists dissented that such political action was inappropriate and not truly representative of the medical profession. Now that some scientists have successfully recruited the support of powerful public spokesmen, whereas others were not successful, there has been dissent from the unsuccessful about the appropriateness of such public partisanship. The fact is that the public is in the middle of all of our affairs, and from this point on what is to be granted by the public will have to have its support before professionals can have their programs. Many scientists, educators, and physicians will be disappointed with the outcome of many of these issues because of the differing viewpoints between professionals. But there is no other recourse. The best next step is for us to actively recruit consumer advocates so as to have a strong partnership in the programs and projects that are important to us all. The public and the professionals are joined in one community; we will have to work well together.

M.D.B.

Autonomic Hyperreflexia in Spinal Cord Injury

To the Editor.—I am grateful to Gotshall for his recent emphais on autonomic hyperreflexia in spinal cord injury.[1] I have been pondering the cause of a patient's sudden hypertension and autonomic hyperreflexia may have been the mechanism.

A 40-year-old woman with widespread osseous metastases from cancer of the breast underwent bilateral adrenalectomy without complications after an 18 month remission induced by oophorectomy. Blood pressures before, during, and immediately after the operation ranged from 90/60 to 150/100 mm Hg. On the first three postoperative days numerous blood pressure determinations varied from 150/80 to 180/110 mm Hg. On the fourth postoperative day blood pressures of 154/94 and 150/94 mm Hg were recorded in the morning. After a pelvic examination, done for investigation of a profuse vaginal discharge, blood pressures of 200/90 and 200/105 mm Hg were recorded within the hour. Blood pressure fluctuations from 130/80 to 180/110 mm Hg were noted during the remainder of the hospital stay, apparently unrelated to fluid, sodium, or cortisone intake. An intravenous pyelogram revealed no changes from the preoperative x-ray films.

Within two months of the adrenalectomy the patient was readmitted for progressive weakness of her legs. A myelogram done with needle introduced into the high cervical area revealed partial blocks from T-2 to T-7 and a complete block at T-12. A few episodes of hypertension with blood pressure up to 170/110 mm Hg were again recorded during the remainder of her terminal illness.

Although factors such as fluid overload, excessive corticosteroid therapy, and renal injury should be considered in this patient, the detection of hypertension soon after pelvic examination suggests autonomic hyperreflexia. Whereas various stimuli can provoke the paroxysm, manipulation of the anogenital area is said to provide the maximal response.[2]

This case suggests that (*a*) autonomic hyperreflexia may be a manifestation of spinal cord metastases, (*b*) spinal cord compression should be considered in cancer patients with paroxysmal hypertension and (*c*) further investigation of the autonomic nervous system in spinal cord metastases is indicated.

CHARLES K. TASHIMA, MD
Honolulu

References

1. Gotshall RA Jr: Blood pressure in spinal cord injury. *Arch Intern Med* **127**:775, 1971.
2. Bors E, French JD: Management of paroxysmal hypertension following injuries to cervical and upper thoracic segments of the spinal cord. *Arch Surg* **64**:803-812, 1952.

Pagophagia

DEAR DR. CROSBY.—I want to express my appreciation for the kind remarks in your editorial (*Arch Intern Med* **127**:960-961, 1971). I have no qualms about any statement that you make in the editorial but could only add additional anecdotes to amplify your remarks.

The first patient I ever saw with pagophagia was an 18-year-old Negro girl who presented herself to my office in a state of sheer panic because she had been convinced by her father that she would die of cancer if she did not stop her ice eating. In spite of her absolute conviction that her father was correct, she had an ungovernable ice consumption. Careful evaluation of the patient revealed only mild iron lack anemia which I treated with iron sulfate given orally. At a follow-up visit a week later, the patient was absolutely ecstatic because she no longer wanted ice and I had "saved her life."

A 35-year-old woman, when questioned in regard to her craving, indicated to me that she had always had an excellent appetite for cold beer. She regularly consumed five to six cans of beer a day but volunteered that if it ever came to a choice between beer and ice she would give up the beer in a moment.

One patient was a chain smoker, whose initial act upon arising was to light a cigarette. With the onset of pagophagia, her initial act was to go to the refrigerator, with her cigarette often delayed to midmorning.

The husband of one pagophagiac, who had destroyed two sets of full dentures with her ice chewing, embraced me in public when he was introduced to me as the doctor who gave his wife iron and saved him from financial ruin.

The Figure illustrates truly pathognomonic "*physical findings*" of pagophagia. As part of my initial study, I requested that each patient bring me a representative ice tray so that I could measure its volume and better estimate their daily ice consumption.

One patient appeared with a brown paper bag clutched beneath her arm

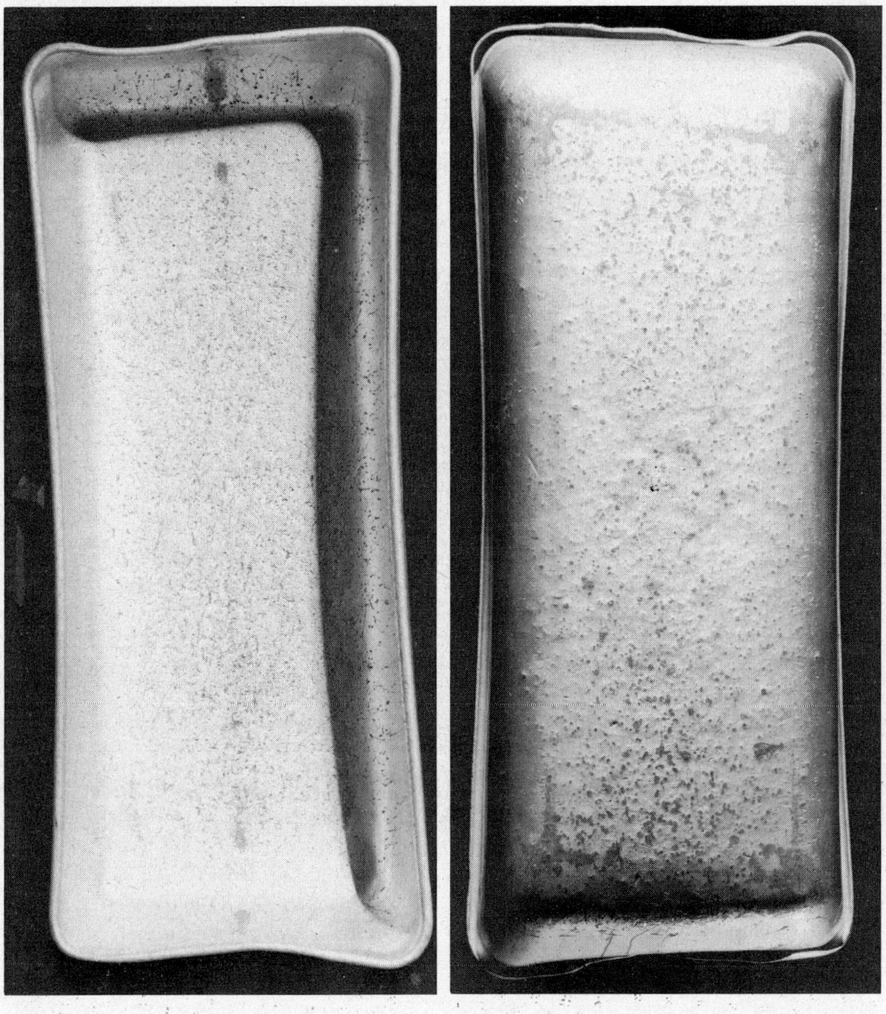

Ice cube tray.

and with great embarrassment, withdrew the ice tray which you see in the Figure. You can readily appreciate that the tray had been severely pockmarked by the ice pick which she used to crush her ice. On a subsequent visit, following cessation of her pagophagia, she presented me with this ice tray as a souvenir, having bought some new ones which she continues to use, unscathed, to the present.

We have seen two carrot eaters; one of whom indicated that she spent most of her waking hours going to and from the grocer to buy carrots. She ate them by the bunch! In spite of her deep orange appearance, which she related to the carrot ingestion, she could not control this appetite. Within five days of the initiation of iron therapy, the mere mental image of carrot made her retch.

Lt Col Charles A. Coltman, Jr, MC, USAF
Lackland Air Force Base, Tex

Combination Therapy

To the Editor.—In the February issue (*Arch Intern Med* **127**:217-227, 1971) a discussion of the medical therapy for lung abscesses included reference to a substantial proportion of patients who were treated with a combination of penicillin and tetracycline. Recently, however, it has become apparent that such combinations are actually inferior to an adequate dose of the more effective agent.[1,2] Tetracycline is currently thought to diminish the bactericidal activity of penicillin, both in vitro and in vivo. This important point is not mentioned in the discussion and may lead the reader to falsely assume that this specific combination is more effective than the single administration of penicillin.

Alan A. Pollock
New York

References

1. Goodman L, Gilman A: *The Pharmacological Basis of Therapeutics.* New York, Macmillan Co, 1969, pp 1183-1184.
2. Interactions of Drugs. *Med Lett Drugs Ther* **12**:93-96, 1970.

Books

AMA Drug Evaluations 1971. Edited by AMA Council on Drugs. Price, $15. Pp 675+. American Medical Association, 535 N Dearborn St, Chicago 60610, 1971.

It is terrible form for an editor to review his own book (!!). But how about a book that has several hundred authors (of whom you are just one)—and you are convinced that this is one of the most important books to appear in recent years—and you want to assure it an eye-catching review in a prominent journal? (And you just happen to be a book review editor.)

The *AMA Drug Evaluations* is the pride and joy of the AMA Department of Drugs and Council on Drugs. In my opinion it represents one of the most significant contributions to American medicine made by the American Medical Association in the past decade.

I will not regale you with the details of blood, sweat, and tears—the dollars and the hours—the anxieties, determination, and dedication that went into this book. But I can assure you that it was a monumental effort from many aspects by many people. And the book reflects this effort; it can only be described as superb. For the purpose for which it was created and the audience for whom it is intended—it is ideal.

Of course it is not without flaws—no first edition ever is—but they are comparably minor and will be expunged from future editions (which will appear every two years).

The book is organized into 90 chapters on the basis of pharmacological action of a group of drugs. It covers 1,200 single item agents. Medications are listed according to the preference of the experts (over 300) who wrote and edited each of the chapters. Each section includes a discussion of the drugs including indications, contraindications, adverse reactions, available forms, and doses. It is heavily indexed, and information can be located quickly. There is an "indications" index, all drugs are listed by generic and trade names, and there is a separate index for adverse reactions.

Of course, there will be areas of disagreement about the recommended drugs, but the statements of *AMA DE* are made by practical clinician-investigators of national reputation and the AMA Council of Drugs stands behind them. Fixed dose combinations are frowned upon, although the use of the word "irrational" sticks a bit in the craw. However, the point is well made, and I feel the semantics may be appropriate for the first edition; I am sure it will be softened in the future. However, the "rationality" of most fixed-dose combinations remains to be proved to the satisfaction of the Council.

As of June 9, 1971, 167,650 copies had been mailed to dues paying members of AMA; 2,835 had been sent out as complimentary copies, and 2,093 were sold at $15 a copy. That leaves 126,046 which are in a warehouse in Wisconsin available for sale. In my opinion, it is the best bargain in textbooks of therapy that has ever appeared.

AMA DE should quell forever the outcries for a "compendium of therapeutics." Gentlemen, it is here.

ROBERT H. MOSER, MD
Wailuku, Maui, Hawaii

Communications to this Department may be sent directly to Robert H. Moser, MD, Maui Medical Group, Maui Professional Center, Wailuku, Maui, Hawaii 96793, or to the Chief Editor for transmittal to him.

Gastroenterologic Medicine. Edited by Moses Paulson, MD. Price, $60. Pp 1,627, with 496 illustrations. Lea & Febiger, 600 S Washington Sq, Philadelphia 19106, 1969.

This is a volume of very large size (67 chapters) written by a very large number of authors (85) and directed at a very ambitious goal: "to fill the need for a single comprehensive volume concerning disorders involving the alimentary canal, liver, gallbladder, and pancreas." Indeed, almost all conceivable aspects of the physiology, pathophysiology, clinical features, diseases, and diagnostic methods relevant to these organs are considered. In general, the chapters are concise and well written by appropriate authorities and contain useful information, as current as possible considering the complicated circumstances of compiling a multiauthored text.

Most of the chapters represent useful contributions. The well written discussions of epidemiologic, genetic, and historical aspects of gastroenterology are unique, and the discussions of the involvement of the gastrointestinal tract in diseases of other systems are welcome. The chapter on the "Roentgenologic Diagnosis of Diseases of the Gastrointestinal Tract" has an extraordinarily complete listing of roentgenographically demonstrable lesions of the gastrointestinal tract and a few well selected examples of the most important lesions.

Nevertheless, there are serious faults. The unavoidable problems of a multiauthored text—repetitiousness, overlapping, conflicts, and omissions—are compounded by the erratic arrangement of the chapters. Chapters 3, 7, and 12 deal with the physiology of the stomach. They are separated from each other by chapters on unrelated and divergent topics. Diagnostic methods in liver disease are discussed in chapters 14 (liver biopsy), 18 (radioisotopes), 22 (hepatic function tests), and 27 (jaundice), while hepatic disease is in chapter 40. Between these scattered chapters, there are, again, numerous unrelated topics. Despite the overlapping contents of several of these chapters, there are still omission or insufficient treatment of important topics. Disorders of blood coagulation in hepatic disease are dealt with too briefly. Serum enzyme levels in hepatic disease, discussed in several chapters (8, 22, 27) are not dealt with adequately in any. This, presumably, is the result of divided responsibility.

Despite the deficiencies, this first edition of *Gastroenterologic Medicine* is a useful source of important information. It's usefulness would be enhanced if, in future editions, the order of chapters were rearranged and a greater effort were made to avoid repetition and to insure more even coverage.

HYMAN J. ZIMMERMAN, MD
Boston

Experimental Cardiovascular Diseases, part 1. By H Selye, CC, MD, PHD, DSC, FRS (C), FICS (hon). Price, $54.50. Pp 611, with 52 figures. Springer-Verlag New York Inc, 175 Fifth Ave, New York 10010, 1970.

This monumental two-volume monograph on experimental cardiovascular disease by Hans Selye is an indispensable reference work and review of the world's literature. As pointed out in the prefatory remarks on the style of the book, it is really a book within a book. From the 9,000 original articles that Selye reviewed, 5,000 of the more relevant abstracts were selected for inclusion in the text and appear in double column, small print. The author's narrative is printed in single column, large type, presenting his interpretation of the literature, his hitherto unpublished observations with numerous illustrations, diagrams, tables, charts, electronphotomicrographs, conventional light photomicrographs, and photographs of gross pathology, a good many reproduced in color.

The chapter headings are "History," "Factors Inducing Cardiovascular Disease," "Factors Influencing Cardiovascular Disease," "Histology and Histochemistry," "Chemical and Functional Changes Accompanying Cardiovascular Diseases," and "Theories."

It is essential for the uninitiated reader to consult the glossary to learn the meaning of many abbreviations that recur throughout the text, such as ARH, C1-COL, COMT, ESCC, ESCH, ESCN, MAD, SSP-G, SSP-L, SSS.

The works and thoughts of Hans Selye have had a profound influence on world medicine during the past three decades. His animal work relating to the adaptation syndrome, diseases of stress, hormonal factors in cardiovascular disease, the influence of electrolytes such as K^+, Cl^-, Mg^{++}, Na^+, and phosphates in ameliorating, preventing, or aggravating these diseases is still an area that has hardly been surveyed by the clinical investigator. This poses a challenge to the clinical investigator to determine which of these forms of experimental cardiovascular disease are most relevant to clinical medicine, and then to clarify their mechanisms of action.

WELDON J. WALKER, MD
Los Angeles

Interferon. Edited by the New York Heart Association. Price, $8.50. Pp 268, with 58 illustrations. Little Brown & Co, 34 Beacon St, Boston 02106, 1970.

Interferons are proteins of cellular origin capable of conferring resistance against viral invasion. The resistance is nonspecific in contrast to that provided by antibody, which is virus-specific. Because of the broad spectrum antiviral effect, interferon has been considered, for a number of years, a prime prospect in viral chemotherapy. With this in mind, extensive search for potent interferon inducers has been carried out by a number of investigators. Indeed, many have been discovered and found to be effective in curing experimental viral diseases.

What happens when these potent inducers are used to treat human viral diseases? Very little. It is a great disappointment.

Why? It has been thought that interferons, not antibodies, are responsible for recovery from viral diseases. Therefore, by inducing interferon production, one could hasten the recovery. It turns out that this concept is debatable. Furthermore, potent inducers which are effective in treating experimental viral infections are also capable of doing many other things. Trying to relate the recovery from viral diseases to interferon production alone is somewhat reminiscent of the story about the six blind men attempting to define the nature of an elephant.

The New York Heart Association arranged a symposium on interferons as the topic of the Association's Symposium on Basic Science. It was held on Dec 5 and 6, 1969, in New York. In spite of the rationalization offered by the sponsors, it is still difficult to visualize at the present time the role of interferon in cardiovascular diseases.

The book is divided into four parts: Interferon Induction, I and II; Purification and Mechanism of Action; and Interferon and its Inducers in Diseases. Viral sensitivity to interferon, however, is not covered. Nineteen experts participated; exactly the same number of papers were presented.

Many disagreements arose when the experts got together. The molecular aspects of interferon induction by viruses, for instance, have not been completely agreed upon. Is it true that only double-stranded RNA is responsible for interferon induction? Does viral protein play a role in the induction at all? Or, perhaps neither nucleic acid nor protein moieties act as inducing molecules?

Nonviral inducers have been discovered in increasing numbers: (*a*) gram-negative bacteria and their endotoxins (curiously, none of the gram-positive and acid-fast organisms are inducers); the active moiety of endotoxin being the lipid portion rather than the side chains or core polysaccharides; (*b*) other organisms such as rickettsiae, *Chlamydia*, and protozoa; (*c*) fungal products such as mannan from *Candida* and neomycin from streptomycetes; (*d*) plant seed extracts such as mitogens; and (*e*) polyanions (multistranded RNA, polynucleotides, plastics, and polysaccharides).

No interferon has so far been prepared in a pure state. The molecular weights of virus induced interferons range from 25,000 to 35,000. Nonviral induced interferons often, but not always, have higher molecular weights.

The antiviral action of interferon requires host RNA and protein synthesis, and the main action of interferon appears to be inhibiting the translation of viral genetic information, probably by inhibiting the initiation of virus protein synthesis.

Finally, some controversial aspects on the role of interferons in host resistance are discussed. The palliative effects of interferon inducers on some experimental malignancies are also presented.

As in many fields of science, the symposium is arranged by interferon people for interferon people. For microbiologists, oncologists, and infectious disease specialists, the new edition of Finter's book appears more useful.

TE-WEN CHANG, MD
Boston

Synopsis of Dermatology. By WD Stewart, MD, FRCP (C); Julius L Danto, MD; Stuart Maddin, MD. Price, $13.85. Pp 445, with 193 illustrations and 49 color plates. CV Mosby Co, 3207 Washington Blvd, St. Louis 63103, 1970.

Conciseness and 193 illustrations, 49 in color, are the major virtues of this practical dermatological text, which is aimed at pediatricians, internists, and generalists; not dermatologists. It is an updated version of the four-year-old first edition.

Deserving of special approval are the sections on differential diagnosis under each disease; the 32 pages on regional diagnosis, with a terse paragraph under each entity so catalogued; and 12 pages devoted to drug reactions, organized under various types of response. These are of practical value and are very well done.

Corticosteroid therapy is handled so gingerly that there is sometimes a real failure to present it in a bright enough light. In Stevens-Johnson syndrome, it is said that "systemic corticosteroids will relieve the symptoms and shorten the course if no infection or underlying disease is found." Actually, they may be so urgently indicated to stave off blindness or death that they should be given anyway. And for acute dermatitis venenata, "20 to 30 mg daily" is said to be the dose "of systemic steroids"—but which steroid and by what route? And for lichen simplex chronicus, it is suggested that steroids be given within the lesion weekly for three or four weeks, whereas, in fact, a single infiltration of the lesion should suffice for many, many months—or, on the ankle or foot, years.

The major drawback of oral 8-methoxypsoralen (methoxsalen) therapy for vitiligo (unsightly hyperpigmentation of normal skin) is not mentioned; nor are the reasons for the decline in popularity of dermabrasion spelled out. Electrodesiccation is suggested for seborrheic keratoses and cellular nevi, whereas nothing more than a styptic should be used for either one, after its removal.

Some editing oversights occurred. On page 85, a vital negative was omitted in a line which reads "tetracycline should be prescribed during pregnancy." Dermabrasion is not in the index. Lichen amyloidosis (for amyloidosus) is joined, on one page, by two uses of lichen spinulosis (for spinulosus) and, on page 327, by "pruritis." Rothman-Makai is spelled (a Scotticism?) "McKay." The statement that "Acne lesions contain no pathogenic organisms" is followed in the next paragraph by "*Corynebacterium acnes* . . . is found in quantity in some acne lesions." Typographical errors, in contrast, I did not see.

The book is handsomely produced, with headings and subheadings in contrasting type faces that make for easy reading and even easier reference use. Overcoat-pocket size, it would be a convenient volume for desk-top use and frequent, easy reference. It will improve the dermatological acumen of any nondermatologist.

HARRY L. ARNOLD, Jr., MD
Honolulu

Origins of Psychopharmacology: From CPZ to LSD. By Anne E Caldwell, MD. Price, $12. Pp 255. Charles C Thomas Publisher, 301-327 E Lawrence Ave, Springfield, Ill 62703, 1970.

Despite the grandiloquent title, this monograph is no more than a publicity puff for chlorpromazine (CPZ to the initiate) and its creator, H. Laborit. By dividing its message into 132 pages of narrative and 59 of notes, with liberal duplication of content and citation throughout, the book succeeds in being longer than it need be and seeming longer than it is.

The style is Press-Agent Breathless. There are 1.2 exclamation points per page in the first chapter, and many more follow. So counter-productive is the insistence upon CPZ as God's (or Laborit's, the distinction not being clear) unsurpassed greatest gift to the 20th century, one may reactively forget that chlorpromazine is, despite this partisan push, still a frequently useful antiemetic, and that, on balance, the chemical bond is probably a more humane restraint than strap and lock.

Priority is of great moment to Caldwell. Distant battles over who first suggested using CPZ alone or in combination, in anesthesia or in psychiatry, echo through her advocacy; victory often turns upon a single soul found in a paragraph heading.

The tone of the work is cavalier. Investigators who miss the ontological distinction between "sedation" and "ataraxy" merit its disdain. Equally scorned is the psychiatrist who welcomes rauwolfia fully a year after CPZ is introduced. The author resolves contradictions in the early literature by weaving chlorpromazine into the emperor's new clothes, the appreciation of which serves as talisman of the investigator's fitness for research. Her favorite, much-repeated, bit of prose, ". . . a drug—such as Pavlov could only dream about and psychoanalysts were ready to give up their dreams for," typifies the depth of her approach to the problem: how openly is any new enthusiasm received by those whose historical relevance it threatens?

An excursion into the first Golden Age of Mythopharmacology as reported by Homer is best enjoyed by those with a well-cultivated taste for whimsy. Unaccountably, without preamble, the antepenultimate chapter cops the plea that even if CPZ's current success is only mythical, it still stands as a remarkable epic in the history of medicine, and well worth the present recounting.

This volume will be welcomed by all clinicians and students who have long felt the saga of chlorpromazine to be insufficiently celebrated.

MYRON C. GREENGOLD, MD
Reseda, Calif

Diagnosis and Management of Common Thyroid Problems. By JI Hamburger, MD. Price, $9.75. Charles C Thomas Publisher, 301-327 E Lawrence Ave, Springfield, Ill 62703, 1969.

This book is not worth $9.75. It is an interesting, but highly personalized and incomplete account of thyroid problems. The same basic information is available in any standard textbook of medicine. Its chief attraction is the profusion of thyroid scans and short case histories. Regrettably, it cannot be recommended.

J. U. MEAKIN, MD
Toronto

Recent Results in Cancer Research: Endoscopy in Gastric Cancer. By Robert S Nelson. Price, $13.20. Pp 85, with 66 figures. Springer-Verlag New York Inc, 175 Fifth Ave, New York 10010, 1970.

We hear a great deal about the unexplained decrease in gastric cancer in this country over the past several years, mainly because it is the only good thing that has happened in gastrointestinal oncology in such a long time. But gastric cancer remains, of course, one of the most frequent forms of tumor, not only in Japan, Iceland, and Chile (where it may actually be on the increase), but also here at home.

Nelson's monograph shows how gastroscopic examination can make diagnostic effort more reliable, although he does not suggest that treatment will thereby become more effective.

The gastroscopist-oncologist is not so naïve as to believe that application of (gastroscopy) on a wide scale would make a great improvement in cancer mortality. However, he cannot help having faith that it would decrease morbidity in many patients in a disease which has resisted all efforts to produce some kind of diagnostic and therapeutic breakthrough.

The main point of the essay is that gastroscopic evaluation is not used enough in examination of the patient who may have gastric cancer. Nelson believes that now, more than in the past, the gastroscopist can be of help, thanks to certain advantages offered by current fiberoptic construction, by efficient endophotographic attachments, and by reliable direct-vision biopsy mechanisms. Today's peroral endoscopist has many technical capabilities, including the ability to carry out continuous inspection from teeth to midduodenum. (Parenthetically, this makes it necessary for him, prior to each examination, to rummage through a closet-full of expensive instruments to select the one that will be of most help for the problem at hand—whatever fiscal disadvantages there may be to this, we can at least agree that there is no longer any point in arguing over which instrumental design represents the optimal all-round peroral endoscope.)

In projecting instrumental requirements for the future, Nelson emphasizes the need for more effective biopsy forceps. The jaws of current forceps can usually be applied accurately to the suspicious point on the mucosa, but often the endoscopist can then do no more than make a feeble pinching gesture at it, hoping to tear enough tissue away to permit a histopathologic opinion. Designing efficient cutting forceps does not seem too tough a problem for instrument makers who have devised truly magical machines for examining the stomach during the past half century.

Nelson writes defensively about gastroscopy, in the fashion of one who knows the method has a great deal to offer the patient, but who is dismayed at continued reluctance of the profession to make full use of it. He must make a pitch for gastroscopy at a time when one might hope that a pitch is no longer needed. The feature of the book that makes the author's position particularly unassailable is the series of gastrophotographs offered to support his claims. The nonendoscopist (and even the antiendoscopist) can see the gross features of gastric cancer better in these photographs than he has ever seen them at the operating table or in the pathology laboratory.

This is an effective and pleasant discussion of an important subject. It would be good for the general surgeon and the oncologist, especially, to take heed. The endoscopist will be delighted by both the philosophy and the seasoned advice.

EDDY D. PALMER, MD
Schooley's Mountain, NJ

Inhalation Therapy Procedure Manual. By Thomas J DeKornfeld, MD; Don E Gilbert, ARIT. Price, $7.25. Pp 102, with 10 illustrations. Charles C Thomas Publisher, 301-327 E Lawrence Ave, Springfield, Ill 62703, 1970.

This is the second edition of a procedure manual for an inhalation therapy service. It sets forth the organization of such a unit with job descriptions for inhalation therapists, including the chief therapist, as well as technicians. It outlines the inhalation therapy procedures and techniques used at the University of Michigan University Hospital. Each description details the steps which are the responsibility of physician, ward clerk, inhalation therapist, and nurse. Oxygen analyzers, humidifiers, nebulizers, various methods of oxygen therapy, and different types of respirators are discussed. Finally, there are sections on drugs used in inhalation therapy, the cleaning and sterilizing of equipment, as well as a presentation of the methods of record keeping and patient rounds employed at the authors' hospital.

It is recommended that all inhalation therapy be done by a therapist registered by the American Registry of Inhalation Therapists. In the second edition, the job description for inhalation therapy technicians is much more realistic than that presented in the first (published in 1968). It is recognized that the shortage of registered inhalation therapists often requires the use of an inhalation therapy technician in many situations where a registered therapist would be preferable.

Each section opens with a short description of the function and principles of operation of each piece of equipment. This is followed by a description of the procedures involved when using such equipment. Occasionally, the advantages and disadvantages of a piece of equipment are discussed, but more of this type of information would have been helpful.

The use of respirators as a form of mechanical ventilatory assistance is made the responsibility of the physician just as it should be. This section would have been strengthened by discussion of methods for recognition of apparatus leaks and equipment malfunction, which should be detected by the nurse or inhalation therapist. There should also be some comment on methods of measuring expired volume while receiving mechanical ventilatory assistance. Finally, it is disappointing in that the most versatile respirator (Engstrom) and the use of an expiratory retard valve are not discussed.

This second edition has a strong statement on the dangers of 100% oxygen and recommends compressed air rather than oxygen for aerosol therapy. Oxygen tents are given less emphasis than in the first edition.

The elimination of some ineffective and harmful agents has strengthened the section on drugs administered as aerosols. The use of steroids and antibiotics via the aerosol route is condemned except for aerosol steroids in treatment of chemical irritation.

The discussion on the cleaning and sterilization of equipment is short, but to the point: gas sterilization is recommended.

This inhalation therapy manual is a very valuable procedural guide for the operation of an inhalation therapy service. It provides a very useful description of the organization and operation of the excellent inhalation therapy service at the University of Michigan University Hospital. It should be in every inhalation therapy service unit.

JAMES H. CULLEN, MD
Albany, NY

Diagnostic Histochemistry. By Frederick T Zugibe, MD, PhD. Price, $15.85. Pp 366, with 41 illustrations. CV Mosby Co, 3207 Washington Blvd, St. Louis 63103, 1970.

The field of histochemistry has grown rapidly in recent years, reflecting the growth of its sister disciplines, biochemistry, molecular biology, and ultrastructure morphology. While several handbooks and stain formularies are available, pathologists and investigators have had need of an adequate reference in histochemistry. *Diagnostic Histochemistry* is an important new work which should receive wide acclaim in the area of laboratory medicine. The major strength of the book is the author's ability to describe specific procedures understandably and to discuss their merits and shortcomings objectively. The text is comprehensive, but not encyclopedic. The reader soon realizes that Zugibe has expended considerable thought and laboratory time in evaluating and analyzing procedures; he has translated broad personal experience into the pages of this textbook.

There are three major sections in the book. The first deals with the theoretical considerations of tissue processing and identification of components. Separate chapters deal with the lipids, carbohydrates, and enzymes, reviewing their basic biochemistry and the problems in processing specimens so that these substances can be demonstrated. Following thorough discussions of these tissue components, there are excellent charts that provide useful schemata for identifying different lipids and enzymes.

The second section deals with diagnostic applications and gives recommendations for establishing a histochemistry laboratory. Procedures are provided for handling renal, liver, muscle, lymph node, bowel, and brain biopsies. Certain special problems are discussed, such as the diagnosis of the pneumoconioses and differentiating pigments. Many other useful procedures are described, including differentiating normal from leukemic myeloblasts, distinguishing proliferating bile ducts, and diagnosing tumors through histochemistry.

In the appendices, a large number of techniques are presented, with the applications of each method stated clearly. There is a very comprehensive treatment of procedures for a variety of cell and tissue components, microorganisms, and pigments and metals. The chapter on enzyme histochemistry is excellent, as is the appendix on immunochemistry. Perhaps the major weakness of the book is neglect of the nucleic acids and proteins. The author does not deal with quantitative histochemistry or electron microscopy at great length. Other topics are presented clearly and concisely in a well-organized format. The book is recommended for the diagnostic pathologist and to the investigator interested in applying biochemistry to tissue sections or smears.

S. L. INHORN, MD
Madison, Wis

Preventive Myocardiology: Fundamentals and Targets. By Wilhelm Raab, MD. Price, $13.50. Pp 227. Charles C Thomas Publisher, 301-327 E Lawrence Ave, Springfield, Ill 62703, 1970.

This monograph by the late Wilhelm Raab is part of the American Lecture Series of publications. The subject matter is certainly timely: an extensive review of myocardial necroses that can occur due to *other* than obstructive coronary artery disease. The author has written on this subject on many previous occasions and he is well-known in this area of interest. At least 37 references in the extensive bibliography are by Raab.

The presentation is interesting and informative but makes difficult reading. Raab's neologisms do not, in my opinion, enhance the presentation or provide clarity (for example "dysionism," "hypoxiating," "catecholamine desensitizing thyrostatic therapy," and "non-coronarogenic" are terms to make the reader pause and ponder). Nonetheless Raab's review of the contribution of electrolyte derangements and adrenal hormone and adrenergic nervous system excesses to the genesis of myocardial damage is important. The concluding review, including specific possibilities for preventive action, is a succinct presentation of the entire book and well worth reading. This book should be available in medical libraries.

LTC William P. Nelson, MC, USA
Denver

Current Psychiatric Therapies, vol 10. Edited by Jules H Masserman, MD. Price, $14.75. Pp 339. Grune & Stratton Inc, 757 Third Ave, New York 10017, 1970.

As the editor of this volume notes in his "Preface to a Decennial," *Current Psychiatric Therapies* each year has chapters by "three- or four-score authorities in various modes of psychiatric therapy (who) have been invited to submit brief reviews of the latest developments in their respective fields and a response of their significant contributions." This year they cover five sections dealing with child therapy, adult techniques, therapy of addictive and deprivation states, institutional therapies, and community therapy.

The most useful chapters have to do with the treatment of alcohol withdrawal states in which several authors present their therapeutic methods, allowing the reader to compare and evaluate various approaches. Some contributions in other sections suffer from too much brevity, lack of references, lack of scientific validation, and "shotgun" approaches with no consideration of underlying etiological factors. Note for example this comment on the use of lithium carbonate:

> Because the word anxiety means different things to different people (including therapists), lithium–like hydrazines, diphenylhydantoin, and propranolol–probably deserves an empirical trial in any "anxiety state" refractory to more traditional therapies. Again, it may be used continuously or intermittently, and alone or with other drugs.

Others are too alloplastic in nature in that they tend to manipulate the environment of the patient rather than bring about more lasting personality changes. The least useful discussion concerns itself with the treatment of transsexuals in which the authors defend "surgical sex reassignment" against all critics and suggest that if a psychiatrist does not agree with their viewpoint (that for some it "offers the prospect of a more adaptive psychosocial and psychosexual adjustment"), he refers the patient to one who does, ie, "another psychiatrist with a more flexible approach based on the requirement of that individual patient."

For those readers interested in an overview of "current" psychiatric therapies, their pitfalls, limitations, and advances, this book may prove of interest.

Harry S. Abram, MD
Nashville, Tenn

Pain and Suffering. Edited by Benjamin L Crue, Jr, MD, Capt (MC) USNR. Price, $12.75. Pp 205. Charles C Thomas Publisher, 301-327 E Lawrence Ave, Springfield, Ill 62703, 1970.

While this small book is actually written for neurosurgeons, I believe it is worthwhile to bring it to the attention of internists, since it shows certain practical methods to relieve pain with which they may not be familiar. This work represents a symposium held at the City of Hope in which various new technical approaches for control of intractable pain were reviewed by experts in such fields as neurosurgery, neurology, cardiology, oncological surgery, psychiatry, psychology, neurophysiology, and legal medicine.

The book limits itself, to a large extent, to the surgical control of intractable trigiminal neuralgia. While the editors state that the main purpose of the book is to attempt to formulate underlying neurophysiological mechanisms for chronic pain, they are unable to achieve their purpose. There is a large chasm between the neurophysiologist studying pain in the laboratory and the clinician treating a patient. There is not even unanimity in regard to definitions.

This book represents a one-day meeting and is not complete or comprehensive. Considering pain as a specific modality is misleading. While it is agreed that small nerve fibers are critical to the transmission of impulses perceived as pain, the central neural mechanisms are not understood. One's choice on what pain is will depend mostly on his profession. For example, any method that reduces anxiety also reduces pain.

The book uses mechanisms similar to epilepsy to explain much of pain. No balanced approach is given for pharmacologic treatment of pain, but only specific and restricted neurosurgical methods are emphasized. While the text is only illustrative and not complete, it reveals some of the great gaps in our knowledge and will help the internist and other nonsurgical professionals to become familiar with certain neurosurgical methods in use today. The participants in this symposium are to be complimented in attempting to use the various disciplines to seek understanding in such a universal and important subject.

Thomas Auerbach, MD
Chicago

Body Fluid Replacement in the Surgical Patient. Edited by Charles L Fox Jr, MD; Gabriel Nahas, MD. Price, $25. Pp 374. Grune & Stratton Inc, 757 Third Ave, New York 10017, 1970.

This book is a compilation of papers presented at an International Symposium held in 1969, sponsored by the departments of surgery and anesthesiology of the College of Physicians and Surgeons, Columbia University, in association with the Division of Medical Sciences, National Research Council. The editors were chairmen of the symposium.

The book is divided into four parts, each consisting of from 9 to 11 papers; the contributors are, therefore, numerous. The participants to the symposium, 95 experts in their fields, were representatives of outstanding medical schools and medical centers from all over the United States as well as Sweden, France, and Switzerland. The four parts of the book cover in considerable detail blood, colloid, water, and electrolyte replacement and parenteral alimentation.

No particular format is followed in the specific chapters since they are made up of individual papers presented. References are adequate and chapters are well supported by numerous tables, graphs, and occasional photographic illustrations. Several chapters are followed by discussions of the participants.

While the book title refers to care of the surgical patient, and reference is made to the burn and trauma patient, the material presented is applicable to most patients in need of fluid replacement. As such, this book serves as an excellent reference for investigator and clinician.

MG CARL HUGHES, MC, USA
Honolulu

The Paranoid. By David W Swanson, MD; Philip J Bohnert, MD; Jackson A Smith, MD. Price, $15. Pp 544, with three illustrations. Little Brown & Co, 34 Beacon St, Boston 02106, 1970.

This book provides very interesting treatment of its subject. It holds wide reading appeal, especially for everyone concerned with the effect of one's mental condition upon all of his activity that may be described as social. To begin with, its unusually effective jacket focuses the localization of paranoid reactions within the individual's own mind, by providing the outline of the figure of a person by verbal description of grievance feelings. The extensive study is helpfully divided into the following four sections: Survey of the Problem, Clinical Aspects, Theoretical Considerations, and The Spheres of Influence. References, numerous and well selected, follow each of the 21 chapters. A workable index is provided.

The authors present richly descriptive accounts of paranoid disorders in a comprehensive, relevant way. Each section is strong in its own area, including readily understandable illustrative material. Every portion of the book is well done. Special attention is given to the human tendency to project one's feeling into one's "external world." The meaning of the individual's mental health in terms of the welfare of his world receives thoughtful consideration. Reader attention is invited to the professional competency inherent in the health worker's identifying with his fellowman's hurt feeling by observing paranoid tendencies in his own living. Each author may feel justly proud of this contribution to appreciating the nature and extent of the health ordeal named paranoia.

JOHN M. DORSEY, MD
Detroit

Laboratory Diagnosis of Diseases Caused by Toxic Agents. Edited by F William Sunderman, MD, PhD, F William Sunderman, Jr, MD. Price, $32.50. Pp 592. Warren H Green Inc, 10 S Brentwood Blvd, St. Louis 63105, 1970.

The increase in knowledge of biological and physical phenomena has led to a need for monographs which treat minutae in exquisite detail and for general texts which provide an overview yet with sufficient detail to make it worthwhile for the specialist. There is a third type of text, the edited proceedings of a seminar or meeting, which allows the reader the privilege of enjoying a wide ranging program, without the inconvenience of physically attending the sessions. This book is a fine example.

As a timely and up-to-date report of a seminar on *Laboratory Diagnosis of Diseases Caused by Toxic Agents* this is excellent. It provides the reader with a view of many toxicologic problems without becoming bogged down in detail. But the reader who needs more depth and detail has best look elsewhere.

The four parts of the book: "General Toxicologic Considerations"; "General Methodologic Considerations"; "Specific Toxic Agents"; and "Clinicopathologic Considerations" are interesting vistas of a particular specialty area. Again, these are fine for an overview but perhaps too brief for indepth understanding. This is not a catalog of toxic actions but a thoughtful approach to the procedures needed to evaluate the action on humans of the chemicals in our environment. The effects of those chemicals are discussed in relation to their modes of action, their analysis in tissue and body fluids, and their clinicopathological effects.

As with any multiauthored text the sections are uneven in quantity and quality. But this is true of any seminar or other meeting. The title is misleading; it is not truly a guide to laboratory diagnosis in the sense we usually use that term. It is a seminar on the effects of toxic agents and their laboratory analysis, and it is well worth reading.

MITCHELL R. ZAVON, MD
Cincinnati

Rational Therapy and Control of Tuberculosis. Edited by Joseph E Johnson III, MD. Price, $8.50. Pp 191, with no illustrations. University of Florida Press, Gainesville, 1970.

During the past several years, the Public Health Service spent money to disseminate modern information about tuberculosis. Much of this money was used to sponsor conferences in various parts of the country. It seems highly likely that the best investment made was in the conference in Gainesville, Fla. This must represent one of the more outstanding presentations of the series and has the distinct advantage of survival in book form.

In a day of increasing complexity, it is delightful to find a volume less than 200 pages which has been prepared so carefully as to include virtually all essential concepts for understanding treatment and control of tuberculosis.

The text material is of very high quality. Outstanding chapters are presented by Riley on "Airborne Transmission," by Mackaness on "Cellular Immunity," by Simon on "Microbial Persistence," and by Edwards on the "Interpretation and Significance of the Tuberculin Test."

One of the most pertinent and enlightening chapters is by Cluff, relating experience in brucellosis and influenza. This chapter points out the difficulty encountered by certain patients with depressive tendencies while they attempt to cope with illness.

The section on therapy is much too casual if the book is to serve as a manual for tuberculosis control. However, the essayists, in general, set a good example for scholarship, and the reader finds ample references to pertinent literature.

All in all, the volume promises to be useful for busy practitioners and house officers alike. It seems to have been released at a time when the medical profession greatly needs it. Teachers must have a copy; those who treat patients with tuberculosis should master the concepts presented. All will appreciate the compact form and the reasonable cost. This little volume is recommended strongly.

JOHN A. PIERCE, MD
St. Louis

The Hepatic Circulation and Portal Hypertension. Edited by Carroll M Leevy, MD, Richard C Britton, MD. Price, $23. Pp 405. New York Academy of Sciences, 2 E 63rd Street, New York 10021, 1970.

Clinicians and investigators interested in hepatology should peruse these proceedings of the conference on the hepatic circulation and portal hypertension held in October 1969, cosponsored by the New York Academy of Sciences and the American Association for the Study of Liver Diseases. Thirty communications by recognized authorities are published; about a third are basically oriented; the remainder clinical. Discussions follow most of the communications. A few give valuable perspective and critical evaluations of a subject.

Anatomical and morphological topics include the gross and microscopic vascular anatomy of the liver, effects of altered oxygen supply on hepatocytes, microcirculatory basis for portal hypertension, and mechanisms of hepatic fibrogenesis. Physiological communications discuss tracer dilution techniques for the study of hepatic membrane transport, the application of Michaelis-Menten kinetics to dye, dilution curves, the pulmonary circulation in portal hypertension and abnormalities of the oxyhemoglobin dissociation curve in cirrhosis. Communications combining a review with experimental work (and offering good source material) are offered on portal hypertension in association with normal liver histology and on the pathogenesis of portal hypertension in schistosomiasis. Four communications deal with the clinical evaluation of the patient by means of roentgenologic techniques, endoscopy, hepatic and umbilicoportal catheterization, and transhepatic pressure measurements. Surgical topics include a discussion of the effects of major hepatic resections, surgical treatment of hepatic encephalopathy, the status, effects and complications of portocaval shunt surgery, and current experience with hepatic transplantation.

The proceedings contain some excellent material on the pathogenesis of ascites and on the origin of renal failure in cirrhosis. Communications and discussions on hepatic and splanchnic lymph flow (Dumont, Witte, and Witte), on renal failure in cirrhosis (Baldus), on intractable ascites (Orloff), and on the alternate theories of reduced "effective" blood volume versus the "overflow" theory of ascited formation (Lieberman, Denison, and Reynolds) throw the current thoughts on these subjects into clear relief. Taken collectively, I believe these communications represent one of the best single sources available on these subjects. And, as Chalmers points out, these theories are far from academic; they bear directly on practical therapeutics.

Finally, important and practical discussions of emergency medical treatment stem from two communications, one by Seymour Schwartz on the influence of vasoactive drugs on the portal circulation, the second on the prognosis and management of bleeding esophegeal varices by Harold O. Conn. Improved techniques for the use of vasopressin seem to herald more effective and safer ways to control variceal hemorrhage; namely, the repeated or continuous infusion of vasopressin intravenously, and the continuous intraarterial infusion of the drug into mesenteric arteries.

These latter discussions reemphasize the devastating effects of portal hypertension and advanced liver disease. Of course, we must strive to understand the vascular effects of liver injury and the pathogenesis, pathophysiology, and treatment of portal hypertension. This volume is a good review and is a valuable reference source on these subjects. But knowing these phenomena are secondary and often irreversible, I am made acutely aware of the cost of unchecked alcoholism and our poor understanding of the etiologic factors causing nonalcoholic cirrhosis.

DON P. JONES, MD
Chicago

Skin Signs of Systemic Disease. Irwin M Braverman, MD. Price, $29.50. Pp 448, with 474 illustrations. WB Saunders Co, 218 W Washington Sq, Philadelphia 19105, 1970.

This is a major new dermatological textbook, indispensable for every dermatologist, rheumatologist, or internist who is serious about keeping sharp professionally.

It is not about treatment; it is about pathogenesis, pathologic physiology, and diagnosis. Illustrations are abundant—more than one per page—and almost every one is outstanding. Nearly 200 are in color.

Style is concise and vivid, presentations forthright, and opinions positive. When there are opposing views they are stated fairly, but the author's preference is made clear. His "lumper" treatment of acanthosis nigricans (with no reference to Curth's publications and only casual and superficial reference to her views) is an exception to this, but there are not many such.

His treatment of the connective-tissue diseases, angiitides, and hypersensitivity syndromes alone would be worth the price of the book to any internist or rheumatologist, let alone any dermatologist. The book is not just a book to refer to now and then. It is a book to read. It is a book to own. I bought *my* copy (sob!) before the review copy arrived.

HARRY L. ARNOLD, JR., MD
Honolulu

Osteoporosis. Edited by Uriel S Barzel, MD. Price, $25. Pp 290. Grune & Stratton Inc 757 Third Ave, New York 10017, 1970.

This book is in essence a compendium of the papers presented at the first International Symposium on Osteoporosis held at the Montefiore Hospital and Medical Center in New York in June 1969. Some of the important papers were not included, but most of the discussion after each presentation and several summaries have been retained. These seem to emphasize the lack of unanimity of opinion as to the cause and most effective forms of therapy for this common metabolic bone disorder.

In some ways this book is similar to the annual volumes "Recent Progress in Hormone Research," which publish the papers and discussions of the Laurentian Hormone Conferences. It is by no means to be considered a textbook for students or general physicians interested in bone disorders since it is not well organized, omits many detailed aspects of the newer forms of treatment of osteoporosis such as fluoride, phosphate and calcitonin, although these agents are mentioned frequently.

The role of growth hormone is not covered. There is an undue stress on the importance of the parathyroid glands in this disorder, and a great deal of speculation as to increased or decreased sensitivity of bone to parathyroid hormone (most of which is not backed with actual measurements). One may well ask why osteoporotic bone does not look like osteitis fibrosa if excessive bone resorption is attributed principally to the action of parathyroid hormone. The interesting suggestion by the editor that the acid ash diet of the carnivorous humans contributes to this high incidence of osteoporosis, leaves doubts about the bone structure of other carnivores such as the lion or tiger.

The important work of Frost using tetracycline labelling of bone, and the technique of microradiography are not covered. The value of this book would have been greatly enhanced by better grouping of papers into sections, rather than into 23 chapters (eg, a section on the etiology and natural history, a section on experimental work-differentiating animal and human research, and last a section on therapeutic approaches).

The last two chapters by Haney and Whedon on "A Unified Concept of Osteoporosis: A Second Look" and "Symposium Comment" point out the deficiencies of a symposium such as this and help the less informed reader to be aware of the many areas of controversy in this field.

The illustrations are clear, the x-ray films are well reproduced, and the appendix of 14 pages of references on osteoporosis enhances the usefulness of this book. A great deal of new information will be forthcoming in this rapidly moving field. One wonders if the title for this hardcover book should not be "Recent Progress in Osteoporosis Research, vol 1," rather than suggesting that it presents a treatise on osteoporosis.

The book is recommended for the informed reader engaged in clinical or animal research in metabolic disorders of bone. It is not recommended for the student or the general internist or orthopedist who wants up to date information on how to manage the osteoporotic patient.

FELIX O. KOLB, MD
San Francisco

Penetrating Wounds of the Abdomen. Edited by James E Pridgen, MD, FACS; J Bradley Aust, MD, FACS; George W Fisher, MD, FACS. Price, $9.75. Pp 126, no illustrations. Charles C Thomas Publisher, 301-327 Lawrence Ave, Springfield, Ill 62703, 1970.

For several years we have turned to the experiences of large city hospitals for guidance in the management of penetrating trauma from low velocity instruments of civilian "warfare." The Robert B. Green Hospital of San Antonio, Tex, has a vast number of cases to study, and this book suggests that their handling of such injuries is especially worthy of our attention. They also included the management of high velocity wounds in Vietnam, which adds significantly to the story of penetrating wounds.

The organization of the book is slightly puzzling since they begin with a chapter on anesthesia before describing the immediate resuscitation and steps in diagnosis.

The chapter on radiological diagnosis provides a good explanation of the diagnosis of full thickness abdominal wall injury by the insertion of a catheter into the wound and injection of contrast medium. Most of the other techniques are more appropriate for blunt trauma than penetrating, since there is less difficulty in deciding in favor of exploration of penetrating wounds. Careful exploration reveals the organs perforated once laparotomy is accomplished. Special x-ray studies such as excretory urography, cystograms, barium enemas, gastrointestinal series, and aortograms are more helpful in blunt trauma. They serve mainly to gather information by techniques which could be obtained as reliably and more expeditiously by exploration of penetrating wounds.

The book's most important contribution is the description of the proper selection of patients with penetrating wounds who can be observed without surgery. This is another instance of the pendulum swing which describes an arc from the days before surgery of the abdomen through the period when all penetrating wounds were explored to now, when we attempt to identify those cases which do not require exploration. They are quick to point out that not all centers accept selective exploration since poor results were obtained when it was attempted. There are a significant number of patients with negative physical findings who later prove to have visceral injury; unnecessary delay and morbidity results from procrastination and observation. The author's indications for exploration in borderline cases are (1) presence of peritoneal irritation as evidenced by tenderness, rebound pain or absent bowel sounds; (2) x-ray evidence of contrast material entering the peritoneal space when injected into the wound; (3) recovery of blood, enteric debris or more than 200 leukocytes per cubic millimeter after instillation of saline at the rate of 20 ml/kg via peritoneal lavage.

The book is superficial in several areas, but taken as a whole the book has most of the necessary tips and safeguards in successful management of penetrating wounds of the abdomen.

This book is a worthwhile contribution to the library of the surgeon or emergency room physician.

DARRELL A. JAQUES, MD, MC, USA
Washington, DC

AUDIOVISUAL MATERIAL

Educational Aids From the Tampa Tracings

Digitalis Intoxication: 45 slides, 60 minutes magnetic tape, 6 pages text. Price, $110.

Introduction to Congestive Heart Failure. By and presented by Henry JL Marriot. 13 slides, 25 minutes magnetic tape, 5 pages text. Price, $40.

Sophisticated Monitoring Slides: 80 slides, 23 pages text. Price, $95.

Pacemakers. 40 slides, 8 pages text. Price, $50.

Introduction to Monitoring. 28 slides, 30 minutes magnetic tape, script. Price, $60.

The Premature Beat. 32 slides, 30 minutes magnetic tape, script. Price, $60. Educational Aids from the Tampa Tracings, Box 636, Oldsmar, Fla 33557.

Special training has become the essential ingredient for success of new facilities for treatment of cardiovascular diseases. In this new situation, the cardiologist may find that his direct personal contribution to his patient's care plays a less decisive role than his direct personal contribution to training the intensive care team which surround his patient day and night. Reversible life-threatening catastrophes are more likely to occur while the cardiologist is absent from the bedside than while he is there. At that moment, the training of his team to recognize the problem promptly and act efficiently may well determine the fate of the patient.

It has been difficult for the cardiologist to shift his thinking to meet the new requirements of his specialty: to devote major attention to the training program. Rapid turnover of the house staff and intensive care nurses and aides requires such frequent repetition of the training program as to virtually overwhelm even the most dedicated attending staff. In this situation, I welcomed the opportunity to review *Tampa Tracings* as summaries of essential material for an instruction program. The prepared slides made it easy to review the material and to present it repeatedly in a standard way. The slide program can be supplemented by adding new material to fit individual hospital needs, while preserving the fundamental framework. Attending cardiologists will find considerable reenforcement for their own lifetime learning program; and may (as I did) find the repetition produces other valuable rewards.

Some colleagues and I first tested the lectures on *Digitalis Intoxication and Congestive Heart Failure* in a 500-bed general community hospital. At first it was used without modification; later it was modified for presentation at a cardiovascular seminar, and still later, it was used with a case presentation at medical grand rounds. During the first presentation, the ideas caught the attention of some visiting medical students and led them to carry out a survey of their own throughout the hospital. They found a disturbingly high incidence of minor digitalis intoxication among patients whose physicians had failed to appreciate its presence. The interaction between students, and attending and house staffs produced rewards in the form of improved therapy for patients and better understanding by the professional staff.

Characteristic of the pithy remarks scattered throughout *Tampa Tracings,* the commentary suggests "Lanatocide is replacing homicide." It goes on to point out "the inexpert use of glycosides . . . is unfortunately all too common." With increased delegation of authority for writing orders to junior house officers, as part of their training program, the risk of intoxication has become particularly great. Occasionally this occurs when a patient is least able to withstand it. Often he is sensitized to the toxic effect of digitalis by the action of potent diuretics which wash potassium out and make the myocardium particularly susceptible. The slides illustrate the wide variety of gastrointestinal, cardiac, neurologic, and other symptoms produced by digitalis, as well as the cardio-depressant and cardio-stimulant electrocardiographic effects.

As prerequisite for studying *The Introduction to Monitoring,* the student needs only to recognize the main waves of the ECG to know where electrodes are applied, and to understand the rudimentary anatomy of the conduction system of the heart. From that beginning the lecture and slides carry him through each of the successive steps necessary to draw a diagnosis out of squiggles appearing on an electrocardiographic monitor. Each step of learning is punctuated by a simple test slide to insure that learning has advanced enough to prepare for the next step. Normal activation, right and left bundle branch block, and right and left ventricular origin of premature beats are explained so simply and logically that a bright student should be able to learn the material in the 30 minutes required to go through the series of 28 slides while listening to the magnetic tape recording. Even a dullard should require little more time and repetition to master it.

The beginning student is advised to seek the QRS complexes first as he looks at the record because they offer the richest source of primary diagnostic information, following, as the lecturer states, the principle of Willy Sutton: "To rob banks because that is where the money is." Only later is the student asked to identify P waves (Cherchez le P) and establish relationships between atrial and ventricular activity (Who's married to whom?).

The Premature Beat identifies the significant features of ventricular and supraventricular beats, the compensatory pause, retrograde conduction, and bigeminy and trigeminy. The lessons show how readily aberrant conduction can mask a supraventricular beat to make it appear to have originated within the ventricle. The lesson extends the learning from that acquired in *The Introduction to Monitoring* in similar steps, punctuated again with test slides that insure the student's progress and reinforce his learning by appropriate repetition. Few cardiologists would choose to review their own understanding in such tiny steps, but the lesson provides a quick painless pathway for that review while the cardiologist uses it to brief his intensive care team on fundamentals. As I went through the exercise myself, I found that I had never quite fully appreciated T. Killip's rule establishing a mathematical probability that a given atrial extrasystole would induce atrial tachyrhythmias and was impressed with the slide that demonstrated induction of atrial fibrillation. Although I had already known about the vulnerable period of the atrium and its mechanisms, I had failed to recognize the importance of whether the beat fell later than a half cycle duration from the preceding P wave, where it rarely induces tachyrhythmia, and within the first half cycle duration, where it usually does. The slide showed fixed coupling of the atrial premature beat at an interval of 0.40 seconds, inducing no response when the preceding cycle length was 0.70 seconds but inducing atrial fibrillation when the preceding cycle length was 0.88 seconds.

The *Sophisticated Monitoring Slide Guide and Commentary* demonstrates a common error of conventional monitoring, particularly the attachment of electrodes in any position that will provide a large R-wave on the oscilloscopic screen. Marriott has emphasized the advantage of special connections (MCL_1, MCL_6, and M_3) designed to identify whether premature beats originate in the right or in the left ventricle and to distinguish aberrantly conducted supraventricular rhythms from idioventricular rhythms. This information may help guide the management of arrhythmias, which have been responsible for about half the deaths following myocardial infarction in ordinary hospital facilities.

Now precise identification of arrhythmias, to facilitate rapid institution of specific management now available in intensive care units, takes on special importance. One rarely loses the patient from an arrhythmia alone, in special care units. But this success deepens our discontent with the very slight improvement in control of cardiogenic shock, the other major cause for death following myocardial infarction. Still, it certainly fans enthusiasm for the quest for better understanding of the mechanism responsible for shock and for better methods of managing it.

In the series of 80 slides, one sees examples not only of all the common supraventricular and idioventricular rhythms but also of types likely to mimic one another. Supraventricular tachycardias and supraventricular premature beats with aberrant conduction may mimic ventricular tachycardias and ventricular premature beats sufficiently to fool experts with long experience unless they pay attention to clues, well illustrated in this series of slides. They help the clinician avoid diagnostic booby traps as they show escape rhythms, pacemaker beats, artifacts, and arteriovenous (A-V) dissociation with and without block.

The Pacemaker Slide Guide and Commentary distinguishes among four types of pacemakers in current use: (1) continuous, asynchronous; (2) demand; (3) atrial triggered; and (4) ventricular triggered. Any type of pacemaker may end up in your coronary care unit now that patients with heart block are able to travel. Peculiar spikes, if you think only of those produced by the pacemaker preferred by your local surgeon, may not indicate pacemaker malfunction. The guide clarifies their mechanism so that you will not confuse normal spikes with those produced by the great variety of malfunctions that must also be clearly recognized.

In the ventricular triggered unit, the spike immediately precedes the QRS-complex when it is pacing but follows it when the ventricle is going on its own. Spontaneous arrhythmias produce many peculiarities, but each produces changes that must conform to precisely measured patterns; these must be familiar to the cardiologist or he will overlook malfunctions when they occur. Controlling the pacemaker rate with a magnet or alteration of the heart's own rhythm by carotid pressure or isoproterenol can create test circumstances appropriate for determining how the pacemaker will function under varying circumstances and whether it is adequate to deal with the situation when it arises spontaneously. The illustrations from actual clinical situations prepare one to deal with these difficult problems when they actually occur in practice.

I can heartily recommend this instruction material and consider it well worth its rather considerable cost. The "Tracings" are useful for training house staff, medical students, and nurses, if one makes appropriate adjustments in techniques of presentation. The attending staff who must present the material can also expect to profit in the form of improved clinical skill.

WILLIAM H. WEHRMACHER, MD
Chicago

Internal medicine at large

Memory and neurotransmitters

Variations in the level of neurotransmitter substances, rather than genetics, may be at the root of poor memory, according to a Philadelphia investigator.

Moreover, Louis B. Flexner, MD, believes that both loss of memory and its restoration can be achieved by the administration of appropriate chemical substances. Dr. Flexner, of the Department of Anatomy of the University of Pennsylvania School of Medicine, told the annual meeting of the Spanish Society of Biochemistry at Barcelona:

"We have recently found that a transient amnesia, experimentally produced and previously ascribed to lack of synthesis of a specific protein, can be prevented by injections of metaraminol, which increases the level of available norepinephrine.

"Thus, it now appears that neurotransmitters, rather than changes in gene expression, may play an important role in memory."

The Philadelphia investigator said that his group has focused its attention on the possible role of norepinephrine in memory because of earlier findings that metaraminol displaces norepinephrine from storage sites in the brain.

"A variety of approaches had been used to test the hypothesis that memory depends on changes in gene expression. But all had failed to give convincing evidence that synthesis of a new type of RNA protein is necessary in the biochemistry of memory," Dr. Flexner asserted.

"For example, memory of maze learning in mice is lost permanently after intracerebral injections of puromycin, which profoundly inhibits protein synthesis. However, this effect is due to formation of abnormal puromycin-peptides and not to interference with protein synthesis. In fact, it was the similarity in structure of the o-methyl tyrosine moiety of puromycin and norepinephrine that suggested to us the possibility that the puromycin-peptides block memory by blocking adrenergic sites."

He added that such memory blocks can be overcome and memory completely restored in animals following injection of a variety of drugs that also displace norepinephrine from binding sites. These agents include imipramine, d-amphetamine and tranylcypromine.

"The use of such agents led to a remarkable restoration of memory. This was accompanied by a significant decrease of the puromycin complex at the nerve endings but the mitochondrial fractions of the brain cells showed no changes."

Norepinephrine

Scientists attending the meeting of the Spanish Society of Biochemistry also heard a warning that the specific functions of norepinephrine remain unclear even though quite a bit is known about norepinephrine transmitter function at peripheral synapses, as well as its (and epinephrine's) peripheral involvement in emotional states.

"In the brain, no biogenic amine has been conclusively shown to be a transmitter. The evidence is indirect

continued

Highlights This Month

Two "slow viruses" linked to cancerous transformation of cells in vitro . . . page 514.

Bone scans with sodium fluoride are helpful in staging lymphomas, but only as an adjunct to roentgenographic examination . . . page 516.

Synthesis of luteinizing hormone-releasing hormone may lead to new advances in fertility control . . . page 516.

Internists in the news . . . pages 521 and 524.

Norepinephrine continued

or inferential but sufficiently extensive and consistent to permit the formulation of hypotheses that central, as well as peripheral actions of biogenic amines mediate arousal and certain emotional states," said Seymour S. Kety, MD, of the Harvard Medical School.

"Catecholamines, as well as serotonin, have been demonstrated throughout the brain and spinal cord—concentrated in the presynaptic varicosities along the terminal axons of particular neurons."

He conceded that there have been many reports consistent with the premise of a release of norepinephrine centrally in association with affective states. Such a phenomenon has been noted particularly in arousal, aggression, and certain types of behavior associated with various types of appetities. At the same time, some of the observations seem more consistent with the possibility that dopamine is the agent with an important role in such states.

"However, there appears to be no simplistic hypothesis compatible with all of the observations to date and it seems quite futile to attempt to account for a particular emotional state in terms of the activity of one or more biogenic amines.

"It may be more likely that these amines may function separately or in concert at crucial nodes of the complex neuronal networks which underlie emotional states," Dr. Kety said at the meeting in Barcelona.

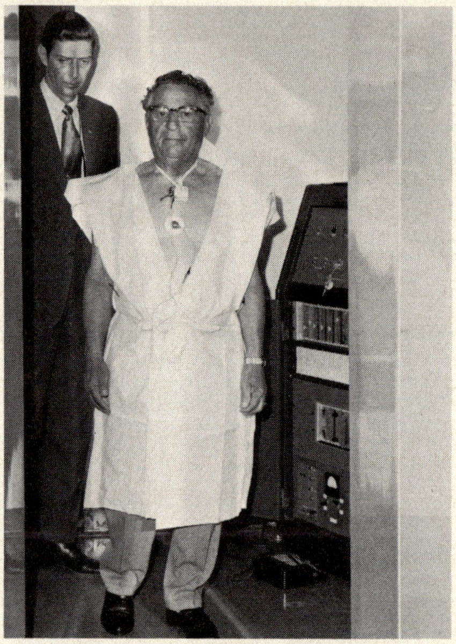

A patient with pacemaker enters the passway where the detection system is located with Oliver C. Hood, MD, of the Federal Aviation Administration, watching close by.

Detector seems 'safe'

The weapon detector—called a magnetometer—is in place. A man starts to walk through its electromagnetic field. The Federal Aviation investigators lean forward.

Their search is not for a potential airline hijacker, but for a possible effect of the magnetism on the man's cardiac pacemaker.

The test device is a recently developed Westinghouse magnetometer. The investigators for the FAA are physicians from George Washington University School of Medicine and the Potomac Fund for Cardiovascular Research, Washington, DC.

Their conclusion: In 53 patients, no effect on unipolar fixed rate, and unipolar or bipolar triggered ventricular pacemakers—the three most widely used types—and minor, clinically insignificant changes in a few special types. Studies continue on other potential sources of pacemaker interruption.

Slow viruses and cancer

National Institutes of Health investigators report that two "slow viruses" associated with slowly progressing diseases in sheep have been shown to cause cancerous transformation in normal mouse cells in vitro. Moreover, these transformed cells, when injected into newborn or irradiated young adult mice, cause fibrosarcomas at the site of inoculation.

Kenneth K. Takemoto, PhD, and Lawrence B. Stone, PhD, both of the National Institute of Arthritis and Metabolic Diseases, said the viruses are the progressive pneumonia virus (PPV) and visna virus, which causes a neurologic disorder in sheep.

The cells transformed by the two viruses were altered in both form and structure, and after two passages the cell cultures consisted entirely of transformed cells. At that time, infectious virus could not be recovered, but when the mouse cells were then co-cultivated with normal sheep testis cells, both viruses were recovered from all cell lines. This indicated that the viral genetic material was associated with transformed cells.

Drs. Takemoto and Stone said there was no evidence that any other oncogenic DNA or RNA viruses were involved in the cell transformation.

These two slow viruses contain RNA-dependent DNA polymerase, the investigators said, lending support to the "protovirus" theory of Howard M. Temin, PhD, of the University of Wisconsin, who has hypothesized that cell transformation by RNA tumor viruses involves a DNA intermediate which becomes integrated with the host cell's genetic material.

John R. Seal, MD, acting director of NIAMD, says that the findings of Drs. Takemoto and Stone may have some bearing on the pathogenesis of slow virus infections. It is suggested that infection of animals hosts by visna virus and PPV involves "integration" of a DNA copy of the viral genome in host cells and virus replication by the DNA template. This may explain the difficulty experienced heretofore in detecting virus in such diseases.

Slow viruses also have been implicated to a degree in other diseases such as multiple sclerosis in man, scrapie in sheep, and Aleutian disease of minks.

Visna virus (× 102,000)

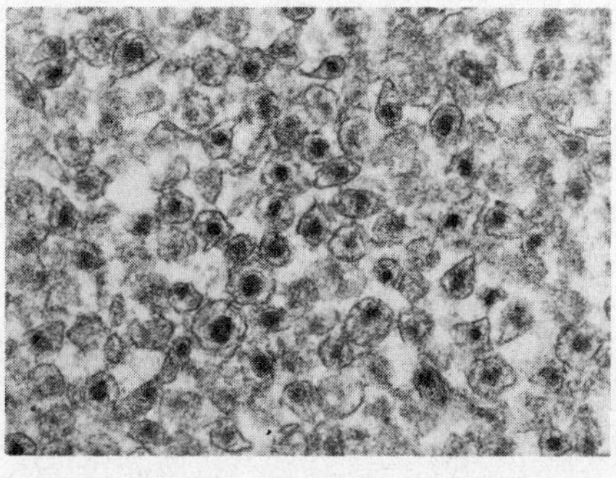

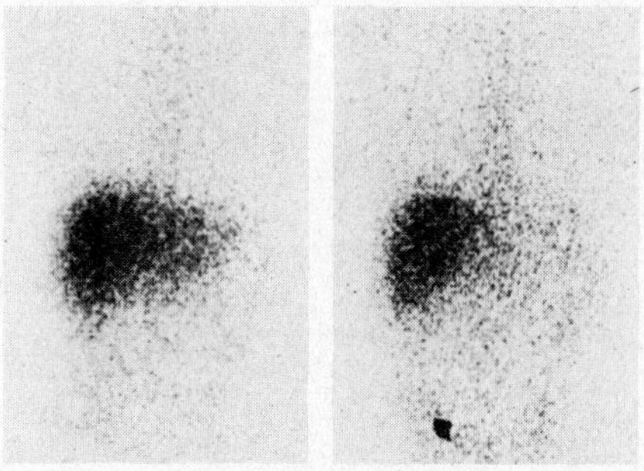

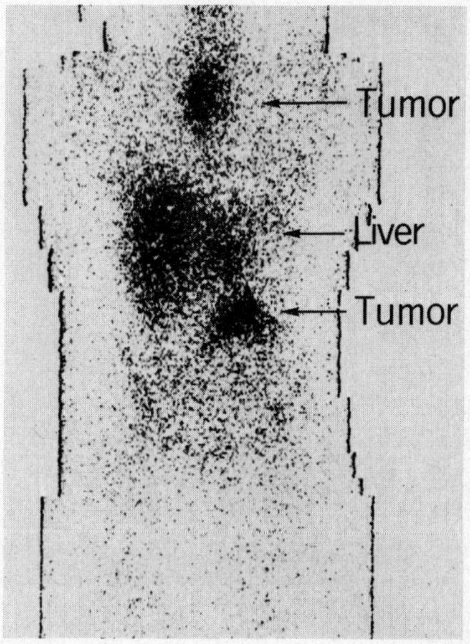

Right anterior (above, left) and posterior gallium 67 citrate scans of a normal person show localization of the isotope in the liver and, to a lesser degree, the vertebrae. The scan (right) of a patient with Hodgkin's disease shows uptake of the isotope by tumor sites in the mediastinum and the abdomen (arrows) as well as by the liver.

Gallium scans

Gallium 67 citrate, a relatively new isotope, tends to localize in the liver—and also in various neoplastic tissues. Investigators say that this property may make it possible to locate all the sites of involvement in patients with Hodgkin's disease. This is important because some specialitists believe that as many as 75% of such patients could be cured if all the loci of neoplasm are found.

Steven M. Pinsky, MD, described the scanning technique at the recent meeting of the Association of University Radiologists in Durham, NC. In one series, Hodgkin's disease had been confirmed by biopsy in 16 patients. Eight had normal gallium scans, indicating no secondary disease sites; this was confirmed by laparotomy. Scans in the other eight patients showed 14 additional sites; all were confirmed by laparotomy, and one more was found during surgery. The series had one false negative—a diffusely involved spleen appeared normal on the scan—and two false positives, also involving the spleen.

Dr. Pinsky said the technique would probably be useful for staging other lymphomatous diseases and for checking the effectiveness of therapy in Hodgkin's and similar diseases.

Dr. Pinsky is a resident in radiology at the University of Chicago. His co-workers were Paul B. Hoffer, MD, chief of the section on nuclear medicine, and Alexander Gottschalk, MD, professor of radiology and director of the Argonne Cancer Research Hospital, Lemont, Ill.

Internal medicine at large

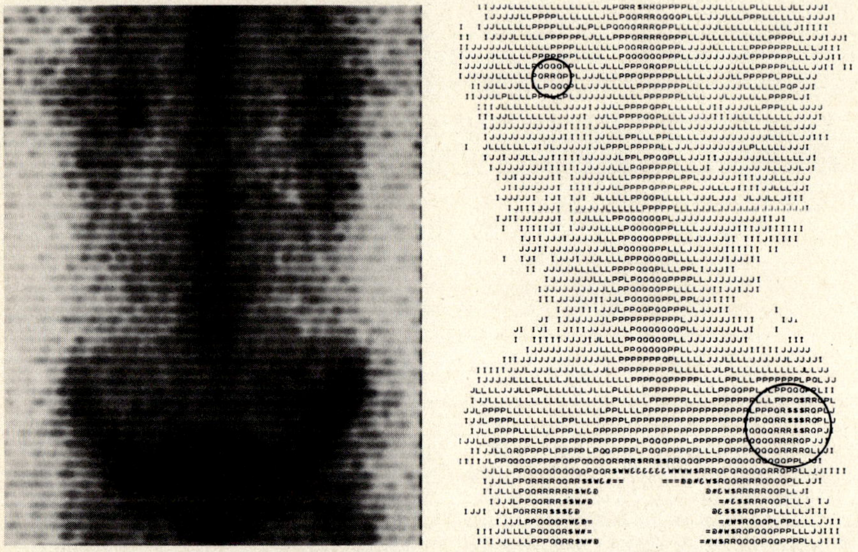

The faint indications of bony lesions in the right thoracic and pelvic regions in the anterior photoscan (left) showing distribution of fluorine-18 become clearer in computer analysis with higher letters (P,Q,R) indicating greater uptake. The scans were made on a 27-year-old woman with Hodgkin's disease.

Bone scans and lymphomas

Bone scans with sodium fluoride F 18 can help in staging a lymphoma, but conventional roentgenograms are still needed to pick up "the occasional lesion that is missed by the bone scan."

Richard S. Benua, MD, chief of the nuclear medicine service at Memorial Hospital of Memorial Sloan-Kettering Institute Cancer Center, New York City, described the use of the radionuclide at the recent meeting of the Society for Nuclear Medicine in Los Angeles. The technique has been used on more than 500 patients.

Apparently, the sodium fluoride replaces hydroxyl ions in bones, and the process is enhanced where bone metabolism is increased to compensate for areas damaged by tumors. Thus, although the radiation dosage is lower than that of a typical roentgenogram, the radionuclide is specifically attracted to areas of bony involvement, and may reveal lesions that could be obscure or invisible on a roentgenogram.

Each of the patients at Sloan-Kettering received 1 mc of cyclotron-produced sodium fluoride 18; 60 of them had lymphomatous diseases, including 39 cases of Hodgkin's disease, 12 patients with lymphosarcoma, and nine with reticulum cell sarcoma. Scans were made two to five hours after administration of the radionuclide. Both photoscans and digital tapes for computer analysis were made.

The bone scans turned up lesions in 21 patients with normal roentgenograms, and found additional bony metastases in eight patients with abnormal roentenograms. But the technique is not foolproof: roentgenograms revealed new lesions in nine patients whose bone scans appeared normal. Two other patients had abnormal bone scans, but roentgenograms showed still more lesions. In four instances, negative bone scans were used to confirm that suspicious bone "islands"—areas of increased density on roentgenograms—were harmless.

Spinal bone scan counts were elevated in 11 patients; six of them had roentgenogram-positive lesions. One of the 11 patients had arthritis, accounting for the elevated scan, but the other four cases remain unexplained.

The technique resulted in changing the stage of the disease in only seven of the 60 patients, but 44 of the group were already at stage IV.

Dr. Benua's co-workers were John S. Laughlin, MD, Burton J. Lee, MD, and Roy S. Tilbury, MD, all of the Memorial Sloan-Kettering Cancer Center.

LH-RH synthesized

After a decade of work, a Tulane University School of Medicine team has synthesized the hypothalamic hormone that stimulates the release of luteinizing hormone from the pituitary gland. The hormone is called luteinizing hormone-releasing hormone or LH-RH.

The team was headed by A. V. Schally, PhD, professor of medicine at Tulane and chief of the endocrine and polypeptide laboratories at New Orleans VA Hospital. He reported the achievement at the annual meeting of the Endocrine Society in San Francisco.

According to Abba Kastin, MD, assistant professor of medicine at Tulane and chief of the endocrinology section at the New Orleans VA Hospital, another member of the team, "one of the remarkable aspects of this study—and in this regard perhaps the real breakthrough—is the recognition that the hypothalamus controls the fertility action of the pituitary. Ten years ago no one would have accepted that statement."

Among the potential consequences of the synthesis of LH-RH are the development of new, cheaper and safer fertility stimulators and contraceptives, said Dr. Schally. For example, synthetic LH-RH might be used in place of gonadotropins or clomiphene to stimulate fertility.

In addition, the development of an LH-RH antagonist is on the horizon. Such an antagonist would induce contraception by blocking the release of luteinizing hormone, thus blocking ovulation.

One of the first steps in the research project was to isolate LH-RH from the hypothalami of 165,000 pigs. Clinical testing of the porcine hormone showed that administration of porcine LH-RH to patients resulted in a rise in plasma values of luteinizing hormone. This demonstrated among other things that the LH-RH is not species-specific.

Subsequent steps involved determination of the molecular structure of LH-RH and then the synthesis, completed in mid-April.

The team also includes Luciano Debeljuk, PhD; R. M. G. Nair, MD; Juergen K. Sandow, PhD; Ichiji Wakabayashi, PhD; Akira Arimura, MD; and Mr. T. W. Redding, all of Tulane University School of Medicine and New Orleans VA Hospital.

The placenta mystery

The placenta, says Robert E. L. Nesbitt, Jr., MD, "has been studied for decades and yet remains somewhat of a mystery in the way it accepts nourishment from the mother and releases what is needed to the unborn child."

At the State University of New York's Upstate Medical Center in Syracuse, where Dr. Nesbitt is professor and chairman of obstetrics and gynecology, a model resembling the uterus in shape has been developed to study the placenta.

Polyethylene tubes lead from the model to a heart pump oxygenator and fluid tank, simulating maternal circulation into the placenta. Placentas from local hospital delivery rooms are placed in the model, the umbilical cord cut, and catheters (leading to a second heart pump and fluid tank) inserted.

Water is injected in the top of the model to simulate amniotic fluid. Then, for up to five hours, blood, oxygen, sugar, and other substances are circulated for studies aimed at improved understanding of prenatal death, miscarriage, maintenance of premature birth, and effects of alcohol, tobacco, and drugs.

"We are studying normal mature placentas taken at the birth of full-term babies from normal pregnancies, says Dr. Nesbitt. "Once we understand what happens in a totally normal situation, we will move on to specific diseases which affect pregnancy, and other factors such as drugs, and study placentas taken at different stages of pregnancy through miscarriages and abortions."

Philip A. Rice, PhD, associate professor of chemical engineering and metallurgy at Syracuse University, heads the research team with Dr. Nesbitt.

Growth rate indicator?

The level of amino acid excretion in the urine appears to reflect changes in the rate of a child's growth.

In reporting this observation, a British physician—Phillip A. Zorab, MD, of London's Brompton Hospital—suggested the assay may prove useful in managing children with curvature of the spine.

Dr. Zorab, who also is consulting physician to several institutions, told the meeting of the Scoliosis Research Society in Hartford, Conn, that the total urine hydroxyproline excretion rate reflects the turnover of bone collagen—itself an indication of the rate of bone growth. A five-year study at London's Institute of Child Health appears to confirm the usefulness of the test.

Home again.

After 2 hours of angina protection.

For up to two hours of protection, your angina patient needs *more* than sublingual nitroglycerin. And Chewable Sorbitrate (isosorbide dinitrate) provides more.

☐ Acts almost as fast as nitroglycerin... lasts about 4 times as long.

☐ More stable in air than sublingual nitroglycerin: it can be stored or carried with no significant loss of potency.

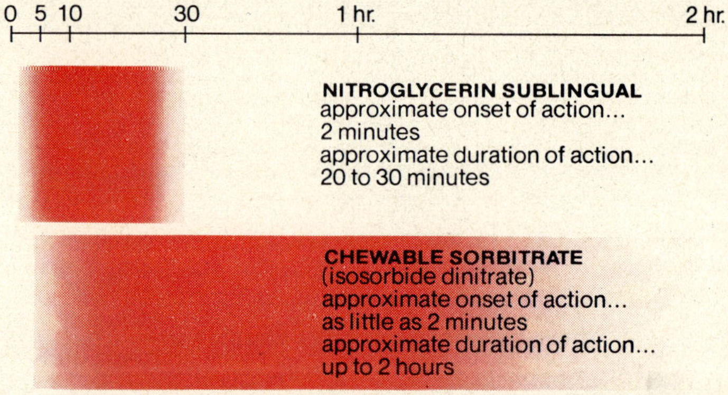

SUMMARY OF PRESCRIBING INFORMATION

Mode of Action: The mechanism of action of SORBITRATE (isosorbide dinitrate) is unknown, although the basic pharmacologic action is to relax smooth muscle. Isosorbide dinitrate reduces in number and severity the incidence of angina pectoris attacks, with concomitant reduction in nitroglycerin intake.

Indications: *Sublingual and Chewable:* For the prevention and treatment of angina pectoris.

Oral: For the relief of angina pectoris. It is not intended to abort the acute anginal episode. SORBITRATE WITH PHENOBARBITAL is indicated for patients in whom the angina pectoris is accompanied by anxiety or its related symptoms.

Contraindications: A history of sensitivity to the drug.

Warnings: Data supporting the use of nitrates during the early days of the acute phase of myocardial infarction are insufficient to establish safety. Phenobarbital may be habit forming.

Precautions: Should be used with caution in patients who have glaucoma. Tolerance and cross tolerance to other nitrates may occur.

Adverse Reactions: Headache which may be severe and persistent. Lowering the dose and using analgesics will help control the headaches which usually diminish or disappear as therapy is continued.

Adverse reactions seen occasionally: Cutaneous vasodilation with flushing; transient dizziness and weakness as well as other signs of cerebral ischemia associated with postural hypotension; individual marked sensitivity to the hypotensive effects of nitrates wherein severe responses can occur even with the usual therapeutic dose (alcohol may enhance this effect); drug rash and/or exfoliative dermatitis.

This drug can act as a physiological antagonist to norepinephrine, acetylcholine, histamine and other agents.

Dosage and Administration: *Route:* Sublingual, oral and chewable tablets.

Individual Dose: To minimize hypotensive responses, which may occasionally be severe with chewable doses as low as 5 mg., the smallest effective dose should be employed. Chewable tablets are generally given in doses of 5 mg. Sublingually or orally, 5 to 10 mg. is the range commonly used although doses of up to 30 mg. have frequently been employed.

Dosage Schedule: Smallest effective dose necessary for the prevention and treatment of pain of an anginal attack. Sublingual SORBITRATE may be taken p.r.n. or at 4 to 6 hour intervals; Oral SORBITRATE may be taken 3 or 4 times daily. Chewable SORBITRATE may be taken for prompt relief of anginal pain 3 or 4 times daily. Although the onset and duration of effect of coronary nitrates may vary, following are the generally reported ranges of these values for SORBITRATE:

Onset of Effect: Sublingual and Chewable: 2 to 5 minutes. Oral: 15 to 30 minutes.

Duration of Effect: Sublingual and Chewable: 1 to 2 hours. Oral: Estimated to be 4 to 6 hours.

It is recommended that the oral dosage be taken on an empty stomach.

STUART PHARMACEUTICALS | Pasadena, Calif. 91109
Division of ATLAS CHEMICAL INDUSTRIES, INC.

goes beyond the benefits of sublingual nitroglycerin.

CHEWABLE SORBITRATE®

ISOSORBIDE DINITRATE 5 mg.

And when indicated: Sorbitrate® (isosorbide dinitrate) Sublingual 5 mg. and 2.5 mg.

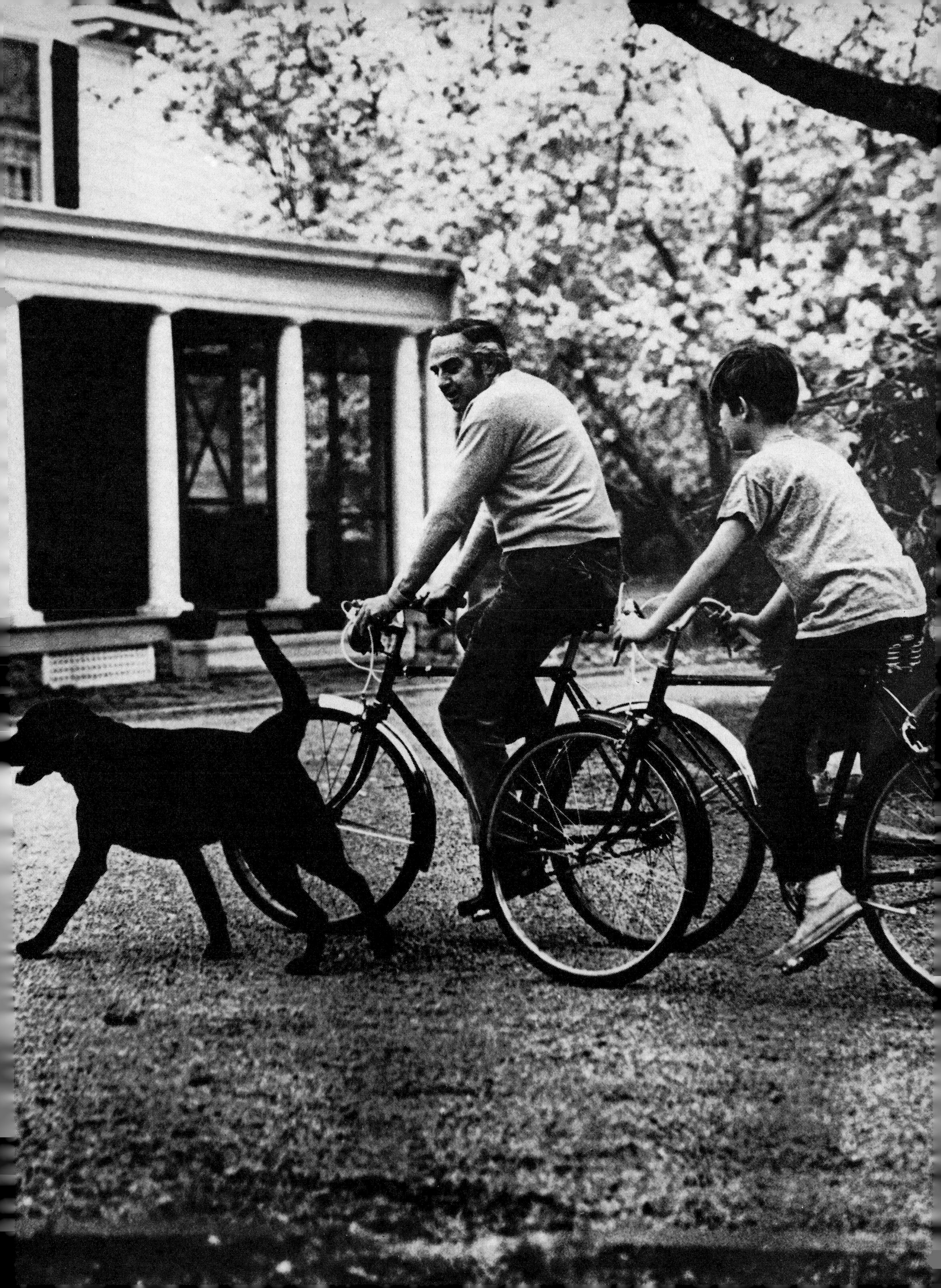

Internal medicine at large

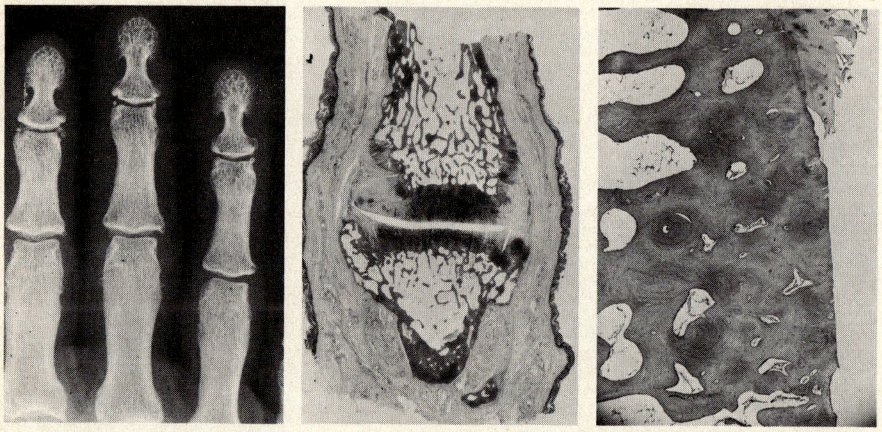

A radiograph of an acromegalic hand (left) shows widened joint spaces due to hypertrophy of cartilage, hooklike extensions of bone and calcinosis of the joint capsule. Histological examination (center) revealed thickened hypertrophied overactive cartilage (darkly stained). The microphotograph shows absence of cartilage in area undercut by fissuring and ulceration.

Acromegalic arthropathy

Clinical, radiological, and histological studies of 42 patients with adult-onset acromegaly and arthropathy have shown that the disease begins with overproduction of joint cartilage due to growth hormone overproduction and becomes self-perpetuating.

Rodney Bluestone, MB, chief of rheumatology at the Wadsworth Veterans Administration Hospital in Los Angeles, told the American Rheumatism Association meeting in New York that affected joints of these patients appeared normal upon clinical examination. There were complaints of pain but little evidence of arthritis and no difficulty in spinal movement.

Joint degeneration with osteophytes and increased cartilage spaces was apparent upon radiological examination, however, and histological study showed that the overstimulated cartilage was deposited irregularly instead of in normal, orderly layers. This resulted in fissures, then ulceration, undermining of cartilage, and subsequent overproduction of more cartilage. The excess fibrocartilage then caused periosteal spurs, osteophytes, and capsule calcinosis.

Dr. Bluestone believes generally that affected joints should be treated with physiotherapy and mild analgesics. Total hip replacement was successful in one patient.

Dr. Bluestone's co-workers were E. G. L. Bywaters, MD, and P. L. Holt, MB, of the Royal Postgraduate Medical School of London, and M. Hartog, MD, of the Royal Infirmary, Bristol University Medical School, England.

Mechanism of CO damage

Carbon monoxide is directly toxic to mammalian cells because it inhibits their consumption of oxygen, a San Francisco investigator has found.

It has been generally accepted that the harmful effects of carbon monoxide were due to hypoxia as a result of the formation of carboxyhemoglobin, said Mitchell L. Rhodes, MD, acting chief of the Pulmonary Section, USPHS Hospital, San Francisco. But the investigator said that his studies show carbon monoxide directly harms slices of lung tissue taken from mice.

When the tissue was incubated with oxygen-enriched air and carbon monoxide was added, oxygen consumption stopped immediately. Study of the cells showed "bizarre configurational changes in the mitochondria," swelling, disruption, and increased formation of bubbles in the cytoplasm of the nonciliated bronchiolar cells. Slices of mouse lung tissue exposed only to oxygen-enriched air were used as controls.

Dr. Rhodes said that because the oxidative metabolic chain is disturbed, energy production and therefore all cellular activity is disrupted. Tissues in the heart and brain are the most severely affected.

Dr. Rhodes spoke at the American Thoracic Society meeting.

Bruce E. Spivey, MD, has been named dean of the School of Medical Sciences of the Pacific Medical Center in San Francisco. He had been on the faculty of the University of Iowa College of Medicine.

William G. Cooper, MD, has been named assistant vice president for health affairs of the University of Colorado Medical Center. Dr. Cooper joined the Colorado faculty in 1955 and was promoted to professor of anatomy in 1966.

Anthony J. Chapman, MD, a former Fort Worth, Texas, pathologist, has succeeded **James L. Luke,** MD, as clinical professor of forensic pathology at the University of Oklahoma Medical Center and Oklahoma's state medical examiner.

The recipient of the 1971 **Gold Medal Award for Excellence in Hospital Administration** is **T. Stewart Hamilton,** MD, executive director of the Hartford, Conn, Hospital. Dr. Hamilton, who has headed the Hamilton Hospital since 1954, received the award at the annual meeting of the American College of Hospital Administrators.

Robert T. McCluskey, MD, former professor and chairman of the Department of Pathology at State University of New York at Buffalo School of Medicine, has been named S. Burt Wolbach Professor of Pathology at Harvard Medical School.

Miguel Dao Dao, MD, head of the Chair of Radiology at the Central University of Venezuela and chief of the Radiological Department of the University Hospital of Caracas, has succeeded **Juan del Regato,** MD, of Colorado Springs, as president of the Interamerican College of Radiology. Dr. Dao is editor of *Radiologia y Medicina Nuclear.*

The new chairman of the Department of Medicine at the Creighton University School of Medicine is **George O. Clifford,** MD, associate professor of medicine at Cornell University Medical College.

Warren Winkelstein, Jr, MD, MPH, is serving as acting dean of the School of Public Health at the Berkeley Campus of the University of California. Dr. Winkelstein, professor and head of the Division of Epidemiology since 1968, was named to his position after **William C. Reeves,** PhD, resigned to return to full-time teaching and research.

John S. Fordtran, MD, is the recipient of the **Distinguished Achievement Award** of the American Gastroenterological Association. Dr. Fordtran is professor of internal medicine and chief of the Gastroenterology Section at the University of Texas Southwestern Medical School.

Betty Geren Uzman, MD, has been promoted to professor of pathology at the Harvard Medical School.

The recipients of the 1971 **Dickson Prize** are two New York scientists, **Solomon A. Berson,** MD, and **Rosalyn S. Yalow,** PhD, who received the $10,000 award presented by the University of Pittsburgh for their introduction of competitive binding and radioimmunoassay in the detection and quantification of hormones. Dr. Yalow is research professor of medicine at Mt. Sinai School of Medicine and Dr. Berson is Murray M. Rosenberg professor and chairman of the Department of Medicine at the same school.

Harry Gold, MD, clinical professor of pharmacology (emeritus) at Cornell University Medical College and one of the first investigators to make double-blind studies, has been named to receive the 1971 **Award of Distinction** of the Cornell University Medical College Alumni Association.

James E. Bowman, Jr, MD, associate professor of pathology and medicine at the University of Chicago Pritzker School of Medicine, has been named director of laboratories at The University of Chicago Hospitals and Clinics.

The new chairman of the Department of Pediatrics of the Faculty of Medicine at the University of Alberta is **Ernest E. McCoy,** MD. Dr. McCoy, who joined the faculty in 1970, succeeds **J.K. Martin,** MD.

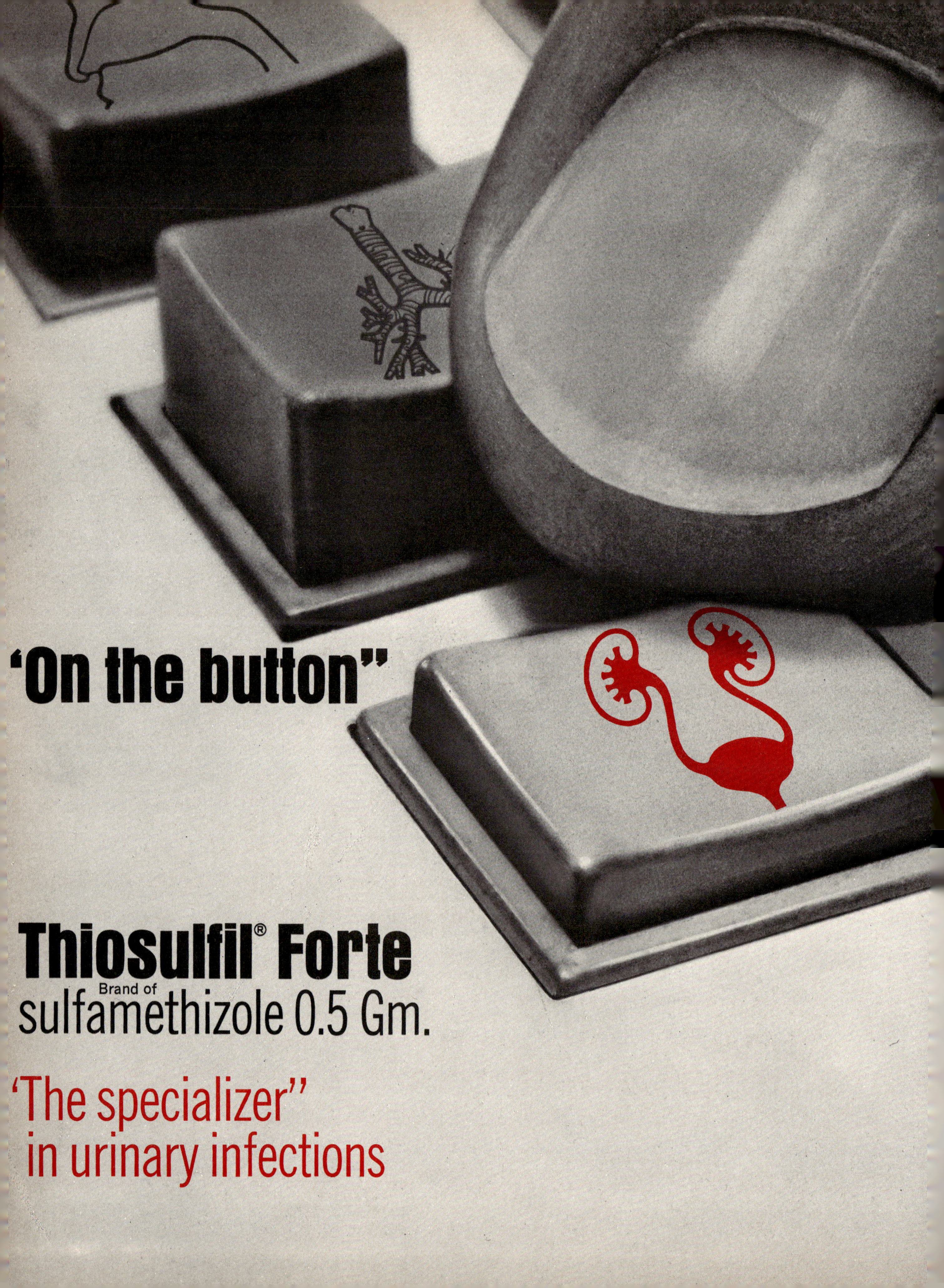
'On the button"
Thiosulfil® Forte
Brand of
sulfamethizole 0.5 Gm.
'The specializer"
in urinary infections

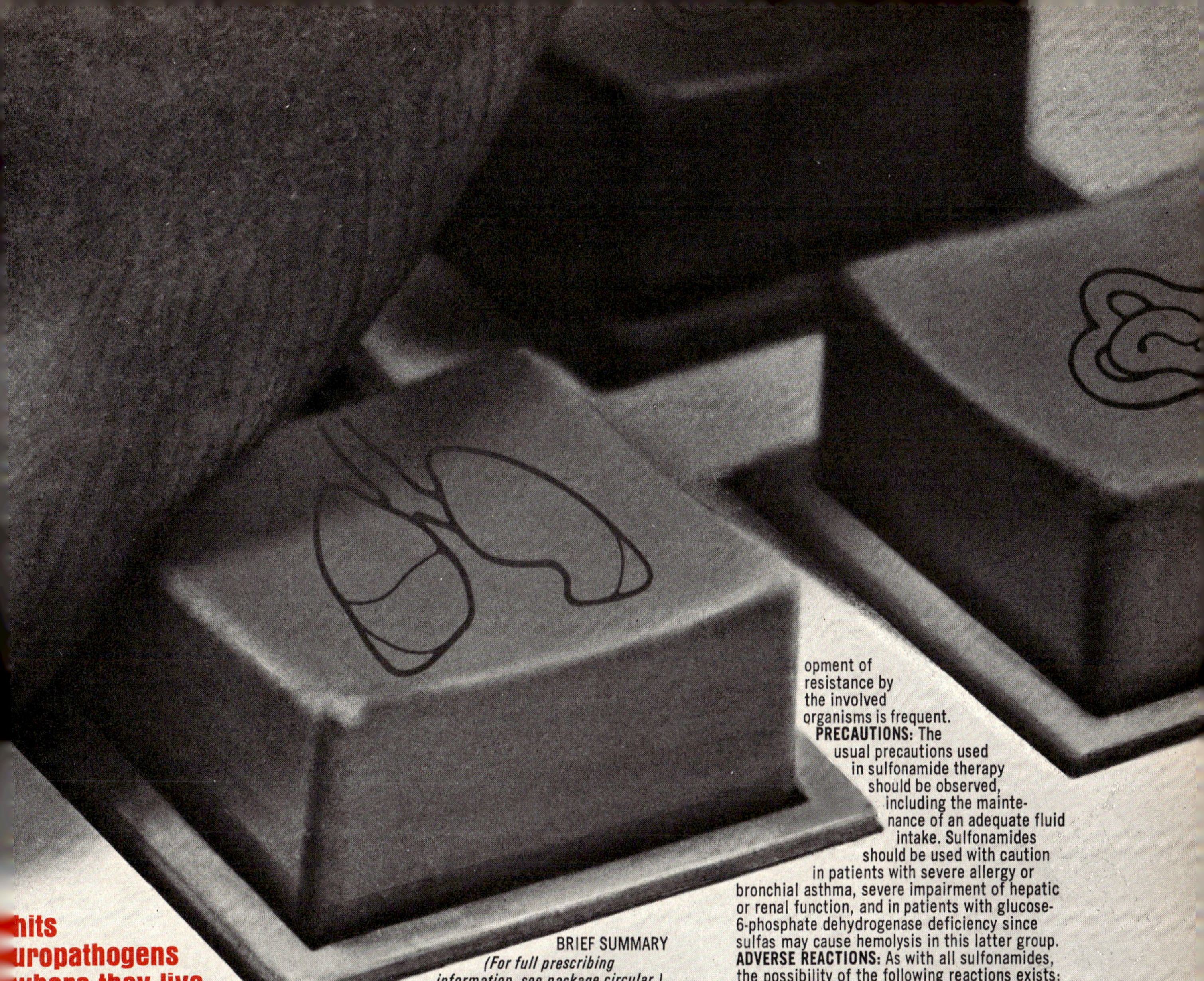

Internal Medicine at large

Anthony M. Bruno, MD, has been appointed assistant director of the National Cancer Institute. Dr. Bruno joined the staff of the National Institutes of Health in 1967.

Alvin P. Shapiro, professor of medicine at the University of Pittsburgh School of Medicine, has been named associate dean for academic affairs. Dr. Shapiro, a consultant to the AMA Council on Drugs, is an associate editor of *Psychosomatic Medicine.*

William Larsen, MD, has been promoted to professor of medicine at the University of Kansas School of Medicine.

Theodore M. King, MD, has succeeded **Alan Barnes,** MD, as professor and chairman of the Department of Gynecology and Obstetrics at the Johns Hopkins University School of Medicine. Dr. King formerly held the corresponding position at Albany Medical College.

The University of Florida College of Medicine has a new faculty member–**S. Leon Israel,** MD, professor of obstetrics and gynecology, who formerly held the same appointment at the University of Pennsylvania School of Medicine. Dr. Israel is editor of the *Journal of Obstetrics and Gynecology,* president of American Gynecological Society, and author of a textbook, *Diagnosis and Treatment of Menstrual Disorders and Sterility.*

Thomas J. Gill III, MD, has been appointed professor and chairman of the Department of Pathology at the University of Pittsburgh School of Medicine. Dr. Gill, a member of the editorial board of *Immunochemistry,* was formerly associate professor of pathology at Harvard Medical School.

Michael Heidelberger, PhD, adjunct professor of pathology at New York University School of Medicine, and **Felix Haurowitz,** MD, DSc, professor of chemistry, emeritus, at Indiana University, were among five scientists who received **Distinguished Service Awards** at the recent First International Congress of Immunology in Washington. The other recipients of the award were **Sir F. Macfarlane Burnet,** MD, of Australia; **Pierre Grabar,** PhD, ScD, of France, and **John Marrack,** MD, of England.

The new chairman of the Department of Radiology at the University of Chicago Pritzker School of Medicine is **Alexander Gottschalk,** MD, a faculty member since 1964 and a specialist in the diagnostic use of radioactive isotopes.

Col Richard H. Ross, MC, USA, has been appointed staff surgeon and head of the US Army Medical Command in Vietnam.

James Lowman, MD, is now professor of pediatrics at the University of Kansas School of Medicine.

Robert T. Manning, MD, associate dean of student affairs at the University of Kansas School of Medicine, has been named dean of the new Eastern Virginia Medical School at Norfolk.

The first woman hospital director in the Veterans Administration system is **Valerija B. Raulinaitis,** MD. Dr. Raulinaitis heads the 951-bed Leech Farm VA Hospital in Pittsburgh.

J.D.R. Miller, MD, clinical professor and acting chairman of the Department of Radiology on the University of Alberta Faculty of Medicine, has been appointed chairman of the department.

Hans Grieble, MD, has been promoted to professor of medicine at the Chicago Medical School. **Parker R. Beamer,** MD, visiting professor of pathology, was appointed professor of pathology, and **William Thomas, Jr,** MD, was promoted to professor of pathology at the school.

Joseph D. Sapira, MD, has joined the faculty of the University of Alabama in Birmingham School of Medicine as professor of psychiatry and associate professor of medicine.

Three members of the faculty of Albany Medical College–**David F. Brown,** MD; **Eugene D. Furth,** MD, and **Frank C. Maxon, Jr,** MD–have been promoted to the rank of professor of medicine.

Volume 128, Number 4, October 1971

Archives of Internal Medicine

Original Articles

"Triiodothyronine (T_3) Toxicosis"

Its Role in Graves' Disease

Horace K. Ivy, MD; Heinz W. Wahner, MD; and Colum A. Gorman, MB, BCh, Rochester, Minn

Eight cases of "triiodothyronine (T_3) toxicosis" in Graves' disease have been identified. All eight patients had normal values for total or free thyroxine or both and significant elevations of T_3. It is important for the physician to be aware of this entity and to suspect it in patients whose condition appears to be thyrotoxic but for whom standard laboratory tests reveal no abnormalities. The diagnosis must be based on laboratory findings, because these patients cannot be distinguished clinically from other patients with Graves' disease. In most instances, the condition is identified in patients with mild clinical toxic reaction, perhaps because the level of only one of the two metabolically active thyroid hormones is elevated. It is recognized that in patients with marked elevations of T_3, severe thyrotoxicosis might be observed.

Since the advent of newer methods for determining serum triiodothyronine (T_3) levels, there has been increased interest in defining the role of this hormone in disorders of thyroid function. Using the method of Sterling and associates,[1] as modified by Wahner and Gorman,[2] the level of T_3 has been determined in numerous patients seen in our Thyroid Clinic. In certain of these patients, conventional laboratory studies did not confirm a clinical diagnosis of thyrotoxic condition. In these patients, elevated levels of T_3 helped explain the clinical findings and suggested that a diagnosis of "T_3 toxicosis" (thyrotoxicosis due to elevated levels of T_3) might be justified. We describe these patients and attempt to place in perspective the role of "T_3 toxicosis" in the general spectrum of Graves' disease.

Received for publication April 27, 1971; accepted May 14.

From the Division of Endocrinology and Internal Medicine (Drs. Ivy and Gorman); and the Department of Clinical Pathology (Dr. Wahner), Mayo Clinic and Mayo Foundation, Rochester, Minn.

Reprint requests to Mayo Clinic, Rochester, Minn 55901 (Dr. Ivy).

Clinical Material and Methods

All patients in this study were referred to the Thyroid Clinic for consultation after an initial general medical examination. They were evaluated by clinicians experienced in thyroid diagnosis; a decision regarding therapy for thyroid disease was made prior to the knowledge of the results of the serum T_3 determination. Even in the patients who had an equivocally toxic reaction (Table), there was enough clinical evidence to warrant radioactive iodine (sodium iodide I 131) therapy, regardless of the presence of normal levels of total or free thyroxine (T_4) or both. Thyroid function was assessed by measuring total T_4 by the method of Murphy and Jachan,[3] and free T_4 as described by Sterling and Brenner.[4] In addition, the basal metabolic rate (BMR), the 6- and 24-hour uptakes of ^{131}I by the thyroid gland, and the levels of thyroxine-binding globulin (TBG) and thyroxine-binding prealbumin (TBPA) were determined when necessary, according to previously described techniques.[2] Thyroid-stimulating hormone (TSH) was determined by a double antibody radioimmunoassay using h-TSH and rabbit anti-h-TSH serum.[5] The T_3 suppression test was performed by observing the decrease in ^{131}I uptake on the fifth day of daily oral administration of 100μg of liothyronine sodium.

Results

The Table lists the results of appropriate laboratory studies and clinical evaluation. Six of the eight patients were women, an expected ratio in any series of patients with Graves' disease. Ages varied from the second through the eighth decade. Autono-

Data on Eight Patients With Graves' Disease and Triiodothyronine (T_3) Toxicosis

Patient	Sex and Age (yr)	T_3 Suppression Test*	BMR† (%)	TBG (mg/100 ml)	TBPA (mg/100 ml)	Total T_4 (μg/100 ml)	Free T_4 (ng/100 ml)	T_3	Weight of Gland (gm)	Clinical Toxic ± Reaction	Eye Findings	Treatment	Follow-up
1	F, 34	50/51	+19	18.8	245.0	10.3	...	580	30	Equivocal	None	^{131}I	None
2	F, 59	25/18	+26	21.9	...	10.8	...	391	35	Toxic	None	^{131}I	Improved (euthyroid)
3	M, 51	34/32	+31	19.4	334.0	11.0	3.5	551	20	Toxic	Equivocal	^{131}I	Improved (post^{131}I myxedema)
4	F, 26	49/43	...	22.0	344.5	10.5	2.8	512	35	Equivocal (Hashimoto's thyroiditis on biopsy)	Minimal	Potassium iodide	Improved (euthyroid)
5	M, 19	36/30	+19	18.0	...	10.6	4.9	556	30	Equivocal (periodic paralysis)	None	^{131}I	Improved (post^{131}I myxedema; no further paralysis)
6	F, 76	30/26	...	20.5	279.0	9.0	2.1	772	25	Equivocal	Muscle paresis	None	Improved (euthyroid)
7	F, 49	77/...	+25	17.5	256.0	11.2	2.6	840	35	Toxic	Equivocal	^{131}I advised	Improved (post^{131}I myxedema)
8	F, 57	71/...	...	25.3	258.0	11.5	2.4	955	35	Toxic	Muscle pareis	^{131}I	Improved (post^{131}I myxedema)
Normal range		>50	−10 to +10	16-24	270 ±70	4.0-11.0	0.8-2.8	240 ±80					

* Percentage uptake of ^{131}I at 24 hours before and after five days of administration of 100μg of liothyronine sodium daily.
† BMR signifies basal metabolic rate; TBG, thyroxine-binding globulin; TBPA, thyroxine-binding prealbumin; and T_4, thyroxine iodine.

mous thyroid function was demonstrated in the six patients in whom a T_3 suppression test was done. In the remaining two patients, the ^{131}I uptake was elevated. The most reliable test that reflected hypermetabolism was that of BMR; the BMR was significantly elevated in each of the five patients in whom the test was performed. The values for TBG and TBPA, when determined, were invariably compatible with normal binding of thyroid hormones. Although two patients had total T_4 values that were slightly elevated, the free T_4 values of these patients were normal. Two other patients had elevated free T_4 values when the total T_4 and TBG values were normal. It can be argued that such patients do not truly have T_3 toxicosis because unbound T_4 could solely account for the clinical findings. However, Arango et al[6] have indicated that the total T_4 value is a more reliable indicator of thyroid status when binding of the hormone is normal, and Sterling and Brenner[4] have found that the free T_4 value may be elevated in illness other than thyrotoxicosis. Certainly, the combined determination of total and free serum T_4 did not provide a clear-cut differentiation from normal. In contrast to the nondiagnostic T_4 values, serum T_3 values were elevated in all of these patients, with values ranging from 391 to 955 ng/100 ml, with the normal range being 240 ± 80 ng/100 ml.

The clinical evaluation of each patient was a diagnostic problem in that the findings suggested thyrotoxicosis, though the usual values for thyroid hormone were normal. Autonomous function of the thyroid gland was a helpful finding, but this does not prove excessive secretion of hormone. All patients had a palpably abnormal thyroid gland, though none had a large goiter. None of the four patients who had a clearly toxic reaction had one which was severe. These patients received sodium iodide I 131 therapy; one patient chose to return to her home community for treatment. Of the four patients who had equivocally toxic reactions, three warranted therapy. Therapy with supersaturated potassium iodide was judged to be adequate treatment in one case (patient 4) because the presence of biopsy-proved Hashimoto's thyroiditis probably would prevent more severe thyrotoxicosis.[7] Only one patient did not receive therapy, and on follow-up, her equivocal toxic reaction subsided.

Each patient presented with only mild toxic reaction, and none had serious opthalmopathy. Three patients had normal eyes, and none had pretibial myxedema or acropachy. One patient had mild lid retraction and minimal unilateral impairment of extraocular muscle function, both of which subsided spontaneously in less than 12 months. Two patients had equivocal findings of "stare" and minimal lid retraction. Two additional patients had significant extraocular muscle paresis; in one, surgical correction was required.

Comment

The concept of "T_3 toxicosis" is not new, having been reported by several authors.[8-11] Because of the limitations of the methods used, the reliability of estimates of T_3 levels has been questioned. In the most recent report by Sterling and associates[8] and by Wahner and Gorman,[2] T_3 has been accurately measured by a simplified method. Sterling and coauthors, unfortunately, personally appraised only a few patients and, therefore, could not clinically characterize them. They clearly demonstrated, however, that there are patients whose clinical condition is thyrotoxic but who have normal T_4 values and elevated T_3 levels. We believe that on clinical evidence the patients in our series cannot be distinguished from other patients with Graves' disease. The only common feature noted was the presence of normal values for total or free T_4, or both, normal levels of TBG, and elevated levels of T_3. The size of the thyroid glands and the presence or degree of infiltrative phenomena (ophthalmopathy, pretibial myxedema) were not remarkable. In general, the patients seemed to have mild toxic reaction, and in some, the effort to demonstrate the existence of thyrotoxicosis presented a distinct clinical challenge.

If the physician suspects thyrotoxicosis, he should proceed with the usual measures of thyroid function, including determinations of ^{131}I uptake, total T_4, and BMR. If elevated levels of T_4 are not found in the presence of a strong clinical suspicion or the obvious presence of thyrotoxicosis, autonomy of thyroid function must be demonstrated by the T_3 suppression test. In addition, normal binding of T_4 should be demonstrated by determining the values for free T_4, TBG, and TBPA. Although not a consistent finding in thyrotoxicosis, decreased levels of TBG and TBPA are observed and can be of a magnitude capable of changing the total T_4 significantly.[12,13] The BMR is the only test of this group that truly reflects hypermetabolism; it is, of course, not a specific test of thyroid function. Autonomy of ^{131}I uptake may exist in patients who are not in a thyrotoxic condition, but when autonomy is demonstrated in the clinical presence of thyrotoxicosis associated with normal T_4 values, if normal hormone binding has been demonstrated, T_3 levels should be determined. If the levels are elevated, a diagnosis of "T_3 toxicosis" is justified, based on the additive metabolic effects of nonsuppressible T_4 formation plus elevated levels of T_3.

No single test of thyroid function proves the presence of thyrotoxicosis, including measurements of thyroid hormones in blood. Patients who are myxedematous or hyperthyroid may have normal levels of T_3 (Figure). In this as well as previous reports, there have been patients with thyrotoxic conditions who have elevated T_3 values associated with normal T_4 levels. Generally, in patients with toxic reactions, however, when both hormones have been measured, the levels of both usually have been elevated. The Figure shows that patients with "typical" Graves' disease, recurrent Graves' disease, or toxic nodular glands all had elevated T_4 values. A complete overlap of T_3 elevation in these patients and those with "T_3 toxicosis" is apparent. It seems reasonable to presume that the mild clinical findings in our patients with T_3 toxicosis were apparent because only one of the two hormones that contribute to toxic reaction was definitely abnormal. It should be apparent that with extreme elevations of T_3, severe thyrotoxicosis might be observed.

The relative contribution of T_3 and T_4 to the metabolic state must be considered. Thyroxine is strongly bound to plasma protein, approximately 30% being associated with TBPA, 60% with TBG, and 10% with serum albumin.[14] Approximately 0.05% of the total plasma T_4 concentration is free or unbound.[6] Triiodothyronine is much less strongly bound than T_4, is associated primarily with TBG and secondarily with serum albumin, and is not bound to TBPA. Triiodothyronine is displaced by T_4 from its binding site on TBG. Consequently, a much larger percentage of T_3 than T_4 will be free in the serum. In addition, the secretion rate of T_3 probably is higher than that of T_4 in hyperthyroidism.[9] The maximal metabolic effect of a single dose of T_3 is three or four times that of T_4, but the duration of the effect is significantly shorter.[15] In addition, the serum half-time of the two hormones is significantly different and is

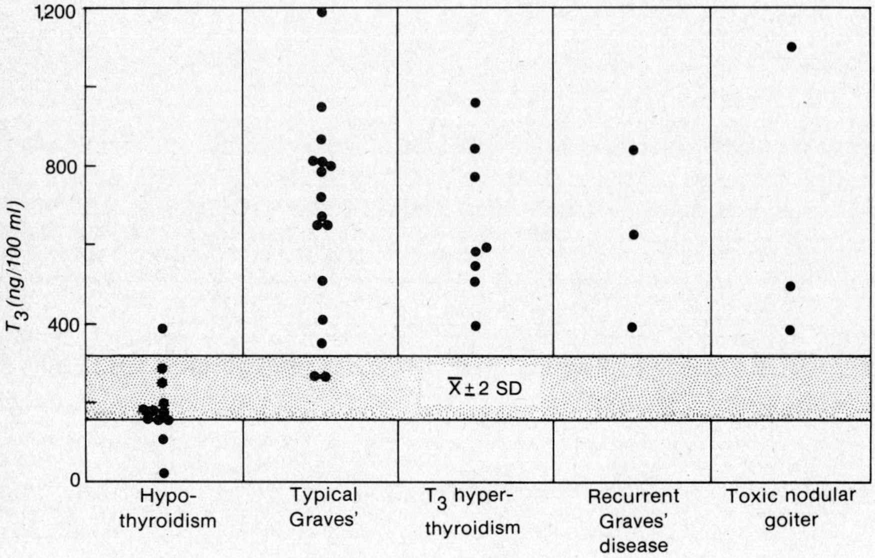

Triiodothyronine (T_3) serum levels in hypothyroidism and in various types of thyrotoxicosis. There is no difference in elevation of T_3 values in "T_3 toxicosis" and in other forms of thyrotoxicosis associated with increase of thyroxine.

affected by the state of thyroid function, being shorter in hyperthyroidism.[9,16] The extrathyroidal iodine pool is increased in thyrotoxicosis, and the degradation rate of T_4 is increased.[16,17] There is no formula to calculate the relative metabolic contribution of each hormone in thyrotoxicosis that takes into consideration all of these variables, but there is no doubt that T_3 can contribute significantly. The elevated levels of T_3, as observed in these patients, when superimposed on a base line of "high normal" T_4 values, seem a ready and obvious explanation for the patient's symptoms of thyrotoxicosis.

The reason for the increased T_3:T_4 ratio in these patients is unknown. Studies in rats[18] that were rendered iodine deficient revealed a progressive increase in T_3:T_4 ratio for the duration of iodine deficiency. In addition, the T_3:T_4 ratio was higher in the thyroid effluent than in the gland itself, reflecting an important adaptive mechanism to iodine deficit. It has been shown that the rat adapts to iodine deficiency with an absolute increase in T_3 in plasma and tissues and a decrease in T_4 concentration in these areas. However, the rat cannot completely suppress T_4 synthesis.[19] Increased percentages of endogenously labeled T_3 were found in patients with thyrotoxic conditions who were iodine deficient and who had normal values for protein-bound iodine.[20] The contribution that iodine deficiency makes in the altered T_3:T_4 ratio observed in "T_3 toxicosis" is conjectural.

With the development of a relatively simple and rapid immunoassay for T_3, this area will undoubtedly be more fully explored and the full physiologic and pathologic impact of T_3 characterized.[21]

Patient Summaries

PATIENT 1.—A 34-year-old saleswoman had symptoms of increased irritability, nervousness, and depression nine months prior to her visit to the Mayo Clinic. Hyperthyroidism was diagnosed, and oral antithyroid therapy with propylthiouracil was started. In spite of this therapy, symptoms became worse, and the patient lost 13 lb in the two months before evaluation.

On physical examination, the thyrotoxic condition could not be diagnosed with certainty. We estimated that the weight of the thyroid gland was about 30 gm. There was no evidence of ophthalmopathy. Antithyroid therapy was discontinued 12 days prior to the ^{131}I studies. The initial 24-hour uptake of ^{131}I was 50%, and after the administration of 100μg of liothyronine sodium for five days, the uptake was 51%, thereby demonstrating autonomy of thyroid function. The BMR was +19%; the TBG and TBPA levels were normal, as was the total T_4 level. On the basis of the patient's symptoms, the elevated BMR, and the demonstration of nonsuppressible thyroid function, sodium iodide I 131 was administered. It was later reported that the serum T_3 level was significantly elevated to 580 ng/100 ml.

Even though hyperthyroidism was suspected clinically, the diagnosis could not be proved by conventional laboratory studies. The elevated T_3 level, however, reinforced our clinical impression of thyrotoxicosis.

PATIENT 2.—For three years prior to her visit to our clinic, this 58-year-old woman had been unsuccessfully treated with digitalis for a "fast heart." On questioning, she admitted that she had increased nervousness and heat intolerance for many months. The patient had gained several pounds but was not aware of unusual weakness or fatigue.

On examination, the patient was moderately stimulated, and had a mild tremor of the outstretched hands. The only eye abnormality noted was lid lag. Because of a heavy neck and a low-lying gland, the thyroid was difficult to palpate, but was believed to be diffusely enlarged, with an estimated weight of 35 gm. The BMR was +26%, and the uptake of ^{131}I was 19% and 25% in 6 and 24 hours, respectively. After the T_3 suppression test, the uptake was 12% and 18% at 6 and 24 hours, respectively. The TBG and total T_4 values were normal. A free T_4 value was not obtained but, in the absence of a TBG abnormality, was assumed to be normal. On the basis of the patient's symptoms, the palpable thyroid abnormality, the elevated BMR, and the nonsuppressible uptake of ^{131}I, therapy was considered justifiable even though the T_4 value was normal. It was later learned that the serum T_3 value was elevated to 391 ng/100 ml.

At reevaluation three months later, the total T_4 level had dropped to 7.4μg/100 ml, and symptomatically the patient had improved. After another three months, the patient was clinically euthyroid, without a palpable thyroid. The total serum T_4 value was 6.0μg, and the free T_4 was 1.0 ng/100 ml.

PATIENT 3.—This 51-year-old maintenance worker was referred for evaluation because of a six-month history of loss of weight, unusual fatigue, excessive sweating, and palpitations.

On examination, the patient seemed tense, tremulous, and moderately stimulated. Atrial fibrillation was present. The thyroid gland was palpable but not enlarged, and was estimated to weigh no more than 20 gm. Specific eye abnormalities were lacking. The BMR was +31%, and the uptake of ^{131}I was 23% and 34% in 6 and 24 hours, respectively. After five days of liothyronine administration, the 24-hour uptake of ^{131}I was 32%. The values for TBG, TBPA, and total T_4 were normal. The value for free T_4 was somewhat elevated (3.5 ng/100 ml), and for T_3 was approximately twice normal (551 ng/100 ml). Sodium iodide I 131 was administered.

During the ensuing weeks, the patient gained 20 lb and lost all signs and symptoms of thyrotoxicosis. The cardiac rhythm reverted to a normal sinus rhythm. Gradually, the patient noted evidence of hypothyroidism and, when reevaluated three months after therapy, he had clinical myxedema, which was confirmed by appropriate laboratory studies. Therapy with levothyroxine sodium was instituted.

The patient had a typical history of Graves' disease, which was supported by clinical signs of thyrotoxicosis. The normal total T_4 value, however, did not confirm such a diagnosis, and the modest elevation of the free T_4 was considered nondiagnostic. The elevated value of serum T_3, however, provided additional evidence supporting the clinical diagnosis.

PATIENT 4.—A 26-year-old teacher was seen at the Mayo Clinic because of lid retraction that had been present for approximately eight months. She had gained weight in spite of a diminished food intake, was unusually nervous (which she attributed to domestic problems), and had a sense of unusual warmth. Clinical thyrotoxicosis was equivocal. The thyroid gland was diffusely but asymmetrically enlarged, with an estimated weight of 35 gm. On the basis of palpation, it was suspected that Hashimoto's thyroiditis was present; this was confirmed by means of a thyroid needle biopsy. The uptake of ^{131}I failed to suppress significantly after the standard T_3 suppression test. The values for both total and free T_4 were in the high range of normal. Because of the equivocal clinical findings, therapy with ^{131}I was avoided and supersaturated potassium iodide was prescribed instead. The T_3 value was later reported to be elevated (512 ng/100 ml).

The patient returned three months later, at which time the eye abnormalities had improved. There seemed little doubt about clinical euthyroidism; the total T_4 level was 10.3μg/100 ml, and the free T_4 level was 2.4 ng/100 ml. It was suggested that the patient discontinue the use of potassium iodide.

The patient was seen once again 12 months after her initial visit. At this time, the eyes were entirely normal. The patient was asymptomatic, and on palpation the thyroid gland seemed essentially unchanged from the initial examination. The total serum T_4 level was only 5.0μg, and the free T_4 level was 0.9 ng/100 ml. The TSH radioimmunoassay revealed a value within the range of normal (4.4 micro-units/ml). This patient was considered to have Graves' disease on the basis of minimal ophthalmopathy and a nonsuppressible uptake of ^{131}I over a diffusely enlarged thyroid gland. The initial symptoms of thyrotoxicosis resulted from the elevated level of T_3. Interestingly, a spontaneous remission occurred.

PATIENT 5.—A 19-year-old student noted the onset of periods of paralysis eight months prior to his examination at our clinic. The episodes became more frequent until they occurred weekly. The weakness was so severe that the patient was unable to move his extremities; the paralysis lasted for 10 to 12 hours before spontaneous recovery occurred. For some years, the patient had averaged 6 to 12 bowel movements daily and admittedly consumed large amounts of food without gaining weight.

Clinically, there was minimal if any stimulation, and ophthalmopathy was lacking. The thyroid gland was estimated to weigh 30 gm and was not unusually firm. A thyrotoxic condition was suspected clinically but could not be established. The BMR was +19%, and the uptake of ^{131}I was 28% and 36% at 6 and 24 hours, respectively. After T_3 suppression, the uptake was 19% and 30% at 6 and 24 hours, respectively. The values for TBG and total serum T_4 were normal; the value for free T_4 was elevated (4.9 ng/100 ml). Neurologic evaluation, including electromyography, revealed abnormalities consistent with a diagnosis of periodic paralysis. Sodium iodide I 131 was administered in December 1968. Though the free T_4 value was elevated, the normal value for total serum T_4 was nonconfirmatory. The finding of an elevated T_3 level was important in reenforcing the clinical diagnosis.

At follow-up three months later, the patient had clinical hypothyroidism confirmed by a total serum T_4 value of only 0.9μg/100 ml. Treatment with levothyroxine was instituted. Interestingly, after treatment with sodium iodide I 131, further episodes of periodic paralysis have been completely absent.

PATIENT 6.—A 75-year-old woman was referred to the Mayo Clinic for evaluation of edema of the right upper lid, dull aching in the right orbit, blurred vision, and diplopia. The thyroid gland was not abnormal to palpation.

Examination failed to reveal specific evidence of thyrotoxicosis. The patient was observed for two months, during which there was no change except for an increase of the previously noted ophthalmopathy. At that time, there was definite evidence of muscle paresis on upward and lateral gaze, as well as edema of all lids. The uptake of ^{131}I was 30% at 24 hours prior to T_3 suppression and 26% after the ingestion of 100μg of liothyronine sodium daily for five days. Additional examination revealed that the skin was unusually warm and soft; there was no evidence of pretibial myxedema or acropachy. The values for total and free T_4 were normal, as were the values for TBG and TBPA. The T_3 value, however, was significantly elevated (772 ng/100 ml). Because of the lack of convincing clinical evidence of thyrotoxicosis, specific antithyroid treatment was not advised. Appropriate eye muscle surgery was performed, with good results.

On subsequent follow-up examinations during the next 12 months, the equivocal evidence of thyrotoxicosis subsided; specific antithyroid treatment was never prescribed. In retrospect, it was obvious that the patient had Graves' disease with ophthalmopathy but clinically never had a clearly toxic reaction in spite of the elevated serum T_3 level.

Minimal elevations of the total T_4 values were noted in patients 7 and 8. However, free T_4 values were within the range of normal. The degree of toxic reaction was probably related more to the pronounced elevations of T_3 than to the equivocal abnormalities in T_4 values.

PATIENT 7.—Until six weeks prior to her first visit to our clinic, this 49-year-old housewife felt well. The onset of symptoms was rather sudden, and in the ensuing six weeks, she lost almost 35 lb, was aware of generalized tremulousness, and had mild heat intolerance.

On initial examination, the patient was stimulated, tachycardia was present, and the thyroid gland was moderately and diffusely enlarged, with an estimated weight of 35 gm. There was a slight stare and minimal lid retraction of the left eye. The skin was soft and warm, and a fine tremor was noted. Clinically, the patient's condition was moderately thyrotoxic. The BMR was +25%, and the uptake of ^{131}I was 76% and 77% in 6 and 24 hours, respectively. The total serum T_4 value was minimally elevated at 11.2μg/100 ml; the free T_4 level was 2.6 ng/100 ml. The levels of TBG and TBPA were normal. On the basis of clinical assessment, treatment with sodium iodide I 131 was advised. Only later was it learned that the serum T_3 value was 840 ng/100 ml.

When reevaluated by her local physician six months later, the patient had myxedema as a result of the sodium iodide I 131 therapy.

PATIENT 8.—A 57-year-old housewife noted the onset of diplopia, photophobia, and excessive lacrimation in October 1969. The symptoms gradually became worse, and she visited the Mayo Clinic nine months later, at which time minimal bilateral conjunctival injection and lid retraction were noted. In addition, there was severe paresis of upward gaze bilaterally. The thyroid gland was diffusely enlarged and estimated to weigh 35 gm. Clinical assessment suggested that the patient's condition was mildly thyrotoxic. The uptake of ^{131}I at 6 and 24 hours was 62% and 71%, respectively; the total serum T_4 level was 11.5μg/100 ml, and the free T_4 level was 2.4 ng/100 ml. The BMR was not determined. On the basis of clinical assessment, sodium iodide I 131 was administered. It was later noted that the levels of TBG and TBPA were normal and that the serum level of T_3 was 955 ng/100 ml.

Myxedema was noted at reevaluation three months later, but there was no significant change in the mild degree of ophthalmopathy.

William M. McConahey, MD, assisted in the evaluation of many of these patients.

The h-TSH and rabbit anti-h-TSH serum were supplied by the National Pituitary Agency.

References

1. Sterling K, Bellabarba D, Newtnan ES, et al: Determination of triiodothyronine concentration in human serum. *J Clin Invest* **48**:1150-1158, 1969.

2. Wahner HW, Gorman CA: Interpretation of serum triiodothyronine levels measured by the Sterling technique. *New Eng J Med* **284**:225-230, 1971.

3. Murphy BP, Jachan C: The determination of thyroxine by competitive protein-binding analysis employing an anion-exchange resin and radiothyroxine. *J Lab Clin Med* **66**:161-167, 1965.

4. Sterling K, Brenner MA: Free thyroxine in human serum: Simplified measurement with the aid of magnesium precipitation. *J Clin Invest* **45**:155-163, 1966.

5. Mayberry WE, Gharib H, Bilstad JM, et al: Radioimmunoassay for human thyrotropin: Clinical value in patients with normal and abnormal thyroid function. *Ann Intern Med* **74**:471, 1971.

6. Arango G, Mayberry WE, Hockert TJ, et al: Total and free human serum thyroxine in normal and abnormal thyroid states *Mayo Clin Proc* **43**:503-516, 1968.

7. Wyse EP, McConahey WM, Woolner LB, et al: Opthalmopathy without hyperthyroidism in patients with histologic Hashimoto's thyroiditis. *J Clin Endocr* **28**:1623,1629, 1968.

8. Sterling K, Refetoff S, Selenkow HA: T_3 thyrotoxicosis: Thyrotoxicosis due to elevated serum triiodothyronine levels. *JAMA* **213**:571-575, 1970.

9. Hollander CS: On the nature of the circulating thyroid hormone: Clinical studies of triiodothyronine and thyroxine in serum using gas chromatographic methods. *Trans Assoc Amer Physicians* **81**:76-91, 1968.

10. Shimaoka K: Toxic adenoma of the thyroid with triiodothyronine as the principle circulating thyroid hormone. *Acta Endocr* **43**:285-293, 1963.

11. Maclagan NF, Bowden CH, Wilkinson JH: The metabolism of thyroid hormones: 2. Detection of thyroxine and tri-iodothyronine in human plasma. *Biochem J* **67**:5-11, 1957.

12. Inada M, Sterling K: Thyroxine transport in thyrotoxicosis and hypothyroidism. *J Clin Invest* **46**:1442-1450, 1967.

13. Braverman LE, Foster AE, Ingbar SH: Thyroid hormone transport in the serum of patients with thyrotoxic Graves' disease before and after treatment. *J Clin Invest* **47**:1349-1357, 1968.

14. Oppenheimer JH: Role of plasma proteins in the binding, distribution and metabolism of the thyroid hormones. *New Eng J Med* **278**:1153-1162, 1968.

15. Blackburn CM, McConahey WM, Keating FR Jr, et al: Calorigenic effects of single intravenous doses of L-triiodothyronine and L-thyroxine in myxedematous persons. *J Clin Invest* **33**:819-824, 1954.

16. Sterling K, Chados RB: Radiothyroxine turnover studies in myxedema, thyrotoxicosis, and hypermetabolism without endocrine disease. *J Clin Invest* **35**:806-813, 1956.

17. Ingbar SH, Freinkel N: Simultaneous estimation of rates of thyroxine degradation and thyroid hormone synthesis. *J Clin Invest* **34**:808-819, 1955.

18. Greer MA, Grimm Y, Studer H: Qualitative changes in the secretion of thyroid hormones induced by iodine deficiency. *Endocrinology* **83**:1193-1198, 1968.

19. Heninger RW, Albright EC: Effect of iodine deficiency on iodine-containing compounds of rat tissues. *Endocrinology* **79**:309-315, 1966.

20. Pineda G, Silva E, Gianetti A, et al: Influence of iodine deficiency upon PBI in hyperthyroidism. *J Clin Endocr* **30**:120-124, 1970.

21. Gharib H, Mayberry WE, Ryan RJ: Determination of triiodothyronine concentration in human serum by radioimmunoassay, abstracted. *J Lab Clin Med* **76**:863, 1970.

Sequential Observations on Pulmonary Functional Derangements in Bagassosis

Daniel E. Jenkins, MD; Suresh K. Malik, MD; Juan C. Figueroa-Casas, MD; and Ralph D. Eichhorn, MD, Houston

Bagassosis developed in three patients following repeated exposure to bagasse handled in the manufacture of mud used for oil drilling operations. Physiologic studies were carried out with prolonged observations. All patients recovered without corticosteroid therapy. Main abnormalities were reduction in lung volumes, diminished diffusing capacity, hypoxemia, and low pulmonary compliance. No airways obstruction or impairment of intrapulmonary gas distribution was noted. Functional defects improved within two months; maximum recovery was achieved after six months. Since all patients were treated symptomatically, the speed and extent of recovery may be considered as a baseline for persons with normal pulmonary function results before and after illness who have had no more than one clinical episode of bagassosis.

The clinical picture of bagassosis is well known and since 1941 has been repeatedly described.[1-6] Recently, more detailed information has been published concerning the pathology and pathogenesis of the disorder.[7,8] An improved understanding of the functional alterations produced by the disease is needed and would be helpful in providing a better insight into symptomatology, the evolution of the disease, and its degree of reversibility once the source of contact with bagasse has been eliminated.

Until recently no detailed studies have been available on the physiologic derangements associated with this disease. Weill et al,[9] in a report on detailed pulmonary function studies in 20 cases of bagassosis, found restrictive ventilatory impairment and reduction in diffusing capacity which normalized a few months following removal from the source of exposure. Pierce et al[10] reported similar pulmonary functional changes during the course of the acute illness, and while the chest roentgenograms returned to normal appearance, the reduction in diffusing capacity persisted even after 12 months of follow-up. The purpose of this report is to present three patients with bagassosis in whom clinical observations and repeat measurements of pulmonary function have been carried out from the beginning of the acute illness until maximal spontaneous recovery was achieved, with a further prolonged follow-up in two of the three patients.

Received for publication Jan 27, 1971; accepted May 6.

From the Pulmonary Disease Section, Department of Medicine, Baylor College of Medicine and the Ben Taub General and Methodist Hospitals, Houston. Dr. Eichhorn is now with the Universidad del Litoral, Rosario, Argentina.

Reprint requests to Department of Medicine, Baylor College of Medicine, 1200 Moursund Ave, Houston 77025 (Dr. Jenkins).

Methods

Spirometric studies were performed using a 13.5-liter spirometer (Collins) and forced vital capacity measurements were carried out on a low resistance, waterless bellows spirometer. Predicted values are those established by Kory et al.[11] The lung volumes were determined by the open circuit method of Darling et al,[12] and the predicted normal values are those of Needham et al.[13] Intrapulmonary gas distribution was evaluated by the single-breath nitrogen method of Comroe and Fowler[14] in which the expired nitrogen concentration was recorded as a function of volume and measurements were made of the difference in nitrogen concentration between 750 and 1,250 ml of expired volume. Diffusing capacity ($D_{L_{CO}}$) was measured by the single ten-second breath-holding technique[15] and prediction values are those in which $D_{L_{CO}}$ is a function of body height (0.344 of the height in centimeters $-31.6 = D_{L_{co}}$).[15] Arterial blood gas determination were performed with the use of the Clark and Severinghaus electrodes and arterial oxygen saturation was calculated by the Severinghaus nomogram.[16]

Dynamic pulmonary compliance values were obtained by dividing the tidal volumes measured during quiet breathing by the differences in pressure between the esophagus and the mouth.[17] The differential pressures were measured by a conventional strain gauge transducer and recorded from an oscilloscopic display of the electrical events. The specific compliance was calculated by dividing the tidal compliance by the functional residual capacity. Instantaneous air flow measurements were recorded during the procedure and nonelastic pulmonary resistance during slow tidal air flow was also calculated.[17,18] Maximal negative recoil pressures were obtained after performance of the vital capacity.

Clinical Material

Details concerning clinical evaluation of each of the patients studied are presented in Table 1. The physiologic data are summarized in Table 2. All three patients worked for a company engaged in the manufacture of drilling mud in which the dried husks of sugar cane, or bagasse, were used as an ingredient. The material

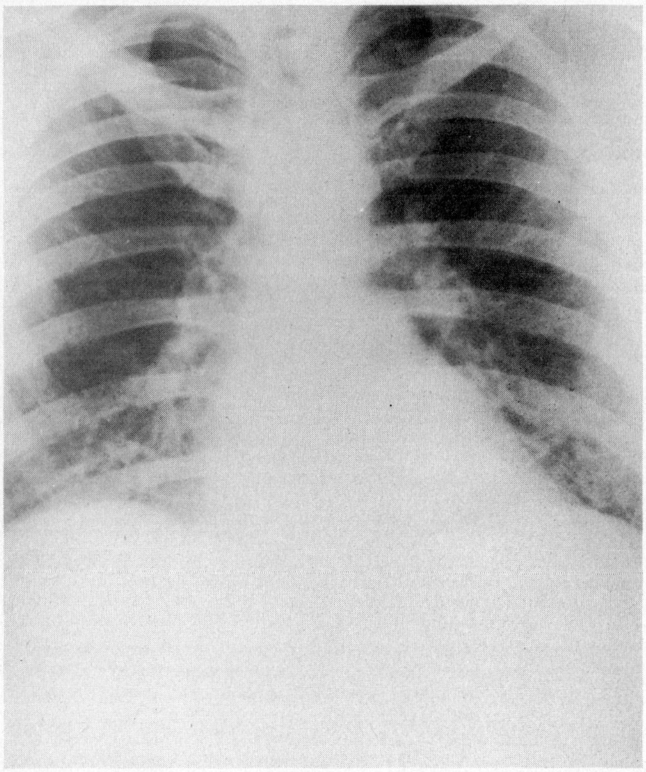

Fig 1.—Patient 3.—The chest roentgenogram of Feb 15, 1965 (posterioanterior view), shows fine reticular densities best seen in the lower portion of both lung fields.

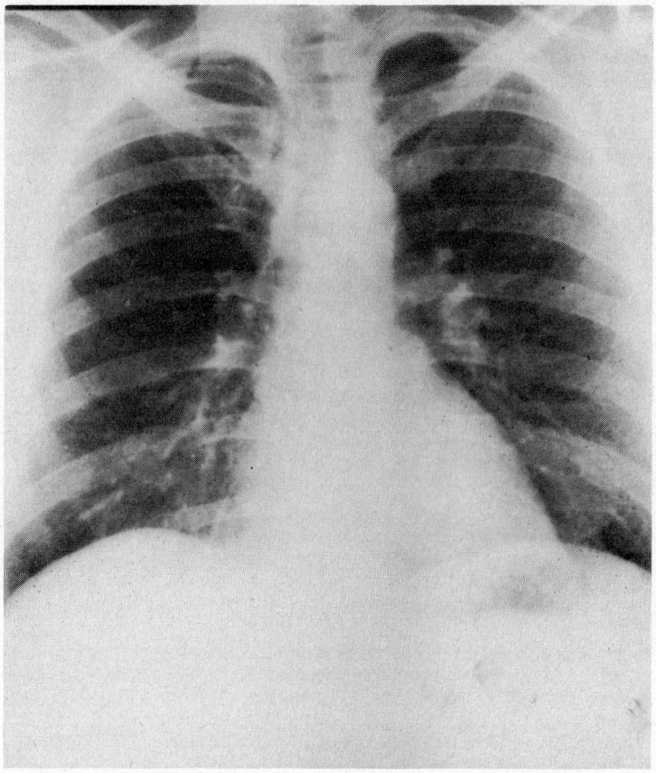

Fig 2.—Patient 3.—April 29, 1965, posterioanterior view shows considerable clearing of the densities in the lower lung fields.

Fig 3.—Patient 2.—February 12, 1965, posterioanterior view reveals very fine reticular densities throughout the lower portion of both lung fields.

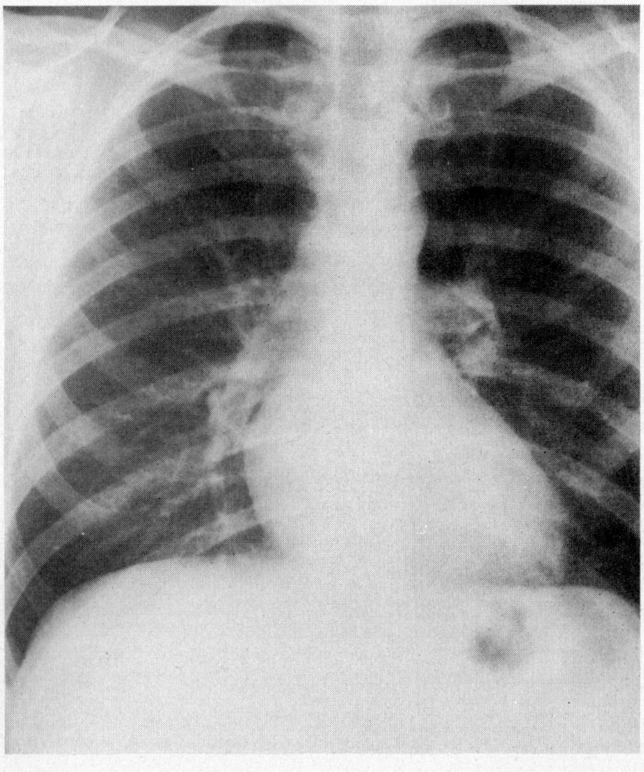

Fig 4.—Patient 2.—Roentgenogram of April 28, 1965, shows nearly complete clearing of the fine densities in both lower lung fields (posterioanterior view).

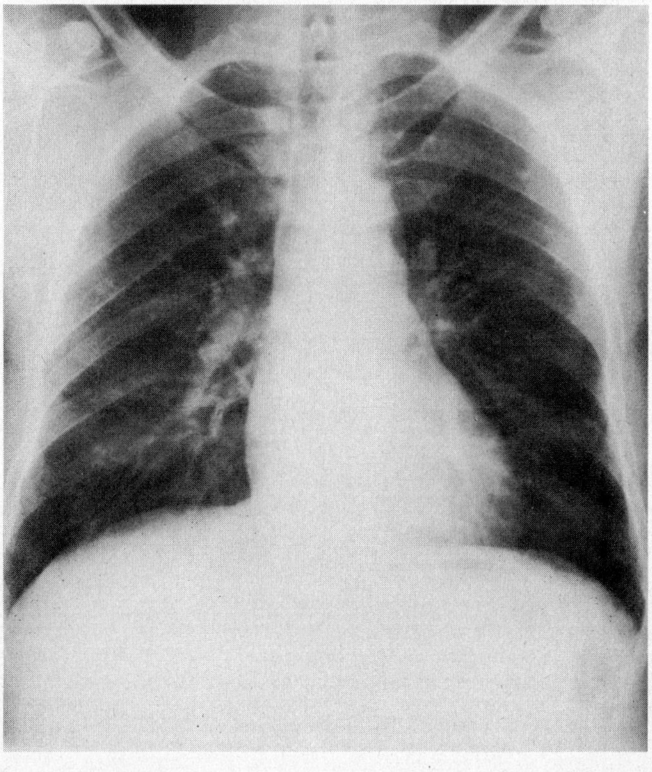

Table 1.—Clinical Findings

Patient No. and Data	Duration of Bagasse Exposure Prior to Acute Illness	Symptoms	Smoking History	Physical Examination	Asymptomatic (Time After Separation From Bagasse)	Time of Persistence of Crepitant Rales
3 42-year-old White Man	90 days	Weight loss, 20 lb Tight feeling chest Dry cough Muscular aching Flushing face Progressive dyspnea Night sweats	30 cigarettes daily for 30 years; inhaled moderately	Fever Bilateral wheezing Moist rales	20 days	4 mo
2 40-year-old White Man	50 days	Weight loss, 15 lb Weakness Chills and fever Muscular aching Cough and sputum Progressive dyspnea	50 cigarettes daily for 22 years; inhaled deeply	Fever Moist rales	20 days	6 mo
1 57-year-old Negro Man	45 days	Weakness Chills and fever Cough Sputum production Progressive dyspnea Cigarettes unpleasant	10 cigarettes daily for 39 years; inhaled slightly	Fever Bilateral wheezing Moist rales	30 days	3 mo

was received in 80-lb bales from a commercial supplier in Lockport, La, close to the center of the sugar cane industry in that state. Following delivery the bagasse was processed through a hammer-mill, the dust extracted, and the fiber sacked into paper bags to be used later in preparation of the drilling mud. The hammer-mill and bagging operations were very dusty inasmuch as 1,000 lb of dust was produced for every ton of bagasse introduced into the system. Analysis of the dust showed a silica content in excess of 5% α-quartz, but no β-quartz was identified. Prior to the illness herein described, none of the workers wore protective masks. All three patients were exposed to the dust of bagasse for a period varying from 45 days to 90 days. The clinical course was characterized by marked constitutional symptoms, bilateral chest wheezing in two patients, and auscultatory crepitant rales in all three patients with gradual return to clinical recovery following the separation from bagasse dust. (See Table 1). Serial follow-up with chest roentgenograms showed fine reticular densities predominantly in the lower lung fields which later improved in a period varying from 6 to 12 weeks after the initial x-ray observation. (Fig 1 to 6)

Results of Physiological Studies

Evaluation of several pulmonary functional indexes was carried out on each of the three patients over the course of nearly a year following clinically manifest bagassosis (Table 2). The first studies were performed within 30 days of the onset of the acute illness and as soon as the patients were capable of cooperation. The second set was obtained within 45 to 60 days and the third after an interval of six months. The fourth set of studies was conducted 9 to 11 months after the original illness, and in two patients prolonged follow-up was obtained at 54 (patient 1) and 56 (patient 2) months, respectively.

At the time of initial studies the vital capacity was either subnormal or in a low-normal range in all three patients with no evidence of significant airways obstruction. The vital capacity improved significantly in two of the patients between the first and second measurement and this improvement continued to be evident in the total evaluation on all three patients. Further improvement in the vital capacity beyond six months was not seen. Lung volume measurements showed a marked initial reduction of residual volume in one patient (3). In all three patients there was a gradual increase in both the residual volume and the total lung capacity between the early and late measurements. Intrapulmonary gas distribution was not significantly impaired in any of the patients and remained essentially unchanged during the entire period of observation.

The diffusing capacity was diminished in all three patients at the time of the initial measurements. This test also showed consistent improvement at the time of the second evaluation, and further gradual improvement was seen between the second and third studies. Hypoxemia was observed in all three patients at the onset with gradual improvement through the follow-up period.

Two determinations of lung compliance were performed on each patient within an interval of four to six months. The initial compliance values were in a low-normal range (patients 1 and 3) or slightly below normal (patient 2) and all three showed improvement on the second evaluation. The specific compliance, which is of value in separating variations due to change in volume from those due to intrinsic alteration of elastic properties, improved in two of the patients. The coefficient of retrac-

Table 2.—Physiologic Findings

Dates Studied	Patient 3* 3/2/65	Patient 3* 4/13/65	Patient 3* 8/17/65	Patient 3* 11/23/65	Patient 2† 2/16/65	Patient 2† 4/16/65	Patient 2† 8/18/65	Patient 2† 1/10/66	Patient 2† 10/2/69
Functions									
Forced volume capacity (liters)§	4.70	4.85	5.60	5.90	3.50	4.30	4.72	4.90	4.63
% Predicted	82	84	97	103	70	86	94	98	92.6
Forced expiratory volume$_{1.0}$/forced volume capacity × 100	80	82	81	76	80	78	76	75	77
Residual volume (liters)§	0.87	1.73	2.04	2.65	1.62	2.10	1.85	1.84	2.09
% Predicted	53	105	124	161	98	127	112	111	126.6
Total lung capacity (TLC) (liters)§	5.37	6.88	7.64	8.15	5.37	6.28	6.28	6.36	6.82
% Predicted	85	109	121	129	85	99	99	100	108
Single-breath N_2 (Rise in % of 750-1,250 ml)	1.13	0.3	1.23	0.63	1.67		0.80	1.2	1.30
Diffusion (D_{LCO}) (ml/min/mm Hg)	17.2	24.5	32.8	32.0	19.1	27.3	30.0	30.0	26.0
% Predicted	48.0	68.4	91.6	89.4	62	89	98	98	84.7
Arterial Blood Gases, Resting, pH	7.46		7.45		7.48		7.45		7.41
Arterial Blood Gases, Resting, P_{CO_2} (mm Hg)	36		31		35.0		34.0		35.0
Arterial Blood Gases, Resting, P_{O_2} (mm Hg)	67		63		74.0		83.5		91.0
Arterial Blood Gases, Exercise, pH	7.48		7.39		7.40		7.44		7.37
Arterial Blood Gases, Exercise, P_{CO_2} (mm Hg)	26		37		35.3		34.0		41.0
Arterial Blood Gases, Exercise, P_{O_2} (mm Hg)	55		70		78.8		87.0		94.0
Compliance (liters/cm of H_2O)§	0.121		0.259		0.110		0.183		0.221
Specific compliance§ (Liters/cm of H_2O/liter)	0.053		0.071		0.035		0.049		0.065
Nonelastic resistance (cm of H_2O/liter/sec)									
Inspiration	0.89		0.41		<1.0		<1.0		<1.0
Expiration	3.47		2.43		6.5		3.96		5.38
Coefficient of retraction (MIP‖/TLC)	8.19 (44/5.37)		6.28 (48/7.64)		6.15 (33/5.37)		4.22 (26.5/6.28)		5.28 (36/6.82)

* Patient 3 was a 42-year-old white man; height = 196 cm, weight = 103 kg.
† Patient 2 was a 40-year-old white man; height = 181 cm, weight = 77 kg.
‡ Patient 1 was a 57-year-old Negro man; height = 173 cm, weight = 77 kg.
§ Body temperature, pressure, saturation.
‖ Maximal inspiratory pressure (transpulmonary).

tion was initially high in two patients (2 and 3) and the values decreased during follow-up. Expiratory nonelastic pulmonary resistance was slightly elevated in all three patients and returned to normal on the second measurement, but in only one patient was the improvement very sizable. Two of the patients (1 and 2) were restudied after 56 and 54 months of observation and the pulmonary functional profile remained in the normal range.

Comment

Bagassosis is one of the vegetable fiber pneumoconioses and is currently thought to be associated with a hypersensitivity state of the lungs. The observations by Selvaggio et al[8] regarding the presence of precipitating antibodies against moldy bagasse in the serum of patients with bagassosis, as well as in bagasse workers who were not affected by the disease, are similar to those reported by Pepys et al[19] in farmer's lung, and by Hargreave et al[20] in the bird-breeder's lung. Also, coniosporosis (Maple bark disease), byssinosis, and sequoiosis have been included in this group of diseases secondary to inhalation of organic dusts.[21]

The clinical picture of a flu-like syndrome following a history of bagasse exposure with progressive worsening of symptoms during continued exposure has been previously described.[22] Associated radiographic findings have usually been those of a fine, diffuse mottling of both lung fields with a "reticulated" appearance which is often indistinguishable from miliary tuberculosis.[22] Both the clinical and radiological features show spontaneous improvement after the subjects are separated from bagasse, although one case[23] has been reported in which bagassosis apparently led to progressive pulmonary fibrosis and death. Persistence of diffuse fibrosis is an outcome which has been recorded by other observers.[24] The three cases described in this paper followed the usual pattern of prompt symptomatic recovery after receiving only supportive treatment. No corticosteroids were administered.

Recent studies from Reynolds and Stembridge[7] under light and electron microscopy revealed characteristic

Patient 1‡				
3/2/65	4/19/65	7/21/65	12/21/65	9/30/69
2.85	3.55	3.85	3.75	3.36
68	85	92	89	80
84	81	65	71	80
1.78	1.47	2.14	2.27	1.82
93	77	113	119	95.7
5.03	5.07	5.82	5.77	5.32
81	81	93	92	86
1.5		0.93	1.33	0.90
16.8	23.6	27.8	25.2	26.3
60.2	84.6	99.6	90.3	94.2
7.46		7.47		7.41
33		36		35.3
74		80		103
7.39		7.45		7.40
28		36		33.0
78		86		96
0.126		0.181		0.169
0.045		0.047		0.042
1.61		1.68		1.64
3.71		1.69		2.66
3.88		3.61		3.76
19.5/5.03)		(21/5.82)		(20/5.32)

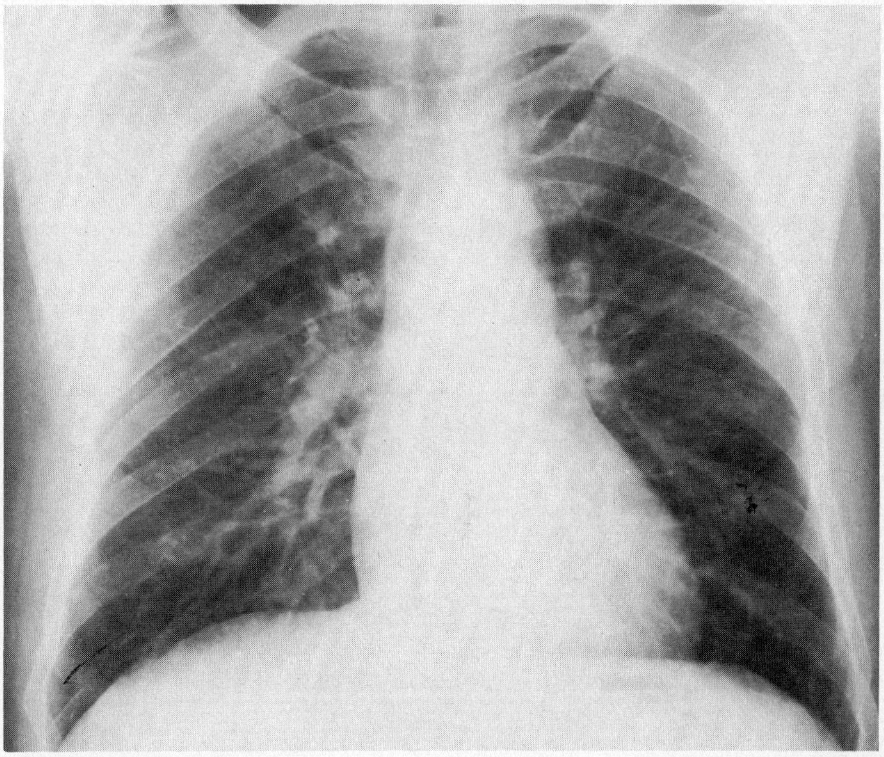

Fig 5.—Patient 1.—March 5, 1965, posterioanterior view shows patchy lobular and fine granular densities throughout the lower two thirds of both lung fields.

Fig 6.—Patient 1.—April 19, 1965, posterioanterior view reveals almost complete clearing of the densities in the lower lung fields.

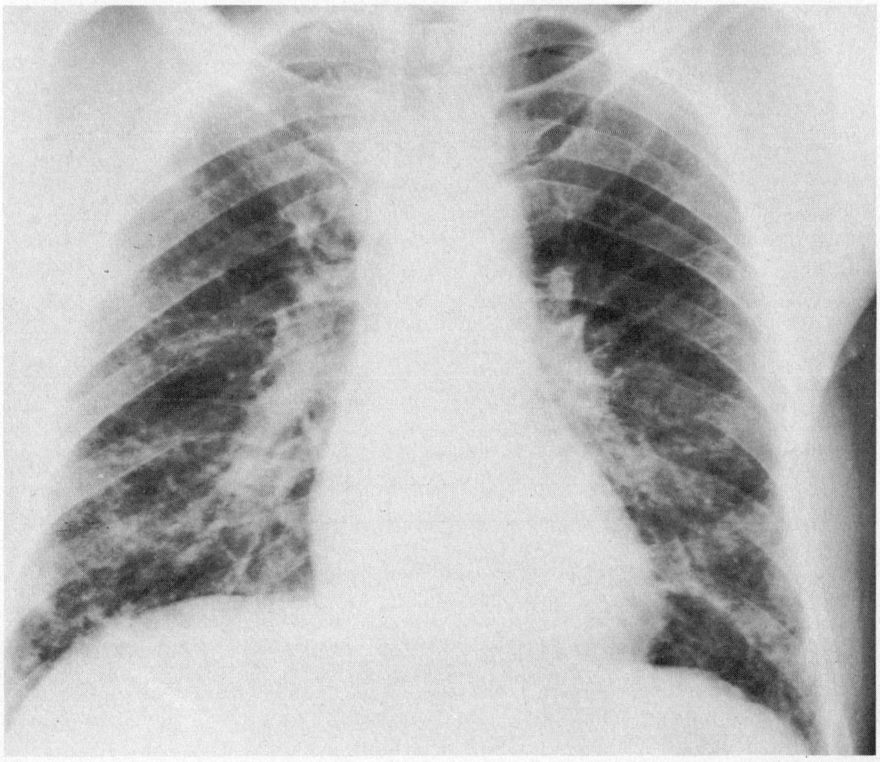

nodular interstitial and epithelial lesions surrounded by zones of chronic inflammation and early fibrosis. Electron microscopy of these nodules showed that the epithelioid cells were derived from the type II alveolar cell.

These few pathologic reports allow a reasonable interpretation of the nature of the physiological impairment shown by the pulmonary function studies. Data presented in Table 2 are in essential agreement with the results reported by Weill et al[9] and Pierce et al.[10] At the beginning of the illness there is usually a reduction in the lung volume without airways obstruction. The initial physiological studies were performed 20 or 30 days after the patient had been separated from bagasse, so it is possible that some degree of reversible airways obstruction had come and gone by the time the first pulmonary function studies were performed. In two of the three patients, wheezing was noted at the time of initial physical examination, so that some degree of airways obstruction might have been present although concomitant physiological data are not available to prove the point. The DL_{CO} was consistently decreased, however, and improved in all patients as the clinical evidence of pulmonary involvement decreased. Pulmonary compliance was in a low-normal or slightly subnormal range and also improved as the pathologic process cleared, which suggests a resolution of the interstitial process rather than a fibrosis. The same interpretation applies to the progressive drop in the coefficient of retraction. The low values of O_2 tension (Po_2) and saturation at rest are consistent with the subnormal DL_{CO} and suggest either a diffusional defect or a ventilation-perfusion imbalance, or both.

In our data and in those reported by other workers,[9,10] the observed restrictive defect was largely reversible and eventually disappeared. Improvement was evident in the first two months, although complete recovery seemed to be achieved in about six months. Beyond six months no further improvement was noted. The roentgenographic manifestations cleared in all three patients within 6 to 12 weeks from the beginning of observation. It is apparent that further improvement in some of the physiologic studies continued beyond 12 weeks so that physiological measurements are a somewhat more sensitive guide to the extent of recovery than is the roentgenogram.

It seems clear that bagassosis may produce serious illness with severe clinical manifestations and physiologic disturbances. Bagasse is now widely used throughout the world and continued reporting of bagassosis is urged since this is an important occupational illness and is largely prevented by processing and controlling the inhalation of dust containing bagasse.[5,25,26] A physiologic baseline of the natural course of the disease needs to be established so that the results of proposed forms of treatment may be evaluated with greater clarity than has hereto been possible. Corticosteroids have been advocated, especially in the treatment of patients severely ill with bagassosis,[22,25] but, as mentioned by Weill,[9] the frequent use of corticosteroids makes difficult a valid description of functional alterations during the natural course of the disease. Since the three patients reported in this study were given no specific treatment and were observed to have a return of physiologic studies to normal or near-normal values, it can be assumed with reasonable accuracy that the pulmonary function studies were normal prior to bagasse exposure. The observations represent a valid study of the natural course of the disease and the speed of recovery in otherwise healthy persons following their first episode of clinical bagassosis.

This investigation was supported in part by Public Health Service research grant UI-00405.

References

1. Jamison SC, Hopkins J: Bagassosis: Fungus disease of lungs: Case report. *New Orleans Med Surg J* **93**:580-582, 1941.
2. Castleden LIM, Hamilton-Paterson JL: Bagassosis: An industrial lung disease. *Brit Med J* **2**:478-480, 1942.
3. Gillison JA, Taylor F: Four cases of bagassosis. *Brit Med J* **2**:577-578, 1942.
4. Sodeman WA, Pullen RL: Bagasse disease of the lungs. *Arch Intern Med* **73**:365-374, 1944.
5. Nicholson D: Bagasse worker's lung. *Amer Rev Resp Dis* **97**:546-560, 1968.
6. Hearn CED: Bagassosis: An epidemiological, environmental and clinical survey. *Brit J Industr Med* **25**:267-282, 1968.
7. Reynolds RC, Stembridge VA: Electron microscopy of bagassosis in humans. *Amer Rev Resp Dis* **92**:327-328, 1965.
8. Selvaggio JE, Buechner HM, Seabury JH, et al: Bagassosis: Precipitins against extract of crude bagasse in the serum of patients. *Ann Intern Med* **64**:748-758, 1966.
9. Weill H, Buechner HM, Gonzalez E, et al: Bagassosis: A study of pulmonary function in 20 cases. *Ann Intern Med* **64**:737-747, 1966.
10. Pierce AK, Nicholson DP, Miller JM, et al: Pulmonary function in bagasse worker's lung disease. *Amer Rev Resp Dis* **97**:561-570, 1968.
11. Kory RC, Callahan R, Boren HG, et al: The Veterans Administration Army cooperative study of pulmonary function: Clinical spirometry in normal men. *Amer J Med* **30**:243-258, 1961.
12. Darling RC, Cournand A, Richards DW: Studies on the intrapulmonary mixture of gases: III. An open circuit method for measuring residual air. *J Clin Invest* **19**:609-618, 1940.
13. Needham CD, Rogan MC, McDonald I: Normal standards for lung volumes, intrapulmonary gas mixing and maximum breathing capacity. *Thorax* **9**:313-325, 1954.
14. Comroe JH, Fowler WS: Lung function studies: VI. Detection of uneven ventilation during a single breath of oxygen. *Amer J Med* **10**:408-413, 1951.
15. Ogilvie CM, Forster RE, Blakemore WS, et al: A standardized breath-holding technique for the clinical measurements of the diffusing capacity of the lung for carbon monoxide. *J Clin Invest* **36**:1-17, 1957.
16. Severinghaus JW: Oxyhemoglobin dissociation curve correction for temperature and pH variation in human blood. *J Appl Physiol* **12**:485-486, 1958.
17. Frank NR, Mead J, Ferris BG: The mechanical behavior of the lungs in healthy elderly persons. *J Clin Invest* **36**:1680-1687, 1957.
18. Terplan M, Fruhmann G: Significance of the dynamic pressure-volume curve in subjects with and without obstructive respiratory disease. *Med Thorac* **20**:372-383, 1963.
19. Pepys J, Riddel RW, Citron KM, et al: Precipitins against extracts of hay and molds in the serum of patients with farmer's lung, aspergillosis, asthma and sarcoidosis. *Thorax* **17**:366-374, 1962.
20. Hargreave FE, Pepys J, Longbottom JL, et al: Bird breeder's (fancier's) lung. *Lancet* **1**:445-449, 1966.
21. American Thoracic Society: Definition and classification of non-infectious reactions of the lung. *Amer Rev Resp Dis* **93**:965-981, 1966.
22. Buechner HA, Prevatt AC, Thompson J, et al: Bagassosis: A review, with further historical data, studies of pulmonary function and results of adrenal steroid therapy. *Amer J Med* **25**:234-247, 1958.
23. Hunter D, Perry KMA: Bronchiolitis resulting from the handling of bagasse dust. *Brit J Industr Med* **3**:64-74, 1946.
24. Buechner HA: Bagassosis: A true pneumoconiosis. *Industr Med Surg* **31**:311-314, 1962.
25. Buechner HA, Aucoin E, Vignes AJ, et al: The resurgence of bagassosis in Louisiana. *J Occup Med* **6**:437-442, 1964.
26. Buechner HW: Bagassosis: Peculiarities of the geographical pattern and report of the first case from Peru and Puerto Rico. *JAMA* **174**:1237-1241, 1960.

Aspergillus Infection Complicating Cardiac Transplantation

Report of Five Cases

Marc J. Gurwith, MD; Edward B. Stinson, MD; and Jack S. Remington, MD, Stanford and Palo Alto, Calif

During the initial two-year period of the cardiac transplant program at Stanford University Hospital, a 28% incidence of invasive pulmonary aspergillosis was observed. The diagnosis was based on postmortem findings in two patients, and on isolation of the fungus from percutaneous lung aspirates or transtracheal aspirates in the other three. *Aspergillus* was isolated from multiple cultures of sputum from four of the five patients. Local or systemic amphotericin B therapy or both was administered to three patients, and in two of them long-term treatment and necessary. Among the multiple underlying predisposing factors responsible for the high incidence of aspergillosis in cardiac transplant patients, pulmonary factors relatively unique to cardiac transplantation as well as immunosuppression appeared to play major roles.

Infection by "opportunistic" organisms in renal transplant patients receiving immunosuppressive therapy is well documented.[1,2] With the advent of transplantation of other organs, infections unique to the transplant procedure and site may be expected. Such infections have been a major cause of morbidity and mortality in 18 cardiac transplant recipients at Stanford in the two-year period from January 1968 to December 1969.[3] The appearance of significant infection with *Aspergillus* in five of these patients was considered remarkable in our hospital population. We describe these five cases and their management, and discuss the factors which may have predisposed to this unusually high incidence.

Eighteen cardiac transplants were performed from January 1968 to December 1969. The patients' ages ranged from 33 to 64 years with an average of 50 years, and 15 were men.

Received for publication Oct 7, 1970; accepted March 22, 1971.

From the departments of medicine (Drs. Gurwith and Remington) and surgery (Dr. Stinson), Stanford University School of Medicine, Stanford, Calif; and the Division of Allergy, Immunology, and Infectious Diseases, Palo Alto Medical Research Foundation (Dr. Remington), Palo Alto, Calif. Dr. Gurwith is a special fellow of the National Cancer Institute and is now with the Bess Kaiser Hospital, Portland, Ore. Dr. Stinson is now with the National Institutes of Health, Bethesda, Md.

Reprint requests to 860 Bryant St, Palo Alto, Calif 94301 (Dr. Remington).

The operative diagnosis was coronary artery disease in 13 patients, and idiopathic cardiomyopathy in five. The surgical techniques, prophylactic antibiotics, and immunosuppressive therapy regimens employed have been previously described.[4]

Preoperative cultures of sputum, urine, and stool for fungi and bacteria were obtained from all patients. Postoperatively, cultures of sputum were obtained at least three times weekly for one month, weekly until discharge, and after discharge as indicated. Percutaneous transtracheal aspiration for bacterial and fungus cultures and gram and methenamine silver stains were performed promptly in all patients upon suspicion of pulmonary infection. In four patients, needle aspiration biopsy of pulmonary infiltrates was performed for culture and histology under fluoroscopic control.[5]

Patient Summaries

PATIENT 1.–A 54-year-old man with a history of postviral cardiomyopathy underwent transplantation on Jan 6, 1968. Reexploration was necessary four hours postoperatively because of hemorrhage. Tracheostomy was performed at the time of initial surgery, and ventilation via the tracheostomy tube on a volume-cycled respirator was required throughout the postoperative survival. Complications included severe thrombocytopenia, renal failure, and gastorintestinal (GI) bleeding appearing on postoperative day three. Peritoneal dialysis was begun on day two and continued daily. On the seventh day acute gallbladder hydrops due to hemobilia developed and emergency cholecystectomy and common duct exploration with T tube placement and liver biopsy were performed. Severe upper GI bleeding on the 12th day led to exploratory laparotomy, vagotomy, and pyloroplasty. The following day, recurrent severe hemorrhage required reoperation; splenectomy was performed at this time. On the eighth day, pneumonia due to *Enterobacter* was diagnosed; despite administration of appropriate antibiotics, it was progressive, and gram-negative septicemia due to *Enterobacter* developed on the 13th day. The patient died on postoperative day 15. Pathologic findings included mild histologic evidence of cardiac rejection.[6] The lungs were congested with severe generalized *Enterobacter* bronchopneumonia. Invasion by *Aspergillus* with widespread peribronchial necroses was noted in the left lung. Dissemination of *Aspergillus* infection was evident in the heart, with multifocal fungal necroses scattered throughout the myocardium. The species was identified as *Aspergillus flavus*.

PATIENT 2.–A 54-year-old woman with a preoperative diagnosis of end-stage ischemic heart disease underwent transplantation on Oct 4, 1968. Severe and recurrent episodes of threatened graft rejection required repeated high-dose immunosuppressive therapy on postoperative days 2 through 4, 8 through 12, 41 through 43, 55 through 56, and 61 through 64. Urinary-tract infection due to *Escherichia coli*, diagnosed on the 34th day, seemed initially to respond to antibiotic treatment but recurred following discontinuation of antibiotics three weeks later. Leukopenia developed on the 46th day and progressed to a minimum white blood cell count (WBC) of 1,600/cu mm with 85% polymorphonuclear cells on day 51. Thereafter, the WBC rose slowly to normal levels within a week. Evidence of progressive hepatic dysfunction, thought to be related to drug toxic reaction, developed on the 44th day, and progressive hepatic insufficiency ensued with terminal elevation of the total serum bilirubin level to 12 mg/100 ml. On the 60th day, chest roentgenograms showed diffuse bilateral infiltrates. *Escherichia coli* was recovered from transtracheal aspirates performed on the 63rd day, and on the next day bacteremia due to *E coli* was documented. Despite treatment with multiple antibiotics, death occurred on the 65th day. Postmortem examination disclosed disseminated cytomegalovirus (CMV) infection in lungs, liver, and kidneys. In addition to *E coli* and CMV, other organisms found in the lungs at autopsy included bacteroides, *Pneumocystis carinii*, and *Toxoplasma gondii*. There was a localized focus of *Aspergillus* infection in the lung, without evidence of dissemination. Postmortem cultures of the lung did not grow any fungi.

PATIENT 3.–A 59-year-old man underwent transplantation on April 13, 1969, for end-stage ischemic heart disease. Treatment for diagnosed rejection was given on postoperative days 8 through 11, and 15 through 17. On day 51 pneumonia in the lower lobe of the left lung due to *Proteus morgani* was diagnosed by transtracheal aspiration was treated successfully with carbenicillin disodium. A concurrent complication was agranulocytosis, which spontaneously resolved following temporary discontinuation of azathioprine. On the 84th day chest roentgenograms showed an enlarging cavitary lesion in the upper lobe of the right lung with an adjacent infiltrate (Fig 1). Needle aspiration biopsy of the cavity revealed hyphae, and cultures of the aspirate grew *A fumigatus*. Intravenous treatment with amphotericin B over the following 35 days (total dose of 865 mg) was given without roentgenographic or clinical evidence of improvement. The cavitary lesion increased progressively in size. On postoperative day 134, cultures of another needle aspiration of the cavity again grew *Aspergillus*, and a No. 50 polyethylene catheter was inserted into the cavity. Intravenous therapy with amphotericin B was then discontinued, and treatment through the catheter with amphotericin B, 25 mg, and 2% sodium iodide, 300 mg, was instituted three times weekly. There was rapid clinical improvement, and serial chest roentgenograms over the following month revealed progressive diminution in size of the cavity; now, 14 months after the operation, a total of 2,000 mg of amphotericin B and 29 gm of sodium iodide have been infused through the endocavitary catheter. The cavitary lesion has decreased to less than one third its original size and mycetoma formation has been observed (Fig 1). No systemic toxic reaction attributable to amphotericin B or sodium iodide injected into the cavity has been noted. The only residual symptom remaining at this time is slight, infrequent hemoptysis.

PATIENT 4.–A 44-year-old woman underwent cardiac transplantation on Sept 3, 1969, for idiopathic cardiomyopathy. Episodes of threatened graft rejection were diagnosed and treated on postoperative days 9 through 12, 29 through 31, and 67 through 69. On the 35th day chest roentgenograms showed multiple bilateral nodular infiltrates (Fig 2). Within one week following their initial appearance, cavitation developed within most of the nodules. *Aspergillus fumigatus* was recov-

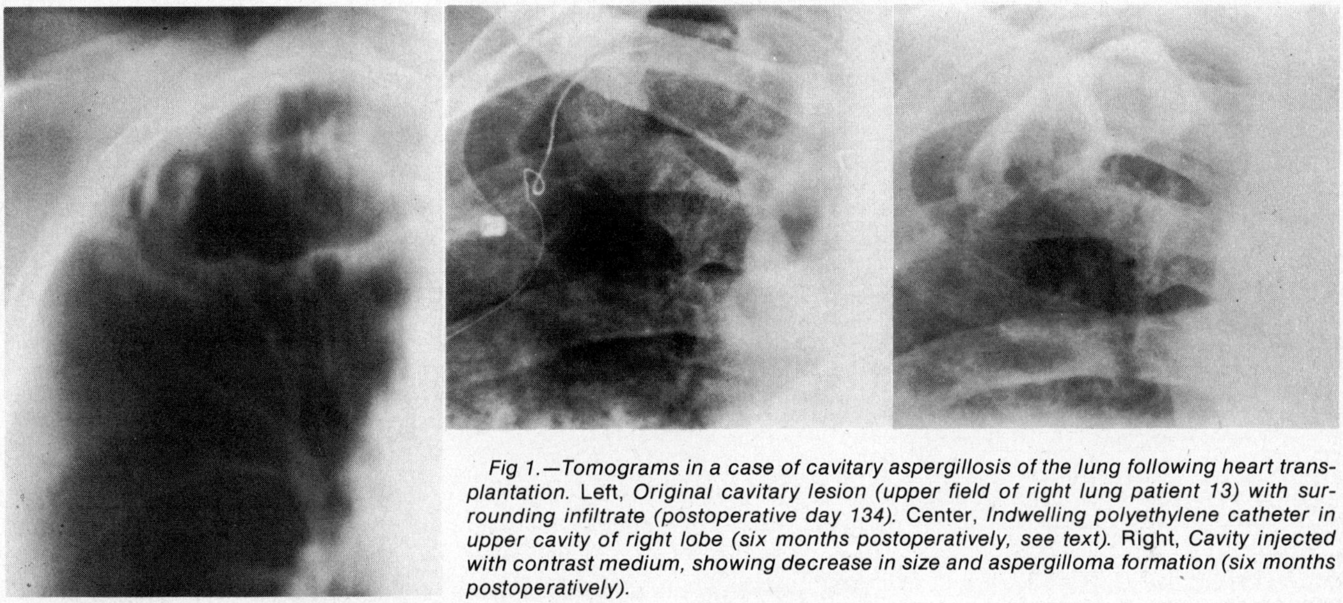

Fig 1.—Tomograms in a case of cavitary aspergillosis of the lung following heart transplantation. Left, *Original cavitary lesion (upper field of right lung patient 13) with surrounding infiltrate (postoperative day 134).* Center, *Indwelling polyethylene catheter in upper cavity of right lobe (six months postoperatively, see text).* Right, *Cavity injected with contrast medium, showing decrease in size and aspergilloma formation (six months postoperatively).*

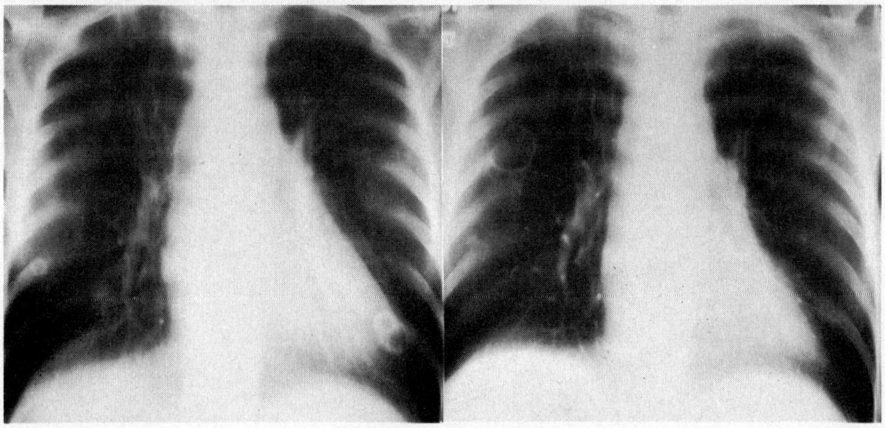

Fig 2.—Tomograms showing multiple cavitary lesions in a case of Aspergillus *of the lung following heart transplantation (patient 17).* Left, *Multiple cavitated nodules in lower lung fields six weeks postoperatively (multiple additional nodules throughout upper lobes demonstrable in tomograms at different depths).* Right, *Resolution of nodules four months following initiation of systemic amphotericin B therapy (thin cyst-like lesion in right midlung field represents residual change following therapy of intercurrent anaerobic bacterial pneumonia).*

ered by direct needle aspiration of one of the nodules on the 42nd day, and intravenous treatment with amphotericin B were initiated, along with nightly nystatin aerosols, on the 44th day. Treatment with amphotericin B has been continued to a total dose of 1,300 mg at nine months postoperatively. The nystatin aerosols were continued for approximately two weeks. During the first month following initiation of amphotericin B therapy, the pulmonary lesions which were now cavitary remained apparently stable. In the ensuing two months they gradually disappeared, as determined by serial chest tomograms (Fig 2). Except for fever and a slight nonproductive cough during the period of initial diagnosis of pulmonary aspergillosis, the patient has experienced no symptoms attributable to pulmonary disease.

Patient 5.—A 64-year-old man underwent cardiac transplantation on Sept 14, 1969, for idiopathic cardiomyopathy. Rejection episodes were diagnosed and treated on postoperative days 10 through 13, 25 through 29, and 36 through 41.

On the 27th day multiple nodular pulmonary infiltrates appeared and transtracheal aspirates showed *A fumigatus*. Treatment with nightly aerosols of nystatin was unsuccessful in halting progress of the infection. On the 43rd day intravenous treatment with amphotericin B was begun. During the following 16 days, a total of 580 mg of amphotericin B was infused, but the clinical and roentgenographic signs of infection did not improve. The patient had signs of increasing fever, productive cough, and hemoptysis. On the 58th day intermittent generalized seizures developed and progressed to status epilepticus. Lumbar puncture disclosed clear and colorless cerebrospinal fluid with a protein content of 123 mg/100 ml and 7 WBC/cu mm. Cultures for fungi were negative. The patient died on the 60th postoperative day. Postmortem examination revealed severe bilateral pulmonary infection due to *Asper-*

gillus, as well as *Klebsiella*, with dissemination of *Aspergillus* to the heart, gastrointestinal tract, pancreas, and brain. There were five separate cerebral abscesses containing *A fumigatus*.

Comment

Each of the five patients presented here had the invasive form of pulmonary aspergillosis.[7] Premortem diagnosis of this form by roentgenographic, serological, or cultural methods is complicated by a number of factors. X-ray diagnosis is difficult because roentgenographic appearance is not specific; aspergillosis may mimic the roentgenographic appearance caused by other pathogens or by the underlying disease itself.[8] Roentgenograms in our patients were helpful because rapid appearance of an infiltrate led to the vigorous diagnostic efforts. Of the four cardiac transplant patients whose sera were assayed in the complement fixation test,[9] only patient 3, with cavitary aspergilloma, had a titer. In contrast, two nontransplant patients with invasive aspergillosis recently studied at Stanford had titers of 1:16 and 1:64 respectively. Repeated administration of high doses of immunosuppressive drugs may have resulted in a failure of serologic response to the fungus in our patients.

Diagnosis of aspergillosis is frequently hampered by the inability to isolate the fungus from clinical sources[10-11] and by the frequent contamination of routine cultures by spores, although *A fumigatus*, the prevalent pathogen, is not a common contaminant.[12] But despite difficulties in interpretation, positive cultures of *Aspergillus* from specimens in our patients have frequently been significant. Four of the five cardiac recipients infected with *Aspergillus* had multiple positive cultures.

Our experience and that of others[11-13] suggest that isolation of *Aspergillus* from immunologically compromised patients with clinical and roentgenographic evidence of active pulmonary infection must be considered as an indication for percutaneous lung aspiration, open lung biopsy or repeated sputum cultures or both, or transtracheal aspirates to confirm the diagnosis.

Evaluation of the outcome of antifungal therapy in cases of aspergillosis is complicated by the fact that spontaneous resolution of disseminated aspergillosis has been reported.[14,15] Because the diagnosis is often established only just prior to death, amphotericin therapy has been instituted in only a minority of cases, and often has been a measure of desperation.[13,16] Two of the patients reported here received both amphotericin B intravenously and aerosolized nystatin; one patient received amphotericin B intravenously shortly after multiple pulmonary infiltrates were noted, and her disease has been controlled. The other patient initially received only aerosolized nystatin; intravenously administered amphotericin B was added 16 days later, but dissemination of *Aspergillus* infection caused death. A third patient received amphotericin B intravenously and amphotericin B and sodium iodide within the cavity. Control of his infection seems most clearly related to intracavitary therapy.

The incidence of *Aspergillus* infections (28%) in our first 18 cardiac recipients appears to be unusually high. During the two-year time period covered by this report, there were only three other cases of aspergillosis at the Stanford University Hospital, and in the previous eight years a total of only six cases.[10] Possible reasons for the high incidence are immunosuppression by corticosteroids and cytotoxic drugs, alterations of microbial flora by antibiotics, pulmonary changes associated with chronic congestive heart failure, postthoracotomy congestion and atelectasis, and exposure to unusually large numbers of *Aspergillus* spores from a common source.

The role of corticosteroids, cytotoxic drugs, antibiotics, and irradiation in predisposing man to fungus infections has recently been reviewed by Hart et al.[10] The increasing incidence of fungal infections in the immunologically compromised host has been noted by many investigators and has been related to such therapy. It is unclear, however, whether such infections are due to direct effects of therapy or to the longer survival of patients with underlying diseases predisposing to opportunistic fungi. The major factor predisposing to infection in organ transplant recipients appears to be the immunosuppressive therapy administered to prevent graft rejection, but it is difficult to implicate specific drugs or side effects of immunosuppression.

Four of the five patients in this series who developed *Aspergillus* infections were receiving antilymphocyte globulin at the time infection with *Aspergillus* had its apparent onset. The significance of this factor is questionable, however, since Starzl et al[17] have reported that in 20 consecutive cases of renal transplantation treated with antilymphocyte globulin and immunosuppressive therapy, rather than previous forms of immunosuppression, infectious complications was reduced.

It is possible that local pulmonary factors played an important role in our heart transplant patients. Pulmonary infections developed in a higher percentage (56%) of our heart transplant recipients[4] than in one renal transplant series in which episodes of pneumonia occurred in only five of 30 patients (17%).[2] Predisposing factors unique to cardiac transplant recipients include the presence of pulmonary abnormalities existing prior to surgery, effects of the thoracotomy, and postoperative respiratory care. Previous experience has shown a relationship between pulmonary edema and bacterial pulmonary infection.[18] Similarly, thoractomy effects on respiratory mechanics and the pulmonary parenchymal changes which follow cardiopulmonary bypass may predispose to pulmonary infection[19,20] but apparently not to *Aspergillus* in the absence of immunosuppressive therapy.

Prolonged mechanical ventilatory assistance is another factor by which cardiac transplant patients differ from other organ transplant recipients. Each of our cases received mechanical ventilatory assistance or intermittent positive pressure breathing exercises, thus enabling *Aspergillus* spores already present in the hospital environment[21,22] or as normal flora in the upper-respiratory tract to be driven into the lungs.

The high incidence of aspergillosis makes the possibility of a heavy exposure to *Aspergillus* spores from a source common to the cardiac recipients a serious consideration. But no environmental or other epidemiologic factors common to our cardiac transplant recipients could be identified.

The causes of the unusual incidence of pulmonary *Aspergillus* infections observed in this study remain unclear. A combination of pulmonary factors unique to cardiac transplant recipients, immunosuppression, and an as yet unrecognized source of exposure to a high concentration of *Aspergillus* spores may provide a possible explanation.

This study was supported by Public Health Service grants HE-08696 and FR-70; and by a grant from John A. Hartford Foundation, Inc.

The serologic tests for aspergillosis were performed by Robert D. Jones and Fred E. Tosh, MD, National Communicable Disease Center, Kansas City Field Station, Mycoses Section, Kansas City, Kansas.

Nonproprietary and Trade Names of Drugs

Azathioprine—*Imuran.*
Carbenicillin disodium—*Pyopen.*

References

1. Hill RB, Rowlands DT, Rifkind D: Infectious pulmonary disease in patients receiving immunosuppressive therapy for organ transplantation. *New Eng J Med* **271**:1021-1027, 1964.

2. Rifkind D, Marchioro TL, Schneck SA, et al: Systemic fungal disease complicating renal transplantation and immunosuppressive therapy: Clinical, microbiologic, neurologic and pathologic features. *Amer J Med* **43**:28-38, 1967.

3. Stinson EB, Bieber CP, Griepp RB, et al: Infectious complications following cardiac transplantation in man. *Ann Intern Med* **74**:22-36, 1971.

4. Stinson EB, Dong E Jr, Iben AB, et al: Cardiac transplantation in man: III. Surgical aspects. *Amer J Surg* **118**:182-187, 1969.

5. Castellino RA, Goldstein HM, Stinson EB, et al: Needle aspiration biopsy technique in pulmonary disease: Application to therapy. *JAMA* **213**:463-464, 1970.

6. Saunders AM, Bieber CP: Pathologic findings in a case of cardiac transplantation. *JAMA* **206**:815-820, 1968.

7. Hinson KFW, Moon AJ, Plummer NS: Bronchopulmonary aspergillosis: A review and a report of eight new cases. *Thorax* **7**:317-333, 1952.

8. Golbert B: Radiological appearance in pulmonary aspergillosis. *Clin Radiol* **13**:106-114, 1962.

9. Walter JE, Jones RD: Serologic tests in diagnosis of aspergillosis. *Dis Chest* **53**:729-735, 1968.

10. Hart PD, Russell E, Remington JS: The compromised host and infection: II. Deep fungal infection. *J Infect Dis* **120**:169-191, 1969.

11. Young RC, Bennett JE, Vogel CL, et al: Aspergillosis: The spectrum of the disease in 98 patients. *Medicine* **49**:147-173, 1970.

12. Wilson JW, Plunkett OA: *The Fungus Diseases of Man.* University of California Press, Berkeley, Calif, 1965, p 202.

13. Young RC, Vogel CL, De Vita VT: *Aspergillus* lobar pneumonia. *JAMA* **19**:1156-1162, 1969.

14. Conen PE, Walker GR, Turner JA, et al: Invasive primary aspergillosis of the lung with cerebral metastasis and complete recovery. *Dis Chest* **42**:88-94, 1962.

15. Vedder JS, Schott WF: Primary disseminated pulmonary aspergillosis with metastatic skin nodules: Successful treatment with inhalation mystatin therapy. *JAMA* **209**:1191-1195, 1969.

16. Heffernan AGA, Asper SP: Insidious fungal disease: A clinicopathological study of secondary aspergillosis. *Bull Johns Hopkins Hosp* **118**:10-26, 1966.

17. Starzl TE, Groth CG, Terasakai PI, et al: Heterologous antilymphocyte globulin, histoincompatibility, matching and human renal transplantation. *Surg Gynec Obstet* **126**:1023-1040, 1968.

18. Robin EP, Thomas ED: Some relations between pulmonary edema and pulmonary inflammation (pneumonia). *Arch Intern Med* **93**:713-724, 1954.

19. Rosky LP, Rodman P: Medical aspects of open heart surgery. *New Eng J Med* **274**:833-840, 1966.

20. Garzon AA, Seltzer D, Karlson JE: Respiratory mechanics following open heart surgery for acquired valvular disease. *Circulation* **33, 34** (suppl 1):57-64, 1966.

21. Sayer WJ, Shean DB, Ghosseiri J: Estimation of airborne fungal flora by the Andersen sampler versus the gravity settling culture plate: I. Isolation frequency and number of colonies. *J Allerg* **44**:214-227, 1969.

22. Noble WC, Clayton YM: Fungi in the air of hospital wards. *J Gen Microbiol* **32**:397-402, 1963.

Salmonellosis in Patients With Neoplastic Disease

A Review of 100 Episodes at Memorial Cancer Center Over a 13-Year Period

Martin S. Wolfe, MD; Donald Armstrong, MD; Donald B. Louria, MD; and Anne Blevins, RN, New York

One hundred *Salmonella* isolations from 95 patients at Memorial Cancer Center over a 13-year period were reviewed. *Salmonella typhimurium* and *Salmonella derby* made up 61% of the isolations. Practically all patients had serious underlying disease, and most were under or had undergone recent adrenocorticosteroid treatment, chemotherapy, radiotherapy, or surgery. The predisposition of patients with recent surgery to salmonellosis was reaffirmed. A striking relationship was found between patients with leukemia and lymphoma and *S typhimurium* septicemia. It is suggested that the hemolytic component in these diseases may predispose to *S typhimurium* septicemia, and these diseases should perhaps be included with sickle-cell disease, bartonellosis, and malaria in having a specific predisposition to associated salmonellosis. A number of unusual *Salmonella* infections were noted.

The relationship between infections with *Salmonella* and various underlying diseases, previous surgery, and extremes of age has been established.[1-10] An association with neoplasms might be expected due to debility and the types of therapy used in the majority of patients with these diseases, and some recent reports have made note of this.[11-13] This report summarizes a review of our cases of *Salmonella* infections at the Memorial and James Ewing Hospitals occurring during the 13 years of 1955 through 1967 and attempts to uncover specific associations.

Materials and Methods

Lactose nonfermenting gram-negative rods that fulfilled the biochemical and cultural characteristics of *Salmonella* and agglutinated with *Salmonella* polyvalent antiserum were typed at the New York Salmonella Center, New York.

The case records of 95 patients with one or more positive cultures for *Salmonella* were reviewed.

Results

Of the 95 patients, 54 were females and 41 males. Seventy-eight were adults and 17 were children (below age 12). Nine patients did not have neoplastic disease: five had recently undergone abdominal surgery for benign conditions; one had aplastic anemia; one, lupus erythematosus; one, duplication of the large bowel; and another had recurrent pleurisy. Of the 86 patients with neoplastic disease, 46 had a leukemia or a lymphoma (Table 1).

Four patients had multiple *Salmonella* infections and isolations of different serotypes (three cases with two serotypes and one with three serotypes), so that a total of 100 different episodes of infection are reported for the 95 patients.

Serotypes Isolated.—Nineteen different serotypes were isolated with two, *S typhimurium* and *S derby*, making up 61% of the isolations. The other 17 serotypes each comprised from 1% to 7% of the total (Table 2). Of the 25 *S derby* isolates, 22 were obtained during the epidemic of hospital-associated infections with this organism in the northeastern United States between March 1963 and August 1964.[14]

Clinical Syndromes.—The illnesses occurring at the time of isolation of the 100 *Salmonella* species were categorized in the usual fashion[2,6]: (1) septicemia; (2) enteritis; (3) focal infection; and (4) carrier state. As indicated in Table 2, 35% were septicemias, 37% enteritis, 16% focal, and 12% were classified as carriers.

Septicemia.—Of the 35 episodes of septicemia, 65% were caused by *S typhimurium.* Only six other species caused septicemia: *S enteritidis* (14.3%), *S derby* (5.7%), *S choleraesuis*

Received for publication Nov 4, 1970; accepted March 22, 1971.

From the Department of Medicine (Microbiology Laboratory), Memorial Cancer Center, New York. Dr. Wolfe is now with the Department of State, Office of Medical Services, Washington, DC.

Read in part before the 49th annual session of the American College of Physicians, Boston, April 3, 1968.

Reprint requests to Office of Medical Services, Department of State, Washington, DC 20520 (Dr. Wolfe).

(5.7%), *S montevideo* (2.8%), *S blockley* (2.8%), and *S heidelberg* (2.8%). Thirty-two of the 35 septicemia episodes were in patients with a neoplastic disease; the other 3 were in patients with aplastic anemia, lupus erythematosus, or perforated bowel. The most common underlying neoplastic diseases were leukemias and lymphomas, and these were associated with 74.3% of the septicemia episodes. Of the 23 episodes of *S typhimurium* septicemia, 19 patients had either a leukemia or lymphoma, 3 had carcinomas, and 1 aplastic anemia (Table 3).

Enteritis.—The leading serotype isolated in these 37 episodes was *S derby* (43.2%), and all but one were associated with the previously mentioned epidemic. *Salmonella typhimurium* made up 13.5% of the isolates and *S thompson* 10.8%, while the remaining episodes were divided among ten other serotypes. Three patients with enteritis did not have underlying neoplastic disease, but two had undergone recent surgery. In contrast to the septicemia episodes, only 13 of the isolations were in patients with leukemia or lymphoma; the majority of the enteritis isolates were in association with patients with carcinomas. Seven of the patients with enteritis had underlying malignant or nonneoplastic disease of the gastrointestinal tract and in five of these infection was caused by *S derby*.

Focal Infections.—There were 16 isolates in this category. In five, *Salmonella* was found only at postmortem examination: three from the lung, one from a left ventricular mural endocardial vegetation, and one from the peritoneal cavity. *Salmonella typhimurium* was responsible for six of the focal infection episodes, *S derby* for three, *S enteritidis* for two, and the others were caused by five different serotypes. Two of the infections were associated with nonneoplastic disease, both following surgery. Six isolates (37.5%) were in patients with leukemia or lymphoma, and three of these infections were caused by *S typhimurium.*

Table 1.—Type of Underlying Condition in 95 Patients With Salmonellosis

Neoplastic Disease	Total	Children	Adults	Adults >65
Leukemia	21	11	10	...
Acute lymphatic	6	4	2	...
Acute myelocytic	6	2	4	...
Acute stem cell	5	5	...	...
Chronic myelocytic	2	...	2	...
Leukolymphosarcoma	2	...	2	...
Lymphoma	25	...	21	4
Hodgkin's disease	9	...	7	2
Lymphosarcoma	7	...	7	...
Reticulum cell sarcoma	8	...	6	2
Mycosis fungoides	1	...	1	...
Gastrointestinal	9	...	3	6
Gynecologic	5	...	5	...
Breast	5	...	4	1
Genitourinary	5	...	3	2
Respiratory	5	...	3	2
Head and neck	2	...	1	1
Miscellaneous	9			
Embryonal cell carcinoma	1	1	...	...
Sarcoma	3	1	2	...
Malignant melanoma	1	...	...	1
Myoblastoma	2	1	1	...
Wilm's tumor	2	2	...	...
Nonneoplastic disease	9	1	7	1
Total	95	17	60	18

Carriers.—Twelve patients were classified as asymptomatic carriers, six being stool carriers and four urinary carriers. The two other patients had *Salmonella* isolated from the nose and throat and from a smear of the cervix. *Salmonella derby* was found in four of the carriers, and two of these isolates were made during the *S derby* epidemic. A variety of serotypes made up the remaining carrier isolates. All but one had neoplastic disease and five (41.7%) had leukemia or lymphoma. The two *S typhimurium* carriers had leukemia or lymphoma.

Previous Surgery.—Twenty-six isolates in this series followed surgery (Table 4). These infections developed after gastrointestinal surgery in 16 cases, three of which were gastric procedures. One patient had a subtotal gastrectomy and gastrojejunostomy in 1955, and in 1960 had two different episodes of infection with *Salmonella;* one an *S panama* enteritis and the other a *S typhimurium* septicemia. Another patient had a subtotal gastrectomy and Billroth II anastomosis in late August 1965, and suffered an *S typhimurium* septicemia in March 1966. The third patient with gastric surgery, performed for a bleeding gastric ulcer, had an *S derby* enteritis 12 days following her surgery.

Two patients had esophagectomy for esophageal carcinoma, followed by pyloroplasty, colon transplant, and gastrostomy, and developed *S cubana* infections during these procedures. Both had negative preoperative stool cultures, and received carmine red dye markers before the *S cubana* isolations. One patient developed an abscess and a secondary cutaneous fistula at the site of his colon transplant (patient 1). The second patient, who had been in the same room, developed an enteritis one week later. The lots of carmine red dye given to these patients were unfortunately not available for subsequent culture.

Table 2.—Types of *Salmonella* and Clinical Category in 100 Different Isolates, in Order of Frequency

Type	Septicemia, %	Enteritis, %	Focal, %	Carrier, %	Total, %
S typhimurium	23	5	6	2	36
S derby	2	16	3	4	25
S enteritidis	5	...	2	...	7
S thompson	...	4	...	1	5
S heidelberg	1	1	...	1	3
S montevideo	1	2	...	...	3
S blockley	1	...	...	1	2
S choleraesuis	2	...	...	...	2
S cubana	...	1	1	...	2
S infantis	...	1	1	...	2
S oranienburg	...	1	...	1	2
S sandiego	...	1	...	1	2
S senftenberg	...	2	...	...	2
S tennessee	...	1	1	...	2
S manhattan	...	...	1	...	1
S muenchen	...	1	...	...	1
S panama	...	...	...	1	1
S saintpaul	...	1	...	...	1
S typhosa	...	...	1	...	1
Total	35	37	16	12	100

The 11 other isolates followed various types of gastrointestinal surgical procedures. The only *S typhosa* infection in this series followed a cholecystectomy and the organism was isolated both from the stool and from a wound infection.

Of the ten patients who developed salmonellosis following surgical procedures not involving the gastrointestinal tract, five isolates were *S typhimurium*. Four *S derby* infections occurred, all during the 1963-1964 epidemic.

The relationship to previous surgery was most apparent in the enteritis isolates; 17 of 37 (45.9%) were in patients who had operations, ten of which involved the gastrointestinal tract. Four of the 16 patients with focal infections had previous surgery, but only five of 35 patients with septicemia and none of the carriers had surgery (Table 5).

Adrenocorticosteroids, Chemotherapy, and Radiation Therapy.—A definite relationship existed between treatment with adrenocorticosteroids, chemotherapy, or radiotherapy and the occurrence of salmonellosis. This was most striking in the septicemia group where 85.7% of the patients were receiving or had recently received one of these forms of treatment. In the categories of enteritis and focal infections, 59.5% and 50% of patients, respectively, were under one or more of these forms of therapy. Among the carriers, 66.7% had received either corticosteroids, chemotherapy, or radiotherapy (Table 5).

Relation to Leukemia or Lymphoma.—Although leukemia and lymphoma account for less than 10% of Memorial Cancer Center admissions,[15,16] 46 patients in this series, representing 50 episodes of salmonellosis, had these underlying diseases (Tables 1 and 3). By far the most frequent serotype found in these patients was *S typhimurium*, present in 12 of 21 isolates in leukemia patients and 14 of 29 isolates in lymphoma patients. In 19 of these 26 *S typhimurium* isolations, septicemia was the form of infection. This association with *S typhimurium* septicemia was most apparent in patients with acute lymphatic leukemia, lymphosarcoma, and reticulum cell sarcoma. Only one of ten episodes of salmonellosis in patients with Hodgkin's disease was an *S typhimurium* septicemia. In contrast to this striking situation in the leukemia-lymphoma patients, *S typhimurium* septicemia occurred in only three of 41 *Salmonella* episodes in patients with other malignancies and only once in nine episodes in patients with nonneoplastic conditions (Table 3). *Salmonella typhimurium* was isolated from two carriers, three focal cases, and two cases of enteritis in the leukemia lymphoma patients. Only six of the leukemia-lymphoma patients had *S derby* infections, only one of which was a septicemia. No other serotype appeared with any unusual frequency in patients with leukemia or lymphoma.

Antibiotic Sensitivities.—All *Salmonella* isolates tested by the disk method were sensitive to chloramphenicol and ampicillin. Sensitivity to other antibiotics was variable. When the diagnosis was established and therapy with chloramphenicol or ampicillin was instituted early, there were some notable responses. The relatively high mortality was more likely due to alterations in host defenses in our patients rather than to antibiotic failure.

Mortality.—In this series of patients, most of whom had a malignancy, there was an expected high mortality. Seventy-one patients died during the period under review, and in ten their *Salmonella* infection was considered the immediate cause of death. All but one of these ten patients were adults, four of whom were above age 60, and serious underlying disease was present in all. Six of the deaths were in patients with lymphoma and one in a patient with acute stem cell leukemia. *Salmonella typhimurium* was the responsible serotype in five of these, four of whom had leukemia or lymphoma.

Table 3.—Underlying Conditions Associated With *Salmonella typhimurium* Episodes

Underlying Disease	No. of Patients	No. of *Salmonella* Episodes	No. of *S typhimurium* Episodes	No. of *S typhimurium* Septicemia Episodes
Acute lymphatic leukemia	6	6	5	3
Acute myelocytic leukemia	6	6	1	1
Acute stem cell leukemia	5	5	3	3
Chronic myelocytic leukemia	2	2	1	1
Leukolymphosarcoma	2	2	2	1
Hodgkin's disease	9	10	3	1
Lymphosarcoma	7	7	4	3
Reticulum cell sarcoma	8	11	7	6
Mycosis fungoides	1	1	...	...
Total	46	50	26	19
Other malignancies	40	41	8	3
Nonneoplastic condition	9	9	2	1

Both *S choleraesuis* infections led to death, and the other deaths were due to *S montevideo*, *S blockley*, and *S heidelberg*. In no case was *S derby* thought to be the direct cause of death.

A number of unusual manifestations of *Salmonella* infections are illustrated in the following case reports.

Patient Summaries

PATIENT 1.—A 67-year-old Negro man with carcinoma of the esophagus underwent a total esophagectomy, cervical esophagostomy, pyloroplasty, and gastrostomy without complication. He then had a special metabolic study, which included the use of a carmine red dye marker. Mild diarrhea occurred during this time, but a stool culture revealed normal flora. Two days later a left colon transplant with cervical esophagocolostomy, colocolostomy, gastrocolostomy, and maintainence of his gastrostomy was performed. Postoperatively, mild diarrhea recurred but no stool culture was done. Shortly thereafter, he developed a neck fistula from which *S cubana* grew. Two days later, a stool culture grew *S cubana* and his sputum was also found to contain this organism. Cultures from the neck fistula and stool were persistently positive for *S cubana*, despite long courses of chloramphenicol and ampicillin. Barium swallow revealed a partial stricture of the esophagocolostomy, and he underwent an exploratory neck operation and laparotomy. At the distal anastomosis site in the neck, stenosis and an abscess which grew *S cubana* were found. His neck wound continued to drain, but *Salmonella* was not cultured. Another neck exploration was performed and a pure culture of *Klebsiella-Aerobacter* grew from a mediastinal abscess. *Salmonella* was not cultured subsequently or following his death six days later.

PATIENT 2.—A 57-year-old white woman with lymphosarcoma was admitted with a six-week history of productive cough and fever, following a course of radiation therapy to the spleen and adrenocorticosteroid treatment. A sputum culture grew *S typhimurium* and chest x-ray films revealed a left hydropneumothorax. A blood culture was negative at this time but one stool culture was positive for *S typhimurium*. A left thoracentesis yielded 350 ml of fecal smelling, thick, brown fluid, positive for *S typhimurium* on culture. She was thought to have a *Salmonella* empyema with a probable bronchopleural fistula, indicated by *Salmonella* in the sputum and the coughing up of methylene blue dye placed in the pleural cavity. A closed thoracotomy with drainage was performed and she was started on a regimen of chloramphenicol. Because of persistence of the empyema, continuously positive for *S typhimurium* after one month of drainage, thoracoplasty was recommended but refused. A right buttock abscess which grew *S typhimurium*, *Staphylococcus aureus* (coagulase positive), *Pseudomonas aeruginosa*, and *Proteus mirabilis* was surgically drained. Four days later the patient suddenly died. At postmortem examination she was found to have disseminated cryptococcosis, and a left bronchopleural fistula with a chronic empyema cavity from which *S typhimurium* was recovered.

PATIENT 3.—A 51-year-old Negro woman with breast carcinoma was admitted with a metastatic pleural effusion, recurrent after introduction of mechlorethamine hydrochloride (nitrogen mustard). She was on a regimen of prednisone at the time. On admission she was afebrile but following thoracentesis her temperature rose to 102 F (38.9 C). Culture of the pleural fluid grew *S enteritidis* and blood and stool cultures were also positive for the same organism. She received a long course of chloramphenicol and remained well for the next six months, maintained on a regimen of prednisone. She then developed a productive cough and *S enteritidis* was found in the sputum. Foul smelling, purulent fluid obtained on thoracentesis grew both *S enteritidis* and *Klebsiella-Aerobacter*. A thoracotomy was done and a large abscess cavity was drained. Again, both stool and blood culture were positive for *S enteritidis*. The patient died two days later, but a postmortem examination was not performed.

PATIENT 4.—A 44-year-old white woman with inoperable metastatic carcinoma of the cervix died of obstructive uremia two months following an exploratory laparotomy. She had been afebrile while hospitalized during this period and no antemorten cultures were obtained. At autopsy, *Streptobacillus moniliformis* was isolated from the heart's blood and *S derby* from vegetations on the left ventricular mural endocardium.

PATIENT 5.—A 4½-year-old Negro girl with acute myeloblastic leukemia treated with steroids and vincristine sulfate developed a persistent fever during bone marrow remission. A source of infection could not be found, but she was treated with chloramphenicol, became afebrile, and was discharged. Shortly thereafter, she was readmitted with fever, intermittent knee

Table 4.—Postoperative Infections

Patient	Age, yr	Sex	Date of Isolation	Serotype	Type of Infection	Underlying Disease	Surgery and Date
Gastrointestinal Procedures							
Gastrectomy							
9	20	M	9/20/60 11/28/60	*S panama* *S typhimurium*	Enteritis Septicemia	Reticulum cell sarcoma Marginal ulcer	Subtotal gastrectomy Gastrojejunostomy, 11/20/55
10	73	F	1/31/64	*S derby*	Enteritis	Bleeding gastric ulcer	70% subtotal gastrectomy & Billroth II, 1/19/64
11	65	F	3/14/66	*S typhimurium*	Septicemia	Metastatic gastric carcinoma	Subtotal gastrectomy & Billroth II, 8/30/65
Esophagectomy and Colon Transplant							
1	63	M	11/8/65	*S cubana*	Neck abscess Cutaneous fistula	Carcinoma esophagus	Total esophagectomy, cervical esophagectomy, pyloroplasty, gastrostomy, 8/10/65; left colon bypass, 10/7/65
12	69	M	11/15/65	*S cubana*	Enteritis	Carcinoma esophagus	Esophagectomy, pyloroplasty, gastrostomy, 8/4/65; left colon transplant, 9/30/65
Other Gastrointestinal Surgery							
13	56	M	2/10/56	*S typhosa*	Abdominal wound Stool	Acute & chronic cholecystitis	Cholecystectomy
14	39	F	5/19/57 (PM)*	*S tennessee*	Abdominal wound Peritoneal cavity	Multiple intestinal adhesions	Enteroenterostomy & colon anastomosis, 5/2/57 (8 previous abdominal operations at another hospital
15	74	M	5/6/59	*S thompson*	Enteritis	Malignant melanoma	Abdominal-perineal resection for melanoma of rectum, 4/28/59
16	35	F	2/6/60	*S sandiego*	Wound infection Enteritis	Ovarian carcinomatosis	Ileotransverse colostomy, 1/31/60
17	61	M	3/21/60 (PM)	*S blockley*	Enteritis Bowel perforation	None	Exploratory laparotomy & ileostomy tube, 3/2/60 (at another hospital)
18	67	M	5/31/63	*S derby*	Septicemia	Carcinoma bladder	Splenectomy, transverse colostomy, 5/13/63

pains, and loose bowel movements. Her left knee was swollen, warm, and tender, and aspiration yielded purulent fluid, from which *S infantis* was cultured. This organism was also grown from a blood culture on the same day, but a stool culture was negative. Following open drainage of the knee and a course of chloramphenicol, her knee improved and became *Salmonella* negative. X-ray films revealed no evidence of osteomyelitis. A sickle-cell preparation was 25% positive, but a hemoglobin electrophoresis was not done.

Patient 6.—A 68-year-old diabetic white woman with a diagnosis of giant follicular lymphosarcoma had been treated intermittently with radiotherapy since 1946. In December 1965, a right axillary mass was noted which was associated with systemic complaints of fever, chills, and a 15-lb weight loss. Aspiration biopsy was attempted but the specimen obtained was not sufficient for diagnosis. No chemotherapy was given. She was admitted to the hospital two months later and at this time had a 5 × 7 cm tender right axillary mass. Blood and urine cultures were negative. Excisional biopsy of the mass yielded purulent material postive for *S typhimurium*. Sections of the mass revealed reticulum cell sarcoma. That night she developed a temperature of 104.5 F (40.3 C) and her blood pressure fell to 80/40 mm Hg. A blood culture grew *S typhimurium*. She recovered following treatment with chloramphenicol and ampicillin.

Patient 7.—A 1-year-old Negro child had been born with a sacrococcygeal mass, and biopsy of a left inguinal node showed embryonal cell carcinoma. Treatment included a course of dactinomycin and radiotherapy. Following this she developed a sacrococcygeal abscess adjacent to the tumor mass which failed to respond to a variety of antibiotics, including chloramphenicol. The abscess was drained surgically and on culture grew *S typhimurium*, *Proteus mirabilis*, and *Escherichia coli*. Blood, stool, and urine cultures were negative for *Salmonella*. She received courses of chloramphenicol and ampicillin, and cultures of the abscess subsequently became negative for *Salmonella*. Nine months later she was found to be an asymptomatic stool carrier of *S heidelberg*.

Patient 8.—A 34-year-old white man with lymphosarcoma, under treatment for cryptococcal meningitis with amphotericin B, developed a perirectal abscess which on aspiration grew *S typhimurium*, *Staphylococcus albus*, and a member of the *E coli-A aerogenes* group. Blood and sputum cultures taken on the same day were also

Table 4.—Postoperative Infections *(Continued)*

Patient	Age, yr	Sex	Date of Isolation	Serotype	Type of Infection	Underlying Disease	Surgery and Date
19	38	F	2/18/64	*S derby*	Enteritis	Adeno carcinoma of common duct	Subtotal colectomy for colitis, 1/17/64; revision of ileostomy & ileosigmoid anastomosis 2/10/64
20	57	M	2/20/64	*S derby*	Enteritis	Carcinoma bladder	Radical cystectomy, ileal conduit 2/12/64
21	51	F	3/20/64	*S derby*	Enteritis	Carcinoma ovary	Resection of pelvic segment of colon, resection of segments of small bowel, 3/15/64
22	60	M	5/6/64	*S derby*	Enteritis	Carcinoma bladder	Radical cystectomy, appendectomy, ileal conduit, 4/19/64
					Other Surgery		
23	64	M	9/1/55	*S typhimurium*	Septicemia	Epidermoid, carcinoma of antrum	Maxillary resection exenteration of orbit, 8/25/55
24	66	F	11/3/55	*S tennessee*	Enteritis	Breast carcinoma metastatic to bone	Hypophysectomy, 10/27/55
25	49	F	4/11/60	*S typhimurium*	Enteritis	Metastatic breast carcinoma	Hypophysectomy, 3/19/60
26	3	F	1/26/63	*S typhimurium*	Enteritis	Cavernous hemangioma	Segmental excision of hemangioma, 1/19/63
27	58	F	5/6/63	*S derby*	Enteritis	Granular cell myoblastoma of chest	Chest wall resection, 4/30/63
28	1	M	6/3/63	*S derby*	Enteritis	Granular cell myoblastoma of tongue	Excision of tumor mass in tongue, 5/22/63
29	83	M	5/20/64	*S derby*	Enteritis	Carcinoma larynx	Total laryngectomy, 4/11/64
30	67	F	2/19/66	*S typhimurium*	Septicemia	Lymphosarcoma	Excisional biopsy right axilla, 2/18/66
31	32	M	10/30/68	*S typhimurium*	Enteritis	Carcinoma lung	Pneumonectomy, 10/26/68
4	44	F	8/10/63	*S derby*	Vegetation in left ventricle	Carcinoma cervix	Laparotomy, 6/6/63

* PM signifies isolated only at postmortem examination.

positive for *S typhimurium*, but no stool or urine cultures were obtained at this time. The perirectal abscess responded well to drainage and chloramphenicol, but stool and sputum cultures two weeks later contained *S typhimurium*. Blood cultures were negative. He received another course of chloramphenicol, and subsequent cultures until the time of his death seven months later were also negative for *Salmonella*.

Comment

During the 13-year period under review, admissions to Memorial Cancer Center ranged from a high of 7,285 in 1955 to a low of 5,844 in 1967 and the yearly average admissions was 6,536. The patient population showed no particular changes, and there were no obvious variables in the levels of skills, interest, and experience in hospital personnel, or in outside environmental conditions during this period. The only variable hospital condition was the *S derby* epidemic which occurred in many hospitals in the northeastern United States in 1963 and 1964, including Memorial Cancer Center.

Unusual and often overwhelming infections have been noted in this and other hospitals caring for patients predominantly having cancer and allied diseases.[15-20] Factors such as debility, anemia, leukopenia, decreased cellular and circulating antibody response, and other less well defined deficiencies in the immunologic mechanism predispose to infections. Chemotherapy, radiotherapy, and the use of adrenocorticosteroids are known to reduce antibody production, depress marrow activity, and produce mucosal alterations, all of which diminish host resistance.[17,21,22] Complicating infection is the leading cause of death in leukemics,[18] and can be expected to increase in other neoplastic diseases with more widespread use of chemotherapy.

This series includes a very large percentage of patients with serious underlying disease, most of whom were receiving treatment with adrenocorticosteroids, chemotherapy, or

Table 5.—Relationship to Forms of Treatment and Associated Conditions in 100 Episodes of Salmonellosis

	Septicemia		Enteritis		Focal		Carrier	
	No.	%	No.	%	No.	%	No.	%
Adrenocorticosteroids	25	71.4	13	35.1	5	31.3	4	33.3
Antineoplastic chemotherapy	19	54.3	15	40.5	4	25.0	6	50.0
Radiotherapy	7	20.0	7	18.9	3	18.8	3	25.0
One or more of above	30	85.7	22	59.5	8	50.0	8	66.7
Previous surgery	5	14.3	17	45.9	4	25.0	...	...
Surgery involving gastrointestinal tract	3	8.6	10	27.0	3	18.8	...	...
Leukemia or lymphoma	26	74.3	13	35.1	6	37.5	5	41.7
Total isolates in each group	35		37		16		12	

radiation therapy, or who had undergone recent surgery. Of the 95 patients, 86 had malignancies and more than half of these had leukemia or lymphoma. Of the remaining nine patients, all but one had some serious underlying condition. Exact figures were not available on the percentage of patients with benign conditions admitted to Memorial Cancer Center for such things as biopsies and general medical care. But the specialized interest of the Center in neoplastic diseases is reflected in the overwhelming predominance of patients with serious neoplastic conditions, which invariably require extensive treatment with one or more of the previously mentioned therapeutic modalities. Prior antibiotic therapy has been related to superinfection with salmonellae in previous reviews,[1,7] and this probably played a role in our patients, who frequently had or were suspected of having infection and had been treated with various antibiotics.

Salmonella typhimurium was by far the most common serotype isolated, comprising 36% of the cases. This percentage approximates the figures from a review of *Salmonella* infections in New York City from 1965 through 1966, in which this serotype accounted for 39.3% of all isolations.[10]

The frequency of *S derby* isolations (25%) is explained by the *S derby* epidemic of 1963 and 1964.[14] Ten of these isolations occurred in post operative cases, six of which followed gastrointestinal surgery. The patients infected with *S derby* during this period, both surgical and nonsurgical, were located in various parts of the Center and became infected at different times. There was no evidence following epidemiological investigations that these *S derby* infections represented a point-source outbreak related to a common location or a specific service. This serotype was presumably introduced, as it was in many other hospitals, through the use of *S derby* contaminated raw or undercooked eggs in egg enriched diet supplements for debilitated patients.[13] Dietary data was not available, but it can be safely presumed that some of the 22 individuals who developed *S derby* infections during the epidemic very likely received egg enriched diet supplements. In this, as well as other hospitals involved in the epidemic, rigid enforcement of both accepted isolation technique and personal hygienic procedures among patients, staff, and employees, seemed to have little effect on the rate of appearance of secondary cases. The perplexing question posed during the course of this outbreak, of what were the mechanics of person-to-person spread of infection, has not been satisfactorily resolved.[14]

Salmonella cubana was found in two patients, who following esophagectomy, and prior to colon transplant for carcinoma of the esophagus, had special physiologic studies which included the use of carmine red dye markers for measurement of bowel transit time. Since it has been recognized that carmine powder, prepared from the insect *Dactylopius coccus costa* can be heavily contaminated with *S cubana*,[23] it is likely that this was the mode of infection in these two cases, since both had negative stool cultures prior to their special studies. We were not, however, able to document this.

Although *S choleraesuis* was isolated from only two patients, both had septicemia and in both death was felt to be directly caused by this organism. This fits well with the characteristic invasiveness of *S choleraesuis* previously described.[24]

An unusual finding in this series was the large percentage (35%) of episodes of septicemia, in contrast to three other larger series, in which this accounted for 6.3% to 8.8% of the cases. In these series, enteritis was recorded as the most common clinical category, including about 70% of cases.[2,3,10] Enteritis occurred in 37% of our episodes, but almost half of these were due to *S derby* during the 1963-1964 epidemic. The number of asymptomatic carriers (12%) was somewhat less than the 19.8% found in the recent large series from the New York *Salmonella* Center.[10] The number of focal infection isolations (16%) was considerably higher than the 2.0% to 7.4% in other series.[2,3,10] However, a strict comparison between our material and these series is not completely valid, since a cancer hospital will have a higher incidence of septicemia compared to a general hospital to which more patients with acute diarrhea would be admitted. Our figures, at least in regard to septicemia, correlate well with a series from another cancer hospital,[11] but cannot be strictly compared due to some differences in classification.

Patients with leukemia and lymphoma, almost all of whom had recent treatment with adrenocorticosteroids, chemotherapy, or radiation therapy, made up the majority of the septicemia cases (74.3%). *Salmonella typhimurium* was by far the commonest serotype isolated in septicemias (65.7%). In other series this serotype has been primarily associated with gastroenteritis (up to 80%) and has caused septicemia in only 2% to 4% of cases.[2,3,6] The reverse was found in our patients: *S typhimurium* accounted for 23 episodes of septicemia, 19 in patients with leukemia and lymphoma; and only 5 episodes of enteritis. In all, 26 of 50 episodes of salmonellosis in patients with leukemia and lymphoma were due to *S typhimurium*, accounting for the majority of the isolates of this serotype. A relationship between *S typhimurium* infection, particularly septicemia, and leukemia and lymphoma has been noted elsewhere.[13,25] In the present investigation, the association of *S typhimurium* with Hodgkin's disease was less striking than in these studies,[13,25] but other diseases of the lymphatic system showed a much higher association with this type infection.

A factor which cannot be overlooked in considering the high incidence of septicemia in lymphoma and leukemia patients as opposed to other neoplastic diseases, is that the majority of the *Salmonella* isolates in lymphoma-leukemia patients occurred while these patients were on the medical service. It is the usual tendency on a medical service to do more blood cultures on fever cases than are done on a surgical service, where solid tumors or carcinomas are usually admitted. Although this is a possible partial explanation for this occurrence, it cannot explain the striking association between septicemia with *S typhimurium* and patients with lymphoma and leukemia, while patients with sickle-cell disease, bartonellosis, and malaria have septicemias with a variety of serotypes.[13]

Other factors mentioned which might account for this relationship include a defect in cellular immunity, hemolysis, the presence of neoplastic tissue, and recrudescence of a latent *Salmonella* infection.[13,25] The first two factors may be the most important. Defective cellular immunity has been discussed in regard to *Listeria* infections complicating lymphatic malignancies.[20,26] A detailed analysis by Simpson et al[26] points out the similarity among *Listeria*, salmonellae, brucellae, the tubercle bacillus, and some pathogenic fungi, in that these organisms are all facultative intracellular parasites. The main host defense mechanism in these infections appears to be mediated by cellular immunity associated with macrophages. Although delayed hypersensitivity is frequently altered in Hodgkin's disease and to a lesser extent in other lymphatic malignancies, macrophage function in ingesting facultative intracellular parasites has not been studied. Since bactericidal mechanisms of the reticuloendothelial system, which operate to eradicate *S typhimurium* and other microorganisms from livers and spleens of normal mice, are severely impaired in animals with hemolysis,[27] it has been postulated that the increased occurrence of *Salmonella* bacteremia in sickle-cell anemia,[28] bartonellosis,[29] and malaria[30] is related to the marked hemolysis occurring in each of these diseases. Overt hemolytic anemia has been described in up to 20% of patients with chronic lymphatic leukemia and lymphosarcoma,[31,32] while varying degrees of hemolysis have been described in other neoplastic diseases, particularly the leukemias and lymphomas.[33-36] Information related to hemolysis in the patients in this series with leukemia and lymphoma was insufficient for analysis. The increased susceptibility to *Salmonella* sepsis of patients with neoplastic disease, especially leukemias and lymphomas, may be in part explained by the hemolytic component of their disease, and these diseases should perhaps be included with sickle-cell disease, bartonellosis, and malaria, in having a specific predisposition to associated salmonellosis. Hemolysis might then be an additional mechanism for altered immune responses in patients with leukemia and lymphoma, and could contribute to the defect in the macrophage system by interfering with the capacity of macrophages to kill salmonellae.[27] Although this hypothesis does not explain the unique association between *S typhimurium* septicemia and patients with leukemia and lymphoma, it is of interest that *S typhimurium* was the serotype used by Kaye et al in establishing a relationship between hemolysis in mice and septicemia with this organism.[27] Further studies obviously are indicated to explain this intriguing association of *S typhimurium* septicemia with leukemia and lymphoma and perhaps specifically with the hemolytic component of these diseases.

The predisposition to *Salmonella* infection postoperative, particularly after gastric or other gastrointestinal procedures,[37,38] was reaffirmed in this study. Over one quarter of the patients had previous surgery, and as in other studies the commonest type of infection in them was enteritis.[37,38]

A number of unusual manifestations of salmonellosis were found in our patients. *Salmonella* is a rare cause of pleuropulmonary disease,[39] but involvement of the lung or thoracic cavity occurred in five of our patients. *Salmonella* endocarditis is also rare, only 24 confirmed cases have been reported between 1936 and 1967.[40] The serotype in the case of mural endocarditis in this series was *S derby* (patient 4), which has not previously been reported as a cause of endocarditis.[40] *Salmonella* arthritis is also a rare manifestation; David and Black were able to find only 84 cases in their review of the literature.[41] Patient 5 in our series, a patient with *S infantis* arthritis of the knee, appears to be the first reported case of arthritis due to this serotype.

Localization of *Salmonella* in carcinomatous tissue also occurs infrequently,[1,11] but in this series *Salmonella* was isolated from an axillary lymph node containing reticulum cell sarcoma (patient 6), and from a sacrococcygeal abscess in an embryonal cell carcinoma (patient 7). The finding of a perirectal abscess (patient 8) and a buttock abscess (patient 2), both due to *S typhimurium*, is also unusual.[42]

All salmonellae included in this investigation were serotyped by Joseph Winter, PhD, New York *Salmonella* Center.

Nonproprietary and Trade Names of Drugs

Amphotericin B—*Fungizone*.
Dactinomycin—*Cosmegen*.
Vincristine sulfate—*Oncovin*.

References

1. Black PH, Kunz LG, Swartz MN: Salmonellosis: A review of some unusual aspects. *New Eng J Med* **262**:811-817, 864-870, 921-927, 1960.
2. MacCready RA, Reardon JP, Saphra I: Salmonellosis in Massachusetts: A 16 year experience. *New Eng J Med* **256**:1121-1128, 1957.
3. Saphra I, Winter JW: Clinical manifestations of salmonellosis in man: An evaluation of 7,779 human infections identified at the New York *Salmonella* Center. *New Eng J Med* **256**:1128-1134, 1957.
4. Eisenberg GM, Palazzolo AJ, Flippen HF: Clinical and microbiologic aspects of salmonellosis: A study of 95 cases in adults and children. *New Eng J Med* **253**:90-94, 1955.
5. Schneirson SS, Herschberger C, Honigsberg R: Salmonellosis at the Mount Sinai Hospital: A ten year survey (1953-1963). *J Mount Sinai Hosp NY* **31**:1-9, 1964.
6. Cohen RA, Geraci JE, Dearing WH, et al: Salmonellosis: Observations on 94 patients. *Proc Mayo Clin* **39**:401-409, 1964.
7. Kough RH, Scichitano DC, Smull CE: Salmonellosis in a rural Pennsylvania hospital: Observations in 100 consecutive cases. *Arch Intern Med* **116**:548-553, 1965.
8. Hook EW: Salmonellosis: Certain factors influencing the interaction of *Salmonella* and the human host. *Bull NY Acad Med* **37**:499-512, 1961.
9. Clyde AW: Salmonellosis in infants and children: A study of 100 cases. *Pediatrics* **19**:175-183, 1957.
10. Cherubin CE, Fodor T, Denmark LI, et al: The epidemiology of salmonellosis in New York City. *Amer J Epidem* **90**:112-125, 1969.
11. Han T, Sokal JE, Neter E: Salmonellosis in disseminated malignant diseases. *New Eng J Med* **276**:1045-1052, 1967.
12. Sinkovics JG, Smith JP: Salmonellosis complicating neoplastic disease. *Cancer* **24**:631-636, 1969.
13. Cherubin CE, Fodor T, Denmark LI, et al: Symptoms, septicemia and death in salmonellosis. *Amer J Epidem* **90**:285-291, 1969.
14. Sanders E, Sweeney FJ, Friedman EA, et al: An outbreak of hospital-associated infections due to *Salmonella derby*. *JAMA* **186**:984-986, 1963.
15. Henkel JS, Armstrong D, Blevins A, et al: Group A beta-hemolytic *Streptococcus* bacteremia in a cancer hospital. *JAMA* **211**:983-986, 1970.
16. Hutter RVP, Collins HS: The occurrence of opportunistic fungus infections in a cancer hospital. *Lab Invest* **11**:1035-1045, 1962.
17. Larsen MC, Diamond HD, Collins HS: *Nocardia asteroides* infection. *Arch Intern Med* **103**:712-725, 1959.
18. Silver RT, Utz JP, Frei E, et al: Fever, infection and host resistance in acute leukemia. *Amer J Med* **24**:35-39, 1959.
19. Louria DB, Blevins A, Armstrong D, et al: Fungemia caused by "non-pathogenic" yeasts. *Arch Intern Med* **119**:247-252, 1967.
20. Louria DB, Hensle T, Armstrong D, et al: Listeriosis complicating malignant disease: A new association. *Ann Intern Med* **67**:261-281, 1967.
21. Miller SP, Shanbrom E: Infectious syndromes of leukemias and lymphomas. *Amer J Med Sci* **246**:420-428, 1963.
22. Miller DG: Pattern of immunological deficiency in lymphomas and leukemias. *Ann Intern Med* **57**:703-716, 1962.
23. Lang DJ, Kunz LJ, Martin AA, et al: Carmine as a source of nosocomial salmonellosis. *New Eng J Med* **276**:829-832, 1967.
24. Harvey AM: *Salmonella suipestifer* infection in human beings: Review of the literature and a report of 21 new cases. *Arch Intern Med* **59**:118-135, 1937.
25. Heineman HS, Jensen WN, Cooper WM, et al: Hodgkin's disease and *Salmonella typhimurium* infection. *JAMA* **188**:632-634, 1964.
26. Simpson JF, Leddy JP, Hare JD: Listeriosis complicating lymphoma: Report of four cases and interpretive review. *Amer J Med* **43**:39-49, 1967.
27. Kaye D, Gill FA, Hook EW: Factors influencing host resistance to salmonella infections: the effects of hemolysis and erythrophagocytosis. *Amer J Med Sci* **254**:205-215, 1967.
28. Hook EW, Campbell CG, Weens HS, et al: Salmonella osteomyelitis in patients with sickle-cell anemia. *New Eng J Med* **257**:403-407, 1957.
29. Cuadra M: Salmonellosis complication in human bartonellosis. *Tex Rep Biol Med* **14**:97-113, 1956.
30. Bennett IL, Hook EW: Infectious diseases (some aspects of salmonellosis). *Ann Rev Med* **10**:1-20, 1959.
31. Norcross JW: Hematologic manifestations of malignant disease. *Med Clin N Amer* **47**:345-352, 1963.
32. Rosenthal MC, Pisciotta AV, Konninos ZD, et al: Autoimmune hemolytic anemia of malignant lymphoma. *Blood* **101**:197-227, 1953.
33. Waggener RE, Pratt PT, Hunt HB: Erythrocyte survival in leukemia, Hodgkin's disease and malignant lymphoma as determined by radiochromate. *Amer J Roentgen* **79**:1045-1049, 1958.
34. Hotchkiss DJ: The anemia of lymphomas and leukemias. *Med Clin N Amer* **48**:1479-1492, 1964.
35. Brain MC, Dacie JV, Hourihane DOB: Microangiopathic hemolytic anemia: The possible role of vascular lesions in pathogenesis. *Brit J Haemat* **8**:358-374, 1962.
36. Stratford EC, Tanaka KR: Microangiopathic hemolytic anemia in metastatic carcinoma. *Arch Intern Med* **116**:346-350, 1965.
37. Waddell WR, Kunz LJ: Association of *Salmonella* enteritis with operations on the stomach. *New Eng J Med* **255**:555-559, 1956.
38. Sokol EM: *Salmonella derby* infections after gastrointestinal surgery. *J Mount Sinai Hosp NY* **32**:36-41, 1965.
39. Weiss W, Eisenberg GM, Flippin HF: *Salmonella* pleuropulmonary disease. *Amer J Med Sci* **233**:487-496, 1957.
40. Schneider PJ, Nernoff J, Gold JA: Acute *Salmonella* endocarditis: Report of a case and review. *Arch Intern Med* **120**:478-482, 1967.
41. David JR, Black RL: *Salmonella* arthritis. *Medicine* **39**:385-403, 1960.
42. Smiley DG, Frank SL, Weil AJ: *Salmonella oranienburg* in a perirectal abscess. *JAMA* **143**:430, 1950.

Potential Hepatotoxicity of Copper in Recurrent Hemodialysis

Jeanette Blomfield, MSc, Sydney, Australia; and Stephen R. Dixon, MB, ChB, MRACP; and David A. McCredie, MD, BSc, MRACP, Melbourne

Tap water acting on copper plumbing contributes up to 1 ppm of copper to dialysis fluid in Australian hemodialysis units. Patients dialyzed against 0.4 ppm of copper show uptake of copper by both plasma and red blood cells during hemodialysis. In experimental dialysis of dogs against 0.4 and 1 ppm of copper, the initial uptake is mainly by the plasma, but copper concentration occurs in the red blood cells and in the liver. The possibility that, in patients on long-term hemodialysis, copper accumulation in the liver might eventually lead to hepatitis and hemolysis is discussed in relation to chronic copper poisoning of sheep and to Wilson's disease.

Acute copper poisoning has been shown to be the cause of severe hemolysis and gastrointestinal disturbances following isolated hemodialysis treatments.[1,2] Retrospective investigation has established a correlation between the hemolytic crises and the formation of acidic water from partially exhausted deionizers which acted on copper components of the artificial kidney machine, resulting in high, and at times lethal, copper concentrations.

The purpose of the present study is to draw attention to the added possibility that copper from relatively low dialysis-fluid copper concentrations derived from untreated tap water, may insidiously accumulate in the liver and eventually present clinically as hepatitis.

In chronic copper poisoning of sheep,[3-6] and in Wilson's disease,[7-10] copper concentrates in the liver without apparent ill-effect until the binding sites are saturated. Then the toxicity is manifested as a necrotic hepatitis or cirrhosis and as a hemolytic crisis due to red blood cell absorption of excessive circulating copper.

Although chronic copper intoxication is virtually unknown in man, hemodialysis supplies an unusual situation in which the blood is subjected to recurrent dialysis against large volumes of fluid over prolonged periods. During hemodialysis, ionic copper in low concentration has been shown to have a one-way flow from the dialysis fluid into the plasma because of protein-binding of the copper.[11] Evidence is presented in this study to show that with slightly higher copper concentrations (within the range encountered in Australian dialysis units), copper transfers from the plasma to the red blood cells and to the liver.

Methods

Samples of dialysis fluid and of tap water used in its dilution were examined from hemodialysis units throughout Australia. One unit used distilled water but no units used deionizers.

The uptake of copper by patients undergoing hemodialysis was assessed in three different units: (1) in four patients dialyzed by a twin-coil machine (Kolff) against a dialysis fluid copper of 15μg/100 ml; (2) in four patients dialyzed by a single-coil of a twin-coil machine (Kolff), with two patients per machine, and a dialysis fluid copper of 40μg/100 ml; and (3) in one patient dialyzed by another dialyzer (Kiil) against a dialysis fluid copper of 40μg/100 ml. The dialyzer was supplied by fluid from a plastic tank with the use of a monitor (Watson Marlow). In each of these three units the established source of the copper in the dialysis fluid was the copper plumbing of the tap water, with the membranes (Cupraphan) providing a possible addi-

Received for publication July 9, 1970; accepted March 22, 1971.

From the Children's Medical Research Foundation, Royal Alexandra Hospital for Children, Sydney, Australia (Miss Blomfield) and the Department of Pediatrics, University of Melbourne and Royal Children's Hospital, Melbourne (Drs. Dixon and McCredie).

Read in part before the Fifth Meeting of the Australasian Society of Nephrology, Sydney, Australia, Oct 10, 1969.

Reprint requests to Children's Medical Research Foundation, PO Box 34, Camperdown, NSW 2050, Australia (Miss Blomfield).

tional contribution in the Kiil dialyzer. No copper-containing parts were detectable in the dialysis machines or delivery systems. Arterial blood was collected before dialysis and samples of blood entering ("arterial") and leaving ("venous return") the dialyzer were collected one hour after commencement and at eight hours, just prior to the end of the dialysis. Simultaneously, dialysis fluid samples from main storage tanks and from the compartment adjacent to the dialysis membranes were also collected.

Liver biopsy specimens were collected from 4 patients and posttransplant 24-hour urine specimens from 12 patients in the unit with dialysis fluid copper of 15μg/100 ml.

Sixteen dogs were also dialyzed with an artificial kidney machine (Travenol-Kolff type) using either cellulose or Cuprophan tubing. Each dog was dialyzed for two hours only and either the dialysis fluid copper level was that of the tap water level of around 40μg/100 ml or copper sulfate solution was added to raise the concentration to approximately 100μg/100 ml (1 ppm). A total of 12 to 24 liters of dialysis fluid was used during the two-hour period. Arterial blood was taken before dialysis and arterial and venous-return samples after ten minutes and again after two hours of dialysis. Two to two and one half liters of 0.9% saline were run through the tubing before commencing dialysis. When indicated this was followed by 500 ml of a degraded gelatin plasma expander, special intravenous gelatin solution (Haemaccel), which was discarded after passing through the tubing. The cellulose tubing coils of the Kolff dialyzer were finally primed with blood from a donor dog prior to dialysis, but the Cuprophan tubing coils, being of lesser capacity, were not. Samples of liver obtained by open biopsy were taken one week prior to dialysis (to avoid bleeding after heparinization) and again at the end of the two-hour dialysis.

The concentration of free ionic copper in tap water, dialysis fluid, plasma, and urine and total copper of red blood cells was measured by the atomic absorption method of Blomfield and MacMahon.[12] Liver copper was estimated by drying liver segments to constant weight over phosphorus pentoxide in a vacuum desiccator, ashing the dried samples in platinum crucibles overnight in a muffle furnace at 450 C, dissolving the ash in copper-free 4N hydrochloric acid, and measuring the copper concentration with an atomic absorption spectrophotometer (Perkin-Elmer).

Liver sections were stained for copper by the method of Mallory and Parker.[13]

Results

Survey of Australian Dialysis Fluid Copper Levels.—Dialysis fluid from most Australian hemodialysis units had a copper concentration lower than 25μg/100 ml, but several had values in the 25μg/100 ml to 100μg/100 ml range. The level in the dialysis fluid closely resembled the level of tap water after the tap had been running for five minutes. With the higher copper levels, tap water values tended to be at least 30μg/100 ml to 40μg/100 ml higher when the tap was first turned on. These results demonstrated that the major source of copper in dialysis fluid was tap water and that this copper was largely derived from copper plumbing. With one machine the dialysis-fluid copper concentration rose by 40μg/100 ml after passing through a copper heat exchanger.

Hemodialysis of Patients.—*Copper Uptake by the Blood.*—1. With patients dialyzed against a copper level of 15μg/100 ml, the venous-return plasma free-copper levels were a little higher than those in the arterial plasma, but there was no increase in red blood cell levels (Fig 1*a*).

2. With a dialysis fluid copper of 40μg/100 ml, there was uptake by both plasma and red blood cells as shown by increased venous-return concentrations, and, after one hour of dialysis, arterial copper levels of both plasma and red blood cells had risen above the predialysis values (Fig 1*b*).

3. With a single patient dialyzed by Kiil dialysis, using Cuprophan membranes, against a dialysis fluid copper of 40μg/100 ml, there was appreciable uptake of copper by both plasma and red blood cells (Fig 1*c*).

Liver Copper.—Liver biopsy specimens for copper measurement have only been available from four patients. Two of these patients had little or no hemodialysis and normal liver copper concentrations of 1.0 and 1.8 mg/100 gm of dry tissue. One patient, after four months of hemodialysis against dialysis fluid with a copper concentration of 15μg/100 ml, had a normal liver copper value of 2.4 mg/100 gm, and one other patient after six months in the same unit showed possible evidence of copper accumulation with a liver copper concentration of 19.6 mg/100 gm. This latter figure is above the normal range of liver copper reported by most workers[10,14-18] (Table). The higher normal ranges found by Levi et al[8] were from children, and the discrepancy in results between the two sample sizes suggests that the yellow color of the copper-diethyldithiocarbamate complex is not sufficiently intense or specific to be reliable with low copper concentrations.

Posttransplant Urine Copper.—Twenty-four hour urine specimens were collected within two weeks of kidney transplantation from 12 patients in a unit with a dialysis-fluid copper concentration of 15μg/100 ml. Four of these patients, who had received prior dialysis with copper-free peritoneal dialysis fluids only, had a urine copper concentration range of 2.5μg/100 ml to 8.0μg/100 ml (mean, 5.6μg/100 ml), and a 24-hour urine copper output of 70μg/day to 130μg/day (mean, 110μg/day). The other eight patients, who had been treated by hemodialysis before receiving the renal transplant, had a urine copper concentration range of 2.3μg/100 ml to 11.7μg/100 ml (mean, 6.8μg/100 ml) and 24-hour urine copper output of 45μg/day to 275μg/day (mean, 145μg/

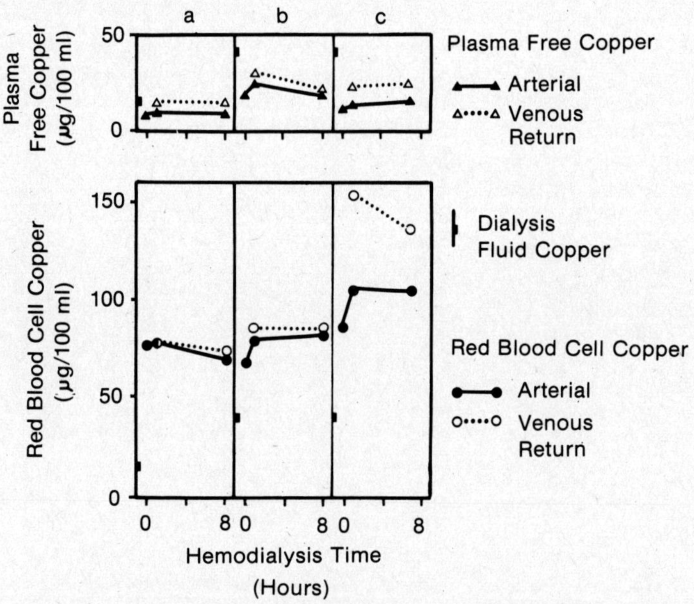

Fig 1.—Uptake of copper by plasma and red blood cells of patients during hemodialysis. (a) *Mean results of four patients on twin-coil Kolff dialyzers.* (b) *Mean results of four patients on single-coil Kolff dialyzers.* (c) *Results of one patient on a Kiil dialyzer.*

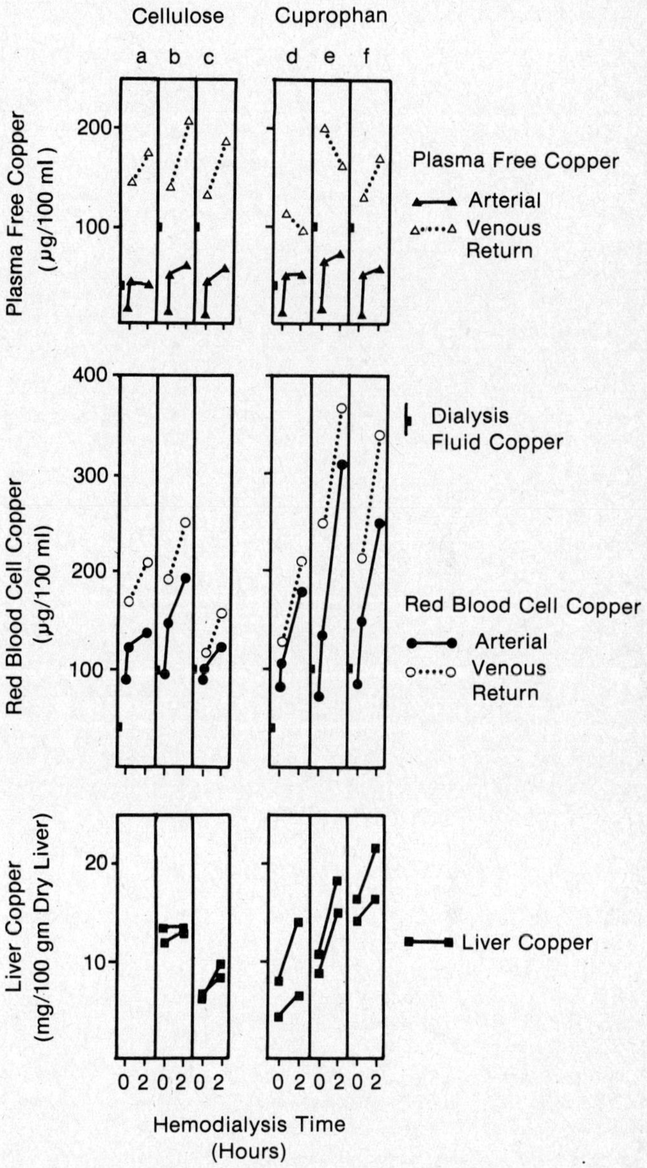

Fig 2.—Uptake of copper by plasma, red blood cells, and liver during hemodialysis of dogs on single-coil Kolff dialyzers. Predialysis gelatin solution primes were used in (c) *and* (f). *Red blood cell and plasma results of* (a) *and* (b) *are means of four dogs and* (c) *to* (f) *of two dogs.*

day). The normal ranges in our laboratory are 1µg/100 ml to 4µ/100 ml (mean, 2.7µg/100 ml) and 10µg/day to 37µg/day (mean, 20µg/day).

Hemodialysis of Dogs.—*Copper Uptake by the Blood.*—Dogs were dialyzed using either cellulose (Fig 2*a* to *c*) or Cuprophan (Fig 2*d* to *f*) dialysis tubing and using the tap water copper concentration of 40µg/100 ml (Fig 2*a* and *d*) or the supplemented copper level of 100µg/100 ml (Fig 2*b*, *c*, *e*, and *f*). All tubing was rinsed with 0.9% saline, and on occasion this was followed by gelatin solution (Fig 2*c* and *f*) to clear copper which was bound to the membranes during the predialysis soaking of the coils.

In all cases the venous-return plasma free-copper levels were considerably higher than the arterial levels. The arterial plasma free-copper concentrations had risen significantly after ten minutes, but, although the elevation was sustained, there was little additional increase during the remainder of the two hours (Fig 2). The copper values of the gelatin solution run through the coil rose from nil to a mean level of 225µg/100 ml, but this preliminary clearing of copper bound to the dialysis membranes failed to prevent the early arterial

Normal Values for Liver Copper								
		Method		Dry Weight of Liver	Copper (mg/100 gm of Dry Liver)			
Author	Year	Sample Preparation	Copper Estimation	Sample	Mean	SD	SE	Range
Butt et al[14]	1954	Drying, 140 C, 16 hr Ashing, 500 C, 24 hr	Emission spectrograph		2.76		0.10	
Levi et al[8]	1967	Ashing, 243 C	? Diethyldithiocarbamate	2-10 mg 10-30 mg	8.07 3.56			1.5-19.5 0.87-11.2
Smallwood et al[15]	1968	Freeze-drying; wet-ashing in nitric: perchloric acid, 9:1	Neutron activation		3.53		1.20	1.5-5.5
Fell et al[16]	1968	? Drying in vacuo; wet-ashing in nitric acid	Neutron activation		2.55	1.15		0.92-4.68
Sternlieb and Scheinberg[10]	1968	Wet-ashing in sulphuric and perchloric acids	Dicyclohexanone-oxalyldihydrazone		3.15	0.68		2.0-4.5
Cumings[17]	1968	?	Atomic absorption		2.76	1.78 (2 SD)	0.26	
Volini et al[18]	1968	Drying, 120 C, 16 hr; preliminary digestion with nitric acid and heat; ashing, 500-550 C 24-hr	Atomic absorption		5.78		0.87	

copper rise.

The red blood cell copper concentrations also increased during the passage of the blood through the dialysis tubing although not to the same degree as the plasma. However, after an initial rise during the first ten minutes, the arterial red blood cell copper values continued to increase progressively over the two-hour period (Fig 2).

Liver Copper Uptake.—Accumulation of copper in the liver was found in nine of the ten liver biopsy specimens in which comparisons were made of the copper concentrations of samples collected one week before dialysis with a further sample collected immediately after the two-hour dialysis period (Fig 2). The predialysis liver copper concentrations of the dogs tended to be higher than the human normal range, but in this study each dog acted as its own control. Goresky et al[19] have reported liver copper concentrations in dogs which ranged from 18.10 to 57.80 mg/100 gm of dry liver, with a mean and standard deviation (SD) of 33.64 ± 16.11 mg/100 gm. Whether the higher copper levels found in dogs' livers are due to a species difference or to environmental accumulation is not known.

Liver Histopathology.—Despite increases in liver copper ranging up to 7.8 mg/100 gm of dry liver, no copper could be detected in the postdialysis liver biopsy sections by histochemical staining.

Dialysis Fluid Copper Loss.—After two hours of hemodialysis, simultaneous samples of dialysis fluid were collected from the main storage tank and from the separate dialysis compartment adjacent to the membranes. With the 1-ppm fluid there was a mean decrease in copper concentration of 15%. The actual copper loss was probably greater than this as some copper contamination occurs within the machine.[11] At the lower copper concentration of 0.4 ppm, the mean loss or gain was nil, presumably because copper contamination equaled blood uptake.

Comparisons of Cellulose and Cuprophan Tubing.—In vitro studies with dialysis tubing showed that Cuprophan membrane not only contained copper (500μg/100 × 40 cm/sheet), but it bound copper more readily than cellulose tubing. When 10 × 10 cm pieces of Cuprophan or cellulose tubing were immersed in 10 ml of aqueous copper sulfate solution with a copper concentration of 100μg/100 ml, at 37 C for ten minutes, the Cuprophan membrane bound 90% of the copper compared with 40% by the cellulose. The original or the bound copper was not significantly released by 0.9% saline, by 10% formaldehyde solution, or by the dextrans (Rheomacrodex, Macrodex, or Intradex), but it was removed by 3% acetic acid, 5% albumin, or by the degraded gelatin polymer.

Comment

Hepatitis is not an uncommon problem in hemodialysis units, and the viral nature of an outbreak is often evident by a high incidence of the disease among staff and close relatives. However, in some units hepatitis has been confined to patients and the possibility that liver dysfunction could be due to hepatotoxic agents such as azathioprine, halothane, or other known hepatotoxic chemicals or insecticides, has been considered.[20-22] Long-term accumulation of copper in the liver has known hepatotoxic consequences in animals and man and has previously been suggested as a potential hazard in hemodialysis.[11]

The strong affinity of the liver for copper has been demonstrated by isotope studies in normal man.[7] Within two hours of the intravenous administration of radioactive copper (^{64}Cu and ^{67}Cu) compounds only 4% remains in the plasma, and a marked localization in the liver can be demonstrated by whole-body profile scanning or by scintiscanning of the abdomen. Some 60% to 80% of the injected dose is still present in the liver after 24 hours.

In our series of dogs, despite continual uptake of copper by the plasma, the arterial plasma free-copper initially rose, then levelled off, forming an inverted L pattern (Γ) (Fig 2). The arterial red blood cell copper concentration, however, rose progressively, tending towards the shape of a stroke (/). The increase of liver copper would, therefore, appear to have been derived mainly from the plasma rather than the red blood cells.

The present investigation of the hemodialysis of patients and of dogs against concentrations of copper up to 1 ppm has shown that copper is taken up by the plasma, the red blood cells, and the liver. One part per million is 1 mg of copper per liter of dialysis fluid, and patients on long-term maintenance hemodialysis are subjected to 200 to 500 liters of dialysis fluid two to three times per week. The total body copper of a normal adult is 75 to 150 mg, and the normal daily oral intake is 2 to 5 mg.[7] When the copper concentration is high in the dialysis fluid and the dialyses are carried on over a long-term period, it is probable that copper accumulation in the liver would occur and that eventually hepatitis and hemolysis might result. The danger levels in terms of copper concentration and time are not known, but some indication of the degree of risk may be obtained by analogy with studies of chronic copper poisoning in sheep and of patients with Wilson's disease.

Chronic copper poisoning of animals, particularly of sheep, has been extensively studied over the past 40 years. Sheep given copper orally in the range 125 to 500 mg per day usually die within one to eight months.[3-6] Copper accumulates in the liver in a clinically benign manner until the sudden onset of an acute hemolytic crisis and severe liver dysfunction, from which the animal usually dies within a few days. The approach of a hemolytic crisis can be predicted biochemically three to eight weeks before the appearance of clinical symptoms by moderate rises in the levels of serum glutamic oxaloacetic transaminase (SGOT) and lactic dehydrogenase (LDH). At the time of the hemolytic crisis there is a sudden massive increase in the levels of SGOT and LDH, and of the more specific liver enzymes, serum glutamic pyruvic transaminase (SGPT) and arginase, and the clearance of sulfobromophthalein (BSP) is abruptly reduced. Blood copper levels are normal to within a few days of hemolysis, when enormous increases in red blood cell and plasma copper occur. With the crisis the hematocrit level drops sharply, hemoglobin is found in plasma and urine, methemoglobinemia may give the blood and liver a brown color, red blood cell glutathione is reduced to very low levels, and a profound hyperbilirubinemia follows. Liver copper concentration shows a 10- to 30-fold increase above normal, the amount of copper retained by the liver being of the order of 100 to 300 mg.

The terminal phase in sheep of intravascular hemolysis and hepatic toxicity resembles acute copper poisoning seen in human subjects,[1,2,23] in which the predominant clinical features are a marked hemolysis occurring 6 to 24 hours after exposure to copper and associated jaundice, methemoglobinemia, hypoglycemia, vomiting, diarrhea, abdominal pain, and liver tenderness. The similarity between chronic copper poisoning in animals and the hemolytic episodes with related hepatic involvement sometimes seen in Wilson's disease, has been emphasized by McIntyre et al.[9] From the normal daily dietary intake of copper, a child with Wilson's disease may accumulate sufficient copper in the liver to present as clinical hepatitis by the age of 5 to 8 years.[7] In presymptomatic Wilson's disease, an increase of SGOT has been found to correlate well with abnormal liver histology and increased liver-copper concentrations.[8]

A direct analogy cannot, of course, be drawn between dialyzed patients and patients with Wilson's disease who have a defect of copper metabolism or with sheep, which are believed to be particularly susceptible to copper poisoning. However, from the evidence presented, we feel that chronic copper accumulation must be regarded as a possible cause of hepatitis and hemolysis in maintenance hemodialysis.

Soft water, where deionizing is not usually felt to be necessary, is the water most likely to dissolve significant amounts of copper. Measurement of tap water and dialysis-fluid copper concentrations should give an indication of the possibility of excessive copper loading. Estimation of plasma free-copper and red blood cell copper in arterial and venous-return samples taken at the end of the dialysis should give some idea of the degree of copper uptake by the patient. It may be noted here that, even with excessive liver copper accumulation, the predialysis plasma free-copper and red blood cell copper are likely to be normal and that measurement of plasma ceruloplasmin has no value as it is unaffected by copper uptake.

Postdialysis urine copper estimations may give some indication of excessive copper uptake but have limited value in patients with impaired renal function. Posttransplant urine copper outputs may give an indication of high liver copper accumulation, although this aspect requires further investigation. All of the posttransplant patients in the present series had urine copper levels above our normal ranges. However, they were all receiving prednisone (1.5 mg/kg/day), and a recent report by Henkin et al[24] has shown that administration of 50 mg of prednisone for five days to normal volunteers caused a more than twofold increase of urine copper excretion. Wiesel[25] also found an increased urinary copper excretion on administration of glucogenic corticosteroids to normal subjects. In the present study liver copper and posttransplant urine copper tended to be slightly higher in dialyzed than in nondialyzed patients, which suggests some degree of copper accumulation, but probably insufficient to cause serious toxicity.

Excessive copper stored in the liver may be bound so that it does not react to copper stains,[8,10] but an accumulation sufficient to cause an acute hepatic reaction would probably give a positive stain. A retrospective survey of liver biopsy and autopsy sections of dialyzed patients by copper staining could reveal the presence of copper as a primary or contributory cause of hepatic dysfunction in some dialysis patients, and, as a prospective study, the more accurate chemical assessment of liver copper levels could prove an invaluable indicator of copper accumulation in patients undergoing hemodialysis.

J.H. Stewart, MB, ChB, of Sydney Hospital, Sydney, Australia, and E. Haywood, MB, of the Royal Perth Hospital, Perth, Australia, assisted with hemodialysis. Mr. K. Curtis and the Department of Pathology, Royal Children's Hospital, Melbourne assisted with hemodialysis of dogs. P. Bale, MB, and Mr. H.J. Mitchell of the Institute of Pathology, Royal Alexandra Hospital for Children, Sydney, performed the liver histopathological examinations. The special intravenous gelatin solution used in the studies was donated as Haemaccel by Hoechst Australia Ltd.

Nonproprietary and Trade Names of Drug

Azathioprine—*Imuran.*

References

1. Ivanovich P, Manzler A, Drake R: Acute hemolysis following hemodialysis. *Trans Amer Soc Artif Intern Organs* **15**:316-320, 1969.

2. Matter BJ, Pederson J, Psimenos G, et al: Lethal copper intoxication in hemodialysis. *Trans Amer Soc Artif Intern Organs* **15**:309-315, 1969.

3. Todd JR, Gracey JF, Thompson RH: Studies on chronic copper poisoning: I. Toxicity of copper sulphate and copper acetate in sheep. *Brit Vet J* **118**:482-491, 1962.

4. Todd JR, Thompson RH: Studies on chronic copper poisoning: II. Biochemical studies on the blood of sheep during the haemolytic crisis. *Brit Vet J* **119**:161-173, 1963.

5. Ross DB: The diagnosis, prevention and treatment of chronic copper poisoning in housed lambs. *Brit Vet J* **122**:279-284, 1966.

6. MacPherson A, Hemingway RG: The relative merit of various blood analyses and liver function tests in giving an early diagnosis of chronic copper poisoning in sheep. *Brit Vet J* **125**:213-221, 1969.

7. Walshe JM: The physiology of copper in man and its relation to Wilson's disease. *Brain* **90**:149-176, 1967.

8. Levi AJ, Sherlock S, Scheuer PJ, et al: Presymptomatic Wilson's disease. *Lancet* **2**:575-579, 1967.

9. McIntyre N, Clink HN, Levi AJ, et al: Hemolytic anemia in Wilson's disease. *New Eng J Med* **276**:493-444, 1967.

10. Sternlieb I, Scheinberg IH: Prevention of Wilson's disease in asymptomatic patients. *New Eng J Med* **278**:352-359, 1968.

11. Blomfield J, McPherson J, George CRP: Active uptake of copper and zinc during haemodialysis. *Brit Med J* **2**:141-145, 1969.

12. Blomfield J, MacMahon RA: Micro determination of plasma and erythrocyte copper by atomic absorption spectrophotometry. *J Clin Path* **22**:136-143, 1969.

13. Mallory FB, Parker F: Fixing and staining methods for lead and copper in tissues. *Amer J Path* **15**:517-522, 1939.

14. Butt EM, Nusbaum RE, Gilmour TC, et al: Use of emission spectrograph for study of inorganic elements in human tissues. *Amer J Clin Path* **24**:385-394, 1954.

15. Smallwood RA, Williams HA, Rosenoer VM, et al: Liver copper levels in liver disease: Studies using neutron activation analysis. *Lancet* **2**:1310-1313, 1968.

16. Fell GS, Smith H, Howie RA: Neutron activation analysis for copper in biological material applied to Wilson's disease. *J Clin Path* **21**:8-11, 1968.

17. Cumings JN: Trace metals in the brain and in Wilson's disease. *J Clin Path* **21**:1-7, 1968.

18. Volini F, de la Huerga J, Kent G: Trace metal studies in liver disease using atomic absorption spectrometry, in Sunderman FW, Sunderman FW Jr (eds): *Laboratory Diagnosis of Liver Diseases.* St. Louis, WH Green Inc, 1968, pp 199-206.

19. Goresky CA, Holmes TH, Sass-Kortsak A: The initial uptake of copper by the liver in the dog. *Canad J Physiol Pharmacol* **46**:771-784, 1968.

20. Evans DB, Millard PR, Herbertson BN: Hepatic dysfunction association with renal transplantation. *Lancet* **2**:929-934, 1968.

21. Eastwood JB, Curtis JR, Wing AJ, et al: Hepatitis in a maintenance hemodialysis unit. *Ann Intern Med* **69**:59-66, 1968.

22. Friedman EA, Thomson GE: Hepatitis complicating chronic hemodialysis. *Lancet* **2**:675-678, 1966.

23. Chuttani HK, Gupta PS, Gulati S, et al: Acute copper sulfate poisoning. *Amer J Med* **39**:849-854, 1965.

24. Henkin RI, Meret S, Jacobs JB: Steroid-dependent changes in copper and zinc metabolism. *J Clin Invest* **48**:38a, 1969.

25. Wiesel LL: Metal chelation in the mechanism of action of glucogenic corticosteroids. *Metabolism* **8**:256-264, 1959.

The urinary excretion of a 17-hydroxycorticosteroids, pregnanetiol, 17-ketosteroids, 11-deoxy-17-ketosteroids, and testosterone were measured in normal men and men with endocrine disorders before and during four days of chorionic gonadotropin administration. Testosterone excretion at least doubled in all normal men and showed the greatest change. Androsterone and etiocholanolone increased to at least 150% of the control. Patients with hypopituitarism and primary testicular disease could not be consistently differentiated on the basis of their response to gonadotropin. Patients with delayed puberty and hypogonadotropic hypogonadism has variable responses. In patients with acromegaly, baseline steroid excretion and response to gonadotropin did not differ from normal men.

The Effect of Chorionic Gonadotropin on Steroid Excretion

Murphy T. Scurry, MD, Galveston, Tex; and
Joseph Bruton, PhD; and Kevin G. Barry, MD, Washington, DC

Chorionic gonadotropin (HCG) has been widely used for the study of testicular physiology, for diagnostic purposes and therapeutically. It specifically stimulates the sex hormone secretion of testicular Leydig cells. This effect has been measured by the urinary excretion of 17-ketosteroids,[1,2] 11-deoxy-17-ketosteroids,[2,3] pregnanetroil,[4] estrogen,[5] testosterone,[6,7] and by plasma testosterone.[2,8]

The purpose of the present study was to determine which of a number of urinary steroids was the most reliable in evaluating the effect of gonadotropin in normal men and to compare these results with stimulation in patients with endocrine disease.

Received for publication July 17, 1970; accepted April 14, 1971.

From the Department of Medicine, University of Texas Medical Branch, Galveston, and the Walter Reed Army Institute of Research, Washington, DC. Dr. Barry is now with Georgetown University Medical Division, DC General Hospital, Washington.

Reprint requests to Department of Internal Medicine, Endocrinology, and Metabolism; University of Texas Medical Branch; Galveston, Tex 77450 (Dr. Scurry).

Methods

Men with normal external genitalia, secondary sexual characteristics, and libido were used as normal subjects. All subjects and patients were studied on a metabolic research ward. Following two 24-hour baseline urine collections, 2,000 units of chorionic gonadotropin were administered intramuscularly every 12 hours for four days with daily urine collections.

17-Hydroxycorticosteroid values were determined by the method of Peterson et al,[9] 17-ketosteroid values by the method of Drekter et al,[10] and pregnanetriol values by the method of Bongiovanni and Eberlein.[11] Androsterone, etiocholanolone, and dehydroepiandrosterone were determined by a modification of the gas chromatography method of Kirschner and Lipsett.[12] Urinary testosterone was measured by a modification of the double-isotope-derivative method of Kliman and Peterson.[13]

The data from normal men were analyzed by a least squares regression method for two-way repeated measurements analysis of variance design with missing data. The baseline steroid data from normal men and the initial baseline value from patients were analyzed by analysis of variance with unequal replication followed by Dunnett's *t*-test.[14] Since the desired comparisons were between the control and the abnormal groups, Dunnett's procedure was selected as the test statistic even though the groups were of unequal size. Although approximate, the probability statements are sufficiently precise to warrant meaningful conclusions.

Results

Normal Subjects.—The excretion of steroids under basal conditions (Table 1) in a group of normal men, age 18 to 40 years, is similar to that reported by others.[5,7,9-11] Eight normal men, aged 23 to 24 years, received gonadotrop and their steroid response is shown in Fig 1 and 2. As determined by the least squares regression method there was no significant change in 17-hydroxycorticosteroid or dehydroepiandrosterone excretion ($P > .05$). The increase in 17-ketosteroid excretion was significant ($P < .05$), but four of the eight subjects had no or only slight increases. Pregnanetriol, androsterone, and etiocholanolone excretion increased significantly ($P < .01$). The rise in pregnanetriol was more variable and the percentage increase less than that seen with androsterone and etiocholanolone. The highest increase in androsterone and etiocholanolone for each subject on the third and fourth day of gonadotropin administration was from 150% to 500% of the baseline values. The most consistent and largest change was seen in testosterone ex-

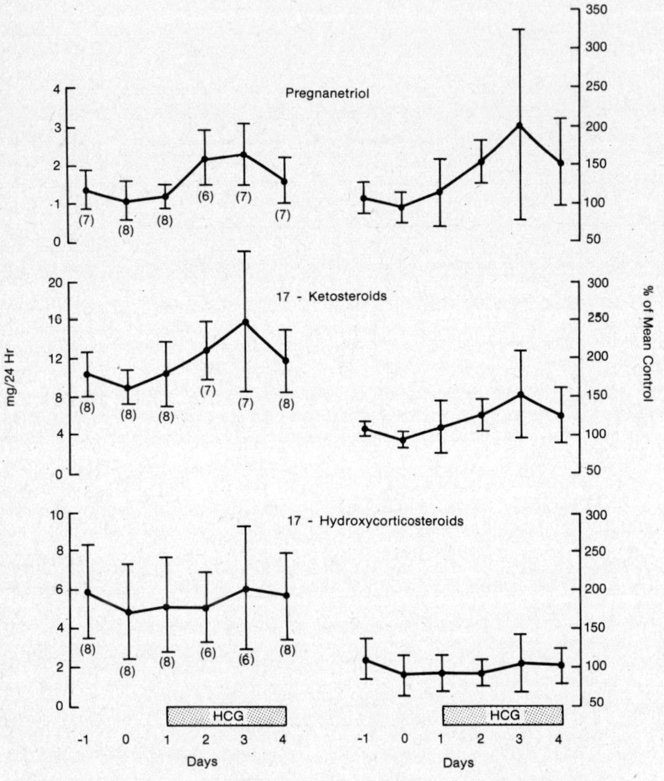

Fig 1.—Urinary excretion of pregnanetriol, 17-ketosteroids, and 17-hydroxycorticosteroids in normal men before and during administration of gonadotropin and expressed as percent of control. Mean with standard deviation of the sample plotted. Number in sample in parenthesis. HCG = chorionic gonadotropin.

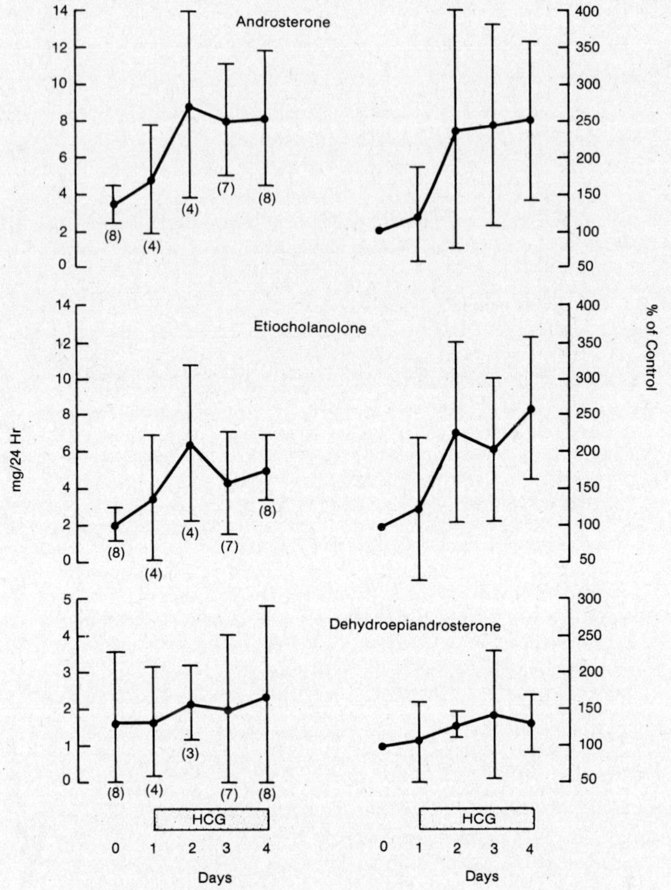

Fig 2.—Urinary excretion of androsterone, etiocholanolone, and dehydroepiandrosterone in normal men before and during administration of gonadotropin and expressed as percent of control. Displayed as in Fig 1. HCG = chorionic gonadotropin.

Fig 3.—Urinary excretion of testosterone in normal men before and during administration of gonadotropin and expressed as percent of control. Displayed as in Fig 1. HCG = chorionic gonadotropin.

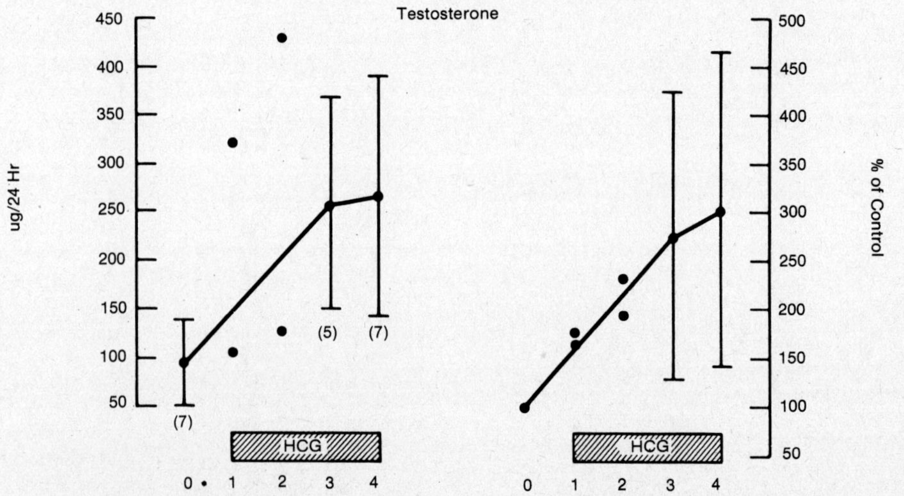

Table 1.—Basal Daily Steroid Excretion in Normal Men

Steroid	No.	Mean±SD
17-Hydroxycorticosteroids	18	5.7±2.6 mg
17-Ketosteroids	18	9.2±2.7 mg
Pregnanetriol	18	1.5±0.8 mg
Androsterone	18	3.2±1.2 mg
Etiocholanolone	18	2.5±1.2 mg
Dehydroepiandrosterone	18	1.2±1.2 mg
Testosterone	18	93±43μg

Table 2.—Male Subjects With Panhypopituitarism*

Patient No.	Age (yr)	Study	17KS	P	A	E	D	T
1	29	Baseline	2.3	0.2	0.4	0.3	<0.1	6
		Baseline	2.4	0.4	0.3	0.3	<0.1	
		HCG, 3rd day	7.0	1.7				
		HCG, 4th day	10.1	1.8	3.2	2.4	0.1	128
2	22	Baseline	4.2	0.6				
		Baseline	3.9	0.2	0.4	0.6	<0.1	13
		HCG, 3rd day	10.8	0.5				
		HCG, 4th day	12.2	1.5	3.3	2.9	0.1	215
3	20	Baseline	0.9	0.5	0.1	<0.1	<0.1	1
		HCG, 3rd day	4.1	1.2				
		HCG, 4th day	2.9	0.9	1.2	0.6	<0.1	4
4	30	Baseline	3.3	0.3	0.9	0.3	<0.1	
		Baseline	3.1	<0.1	0.7	0.2	<0.1	21
		HCG, 3rd day	3.2	0.4	0.6	0.2	<0.1	
		HCG, 4th day	4.0	0.4	0.8	0.3	<0.1	17
5	19	Baseline	3.0	0.3	0.5	0.4	0.1	
Mean baseline value			2.7	0.4	0.5	0.3	<0.1	10
P (vs normal baseline value)			<0.01	<0.05	<0.01	<0.05	<0.05	<0.01

* 17KS=17-ketosteroids, P=pregnanetriol, A=androsterone, E=etiocholanolone, D=dehydroepiandrosterone, T=testosterone, and HCG=chorionic gonadotropin.

Table 3.—Male Subjects With Delayed Puberty or Hypogonadotropic Hypogonadism*

Patient No.	Age (yr)	Study	17OHCS	17KS	P	A	E	D	T
6	16	Baseline	3.5	6.4	0.7	1.3	0.7	0.1	
		Baseline	6.2	6.2	0.6	1.7	0.7	<0.1	31
		HCG, 3rd day	2.8	4.9	0.7	1.4	0.3	<0.1	
		HCG, 4th day	4.9	5.9	1.0	1.7	0.7	<0.1	36
		After 6 weeks of HCG therapy 2,000 units three times a week							
		Baseline	5.2	6.1	0.4				
		Baseline	4.5	5.6	0.5	1.4	0.4	<0.1	13
7	17	Baseline	0.6	1.1	0.1	0.2	0.1	<0.1	
		Baseline	0.8	1.2	0.4				9
		HCG, 3rd day	1.2	3.1	0.9				
		HCG, 4th day	0.7	2.1	0.6	0.7	0.6	<0.1	57
		After 6 weeks of HCG therapy 2,000 units three times a week							
		Baseline	0.8	2.5	1.6				
		Baseline	0.4	1.0	1.2	1.9	0.7	<0.1	278
		HCG, 3rd day	1.0	17.1	3.2				
		HCG, 4th day	1.2	12.3	1.7	5.8	2.1	<0.1	340
8	17	Baseline	3.8	3.6	0.2				
		Baseline	3.4	2.9	0.1	1.6	0.6	0.2	5
		HCG, 3rd day	3.0	3.6	0.4				
		HCG, 4th day	3.3	4.3	0.3	1.2	0.4	0.5	14
		After 6 weeks of HCG therapy 2,000 units three times a week							
		Baseline	3.5	2.5	0.1				
		Baseline	3.0	2.1	0.1	0.7	0.2	0.6	5
		HCG, 3rd day	3.4	6.0	0.8				
		HCG, 4th day	3.4	6.1	1.0	2.3	0.8	0.1	37
9	16	Baseline	1.3	0.5	0.5				
		Baseline	1.2	0.5	<0.1	0.4	0.2	<0.1	2
		HCG, 3rd day	1.8	1.7	0.2	0.3	0.4	<0.1	
		HCG, 4th day	1.3	2.1	0.4				15
Mean baseline value			2.3	2.9	0.4	0.9	0.4	0.1	12
P (vs normal baseline value)			NS	<0.05	<0.05	<0.01	<0.05	NS	<0.01

*17OHCS=17-hydroxycorticosteroids, 17KS=17-ketosteroids, P=pregnanetriol, A=androsterone, E=etiocholanolone, D=dehydroepiandrosterone, T=testosterone, HCG=chorionic gonadotropin, and NS=not significant.

cretion ($P < .01$) (Fig 3). All normal subjects had at least a doubling in testosterone excretion and the greatest response seen was an increase of six times the control.

Men With Panhypopituitarism.—Observations were obtained on five men with space occupying lesions of the sella turcica and clinical and laboratory evidence of panhypopituitarism (Table 2). All were on a regimen of replacement amounts of adrenal steroids and desiccated thyroid replacement at the time of study. Two of the four patients who were stimulated with gonadoptropin showed a marked increase in steroid excretion, which was of greater percentage magnitude than that found in normal men. One individual (patient 3), who had never gone through pubertal development, had an increase in all steroids with only a slight rise in testosterone. Patient 4, who had a nine year history of hypopituitarism without sex steroid replacement, had no response to gonadotropin. The mean baseline excretion of all the steroids was significantly lower in this group as compared to the normal subjects, but all patients were receiving replacement glucocorticoids.

Delayed Puberty of Hypogonadotropic Hypogonadism.—These patients with normal buccal smears had no detectable urinary gonadotropin by rat uterine weight bioassay. Of the four patients studied with at least two-year follow-up (Table 3) only one (patient 6) has subsequehtly gone through pubertal development without additional medication and can be definitely classified as having delayed puberty. The other three did not sustain the clinical changes of puberty that occurred after six weeks of gonadotropin treatment. No consistent response to four days of gonadotropin administration was seen. Only one patient (7) had a definite response in steroid excretion to the initial four days of gonadotropin therapy and this response was augmented after six weeks of gonadotropin administration. Another patient (8) also had increased responsiveness to short-term gonadotropin therapy after six weeks of treatment.

Klinefelter's Syndrome.—Eight patients with chromatin-positive Klinefelter's syndrome were studied (Table 4). Baseline steroid excretion was not significantly different from normal subjects. With stimulation with gonadotropin there was a small increase in testosterone excretion in two patients and in pregnanetriol, androsterone, and etiocholanolone in a third.

Acromegaly.—Data were obtained on seven men with acromegaly of whom four had previously received external radiation treatment (Table 5). Of the five patients stimulated with gonadotropin, one (patient 16) failed to respond. His baseline excretion of 17-ketosteroids and 11-deoxy-17-ketosteroids was considerably higher than that of the normal men. Baseline steroid excretions for the group were not significantly different from normal subjects, but marked variability was seen within the group.

Table 4.—Male Subjects With Klinefelter's Syndrome*

Patient No.	Age (yr)	Study	17OHCS	17KS	P	A	E	D	T
10	23	Baseline	2.4	7.4	0.9				
		Baseline	5.6	7.2	1.5	2.3	2.7	<0.2	61
		HCG, 3rd day	4.2	9.3	1.7				
		HCG, 4th day	4.0	8.8	1.6	2.4	3.5	<0.2	91
11	19	Baseline	4.2	6.5	0.6				
		Baseline	3.6	7.3	0.7	1.7	1.5	0.2	11
		HCG, 3rd day	4.8	7.4	1.5				
		HCG, 4th day	4.6	8.4		2.4	2.1	0.6	36
12	24	Baseline	3.1	7.6	0.2				
		Baseline	5.2	6.3	0.4	3.6	1.0	0.2	
		HCG, 4th day	2.4	7.4	1.0	7.8	3.7	0.4	
13	18	Baseline	9.2	7.1	1.6	3.4	3.8	0.6	85
14	50	Baseline	3.4	5.7	1.6	2.2	1.6	0.2	15
15	20	Baseline	7.7	8.0	3.0	1.6	3.4	0.6	
16	25	Baseline	7.3	9.9	2.2	3.3	3.6	0.6	
17	46	Baseline	7.4	7.7	2.6	0.2	1.8	0.2	
Mean baseline value			5.6	7.5	1.6	2.3	2.3	0.3	43
P (vs normal baseline value)			NS	NS	NS	NS	NS	NS	NS

*17OHCS=17-hydroxycorticosteroids, 17KS=17-ketosteroids, P=pregnanetriol, A=androsterone, E=etiocholanolone, D=dehydroepiandrosterone, T=testosterone, HCG=chorionic gonadotropin, and NS=not significant.

Table 5.—Male Subjects With Acromegaly*

Patient No.	Age (yr)	Study	17OHCS	17KS	P	A	E	D	T
18	38	Baseline	6.4	12.4	2.0	1.6	2.8	<0.2	
		Baseline	9.3	12.5	2.5	3.2	5.3	<0.2	183
		HCG, 3rd day	6.7	17.1	3.2				
		HCG, 4th day	8.1	16.9	2.7	5.1	9.3	0.4	323
19	46	Baseline	5.6	7.7	0.6	2.4	2.8	2.8	90
		Baseline	4.8	6.5	0.8	1.7	2.8		
		HCG, 3rd day	5.2	17.3	4.1	7.8	12.5	2.3	
		HCG, 4th day	6.4	18.9	3.4	7.1	9.6	2.4	426
20	27	Baseline	8.3	23.7	2.7	5.9	10.1	7.8	
		Baseline	7.1	23.9	2.4	5.6	12.0	6.8	80
		HCG, 3rd day	8.6	26.7	3.9	5.9	9.6	5.9	
		HCG, 4th day	7.6	29.4	3.6	7.4	9.9	8.4	115
21	25	Baseline	8.2	24.4	1.6	2.8	4.1	3.0	104
		HCG, 3rd day	10.2	23.7	2.1				
		HCG, 4th day	7.5	44.4	1.9	3.8	9.6	3.8	350
22	35	Baseline	5.2	7.5	1.1	1.5	1.9	0.3	
		Baseline	2.3	6.4	1.1				21
		HCG, 3rd day	5.5	13.0	1.2				
		HCG, 4th day	5.3	11.3	1.8	1.8	3.6	0.2	135
23	51	Baseline	3.1	5.9	1.0	1.2	1.1	0.2	47
24	46	Baseline	6.2	12.6	2.6	1.3	1.5	1.3	78
Mean baseline value			6.1	13.5	1.7	2.4	3.5	2.2	86
P (vs normal baseline value)			NS	NS	NS	NS	NS	NS	NS

*17OHCS=17-hydroxycorticosteroids, 17KS=17-ketosteroids, P=pregnanetriol, A=androsterone, E=etiocholanolone, D=dehydroepiandrosterone, T=testosterone, HCG=chorionic gonadotropin, and NS=not significant.

Comment

The lack of significant change in 17-hydroxycorticosteroids and dehydroepiandrosterone excretion following four days of gonadotropin administration in normal men indicates that gonadotropin has no measureable effect on adrenal steroid secretion in this short period of time in a group in this size. This is in agreement with most previous studies.[1,3] Of the steroids measured, testosterone was the best indicator of Leydig cell response to gonadotropin. Androsterone and etiocholanolone increased to a lesser extent than testosterone but can be used as a good measure of Leydig cell response. Estrogen excretion has also been used to measure the response to gonadotropin[5] but was not measured in these studies.

Short-term administration of gonadotropin has been used by several workers[1,2,6] as a clinical test. In the present study the response to gonadotropin was not a dependable guide for differentiating primary testicular disease from gonadotrophin deficiency. One of four patients with hypopituitarism had no response to gonadotropin. Bardin et al[15] also found variability in the response of plasma testosterone to gonadotropin in hypopituitary patients. The atrophic testes of long-standing hypopituitarism may require much longer periods of gonadotrophin stimulation to increase steroid synthesis and secretion. The variable rise in steroid excretion after gonadotropin administration which was seen in the patients with Klinefelter's syndrome has been observed by others.[5,8] It is not clear why these patients with high gonadotropin excretion can respond to the drug.

The differentiation in hypogonadal boys between delayed puberty and a permanent lack of gonadotropin is a difficult clinical problem. In the small group of patients studied the four days of gonadotropin administration did not prove useful in separating these two types of patients nor did the steroid response to six weeks of gonadotropin therapy. The one patient who later went through pubertal development had no response in steroid excretion to four days or six weeks of gonadotropin administration. Only one of these four patients had a poor testosterone response to gonadotropin as compared to the poor response to gonadotropin found by Bardin et al[15] in patients with hypogonadism and hyposmia.

17-Ketosteroid excretion in acromegaly has been usually reported as normal.[16] Lim and Dingman[17] found that the basal excretion of the individual 11-deoxy-17-ketosteroids was normal in acromegaly. The present study is in accord with those results and with normal basal testosterone excretion in addition. The range of values for these steroids was considerably wider in the patients with acromegaly than in the normal subjects. The values suggest that one of the patients may have partial hypogonadism while others have increased 17-ketosteroid and 11-deoxy-17-ketosteroid excretion. One patient (16) had high 11-deoxy-17-ketosteroid excretion with normal testosterone which suggests an increase primarily in dehydroepiandrosterone and possibly androstenedione secretion of adrenal origin. This is in agreement with the finding of greater than normal increase in 11-deoxy-17-ketosteroids after administration of corticotropin in acromegaly.[17] The response to gonadotropin was similar in these patients to the normal subjects.

Nonproprietary and Trade Names of Drugs

Chorionic gonadotropin—*Antuitrin S, APL, Pregnyl, Follutein.*

Corticotropin—*Actest, Acthar, Actrope, Cortigel, Cortrophin, Depo-Acth, Duracton.*

References

1. Hibbitt LL, Starnes WR, Hill SR Jr: Studies in man on testicular and adrenal response to adrenocorticotrophin and human chorionic gonadotrophin. *J Clin Endocr* **18**:1315-1332, 1958.
2. Stuiver PC, Thijssen JHH, van der Molen HJ: Plasma testosterone, urinary excretion of 17-ketosteroids fractions and urinary total 17-ketosteroids before, during, and after stimulation with HCG in patients with deficient testicular function, in Vermeulin A (ed): *Androgens in Normal and Pathological Conditions.* Amsterdam, Excerpta Medica, 1966, p 87.
3. Cleveland WW, Ahmad N, Sandberg DH, et al: Excretion of testosterone and 17-ketosteroids following administration of HCG and ACTH to normal adult males. *Steroids* **8**:149-156, 1966.
4. Landau RL, Laves ML: Urinary pregnanetriol of testicular origin. *J Clin Endocr* **19**:1399-1404, 1959.
5. Paulsen CA: Hypogonadism (Klinefelter's syndrome)—Leydig cell function: Effect of chorionic gonadotrophin, in Paulsen CA (ed): *Estrogen Assays in Clinical Medicine.* Seattle, University of Washington Press, 1965, p 274.
6. Futterweit W, Freeman R, Siegel GL, et al: Measurement of urinary testosterone and epitestosterone glucuronide as a test of gonadal reserve. *Fertil Steril* **18**:659-665, 1967.
7. Guerra-Garcia R, Velasquez A, Coyotupa J: A test of endocrine gonadal function in men: Urinary testosterone after the injection of HCG: II. A different response of the high altitude native. *J Clin Endocr* **29**:179-182, 1969.
8. Lipsett MB, Wilson H, Kirschner MA, et al: Studies on Leydig cell physiology and pathology: Secretion and metabolism of testosterone. *Recent Progr Hormone Res* **22**:245-281, 1966.
9. Peterson RE, Wyngaarden JB, Guerra SL, et al: The physiology disposition and metabolic fate of hydrocortisone in man. *J Clin Invest* **34**:1779-1794, 1955.
10. Drekter IJ, Pearson S, Bartczak E, et al: A rapid method for the determination of total urinary 17-ketosteroids. *J Clin Endocr* **7**:795-800, 1947.
11. Bongiovanni AM, Eberlein WR: Critical analysis of methods for measurement of pregnane-3-alpha, 17-alpha, 20-alpha triol in human urine. *Anal Chem* **30**:388-393, 1958.
12. Kirschner MA, Lipsett MB: Gas-liquid chromatography in the quantitative analysis of urinary 11-deoxy-17-ketosteroids. *J Clin Endocr* **23**:255-260, 1963.
13. Kliman B, Peterson RE: Double isotope derivative assay of aldosterone in biological extracts. *J Biol Chem* **235**:1639-1648, 1960.
14. Steel RGD, Torrie JH: *Principles and Procedures of Statistics.* New York, McGraw Hill Book Co Inc, 1960.
15. Bardin CW, Ross GT: Rifkind AB, et al: Studies of the pituitary-Leydig cell axis in young men, prepuberal boys and hypopituitary patients. *J Clin Invest* **48**:2046-2056, 1969.
16. Hamwi GJ, Skillman TG, Tufts KC Jr: Acromegaly. *Amer J Med* **29**:690-699, 1960.
17. Lim NY, Dingman JF: Androgenic adrenal hyperfunction in acromegaly. *New Eng J Med* **271**:1189-1194, 1964.

Effect of Azathioprine on Renal Histology and Function in Lupus Nephritis

Weldon D. Shelp, MD; J. M. B. Bloodworth, Jr., MD; and Richard E. Rieselbach, MD, Madison, Wis

The effectiveness of azathioprine was assessed in a longitudinal study of 12 selected patients with varying degrees of lupus nephritis. All had substantial histological evidence of disease (five with lupus glomerulitis and seven with lupus glomerulonephritis), and eight had an initial glomerular filtration rate of less than 80 ml/min 1.73 sq m. Clinical improvement or stability was observed in all patients and confirmed by serial renal clearance studies and protein excretion rates. Histologic evidence of acute glomerular involvement diminished in all patients, in association with the evolution of glomerulosclerosis. Seven patients were able to discontinue corticosteroids without clinical deterioration. Eight patients with initial renal insufficiency remained clinically stable with a mean survival of 32.5 months. Thus, azathioprine appears to offer considerable therapeutic benefit to selected patients with lupus nephritis.

Approximately 50% of patients with systemic lupus erythematosus (SLE) develop clinical evidence of renal disease, and about half of these succumb to uremia resulting from lupus nephritis (LN).[1] Considerable controversy exists concerning the efficacy of therapeutic measures directed against LN. One school believes that corticosteroid treatment sufficient to control the systemic manifestations of SLE prevents progression of LN in most instances.[2] In contrast, others contend that selected patients with severe LN benefit from a course of high-dose corticosteroid therapy with respect to prolongation of survival, particularly when renal failure is not advanced.[3] That steroid medication administered in such fashion frequently results in serious and at times fatal complications is well known, and has prompted the search for less toxic and hopefully more effective modalities of LN therapy.

It is now apparent that the natural history of LN may be divided into three clinical and histological entities.[4] Patients with focal or lupus glomerulitis (LG) rarely develop renal insufficiency or the nephrotic syndrome and the lesion does not appear to be altered by immunosuppressive therapy. Subjects with membranous glomerulonephritis commonly manifest the nephrotic syndrome and may gradually develop renal failure but active or diffuse glomerulonephritis does not supervene, nor is the lesion apparently responsive to immunosuppressive therapy. The final category, diffuse lupus glomerulonephritis (LGN), commonly progresses to renal failure, and is the group to which therapeutic attention has been and should be directed.[3,4]

The present study was conducted to elucidate and compare the effect of azathioprine on renal histology and function in patients with LG or LGN.

Material and Methods

The study population consisted of ten women and two men, all white, ranging in age from 12 to 45 years at the time azathioprine therapy was started. The diagnosis of SLE was substantiated in all patients by the presence of a positive lupus erythematosus (LE) preparation and in some instances a positive antinuclear antibody titer early in their clinical course. Initially, none of the patients manifested severe renal insufficiency (glomerular filtration rate [GFR] < 20 ml/min), but eight of the 12 demonstrated moderate renal insufficiency, arbitrarily define as a GFR of < 80 ml/min/1.73 sq m.

A summary of pertinent clinical observations at the time azathioprine therapy was initiated is presented in Table 1. With two exceptions, all patients had clinical evidence of SLE for at least six months prior to initiating azathioprine therapy. Five of the 12 patients demonstrated persistent renal disease activity with the concomitant development of significant toxic reaction to steroids while receiving 30 to 60 mg of prednisone per day for at least one month. (Patient 3 had received 40 mg of prednisone daily for six months; the dose had been tapered to 12.5 mg at the time of initial evaluation). Two of the patients developed severe steroid toxic reaction (toxic psychosis in patient 7 and debilitating steroid myopathy in patient 10), necessitating a reduction in steroid dosage in the presence of active renal disease and moderate renal insufficiency.

The remaining five patients were judged to be poor candidates for prolonged treatment with high dosage of steroids, either because of emotional lability (patients 9, 2, and 1), or significant diastolic hypertension (patient 4). Although a diagnosis of LG was made in the case of patient 5, she required 30 mg of prednisone daily for control of anemia and leukopenia and was manifesting significant toxic reaction to corticosteroids, leading to the decision to initiate azathioprine therapy as a substitute for corticosteroids, primarily in an attempt at hematological control, with the assessment of its effect on renal function and structure being of secondary importance.

With the exception of patient 12, who was considered too ill to tolerate the procedure at the onset of his therapeutic trail, percutaneous renal biopsies were obtained according to the procedure of Kark and Muehrcke[5] within two weeks of the initiation of azathioprine therapy.

Renal biopsy tissue was divided into two

Received for publication April 23, 1970; accepted Jan 15, 1971.

From the departments of medicine (Drs. Shelp and Rieselbach) and pathology (Dr. Bloodworth), University of Wisconsin Medical School, Madison.

Reprint requests to 1300 University Ave, Madison, Wis 53706 (Dr. Shelp).

Table 1.—Clinical and Therapeutic Data of Patients With Lupus Nephritis

		At Time Azathioprine Was Started								
Patient	Sex	Duration SLE*	Age	Chief Manifestations	Renal Histology	Prednisone Dose (mo)	Azathioprine Indications	Azathioprine (mg/kg/Day)	Prednisone Stopped (Daily Dose)	Azathioprine Therapy (mo)
1	F	6 yr	24	Dermatitis	LG	45 mg(¼)	c	2.0	Yes	27
2	F	5 mo	15	Dermatitis, myalgia	LG	40 mg(2)	c	3.0	No (15 mg)	26
3	M	5 yr	14	Proteinuria, hematuria	LG	12.5 mg(2)	a	2.5	No (7.5 mg)	14
4	F	10 mo	32	Peritonitis	LG	30 mg(1)	c	2.0	Yes	15
5	F	5 mo	17	Anemia, arthralgia	LG	30 mg(1)	c	1.0-3.0	Yes	14
6	F	6 yr	20	Hypertension, edema	LGN	60 mg(2)	a	2.0	Yes	1 15 2 21
7	F	7 yr	28	Edema	LGN	60 mg(2)	b	2.0	Yes	43
8	F	7 yr	43	Edema	LGN	40 mg(1)	a	1.5	No (5 mg)	36
9	F	5 yr	45	Edema, hematuria	LGN	10 mg(6)	c	1.0-2.0	No (10 mg)	28
10	F	7 yr	26	Steroid myopathy, myocarditis	LGN	90 mg(1)	b	2.5	Yes	24
11	F	1 yr	12	Dermatitis, hematuria	LGN	30 mg(3)	a	2.0	No (10 mg)	34
12	M	19 mo	16	Edema, hematuria	LGN	40 mg(2)	a	3.0	Yes	21

* SLE signifies systemic lupus erythematosus; LG, lupus glomerulitis; LGN, lupus glomerulonephritis; a, LN resistant to high dose steroids; b, proven intolerance to high dose steroids; and c, projected intolerance to high dose steroids.

Table 2.—Longitudinal Graded Renal Histologic Changes Observed During Courses of Azathioprine Therapy

Patient	Azathioprine Treatment (mo)	C_{IN}* (ml/min)	Intrinsic Cell Proliferation	Polymorphonuclear Leukocyte Infiltration	Crescents	Osmiophilic Deposits (EM)	Glomerulosclerosis
1	0	79.3	++†	++	+	+	+
	4	71.6	++	+	+	+	+
	9	83.3	+	0	0		
2	0	65.3	++	0	0	+	++
	4	110.0‡	+	0	0	+	+
	13	114.0	+	0	0	0	0
3	0	91.1	+++	+	0	++	++
	6	73.4	+++	0	0	+++	++
	12	87.8	++	0	0	+++	++
4	0	86.0‡	++	+	0	++	+
	7	79.5	++	+	0	+	++
5	0	80.0‡	+++	0	0	+++	+
	8	110.0	++	0	0	+	+
	11	103.0	++	0	0	+	++
6	0	54.0‡	++	++	+	+++	++
	7	60.7	+	+	0	+	+
	13	61.9	+	0	0	+	+
	31	57.9	++		0	+	++
7	0	63.0‡	+++	+	0	+++	+++
	4	82.2	++	+	0	+	++
	10	128.0	++	0	0	+	+++
	17	102.0	+	0	0	+	++++
8	0	38.7	++	+	0	+++	0
	5	53.9	++	0	0	+++	+
	17	75.2	++	0	0	+++	+
	29	81.2	+	0	0	++	+
9	0	62.1	++	+	0	+++	++
	5	51.8	++	+	0	+++	++
	11	40.8	+	0		+	+++
10	0	59.4	+	+	0	+	++
	11	56.2	0	0	0	0	+
11	0	64.0	+++	+	+	+	+
	7	79.3	++	0	0	++	++
	25	80.7	++	+	0	+++	+++
12	7	47.4	++	0	0	+	+++
	12	45.2	++	0	0	+	++++

* C_{IN} signifies inulin clearance.
† Changes were classified on a scale of + to ++++. For details, see text (results).
‡ 12 or 24 hour creatinine clearance.

portions. The first portion was diced into 1 mm cubes and fixed either for one hour in osmium tetroxide or overnight in glutaraldehyde. Glutaraldehye-fixed tissues were postfixed in osmium tetroxide. These blocks were dehydrated, embedded in Epon 812 according to the method of Craig et al,[6] sectioned on an ultramicrotome, and examined in an electron microscope. The second portion was fixed in 10% buffered neutral formaldehyde solution, embedded in paraffin, and stained with hematoxylin-eosin, trichrome, and PAS techniques. The paraffin sections were cut at 3μ thickness, as well as the conventional 6μ to 8μ thickness.

Within two weeks of biopsy, voiding renal clearance studies were performed following ingestion of a water load calculated to assure urine flows of 5 to 10 ml/min. All medications except steroids were withheld at least 24 hours prior to study. Following an appropriate priming dose of inulin and aminohippurate sodium (PAH), a sustaining infusion of these substances in normal saline was initated at a rate of 5 ml/min. Following a 40 to 50 minute equilibration period, three to five 20 to 30 minute urine collections with midpoint venous blood samples were obtained. Urine volume was not precisely replaced. Patients remained at bed rest except to void. Standard formulas were used to calculate the clearance of inulin ($C_{IN} = U_{IN} \times V/P_{IN}$) and aminophippurate ($C_{PAH} = U_{PAH} \times V/P_{PAH}$) in milliliters per minute and filtration fraction ($FF = C_{IN}/C_{PAH} \times 100$). Since several subjects were edematous at the time of study, values obtained were not corrected for body surface area; however, these data are included in the table for reference. Inulin was determined by the method of Roe et al[7] and PAH by the method adopted for the multichannel blood analyzer.[8] In five subjects the initial glomerular filtration rate was estimated by 24-hour endogenous creatinine clearance. Quantitative urine protein was estimated by the sulfosalicylic acid technique. Routine studies were performed in the clinical laboratories.

Following the initial renal biopsy and clearance studies, and complete hematologic studies including hematocrit, hemoglobin, leukocyte count with differential cell count, platelet count, and reticulocyte count, therapy with azathioprine at a dose between 1 and 3 mg/kg of body weight was begun. Prednisone dosage was maintained at admission levels (Table 1) for three to six weeks and then gradually tapered by approximately 5 mg every two weeks. During this time the patients were followed-up at weekly intervals with a careful clinical assessment, hemogram, and urinalysis. Renal biopsies and function studies were repeated at 3- to 12-month intervals depending on the clinical course. Follow-up visits for purpose of the study were terminated as of September 1969.

Table 3.—Longitudinal Renal Function Studies During Courses of Azathioprine

Patient	Time After Starting Azathioprine (mo)	Body Surface Area (sq m)	C_{IN}* (ml/min)	C_{PAH} (ml/min)	FF(%)	Protein Excretion (gm/24 hr)
1	0	1.39	79.3	479	16.50	8.70
	4	1.47	71.6	528	13.60	5.40
	9	1.47	83.8	575	14.60	1.20
	21	1.46	90.6	598	15.20	0.60
2	0	1.43	65.3	475	13.70	1.40
	4	1.53	110.0†	...	...	0.00
	13	1.47	114.0	637	17.90	0.00
3	0	1.33	91.1	697	13.20	3.00
	6	1.34	73.4	796	9.22	2.50
	9	1.39	78.4	577	13.60	2.60
	12	1.37	87.8	717	12.20	2.00
4	0	1.88‡	86.0†	...	...	1.00
	1	1.83	80.4	559	14.50	1.70
	7	1.98	79.5	754	10.50	0.40
	13	1.93	94.5	510	18.50	0.40
5	0	1.67	80.0†	...	...	0.30
	3	1.73	87.2	602	14.70	0.90
	8	1.68	110.0	667	16.20	0.00
	11	1.68	103.0	592	17.40	0.00
6	0	1.54‡	54.0†	...	...	1.30
	7	1.63	60.7	327	18.60	0.20
	13	1.67	61.9	385	16.10	0.15
	31	1.65	57.9	447	13.00	0.50
7	0	1.52‡	63.0†	...	...	4.00
	4	1.58	82.2	397	20.70	1.50
	10	1.57	128.0	...	...	3.40
	17	1.60	102.0	543	18.90	3.20
	29	1.60	100.0	479	21.30	3.50
	41	1.60	94.2	358	26.30	2.00
8	0	1.56‡	38.7	566	6.83	11.30
	5	1.61	53.9	...	...	3.30
	11	1.64	69.5	557	12.50	0.40
	17	1.66	75.2	616	12.50	...
	29	1.67	81.2	497	16.30	0.14
9	0	1.66	62.1	493	8.06	0.60
	5	1.66	51.8	440	11.80	5.40
	11	1.72	40.8	379	10.80	1.80
	23	1.75	63.8	290	22.00	0.60
10	0	1.32	59.4	209	28.50	1.10
	5	1.37	74.2	262	28.30	0.60
	11	1.36	56.2	258	21.80	0.00
11	0	1.56‡	64.0	718	8.91	6.00
	7	1.55	79.3	671	11.90	...
	25	1.62	80.7	593	13.60	1.20
12	0	1.67‡	27.0†	...	...	4.00
	7	1.55	47.4	311	15.20	7.00
	12	1.53	45.2	359	12.60	4.80

* C_{IN} signifies inulin clearance; C_{PAH}, p-aminohippuric acid clearance; and FF, filtration fraction.

† 12 or 24-hour creatinine clearance.

‡ Edematous at time of study.

Results

Histopathologic and Electron Microscopic Findings.—Table 2 presents in tabular form the renal histologic changes present in each case prior to

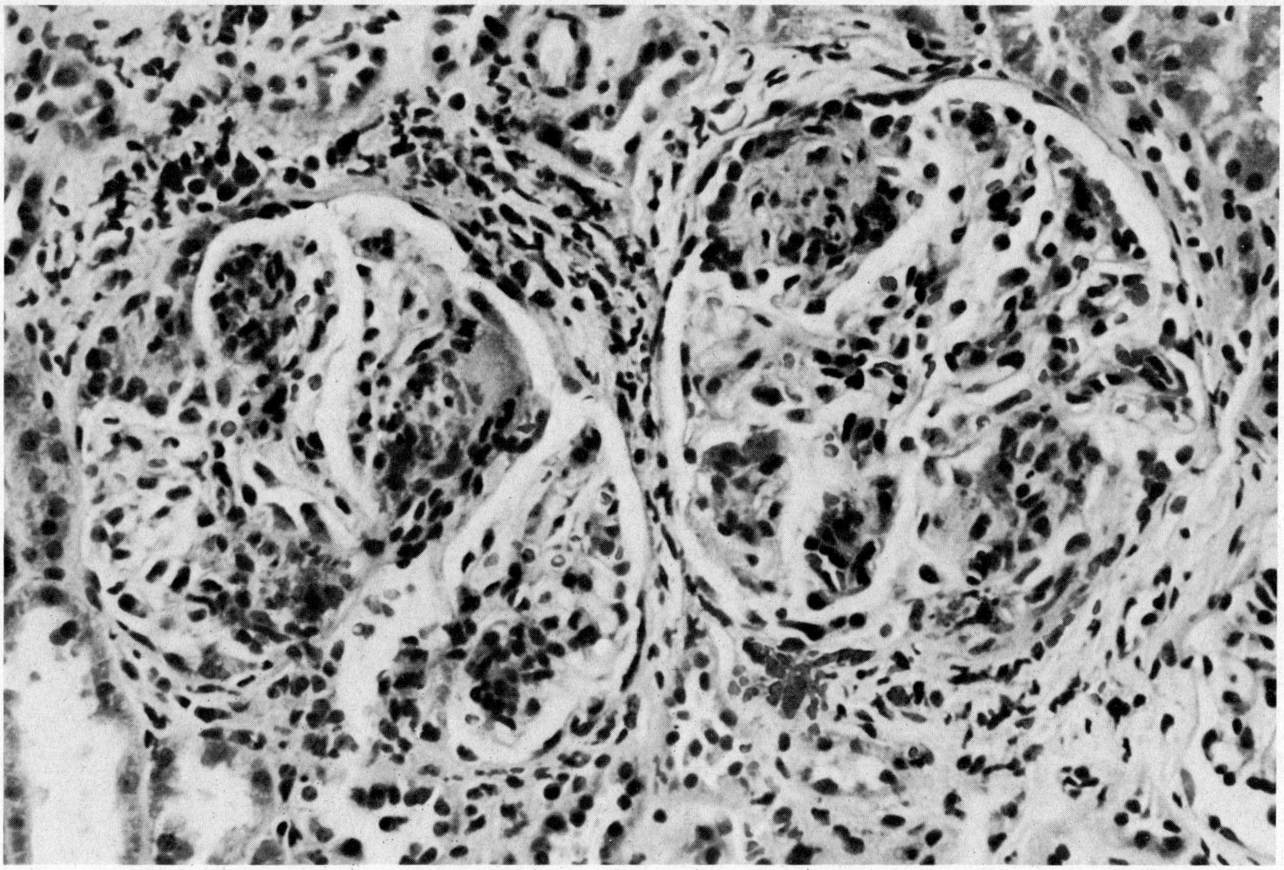

Fig 1.—Light micrograph of glomeruli from patient 11 prior to azathioprine treatment. Note nodules of proliferating intrinsic cells, trapped polymorphonuclear leukocytes, and nuclear debris from degenerating cells. Interstitial acute and chronic inflammation is also evident.

Fig 2.—Light micrograph of a glomerulus from patient 11 prior to azathioprine treatment. N *represents a typical nodule of proliferated intrinsic cells, with fragmentation of nuclei. Note the epithelial crescent* (arrow) *with adjacent acute and chronic inflammatory cells.*

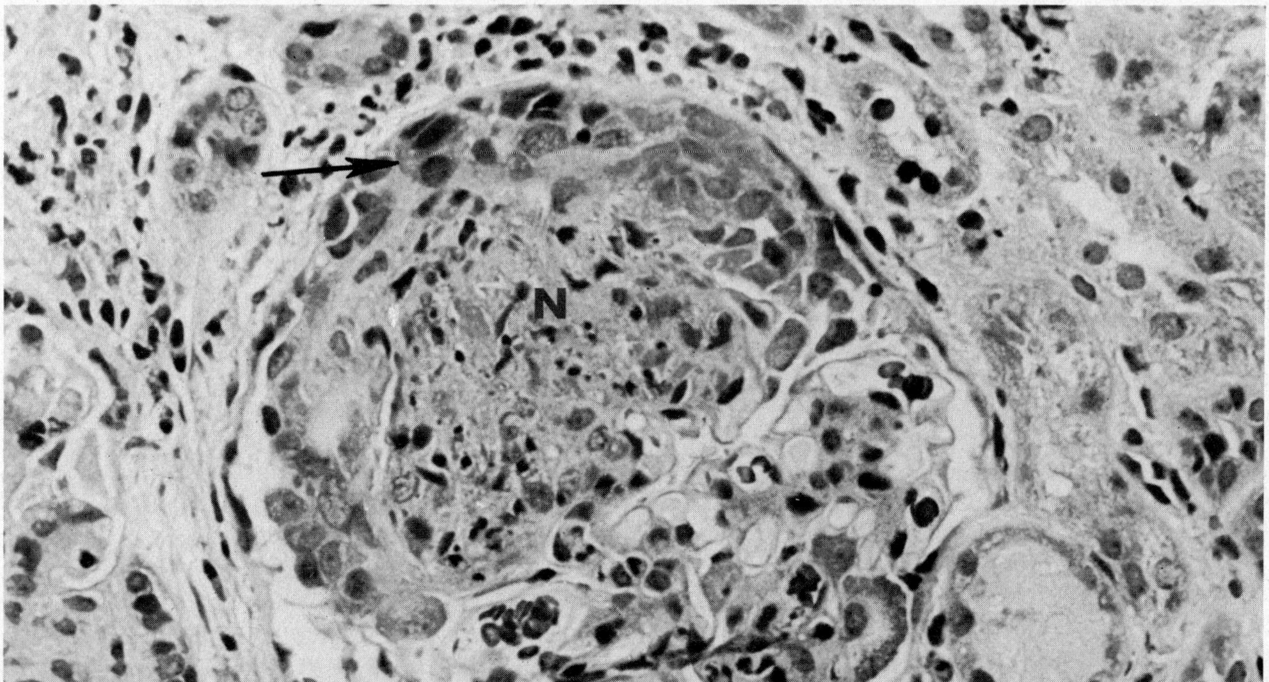

azathioprine therapy and the course following initiation of this therapy. Also included are the concomitant GFRs. Column 4 is an evaluation of the intrinsic cell proliferation based on a scale of + to + + + +. Column 5 lists the degree of polymorphonuclear leukocyte infiltration, again on a scale of + to + + + +. In both columns 4 and 5, a + + + + finding would indicate that there was a massive filling-up of the glomerulus by the cell type involved. Column 7 indicates the degree of osmiophilic granular deposits, as visualized by electron microscopy, on a scale of + to + + + +. A + + + + listing would indicate that massive involvement of almost all capillary loops was present sufficient to give a light microscopic appearance of a "wire loop." Column 8 lists the degree of glomerulosclerosis, on a + to + + + + scale, + + + + indicating essentially complete obliteration of the glomerulus (hyaline ball) with absence of capillary blood flow.

The progressive histologic changes are well represented by patient 11 (Fig 1-5) who over a period of 25 months demonstrates a diminution of findings suggestive of acute glomerular disease, with resolution of deposits and some increase in glomerulosclerosis.

Renal Function Studies.—A summary of these results is presented in Table 3. Glomerular filtration rates remained stable or improved in all patients during the observation period. Effective renal plasma flow (RPF), although showing a wider variance, in general paralleled changes in GFR. In this regard an almost uniform finding (10 of 12 subjects) was a relatively elevated RPF when compared to GFR, resulting in a filtration faction less than normal. Although unpredictable, this factor tended to improve with therapy.

Protein excretion appeared to decrease significantly in eight patients and remained unchanged in four. This improvement is emphasized by the fact that all eight patients did so despite a corresponding stable or improving GFR. One of the subjects with stable protein excretion rates (patient 7) manifested subsequent GFRs higher than baseline determinations; this could be interpreted as a relative decrease in protein filtration and excretion per nephron. However, since protein excretion rates from the diseased kidney vary considerably from day to day, and since sequential 24-hour collections were not obtained in any subject conclusions relative to these data must be tentative.

Complications Observed During Azathioprine Administration.—Patient 10 experienced fever following pelvic surgery while receiving only azathioprine. Steroids were administered parenterally during surgery because of a history of adrenal insufficiency ten months previously. This therapy was continued because of the suspicion that the fever was due to SLE. However, defervescence occurred following antimicrobial therapy for a urinary tract infection. At the time of last follow-up, patient 10 was receiving azathioprine alone without symptoms.

Patient 2 developed oral moniliasis 20 months after starting therapy with azathioprine; prednisone had been discontinued 17 months previously. Treatment with azathioprine was discontinued and oral therapy with nystatin (Mycostatin) begun. However, the moniliasis progressed to include esophagitis, and in three weeks florid SLE became apparent, with dermatitis, myositis, myocarditis, pleuritis, seizures, proteinuria, hematuria, and conversion to positive LE preparations. Therapy with prednisone and azathioprine was reinstituted, and following a very stormy six weeks of hospitalization, she again developed partial remission. Prednisone (10 to 15 mg/day) is still required to control systemic manifestations of SLE, primarily arthritis and dermatitis.

Patients 6, 9, 4, and 5 have experienced significant leukopenia (white blood cell count [WBC] 4,000/cu mm) at some period during azathioprine therapy. This promptly responded to reduction in dosage, although at times it has been difficult to differentiate drug-induced leukopenia from that related to SLE. Patient 5 demonstrated leukopenia (range, 3.1 to 3.8×10^3/cu mm) at time of diagnosis which improved to normal range while she was receiving 30 mg prednisone per day for three months. Following cessation of steroid therapy, the leukocyte count decreased to a low of 2.3×10^3/cu mm accompanied by a normal differential cell count. Azathioprine therapy was discontinued for one month with return of leukocyte counts to normal range. At present, she is receiving azathioprine, 2 mg/kg per day, without complications.

Patient 6 developed daily fever of 104 F (40.0 C), chills, and malaise after receiving azathioprine for 15 months. Extensive studies failed to determine an etiology and LE preparations were negative. Fever disappeared by lysis, but because of leukopenia of 1.8×10^3/cu mm and platelet count of 22×10^3/cu mm, azathioprine therapy was discontinued for a period of 12 months, when obvious evidence of SLE recurred. Remission again occurred with 2 mg/kg of azathioprine and 10 mg of prednisone per day; the latter was discontinued in six months without

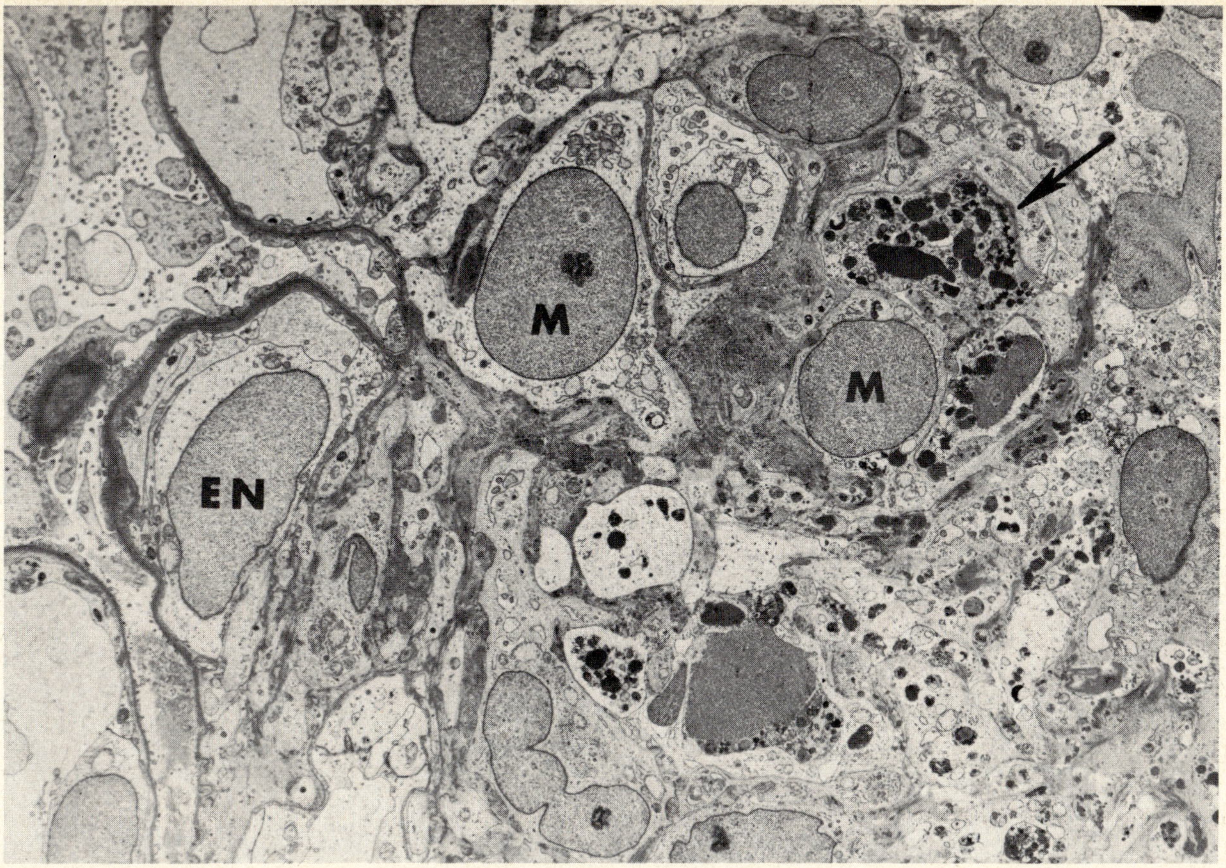

Fig 3.—Electron micrograph of a glomerulus from patient 11 before azathioprine therapy. Mesangial (M), *epithelial, and endothelial* (EN) *cells are increased in number. Trapped polymorphonuclear leukocytes* (arrow) *contain black granules representing nuclear debris related to degeneration (×3,400).*

Fig 4.—Light micrograph of a glomerulus from patient 11 after 25 months of azathioprine treatment. As compared to Fig 1 and 2, intrinsic cells appear normal in number. The mesangium (M) *appears increased and adhesions are present* (arrows) *(PAS stain, ×700).*

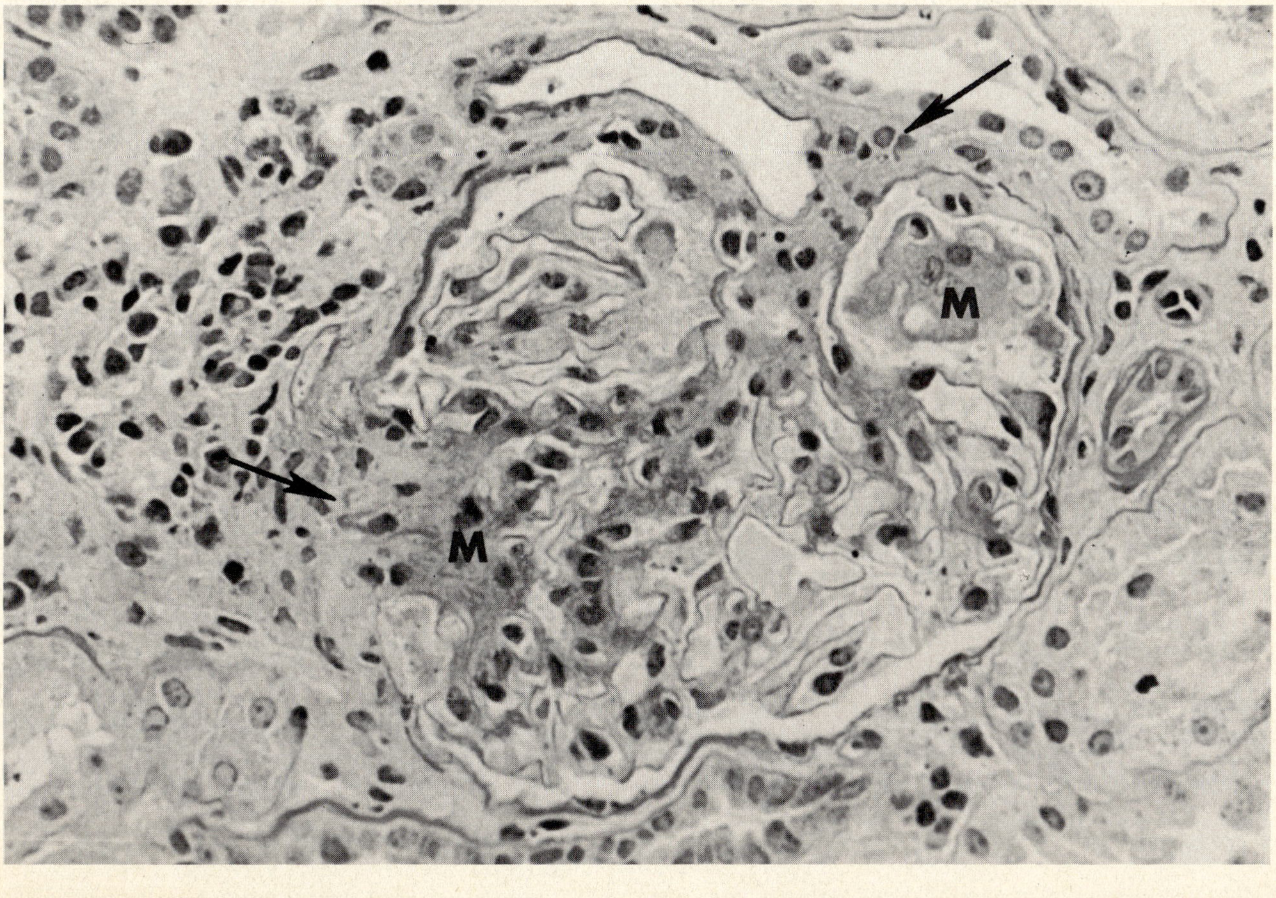

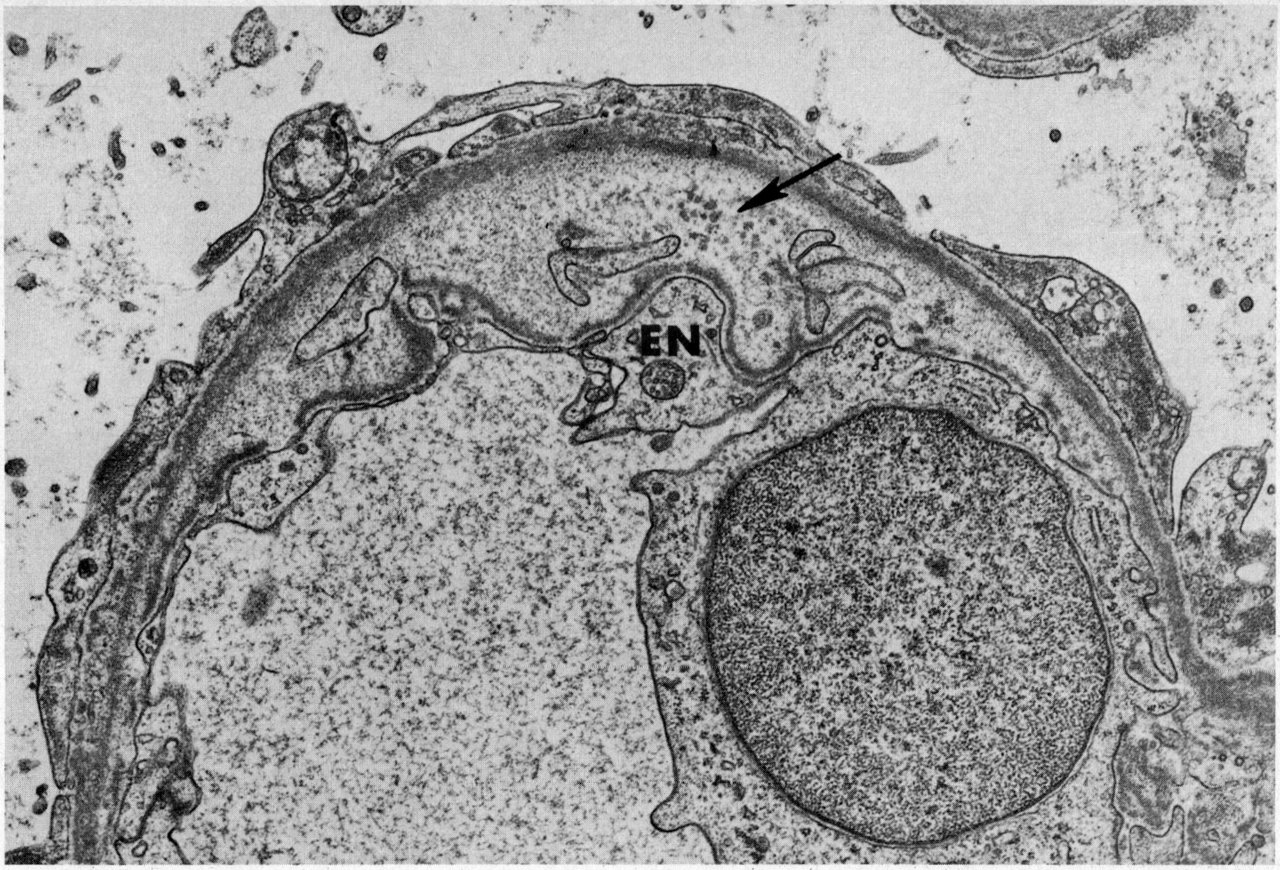

Fig 5.—Electron micrograph of a glomerular capillary loop from patient 11 after seven months of azathioprine therapy. Subendothelial granular deposits are undergoing resolution, with clumping (arrow). *Note new basement membrane formation adjacent to the endothelial cell* (EN) *(X14,600).*

evidence of relapse. Patients 6, 7, and 12 developed herpes zoster 1, 9, and 11 months, respectively, after initiating azathioprine therapy. Patient 7 developed herpes zoster ophthalmocus of the right eye with trigeminal nerve involvement. Azathioprine was continued at the same dosage, and she responded to topical steroid and mydriatic therapy with complete resolution. The other two patients had thoracic wall involvement which resolved without change in medication. Patient 9 has had recurrent urinary tract infections, due to *Escherichia coli*, which responded satisfactorily to appropriate antimicrobial therapy.

There have been no instances of mouth ulceration or gastrointestinal symptoms during the therapeutic trials.

Comment

Students of SLE are in near unanimous agreement concerning the difficulty in evaluating the therapy of a chronic, spontaneously remitting disease such as SLE. The excellent study of Zweimen et al underscores this point well.[9] Their results would suggest that the clinical course of the majority of LN patients is quite unpredictable and, in general, appears not to be influenced by duration or quantity of corticosteroid therapy. If these conclusions are correct, it would appear to be extremely difficult, if not impossible, to design a properly controlled therapeutic study of SLE with LN.

The authors are well aware of the deficiencies of this study, particularly in regard to the absence of a well matched control group receiving either placebo or corticosteroids alone. We are also aware of the significant differences of opinion on the part of pathologists attempting to analyze renal biopsy specimens. It was unfortunate that it was not possible to perform sequential immunofluorescent studies of the biopsy specimens, a technique that was not available to us at the initiation of the study. Because of the availability of electron microscopy for the majority of biopsy specimens, which can define the presence or absence of nonspecific immune deposits, we chose not to add the immunofluorescent technique to the protocol.

Finally, one might question the desirability of including alterations in quantitative measurements of immune globulins and complement during azathioprine therapy. These determinations, along with serial LE preparations, were performed on several of the patients, but it was not possible to correlate the degree of histologic disease activity and alterations in renal function with changes in the aforementioned serologic indices.

This study differs from those previously reported in that a comparison of alterations in renal structure and function observed during a specified azathioprine trial period has been made between patients with LG and those with LGN.[10-12]

Patients 1, 2, 3, 4, and 5 would appear to satisfy the criteria of LG with essentially normal renal function. Although Patient 2 had a significantly depressed GFR initially, this was probably related to acute glomerulitis, subsequent histologic studies showed minimal focal involvement of glomeruli, and the GFR returned to normal. These subjects have received azathioprine for a mean of 19.2 months. Protein excretion has decreased or remained stable in all, renal function has remained stable, and histologic changes have suggested a decrease in disease activity. Patients 2 and 3 appear to require prednisone for control of arthralgias and dermatologic manifestations of SLE.

The remaining seven patients appear to fulfill the criteria for LGN with renal functional impairment. They have received azathioprine an average of 32 months and have survived a mean of 33 months. Renal function has remained stable or, in the cases of patients 7 and 8, has significantly improved. At the time of initial study, contraction of the intravascular volume was present in five patients due to hypovolemia related to the nephrotic syndrome. Therefore, observed improvement in GFR may have been influenced by restoration of blood volume due to amelioration of the nephrotic syndrome. The depressed filtration fraction was considered to be compatible with significant glomerular pathology resulting in impaired filtration across the capillary basement membrane in the absence of significant intrarenal vascular disease. It is of interest that the two patients with consistently normal or elevated filtration fractions (patients 7 and 10) demonstrated significant renal arteriolar disease on serial histologic examination.

The degree of histological disease activity in LGN patients has decreased or remained stable, although glomerulosclerosis has tended to progress. Protein excretion has stabilized or decreased in all except patient 12. Three of the subjects require small doses of prednisone for control of systemic manifestation of SLE, primarily arthralgias.

These results compare very favorably with those described by Pollack et al for a much larger series of patients with LGN who arbitrarily received high doses of prednisone for an average of six months.[4] Fourteen of 31 patients were alive an average of 31 months following initiation of treatment and only 1 was in renal failure. The majority of the renal deaths occurred within the first six months of treatment, suggesting that renal failure was more advanced in a significant number of Pollack's series as compared to these patients, with the possible exception of patient 12.

It is not our intent to offer azathioprine as a superior therapeutic approach for all patients with SLE and LN, particularly in view of the disturbing reports of lymphoproliferative disorders developing in transplantation recipients receiving long-term azathioprine.[13] However, the results of this study do suggest that carefully selected SLE patients with significant renal involvement may achieve histological, functional, and clinical stability with this mode of therapy at least comparable to that achieved with large doses of corticosteroids. In terms of patient acceptance and degree of toxic reaction azathioprine appears to be more satisfactory than corticosteroids. Only a longer treatment period with a larger number of patients possibly studied in a controlled manner will establish the ultimate role of azathioprine in the therapy of lupus nephritis.

This study was supported in part by Public Health Service grants AM-05630, AM-09659, AM-09943-03, and FR 5435-05. Additional support was provided by the Wisconsin Heart Association and Veterans Administration. Dr. Rieselbach was supported by Public Health Service career development award 1KO4AM18231 and is a Markle Scholar in Academic Medicine.

Azathioprine was supplied as Imuran through Peter Mawdsley, MD, of Burroughs Wellcome & Co., Inc.

Nonproprietary and Trade Names of Drugs

Azathioprine—*Imuran.*

References

1. Dubois E: *Lupus Erythematosus.* New York, McGraw-Hill Book Co Inc, 1966, p 135.
2. Rothfield NF, McCluskey RT, Baldwin DS: Renal disease in systemic lupus erythematosus. *New Eng J Med* **269**:537-544, 1963.
3. Pollack VE, Pirani CL, Kark RM: Effect of large doses of prednisone on the renal lesions and of life span of patients with lupus glomerulonephritis. *J Lab Clin Med* **57**:495-511, 1961.
4. Pollack VE, Pirani CL, Schwartz FD: The natural history of the renal manifestations of systemic lupus erythematosus. *J Lab Clin Med* **63**:537-550, 1964.
5. Kark RM, Muehrcke RC: Biopsy of kidney in prone position. *Lancet* **1**:1047-1049, 1954.
6. Craig EL, Frajola WJ, Greider MH: An embedding technique for electron microscopy using Epon 812. *J Cell Biol* **12**:190-194, 1962.
7. Roe JH, Epstein JH, Goldstein NP: A photometric method for the determination of inulin in plasma and urine. *J Biol Chem* **178**:839-845, 1949.
8. Harvey RB, Brother AJ: Renal extraction of para-aminohippurate and creatinine measured by continuous in vivo sampling of arterial and renal vein blood. *Ann NY Acad Sci* **102**:46-54, 1962.
9. Zweiman BZ, Korblum J, Cornog J, et al: The prognosis of lupus nephritis. *Ann Intern Med* **69**:441-462, 1968.
10. Corley CC, Lessner HE, Larsen WE: Azathioprine therapy of "autoimmune" diseases. *Amer J Med* **41**:404-412, 1966.
11. Adams DA, Gordon A, Maxwell MH: Azathioprine treatment of immunological renal disease. *JAMA* **199**:459-463, 1967.
12. Maher JF, Schreiner GE: Treatment of lupus nephritis with azathioprine. *Arch Intern Med* **125**:293-298, 1970.
13. Immunosuppression and cancer, editorial. *Lancet* **1**:505-506, 1969.

Nerve Conduction Velocity in the Assessment of Hypertension

Reuven J. Viskoper, MD; Joshua Chaco, MD;
and Alexander Aviram, MD, Jerusalem, Israel

Motor nerve conduction velocity was measured in 52 hypertensive and 10 control subjects. Reduction of nerve conduction velocity paralleled elevation of blood pressure and retinal changes. No correlation was found between nerve conduction velocity and the duration of hypertension. Nerve conduction velocity can provide us with an objective measurable index of the severity of hypertension.

Peripheral neuropathy may accompany a number of diseases of varying etiology. It is noted frequently in diabetes mellitus, uremia, and malignant tumors. Measurements of motor nerve conduction velocities in these conditions revealed that a functional conduction defect may precede the overt clinical manifestations of peripheral neuropathy.[1] Reduced motor nerve conduction velocity is therefore an early indicator of subclinical nerve involvement. The exact nature and pathogenesis of the neural lesions is unknown. There is, however, some evidence, derived mainly from studies in diabetes, which suggests that degenerative vascular changes in the vasa nervorum may be responsible for the neuropathy.[2] As these changes reflect the more generalized proneness of the diabetic vascular system to atherosclerosis, it was reasonable to expect peripheral neuropathy also in hypertension, another condition which intensifies atherogenesis. A case of clinical neuropathy attributed to hypertension was recently described by Popovtzer et al,[3] and in preliminary studies we found reduced motor nerve conduction velocity in hypertensive patients.

In the present study an attempt is made to correlate the reduction in motor nerve conduction and the severity of the hypertensive disease, as judged by the more conventional indexes, such as the level of blood pressure and retinal changes.

Received for publication Oct 8, 1970; accepted Feb 8, 1971.

From the Nephrological Service and the Department of Physical Medicine, Hadassah University Hospital, Jerusalem, Israel.

Reprint requests to Nephrological Service, Hadassah University Hospital, Jerusalem, Israel (Dr. Viskoper).

Material and Methods

The study group included 52 patients (33 men and 19 women), aged 41 to 66 years, with established essential hypertension. In all of them the diastolic blood pressure was higher than 100 mm Hg on repeated occasions. Routine clinical and laboratory examinations excluded diabetes mellitus, renal insufficiency, and neurologic disorders. The peripheral pulses were normal and the vessel walls not obviously arteriosclerotic on palpation. All but three of the patients were being treated with methyldopa and chlorothiazide.

Measurements of motor nerve conduction velocity of the right ulnar and left median nerves were performed in the 52 patients and in ten age-matched healthy subjects. An apparatus (Medelec EMG) with bicoaxial needle electrodes was used. Electrodes were inserted into the right musculus abductor digiti minimi and into the left musculus opponens pollicis for determination of the motor nerve conduction velocity of the ulnar and median nerves respectively.

The nerves were stimulated through the skin in the elbow region and the wrist region. The stimulus had a voltage of 150 v, a duration of 0.1 msec.[4]

As differences in conduction velocity between median and ulnar nerves in the same subject were found to be negligible, both in patients and normal controls, we shall refer here to the mean of the two measurements.

Results

The average motor nerve conduction velocity for all hypertensive patients was 45.4 m/sec, ranging from 29.5 to 60 m/sec, the range in our control subjects being 54 to 60 m/sec.

The reduction in motor nerve conduction velocity showed a direct correlation with the height of the diastolic blood pressure (Fig 1 and 2, *top left*). Similar results were obtained when mean or systolic blood pressures were used.

Correlation of nerve conduction velocity with fundoscopic findings in the hypertensive patients shows that the mean conduction velocity was normal (54.9 m/sec) when retinal changes did

Fig 1.—Correlation between nerve conduction velocity and diastolic blood pressure in 52 patients with essential hypertension.

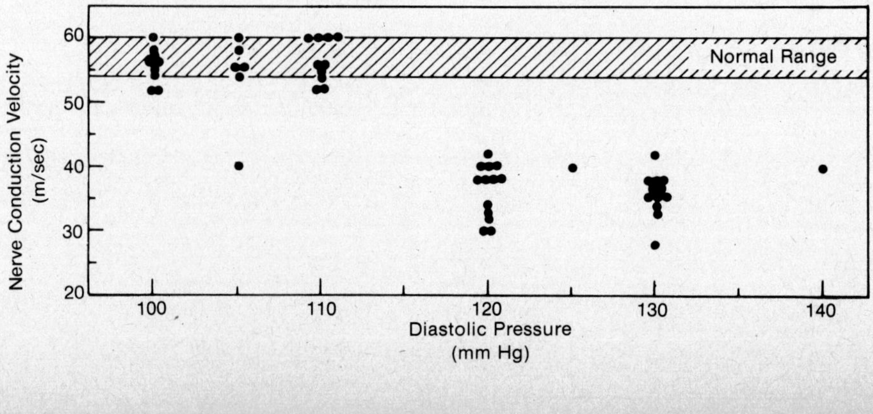

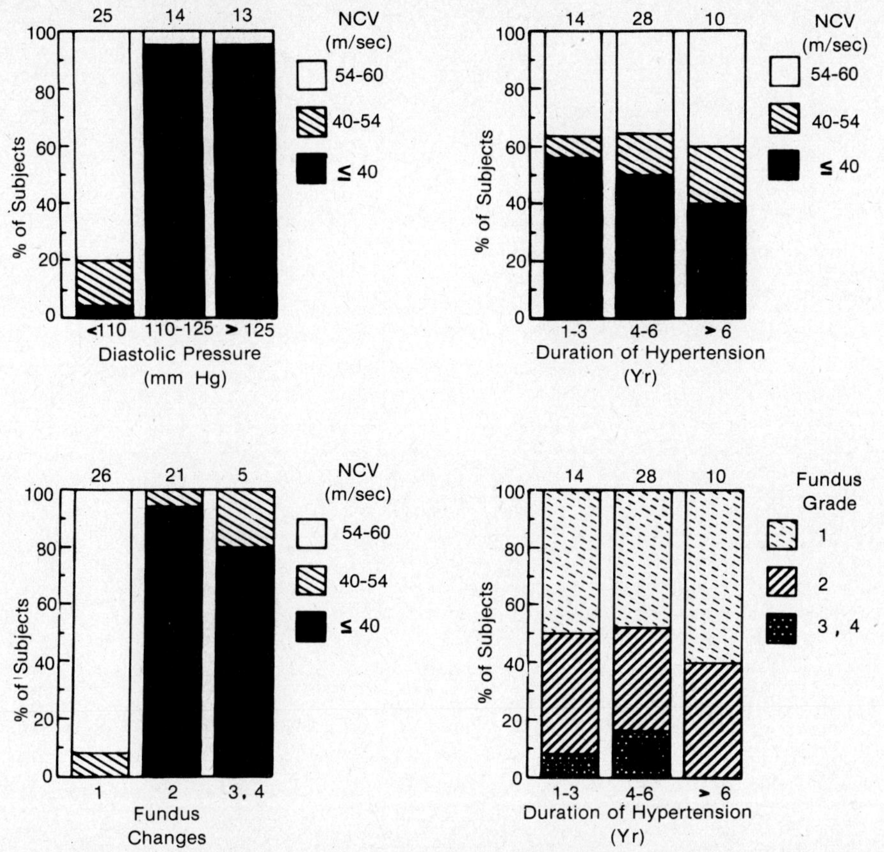

Fig 2.—Correlation between motor nerve conduction velocity and diastolic blood pressure (top left), *duration of hypertension* (top right), *and retinal changes* (bottom left). Bottom right, *Correlation between retinal changes and duration of hypertension. The figures above the columns indicate the number of patients in each subgroup.*

not exceed grade 1. Only six out of 26 patients in this group had a moderate reduction in nerve conduction velocity. In all 26 patients with more severe retinal changes (grade 2, 21; grade 3, 4; and grade 4, 1) there was reduced conduction velocity, with a mean value of 36 m/sec. Reduction in velocity was severe in 18 and moderate in eight of these patients (Fig 2, *bottom left).*

There was no correlation between the nerve conduction velocity and the duration of the hypertension (Fig 2, *top right).* Neither could a correlation be found between the retinal findings and the duration of the hypertension (Fig 2, *bottom right).*

Nerve conduction velocity is not related to age, neither in the present study group, nor in a very large number of normotensive subjects examined routinely in our laboratory. Drug effect was also excluded as all patients received the same treatment with only minor dose differences.

Comment

The above findings support previous impressions that hypertensive patients suffer from subclinical peripheral neuropathy which can be detected only by measurement of motor nerve conduction velocity. They also indicate that this electrophysiological disturbance is related to the severity of the disease. It seems that an "all or none" type of correlation exists: When the blood pressure is only moderately elevated, with only minimal secondary vascular changes, motor nerve conduction velocity is not reduced. However, when the hypertension is severe, which causes more advanced vascular changes, motor nerve conduction is markedly disturbed. Popovtzer et al[3] suggested that the peripheral neuropathy in their case was the result of nerve ischemia caused by the severe arteriospasm. Our results tend to support this assumption, although it is not clear whether severe arteriospasm is sufficient to cause the electrophysiological derangement or whether the latter appears only after the development of organic destructive changes in the vasa nervorum. Moreover, it is not yet known whether the conduction defects will be reversible when the blood pressure is reduced.

It was demonstrated that the changes in nerve conduction go in parallel with the vascular changes in the retina. The examination of the fundus is markedly prone to subjective observation and interpretation errors,[5] whereas nerve conduction velocity is a measurable index. It thus may contribute to an objective assessment of the severity of the hypertensive disease.

Nonproprietary and Trade Names of Drug

Methyldopa—*Aldomet.*

References

1. Licht S: *Electro Diagnosis and Electromyography.* New Haven, Conn, Elizabeth Licht Publisher, 1961, pp 385-395.

2. Raff MC, Sangalang V, Asbury AK: Ischemic mononeuropathy multiplex associated with diabetes mellitus. *Arch Neurol* **18**:487-499, 1968.

3. Popovtzer MM, Rosenbaum BJ, Gordon A, et al: Relief of uremic polyneuropathy after bilateral nephrectomy. *New Eng J Med* **281**:949-950, 1969.

4. Chaco J: Electromyography and motor nerve conduction velocity in peripheral atherosclerosis obliterans. *Angiology* **20**:195-199, 1969.

5. Michaelson IC, Eliakim M, Avshalom A, et al: An approach to the investigation of the vascular changes in the fundus of the eye in hypertension and arteriosclerosis, in Proceedings of the 20th International Congress of Ophthalmology, Munich, 1966, abstracted. *Excerp Med Int Cong Ser* **146**:207-219, 1966.

Allergic Bronchopulmonary Aspergillosis

Report of Two Cases and Evaluation of Tests for Hypersensitivity

M. Colin Jordan, MD; C. Warren Bierman, MD; and Paul P. VanArsdel, Jr., MD, Seattle

In recent years increasing attention has been devoted to a group of pulmonary diseases characterized by a host reaction to the inhalation of various organic dusts. Thermophilic actinomycetes have been implicated as respiratory allergens in bagassosis and farmers' lung[1,2] while avian and animal proteins have been found to be etiologically important in pigeon breeders' disease and pituitary snuff-takers' lung.[3,4] Although these disorders are well-known in this country, reports of a similar but more complex syndrome, allergic bronchopulmonary aspergillosis, have come primarily from Great Britain.[5] The reason for this is unclear since spores of the causative fungus, *Aspergillus fumigatus* (Fig 1) are frequently inhaled by the population at large and are a relatively common cause of allergic bronchial asthma in the United States.[6,7] This report describes two patients with allergic bronchopulmonary aspergillosis and evaluates the role of immunologic tests in the diagnosis of fungal hypersensitivity.

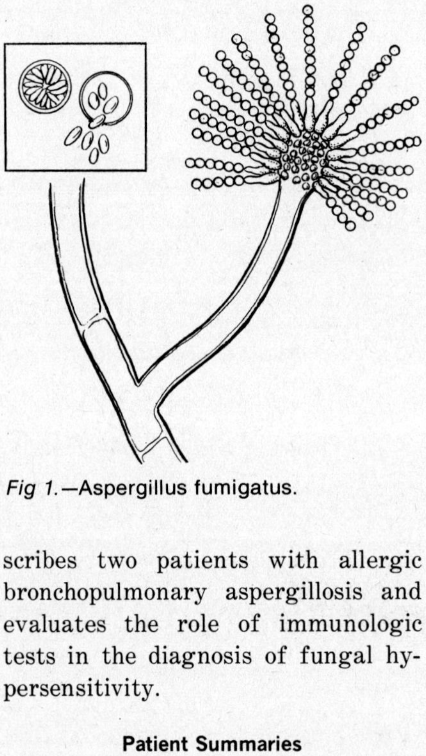

Fig 1.—Aspergillus fumigatus.

Received for publication Oct 21, 1970; accepted Jan 22, 1971.

From the departments of medicine (Drs. Jordan and VanArsdel) and pediatrics (Dr. Bierman), University of Washington School of Medicine, and the Department of Pediatrics, Children's Orthopedic Hospital and Medical Center, Seattle (Dr. Bierman). Dr. Jordan is now with the National Communicable Disease Center, Kansas City, Kan.

Reprint requests to Department of Medicine, BB-509, University Hospital, Seattle 98105 (Dr. VanArsdel).

Patient Summaries

PATIENT 1.–A 15-year-old boy with a history of bronchial asthma was admitted to a hospital in December 1968 because of wheezing, cough, purulent sputum, and fever. A roentgenogram of the chest revealed infiltrates in both upper lobes of the lungs, including the lingula. Although his symptoms improved after treatment with ampicillin trihydrate, the roentgenographic abnormalities persisted. During the next four months the patient experienced recurrent bouts of wheezing and productive cough. At the time of admission to the Seattle Children's Orthopedic Hospital and Medical Center in May 1969, he appeared chronically ill. Wheezes and rales were audible throughout the chest and the fingers were moderately clubbed. An x-ray film of the chest (Fig 2, *top*) revealed infiltrates in both upper lobes and in the lower lobe of the right lung; cystic changes were noted in the lingula. The absolute eosinophil count ranged from 399 to 540/cu mm. The patient expectorated copious, greenish sputum containing numerous brown flecks 1 to 2 mm in diameter. Cultures of the sputum repeatedly contained *A fumigatus* but no bacterial pathogens. Pulmonary function tests demonstrated significant obstructive and restrictive disease and a lowered diffusion capacity (Table 1). The results of cutaneous and immunologic tests will be described later.

Because the nature of the patient's illness was unclear, an open lung biopsy was performed. At surgery the left lung appeared congested and had a firm consistency. Microscopic examination of the excised tissue revealed marked peribronchial and alveolar infiltration with plasma cells, eosinophils, and mononuclear cells. Dense collagenous thickening was noted beneath the pleura. There was no evidence of vasculitis although considerable medial thickening of arterioles was present. No fungi were identified. Pathologic diagnosis was "allergic granulomatous disease of the lung." Culture of the resected tissue contained *A fumigatus.*

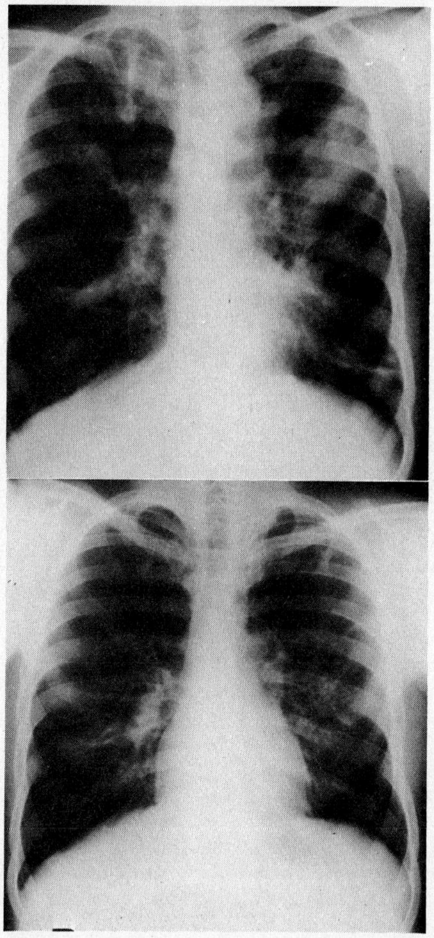

Fig 2.—Roentgenogram of the chest of patient 1 at time of admission to hospital (top) *and after corticosteroid therapy* (bottom).

Shortly after surgery, treatment was begun with prednisone (60 mg/day) and the dosage was rapidly decreased during the following two weeks. There was dramatic improvement, with marked diminution in the amount and purulence of the sputum, as well as cessation of wheezing. Follow-up x-ray film of the chest two months after discharge revealed nearly complete resolution of the pulmonary infiltrates (Fig 2, *bottom*). Pulmonary function studies demonstrated gradual improvement in vital capacity and single-breath diffusing capacity while forced expiratory volumes (FEV) remained unchanged (Table 1). During the next seven months the patient gained 13.6 kg (30 lb) in weight, and he is now participating in school athletic activities. Periodic episodes of bronchospasm still occur, however. Current prednisone dosage is 5 mg daily.

PATIENT 2.—A 31-year-old boilermaker was in good health until March 1967 when he developed a persistent productive cough. In May 1968, a roentgenogram of the chest revealed partial consolidation of the upper lobe of the right lung. When no improvement was noted after several days of antimicrobial therapy, he was admitted to a local hospital for further evaluation. Bronchoscopy and a scalene lymph node biopsy were unrewarding. At thoracotomy the upper lobe of the right lung was consolidated and adherent to the mediastinum. Numerous rubbery lymph nodes were present in the paratracheal region. The upper lobe of the right lung bronchus contained a large mucus plug and whitish, purulent material which could be expressed with gentle pressure. The lobe was removed and the patient was discharged several days later. Cough and production of purulent sputum returned in December 1968. Despite treatment with antibiotics no improvement occurred and intermittent wheezing was noted. The sputum was said to contain "brown spirals" and had a "gritty" consistency. The patient was first seen at the University of Washington Hospital in August 1969. On admission to the medical service, rales and expiratory wheezes were heard over the left lung. The white blood cell count was 16,700/cu mm, with 3,200 eosinophils/cu mm. Roentgenograms of the chest demonstrated confluent densities in the lingula interspersed with small cystic areas. The sputum was thick and tenacious with a greenish color; numerous small white and brown flecks were readily visible. Multiple cultures contained "normal bacterial flora" and *A fumigatus*. Bronchograms demonstrated a complete occlusion of the lingular bronchus, presumably due to a mucus plug (Fig 3). Results of pulmonary function tests revealed a normal vital capacity with mild airway obstruction which did not change after the inhalation of isoproterenol sulfate (Table 1).

Microscopic examination of the lung tissue removed during the first hospitalization revealed changes similar to those described in patient 1. In addition, numerous mycelial forms of *A fumigatus* were visible within the involved bronchi. The results of cutaneous and immunologic tests will be described later.

Shortly after treatment was begun with prednisone, the patient expectorated a large mucus plug. The sputum lost its purulent character and significant improvement in exercise tolerance was noted. Results of pulmonary function tests and the eosinophil count returned to normal. One month after discharge the lingular infiltrate had cleared, but a partially fluid-filled cavity remained in that area. The patient was treated with postural drainage and maintained free of symptoms with 7.5 mg/day of prednisone. There was no significant decrease in the cavity size during the next seven months, though it no longer contained fluid (Fig 4). Ten months after discharge the cavity was significantly smaller. Several sputum cultures have been negative for *Aspergillus*.

Materials and Methods

Study Population.—Twenty-six subjects were studied to assess the value of immunologic and cutaneous tests in the diagnosis of hypersensitivity to fungi. The study population included (1) 12 normal volunteers (four mothers with their newborn infants and four laboratory technologists); (2) ten asthmatic adults and children specifically sensitive to *Aspergillus* or *Helminthosporium* as demonstrated by previously described methods[7]; (3) one adult with chronic bronchitis and a sputum culture positive for *A fumigatus;* (4) one patient with congenital absence of serum beta lipoprotein (familial acanthocytosis); and (5) the two reported patients with allergic bronchopulmonary aspergillosis. Helminthosporium was included in the study as a representative of other common fungi in order to test the specificity of positive responses to *Aspergillus*, and also because *Helminthosporium* extract gave interesting nonspecific reactions with serum as described here.

Cutaneous Tests.—Tests for cutaneous hypersensitivity were performed by intradermal injection of 0.02 ml of *Aspergillus* and *Helminthosporium* extracts (both 5μg protein nitrogen/ml) into separate sites. The development of a wheal 5 mm or greater in diameter than the control within 15 minutes of injection was considered a positive response. Skin test sites were observed for 48 hours for the development of a late reaction. Subjects with negative immediate responses were also tested for late reactions by intracutaneous administration of 0.1 ml of the same antigens.

Immunologic Tests.—The serum of all subjects was tested by double diffusion in agar for precipitin reactions to extracts of *Helminthosporium* and *Aspergillus* (aqueous solutions prepared by grinding and extracting broth culture pellicles, composed primarily of mycelia[5]). All serum specimens demonstrating precipitins were further tested by immunoelectrophoresis in agar against the reacting extracts. The location and character of the precipitin bands were then compared to reactions obtained with standard immunoelectrophoresis with goat antiserum to human immunoglobulin G.

Results

Cutaneous Tests.—As expected, all ten patients with asthmatic sensitivity to *Helminthosporium* or *Aspergillus* species had a positive immediate skin reaction when challenged intradermally with their respective allergens (Table 2). Both patients with allergic bronchopulmonary aspergillosis also had marked immediate reactions to *Aspergillus* extract. In addition, patient 2 had a lesser response to *Helminthosporium.* The remaining subjects had negative cutaneous responses to both antigens. In patient 2 an area of erythema and edema 30 mm in diameter developed six hours after the *Aspergillus* skin test had been applied and gradually diminished during the next 48 hours. Patient 1 and all other subjects failed to demonstrate this "dual response" and no subject developed the late reaction alone.

Table 1.—Pulmonary Function Tests in Two Patients With Allergic Bronchopulmonary Aspergillosis

Patient	Date	Vital Capacity, Liters	Forced Expiratory Volume 1 sec (FEV_1), Liters	FEV_1 as Percent of Vital Capacity, %	Diffusing Capacity* ml/min/mm Hg
1					
	6/9/69†	2.4	1.6	67	19.7
	6/23/69	3.1	2.1	68	...
	10/15/69	3.5	2.3	67	28.7
2					
	7/6/69†	5.0	3.1	62	...
	12/12/69	5.0	4.4	88	...

* Single breath carbon monoxide; normal = 24 ml/min/mm Hg.
† Prior to corticosteroid therapy.

Table 2.—Summary of Cutaneous and Immunologic Studies

Diagnosis	Number of Patients	Positive Immediate Skin Test		Positive "Late" Skin Test		Serum Precipitins	
		Asper*	Helmin	Asper	Helmin	Asper	Helmin
Asthma: allergic to fungi	6	3	3	0	0	0	6
Asthma: allergic to fungi (hyposensitized)	4	4	4	0	0	0	4
Chronic bronchitis: *Aspergillus* in sputum	1	0	0	0	0	0	1
Allergic bronchopulmonary aspergillosis	2	2	1	1	0	2	2
Familial acanthocytosis†	1	0	0	0	0	0	0
Normal volunteers	12	0	0	0	0	0	11

* Asper = *Aspergillus* extract; Helmin = *Helminthosporium* extract.
† Congenital absence of serum beta lipoprotein.

Immunologic Tests.—Precipitin reactions to *Aspergillus* extract were demonstrated with the serum samples of both patients with allergic bronchopulmonary aspergillosis by microouchterlony technique. The best results were obtained by placing the undiluted serum in the center well and dilutions of antigen in the peripheral wells (Fig 5). The reaction was positive to an antigen concentration as low as 90μg protein nitrogen/ml with serum for patient 1 and as low as 11μg protein nitrogen/ml with serum from patient 2. When antigen in concentration of 90μg protein nitrogen/ml was placed in the center well and dilutions of serum in the peripheral wells, the reaction was positive to a serum dilution of 1:4 with serum from patient 1 and of 1:8 from patient 2. In both instances the precipitin bands appeared in the same area as immunoglobulin G on immunoelectrophoresis. Absorption studies for C substance-C reactive protein interactions were negative.[8] The serum samples from all other subjects failed to develop precipitin reactions with *Aspergillus* extract (180μg protein nitrogen/ml).

Precipitin lines against a relatively high concentration of *Helminthosporium* extract (25 mg protein nitrogen/ml) unexpectedly developed with the serum samples of all subjects with bronchial hypersensitivity to this organism. However, these reactions were also noted with serum samples from all asthmatic subjects allergic to *Aspergillus*, both patients with allergic bronchopulmonary aspergillosis, and all control subjects except for one newborn infant. On immunoelectrophoresis, the precipitins with *Helminthosporium* developed in the β-globulin rather than the γ-globulin region. These reactions appeared identical to those resulting between human beta lipoprotein and goat antiserum against human lipoprotein. The impression that the *Helminthosporium* precipitin reactions were artifactual (ie, not γ-globulin) was strengthened when serum from the patient with congenitally absent beta lipoprotein failed to form precipitin bands with this antigen.

Comment

In their descriptions of the various forms of aspergillosis Louria[9] and Wahrner et al[10] have distinguished between invasive and noninvasive pulmonary infection. Tissue invasion occurs almost exclusively in patients with impaired host defenses or as a superinfection following the administration of antibiotics. On the other hand, a noninvasive infection usually represents colonization of a preexisting pulmonary lesion (such as bronchiectasis) and often occurs as a mycetoma in situ (aspergilloma). Although airborne spores of this fungus are ubiquitous and frequently in-

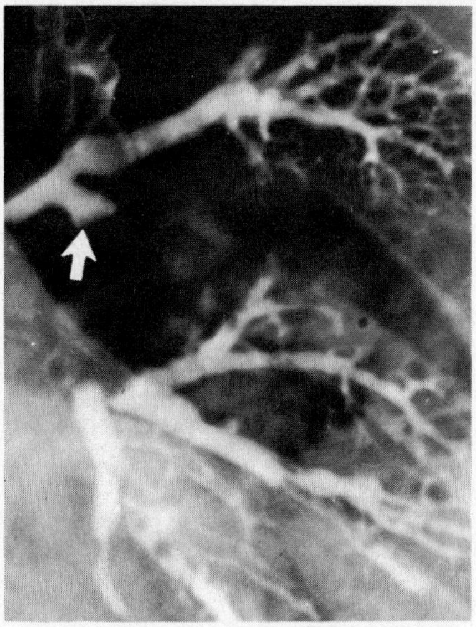

Fig 3.—Bronchogram of patient 2. Complete occlusion of left lingular bronchus (arrow).

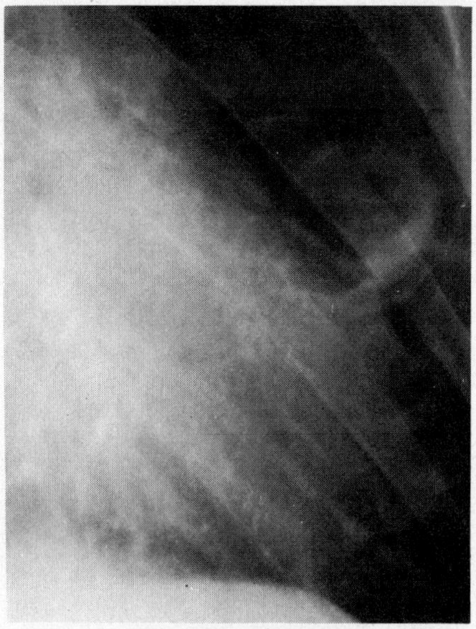

Fig 4.—Right anterior oblique roentgenogram of patient 2 in April 1970. Cavity in lingular segment.

duce bronchial asthma in allergic subjects, they rarely germinate to produce infection in such patients.[6,7] However, a characteristic host reaction occurs in allergic bronchopulmonary aspergillosis which involves the antigenically similar—but more massive-mycelial form of the fungus.[5] An allergic basis for this response was first postulated by Hinson et al,[11] but it was not until after the demonstration of circulating precipitins against *Aspergillus* extract by Pepys et al[5] in 1959 that evidence for specific hypersensitivity began to accumulate.

Allergic bronchopulmonary aspergillosis is usually described in patients with preexisting asthma which may or may not be related to fungal allergens. A personal or family history of other atopic illnesses is often present.[5,6,12] Wheezing, dyspnea, and cough with tenacious purulent sputum containing brown flecks barely visible to the naked eye are commonly noted. Many patients expectorate mucus plugs consisting of aggregates of fibrin, eosinophils, Curschmann spirals, and Charcot-Leyden crystals. Fungal mycelia are often visible microscopically within these plugs. Intermittent febrile episodes accompanied by pulmonary infiltrates are a hallmark of the syndrome.[5] The infiltrates are usually segmental in nature and may give the appearance of consolidation or collapse.[5,6] New lesions often appear prior to the resolution of existing shadows. Most patients have peripheral eosinophilia in excess of 1,000 cells/cu mm unless catecholamines or corticosteroids have been administered.

The following tests may be used to establish a diagnosis of allergic bronchopulmonary aspergillosis: (1) intradermal challenge with *Aspergillus* extract; (2) agar diffusion studies for the presence of serum precipitins; and (3) inhalation challenge with a dilute *Aspergillus* solution.

Intradermal testing with *Aspergillus* extract results in an immediate wheal and flare response in asthmatic patients with specific bronchial hypersensitivity reactions (bronchospasm) to the organism.[5,6] This reaction is identical to that seen in individuals allergic to pollens and danders and has been termed "type I allergy" by Coombs and Gell.[13] Available evidence indicates that it is mediated by a circulating reaginic antibody, probably of the immunoglobulin E class.[14] In patients with allergic bronchopulmonary aspergillosis, however, a delayed component to the skin test may also be present.[5] Several hours after the immediate reaction has subsided, erythema and edema develop within the border of the original response. The second component usually subsides within 24 to 36 hours and is thought to represent a precipitin-mediated Arthus-like phenomenon (type III reaction). Biopsy specimens of these "late" skin reactions have shown perivascular infiltration with eosinophils and polymorphonuclear leukocytes.[6,15] While these findings suggest that precipitating antibodies are responsible for the lesions, the presence of antigen, specific antibody, and complement together has not yet been shown. Better evidence for the pathogenic role of these antibodies has recently been reported by Golbert and Patterson, who induced pulmonary lesions in a monkey by inhalation of *Aspergillus* antigen after passive sensitization with serum from a patient with pulmonary allergic aspergillosis.[16]

The serum samples of most patients with allergic bronchopulmonary aspergillosis contain specific precipitins against *A fumigatus*. In one study 63% of patients with asthma, pulmonary infiltrates, peripheral eosinophilia, and *Aspergillus* in the sputum had circulating precipitins.[8] When the serum was concentrated threefold or fourfold, more than 90% of these patients had precipitins.[15] However, positive reactions to precipitin tests must be interpreted with caution since serum C-reactive protein may precipitate in agar with the somatic C-substance of the fungus.[8] No such reactions were noted in our study, but it was found that serum lipoprotein may cause a nonspecific reaction with some fungal extracts, specifically *Helminthospo-*

rium. Because these false-positive reactions occur, all precipitins must be shown by immunoelectrophoresis to involve γ-globulin. Nevertheless, even true γ-globulin precipitins are not specific for allergic bronchopulmonary aspergillosis since virtually all patients with aspergilloma have such circulating antibodies.[17] However, these patients rarely show positive cutaneous or bronchial responses.

Inhalation of dilute *Aspergillus* extract by hypersensitive asthmatic individuals results in a marked and specific increase in airways resistance. The patient reported by Slavin et al[6] experienced a reduction from his baseline FEV_1 of 43% to 23% within 15 minutes of inhalation. It should be pointed out that a positive bronchial response (bronchospasm) is a type I reaction and would be expected in asthmatic patients with reaginic antibody, whether or not circulating precipitins are present. Pepys[15] has described "dual" bronchial reactions in some patients manifested by a recurrence of wheezing several hours after inhalation of antigen. Neither of our patients had inhalation challenge testing because a constant state of provocation was already present, due to the heavy growth of *Aspergillus* in the sputum. These studies could have been performed after corticosteroid therapy, but provocation of symptoms was not felt to be justified.

Although differing in degree, the clinical features of both of our patients are typical of allergic bronchopulmonary aspergillosis. Despite the fact that patient 1 was more severely ill, patient 2 had greater peripheral eosinophilia, a higher precipitin titer, and a "late" skin reaction to *Aspergillus*. The reason for the absence of this type III cutaneous response in patient 1 is not clear. It is conceivable that an insufficient amount of antigen was injected (0.1μg). Another possibility relates to the recent demonstration by Brostoff and Roitt[18] of the fact that skin test antigens may be diluted and dispersed by fluid exudation occurring as a result of the immediate response. Delayed (tuberculin-type) skin reactions developed in four of their six patients with pollen sensitivity only when the type I reactions were suppressed by antihistamines.

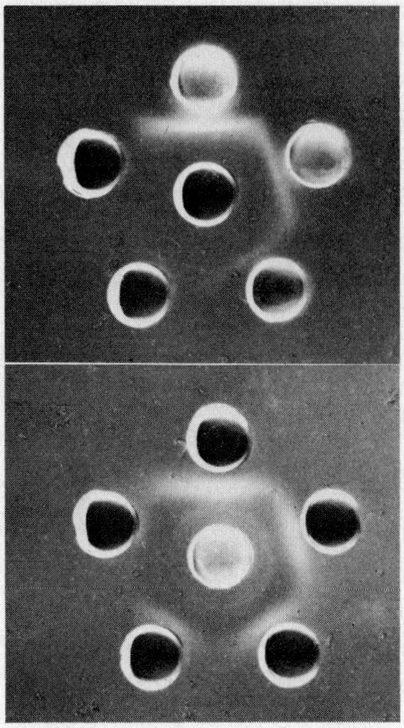

Fig 5.—Double diffusion test with serum of patient 2 and Aspergillus *extracts.* Top, *Center well* Aspergillus *9μg/ml. Peripheral wells clockwise: patient's serum undiluted* (top), *diluted 1:2, 1:8, and 1:16.* Bottom, *Central well: patient's serum undiluted. Peripheral wells clockwise:* Aspergillus *9μg/ml* (top), *4.5μg/ml, 2.25μg/ml, 1.12μg/ml and 0.6μg/ml.*

The etiology of the pulmonary infiltrates in allergic bronchopulmonary aspergillosis is not known. Their frequent occurrence in a segmental distribution suggests that intermittent bronchial occlusion by mucus plugs predisposes to bacterial infection within the obstructed segment.[10] However, this hypothesis cannot explain the presence of infiltrates in patients without mucus plugs.[12] Several workers feel that the infiltrates represent an intrapulmonary precipitin-mediated Arthus-like phenomenon analogous to the "late" cutaneous response.[6,12,15] The histopathology of lung tissue resected from our patients supports this view since the abnormalities observed closely resemble those seen in biopsy specimens of positive "late" skin reactions.[12,15] On the other hand, Campbell and Clayton[17] have pointed out that precipitins are almost always present in the serum of patients with aspergilloma who have no clinical evidence of allergy. It may be that both reaginic and precipitating antibodies are required for the production of pulmonary infiltrates as has been suggested by Pepys.[15] Certainly the coexistence of type I with type III allergy appears to result in greater peripheral and pulmonary eosinophilia than occurs in disorders characterized by pure type III hypersensitivity. Diseases of the latter group, such as farmers' lung and pigeon breeders' disease, have been termed "extrinsic allergic alveolitis" by Pepys[15] because they involve primarily the peripheral gas-exchanging tissues of the lung and produce the roentgenographic appearance of a diffuse interstitial pneumonitis. Although the pulmonary infiltrates in allergic bronchopulmonary aspergillosis are mainly due to peribronchial involvement,[15] patient 1 demonstrates that alveolar infiltration sufficient to produce diffusion abnormalities may also be present.

Therapeutic efforts have been directed primarily at reducing the hypersensitive reaction to the fungus, although attempts have been made to eradicate the organism from the respiratory tree by inhalation of fungistatic agents.[6,12] Stark[19] successfully treated one patient with allergic aspergillosis in this manner, but most patients have required corticosteroids for control of their symptoms.[12] Both of our patients experienced rapid improvement with clearing of pulmonary infiltrates, fall in eosinophil count, and improved pulmonary function tests with corticosteroids, although patient 1, who had severe preexisting asthma, is still plagued by intermittent episodes of bronchospasm. Treatment with corticosteroids is often cited as a predisposing factor in patients who develop invasive or disseminated aspergillosis,[10] but this complication has not been reported in patients with allergic bronchopulmonary aspergillosis.

The reason for the apparent rarity of this syndrome in North America is unclear. In a 1967 report on 53 unselected chronic asthmatic patients in Maryland, Agbayani et al[20] described two patients with clinical histories compatible with allergic bronchopulmonary aspergillosis, but neither precipitins nor "late" cutaneous responses were demonstrated. However, a few well-documented cases have been reported since then.[6,12,16] The paucity of these cases probably reflects a low index of suspicion, with other diagnoses being invoked as an explanation of the patient's symptoms. The fact that both of our patients underwent diagnostic thoracotomy prior to recognition of their illness supports this view. Sputum cultures containing *Aspergillus* can easily be regarded as contaminated and pulmonary consolidation with fever is more radily attributable to bacterial pneumonia. Only a more acute awareness of allergic bronchopulmonary aspergillosis can lead to its early recognition and obviate the need for potentially hazardous diagnostic procedures.

Summary

Allergic bronchopulmonary aspergillosis has been reported infrequently in the United States. Two patients with this syndrome are described. Both had pulmonary infiltrates, peripheral eosinophilia, positive immediate skin responses to *Aspergillus*, and serum precipitins against *Aspergillus* extract. One patient also developed a "late" Arthus-type skin reaction. Lung biopsy specimens of both patients showed peribronchiolar and alveolar infiltration with plasma cells and eosinophils. Excellent clinical responses to corticosteroids were observed and the fungi were eliminated from the sputum.

The specificity of immunologic and cutaneous tests in fungal hypersensitivity was investigated in 26 subjects, ten of whom had asthma related to fungal allergens. No false-positive reactions to *Aspergillus* occurred. However, serum samples from 25 subjects demonstrated precipitin reactions with *Helminthosporium* extract. Immunoelectrophoresis revealed that these precipitins were nonspecific reactions with serum beta lipoprotein and did not involve γ-globulin.

This investigation was supported by Public Health Service training grant AI-00011.

Robert F. Dunlop, MD, referred patient 2 to us. William E. Pierson, MD, and Gerald J. Roth, MD, assisted with the clinical and laboratory studies. Bruce Beckwith, MD, and Victor Goldenberg, MD, interpreted the pathologic specimens.

References

1. Salvaggio J, Arquembourg P, Seabury J, et al: Bagassosis: IV. Precipitins against extracts of thermophilic actinomycetes in patients with bagassosis. *Amer J Med* **46**:538-544, 1969.
2. Pepys J, Jenkins PA, Festenstein GH, et al: Farmers' lung: Thermophilic actinomycetes as a source of "farmers' lung hay" antigens. *Lancet* **2**:607-611, 1963.
3. Fink JN, Sosman AJ, Barboriak JJ, et al: Pigeon breeders' disease: A clinical study of a hypersensitivity pneumonitis. *Ann Intern Med* **68**:1205-1217, 1968.
4. Pepys J: Pulmonary hypersensitivity disease due to inhaled organic antigens. *Ann Intern Med* **64**:943-948, 1966.
5. Pepys J, Riddell RW, Citron KM, et al: Clinical and immunologic significance of *Aspergillus fumigatus* in the sputum. *Amer Rev Resp Dis* **80**:167-180, 1959.
6. Slavin RG, Stanczyk DJ, Lonigro AJ, et al: Allergic bronchopulmonary aspergillosis—A North American rarity. Clinical and immunologic characteristics. *Amer J Med* **47**:306-313, 1969.
7. Colen J, Vanarsdel PP Jr, Pasnick LJ, et al: Observations on the experimental reproduction of asthma with mold antigens. *J Allerg* **35**:331-338, 1964.
8. Longbottom JL, Pepys J: Pulmonary aspergillosis: Diagnostic and immunologic significance of antigens and C-substance in *Aspergillus fumigatus*. *J Path Bact* **88**:141-151, 1964.
9. Louria DB: Deep-seated mycotic infections, allergy to fungi, and mycotoxins. *New Eng J Med* **277**:1065-1071, 1126-1134, 1967.
10. Wahrner HW, Hepper N, Anderson H, et al: Pulmonary aspergillosis. *Ann Intern Med* **58**:472-485, 1963.
11. Hinson KFW, Moon AJ, Plummer NS: Bronchopulmonary aspergillosis: A review and a report of eight new cases. *Thorax* **7**:317-333, 1952.
12. Warren WP, Rose B: Hypersensitivity bronchopulmonary aspergillosis. *Dis Chest* **55**:415-421, 1969.
13. Coombs RRA, Gell PGH: Classification of allergic reactions responsible for clinical hypersensitivity and disease, in Gell PGH, Coombs RRA (eds): *Clinical Aspects of Immunology*, ed 2. Philadelphia, FA Davis Co, 1968, pp 575-596.
14. Ishizaka K, Ishizaka T, Hornbrook MM: Physicochemical properties of human reaginic antibody: IV. Presence of a unique immunoglobulin as a carrier of reaginic antibody. *J Immun* **97**:75-85, 1966.
15. Pepys J: *Hypersensitivity Diseases of the Lungs due to Fungi and Organic Dusts, Monographs in Allergy*. White Plains, NY, S Karger AG, 1969, vol 4.
16. Golbert TM, Patterson R: Pulmonary allergic aspergillosis. *Ann Intern Med* **72**:395-403, 1970.
17. Campbell J, Clayton YM: Bronchopulmonary aspergillosis. A correlation of the clinical and laboratory findings in 272 patients investigated for bronchopulmonary aspergillosis. *Amer Rev Resp Dis* **89**:186-196, 1964.
18. Brostoff J, Roitt IM: Cell-mediated (delayed) hypersensitivity in patients with summer hay-fever. *Lancet* **2**:1269-1272, 1969.
19. Stark JE: Allergic pulmonary aspergillosis successfully treated with inhalations of nystatin. *Dis Chest* **51**:96-99, 1967.
20. Agbayani BF, Norman PS, Winkenwerder WL: The incidence of allergic aspergillosis in chronic asthma. *J Allerg* **40**:319-326, 1967.

Shiga Bacillus Dysentery Acquired in Nicaragua

George W. Counts, MD; Joel L. Nitzkin, MD, MPH; Miami, Fla;

Charles H. Hennekens, Jr., MD, Atlanta; and N. Joel Ehrenkranz, MD, Miami, Fla

At present there is a widespread epidemic of dysentery caused by *Shigella dysenteriae*, type 1, (the Shiga bacillus), in Central America.[1] Gangarosa et al estimate some 112,000 cases with 8,300 deaths occurred in Guatemala in the first ten months of 1969. The severity of this outbreak is indicated by the mortality of 17 deaths per 10,000 persons, in contrast to a previous rate of 3.9.[2]

In the past 18 months there has been a substantial increase in the number of Shiga bacillus strains from persons who had been recent visitors to Mexico or Central America.[3] In a recent 11-week period, two adults with shigellosis acquired in Nicaragua were seen in Miami, Fla. They presented with an illness resembling ulcerative colitis. Since infection with Shiga bacillus can mimic severe noninfectious enteric diseases, awareness of the seriousness of infection with this particular strain of *Shigella* is important to insure agressive therapy for the patient, and prevention of spread to his contacts. These cases are presented in detail in order to alert physicians serving patients from Central America, or their contacts, of the possibility of Shiga bacillus dysentery as a cause of life-threatening disease.

Received for publication April 14, 1971; accepted April 16.

From the Department of Epidemiology and Public Health, University of Miami School of Medicine and the Jackson Memorial Hospital (Drs. Counts and Ehrenkranz), the Dade County Department of Public Health, Miami, Fla (Dr. Nitzkin), and the Epidemiology Program, Center for Disease Control, Atlanta (Dr. Hennekens).

Reprint requests to 1700 NW Tenth Ave, Miami, Fla 33136 (Dr. Counts).

Patient Summaries

PATIENT 1 (JMH-455766).—A 78-year-old woman was admitted in May 1970 because of persistent bloody diarrhea. She was born in Nicaragua and had lived there until 15 years ago when she moved to Miami. On March 31, 1970, she went to Granada, Nicaragua, for her yearly visit and was in her usual state of good health. She remained healthy until approximately one week later, when she had the abrupt onset of bloody diarrhea, with as many as 20 bowel movements per day. The patient was treated with tetracycline and another antibiotic for several days, along with intravenous administration of fluids. Because of lack of improvement she was flown back to Miami on May 7, 1970. There was no history of previous episodes of diarrhea in the patient or her family, although epidemic diarrheal disease was occurring in Granada at that time. On admission her blood pressure was 98/60 mm Hg, pulse rate, 80 beats per minute; temperature, 97 F (36.1 C). She was obtunded but could be aroused. The serum sodium level was 110 mEq/liter; hematocrit value, 40%; and blood urea nitrogen (BUN) level, 90 mg/100 ml; white blood cell count (WBC) was 13.200/cu mm. The diarrheic feces contained mucus and blood. X-ray films of the chest and abdomen and results of other laboratory studies were within normal limits. The initial clinical impression was "possible ulcerative colitis, with amebic colitis and bacillary dysentery to be excluded." Sigmoidoscopic findings included a friable ulcerated rectosigmoid. No ova or parasitic forms were seen in examination of three stool specimens; culture of feces on three occasions yielded neither *Salmonella* nor *Shigella.* Rectal tissue taken by biopsy showed only nonspecific ulceration. A barium enema revealed spasm of the left colon and sigmoid diverticuli. The patient was initially treated with intravenous administration of fluids, two doses of chloramphenicol, and metronidazole. After 48 hours there was little improvement. Her WBC rose to 16,400/cu mm. Intravenous administration of penicillin G sodium, 18 million units/day, and kanamycin sulfate, 500 mg/day intramuscularly, were then added to her therapy, and four days later salicylazosulfapyridine therapy was begun. Dexamethasone was added on the eleventh hospital day.

The patient's temperature remained below 100.6 F (38.1 C) rectally until the tenth hospital day when she developed lower lobe bronchopneumonia. Her temperature reached 103 F (39.4 C). She died on the twelfth hospital day following a cardiac arrest. No autopsy was performed. *Shigella dysenteriae,* type 1, was grown from one of three blood cultures drawn on admission. Thirty-seven family members and contacts were interviewed, fecal cultures made, and blood taken from hemagglutinating antibody to *S dysenteriae,* type 1. No Miami family contacts had diarrheal disease, no carriers were found, and none had antibodies to Shiga bacillus.

PATIENT 2 (MH-275187).—A 22-year-old Dutch merchant seaman was in good health until July 21 when he had the abrupt onset of diarrhea and abdominal pain while onboard ship. The patient's last visit ashore was on July 16, in Corinto, Nicaragua, where he had eaten dinner. Prior to that the ship made several brief visits to other Central American ports.

On admission he appeared acutely ill and dehydrated. He was afebrile; pulse rate was 112 beats per minute. His abdomen was soft and tender to palpation of both lower quadrants and hypogastrium. Bowel sounds were hypoactive. Rectal examination evoked considerable tenderness. The WBC was 12,000/cu mm, x-ray films and results of other laboratory studies were normal. Ulcerative colitis, amebiasis, and appendicitis were considered as diagnostic possibilities. During the first 18 hours he had profuse watery diarrhea containing mucus and blood. Sigmoidoscopy showed a friable and hyperemic rectal mucosa. The WBC reached 18,000/cu mm and temperature was 102.4 F (39.1 C), during the first 48 hours. At first, he was treated with 2 gm of ampicillin sodium intravenously per day. Because of lack of clinical improvement after 48 hours, the ampicillin was increased to 12 gm/day and kanamycin, 1 gm/day intramuscularly, was added. Thereafter, his course was one of rapid improvement and he was discharged 13 days later after stool cultures revealed no pathogens. *Shigella dysenteriae,* type 1, was recovered from the initial stool culture. The patient's serum, obtained on July 28, had a hemagglutination titer of 1:64 against Shiga bacillus. Rectal swabs taken from the remaining 23 men on the ship yielded on *Shigella* and none of the men had antibodies against Shiga bacillus.

Comment

Our previous experiences with the diagnosis and management of shigellosis in adults have shown it to be generally a mild disease. A common-source hospital outbreak of *Shigella sonnei* infection in 1957 resulted in 78 cases but no deaths.[4] In 30 sporadic cases of *Shigella* infection in adults between 1962 and 1965, there were two deaths, but both were in previously debilitated persons.[5] In these 30 patients there seemed to be little difference in the clinical responses of those treated with antibiotics and those who were not. None of these infections was caused by *S dysenteriae.* By contrast both patients in this report had been in prior good health and were acutely ill when seen here. In both cases, ulcerative colitis and amebiasis were diagnostic considerations. Delay in diagnosis and institution of proper therapy, or increased severity of disease associated with this type of *Shigella,* or both, may have contributed to the fulminant disease seen in these cases.

The finding of shigellae in blood but not feces of patient 1 merits comment. While *Shigella* usually remains localized in the gut wall, bacteremia has been amply documented on rare occasion for all four *Shigella* species.[6,7] The recovery of *Shigella* from blood in the face of negative stool cultures has also been previously described.[8,9] Failure to recover *S dysenteriae* from feces may be related in part to the fragility of this organism. Mata et al[1] found that 70% of 49 strains of Shiga bacillus failed to grow on *Salmonella-Shigella* agar. These grew well on tergitol 7 agar containing triphenyl tetrazolium chloride (T7T). It is recommended by workers at the Center for Disease Control that T7T, xylose-lactose-desoxycholate (XLD), or MacConkey's bile salt agar, in addition to routine media, be used for culturing when this organism is being sought.[10]

Supportive measures, including replacement of fluids and electrolytes lost in the stool, are necessary in all cases of dysentery. In addition, in Shiga infection, antibiotic therapy is of prime importance. Antibiotic sensitivity testing is clearly necessary as a guide to selection of therapy since resistance to commonly used antibiotics may occur. Episomal transfer of antibiotic resistance is a well described phenomenon among shigellae[11,12] and may limit usefulness of a number of therapeutic agents.[13] Thus far, all strains from Central America have had a similar pattern of antibiotic susceptibility. Fifty-three strains from Guatemala were sensitive to cephalothin sodium, ampicillin, kanamycin, nalidixic acid, and nitrofurantoin. All were resistant to sulfathiazole and 52 were resistant to chloramphenicol, tetracycline, and streptomycin.[1] Patients who are acutely ill could be treated initially with ampicillin, 4 to 6 gm/day, or kanamycin, 15 mg/kg/day, or both until antibiotic sensitivity is known and renal function is assessed. In a recent study from Vietnam, while ampicillin was effective, kanamycin appeared to be of no value in the treatment of shigellosis.[14] However, only 8 of 90 patients were infected with *S dysenteriae* (types not mentioned) and all eight strains were sensitive in vitro to ampicillin and kanamycin. It would seem to us that the results of that report further stress the need to use sensitivity testing in the selection of antibiotic therapy for shigellosis.

The level of sanitation and personal hygiene in the United States is such that a major epidemic is unlikely to occur. However, physicians who have the opportunity to treat patients with dysentery who have been recent travelers to Mexico or Central America, or contacts of such persons, should consider Shiga bacillus as a definite possible etiology. They should be aware of the laboratory cultural requirements of this organism and the antibiotic sensitivities of the previously isolated strains from that region. There have been 25 common-source outbreaks of shigellosis in the United States in the past five years, and an additional 23 outbreaks thought to be person-to-person spread.[15] Although the asymptomatic carrier state occurs less often with *Shigella* than with *Salmonella*,[16] contamination of food or water by undetected carriers who have acquired Shiga bacillus in Central America could occur. Indeed, one secondary case of dysentery associated with the current epidemic in Central America has already been reported in the United States in a contact of a person who had acquired Shiga bacillus dysentery in Leon, Nicaragua.[10] A second indigenously acquired case was recently reported from California in a child whose contact probably acquired the disease in Mexico.[17] These cases illustrate the need for thorough epidemiologic studies in each instance where the organism is found. Local and state health authorities should be notified in each case.

Summary

Two acutely ill patients who acquired dysentery in Nicaragua were recently seen in Miami, Fla, hospitals. The clinical picture was similar to fulminating ulcerative colitis. *Shigella dysenteriae*, type 1 (the Shiga bacillus), was recovered from the blood of one and from the stool of the other. This organism is currently associated with an epidemic of dysentery in Central America and has been responsible for unusually severe disease. Antibiotic therapy for shigellosis caused by this organism is mandatory. The organism has been generally resistant to chloramphenicol, tetracyclines, and sulfonamides, and sensitive to ampicillin and kanamycin.

This investigation was supported by Public Health Service general research support grant FA-5363.

Nonproprietary and Trade Names of Drugs

Metronidazole—*Flagyl*.
Salicylazosulfapyridine—*Azulfidine*.
Ampicillin sodium—*Alpen-N Amcil-S, Omnipen-N, Penbritin-S for Injection, Polycillin-N for Injection, Principen/N, Totacillin-N*.
Cephalothin sodium—*Keflin*.

References

1. Mata LJ, Gangarosa EJ, Caceres A, et al: Epidemic Shiga bacillus dysentery in Central America: I. Etiologic investigations in Guatemala, 1969. *J Infect Dis* **122**:170-180, 1970.
2. Gangarosa EJ, Perera DR, Mata LJ, et al: Epidemic Shiga bacillus dysentery in Central America: II. Epidemiologic studies in 1969. *J Infect Dis* **122**:181-190, 1970.
3. Shigellosis—United States 1969. *Morbidity Mortality Weekly Rep* **19**:142-143, 148, 1970.
4. Ehrenkranz NJ, Takos MJ, Hoffert WR, et al: An epidemic of *Shigella sonnei* dysentery arising in a general hospital. *New Eng J Med* **259**:375-377, 1958.
5. Barrett-Connor E: Shigellosis in the adult. *JAMA* **198**:717-720, 1966.
6. Faucon R, Ducloux M: Septicémies á *Shigella*. *Med Trop* **24**:537-545, 1964.
7. Barrett-Conner E, Conner JD: *Shigella boydii* bacteremia. *J Pediat* **75**:298-300, 1969.
8. Robertson HC: Outbreak of shigellosis resembling enterovirus. *Southern Med J* **56**:662-665, 1963.
9. Graber CD, Browning D, Davis JS: Shigellemia without *Shigella* diarrhea. *Amer J Clin Path* **46**:221-224, 1966.
10. Indigenously-acquired Shiga bacillus dysentery. *Morbidity Mortality Weekly Rep* **19**:381-382, 1970.
11. Watanabe T: Infective heredity of multiple drug resistance in bacteria. *Bact Rev* **27**:87-115, 1963.
12. Lewis MJ: Multiple transmissable drug resistance in the outbreak of *Shigella flexneri* infection. *Lancet* **2**:953-956, 1967.
13. Farrar WE, Dekle LC: Transferable antibiotic resistance associated with an outbreak of shigellosis. *Ann Intern Med* **67**:1208-1215, 1967.
14. Tong MJ, Martin DG, Cunningham JJ, et al: Clinical and bacteriological evaluation of antibiotic treatment in shigellosis. *JAMA* **214**:1841-1844, 1970.
15. Reller LB, Gangarosa EJ, Brachman PS: Shigellosis in the US, 1964-1968. *J Infect Dis* **120**:393-396, 1969.
16. Felsen J: *Bacillary Dysentery, Colitis and Enteritis*. Philadelphia, WB Saunders Co, 1945, p 49.
17. Shiga dysentery—California. *Morbidity Mortality Weekly Rep* **20**:75, 1971.

Successful Defense Against *Histoplasma capsulatum* in Hypogammaglobulinemia

W. Douglas Biggar, MD; Hilaire J. Meuwissen, MD; and Robert A. Good, MD, PhD, Minneapolis

The mechanisms of bodily defense against fungal diseases remain largely unknown. Circulating antibodies are frequently demonstrable during infections with *Histoplasma capsulatum* and *Candida albicans*, for instance, but this may reflect activity of the infectious process rather than specific immunity.[1]

It has been suggested that cellular immunity plays an important role in killing and eliminating facultative intracellular bacterial pathogens, for exampe, BCG *Brucella* and *Listeria monocytogenes* as well as certain fungi. Thus far, data have been obtained largely from experimental animals. Nonetheless, observations of both animals and humans lacking cell-mediated immune functions indicate that deficiencies of the thymus-dependent immune system are associated with markedly enhanced susceptibility to fungus infection,[2,3] infection with facultative intracellular bacteria pathogens, and even some viral agents.[4]

In this report, we present a patient with nonlymphopenic hypogammaglobulinemia (HGG) who appears to have had an adequate immunological defense against *H capsulatum*, despite a severe deficit in humoral immunity. This case, we believe, illustrates the importance of the cellular immune processes in the defense against this fungal pathogen.

Patient Summary

A 46-year-old white man with late onset, nonlymphopenic HGG, was admitted to the University of Minnesota Hospitals, Minneapolis, for removal of an asymptomatic pulmonary mass, found on routine x-ray film of the chest (Fig 1). The patient had suffered from multiple pulmonary infections since the age of 13 years. One year prior to admission, quantitative immunoglobulin levels were (in mg/100 ml) IgG, 42; IgA, 4.7; and IgM, < 6. The patient was of blood group O, Rh+, but had no isohemagglutinins. The Schick test was positive despite repeated immunizations with diphtheria toxoid and little or no antibody response was observed after repeated immunizations with typhoid and paratyphoid antigens. Peripheral lymphocyte count was normal, and numerous small lymphocytes were seen on peripheral blood films. Skin test for delayed hypersensitivity (DHS) to histoplasmin antigen was negative; but the patient had positive DHS responses to mumps, *Candida* antigens, and to a challenging dose of dinitrofluorobenzene after prior sensitization. The peripheral lymphocytes responded normally to stimulation with phytohemagglutinin as well as to allogeneic cells. The inflammatory cycle, as studied by the Rebuck skin window technique, was normal.

On admission the patient appeared to be a vigorous man in good general health, who was afebrile and normotensive. The axillary lymph nodes were enlarged bilaterally, but were not tender or fixed; otherwise, the results of physical examination and routine laboratory tests were unremarkable. Tomograms of the chest lesion revealed a round homogeneous mass in the left lower lobe of the lung 2.5 cm in diameter with an irregular inferior margin. The DHS response to *H capsulatum* was now strongly positive (induration, 15 mm; erythema, 30 mm at 48 hours), while the DHS skin tests to old tuberculin, blastomycosis, and coccidiocomycosis antigens were negative. The diagnosis of pulmo-

Received for publication Oct 21, 1970; accepted Nov 10.

From the Department of Pediatrics, University of Minnesota Research Laboratories of the Variety Club Heart Hospital, Minneapolis. Dr. Meuwissen is now with the Kidney Disease Institute, Albany, NY.

Reprint requests to University of Minnesota Hospitals, Mayo Box 494, Minneapolis 55455 (Dr. Biggar).

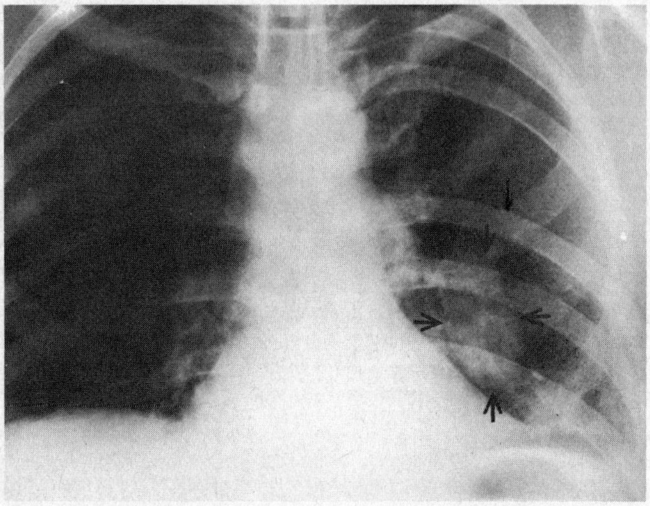

Fig 1.—Roentgenogram of the chest demonstrating a round homogeneous mass in the left lower lobe of the lung.

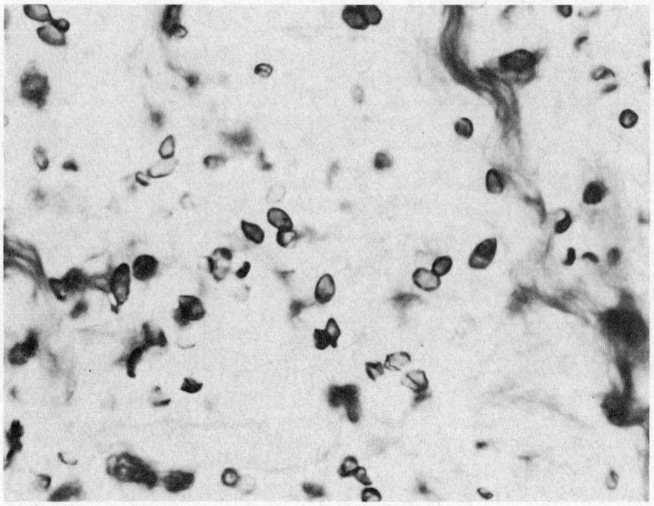

Fig 2.—High-power photomicrograph of a section of pulmonary lesion from time of surgery in 1968. Note yeast-like organisms ovoid in shape and without budding (methenamine silver × 1,000, oil immersion).

nary histoplasmosis was considered likely, but since a neoplasm could not be excluded, the pulmonary mass and left axillary lymph node were excised. The pulmonary lesion was firm and necrotic and on histologic examination contained a central area of necrosis surrounded by a narrow zone of fibroblasts, mononuclear cells, and small lymphocytes. In the central part of the necrotic area clusters of yeast-like organisms were present; these were ovoid in shape, without budding, and on morphological analysis seemed most compatible with *H capsulatum* (Fig 2). No acid-fast bacilli were seen. The left axillary lymph node had normal-appearing, thymus-dependent areas, but lacked germinal centers and plasma cells. Serum specimens taken at the time of surgery and at regular intervals thereafter, failed to show complement-fixing antibodies directed against *H capsulatum, Coccidioides immitis,* or *Blastomyces dermatitides.* Convalescence from surgery was uneventful and with γ-globulin and antibiotic prophylaxis, the patient has remained well and free from pulmonary disease in the two years following this episode.

Comment

Patients with nonlymphopenic HGG are deficient in humoral immunity and are susceptible to infections caused by encapsulated extracellular pyogenic pathogens.[4] Immunity to fungal and viral agents, with the exception of the hepatitis virus appears to be normal in many such patients.[5]

Our patient illustrates the features characteristic of nonlymphopenic HGG. Humoral immunity, evaluated by serum immunoglobulins, the capacity to form antibodies, and the absence of plasma cells and germinal centers, was severely impaired. By contrast, the cellular immune defenses as demonstrated by the normal number of lymphocytes, presence of small lymphocytes, normal DHS responses, the in vitro lymphocyte tests, and the presence of intact thymus-dependent areas in the lymph node were normal.

The recent conversion from a negative to a positive DHS response to *H capsulatum,* the microscopic appearance of the organism and the absence of serological and DHS reactivity to other fungi strongly suggest that in this instance we were dealing with an infection caused by *H capsulatum.* The patient was clinically well and had no weight loss, cough, or dyspnea. He did not have fever, anemia, hepatosplenomegaly, or bone marrow abnormalities. The pulmonary lesion was well demarcated on roentgenographic examination and had a definite capsule; no evidence of pulmonary or systemic dissemination of fungus infection was found. Surgical extirpation of the pulmonary mass resulted in a complete cure without drug therapy. We consider, therefore, that the patient had an adequate defense against *H capsulatum.*

Bodily defense against *H capsulatum* appears to be unrelated to the presence or absence of anti-*H capsulatum* antibodies in the blood.[1] Although circulating anti-*H capsulatum* antibodies are frequently demonstrable during infections caused by *H capsulatum,* their role in the defense against it is uncertain. High titers of complement-fixing, agglutinating, and precipitating antibodies against *H capsulatum* are often found in patients dying of disseminated *H capsulatum* infection.[1]

A similar paradox has been observed in experimental and human infections caused by facultative intracellular pathogens.

One might even reason from these observations that patients with high titers of circulating antibodies against *H capsulatum* have a poorer prognosis than do patients with low titers. It is difficult here, however, to sort out cause and effect. Our patient, who had adequate defenses against *H capsulatum* while lacking demonstrable circulating anti-*H capsulatum* antibodies supports the view that circulating antibodies play little role in the bodily defense against *H capsulatum*.[1] It seems likely that, in this instance, defense was related primarily to the integrity of cell-mediated immunity. In the normal person, following exposure to *H capsulatum*, the population of lymphocytes of the thymic-dependent system carrying specificity for *H capsulatum* is expanded and sensitization occurs. In addition, lymphocytes of the thymus-independent system are stimulated and this response results in production of a variety of antibodies including some cytophilic for macrophages.[6] The macrophages proliferate, become metabolically active, and seem to participate in the inflammatory process which acts as a defense against the offending pathogen. Mackaness and his associates have recently brought forward evidence indicating that the macrophage activation to the bodily defense in cell-mediated immunity is largely nonspecific.[7-9] In these studies, Mackaness et al have defined the macrophages stimulated nonspecifically by sensitized lymphocytes as "activated macrophages"[9] ("angry macrophages"). Such activated macrophages are more capable of phagocytizing and killing a variety of organisms than are macrophages, which are not so activated. In the normal host, specificity of the "angry macrophages" in the bodily defense may be further facilitated by participation of cytophilic antibody which has adhered to the macrophage. Our patient, unable to form circulating antibody in significant amounts against the pathogen, demonstrates that the host defense in this complex interaction may be based primarily on cell-mediated sensitization. Effective defense against the pathogen could be attributed in this instance largely, if not entirely, to delayed hypersensitivity and the nonspecific contributions initiated by these reactions.

Indeed in some situations, certain antibodies produced in response to the sensitizing antigen may interfere with the defense afforded by delayed hypersensitivity. Numerous phenomena based on such enhancing or blocking antibodies have been well studied in tumor systems.[10,11]

Our patient, interpreted as an experiment of nature seems to demonstrate clearly the efficiency of cell-mediated immunity without humoral immunity in the bodily defense against a facultative intracellular parasite of man, *H capsulatum*.

Summary

A 46-year-old white man with nonlymphopenic hypogammaglobulinemia developed clinically and pathologically typical pulmonary histoplasmosis. Convalescence following surgical removal of the pulmonary lesion was uneventful in the two years following this episode. The association of *Histoplasma capsulatum* infection in a patient who appears to have had an adequate immunological defense against the organism despite a severe deficit of humoral immunity illustrates the importance of cellular immunity in the defense against *H capsulatum*.

This investigation was supported by grants from the National Foundation March of Dimes, Public Health Service grants HE-06314, AI-08677, and AI-00798, and the American Heart Association.

Dr. Biggar is a Queen Elizabeth II research fellow.

References

1. Furcolow ML: Histoplasmosis, in Samter M (ed): *Immunological Diseases.* Boston, Little Brown & Co, 1965, pp 448-454.
2. Salvin SB, Peterson RDA, Good RA: The role of the thymus in resistance to infection and endotoxin toxicity. *J Lab Clin Med* **65**:1004-1022, 1965.
3. Kushner DS, Dubin A, Donlon WP, et al: Familial hypogammaglobulinemia, splenomegaly and leukopenia. *Amer J Med* **29**:33-42, 1960.
4. Good RA, Kelly WD, Rotstein J, et al: Immunological deficiency diseases. *Progr Allerg* **6**:187-320, 1962.
5. Good RA, Bridges RA, Condie RM: Host parasite relationships in patients with dysproteinemias. *Bact Rev* **24**:115-132, 1960.
6. Boyden SV: Cytophilic antibody in guinea pigs with delayed-type hypersensitivity. *Immunology* **7**:474-483, 1964.
7. Blanden RV, Lefford MJ, Mackaness GB: The host response to Calmette-Guerin Bacillus infection in mice. *J Exp Med* **129**:1079-1101, 1969.
8. Mackaness GB: The immunological basis of acquired cellular resistance. *J Exp Med* **120**:105-120, 1964.
9. Mackaness G, Blanden RV: Cellular immunity. *Progr Allerg* **11**:89-140, 1967.
10. Kaliss N: Immunological enhancement: Conditions for its expression and its relevance for graft of normal tissues. *Ann NY Acad Sci* **129**:155-163, 1966.
11. Chantler SM, Batchelor JR: Changes in the host response following treatment with lyophilized tissue. *Transplantation* **2**:75-81, 1964.

Earth Day Histoplasmosis

A New Type of Urban Pollution

Robert J. Fass, MD, and Samuel Saslaw, MD, PhD, Columbus, Ohio

In the United States, histoplasmosis is endemic in the Mississippi-Missouri-Ohio River Valley where a warm, moist environment provides optimal conditions for the growth of *Histoplasma capsulatum* in a favorable soil. Infection is not limited to this geographic area, however, and in both endemic and nonendemic areas, microenvironments of both high and low incidence of infection exist. These microenvironments are related to local recovery rates of the fungus from the soil; high rates have been particularly associated with areas where birds or bats or both congregate, roost, and hibernate.[1,2] While naturally infected birds are not known to exist, their droppings and feathers apparently provide nutrients which facilitate growth in an appropriate soil under favorable environmental conditions.[3] Bat droppings provide similar nutrients but, in addition, may contain the fungus and could conceivably serve as a source for direct transmission to man or provide a method of dissemination of spores from one location to another.[4]

In the epidemic form of histoplasmosis, two or more persons are simultaneously exposed to a sufficient number of airborne spores to become infected. The inoculum is usually large and, unlike endemic histoplasmosis which is usually asymptomatic, the majority of infected individuals become ill 7 to 16 days later with an acute influenza-like illness; fever, malaise, myalgia, cough, and a chest roentgenogram which shows patchy nodular pulmonary infiltrates and hilar adenopathy are the common findings. The disease is benign and self-limited in most instances, with less than 1% of cases progressing to severe generalized disease.[2,5] In those who develop chronic pulmonary or disseminated histoplasmosis, however, the prognosis is poorer; recovery is hastened and mortality reduced with amphotericin B therapy.[6]

Received for publication Dec 9, 1970; accepted Jan 28, 1971.

From the Division of Infectious Diseases, Department of Medicine, Ohio State University College of Medicine, Columbus.

Reprint requests to University Hospital, 410 W 10th Ave, Columbus, Ohio 43210 (Dr. Fass).

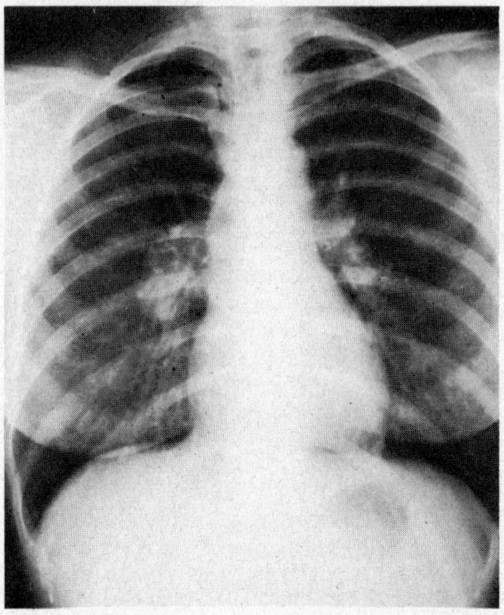

Bilateral hilar adenopathy and patchy reticular infiltrates in patient with acute histoplasmosis.

On May 22, 1970, a schoolteacher from the Willis Intermediate School in Delaware, Ohio, was referred to the Ohio State University Hospital. The prompt diagnosis of acute pulmonary histoplasmosis established the correct etiology of the "Willis flu" which represented one of the largest epidemics of histoplasmosis recorded.

Report of a Case

The patient, an otherwise healthy 35-year-old white woman, became acutely ill early in the second week of May 1970. She complained of fever, chilliness, headache, myalgia, malaise, dry hacking cough, anorexia, and nausea.

Treatment with ampicillin trihydrate and codeine did not result in improvement and she was hospitalized in Delaware, Ohio. A chest roentgenogram showed bilateral nodular patchy pulmonary densities and hilar adenopathy (Figure). Doxycycline hyclate was administered but she remained symptomatic, developed a rash, and eventually was referred to University Hospital. When admitted, she was acutely ill. Her temperature was 102 F (38.9 C); pulse rate, 96 beats per minute; respirations, 24 per minute; and blood pressure, 100 systolic, 70 diastolic. Findings on physical examination were otherwise normal except for the presence of a maculopapular eruption and an erythematous flush on her trunk, proximal extremities, and face, which were felt to be related to her antibiotic therapy.

Complete blood count, urinalysis, blood urea nitrogen level, creatinine value, serum glutamic pyruvic transaminase value, alkaline phosphatase value, and blood glucose level were within normal limits. Sputa smears and cultures were negative for pathogenic bacteria, fungi, and acid-fast bacilli. Chest roentgenogram again showed bilateral hilar adenopathy and spotty bilateral reticular infiltrates. Serial serologic data for *H capsulatum* are shown in Table 1.

The clinical and serologic picture was felt to be consistent with acute histoplasmosis and the patient was treated conservatively with bed rest. By June 6 she had recovered sufficiently to be discharged from the hospital, and by July 8 she felt well and had gained the 20 lb which she lost during her acute illness.

The Epidemic

From the patient's history and information obtained from the referring physician, it was learned that many of the students, faculty, and staff at the Willis Intermediate School had a similar illness during the first two weeks in May which was referred to as the "Willis flu." The extent of the involvement was sufficient to close the school.

Serologic data obtained in our laboratory on 11 patients (Table 2), with clinical and roentgenographic findings similar to those of our patient, and nine additional patients in the community, indicated titers compatible with recent infection with *H capsulatum*.

Subsequent epidemiologic investigation by a team from the Communicable Disease Center[7] revealed that 294 (31%) of the 949 students and faculty were ill enough with an influenza-like illness to be absent from school. An additional 89 individuals were similarly symptomatic but continued in attendance; 79.4% of sera from students tested with yeast phase or histoplasmin complement fixation techniques and gel diffusion techniques had titers of 1:64 or greater or a positive agar gel precipitin band or both. Onset of symptoms, as in our patient, occurred on or about May seventh and did not involve the surrounding community. By analysis of absenteeism data for the period preceding the epidemic, it was determined that common exposure occurred April 22 to 25. At that time, groups of students were involved in a series of clean-up activities associated with Earth Day. These activities included raking and sweeping around the school where blackbirds and pigeons were known to frequent, where the air intakes for the school ventilation system are located, and where *H capsulatum* was eventually recovered from the soil.

Table 1.—Serial Studies With Histoplasmin Collodion Agglutination Tests and Yeast Phase Complement Fixation Tests

Date	Histoplasmin Collodion Agglutination	Yeast Phase Complement Fixation
5/22/70	1:320	1:160
5/27/70	1:320	1:160
6/1/70	1:160	1:160
6/4/70	1:160	1:160
7/8/70	Negative	1:160

Comment

A high index of suspicion based on previous experiences[8-10] in this area resulted in the early diagnosis of epidemic histoplasmosis. Recognition tempered the further empiric use of antibiotic therapy and community concern about a "mysterious communicable disease." Specific antifungal therapy was not instituted since the illnesses were relatively mild. All patients convalesced uneventfully without evidence of dissemination or progression toward chronicity.

The evidence which established *H capsulatum* as the specific etiologic agent was indirect and based on serologic data. The histoplasmin collodion agglutination test[11,12] becomes positive early, usually within two to three weeks of infection; the titer elevation is transient and character-

Table 2.—Clinical and Serologic Data on Patients Afflicted With "Willis Flu"

Patient No.	Age and Sex	Date of Onset	Major Symptoms	Physical Findings	Chest Roentgenogram: Infiltrates	Chest Roentgenogram: Hilar Adenopathy	Histoplasmin Serologic Titer*: CA†	Histoplasmin Serologic Titer*: CF‡
1	11 F	5/8/70	Fever, cough, chest pain	None	Yes	Yes	640	160
2	26 F	5/8/70	Fever, cough	None	ND§		80	20
3	28 F	5/8/70	Fever, chest pain	None	ND		160	160
4	25 F	5/7/70	Fever, myalgia, cough	None	Yes	Yes	160	10
5	26 F	5/8/70	Fever, cough	None	Yes	Yes	160	80
6	14 M	5/5/70	Fever, cough, chest pain	Rales	Yes	Yes	160	160
7	13 M	5/6/70	Fever, cough, chest pain	None	No	Yes	80	160
8	15 M	5/7/70	Fever, cough, chest pain	None	ND		40	80
9	11 F	5/7/70	Fever, sore throat	None	ND		80	320
10	12 M	5/8/70	Fever cough	None	Yes	Yes	160	160
11	36 F	5/10/70	Malaise, cough, chest pain	None	Yes	Yes	160	80

* Sera obtained two to three weeks after onset of symptoms.
† CA = histoplasmin collodion agglutination test.
‡ CF = yeast phase complement fixation test.
§ ND = not done.

istically becomes negative during convalescence two to six months later. The complement fixation titer, utilizing yeast phase antigen, regresses more slowly and may be positive for one year or longer.[12,13]

Recovery of the fungus from biologic specimens such as sputum, blood, or bone marrow is necessary to make an unequivocal diagnosis of histoplasmosis, but cultures require a minimum of seven to ten days of incubation and frequently are negative in the acute pulmonary form of the disease. The recovery from soil provides important circumstantial etiologic evidence but may likewise be unsuccessful. As in the present epidemic, the etiology of epidemic histoplasmosis is frequently determined on the basis of clinical, epidemiologic, and serologic data or skin test conversion and supported by recovery of the organism from the suspected point source of infection.[2,5]

Most epidemics of urban histoplasmosis have resulted from exposure to soil contaminated with bird droppings and the spores of *H capsulatum*. Visits to farms, rural areas, open wooded areas, or old buildings disturbed by renovation or demolition, or the importation of contaminated soil have been implicated.[14] The association of school children sharing a wooded schoolyard with starlings has also been documented as a setting conducive to histoplasma infection[15]; in the present epidemic, a similar setting existed. While such an epidemic might be difficult to anticipate in a given location, its occurrence makes the desirability of eradicating *H capsulatum* from the soil obvious. The report of a second epidemic of histoplasmosis from the same site in Mason City, Iowa[16] emphasizes the potential public health hazard of such contaminated areas. While early attempts to eliminate the fungus from known positive sites were either unsuccessful or rendered the soil unfit for growth of vegetation, the large-scale use of 3% formalin for soil decontamination was at least temporarily effective in destroying the fungus on the surface of the soil in Mason City[17]; a similar procedure is currently being implemented in Delaware. It is ironic that the antipolution spirit of Earth Day was the motivating factor which resulted in the inadvertent contamination of the atmosphere around the school with the spores of *H capsulatum*. Those infected suffered the consequences of this specific type of air pollution in a very tangible way.

Summary

Diagnosis of a case of histoplasmosis in a schoolteacher led to the clarification of the etiology of an epidemic of an influenza-like illness involving an intermediate school in Delaware, Ohio. The onset of the illness in those involved occurred within a several day period. The common denominator was the Earth Day activities of students and faculty in their clean-up program two weeks earlier on April 22, 1970.

Robert Caulkins, MD, submitted the clinical summaries of and sera for patients in Table 2.

Nonproprietary and Trade Names of Drugs

Amphotericin B—*Fungizone.*

Ampicillin trihydrate—*Alpen, Amcill, Am-pen, Amplin, Polycillin, Principen, Supen, Totacillin.*

Doxycycline hyclate—*Vibramycin Hyclate.*

References

1. Furcolow ML: Recent studies on the epidemiology of histoplasmosis. *Ann NY Acad Sci* **72**:127-164, 1958.

2. Lehan PH, Furcolow ML: Epidemic histoplasmosis. *J Chron Dis* **5**:489-503, 1957.

3. Ajello L: Relationship of *Histoplasma capsulatum* to avian habitats. *Public Health Rep* **79**:226-270, 1964.

4. Klite PD, Young RV: Bats and histoplasmosis: A clinico-epidemiologic study of two human cases. *Ann Intern Med* **62**:1263-1271, 1965.

5. Wilcox KR Jr, Waisbren BA, Martin J: The Walworth, Wisconsin, epidemic of histoplasmosis. *Ann Intern Med* **49**:388-418, 1958.

6. Furcolow ML: Comparison of treated and untreated severe histoplasmosis: A Communicable Disease Center cooperative mycoses study. *JAMA* **183**:823-829, 1963.

7. *National Communicable Disease Center Morbidity and Mortality Weekly Report.* Atlanta, Georgia, Public Health Service, Health Services, and Mental Health Administration, **19**:242, 1970.

8. Prior JA, Saslaw S, Cole CR: Experiences with histoplasmosis. *Ann Intern Med* **40**:221-244, 1954.

9. Conrad FG, Saslaw S, Atwell RJ: The protean manifestations of histoplasmosis as illustrated in 23 cases. *Arch Intern Med* **104**:692-709, 1959.

10. Perkins RL, Saslaw S, Ockner SA: Migration histoplasmosis. *Ann Intern Med* **57**:363-372, 1962.

11. Saslaw S, Campbell CC: A collodion agglutination test for histoplasmosis. *Public Health Rep* **64**:424-429, 1949.

12. Saslaw S, Campbell CC: Serologic studies in histoplasmosis. *Amer J Public Health* **40**:427-435, 1950.

13. Saslaw S, Campbell CC: The use of yeast phase antigens in a complement fixation test for histoplasmosis: I. Preliminary results with rabbit sera. *J Lab Clin Med* **33**:811-818, 1948.

14. Furcolow ML, Tosh FE, Larsh HW, et al: The emerging pattern of urban histoplasmosis: Studies on an epidemic in Mexico, Missouri. *New Eng J Med* **264**:1226-1230, 1961.

15. Dodge HJ, Ajello L, Engelke OK: The association of a bird-roosting site with infection of school children by *Histoplasma capsulatum*. *Amer J Public Health* **55**:1203-1211, 1965.

16. Tosh FE, Doto IL, D'Alessio DJ, et al: The second of two epidemics of histoplasmosis resulting from work on the same starling roost. *Amer Rev Resp Dis* **94**:406-413, 1966.

17. Tosh FE, Weeks RJ, Pfeiffer FR, et al: The use of formalin to kill *Histoplasma capsulatum* at an epidemic site. *Amer J Epidem* **85**:259-265, 1967.

Pseudomonas Septicemia

Illustrated Evolution of Its Skin Lesion

Gerald J. Dorff, MD; Nicholas F. Geimer, MD;
Dorothy R. Rosenthal, MD; and Michael W. Rytel, MD, Milwaukee

Pseudomonas aeruginosa infections continue to present a formidable challenge because of the high incidence in patients with chronic disease and impaired defense mechanisms, and the resistance of the organism to most antibiotics. In particular, *Pseudomonas* septicemia is a dread complication which can be effectively treated only if recognized early. A feature that is helpful in making the diagnosis of *Pseudomonas* septicemia is the presence of a characteristic skin lesion commonly known as ecthyma gangrenosum. This lesion was first described by Barker[1] in 1897 and subsequently noted by other authors to be pathognomonic of *Pseudomonas* septicemia.[2-4] Illustrated descriptions of the clinical and microscopic features of this lesion are sparse. We recently saw a patient with multiple myeloma who developed striking skin lesions associated with *Pseudomonas* septicemia. The clinical and histopathological observations of this case provide the basis for this report.

Received for publication Aug 26, 1970; accepted Dec 8.

From the sections of infectious disease and hematology, departments of medicine and pathology, Milwaukee County General Hospital, Medical College of Wisconsin, Milwaukee.

Reprint requests to 7400 Harwood Ave, Wauwatosa, Wis 53226 (Dr. Dorff).

Patient Summary

A 60-year-old man with multiple myeloma was admitted because of sudden onset of headache, malaise, chills, and fever eight hours prior to admission. The diagnosis of multiple myeloma was made three years previously on the basis of serum protein monoclonal gammopathy and plasma cell infiltration of the bone marrow. Treatment had consisted of melphalan 2 mg/day for two weeks with intervening periods of two weeks without treatment. Melphalan therapy was discontinued two months before admission because of pancytopenia and hypoplastic bone marrow. He did not receive corticosteroid therapy. The patient was accustomed to taking tetracycline intermittently at home for frequent minor febrile illnesses. On the morning of admission, the patient took four 250-mg capsules of tetracycline during a six-hour period for these symptoms.

The patient was well-nourished, alert,

and cooperative; blood pressure was 120/70 mm Hg; pulse rate, 120 beats per minute; respiration rate, 24 per minute; temperature, 103.6 F (39.8 C) orally. Pertinent physical findings consisted of warm dry skin without lesions, small nontender lymph nodes in the left axilla, clear lungs, normal sized heart without murmurs, soft abdomen without organomegaly or masses, no nuchal rigidity, and no bony tenderness.

Hematocrit level was 22%, white blood cell count 2,000/cu mm, differential count, 54% bands, 24% segmented neutrophils, 13% lymphocytes, and 3% monocytes with 6% metamyelocytes. Platelet count was 58,000/cu mm. Routine urinalysis showed protein (2+) with normal results of microscopic examination. No Bence Jones protein was found in the urine. Blood urea nitrogen level was 20 mg/100 ml. Total serum protein levels were 11.6 gm/100 ml; albumin, 1.8 gm/100 ml; γ-globulin, 6.8 gm/100 ml. The electrophoretic pattern was characterized by a large monoclonal peak in the γ-globulin area. A x-ray film of the chest and electrocardiogram were normal. Cerebral spinal fluid was normal. Blood cultures were obtained on admission. *Pseudomonas aeruginosa*, sensitive to gentamicin sulfate by the Kirby-Bauer technique, was isolated four days later. *Pseudomonas* was also recovered from the stool.

Treatment with nafcillin sodium, 6 gm/day and gentamicin sulfate, 240 mg/day was begun after cultures were obtained. The patient received three units of packed cells and 20 ml of pooled γ-globulin intramuscularly. On the second hospital day, the patient complained of severe generalized bone pain and had four watery stools. He was febrile and confused and appeared more toxic, dyspneic, and slightly cyanotic. The rest of the examination was unchanged. On his third hospital day, multiple painful pruritic edematous skin lesions measuring 1 cm in diameter were noted. They were prominent on the distal extremities and pelvic area. The lesions over the anterior tibial surfaces resembled those of erythema multiforme. His face was spared but periorbital edema was present. In a few hours some of the skin lesions developed an intense erythematous center with some lesions proceeding on to hemorrhagic bullous formation and then on to full central hemorrhagic necrosis. By the middle of his third hospital day, the patient had skin lesions in all stages and at that time he developed signs of gram-negative bacillary shock. A regimen of hydrocortisone given intravenously, 500 mg every six hours, was begun. Fluids were given intravenously and gentamicin was continued at a reduced dose. The level of gentamicin in the blood on that day was 25μg/ml (accepted therapeutic range is 6 to 12μg/ml). He deteriorated rapidly, and died early the next morning.

Autopsy Findings

Gross and microscopic examinations disclosed minimal evidence of myeloma. Osteoporosis was present and the marrow was hypocellular. The liver, adrenals, and prostate contained necrotic infarcts almost identical to those in the skin, to be described. Gram-negative rods were identified in the radicals of the portal vein supplying the infarcted areas, with necrosis of the vessel wall, thrombosis of the vein, and surrounding abscess formation. No lesions were found in the lungs. Postmortem cultures of blood and skin lesions grew *P aeruginosa.*

Description of Skin Lesions

The skin lesion progressed through a characteristic pattern: edema, erythema, hemorrhagic bullae, and frank necrosis. The entire sequence evolved during less than 12 hours with lesions of varying ages simultaneously present. The edematous phase resembled a local histamine reaction, being raised, well circumscribed, and quickly progressed to the flattened erythematous phase, (Fig 1). Central hemorrhage soon became apparent as the lesion spread to well over 1 cm and then became bullous, and filled with blood, (Fig 2 and 3). The blister quickly collapsed, and the final stage persisted as a large lesion, up to 3 cm (Fig 4). Concentric zones characterized this stage with a central disk of hemorrhage, surrounded by a halo of uninvolved skin, and finally rimmed by a narrow violaceous ring resembling the center. The latter two stages have been identified by many authors as ecthyma gangrenosum.

The microscopic features of this lesion had three hallmarks: vein wall invasion by the bacteria, little accompanying inflammation, and no intimal involvement, (Fig 5). Occasionally fibrin thrombi were seen in small vessels, but these did not appear to be the result of primary intimal damage. Instead, the fibrin was part of an evolving process that seemed to begin with deep, subdermal vein wall invasion by bacteria, which caused subsequent obstruction. The deep dermis and subdermis responded with marked fibrin exudation, which accounted for the edema seen grossly. As more superficial and smaller veins were invaded by bacteria, the fibrin exudation progressed; diapedesis and frank hemorrhage ensued and produced the erythematous phase. The upper dermis ballooned as the engorged lymphatics and hemorrhage expanded, the upper epidermis lifted off, and the third hemorrhagic bullous stage was entered, (Fig 6). Finally, necrosis of the involved dermis resulted. Remarkably, almost no inflammatory cells were encountered at any stage, (Fig 7). A few polymorphonuclear leukocytes were noted very early and only at the vessels invaded by bacteria. The bacteria appeared mainly in the media and adventitia with the intima being affected only in the late stages of the lesion, (Fig 8). Arteries of any size were involved only when the entire region was necrotic and did not appear to be the primary sites of involvement.

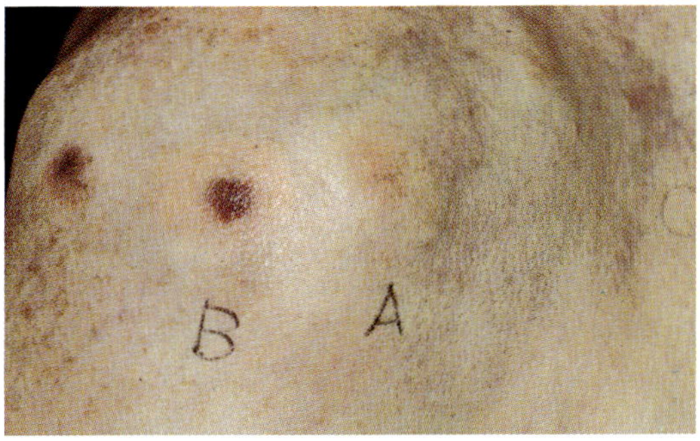

Fig. 1.—Early edematous lesion (A) with slight erythema. Second stage (B) is markedly erythematous. Note varying stages in same geographic location (shoulder).

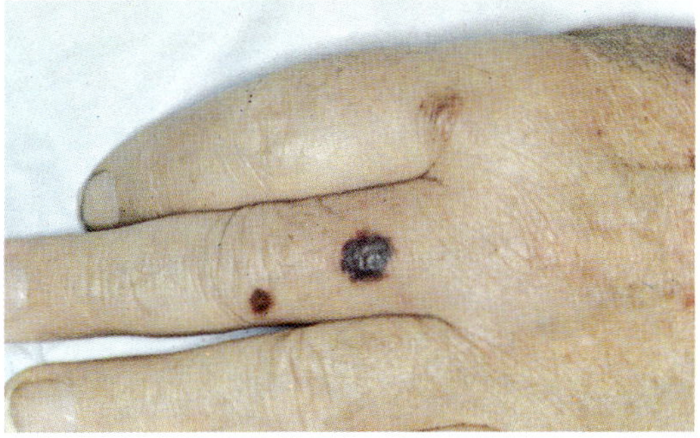

Fig 2.—Hemorrhagic bullous, third stage, on proximal phalanx, second stage on proximal interphalangeal joint, and earlier stage on fifth metacarpo-phalangeal joint.

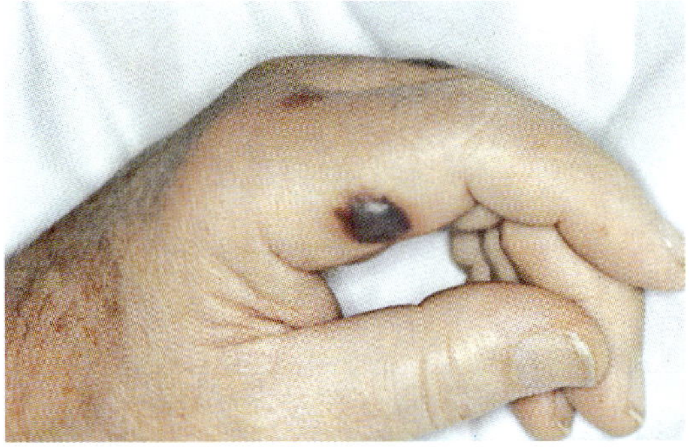

Fig 3.—Fully developed third stage, hemorrhagic bullous. Note rim of hyperemia and spreading border.

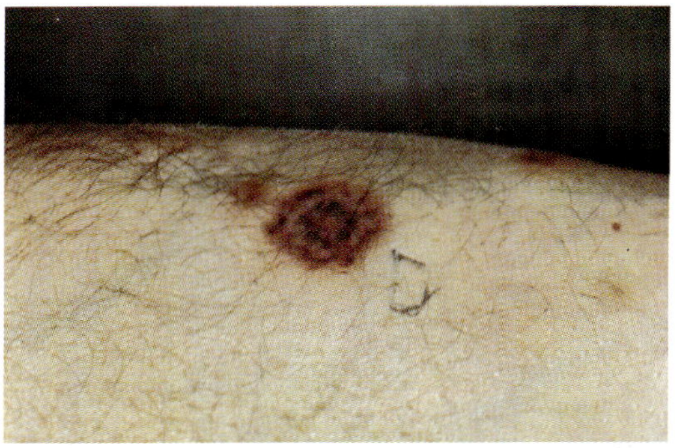

Fig 4.—Final stage (large lesion) with concentric ring configuration and central necrosis. Note smaller adjacent early lesion.

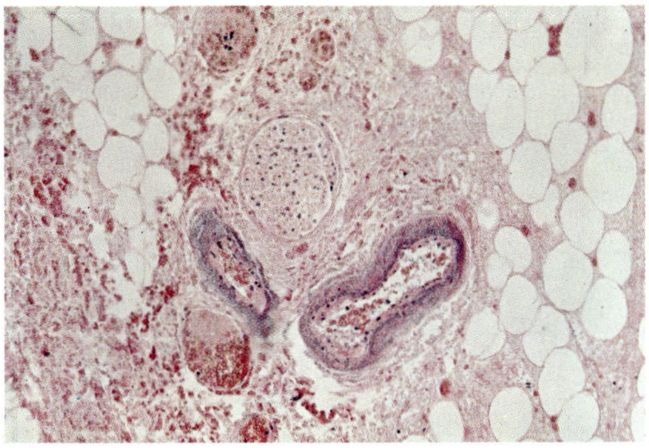

Fig 5.—Bacilli in vessel walls stain blue. Surrounding tissue is undergoing coagulation necrosis (hematoxylin — eosin, ×400).

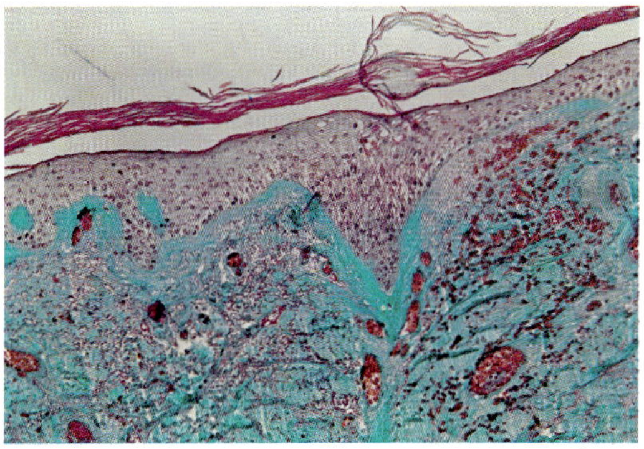

Fig 6.—Bullous third stage with engorged dermal lymphatics filled with fibrin (pink stain, right side of field). Diapedesis of red blood cells in upper dermis on left hand of field (Lendrum fibrin stain, ×100.)

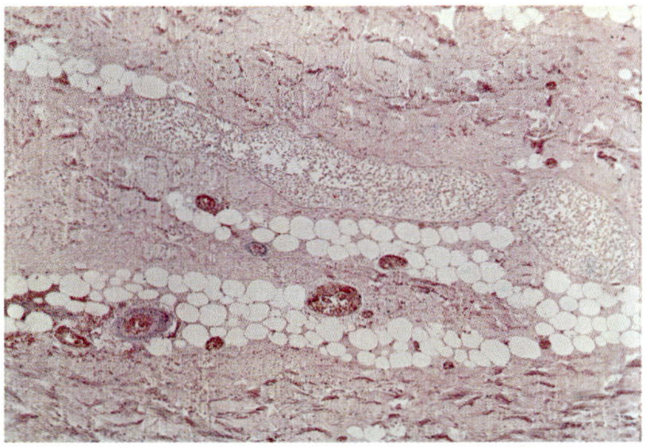

Fig 7.—Markedly dilated dermal lymphatic. Surrounding tissue is necrotic, but devoid of neutrophils. Vessel walls contain bacilli (hematoxylin — eosin, ×100).

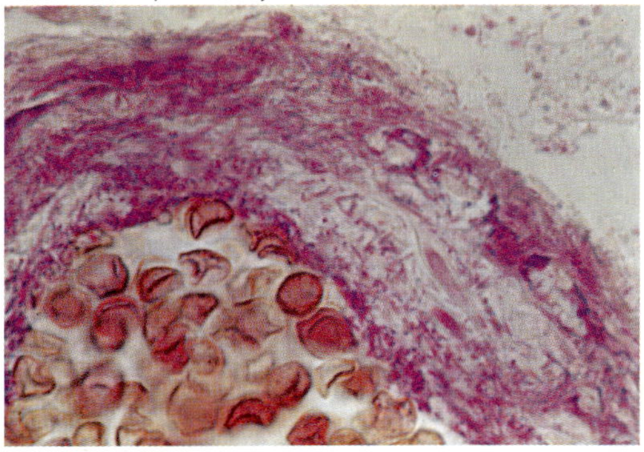

Fig 8.—Bacilli seen in vein wall as purple rods. Note absence of bacilli in lumen. Vessel is part of advanced lesion so intima is now involved (Goodpasture's stain, ×1,000).

Comment

Historically, this lesion has been described numerous times[4-6] and labeled ecthyma gangrenosum. This lesion occurs with variable frequency in *Pseudomonas* infections depending on degree of bacteremia, predisposing diseases, and concomitant antibacterial or immunosuppressive therapy. Its natural history and peculiarities are particularly well illustrated by this patient. Many authors have assumed that because veins were involved, arteries were also involved.[5,7] Dramatic dermal lymphatic engorgement secondary to postcapillary venule thrombosis accounts for many features and to our knowledge has not been previously described. In other forms of bacterial vasculitis, eg, meningococcal vasculitis, septic intraluminal thrombi attach to bacteria and invade the endothelium. Vein wall invasion by *P aeruginosa* involves the adventitia and media, and spares the intima and the lumen. The mechanism of this invasion is unknown. The most remarkable finding which has been noted by all authors is the paucity of leukocytic exudation. Our patient was neutropenic. But in animals with normal neutrophilic counts, Teplitz[7] described similar lesions, also without neutrophilic response. He and others[8] have postulated that either local tissue neutropenia or toxic bacterial products repelling or destroying neutrophils may be responsible for the acellular necrosis.

It should be emphasized that this lesion seems to be associated specifically with systemic *Pseudomonas* infections. Other conditions associated with cutaneous vasculitis, such as polyarteritis nodosa, hypersensitivity angitis, and other forms of bacterial septicemia, may present a similar appearance clinically, but histologic distinction is usually possible. Similarly, the lesion must be distinguished from nonspecific cutaneous lesions occasionally associated with *Pseudomonas* infections, such as pyoderma gangrenosum, the green nail syndrome, erythema nodosum, and other purpuric and erysipeloid lesions.[4] The lesions of ecthyma gangrenosum may be single, but are usually multiple and isolated, and occur most frequently over the lower trunk and the extremities. The palmar, plantar, and mucosal surfaces are usually spared. The organism may be demonstrated in scrapings from the base of the vesicular lesion.[4]

It seems likely that the self administration of tetracycline was an important factor in our patient's illness. Probable alteration of his gastrointestinal flora resulted in overgrowth of *Pseudomonas*. The four day delay in the growth of his cultures might also be attributed to tetracycline ingestion. His underlying disease and his earlier melphalan therapy undoubtedly left him with an impaired ability to respond to overwhelming infection. This may explain why he failed to improve despite high levels of gentamicin in the blood.

We conclude that the skin lesion observed in this patient is an important manifestation of *Pseudomonas* septicemia. Because this lesion may appear before organisms are isolated from the blood, the recognition of this lesion constitutes an indication for therapy even in the absence of positive blood cultures.[4,6,9]

Summary

We have had the opportunity to observe and document the characteristic features of the skin lesion seen in systemic *Pseudomonas* infections. Recognition of this lesion by clinicians should facilitate earlier diagnosis and hopefully, more favorable treatment of *Pseudomonas* septicemia.

George Hensley, MD, assisted with the photomicrographs and the patient was the private patient of Anthony Pisciotta, MD.

Nonproprietary and Trade Names of Drugs

Melphalan—*Alkeran.*
Gentamicin sulfate—*Garamycin.*
Nafcillin sodium—*Unipen.*

References

1. Barker LF: The clinical symptoms, bacteriologic findings, and postmortem appearances in cases of infection of human beings with the *Bacillus pyocyaneus. JAMA* **29**:213-216, 1897.

2. Heffner RW, Smith GF: Ecthyma gangrenosum in *pseudomonas* septicemia. *Amer J Dis Child* **99**:524-528, 1960.

3. Curtion JA, Petersdorf FG, Bennett IL Jr: *Pseudomonas* bacteremia: Review of 91 cases. *Ann Intern Med* **54**:1077-1107, 1961.

4. Hall JH, Callaway JL, Tindall JP, et al: *Pseudomonas aeruginosa* in dermatology. *Arch Derm* **97**:312-323, 1968.

5. Stanley MM: *Bacillus pyocyaneus* infections. *Amer J Med* **2**:253-277, 1947.

6. Forkner CE Jr, Frei E III, Edgecomb JH, et al: *Pseudomonas* septicemia: Observations on 23 cases. *Amer J Med* **25**:877-889, 1958.

7. Teplitz C: Pathogenesis of *Pseudomonas* vasculitis and septic lesions. *Arch Path* **80**:297-307, 1965.

8. Fetzer AE, Werner AS, Hagstrom JW: Pathologic features of pseudomonal pneumonia. *Amer Rev Resp Dis* **96**:1121-1130, 1967.

9. Case records of the Massachusetts General Hospital (case 35—1970). *New Eng J Med* **283**:420-427, 1970.

Psychosis in Vitamin B_{12} Deficiency

Richard J. Hart, Jr., MD, and Paul R. McCurdy, MD, Washington, DC

Vitamin B_{12} deficiency may present with a psychosis which is curable if treated promptly.[1-8] Although this fact is not new and is described in various textbooks,[9,10] it seems that it is often forgotten, which results in prolonged suffering from irreversible brain damage.[1] Accordingly, the following case report is presented to reemphasize the value of recognizing and promptly treating "megaloblastic madness."

Patient Summary

A 53-year-old Negro woman was admitted to the District of Columbia General Hospital for the first time on Sept 12, 1968, because of psychosis and anemia. She had become increasingly anorectic for two months before admission and lost 13.6 kg (30 lb). During the last month she had become unmanageable at home by refusing all food, defecating and urinating in bed, and failing to recognize her husband. She was fearful that various unknown persons would harm her and had to be led by the hand around the house and to the bathroom. During the last week she had hallucinated butterflies in the house and had fainted four times. She had not complained of numbness, tingling, or sore tongue.

There was no family or personal history of anemia, neurologic, or psychologic disorders. She had late onset diabetes.

Vital signs on admission were normal without orthostatic changes. She was obese and disoriented to time and place. She could name objects but had slow mentation and both recent and past memory loss. There were new and old hemorrhages and hard, small waxy exudates in both optic fundi, but there was no papilledema and only minimal arteriolar narrowing. Mucosal and conjunctival membranes were pale, but the tongue was well papillated without glossitis. Neuromuscular examination showed normal cranial nerves and no loss or decrease in the senses of vibration (256 cycles per second) or touch. Deep tendon reflexes were 2+/4+ and equal for both triceps and biceps but were absent at the knees and ankles. Motor strength and cerebellar function including gait and stereognosis were normal. Before the admission examination was completed, she became combative and paranoid.

The values obtained from laboratory tests included negative results for stool blood (Hematest); greater than 100,000 *Escherichia coli* per milliliter of urine; normal cerebrospinal fluid (including negative results to a test for syphilis); protein-bound iodine (PBI), 7.9 mg/100 ml; T_3 test (triiodothyronine), 32%; serum glutamic oxaloacetic transaminase, 10 units/ml; serum lactic dehydrogenase (LDH), 1,230 units/ml (colormetric technique); total bilirubin, 1.95 mg/100 ml (0.97 mg/100 ml direct); and alkaline phosphatase, 7.5 King-Armstrong units. The hematocrit value was 19.5%; reticulocytes, 1.1%; platelets, 220,000/cu mm; and leukocyte count, 5,900/cu mm. On the peripheral smear the red blood cells were macrocytic and there were hypersegmented neutrophils. There was typically megaloblastic maturation of eryth-

Received for publication Oct 8, 1970; accepted Dec 15.

From the Georgetown Medical Division of the District of Columbia General Hospital, Washington. Dr. Hart is now with the Brooke Army Medical Center, San Antonio, Tex.

Reprint requests to 19th St and Massachusetts Ave, SE, Washington, DC 20003 (Dr. McCurdy).

roid and myeloid cells in the bone marrow. Marrow iron was grade 4/6.[11] Assay and starch gel electrophoresis of erythrocyte glucose-6-phosphate dehydrogenase[12] were normal as was hemoglobin electrophoresis. Direct and indirect Coombs' tests were negative and her red blood cells were group O Rh_0(D) positive. There was no free gastric hydrochloric acid after betazole hydrochloride (Histalog) stimulation. A series of roentgenograms of the upper gastrointestinal tract were normal. An electroencephalogram, done three weeks after therapy was started, was normal. "Serum only" tests showed very poor absorption of cyanocobalamin Co 57 (4 cpm/4 ml serum) which became normal upon addition of intrinsic factor (31 cpm/4 ml serum).[13] Assay for folate[14] of serum obtained while she was fasting at the time of admission was high normal. Serum vitamin B_{12} was not measured. The psychiatric consultant doubted that her mental status could be explained by pernicious anemia alone and asked that syphilis and chronic brain syndrome be ruled out.

Intramuscular therapy with cyanocobalamin was begun with 100μg daily and within eight days her paranoid ideation disappeared. No transfusions were given and the patient received a regular diet. She took no other medications except an antibiotic for the asymptomatic urinary tract infection. The reticulocyte count rose to 9% eight days after cyanocobalamin therapy was started, then declined. The hematocrit reading climbed slowly to 32% after three weeks and stabilized at 43% within two months. Within three weeks the serum LDH value fell to 400 units/ml and the total bilirubin value to 0.30 mg/100 ml. In the opinions of all observers, including the family and the psychiatric consultant, her psychosis cleared completely with the full return of memory. The fundal hemorrhages resolved, but hypertension became manifest and later required therapy.

Comment

This patient had pernicious anemia with psychosis as the major presenting complaint. Psychosis from vitamin B_{12} deficiency per se rather than severe anemia has been previously reported,[2] but the mechanism is not known. In one series 14 of 25 cases pernicious anemia had well-marked cerebral symptoms.[1] Indeed, 4 of the 14 had these symptoms for 2 to 8 years before the onset of anemia. A number of authors,[1-7] stress the cerebral symptoms in vitamin B_{12} deficiency. Many of their patients were discovered in mental institutions where the diagnosis of pernicious anemia had been overlooked or delayed. In a recent survey, nearly 1% of more than 1,000 psychiatric patients were found to have undetected vitamin B_{12} deficiency.[15] Indeed, this deficiency may be a more common cause for mental symptoms than syphilis.[5] Prompt therapy is essential and the presence of psychosis for no more than one month probably explains the rapid improvement in our patient following vitamin B_{12} therapy. To miss the diagnosis and consign the patient to permanent custodial care is unconscionable. Hence, anemia in a psychotic patient should be carefully investigated to determine its cause. It may even be desirable to measure serum vitamin B_{12} routinely in all newly mentally disturbed patients.[15]

Summary

A Negro woman with pernicious anemia, whose presenting complaint was psychosis, demonstrates the relationship of mental symptoms to vitamin B_{12} deficiency. This eminently treatable cause for psychosis should not be overlooked.

This investigation was supported in part by Public Health Service research grant AM-09307 from the National Institute of Arthritis and Metabolic Diseases.

References

1. Holmes J: Cerebral manifestations of vitamin B_{12} deficiency. *Brit Med J* **2**:1394-1398, 1956.

2. Shulman R: Psychiatric aspects of pernicious anemia: A prospective controlled investigation. *Brit Med J* **3**:266-270, 1967.

3. Wiener JS, Hope JM: Cerebral manifestations of vitamin B_{12} deficiency. *JAMA* **170**:1038-1041, 1959.

4. Smith ADM: Megaloblastic madness. *Brit Med J* **2**:1840-1845, 1960.

5. Hunter R, Matthews DM: Mental symptoms in vitamin B-12 deficiency. *Lancet* **2**:738, 1965.

6. Strachan RW, Henderson JG: Psychiatric syndromes due to avitaminosis B_{12} with normal blood and marrow. *Quart J Med* **34**:303-317, 1965.

7. Girdwood RH: Abnormalities of vitamin B_{12} and folic acid metabolism: Their influence on the nervous system. *Proc Nutr Soc* **27**:101-107, 1965.

8. Smith R, Oliver RAM: Sudden onset of psychosis in association with vitamin B_{12} deficiency. *Brit Med J* **3**:34-36, 1967.

9. Wintrobe MM: *Clinical Hematology.* Philadelphia, Lea & Febiger, 1967, pp 511-512.

10. Herbert V: *The Megaloblastic Anemias: Modern Medical Monographs.* New York, Grune & Stratton Inc, 1959, pp 1-162.

11. Rath CE, Finch CA: Sternal marrow hemosiderin: Method for determination of available iron stores in man. *J Lab Clin Med* **31**:81, 1948.

12. Kirkman HN, Hendrickson EM: Sex-linked electrophoretic difference in glucose-6-phosphate dehydrogenase. *Amer J Human Genet* **15**:241-258, 1963.

13. McCurdy PR: The detection of intestinal absorption of Co^{57} tagged vitamin B_{12} by serum counting. *Ann Intern Med* **62**:97-102, 1965.

14. Herbert V: Aseptic addition method for *Lactobacillus casei* assay of folate activity in human serum. *J Clin Path* **19**:12-16, 1966.

15. Henderson JG, Strachan RW, Beck JS, et al: The antigastric-antibody test for vitamin B_{12} deficiency in psychiatric practice. *Lancet* **2**:809-813, 1966.

Palmar Varices and Gastrointestinal Bleeding

William C. Sherwood, MD, Philadelphia

In patients with gastrointestinal bleeding, a close inspection of the skin and mucous membranes may produce rewarding diagnostic possibilities.[1] Vascular lesions such as telangiectases, hemangiomas, and phlebectasia may have gastrointestinal counterparts.[2-4]

The present communication describes a patient with repeated gastrointestinal bleeding from isolated gastric varices, without evidence of portal or splenic vein hypertension, who also demonstrated striking variceal changes of the veins of the hands.

Patient Summary

A 69-year-old white man was hospitalized the second time for gastrointestinal bleeding. Fourteen months earlier, upper-gastrointestinal tract bleeding prompted exploratory laparotomy. Results of an x-ray series of the upper gastrointestinal tract performed preoperatively were normal. A large bleeding varix of the antrum was found (Fig 1), and partial gastrectomy was performed. The splenic and portal veins appeared normal and patent. Esophageal varices could not be identified.

On the second admission, repeated exploration revealed a bleeding varix on the greater curvature of the gastric remnant which required further excision. Again, no evidence of portal hypertension was apparent. The spleen and pancreas appeared normal, and liver biopsy specimens were normal. Physical examination following blood replacement revealed numerous cirsoid varices of the palms and fingers of both hands (Fig 2). There was no evidence of venous obstruction, and the veins collapsed with elevation. The skin of the palms was thin and parchment-like, with loss of the normal dermatoglyphic pattern. The venous pressure of an antecubital vein was normal bilaterally. The patient had noted the veins five years earlier, and they had caused him no difficulty. An arteriogram of the left hand (Fig 3) revealed multiple saccular deformations of the veins of the fingers and palm. There was no evidence of arteriovenous communications. Mild, superficial varicosities of the lower portions of both legs were present. The deep venous systems were patent. No other abnormal vascular lesions were noted.

Comment

Varices arise as a result of either prolonged increase in the intraluminal pressure of the veins, or the loss of venous supportive structures.[5] It has been postulated both that the latter phenomenon may arise as an hereditary defect[6] and that it may be associated with a change in connective tissue coincident with aging.[7] In patients with primary varicose veins of the legs, abnormal venous distensibility of forearm veins has been noted,[8] suggesting a diffuse venous abnormality.

Fig 1.—Histologic section of stomach at bleeding margin, demonstrating dilated venous channels and submucosal hemorrhage (×40).

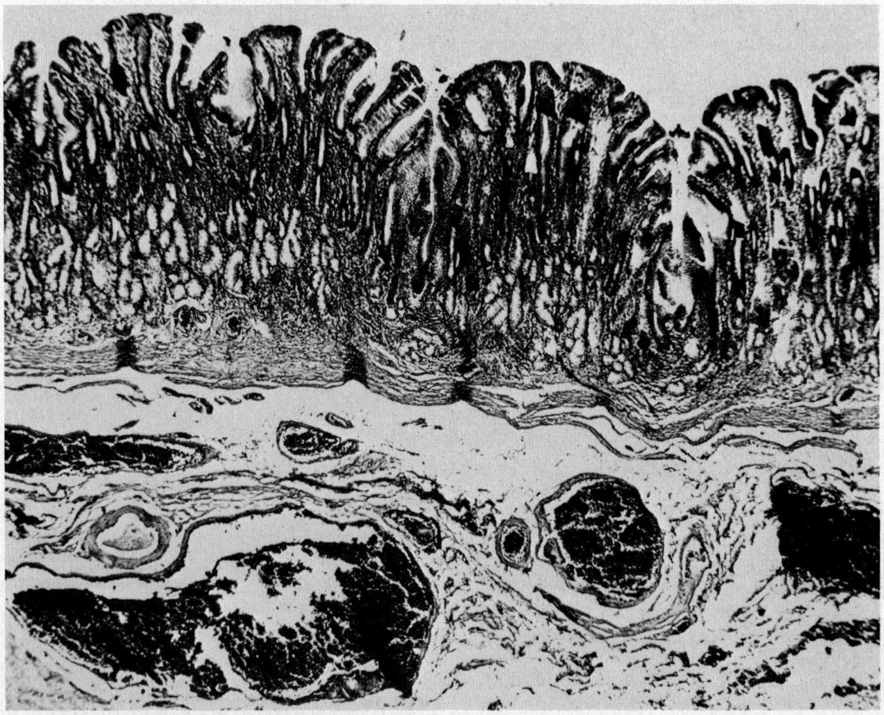

Received for publication Sept 23, 1970; accepted Jan 14, 1971.

From Philadelphia General Hospital, Jefferson Medical College of Philadelphia, and the Cardeza Foundation for Hematologic Research, Philadelphia.

Reprint requests to 1025 Sansom St, Philadelphia 19107 (Dr. Sherwood).

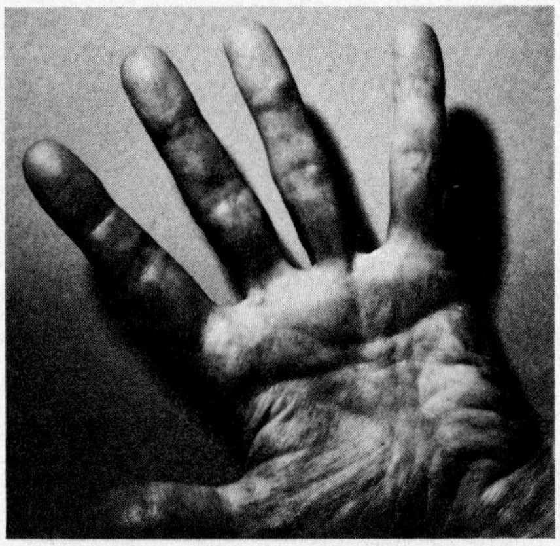

Fig 2.—Left hand of patient, demonstrating numerous cirsoid varices.

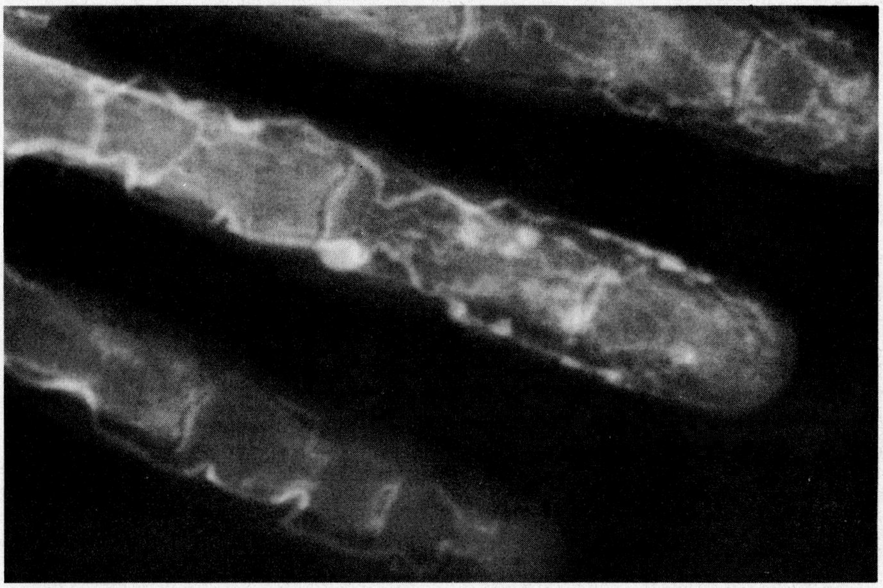

Fig 3.—Early venous phase of arteriogram of left hand, disclosing numerous small venous lakes of fingers.

Gastric varices, isolated or associated with esophageal varices, are regarded as occurring secondary to portal or splenic vein hypertension. Their occurrence unrelated to obstructive factors is not common. Palmer and Brick have described varices of the distal esophagus in the apparent absence of portal hypertension,[9] and Tisdale et al have described gastric and esophageal varices occurring in patients with portal vein hypertension but without obstruction of the portal venous system.[10] Reports of gastric varices in association with pancreatic disease describe local obstructive phenomena of the veins.[11,12]

In their description of multiple phlebectasia, Rappaport and Shiffman postulated that the syndrome occurs as an aging process.[4] With the loss of supportive connective tissue in many organs, saccular dilatation of the venules occurs in a scattered fashion. In the described cases, the venous lesions of the digestive tract have occurred exclusively in the mouth, jejunum, and ileum.[4,13,14] This cause has been applied to other vascular lesions which increase in occurrence with aging, such as Fordyce spots, caviar lesions, venous lakes, and capillary telangiectases.[3]

Bean has said that varices of the hands are rare[3] and also that they occur exclusively in the aging. He attached no particular significance to their presence, and there has been no comment on an association with other vascular lesions. In our patient, an underlying cause was not apparent. Atrophy of the skin and subcutaneous tissues of the hands with normal venous pressures suggests the etiology to be a defect of venous support.

This case contributes supportive evidence to the postulation that gastric varices may occur unrelated to venous obstructive factors. Although coincidence cannot be excluded, the association of palmar varices may be a clue toward an etiology as well as an important clinical signpost.

References

1. Bartholomew LG: Cutaneous manifestations of gastrointestinal disease. *Postgrad Med J* **36**:247-259, 1964.
2. Osler W: On a family form of recurring epistaxis associated with multiple telangiectases of the skin and mucous membrane. *Bull Johns Hopkins Hosp* **12**:333, 1901.
3. Bean WB: *Vascular Spiders and Related Lesions of the Skin.* Springfield, Ill, Charles C Thomas Publisher, 1958, p 190.
4. Rappaport I, Shiffman MA: Multiple phlebectasia involving jejunum, oral cavity, and scrotum. *JAMA* **185**:437-440, 1963.
5. Allen EV, Barker NW, Hines EA: *Peripheral Vascular Diseases,* ed 2. Philadephia, WB Saunders Co, 1955, pp 543-556.
6. Gundersen J, Hauge M: Hereditary factors in venous insufficiency. *Angiology* **20**:346-355, 1969.
7. Svejcar J, Prerovsky I, Linhart J, et al: Biochemical differences in the composition of primary varicose veins. *Amer Heart J* **67**:572-574, 1964.
8. Zsoter T, Cronin RFP: Venous distensibility in patients with varicose veins. *Canad Med Assoc J* **94**:1293-1297, 1966.
9. Palmer ED, Brick IB: Varices of the distal esophagus in the apparent absence of portal and of superior caval hypertension. *Amer J Med Sci* **230**:515-519, 1955.
10. Tisdale WA, Klatskin G, Glenn WWL: Portal hypertension and bleeding esophageal varices. *New Eng J Med* **261**:209-218, 1959.
11. Samuel E: Gastric varices. *Brit J Radiol* **21**:519-522, 1948.
12. Rossi NP, Cohen WN, Gulesserian H, et al: Isolated varices of the gastric fundus. *Ann Surg* **165**:640-643, 1967.
13. Shiffman MA, Rappaport I: Multiple phlebectasia. *Arch Surg* **94**:771-775, 1967.
14. Miller DA, Akers WA: Multiple phlebectasia of the jejunum, oral cavity, and scrotum. *Arch Intern Med* **121**:180-182, 1968.

Postmeningitic Selective Hypopituitarism With Suprasellar Calcification

Barry M. Sherman, MD; Phillip Gorden, MD; and Giovanni di Chiro, MD, Bethesda, Md

The finding of suprasellar calcification in a young male with diabetes insipidus and selective anterior putuitary insufficiency suggests the presence of a craniopharyngioma. However, calcifications at the base of the brain are common in patients successfully treated for tuberculous meningitis[1-5] and both pituitary insufficiency and precocious puberty have been described as sequelae to cured tuberculous meningitis.[6-8]

Haslam et al[9] have recently reported a patient with suprasellar calcifications who developed diabetes insipidus, growth failure, and hypogonadism following the successful treatment of tuberculous meningitis. We have studied a patient with similar hormonal deficiencies and intracranial calcifications occurring several years after the successful treatment of tuberculous meningitis. A suprasellar mass and hydrocephalus were excluded as causes of the hormonal deficiencies. This case further documents localized involvement by the tuberculous process as the cause of the endocrine syndrome.

Patient Summary

A 17-year-old Potawatomi Indian boy was referred to the Clinical Center of the National Institutes of Health for evaluation of short stature, lack of sexual development, and diabetes insipidus.

Received for publication Oct 6, 1970; accepted Dec 30.

From the Diabetes Section, Clinical Endocrinology Branch, National Institute of Arthritis and Metabolic Diseases (Drs. Sherman and Gorden) and the Section on Neuroradiology, National Institute of Neurological Diseases and Stroke, National Institutes of Health (Dr. di Chiro), Bethesda, Md.

Reprint requests to Diabetes Section; Department of Health, Education, and Welfare; National Institutes of Health; Bethesda, Md 20014 (Dr. Gorden).

Birth weight was 3,091 gm (6 lb 13 oz) and early development was normal. At the age of 3½ years he was admitted to the public health service facility at Lawton, Okla, with a two-week history of fever, headache, and vomiting. A chest roentgenogram showed diffuse miliary infiltrates and enlarged tracheobronchial lymph nodes. The spinal fluid was cloudy and contained 260 cells/cu mm with 255 lymphocytes, a total protein value of 165 mg/100 ml, and glucose value of 14 mg/100 ml; a culture was positive for acid-fast bacilli. Bone age was 3½ years and skull roentgenograms were normal. He was treated intramuscularly and intrathecally with streptomycin and orally with isoniazid. Corticosteroids were not administered. Spinal fluid and chest roentgenogram were normal at the time of discharge one year later.

He apparently was asymptomatic until the age of 10 years when he first noted polyuria and clearly recalls leaving his classroom hourly because of urinary frequency or thirst. These symptoms continued undiagnosed until he was seen because of an upper respiratory tract infection at the age of 16. He was noted to be short, obese, sexually undeveloped, and polyuric.

When admitted to the clinical center in August 1968, the patient claimed he had not grown for at least the past five years. His father is 183 cm (6 ft) tall and mother, 178 cm (5 ft 10 in); nine siblings are all taller than the patient and had experienced normal puberty, whereas he had not had voice change and denied libido, erections or ejaculation. He had not been troubled by headaches, seizures, or visual disturbances other than myopia. Performance in school was above average although he admitted to easy fatigability.

On examination the patient was short (153.5 cm [5 ft ½ in]) and obese (82.5 kg [182 lb]) with a high-pitched voice. Span (160.5 cm [5 ft 3 in]) was greater than height and upper segment (79.5 cm [2 ft 8 in]) greater than lower segment (74 cm [2 ft 5 in]). There was no facial or axillary hair and sparse pubic hair. Fat accumulation was particularly notable in the breasts and hips. Visual fields were normal on tangent screen testing. On funduscopic examination there was chorioretinal scarring attributed to prior tuberculous infection. A systolic ejection murmur radiating to the apex was detected; there was no organomegaly. The penis measured 2.5 cm in length and the testes, 1 cm x 1 cm. Results of neurologic examination were normal.

Results of routine hematologic and chemical evaluation, including serum electrolytes, were normal. Several liver function test results were abnormal: alkaline phosphatase, 197 international units (IU) (normal, 75 to 115 IU), serum glutamic pyruvic transaminase (SGPT) 60 Karmen Units (KU) (normal, 5 to 35 KU), and bromsulphthalein (BSP) retention, 27% and 30% at 45 minutes. An oral cholecystogram and liver scan were normal. A percutaneous liver biopsy revealed fatty metamorphosis but no granulomatous changes. Spinal fluid obtained at the time of pneumoencephalography was normal and culture for mycobacteria was negative. Bone age was 15½ years ± 13 months as determined by the standards of Greulich and Pyle.[10] A chest roentgenogram, electrocardiogram, and electroencephalogram were normal. Review of a testicular biopsy performed in February 1968 at Creighton Memorial Hospital, Omaha, Neb, showed small seminiferous tubules consistent with the prepubertal state.

The diabetes insipidus has been treated and adequately controlled with 5 units of vasopressin (Pitressin) tannate in oil every 48 hours.

The hypogonadism was treated with a single weekly injection of 10,000 units of chorionic gonadotropin which increased the plasma testosterone into the normal range. There has been insufficient time to evaluate the efficacy of this therapy with respect to virilization.

His growth retardation is not of sufficient severity to warrant treatment with human growth hormone.

Endocrine Evaluation.—Diabetes insipidus was documented by a 14-hour dehydration study (Table 1) and the patient required vasopressin therapy. There was no increase in immunoassayable growth hormone after insulin-induced hypoglycemia or pyrogen stimulation (Table 2). The diagnosis of hypogonadotropic hypogonadism was consistent with the findings of concentrations of plasma luteinizing hormone (LH) and follicle stimulating hormone (FSH) below the sensitivity of the radioimmunoassay[12,13] and failure of plasma gonadotropins to rise after stimulation with clomiphene[14] (Table 3). Thyroid func-

Table 1.—Dehydration Study

Hour	Weight (kg)	Serum Na (mEq/Liter)	Serum Cr (mg/100 ml)	Creative Clearance (ml/min)	Plasma (mOsm/Liter)	Urine (mOsm/Liter)	Cumulative Urine Volume (ml)
−64	5 units vasopressin tannate in oil						
0	83.7	140			295		
10	81.7	146	0.8	88		245	1,622
12	81.0	150	0.8	65		138	2,512
14	81.0	157	0.8	61	302	154	3,042

Table 2.—Growth Hormone*

Time	Insulin 0.1 Units/kg Glucose (mg/100 ml)	HGH† (ng/ml)	Insulin 0.3 Units/kg Glucose (mg/100 ml)	HGH (ng/ml)	Lipexal‡ (ng/kg) HGH (ng/ml)
000	85	<2	87	<2	1
020	52		44		
030	55	<2	42	<2	
045	61		36		
060	75	<2	54	<2	<1
090	85	<2	65	<2	
120	85	<2	71	<2	<1
180					<1
240					2

* White blood cell count = 12,000 to 23,000/cu cm.
† Growth hormone measured by radioimmunoassay.[11]
‡ Temperature = 36.8 to 38.6 C.

Fig 1.—One hundred gram oral glucose tolerance test. The blood glucose (open circles) *and total plasma insulin* (solid circles) *in the upper panel, and the percent "big" insulin* (hatched bars) *and the "big" insulin concentration* (solid triangles) *in the lower panel, are plotted as a function of time after the administration of glucose.*

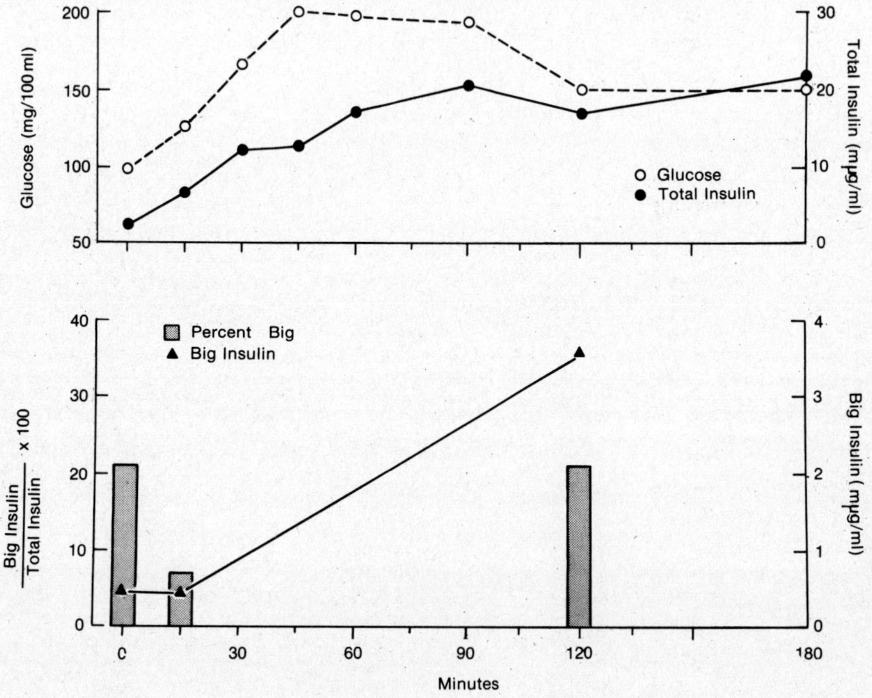

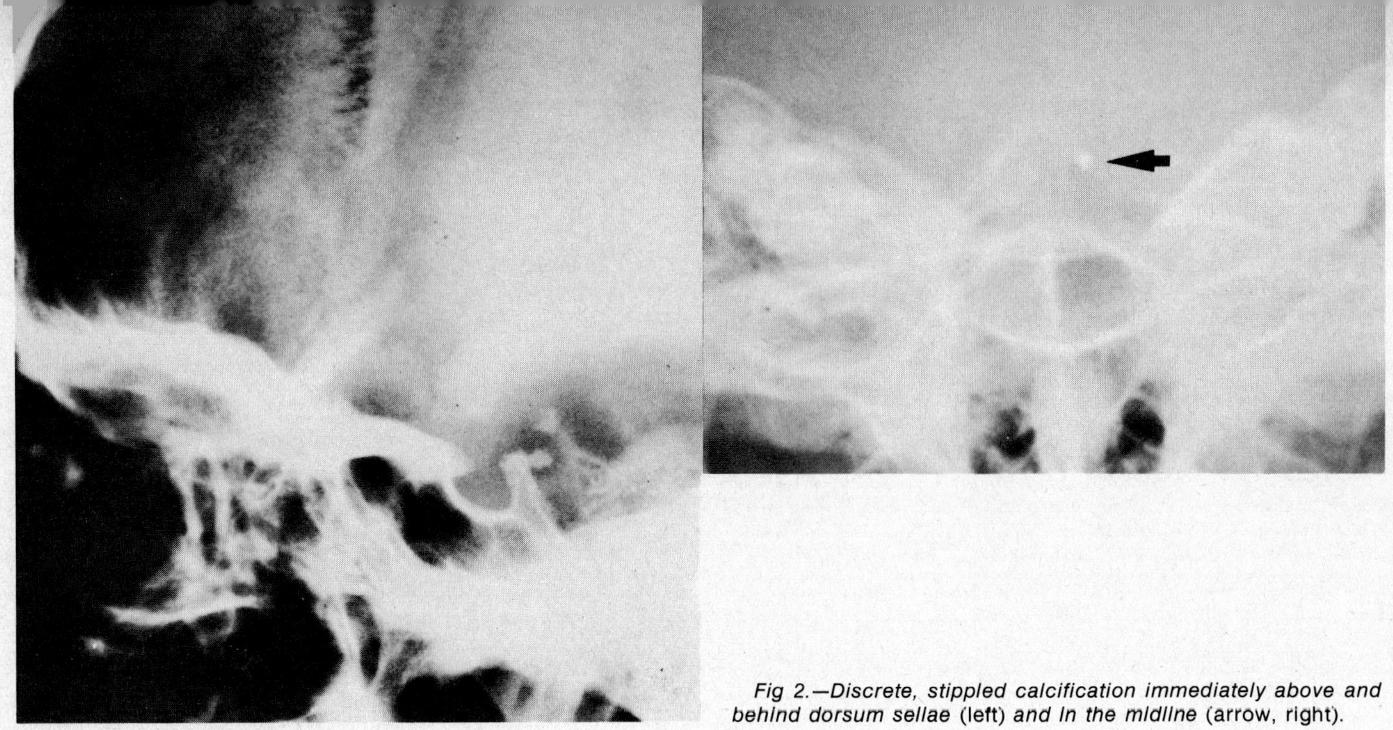

Fig 2.—Discrete, stippled calcification immediately above and behind dorsum sellae (left) and in the midline (arrow, right).

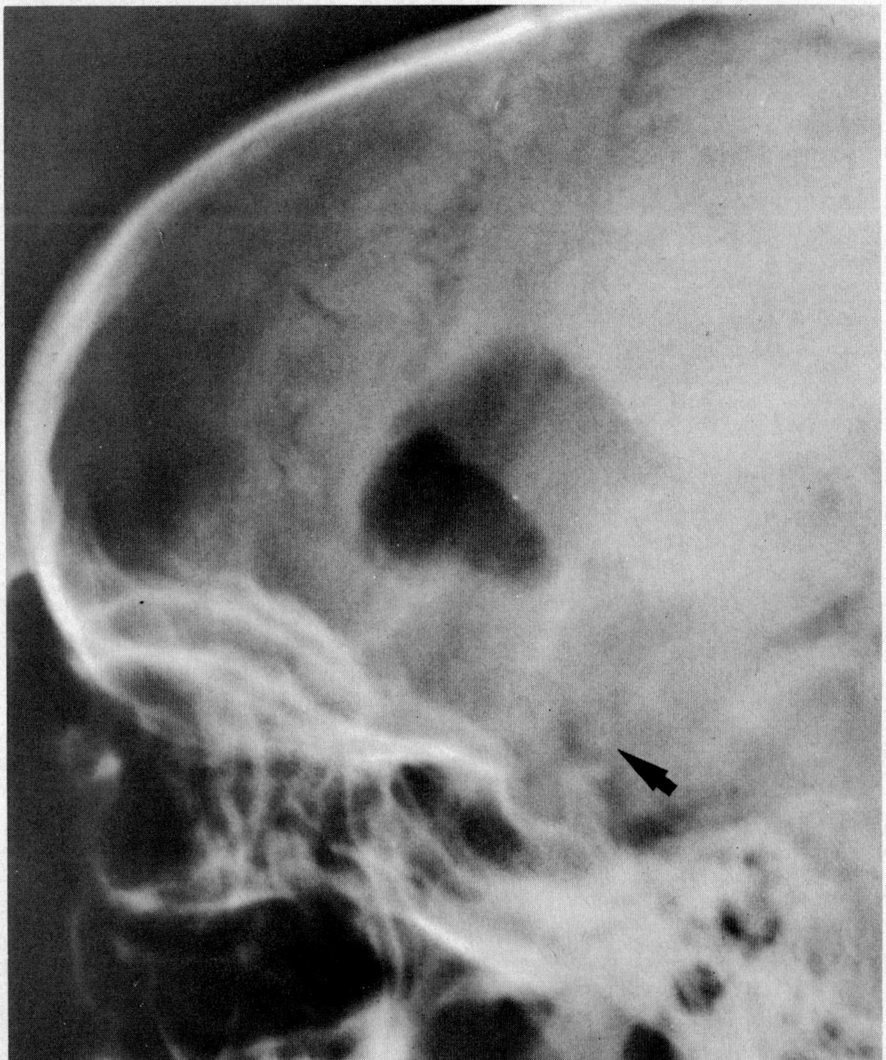

Fig 3.—Calcification in direct contact with tuber cinereum (arrow) behind gas filled anteroinferior part of third ventricle.

tion test results were normal:

Protein bound iodine	5.9μg/100 ml
Thyroxine by column	5.7μg/100 ml
Free thyroxine	1.3μg/100 ml
Thyroid binding globuline	26.0μg/100
Radioactive iodine uptake	4 hours 11%
	24 hours 24%

and the pituitary-adrenal axis was intact (Table 4).

A standard 100-gm oral glucose tolerance test was done after a high carbohydrate diet. Glucose tolerance was abnormal in spite of significant hyperinsulinemia (Fig 1). The "big" and "little" insulin fractions found after filtration of plasma on Sephadex G-50 were not different from fasting[18] and stimulated[19] values observed in other obese patients.

Neuroradiologic Findings.—Routine skull roentgenograms and tomograms of the sella turcica showed a discrete area of dense, stippled calcification immediately above and behind the dorsum sellae (Fig 2, *left*) in the midline (Fig 2, *right*). There was no enlargement or erosion of the sella turcica.

During pneumoencephalography difficulty was encountered in obtaining penetration of air into the ventricular system and ventricular air filling was achieved only after the use of urea intravenously.[20] There was some dilatation of the lateral and third ventricles. The septum pellucidum and third ventricle were in the midline and the aqueduct and fourth ventricle were normal. There was sparse gas filling of the pontine, interpeduncular, and suprasellar cisterns and only a limited amount of air reached the convexity cisterns and sulcuses. The calcification was in the interpeduncular cistern and its upper part was in direct contact with the tuber cinereum (Fig 3). No blunting of the infundibular recess of the third ventricle was noted.

Radioisotope cisternography demonstrated normal ascent of the tracer iodinated I 131 serum albumin[21,22] toward the convexity of the brain and by 24 hours (Fig 4), the isotope had reached the parasagittal area.

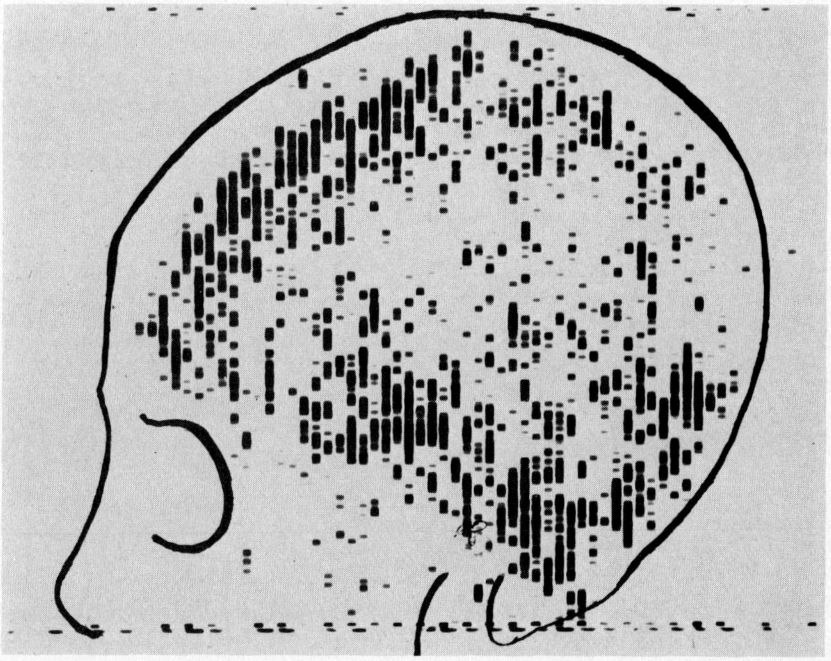

Fig. 4.—Cisternography 24 hours after administration of iodinated I 131 serum albumin. Normal radioactivity distribution rules out communicating hydrocephalus.

Comment

Diabetes insipidus, hypogonadism, obesity, growth retardation, and precocious puberty have been observed singularly and in various combinations in patients surviving tuberculous meningitis. Haslam et al in their recent review of the literature found 18 examples of hypothalamic-pituitary dysfunction.[9] Six of the 18 patients had precocious puberty while five had isolated diabetes insipidus and two of seven had diabetes insipidus in addition to selective anterior pituitary insufficiency.

Our patient had the clinical onset of diabetes insipidus and growth failure approximately six years after treatment of tuberculous meningitis. By the age of 17 years he had no evidence of sexual maturation and low plasma gonadotropin concentration. Delayed puberty may occur in patients with growth hormone deficiency,[23] and low concentrations of plasma LH and FSH, as well as failure to respond to clomiphene, are consistent with delayed onset of puberty.[24] However, the presence of other pituitary deficiencies suggests that he has a permanent gonadotropin deficit and during two years of follow-up, there has been no evidence of sexual maturation.

The intracranial calcifications seen in our patient are identical to those described by Lorber, Haslam et al, and others.[2,5,7,9] The neuroradiologic finding of discrete calcification with no impingement on the anterior-inferior part of the third ventricle essentially rules out the presence of a craniopharyngioma or other space occupying lesion.[25,26] The demonstration of the anatomical detail in the suprasellar and retrosellar area by pneumoencephalography is quite accurate[27] and we were able to localize the area of hypothalamic involvement specifically to the tuber cinerum just in front of the mammillary bodies.

The mechanism of interference with normal endocrine function in these patients with hypothalamic calcification is not known. The interval between meningitis and the development of diabetes insipidus and growth failure in our patient suggests a chronic process of scarring or of necrosis secondary to devascularization. The calcification may, in fact, represent only a small portion of a much larger lesion. However, even with precise localization of the calcification and the physiologic distinction between vasopressin, growth hormone, and gonadotropin deficit in the presence of normal thyroid and adrenal function, present knowledge of functional human hypothalamic anatomy does not permit definition of the hypothalamic areas involved. Moreover, although the calcification focuses our attention on the hypothalamus, in the absence of releasing factors or the ability to assay for releasing factors, it is impossible to exclude the anterior pituitary as a site of involvement. We cannot offer a satisfactory explanation for the lack of penetration of gas into the ventricular system prior to the use of urea. It may be that some adhesions around the lower fourth ventricle foramina were present, and the gas could only pass through these foramina after the brain shrinkage caused by the urea. Although some dilatation of the ventricular system was evident, and the subarachnoidal filling is some-

Table 3.—Gonadotropins

Day	LH (ng/ml) LER 907[15]	FSH (ng/ml) LER 907[15]	Testosterone (μg/100 ml)
1 Baseline	<2.0	<18.0	0.05
2	<2.0	<18.0	
3	<2.0	<18.0	
4 Clomiphene (50 mg/day)	<2.0	<18.0	
5	<2.0	<18.0	
6	<2.0	<18.0	
7	<2.0	<18.0	
8	<2.0	<18.0	
9	<2.0	<18.0	0.10

Table 4.—Pituitary-Adrenal Axis

Day	Comment	Urine 17 OHCS* (mg/24 hr)	Urine 17 KS† (mg/24 hr)	Plasma F (μg/100 ml)	Plasma S (μg/100 ml)	Tetrahydro S (mg/100 ml)
1	Baseline	16.0	10.8	13.2	0.1	1.9
2	Metyrapone (750 mg × 6)	15.9	9.7			
3		47.3	26.2	1.4	12.8	16.0
1	Baseline	5.5	4.1			
2	Dexamethasone (2 mg/day)	7.7	6.4			
3		1.7	2.8			
4		1.9	5.7			
5		1.3	2.2			
6		1.1	5.4			

* Urine 17 hydroxycorticosteroids by method of Peterson.[16]
† Urine 17 ketosteroids by method of Peterson and Pierce.[17]

what deficient, the normal radioisotope cisternography rules out, in our case, the possibility of a communicating hydrocephalus. Thus, an indirect compression on the hypothalamic centers caused by increased pressure into the ventricular system cannot be considered the mechanism responsible for the hypothalamic involvement in this particular instance.

Although only a few cases have been reported from the United States, healed tuberculous meningitis must be considered in the differential diagnosis of anterior or posterior pituitary insufficiency or both.

Summary

A 3-year-old boy was successfully treated for tuberculous meningitis. He developed symptoms of diabetes insipidus at the age of 10 years and when evaluated at 17 was found to have deficiencies of vasopressin, growth hormone, LH and FSH. Suprasellar calcifications were found on skull roentgenograms. The hormonal deficiencies appear to be secondary to localized involvement of the hypothalmic-pituitary axis by the tuberculous process.

Saul W. Rosen, MD, performed the luteinizing hormone and follicle stimulating hormone radioimmunoassay.

Nonproprietary and Trade Names of Drugs

Chorionic gonadotropin—*Antuitrins, APL, Follutein, Pregnyl.*

References

1. Lorber J: The incidence and nature of intracranial calcifications after tuberculous meningitis. *Arch Dis Child* **27**:542-551, 1952.
2. Lorber J: Intracranial calcification following tuberculous meningitis in children. *Amer Rev Tuber Pul Dis* **78**:38-61, 1958.
3. Lincoln EM, Sordillo SVR, Davies PA: Tuberculous meningitis in children. *J Pediat* **57**:807-823, 1960.
4. Wasz-Hockert O, Donner M: A follow-up of 103 children recovered from tuberculous meningitis. *Acta Pediat* **51**(suppl 141):26-33, 1965.
5. Todd RM, Neville JG: The sequelae of tuberculous meningitis. *Arch Dis Child* **39**:213-225, 1964.
6. Lorber J: Diabetes insipidus following tuberculous meningitis. *Arch Dis Child* **33**:315-319, 1958.
7. Asherson RA, Jackson WPU, Lewis B: Abnormalities of development associated with hypothalamic calcification after tuberculous meningitis. *Brit Med J* **2**:839-843, 1965.
8. Summers VK, Hipkin LJ, Hughes RO, et al: Panhypopituitarism after cured tuberculous meningitis. *Brit Med J* **1**:359, 1968.
9. Haslam RHA, Winternitz WW, Howieson J: Selective hypopituitarism following tuberculous meningitis. *Amer J Dis Child* **118**:903-908, 1969.
10. Greulich WW, Pyle SI: *Radiographic Atlas of Skeletal Development of the Hand and Wrist.* Stanford, Calif, Stanford University Press, 1959.
11. Glick S, Roth J, Yalow R, et al: Immunoassay of human growth hormone in plasma. *Nature* **199**:784-787, 1963.
12. Albert A, Rosenberg E, Ross GT, et al: Report of the National Pituitary Agency collaborative study on the radioimmunoassay of FSH and LH. *J Clin Endocr* **28**:1214-1219, 1968.
13. Odell WD, Ross GT, Rayford PL: Radioimmunoassay for luteinizing hormone in human plasma or serum: Physiologic studies. *J Clin Invest* **46**:248-255, 1967.
14. Faiman C, Rayan RJ: Radioimmunoassay for human follicle stimulating hormone. *J Clin Endocr* **27**:444-447, 1967.
15. Bardin CW, Ross GT, Lipsett MB: Site of action of clomiphene citrate in men: A study of the pituitary-leydig cell axis. *J Clin Endocr* **27**:1558-1564, 1967.
16. Peterson RE, Karrer A, Guerra SL: Evaluation of Silber-Porter procedure for determination of plasma hydrocortisone. *Anal Chem* **29**:144, 1957.
17. Peterson RE, Pierce CE: in Sunderman FW, Sunderman FW Jr (eds): *Lipids and Steroid Hormones in Clinical Medicine.* Philadelphia, JB Lippincott Co, 1960, p 158.
18. Gorden P, Sherman B, Roth J: "Big" insulin (circulating proinsulin like components): A high proportion of the basal insulin, abstracted. *Diabetes* **19**(suppl 1):360, 1970.
19. Gorden P, Roth J: Plasma insulin: Fluctuations in the "big" insulin component in man after glucose and other stimuli. *J Clin Invest* **48**:2225-2234, 1969.
20. Engeset A, Hauge T: Urea as an aid in encephalography. *Acta Radio (Diagn)* **1**:565-568, 1963.
21. Di Chiro G, Reames PM, Matthews WB: RISA-ventriculography and RISA-cisternography, *Neurology* **14**:185-191, 1964.
22. Di Chiro G: Observations on the circulation of the cerebrospinal fluid. *Acta Radio (Diagn)* **5**:988-1002, 1966.
23. Rimoin DL, Holzman GB, Merimee TJ, et al: Lactation in the absence of human growth hormone. *J Clin Endocr* **28**:1183-1188, 1968.
24. Kulin HE, Grumbach MM, Kaplan SL: Changing sensitivity of the pubertal gonadal hypothalamic feedback mechanism in man. *Science* **166**:1012-1013, 1969.
25. Lindgren E, Di Chiro G: Suprasellar tumours with calcification. *Acta Radiol* **36**:173-195, 1951.
26. Di Chiro G: *An Atlas of Pathologic Pneumoencephalographic Anatomy.* Springfield, Ill, Charles C Thomas Publisher, 1967.
27. Di Chiro G: *An Atlas of Detailed Normal Pneumoencephalographic Anatomy.* Springfield, Ill, Charles C Thomas Publisher, 1961.

Pasteurella pseudotuberculosis

Acute Sepsis With Survival

Kenneth M. Yamashiro, MD;
Robert H. Goldman, MD;
and Dean Harris, MD, Stanford, Calif;
and Charles T. Uyeda, PhD,
Palo Alto, Calif

There are two clinical patterns of human infection with *Pasteurella pseudotuberculosis*, an animal pathogen having a wide distribution. The more common form presents as a mesenteric lymphadenitis and has been well reported in Europe[1] and Canada.[2] The second form occurs less commonly, presents an acute septic course, and usually ends fatally. There have been three reported cases of the septic form in the United States,[3-5] while two other cases have been alluded to in personal communications.[6,7] There have been no published reports of sepsis with *P pseudotuberculosis* in the United States in over 25 years. Recently, in the European literature, autopsy findings in two cases of diabetes mellitus, cirrhosis, and sepsis due to *P pseudotuberculosis* have been reported.[7,8] We have recently seen a patient with diabetes mellitus and hemochromatosis who developed the septicemic form of *P pseudotuberculosis* and who survived following intensive antibiotic therapy.

Patient Summary

A 64-year-old retired Marine sergeant was admitted to the Palo Alto Veterans Administration Hospital on April 16, 1969, with a chief complaint of epigastric pain, malaise, high fever, and diarrhea of three weeks' duration. In mid-March 1969 he noted the sudden appearance of severe sharp nonradiating epigastric and back pain followed later that day by chills, fever, and diarrhea with 15 to 20 motions per day. He saw his private physician who noted his temperature to be 104 F (40 C) and treated him with a penicillin preparation and antacids. Although his diarrhea decreased to six to ten times per day, the epigastric pain, malaise, and fever persisted. On April 12, 1969, he noted ankle edema and was seen at a Naval infirmary where he was treated symptomatically. On the day before admission he noted that his urine turned dark and because of the persistence of his other symptoms was referred to this hospital. Diabetes mellitus had been diagnosed in 1962 and he was being treated with tolbutamide, 500 mg three times daily. He had undergone an appendectomy in 1921. Social history was negative for alcoholism. Physical examination revealed a blood pressure of 150/80 mm Hg; pulse rate, 88 beats per minute; temperature 102 F (38.9 C). Scleral icterus was noted. Breath sounds were diminished. A grade 2/6 nonradiating holosystolic murmur was noted at the apex. Diffuse abdominal tenderness was noted without rebound. The liver was firm, tender, and palpable 5 cm below the right costal margin. There was ankle edema (3+) and presacral edema (1+). Stool guaiac was 4+. Laboratory studies revealed a hematocrit value of 38%; white blood cell count, 14,000/cu mm with 82% polymorphonuclear cells; riticulocyte count, 2.6/cu mm; and erythrocyte sedimentation rate, 105 mm/hr (Westergren method). There was proteinuria (4+), glucosuria (4+), and moderate amounts of acetone in the urine. The shake test for bilirubin was positive. Microscopic exam-

Received for publication Aug 28, 1970; accepted Nov 20.

From Stanford (California) University School of Medicine (Drs. Yamashiro, Goldman, and Harris) and Palo Alto Veterans Administration Hospital, Palo Alto, Calif (Dr. Uyeda). Dr. Harris is now with the School of Submarine Medicine, US Naval Submarine Medical Center, US Naval Sub Base, New London, Groton, Conn.

Reprint requests to Department of Medicine, Stanford University School of Medicine, Stanford, Calif 94305 (Dr. Goldman).

ination of the urine revealed occasional granular casts and 3 to 5 white blood cells per high power field. The serum glucose level was 284 mg/100 ml and serum was negative for acetone. Serum electrolyte values were as follows: sodium, 124 mEq/liter; potassium, 4.9 mEq/liter; chloride, 93 mEq/liter; bicarbonate, 21 mEq/liter; and blood urea nitrogen, 20 mg/100 ml. Liver function studies showed the following values: total bilirubin, 4.0 mg/100 ml; direct, 2.9 mg/100 ml; alkaline phosphatase, 10.0 Bodansky units; total protein, 6.3 gm/100 ml; serum albumin, 1.8 gm/100 ml; serum glutamic oxaloacetic transaminase (SGOT), 64 units/ml; serum glutamic pyruvic transaminase (SGPT), 42 units/ml; and lactic dehydrogenase (LDH), 320 units/ml. The x-ray film of the chest showed small bilateral pleural effusions and an abdominal roentgenogram was interpreted as normal. His electrocardiogram showed a right bundle branch block pattern.

The patient was initially thought to have a cholangitis secondary either to cholelithiasis and cholecystitis or to carcinoma of the pancreas and was treated symptomatically with fluids intravenously and nasogastric suction. Forty-eight hours after admission his temperature rose to 105.2 F (40.7 C) and after repeated blood cultures were obtained he was placed on a regimen of kanamycin sulfate, 1 gm intramuscularly initially and 0.5 gm every 12 hours, and ampicillin sodium, 2 gm intravenously every 2 hours. During the next two days his temperature returned to normal by lysis.

A lung scan showed areas of decreased uptake in multiple areas of both lung fields. A liver scan with 0.5 millicuries indium phosphate ^{113}In showed a normal sized liver with decreased uptake of radioactivity, increased uptake in the bone marrow, and an enlarged spleen. This reading was compatible with cirrhosis. Blastomycin, coccidioidin, mumps, and intermediate purified protein derivative (PPD) skin tests were negative at 48 hours. Febrile agglutinins were negative and a cold agglutinin titer was 1:4. Stool cultures were negative and stool examinations for ova and parasites were negative × 3. On April 21 gram-negative *Coccobacilli* were reported to be growing from five of five blood cultures taken while the patient's temperature was 105.2 F. Three subsequent cultures taken while the patient was febrile and receiving antibiotic therapy were negative. The organism was sensitive to ampicillin sodium, sodium cephalothin, chloramphenicol (Chloromycetin), kanamycin sulfate, penicillin G sodium, streptomycin sulfate, and tetracycline hydrochloride but was resistant to colistin sulfate by the simple disk method.[9]

Sigmoidoscopy was performed on April 23 and normal mucosa was seen to 15 cm. Black, guaiac positive stool was present. Serial x-ray films of the upper gastrointestinal tract two days later with small bowel follow-through revealed a duodenal ulcer and morphologically normal small bowel. Serial x-ray films of the upper gastrointestinal tract taken four weeks later showed healing of the ulcer.

On April 29, a liver biopsy was performed and microscopic examination showed portal fibrosis and iron pigment in parenchymal cells mainly in periportal areas, in portal scar, and in bile ductular epithelium. Because of the excessive iron pigment present, serum iron per total iron-binding capacity ratios were obtained on May 22, June 10, Sept 16, 1969, and Feb 3, 1970, and were 185:375, 255:465, 230:364, and 235:388, respectively. A ferrikinetic study showed decreased sacral incorporation of iron on day 1 and increased incorporation into the liver. Other data were plasma half-life of iron, 163 minutes (normal 60 to 120 minutes); plasma iron turnover, 1.6 ml/day/100 ml plasma (normal 0.7 to 0.8 ml); daily hemoglobin formation, 0.08 gm/day/100 ml whole blood (normal 0.11 to 0.13 gm); daily hemoglobin percent iron utilized by red blood cells 30% (normal 80%). These findings suggest that iron was being incorporated into the liver and was not available for hemoglobin formation. The patient has undergone weekly phlebotomies from September 1969 to June 1970 with maintenance of his hematocrit value at 42% to 45%.

Microbiological Findings

Gram negative small coccobacilli were repeatedly isolated from blood in brain heart infusion medium containing 0.1% agar. It exhibited an alkaline slant and acid butt with no gas or hydrogen sulfide in triple sugar iron and was indole, Voges-Proskauer, citrate, phenylalanine, and oxidase negative but urease and methyl red positive. The organism grew well on MacConkey and *Salmonella-Shigella* agars, was slightly hemolytic on sheep blood agar, and nonmotile and grew better at room temperature than at 37 C. The tentative identification of *P pseudotuberculosis* was confirmed by the National Communicable Disease Center using phage typing and additional biochemical tests.[10] In Andrade's basal medium the isolate produced acid from glucose, xylose, mannitol, and maltose but not from lactose and sucrose. It was fermentative with glucose (oxidative fermentation tests), catalase positive; nitrate was reduced and esculin was hydrolyzed. Serologic survey workup was done on June 21, 1969, on *P pseudotuberculosis* and showed evidence of *P pseudotuberculosis* serotype I/V infection:

Group	Titer
I (A and B)	1:1,024
II (A and B)	1:256
III	Nil
IV (A and B)	Nil
V	1:1,024

Comment

Pasteurella pseudotuberculosis is an animal pathogen with only occasional human infection. Mair[11] isolated 169 strains of this organism in Great Britain during a four-year period from 13 species of mammals and 26 species of birds. During this time only eight strains were isolated from humans. Epizootics have been reported in guinea pigs and turkeys while sporadic infections have been reported in rodents, sheep, goats, rabbits, cats, dogs, pigeons, canaries, hens, and ducks.[12]

In 1954 the etiologic agent of a pe-

Summary of Symptoms, Source of Diagnosis, and Associated Chronic Liver Disease in Cases of Systemic Infections With *Pasteurella pseudotuberculosis*

Author yr	Country	Age (yr)	Symptoms	Culture Source of Diagnosis*	Associated Liver Disease
Lorey 1911†	Germany	53	Fever, jaundice, diarrhea	Blood	...
Saisawa 1913†	Japan	21	Tonsillitis, fever, jaundice, abdominal distension, diarrhea	Blood	...
Roman 1916†	Czechoslovakia	46	Anorexia, abdominal pain	Liver, spleen	...
Umlauft 1933‡	Germany	48	Fever, jaundice, diarrhea	Blood	Hemochromatosis
	Germany	64	Fever, diarrhea, cough, vomiting	Liver examined at autopsy; no culture taken	Hemochromatosis
Neugebauer 1933†	Czechoslovakia	45	Cough, neck stiffness	Liver, spleen	...
Paul and Weltmann 1934†	Austria	31	Jaundice, liver, spleen enlargement	Spleen	...
Dujardin-Beaumetz et al 1938[13]	France	32	Fever, diarrhea, delirium, coma	Blood	...
Topping et al 1938[3]	United States	29	Fever, chills, jaundice, diarrhea	Blood	...
Macchiavelli 1941‡	Brazil	18	Fever, chills, jaundice, diarrhea	Liver	...
Moss and Battle 1941[4]	United States	34	Headache, chills, abdominal pain, fever	Blood	...
Snyder and Vogel 1943[5]	United States	41	Fever, headache, chills, pain in left sacroiliac joint	Blood	...
Hassig 1949‡	Switzerland	60	Fever, jaundice	Liver, spleen	Pigment cirrhosis
	Switzerland	69	Fever, cough, vomiting, diarrhea		Pigment cirrhosis
Burianek 1949‡	Czechoslovakia	36	Fever, metrorrhagia, spleen and cervical node enlargement	Blood	...
Sachdeva et al 1956[19]	India	22	Fever, abdominal pain	Lymph node	...
Molleret et al 1964[7]	France	67	Fever, liver enlargement	Blood	Cirrhosis
Maccauley et al 1967[8]	Great Britain	51	Drowsiness, confusion, anorexia, jaundice	Liver	Cirrhosis

* Blood cultures taken antemortem; liver, spleen, and lymph nodes cultured at autopsy.
† Summarized by Dujardin-Beaumetz et al.[13]
‡ Summarized by Knapp.[14]
§ Patient survived.

culiar form of mesenteric lymphadenitis with abscesses was found to be *P pseudotuberculosis*.[1] From 1954 to 1957, 117 cases of mesenteric lymphadenitis due to this organism were reported in children from Germany. In Canada Hnatko and Rodin[2] found that five of 66 consecutive patients operated on for acute appendicitis had increased titers of type IA or IIB strains of *P pseudotuberculosis* with subsequent decrease in the titers following the operation.

The septicemic form of human infection with *P pseudotuberculosis*, though described earlier, is much more rare. Since 1911 there have been 18 reported cases in the world literature. Most of the cases have been summarized by Dujardin-Beaumetz et al[13] and Knapp.[14] In addition two individual reports have been made by Molleret et al[7] and Maccauley et al.[8] Most of the cases are described in the European literature and only five cases have been reported in the English language. All reported cases are summarized in the Table.

Six of the patients had accompanying liver disease.[7,8,14] Two had alcoholic cirrhosis while the others were thought to have hemochromatosis. The diagnosis of hemochromatosis was made on histologic examination of the liver at autopsy. Portal fibrosis with iron pigment in both liver parenchymal and Kupffer cells were described. The histological findings in the present patient's liver biopsy were highly suggestive of hemochromatosis. In addition a ferrikinetic study showed a high incorporation of iron into the liver. Finally, the diagnosis of hemochromatosis was substantiated by the patient's response to phlebotomy. The low serum iron to total iron-binding capacity ratio probably reflects the fact that he bled from a duodenal ulcer.

The high incidence of cirrhosis in these patients suggests that chronic liver disease may predispose patients to systemic illness with *P pseudotuberculosis*. The normal liver can clear bacteremia in subacute bacterial endocarditis and in ulcerative colitis.[15,16] On the other hand, cirrhotic rats have been shown to have an impaired ability to destroy bacteria.[17] Partly on the basis of the preceding findings Conn[18] suggested that cirrhotic livers may permit bacteria to bypass the liver's reticuloendothelial system hence causing a bacteremia enabling the infecting organism to establish metastatic foci from which to perpetuate septicemia. It is attractive to postulate that systemic instead of mesenteric lymph node infection with *P pseudotuberculosis* occurs on this basis.

Once established the *P pseudotuberculosis* septicemia if untreated progresses, causing metastatic abscesses and serous effusions.[5] In addition duodenal ulcer[13] and small intestinal ulcers[13,19] have also been described. In our patient the pleural effusions and abnormal lung scan can be attributed to metastatic abscesses. The exact cause of the duodenal ulcer remains unknown.

Fever, jaundice, and diarrhea were present in nearly all patients who had *P pseudotuberculosis* septicemia. Abdominal pain was less frequently noted. Our patient exhibited all of these symptoms. The diagnosis was established in the present case on the basis of positive blood cultures taken at the height of his fever. Of note is that positive blood cultures were noted in ten of the previously reported cases.

Treatment of patients with this disease is lifesaving. Two out of four previous patients treated with antibiotics survived. All the untreated patients died. Intensive treatment with antibiotics produced a dramatic cure in the present case. To our knowledge this is the first patient with hemochromatosis and infection with *P pseudotuberculosis* who survived following antibiotic therapy.

Summary

Septicemia with *Pasteurella pseudotuberculosis*, usually an animal pathogen, occurred in a 64-year-old man with hemochromatosis. His symptoms were jaundice, fever, diarrhea, and abdominal pain. The diagnosis was made on the basis of positive blood cultures. Serologic studies confirmed the presence of *P pseudotuberculosis* type I/V infection. Intensive antibiotic therapy produced a dramatic cure.

This work was supported in part by Public Health Service training grant AM-05418 from the National Institutes of Health. Theodore F. Wexler, PhD, University of Michigan, School of Public Health, Ann Arbor, Mich, performed the serotyping.

References

1. Knapp W: Mesenteric adenitis due to *Pasteurella pseudotuberculosis* in young people. *New Eng J Med* **257**:776-778, 1958.
2. Hnatko SK, Rodin AE: *Pasteurella pseudotuberculosis* infection in man. *Canad Med Assoc J* **88**:1108-1112, 1963.
3. Topping NH, Watts CE, Lillie RD: A case of human infection with *B pseudotuberculosis rodentium*. *Public Health Rep* **53**:1340-1352, 1938.
4. Moss ES, Battle JD Jr: Human infection with *Pasteurella pseudotuberculosis rodentium* of Pfeiffer. *Amer J Clin Path* **11**:677-699, 1941.
5. Snyder GAC, Vogel NJ: Human infection by *Pasteurella pseudotuberculosis*. *Northwest Med* **42**:14-15, 1943.
6. Meyer KF: Animal kingdom reservoir of human disease. *Ann Intern Med* **29**:326-346, 1948.
7. Molleret HH, Temkine J, Prade JM, et al: Les septicemies humaines a bacille de Mallassez et Vignal. *Presse Med* **72**:2671-2674, 1964.
8. Maccauley JD, Wilson JAC, Abbott JD, et al: Fatal case of *Pasteurella pseudotuberculosis* infection associated with hepatic cirrhosis. *Brit Med J* **2**:553-554, 1967.
9. Bauer AW, Kirby WMM, Sherris JC, et al: Antibiotic susceptibility testing by a standardized single disc method. *Amer J Clin Path* **45**:493-496, 1966.
10. King EO: *The Identification of Unusual Pathogenic Gram Negative Bacteria*, Atlanta, Communicable Disease Center, 1967.
11. Mair NS: Sources and serological classification of 177 strains of *Pasteurella pseudotuberculosis* isolated in Great Britain. *J Path Bact* **90**:275-278, 1965.
12. Knapp W: *Pasteurella pseudotuberculosis*, in *Bacterial and Mycotic Infections of Man*, ed 3. Dubos RJ, Hirsch JG (eds): Philadelphia, JB Lippincott Co, 1965, pp 677-681.
13. Dujardin-Beaumetz E, Ballet B, Cebron J: Pseudotuberculose chez l'homme. *Presse Med* **46**:43-45, 1938.
14. Knapp W: *Pasteurella pseudotuberculosis* unter besonderer Berueckscichtigung ihrer human medizinischen Bedeutung. *Ergebn Mikrobiol* **32**:196-296, 1959.
15. Beeson PB, Brannon ES, Warren JV: Observations on the sites of removal of bacteria from the blood in patients with bacterial endocarditis. *J Exp Med* **81**:9-23, 1945.
16. Eade MN, Brooke BM: Portal bacteraemia in cases of ulcerative colitis submitted to colectomy. *Lancet* **1**:1008-1009, 1969.
17. Rutenberg AM, Sonnenblick F, Koven EI, et al: Comparative response of normal and cirrhotic rats to intravenously injected bacteria. *Proc Soc Exp Biol Med* **101**:279-281, 1959.
18. Conn HO: Spontaneous enteritis and bacteremia in Laennec's cirrhosis caused by enteric organisms. *Ann Intern Med* **60**:568-580, 1964.
19. Sachdeva LD, Kalra SL, Taneja BL: A case of human infection with *Pasteurella pseudotuberculosis rodentium* in India. *Indian J Med Sci* **10**:114-121, 1956.

Epidermoid Carcinoma of the Lip After Renal Transplantation

Report of Two Cases

Hermes M. Berger, MD; Ralph Goldman, MD;
Harvey C. Gonick, MD; and Jerry Waisman, MD, Los Angeles

There is evidence that the immunologic system provides a "surveillance" function[1] by which neoplastic cells are identified and either eliminated or restricted. Tumor-specific antigens identify the cells as foreign. Patients on immunosuppressive therapy might not recognize these antigens and, thus, have a greater risk of neoplasia. This theoretical consideration has support in the study of McKhann,[2] who found an incidence of malignancy "de novo" in patients who had renal transplants of 13:2000. He compared this with an incidence of 8.2:100,000 in the population at large under the age of 40 years. Several reports of malignancy (lymphomas and carcinomas) in renal homotransplants have been published,[2-11] and in these instances, it was possible to rule out transplanted neoplasia which has also been described.[12-17] The following is a description of two instances of carcinoma of the lower lip in renal homotransplant recipients.

Received for publication Sept 9, 1970; accepted March 2, 1971.

From the departments of medicine (Drs. Berger, Goldman, and Gonick) and pathology (Dr. Waisman), UCLA School of Medicine, Center for the Health Sciences, Los Angeles. Dr. Berger is now with the Federal University of Rio Grande do Sul, Brazil.

Reprint requests to School of Medicine of Porto Alegre, Federal University of Rio Grande do Sul, Porto Alegre, RS, Brazil (Dr. Berger).

Patient Summaries

PATIENT 1.—A 27-year-old man was well until April 1965, when he developed a sore throat and fever which remitted without antibiotic therapy. In June 1965 he presented facial edema and gross hematuria. These symptoms recurred in August with the addition of nausea with vomiting. He was hospitalized with uremia and severe oliguria, and a diagnosis of acute glomerulonephritis was made. There was no improvement, so in September 1965 treatment was begun with prednisone (60 mg daily) and methotrexate (in increasing doses to 5 mg three times per week). The

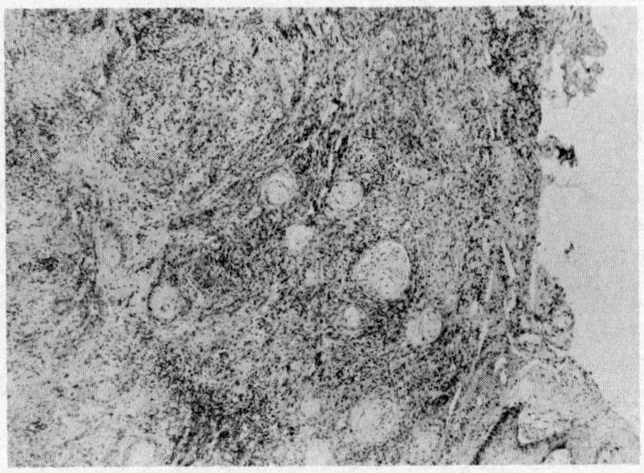

Fig 1.—Ulcerated neoplasm from lip of first patient extends deeply into underlying tissue including striated muscle cells (hemotoxylin-eosin ×30).

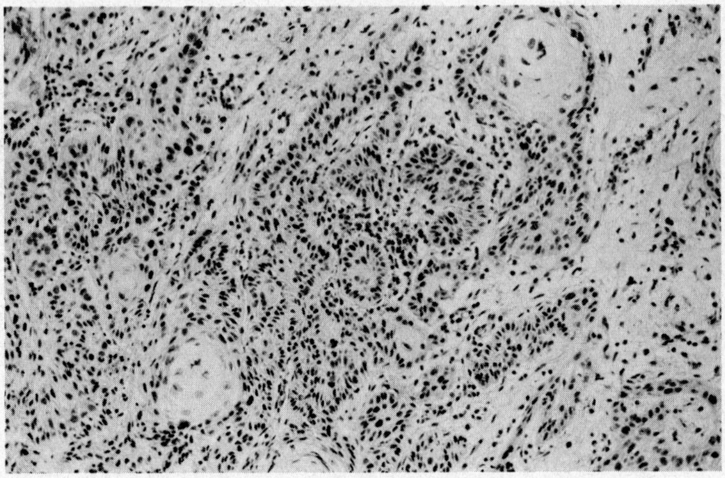

Fig 2.—Seen at higher magnification, cords and sheets of neoplastic epidermoid cells with focal keratinization are irregularly placed in loose fibrous stroma (hematoxylin-eosin ×125).

Fig 3.—In the second patient, neoplasm is more superficial and is not ulcerated (hematoxylin-eosin ×30).

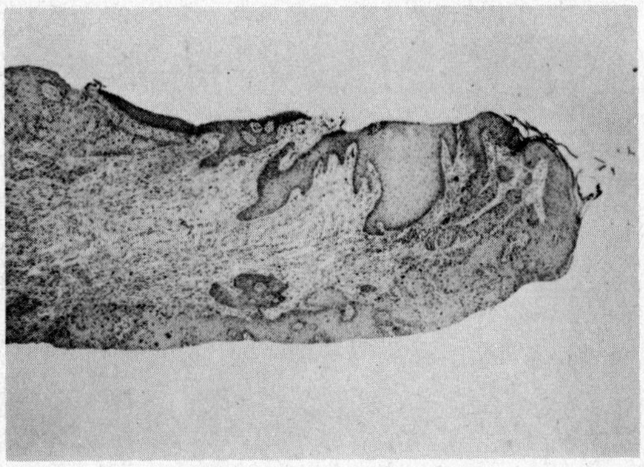

Fig 4.—Nuclear hyperchromatism, abundant mitotic figures, and cellular disorganization are prominent features of this neoplasm (hematoxylin-eosin ×125).

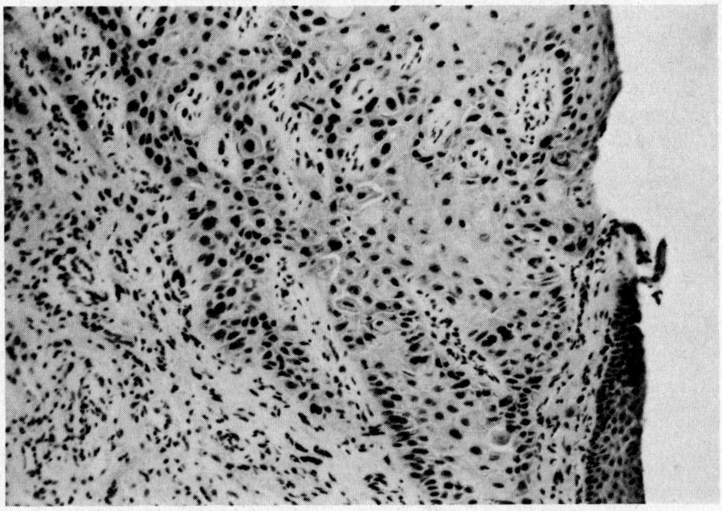

patient received intermittent peritoneal dialysis and hemodialysis. In October 1965 an open renal biopsy disclosed proliferative glomerulonephritis.

The patient's condition remained unchanged until December 1965 when he received a renal transplant from his mother. He received extracorporeal irradiation of blood via the dialysis shunt and was maintained on a regimen of prednisone (100 to 200 mg daily) and azathioprine (200 mg daily). A six-day course of actinomycin (200 to 300 mg daily) was also administered. The patient was discharged in January 1966 with a serum creatinine level of 1.5 mg/100 ml.

In January 1968 an irregular ulcer with raised, firm borders and indurated base appeared on the lower lip. A biopsy revealed nonmalignant epithelial hyperplasia. The lesion persisted and was finally resected in January 1969. Microscopic examination revealed an ulcerated, keratinized epidermoid carcinoma at the mucocutaneous junction (Fig 1). The neoplasm extended into superficial striated muscle. Individual cells were hyperchromatic and pleomorphic (Fig 2). Recurrence of the carcinoma was noted one year later and was treated surgically. The patient smoked 20 to 30 cigarettes a day but denied use of alcohol. When last seen in April 1970 he had a normal blood pressure and a serum creatinine level of 1.3 mg/100 ml. He presently receives 200 mg of azathioprine daily and 15 mg of prednisone every other day.

PATIENT 2.—A 17-year-old girl had an episode of pharyngitis followed by transient facial edema in 1958. In the same year, she developed edema of the lower extremities and was found to have nephrotic syndrome. She was treated intermittently with steroids and diuretics, and in March 1965 was admitted to the UCLA Medical Center with nephrotic syndrome, hypertension, and azotemia. Renal biopsy revealed chronic glomerulonephritis. The patient was maintained on hemodialysis until August 1966 when she received a renal transplant from her brother. Treatment included azathioprine (100 mg daily) and prednisone (30 mg daily). At the time of discharge, 16 days later, the serum creatinine level was 1.3 mg/100 ml. There were several mild episodes of rejection which were controlled with high doses of steroids and irradiation of the kidney. Later the nephrotic syndrome recurred due to either chronic rejection or glomerulonephritis in the transplant.

In July 1969 the patient noted a lesion on the lower lip, which on biopsy proved to be an epidermoid carcinoma. Following the biopsy, an infection of the operative site required systemic antibiotic therapy. In October 1969 the lesion was excised and the microscopic examination revealed a superficially invasive epidermoid carcinoma (Fig 3). The neoplasm was characterized by cytologic variability and abundant mitotic figures (Fig 4). The patient denied the use of tobacco or alcohol. Renal function continued to deteriorate, and the kidney was removed in May 1970, four years after transplantation. Hemodialysis is presently required.

Comment

Carcinoma of the lip is most frequent in older individuals with a history of smoking and alcohol consumption. Chierici et al[18] reviewed 874 cases of oral malignancy and found that oral cancer represented 5.4% of all malignancies. Squamous-cell carcinoma comprised 85.8% of the total number. The average age of patients given the diagnosis of oral cancer was 61 years, with 90% of these patients over the age of 45 years. While the lip was the most common site of oral neoplasia in men, the tongue was the most frequent localization in women. In this survey, 83% of the patients with carcinoma of the lip were smokers and 84% used alcohol.

Several theories have been proposed to explain the occurrence of neoplasms after transplantation. It is believed that cell-mediated immune response plays an important role as a defense mechanism in preventing the growth of spontaneous tumors.[19] In conditions of impaired immunity such as produced by an immunosuppressive regimen for transplantation, tumors may develop. Accidentally transplanted neoplasms from cadaveric renal donors have flourished in recipients.[12-17] In two such cases,[16,17] there was a rapid regression of the malignancy when the immunosuppressive therapy was stopped. Patients with chronic uremia also have impaired delayed hypersensitivity. This impairment is corrected when the uremia disappears after successful kidney transplantation,[20] although immunosuppressive agents employed after transplantation cause abnormal immune response.[21] There is experimental support for the theory that altered immune defenses may favor the development of neoplasia. The administration of azathioprine to NZB and NZB/NZW F_1 hybrid mice is associated with a high incidence of malignant lymphomas.[22,23]

Another hypothesis relates neoplasia to viral infection. Patients with transplanted organs are particularly susceptible to cytomegalovirus disease and herpes simplex. Common warts (verrucae vulgaris) occur in 61% of patients one year after transplantation, compared with normal school children whose incidence is 11% to 16%.[24] Decreased immune response produced by immunosuppressive drugs may permit proliferation of oncogenic viruses, normally resident, but quiescent, in cells of the host.

There is a theory that involves induced chromosomal abnormalities. Azathioprine and methotrexate produce structural chromosomal abnormalities in man.[25] Agents with chromosome-breaking effect may introduce a potential carcinogenic and teratogenic risk. Azathioprine has a significant teratogenic effect in mice.[26] "Immunologic" oncogenesis[27] may be mediated in part by chromosomal aberrations. These aberrations could act directly to promote neoplasia or proliferation of cells consequent to the chromosomal abnormalities which could promote other mutational events. The chromosomal changes themselves may not be sufficient for oncogenesis, but may potentiate malignant transformation by other agents as viruses. Chromosome-breaking agents render mammalian cells in tissue culture more susceptible to transformation by oncogenic virus.[28]

Another explanation for the occurrence of lymphomas in transplanted patients involves lymphoid hyperplasia. The continuous antigenic stimulation from the homograft may cause proliferation of antibody-producing cells. This proliferation eventually results in a group of cells with malignant characteristics. Prolonged antigenic stimulation in mice using *Salmonella* flagellar antigen or bovine serum albumin results in a moderate increase in the incidence of lymphoid leukemia, reticulum cell sarcoma, and plasma cell neoplasia.[29]

We have indicated an unusual occurrence of neoplasia in young patients with renal disease and subsequent renal homotransplantation with attendant immunosuppressive therapy. Possible factors leading to the development of neoplasia in these patients are complex, and we cannot offer a clear explanation for the neoplastic alteration. Regardless of cause, risk of malignancy is significant. In addition to these two cases of carcinoma of the lip, we had one case of lymphoma involving the brain and another case of carcinoma in situ of the uterine cervix and anterior vaginal wall. These four cases represent an incidence of 6% in a total population of 66 renal homotransplants functioning more than one year, performed at the UCLA Medical Center up to June 1970. We urge careful evaluation of these patients for early detection of malignant growths.

Summary

Two young adults received successful related living donor renal transplants, and, at two and three years postoperatively, each developed an epidermoid carcinoma of the lip. The statistical improbability of carcinoma of the lip at this age suggests that the neoplasms are related to transplantation, or immunosuppressive therapy, or both. These observations support the reports of an increased incidence of neoplasia in patients with transplants.

This investigation was supported in part by Public Health Service training grant AM05383 and the Sony Superscope Fellowship in Nephrology.

Nonproprietary and Trade Names of Drug

Azathioprine–*Imuran.*

References

1. Burnett FM: Immunological aspects of malignant disease. *Lancet* **1**:1171-1174, 1967.
2. McKhann CF: Primary malignancy in patients undergoing immunosuppression for renal transplantation. *Transplantation* **8**:209-212, 1969.
3. Zukoski CF, Simmons JL, Killen DA, et al: Cancer in patients on immunosuppressive therapy: Transplanted and spontaneous. *JAMA* **204**:537, 1968.
4. Doak PB, Montgomerie JZ, North JDK, et al: Reticulum cell sarcoma after renal homotransplantation and azathioprine and prednisone therapy. *Brit Med J* **4**:746-748, 1968.
5. Penn I, Hammond W, Brettschneider L, et al: Malignant lymphomas in transplantation patients. *Transplant Proc* **1**:106-112, 1969.
6. Woodruff MFA: Antilymphocyte serum. *Antibiot Chemother* **15**:234-249, 1969.
7. Hume DM: Progress in clinical renal homotransplantation, in Welch CE, (ed): *Advances in Surgery,* vol 2. Chicago, Year Book Medical Publishers Inc, 1966, p 419-498.
8. Seigel JH, Janis R, Alper JC, et al: Disseminated visceral Kaposi's sarcoma: Appearance after human renal homograft operation. *JAMA* **207**:1493-1496, 1969.
9. Deodhar SD, Kuklinka AG, Vidt DG, et al: Development of reticulum-cell sarcoma at the site of antilymphocyte globulin injection in a patient with renal transplant. *New Eng J Med* **280**:1104-1106, 1969.
10. Good RA: Experimental and clinical experiences with chemical suppression of immunity: A personal review, in Miescher PA, Garbar P (eds): *Immunopathology, Fifth International Symposium.* New York, Grune & Stratton Inc, 1967, p 366-417.
11. Schneck SA, Penn I: Cerebral neoplasms associated with renal transplantation. *Arch Neurol* **27**:226-233, 1970.
12. Martin DC, Rubini M, Rosen VJ: Cadaveric renal homotransplantation with inadvertent transplantation of carcinoma. *JAMA* **192**:752-754, 1965.
13. McIntosh DA, McPhaul JJ Jr, Peterson EW, et al: Homotransplantation of a cadaver neoplasm and a renal homograft. *JAMA* **192**:1171-1173, 1965.
14. MacLean LD, Dossetor JB, Gault MH, et al: Renal homotransplantation using cadaver donors. *Arch Surg* **91**:288-306, 1965.
15. Muiznieks HW, Berg JW, Lawrence W Jr, et al: Suitability of donor kidneys from patients with cancer. *Surgery* **64**:871-877, 1968.
16. Wilson RE, Hager EB, Hampers CL, et al: Immunologic rejection of human cancer transplanted with a renal allograft. *New Eng J Med* **278**:479-483, 1968.
17. Zuboski CF, Killen DA, Ginn E, et al: Transplanted carcinoma in an immunosuppressed patient. *Transplantation* **9**:71-74, 1970.
18. Chierici G, Silverman S Jr, Forsythe B: A tumor registry study of oral squamous carcinoma. *J Oral Med* **23**:91-98, 1968.
19. Smith RT: Tumor-specific immune mechanism. *New Eng J Med* **278**:1207-1214, 1268-1275, 1326-1331, 1968.
20. Merrill JP: The immunologic capability of uremic patients. *Cancer Res* **28**:1449-1451, 1968.
21. Swanson MA, Schwartz RS: Immunosuppressive therapy: The relation between clinical response and immunologic competence. *New Eng J Med* **277**:163-170, 1967.
22. Casey TP: Azathioprine (Imuran) administration and the development of malignant lymphomas in NZB mice. *Clin Exp Immun* **3**:305-312, 1968.
23. Casey TP: The development of lymphomas in mice with autoimmune disorders treated with azathioprine. *Blood* **31**:396-399, 1968.
24. Spencer ES: Immunosuppression and cancer. *Lancet* **1**:777-778, 1969.
25. Jensen MK: Chromosome studies in patients treated with azathioprine and amethopterin. *Acta Med Scand* **182**:445-455, 1967.
26. Githens JH, Rosenkrantz JG, Tunnock SM: Teratogenic effects of azathioprine (Imuran). *J Pediat* **66**:959-961, 1965.
27. Fialkow PJ: "Immunologic" oncogenesis. *Blood* **30**:388-394, 1967.
28. Todaro GJ, Green H: Enhancement by thymidine analogs of susceptibility of cells to transformation by SV 40. *Virology* **24**:393-400, 1964.
29. Metcalf D: Induction of reticular tumors in mice by repeated antigenic stimulation. *Acta Un Int Cancr* **19**:657-659, 1963.

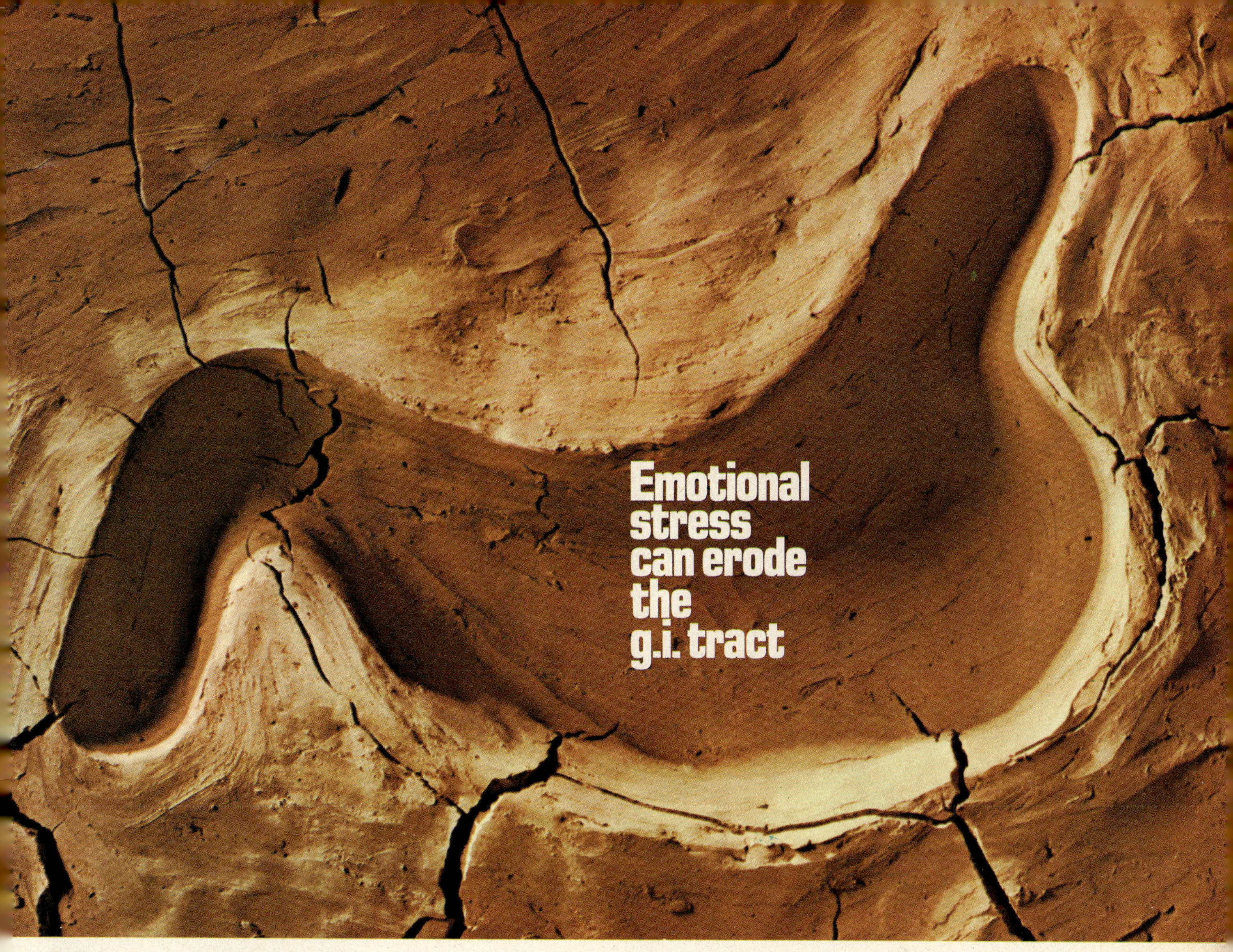
Emotional
stress
can erode
the
g.i. tract

Interface

Chronic Lesions of the Vertebral Column and Joints in Older Mice

Induction by an Active Agent From Rheumatoid Synovial Tissue

Stafford L. Warren, MD; Leonard Marmor, MD; and Dorothy M. Liebes, Los Angeles

Short- and long-term changes in the vertebral column and other joints of mice are induced after injection of saline solution homogenates of human chronic rheumatoid arthritis (RA) synovial tissue; and congenitally in subsequent litters. Immature mice develop abnormalities of short duration. Young adult mice develop painful, reducible kyphosis which becomes a fixed kyphotic deformity with paralysis of the legs in older adults. Generalized atrophy and degeneration of the joint structures occur in the extremities. Bony eburnation, atrophy of the cartilages and disks, with intervertebral capsule rupture and angulation, is common in advanced kyphotic lesions. From the types and sequence of the changes observed, we presume that an experimental acute and chronic rheumatoid arthritis has been induced in mice by the transmission of the active agent present in human rheumatoid arthritis synovial tissues.

In previous reports we have presented evidence for a transmissible agent from human rheumatoid synovial tissue to newborn Swiss Webster mice.[1-3] Intraperitoneal injection of saline solution homogenates of rheumatoid arthritis (RA) tissue induced acute vascular lesions in the paws of mice. Injected joint tissue from nonrheumatoid patients produced no effects.

Received for publication April 19, 1971; accepted April 30.

From the Orthopedic Division, Department of Surgery, UCLA School of Medicine, Los Angeles.

Reprint requests to Orthopedic Division, Department of Surgery, UCLA School of Medicine, Los Angeles 90024 (Dr. Warren).

Determination of the presence of lesions was based on observation, at 100× magnification, of a characteristic pattern of swelling, irregular blood vessels, and sheets of extravasated red blood cells around the small bones and joint capsules of the extremities of the affected mice. This extravasation appeared to be the result of damage to the blood vessel and capillary endothelium. It was accompanied by an infiltration of lymphocytes and macrophages and swelling of the local connective-tissue cells.

Similar abnormalities were passed on to the subsequent litters of injected pregnant mothers and was presumed to be transmitted congenitally through a number of generations. The reaction was enhanced in subsequent litters of mice which had received two to three injections.

The purpose of this report is to extend the range of previous observations and report on the sequential short- and long-term changes in the vertebral column and other joints in Swiss Webster mice of various age groups. The mice were examined at regular intervals for evidence of abnormality. Symptoms of vertebral abnormality included lack of mobility of the spine, abnormal posture, and a fixed kyphosis with weakness or paralysis of the hind legs. These examinations were extended by roentgenography, dissection, and histological study. The control mice were examined in a similar manner and no abnormality was noted.

Materials and Methods

As previously described, synovial granulation tissue was removed surgically from patients with severe subacute and chronic RA. Material used for the controls was removed during reparative surgery from normal patients without a history of RA. The materials were dissected free of fat, minced with scissors, and homogenized with a minimal amount of physiological saline solution. Newborn mice were injected intraperitoneally with 0.025 ml of the material or midterm pregnant mice were injected with 0.2 ml of the material.

Observations.—The abnormalities in these mice varied progressively with age from an acute to a subacute and a chronic phase. Therefore, for this study, the mice were divided into three groups (Table).

In the *immature group* of 557 mice (under 4 weeks of age) 68% were affected by acute lesions with swelling and extravasation of blood in the bony areas of the extremities. Approximately half of these (32%) developed an abnormal waddling gait which suggested vertebral involvement. In both cases these symptoms usually subsided within a week to recur in about half of the adult mice.

In the *young adult group* of 412 mice (4 to 16 weeks of age) 36% were affected with subacute and chronic lesions. Lesions in the extremities involved 45% of these mice. However, there was a decided increase in the percentage (55%) of mice affected with obvious clinical but often transient gait and postural abnormalities which sug-

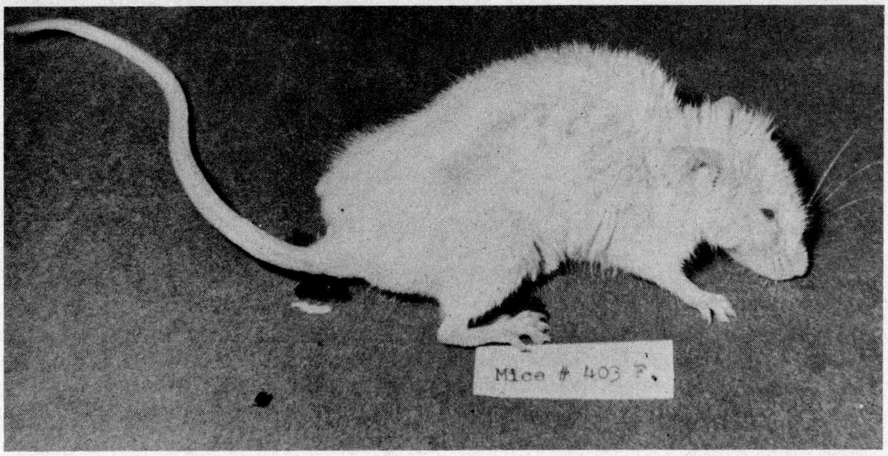

Fig 1.—Advanced kyphosis of thoracic and lumbar spine in 4-month-old RA female mouse. She was injected at 2 and 2½ months with human RA slurry, and delivered an abnormal litter (7:9). She rapidly developed acute and chronic spinal lesions and finally, at 4 months, the fixed hump.

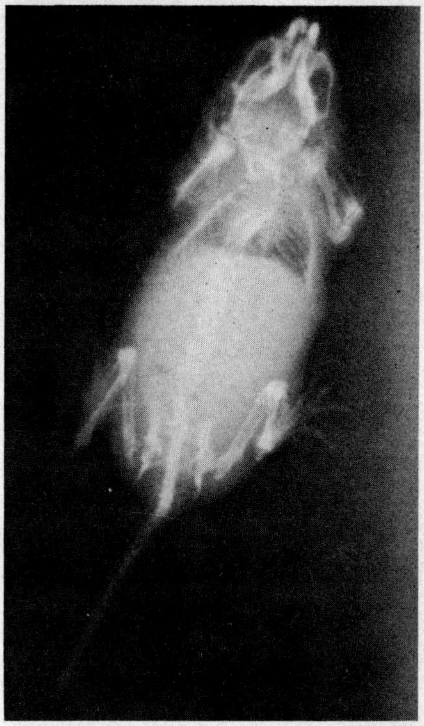

Fig 2.—Posteroanterior roentgenogram of a 5-month-old RA mouse with severe kyphosis and scoliosis in middle of thoracic spine and angulation of tail.

First Appearance of Abnormality of the Vertebral Column and Extremities in Mice of Three Age Groups

	Abnormality						
	Extremities		Vertebral Column		Total		
Groups	No. With Abnormality	Group, %	No. With Abnormality	Group, %	No. In Group	No. With Abnormality	Group, %
Immature*	285	68	134	32	557	419	75
Young adult†	68	45	82	55	412	150	36
Adult‡	24	49	25	51	140	49	35

* Of short duration.
† May wax or wane.
‡ Permanent lesion.

Fig 3.—Four 7-month-old mice injected at birth with human RA tissue. Three show large fixed hump in thoracic spine as contrasted to unaffected mouse No. 4 of the same series.

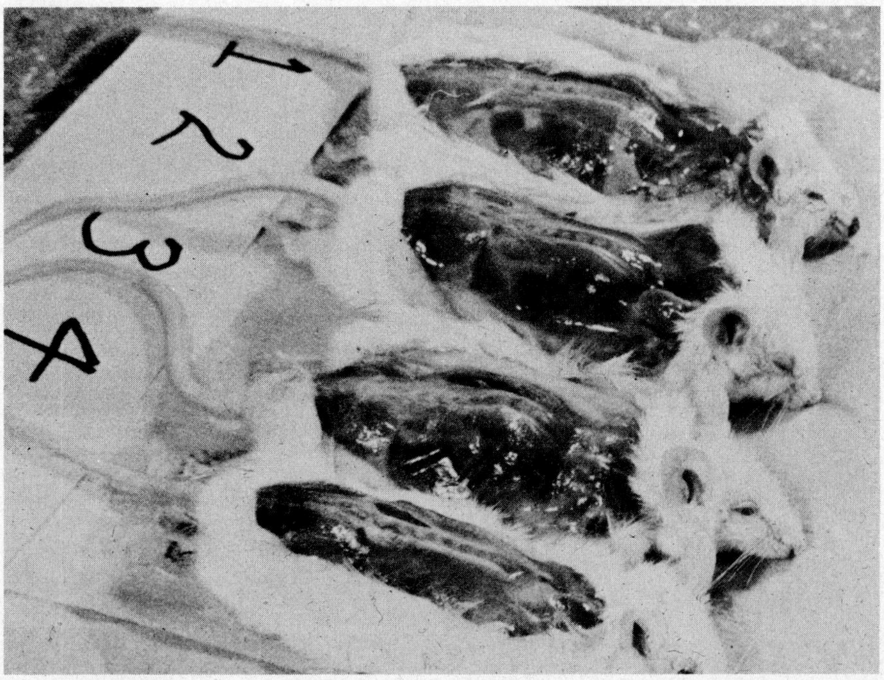

Fig 4.—Four-month-old RA mouse. Posteroanterior view of dorsolumbar vertebrae below kyphosis showing erosion of cartilaginous plates and rotation above the third lumbar as shown by the spinous process (Alizarin red stain, ×15).

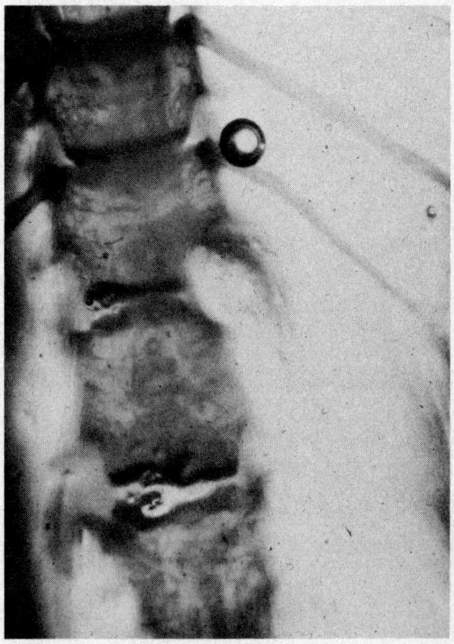

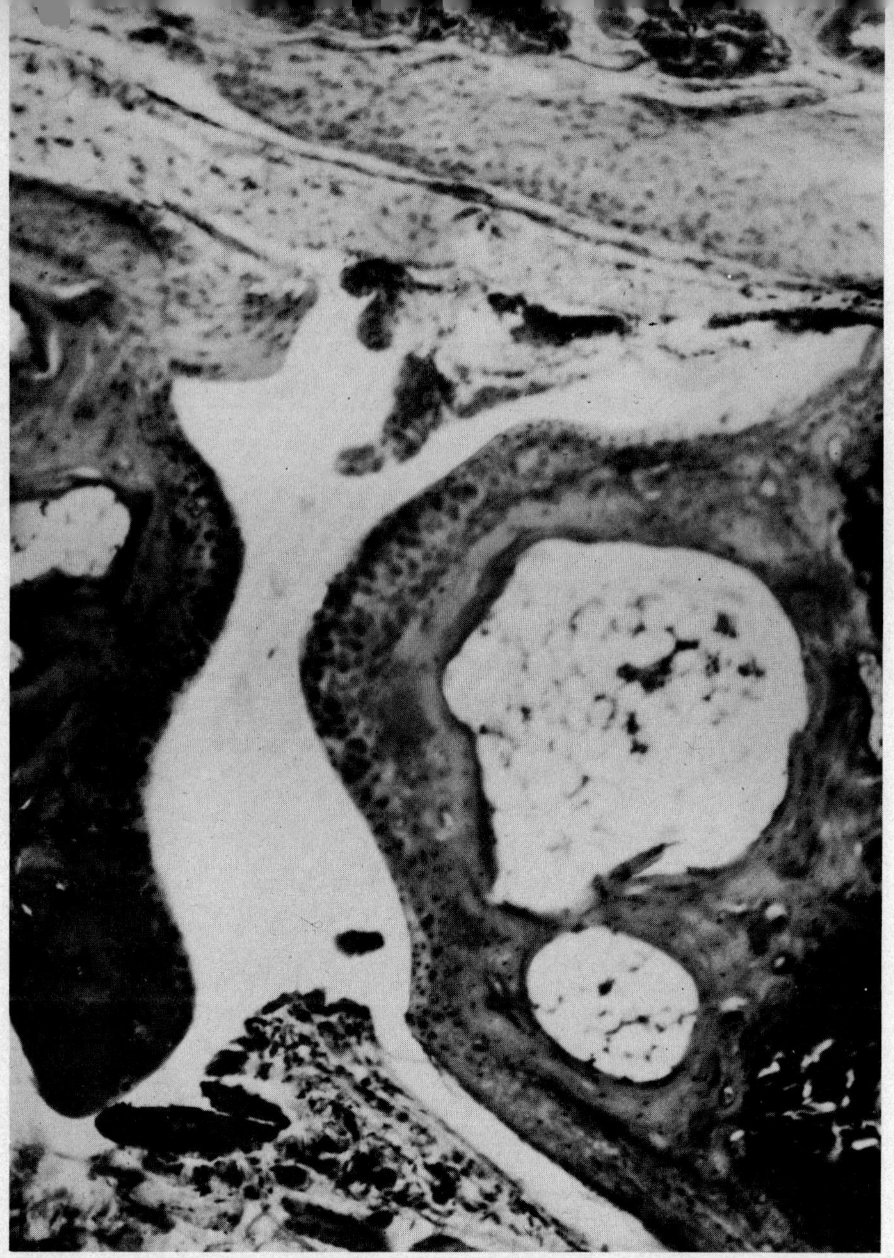

Fig 5.—Nine-month-old RA mouse showing marked stiffness. Intercuneiform joint showing eburnated bone. Cartilage and capsular and ligamentous structures are atrophic. Synovium, where present, is hyperplastic and apparently folded (hematoxylin-eosin stain, ×450).

gested vertebral involvement. Young adults often showed a peculiar stance and stiffness of the joints in the extremities. Kyphosis of the thoracic spine was often visible and painful to palpation. The spine would straighten out when the mouse was suspended by the tail.

In the *adult group* of 140 mice (16 to 44 weeks of age) 35% were afflicted with severe chronic lesions. In 51% of these the vertebral involvement produced a degenerative and irreversible chronic crippling condition and a fixed kyphosis which was no longer painful upon palpation (Fig 1). Progressive weakness and paralysis of the hind legs frequently developed in mice with a fixed kyphosis. There was usually a progressive stiffness and wasting of the tissues. Involvement of both the joints of the extremities and spine was infrequent. The dorsal and lateral curvature of the thoracic or lumbar spine and the rotation of several vertebral bodies could be clearly seen by roentgenography (Fig 2) and in dissected specimens (Fig 3), or in cleared specimens stained with Alizarin red S (Dawson's method)[4] (Fig 4). In the adult mice there were many areas of destruction at the vertebral body and joint articulation margins in various locations in the thoracic, lumbar, sacral, and caudal vertebrae. The cervical vertebrae seemed to be little affected.

An unusual example of severe involvement of both an extremity and the vertebral column occurred in a second-generation mouse born to a female previously injected at birth with human RA slurry. At 2 weeks of age, the suckling mouse developed a severe swelling and contracture of the left forepaw. The lesion of the forepaw subsided and recurred throughout the next five months. By 2 months of age, a marked kyphosis, sensitive to palpation, developed just caudal to the scapulae. When the mouse was suspended by the tail, the hump would straighten out. Roentgenograms at this stage showed some haziness of the lower thoracic vertebrae and of two lower

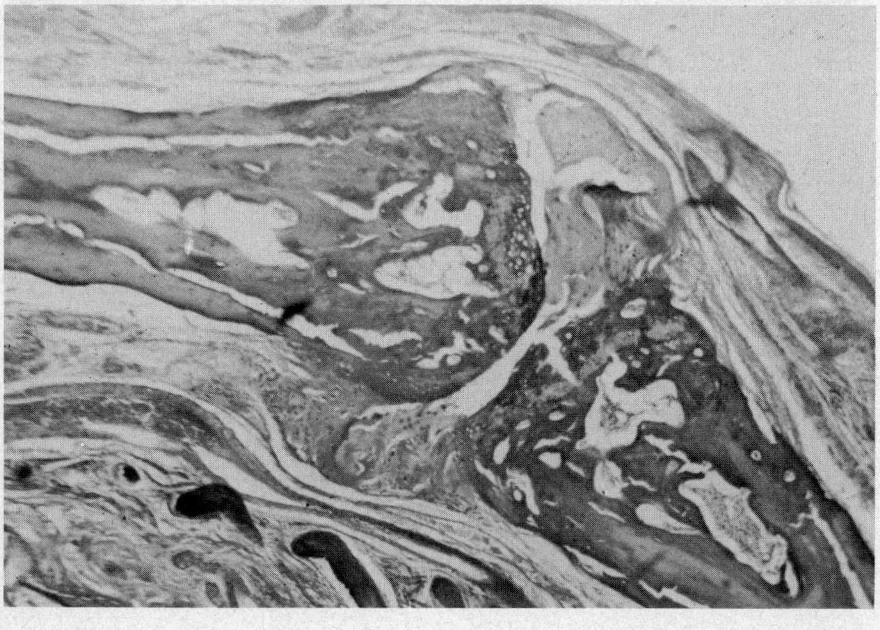

Fig 6.—Tail vertebrae show necrosis and rupture of nucleus pulposus and capsule. Cartilaginous plates are almost destroyed. Bones are eburnated and dislocated. A few mononuclear leukocytes and macrophages line capillaries of interstitial spaces. (hematoxylin-eosin stain, ×450).

lumbar vertebrae. By 5 months of age, the hump in the thoracic vertebrae was fixed and did not straighten out upon suspension by the tail. The left paw was still inflamed, painful, and caused the mouse to limp. The extensor muscles of the hind legs became weak and the leg motion was oar-like. Roentgenograms made at the age of 5 months showed an increase in density in the fourth to eighth thoracic vertebrae throughout the kyphotic curve. There was an acute curvature of the kyphotic portion to the left and some rotation of the vertebral bodies of the lower thoracic and first lumbar vertebrae. There was increased density in the last sacral vertebral body and the first three caudal vertebrae at the angle of the base of the tail. The details of the left paw as seen in Fig 2 are indistinct. This combination of severe, chronic, progressive involvement of both the extremity and spine illustrates the two types of abnormality.

Roentgenograms of other adult mice with fixed kyphosis showed similar increased calcification and distortion of the thoracic vertebrae localized in the kyphotic and scoliotic lesions. In general, the adult mice either developed lesions in one or more extremities or the kyphosis and scoliosis. Control mice of the same age showed none of the lesions described here.

Histological Study (Adult Mice).—A 9-month-old, second-generation mouse had shown stiffness and wasting of the extremities. There was no gross evidence of spinal involvement. Histological examination of the forepaw revealed atrophy of the muscles and subcutaneous structures, and almost complete absence of fat. Occasionally, there were foci of a few mononuclear cells in the muscles and areolar tissues adjacent to ragged capillaries near the joint capsules of the paw bones. The endothelial nuclei of these capillaries were enlarged and densely stained.

The joint areas of the forepaws showed discernible atrophy with reduction of the thickness of the cartilage. The bones were eburnated and sclerotic. Occasionally, the cartilaginous surfaces of the joint space were rough with no synovial covering. The synovium was scattered about in small, densely stained sheets several cells thick, on the capsule side. It often intruded into the joint space (Fig 5). The underlying connective tissue was swollen and almost amorphous in places. A few mononuclear leukocytes and macrophages were ob-

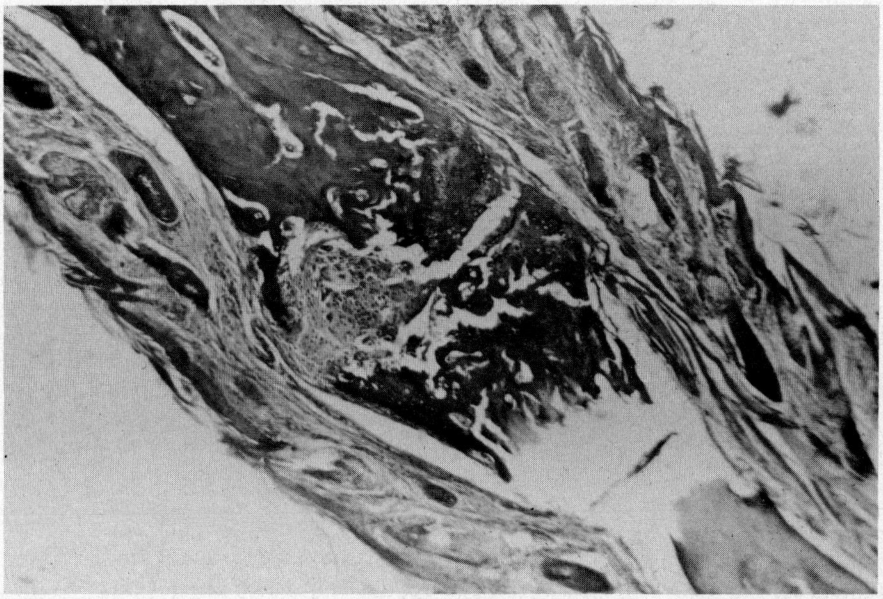

Fig 7.—Vertebral joint caudad to the angulation shows almost complete destruction of cartilaginous plates with erosion of bone. Nucleus pulposus and capsular structures are necrotic. Vertebral bones are in contact and probably incapable of motion (hematoxylin-eosin stain, ×450).

Fig 8.—Typical aspect of other affected intervertebral joints showing eburnation of bones, and atrophy and degeneration of cartilaginous plates, nucleus, and capsule. Little or no cellular reaction is present (hematoxylin-eosin stain, ×450).

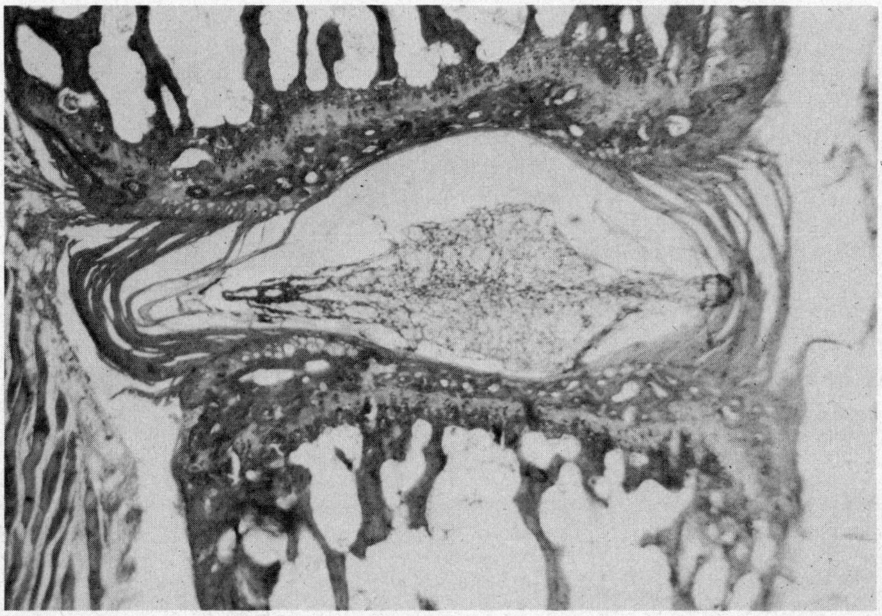

served beneath the synovium fragments. The edge of the cartilage was often undermined. The periosteum was absent near the capsular attachments for some distance where the end of the bone had eroded. Here the nearby connective-tissue fibrils were swollen and were denser than those of the less affected capsular areas. The endothelium, in the capillaries of the capsule and in the undermined area, was swollen and the nuclei were dense but the walls were intact.

Histological study in adult mice was hampered by the extreme hardness of the bones, even after prolonged decalcification. It was difficult to obtain intact sections. However, specimens of affected tails were more readily sectioned. These demonstrated the various degrees of long-term change and damage seen elsewhere in the spine.

Figures 6, 7, and 8 show the typical generalized degenerative process at the site of several intervertebral disks in the tail of a 5-month-old mouse. The lesions were observed to be most advanced at the site of the greatest angle in the tail (or spine). Here there was disintegration and rupture of the nucleus pulposis and capsular fibers accompanied by an angular displacement of the vertebral bodies (Fig 6). The cartilaginous plates of the vertebrae were narrow, degenerated, and bone-like. The synovium could not be identified. These plates were often eroded. In some cases a cavity formed which contained the amorphous remnants of the nucleus pulposus as well as the cartilage and bone of the nearby vertebral bodies (Fig 7). The bone elsewhere was eburnated and seemed to crowd the marrow as well as the degenerated cartilaginous plates.

The nucleus pulposus was generally devoid of nuclei and made up of an amorphous mesh which was often deformed. The capsule fibers were atrophic. Their insertions in the cartilaginous plates seemed to end in abnormal cartilage which contained many spaces (Fig 8). Nuclei were sparse.

There was very little cellular reaction in the atrophic periarticular structures. A few mononuclear leukocytes and macrophages could be seen along the blood vessels in the areolar tissues against the periosteum and occasionally outside the capsule. These were not numerous which suggested that the pathological process was quiescent.

Comment

The injection in mice of saline solution homogenates of RA synovial tissue induced acute and chronic changes in the extremities and, as the mice aged, it particularly induced extensive and severe acute and chronic changes in the vertebral column. Throughout the life of the mouse, it was evident that the abnormality had continued to be the joints and related structures. After the subsidence of the short-term reaction in the immature and young adult mice, the lesions may never recur or may recur after a few months. Fifty-one percent of the adult mice were permanently crippled by lesions of either the extremities, vertebral column, or both. Kyphosis and scoliosis in the thoracic and lumbar vertebral region were the result of extensive damage to the intervertebral disks and to the cartilage associated with the vertebral plates. The rupture of the disk or destruction of part of the vertebral disk region, as well as erosion of the cartilage, seemed to account for the rotation of the vertebral bodies and the angulation of the thoracic spine or tail. In severely damaged adult mice, when the kyphosis had become fixed for some time, the cellular reaction had almost disappeared.

The general emaciation and stiffness which developed in older adults suggested that the atrophy of connective tissue and muscles seen in the joint areas was a generalized process.

The paws and the thoracic, lumbar, and caudal spine seemed to be the most seriously and frequently involved. The cervical vertebrae seemed to have been less affected. None of the controls developed any lesions and at one year of age were normal in appearance.

It is presumed that the acute and chronic abnormalities of the extremities and spine of these mice has been induced by the same active agent which was residing in the synovial-granulation tissue removed from joints of patients with severe subacute and chronic RA.

This work was supported by the Lil and Mel Simmonds Fund.

References

1. Warren SL, Marmor L, Liebes DM, et al: Congenital transmission in mice of an active agent from human rheumatoid arthritis. *Nature* **223**:646-647, 1969.

2. Warren SL, Marmor L, Liebes DM, et al: An active agent from human rheumatoid arthritis which is transmissible in mice. *Arch Intern Med* **124**:629-634, 1969.

3. Warren SL, Marmor L, Liebes DM, et al: Congenital deformities of mice transmitted by a human rheumatoid synovium agent. *Clin Orthop* **70**:216-219, 1970.

4. Gurr E: *Staining, Practical and Theoretical.* Baltimore, Williams & Wilkins Co, 1962, p 125-126.

Transmission of an Active Agent From Rheumatoid Arthritis Synovial Tissue to Chicks

Stafford L. Warren, MD; Leonard Marmor, MD;
Ruth Boak, MD, PhD; and Dorothy M. Liebes, Los Angeles

In order to confirm and amplify the evidence of a transmissible agent in human rheumatoid arthritis (RA) tissue reported in mice experiments, data are presented indicating the transmission of the RA agent from this tissue to chicks as well as from chick to chick and by congenital transmission. Chicks hatched from injected embryonated eggs show clearly identifiable redness of the feet, talipes deformities, and dislocation of the hip. Control embryonated eggs hatched normal chicks. Roentgenograms showed developmental defects of the cervical, thoracic, lumbar, and sacral vertebrae. The chick embryo may provide an avenue to further examine the infectious etiology of RA.

In an effort to identify an active agent in rheumatoid in rheumatoid arthritis (RA), we[1-3] presented evidence for a transmissible agent from human rheumatoid synovial tissue to newborn Swiss-Webster mice. Briefly, intraperitoneal injection of saline solution homogenates of rheumatoid synovium induced a vascular lesion in paws of injected mice whereas joint tissue from nonrheumatoid patients was innocuous. Congenital transmission of the agent was presumed because the pathologic changes could be seen in subsequent litters of injected mice through six generations. In addition to the endothelial lesion in the capillaries of the joint capsules and small bones of the paws seen in the newborn animals, older mice developed a progressive kyphosis of the thoracic and lumbar spine and associated paralysis of the hind limbs.

To confirm and amplify these observations, chicken embryos were injected with similar materials used in the mice experiments. This report presents the data indicating the transmission of an agent from rheumatoid synovial tissue to chicks, as well as chick to chick and congenital transmissions.

Received for publication April 19, 1971; accepted April 29.

From the Orthopedic Division, Department of Surgery (Drs. Warren and Marmor and Mrs. Liebes), the departments of medical microbiology and immunology, and pediatrics, School of Medicine, and the School of Public Health (Dr. Boak), Center for the Health Sciences, University of California, Los Angeles.

Reprint requests of Orthopedic Division, Department of Surgery, UCLA School of Medicine, 1000 Veteran Ave, Los Angeles 90024 (Dr. Warren).

Materials and Methods

Embryonated Eggs.—Fertilized eggs from Single Comb White Leghorn chickens were obtained in batches of two to six dozen from a commercial hatchery and transported to the laboratory for incubation in a standard egg incubator at 38 C. The commercial hatchery experienced a 15% mortality of embryos and reported an incidence of talipes and other abnormalities of 0.15% of 30,000 newly hatched chickens per day. The eggs were candled on the tenth day and all nonviable embryos discarded. The position of the chicken embryo was outlined on the eggshell with pencil preliminary to injections of the chicken embryos. The shell was cleaned with iodine tincture and 70% ethanol and punctured above the air sac. The embryo site was injected with 0.1 ml of material. The puncture site was sealed with paraffin and the eggs incubated until hatched.

Materials for Injection.—Synovial tissue was surgically removed from five patients with a long history of subacute and chronic rheumatoid arthritis (patients 1, 2, 3, 4, and 5). "Control" human joint tissue was removed from young patients who lacked a history of any joint disease and had sustained acute traumatic joint lesions requiring surgery (patients 6, 7, and 8). In a separate experiment, the scarlet contracted feet of two mature unhatched chicks previously injected with rheumatoid tissue from patient 3 were removed aseptically on the 23rd day of incubation. Saline solution homogenates of the tissues were prepared as previously reported. Cultures for bacterial and mycoplasmas failed to yield growth.

Controls.—In addition to injections of nonrheumatoid saline solution extracts, 15 embryonated eggs were candled, punctured, and sealed, but not injected, and 52 embryonated eggs were incubated without experiment manipulation.

Congenital Transmission.—A normal rooster and two hens with severe talipes deformity derived from embryos injected with human rheumatoid synovium were raised under isolated conditions. At maturity the hens produced 69 fertile eggs from which 49 viable chicks were hatched.

Results

The overall mortality of embryos injected with human rheumatoid synovium was 42% as compared with 24% for embryos injected with nonrheumatoid joint tissue and less than 19% for uninjected embryos (Table 1).

A striking observation was that the great majority of surviving newly hatched chicks from embryos injected with RA material had clearly identifiable talipes deformities, redness of the feet, or dislocation of the hip joint, while none of the controls demonstrated any abnormality. All unhatched eggs were opened on the second or third posthatching day and no gross abnormalities were seen in the control dead embryos. One of four un-

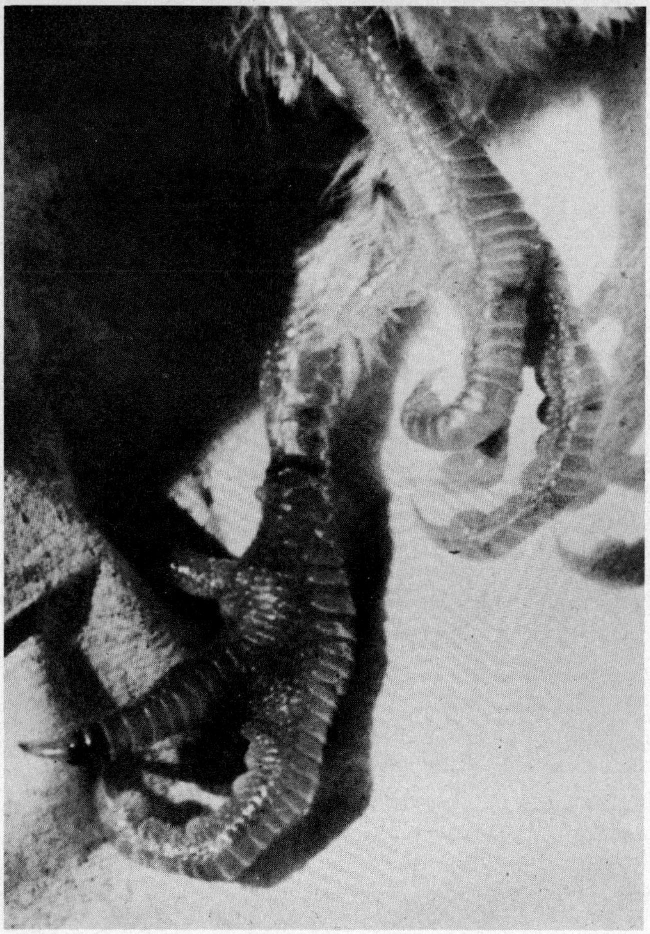

Fig 1.—Bilateral clenched and swollen feet one hour after hatch. Left foot and metatarsal areas are scarlet, right side is pink. Both feet show bright hemorrhagic spots. Upon standing these feet flatten out into talipes as seen in Fig 2 and 3.

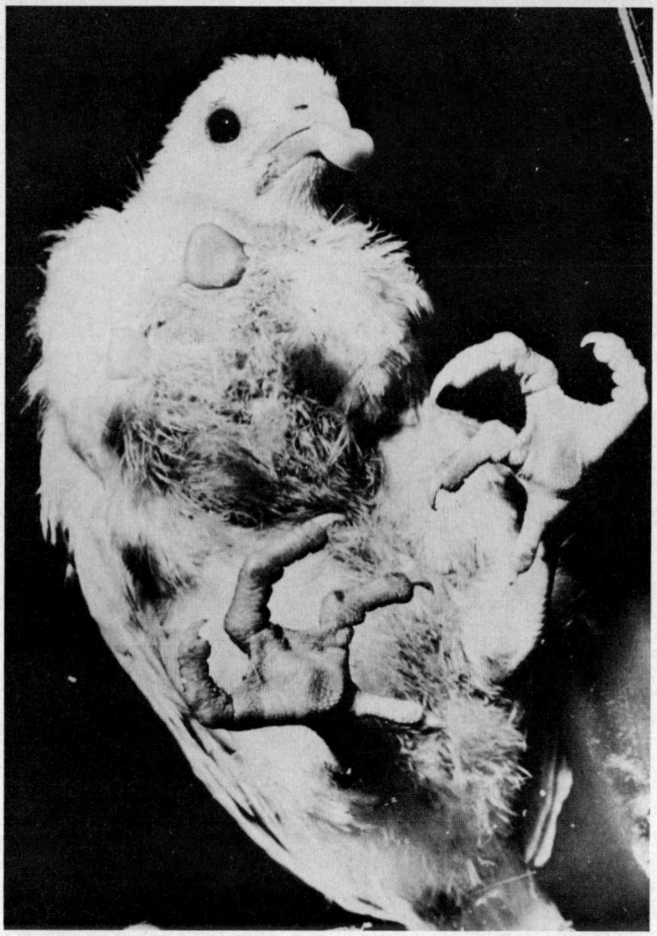

Fig 2.—Plantar view of typical bilateral fixed talipes with medial deflection of the toes of both feet. Pressure points on glass are visible on all toes. Configuration remained the same after 18 months (age 2 weeks).

Fig 3.—Dorsal view of bilateral fixed talipes showing joints of toes severely flexed to the left. Toes and metatarsal joints are still swollen and dark-colored (7-day-old chick).

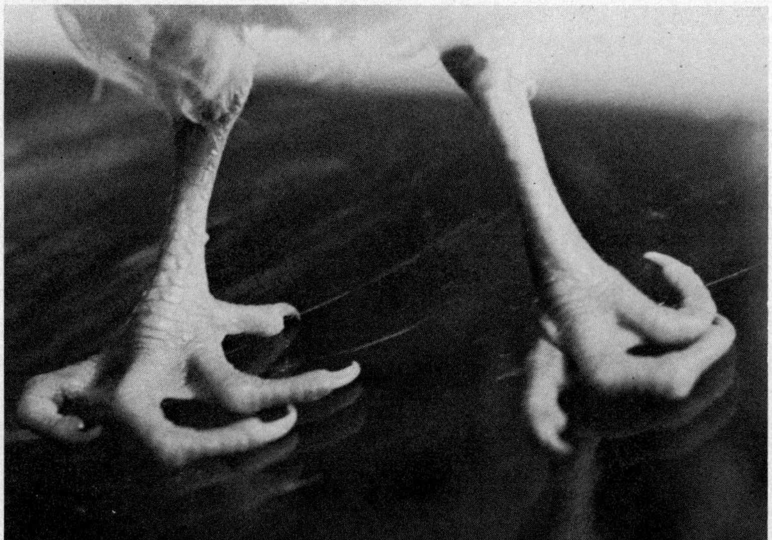

Fig 4.—Twelve-hour-old chicks showing swollen, weak, flattened feet with curved toes which generally straighten within seven days. Tips of toes are often bright red or brown as seen in chick on the right. The fourth toes of chick on the left usually will not straighten out.

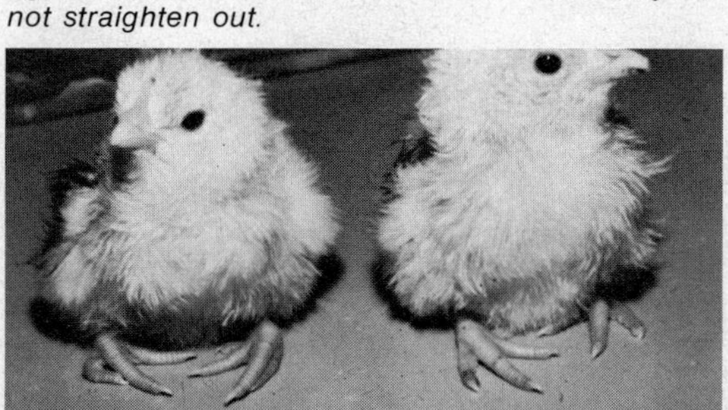

hatched eggs injected with synovial extract from patient 3 contained a mature chick with scarlet-colored "clenched feet" and was the subject of further studies.

The abnormal feet of the embryo described here were aseptically removed and homogenized. The homogenate was injected into 24 embryonated eggs. There was a 37% mortality and 73% of the newly hatched chickens developed abnormalities of the limbs. This observation suggested chick to chick transmission of the presumed active agent.

Sixty-nine fertile eggs were obtained from the two hens with severe talipes derived from embryos injected with human rheumatoid synovium. A mortality of 33% was observed in the embryos. Of 46 hatched chicks, 73% (34:46) had identifiable abnormalities with talipes, etc. This suggested congenital transmission of the "agent."

Essentially all of the 68 surviving embryos of the control group hatched normal chicks on the 21st day of incubation. Unaffected chicks from experimental groups also hatched on the 21st day and remained normal during two months of observation. Abnormal chicks hatched three to four days later than controls or unaffected chicks and showed four major defects (Table 2). At hatch, chicks with marked, fixed talipes of one or both feet exhibited swelling and redness of the clenched, deformed foot (Fig 1). Within a few hours, the chicks were able to stand and walk but the contracted toes deflected either to the right or left and maintained the talipes deformity (Fig 2 and 3). These toes could not be actively straightened by the chick or passively straightened by the examiner for the rest of the life of the chickens. While all three toes were usually involved, some chicks exhibited the angulation deformity in only a single toe with slight fixed dorsal contracture at the metatarsal junction. The redness and swelling subsided within seven days.

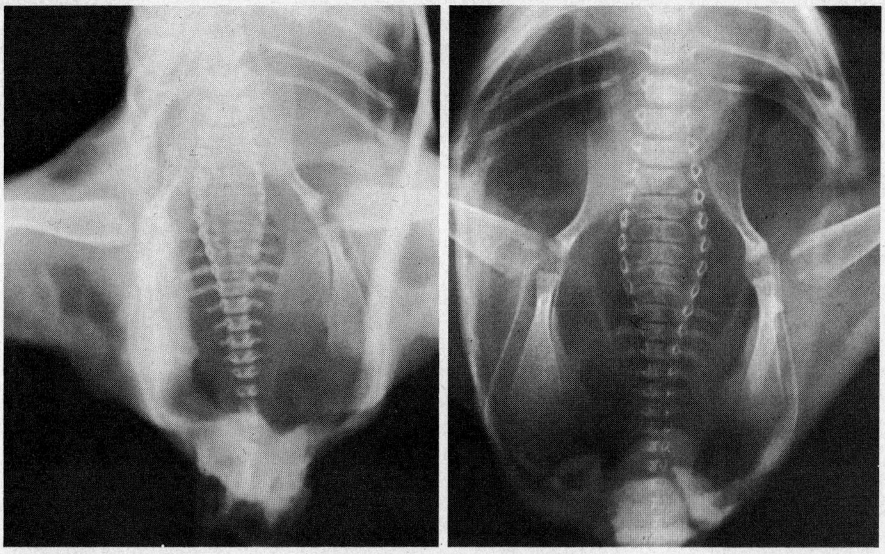

Fig 5.—Fine-grain anteroposterior roentgenograms of dissections of the lumbo-sacral vertebrae of 1-day-old chicks. Left, *Normal chick.* Right, *Extensive developmental and positional anomalies of the bodies and lateral processes in chick with bilateral club feet (× 70).*

Table 1.—Mortality and Morbidity in Chicks From Injection of 10-Day-Old Embryos With Saline Solution Extracts of Rheumatoid Arthritis and Nonrheumatoid Joint Tissues

				Newly Hatched Chicks			
		Mortality		Hatched		Abnormal	
Material	No. of Eggs	Ratio	%	Ratio	%	Ratio	%
RA patients							
1	4	1:4	25	3:4	75	3:3	100
1	5	2:5	40	3:5	60	3:3	100
1	4	3:4	75	1:4	25	1:1	100
1	6	3:6	50	3:6	50	3:3	100
1*	9	0:9	0	9:9	100	9:9	100
2	4	1:4	25	3:4	75	3:3	100
3	4	4:4	100	0:4†	0	...	...
4	8	2:8	25	6:8	75	3:6	50
5	13	8:13	61	5:13	39	5:5	100
Total	57	24:57	42	33:57	58	30:33	91
Non-RA patients							
6	5	2:5	40	3:5	60	0:3	0
7	4	1:4	25	3:4	75	0:3	0
7 (0.05 ml)	4	1:4	25	3:4	75	0:3	0
8	4	0:4	0	4:4	100	0:4	0
Total	17	4:17	24	13:17	76	0:13	0
Control eggs							
Punctured, uninjected	15	2:15	13	13:15	87	0:13	0
Unpunctured	52	10:52	19	42:52	81	0:42	0

* Diluted 1:10.
† Unhatched mature chick with red feet.

The feet apparently were not tender or painful with motion but perching was difficult because of the deformity.

Twenty-nine chicks (30%) showed redness of the digits with swelling and curved and flexed toes (Fig 4). These toes could be actively straightened by the chick and passively extended by the examiner. Perching was possible but difficult to maintain—possibly due to weakness of the toe flexors. Twenty-two chicks (29%) showed mainly extravasation of blood in the tissues of the toes which disappeared within seven days. Usually swelling and some weakness of the toes was also present. Six chicks (9%) not only had the "scarlet clenched" feet but had dislocation of the hip with extreme spasm of the leg mus-

Table 2.—Distribution of the Lesions in the Feet of the 75 Abnormal Chicks as a Result of Injection of RA Materials

Type of Lesion	No. Chicks	%
Permanent talipes	24	32
Weak and deflected toes	23	30
Scarlet lesions only	22	29
Fixed dislocated hip	6	9
Total	75	100

cles. Early fatal dislocation of the neck was common in this group because of extreme anatomical defects of the cervical vertebrae.

Roentgenograms.—Fine grain roentgenograms of several chicks with RA and unstable neck action showed an abnormal development and reduced density of the upper third and fourth thoracic vertebrae. Severe angulation occurred at the junction of the cervical thoracic vertebrae. There was some rotation of the thoracic vertebrae distal to this level. A few chicks had irregularities in the cartilaginous plates of the thoracic vertebrae. Neural arches and lateral processes in various parts of the spine often were absent on one side. The details of the lumbar and sacral regions were obscured by overlying shadows but there were suggestions of failure of development of the bodies and neural arches in the upper sacrum and lower lumbar vertebrae (Fig 5). Several chicks with displaced legs showed the unaffected femoral heads to be displaced upward, apparently resting on the rim of the normally developed acetabulum. This displacement appeared to be the result of the severe muscular spasm rather than joint destruction.

Roentgenograms of these abnormal feet did not disclose bony changes even when there was extreme and rigid flexion of the toes. Roentgenograms of the feet with severe talipes taken at 11 months of age showed considerable damage of the phalangeal joints which could be the result of either RA involvement or long-sustained trauma resulting from the malposition of the toes.

Comment

The injection of chicken embryos with a saline solution homogenate of rheumatoid synovial tissue induced a series of abnormalities in hatched chicks in contrast to the control embryos. Furthermore, the ability to induce these abnormalities could apparently be transferred from involved chicks to embryos and also could occur in a congenital transmission (involved hens to offsprings). Three observations would be consistent with the presence of a self-replicating transmissible agent associated with human rheumatoid synovium. The possibility of traumatically induced lesions seemed improbable as the injection with nonrheumatoid tissues failed to induce the lesions. Furthermore, the probability that these observations would result from genetic abnormalities is improbable because of their absence in the controls and the reported spontaneous occurrence of 0.15% in the hatchery chicks. Cultures of the saline slurries were negative for growth of bacteria, fungi, or mycoplasma and contamination with an unidentified agent seems remote inasmuch as each specimen was collected separately and processed individually.

We have reported pathologic changes in mice injected with human rheumatoid synoviums but the lesions were far less striking, thus the sensitivity of chick embryos to injection of this material may have greater utility in the search for an infectious agent in rheumatoid arthritis. Despite the variable success of others in identifying an agent in rheumatoid arthritis, this new observation on the induction of lesions in chicks by injection of the embryo would appear to confirm the earlier reports of induction of lesions in mice.

There were three basic lesions observed in the chicks: (1) redness and swelling of the feet; (2) foot deformities; and (3) developmental anomalies of the spine and dislocation of the hip. Only the inflammatory vascular type lesions in the feet were reversible, disappearing within seven days, and were comparable to the lesions reported in mice. The anomalies of the spine will require further study to classify, but we have also observed late-appearing spinal involvement in affected mice (unpublished observations). The talipes and other foot deformities could result from neural involvement at a special level but further studies are required to identify the pathogenesis.

To date we have not characterized, isolated, or cultured the presumed agent in an in vitro system. Further studies are needed to confirm and extend these observations, particularly in view of the failure of others to identify an agent of rheumatoid arthritis. Nonetheless, the utilization of the chick embryo may provide the avenue to further examine the infectious agent of rheumatoid arthritis in the human and various other species.

This work was supported by the Lil and Mel Simmonds Fund.

Andrew H. Dowdy, MD, supplied the fine-grain roentgenograms for Fig 4.

References

1. Warren SL, Marmor L, Liebes DM, et al: Congenital transmission in mice of an active agent from human rheumatoid arthritis. *Nature* **223**(5206):646-647, 1969.

2. Warren SL, Marmor L, Liebes DM, et al: An active agent from human rheumatoid arthritis which is transmissible in mice. *Arch Intern Med* **124**:629-634, 1969.

3. Warren SL, Marmor L, Liebes DM, et al: Congenital deformities of mice transmitted by a human rheumatoid synovium agent. *Clin Orthop* **70**:216-219, 1970.

The Mode of Action of Antibiotics on Gram-Negative Bacilli

Victor Lorian, MD, New York

The mode of action of any antibiotic is essentially the same, whether it is against gram-positive or gram-negative microorganisms.[1,2]

In order to present a schematic version of the modes of action, I will try to give just enough molecular and biochemical information to facilitate understanding without burdening the reader with unnecessary details. The illustrations are more diagrammatic than the expression of the real stereomodel of the many biochemical reactions described. Data presented in this manner is more relevant to the practical aspects of antibiotic tests in vitro as well as in the treatment of patients.

As the mode of action of antibiotics is conditioned in part by the bacterial anatomy of the microorganism and its chemical constituents, let me point out a few essential differences between the gram-positive and gram-negative organisms.

Figure 1 schematically pictures a gram-positive coccus and a gram-negative bacillus. The gram-positive organism has a thick cell wall which contains a strong rigid layer of mucopeptides, representing about 60% or more of the cell wall; this is entangled with teichoic acid,[3] and coated with magnesium ribonucleate, both substances characteristic of gram-positive organisms. The gram-negative bacillus has a very thin layer of this rigid component of the cell wall—10% or less. The lipopolysaccharides and lipoproteins constitute the main element forming the wall.[4] The osmotic pressure is about 20 atmospheres in the gram-positive microorganisms but only about 5 atmospheres in the gram-negative organisms.[5] We will see in a short while the importance of these differences.

Some agents first attach to the cell surface.[6,7] In many instances, the sensitive cells bind more antibiotic than the resistant cells.[6,7] The antibiotic has to penetrate to its point of action; therefore, the drugs must be able to go through the cell wall and most of them through the cytoplasmic membrane as well (Fig 2). There is a difference in antibiotic penetrability comparing gram-positive and gram-negative organisms. For instance, polymyxin is inactive on gram-positive organisms mainly because it is stopped by the magnesium ribonucleate coating on the cell wall, while it is very active on gram-negative organisms in which this substance is absent. There is some correlation of membrane or envelope lipid composition and the antibiotic sensitivity of gram-negative organisms.[8]

Figure 3 schematically pictures four groups of antibiotics with their four mechanisms of action which relate each to a different anatomical part of the bacterium. The penicillin group interferes with cell wall synthesis; the polymyxin group acts on the cytoplasmic membrane; chloramphenicol and tetracycline and the others mentioned in the third group act on protein synthesis; and finally, the nalidixic acid (which is not an antibiotic) acts on DNA while rifampin inhibits RNA synthesis.

Practically all the antibiotics, although they have a certain specific primary mode of action, also interfere at least secondarily in other areas of the anatomy or the physiology of organisms. At lower concentrations,

Received for publication Aug 28, 1970; accepted Dec 4, 1970.

From the Bronx-Lebanon Hospital Center, Bronx, New York.

Read before the American Society for Microbiology, Boston, April 1970.

Reprint requests to Bronx-Lebanon Hospital Center, 1276 Fulton Ave, Bronx, NY 10456 (Dr. Lorian).

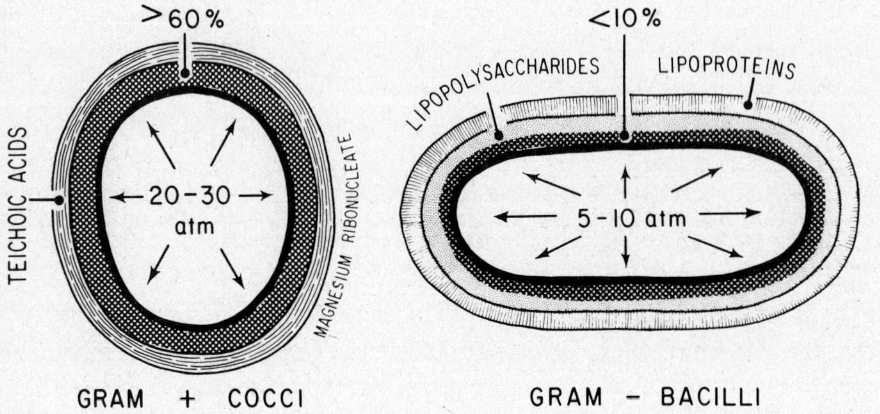

Fig 1.—Comparative anatomy of gram-positive cocci and gram-negative bacilli. Drawings show proportion of cell wall which is mucopeptide and osmotic value.

their effect can be more or less restricted to their primary action; at higher concentrations, multiple vital functions of the microorganism may be affected. Also, because of the close interrelation among the different elements in the bacterial cell, antibacterial agents can produce indirect side effects on sites which they do not affect directly.

In quite a few instances the antibacterial agents act as analogues of essential substances of the normal metabolism in the bacterial cell. For instance, sulfonamides are analogues of *p*-aminobenzoic acid; penicillin is a structural analogue for the D-alanyl-D-alanine end of the pentapeptide chain; cycloserine is an analogue for D-alanine; and chloramphenicol is regarded by some investigators as an analogue of uridylic acid.

The mode of action of the penicillins is illustrated in Fig 4. As pictured, the cell is in the process of division, during which it increases its cytoplasmic volume, and mucopeptides accumulate diffusely in the rigid layer.[9] In gram-positive cocci a small accumulation of mucopeptides takes place in the splitting area.[10] In a normal growing cell there is a certain equilibrium between cell wall synthesis and cell wall lysis so that cell division without cell destruction can be achieved.[11] The lysis is produced by autolytic enzymes in the cell wall, one of which is acetylmuramidase. When an antibiotic of the penicillin group is added during growth, the cell wall synthesis stops very quickly. Protein synthesis and increase of cell volume, however, continue. The autolytic enzymes also continue to lyse, eroding the existing cell wall so that it becomes defective. The rigid layer of the cell wall ceases to be adequately protective and, because the interior osmotic pressure is higher than that of the environment, the cell lyses in the absence of a complete wall.

Figure 5 shows a schematic outline of the chemical structure of the mucopeptide, or rigid layer of the cell wall of *Staphylococcus aureus*.[12] The exact structure varies considerably depending on the species of bacteria. Most bacteria only cross-link about half of the potential D-ala-NH_2-sites. The first stage of the synthesis (Fig 5–1) of the rigid layer occurs in the cytoplasm and consists of the biosynthesis of the uridine nucleotide precursors. Cycloserine, which is a competitive inhibitor of two sequential reactions catalyzed by alanine racemase and D-alanyl-D-alanine-synthetase, deprives the bacteria of the elements necessary for the synthesis of the complete cell wall precursors. A second stage of cell wall synthesis (Fig 5–2) is represented by the addition of new pentapeptides. This takes place also in the cytoplasm through a mechanism involving the cytoplasmic membrane. Vancomycin, ristocetin, and bacitracin inhibit this second stage. The rigid cell wall layer synthesis is almost accomplished, but at this point the net form of this layer is still incomplete, still elastic, and quite soluble.

The main step that confers the rigidity and the insolubility of this layer of the cell wall is the cross-linking of the linear peptide strands which are formed as just described.[13] This is accomplished outside the cytoplasmic membrane (Fig 5–3). The penicillins and the cephalosporins stop this last and essential step of the cell wall synthesis.[14]

Cycloserine, vancomycin, and ristocetin act inside of the cytoplasmic membrane; therefore, they must first penetrate the cell wall if they are to act. As previously indicated, the penicillins block the transpeptidase enzyme that affects the final cross-linking. This enzyme is on the outer side of the cytoplasmic membrane and, therefore, the penicillins are closer to their target and independent of the membrane permeability.[15]

At low concentration, penicillin G potassium or vancomycin is more effective on gram-positive than on gram-negative organisms. The insensitivity of gram-negative bacilli is due not to any lack of sensitive enzymes, but probably to the fact that the antibiotics cannot penetrate to the site of these enzymes in the gram-negative bacterial cell. The intact cells of *Escherichia coli* are not

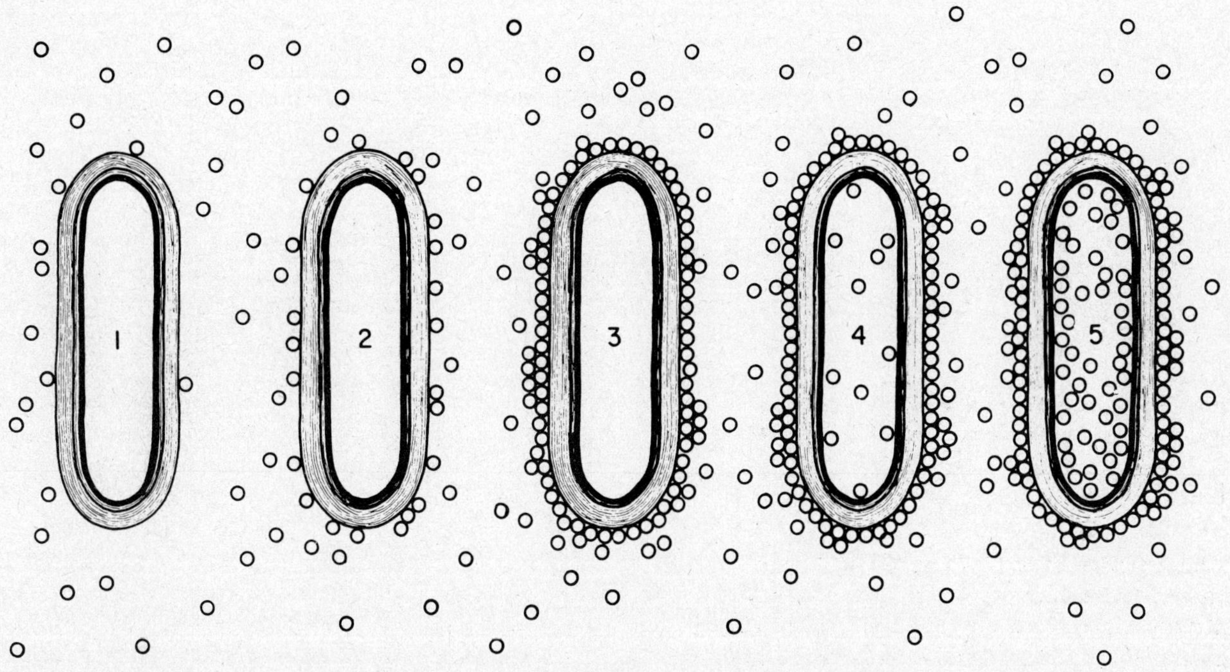

Fig 2.—Attachment on the surface and penetration of antibiotics in gram-negative bacilli.

sensitive to low concentrations of penicillin or vancomycin, but the enzyme obtained from these cells is just as sensitive to these antibiotics as the enzyme of a sensitive staphylococcus.[16] Ampicillin, carbenicillin, and cephalosporin are also active on both types of bacteria, but have greater use against gram-negative bacilli than penicillin G. The essential difference from penicillin G, although resistance to β-lactamase may play some role, consists of penetration capability of these antibiotics through the lipopolysaccharide layer of the gram-negative bacteria.[17]

The penicillin antibiotics, acting on the cell wall synthesis of gram-negative bacilli, have little opportunity to damage the gram-negative bacilli.[18] Although they stop the mucopeptide synthesis, the other constituents of the cell wall which predominate in the gram-negative organisms will preserve for a longer period of time the physical integrity and the protective function of the cell wall. Because the osmotic pressure is lower in gram-negative bacilli, the breaking of the crytoplasmic membrane in a cell with defective cell wall is also retarded.

Figure 6 shows morphological changes produced by penicillin on gram-negative bacilli. The bacilli grow longer (lower left) and then take filamentous forms (center). Although it has been known since 1940 that penicillin produces filamentous forms from gram-negative bacilli,[19] it is not yet explained why it inhibits the septa formation and cell division when, at the same time, it allows the synthesis of sufficient material to produce the walls for the filamentous forms.[20] The cell wall becomes progressively more defective and globular forms appear (right). Finally, the bacilli lyse.

Most of the broad spectrum antibiotics interfere with the protein synthesis of bacteria.[21] The mechanism of protein synthesis is reviewed in Fig 7. During transcription, the DNA, which stores the information for protein synthesis, transmits it to the messenger RNA. On the ribosome the messenger RNA comes in contact with the transfer RNA which forwards the amino acids needed for the synthesis of the coded polypeptides.[22] The messenger RNA, according to the information received from the DNA by transcription, will attract those needed amino acids which will be linked together producing polypeptides and eventually proteins. Figure 8 depicts in close-up what happens at the ribosome level. The amino acids located around the ribosome are activated by enzymes which attach them to the transfer RNA. This complex is then attached to the ribosome. Trans-

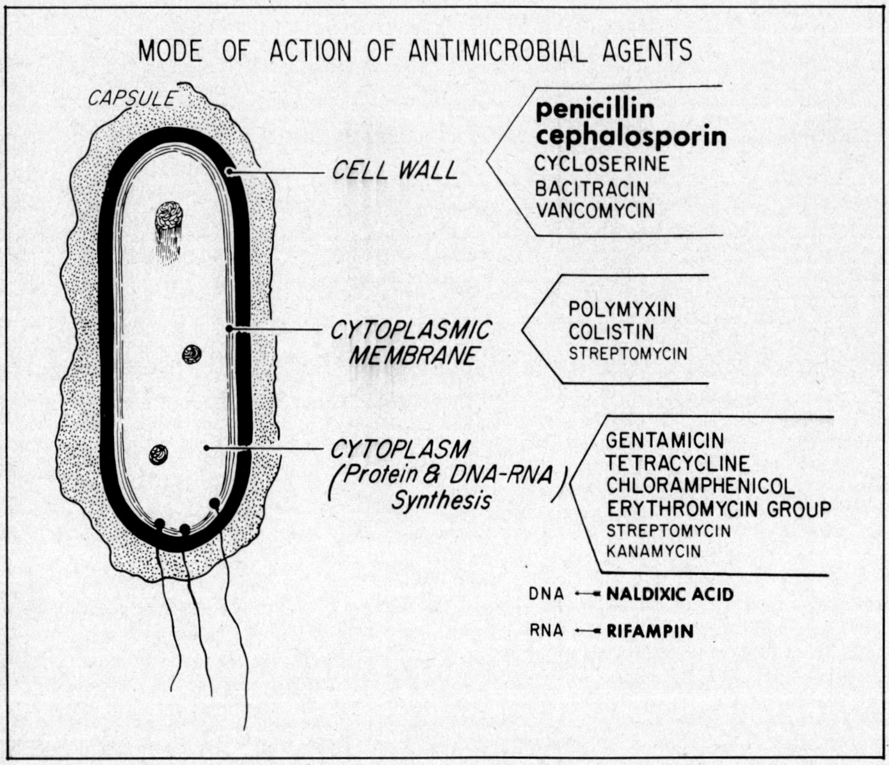

Fig 3.—Site of action of the four groups of antibiotics on a gram-negative bacillus.

Fig 4.—Mode of action of penicillin in a dividing organism.

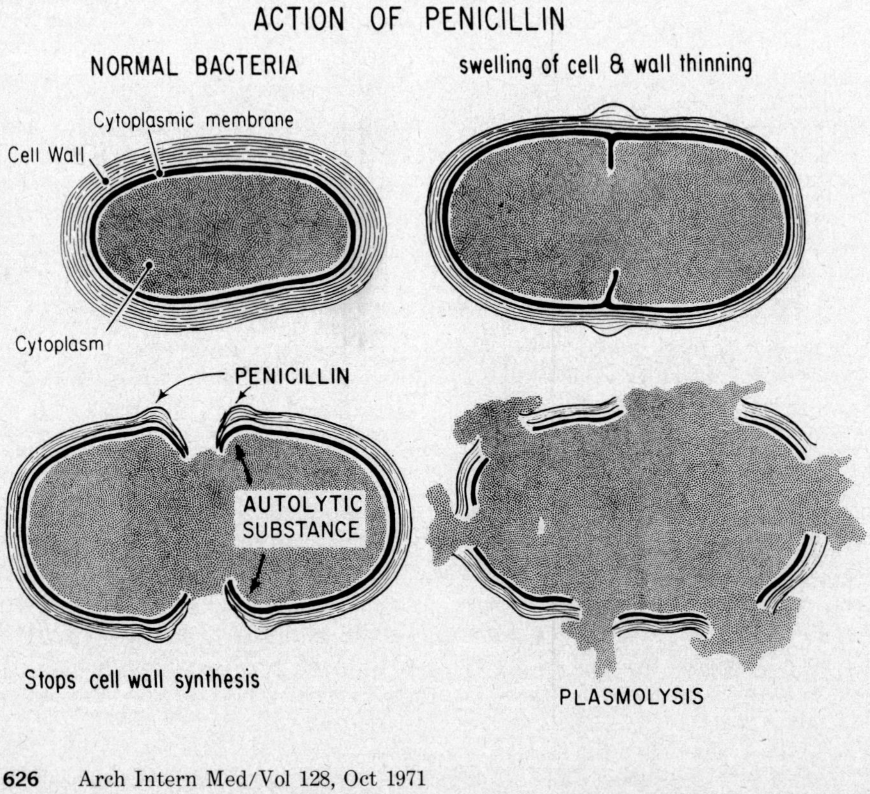

lation occurs when the messenger RNA on the ribosome (on its 30 S part) makes contact with the transfer RNA to which the amino acid is attached, and, according to its code, the messenger RNA picks up the amino acids needed for the polypeptide synthesis.

The site of action of three major antibiotics lies in this area. Tetracycline blocks the binding of the transfer RNA-amino acid complex to the ribosome.[23] Thus, no amino acid is available to the messenger RNA and no polypeptides can be produced.

Chloramphenicol acts by blocking the transfer of the amino acids onto the growing polypeptide chain.[24] Some evidence suggests that chloramphenicol can also block the contact of the messenger RNA with the ribosome so that no amino acid can be selected for the synthesis of polypeptides.[25] In both instances, chloramphenicol stops polypeptide synthesis and, as with tetracycline, no protein synthesis can take place. Both tetracycline and chloramphenicol stop the normal process of protein synthesis, but without producing any irreversible damage to the cell. Consequently, both antibiotics are bacteriostatic drugs. If they are eliminated, the cell can resume its normal protein synthesis and continue after a short while to reproduce.

Streptomycin,[26] gentamicin,[27,28] and kanamycin interfere with the function of the messenger RNA. These antibiotics interfere with the translation mechanism, producing a misreading so that the messenger RNA continues its activity, but in a distorted way. Amino acids will be aligned and transferred into polypeptides, but the messenger RNA will couple incorrect transfer RNA-amino acids and insert them in an erroneous order. The result will be a nonsense

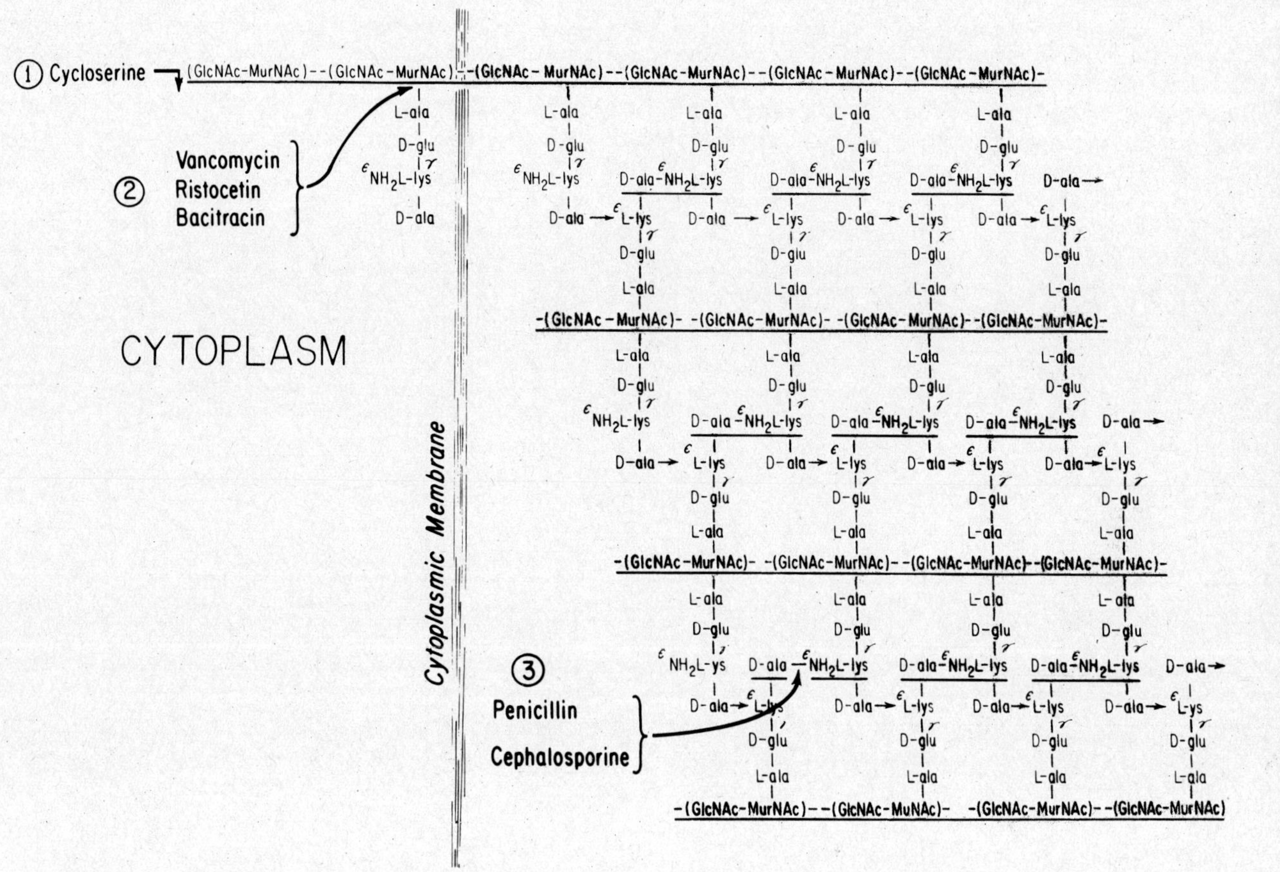

Fig 5.—Site of action of the "cell wall inhibiting" antibiotics during the mucopeptide synthesis.

polypeptide which is obviously nonfunctional and will finally produce a faulty protein. It is possible this might kill the microorganism. Although the streptomycin group of antiotics is bactericidal, the mechanism causing cell death is not yet adequately determined.

All the antibiotics mentioned up to now—the penicillins, chloramphenicol, tetracycline and the streptomycin group—interfere with some active process of the cell. If there is no activity, there is nothing to be stopped or nothing to be interfered with and, therefore, all these drugs in their usual concentration are inactive against resting cells.

The polymyxins act on the cytoplasmic membrane. This membrane has three layers: a middle layer of lipids, and two protein layers, one on each side of this lipid layer.[29] All three layers together are about 80 Angstroms thick. The polymyxin molecule is a peptide of which one end is lipid-soluble and the other end is water-soluble. When polymyxin reaches the plasmic membrane, these molecules will insert themselves between the lipid layer and the protein layers[30] (Figure 9). The lipid-soluble end of the molecule will be buried into the lipidic layer and the water-soluble end will be buried into the protein layer. This will produce a cleavage between the layers which finally leads to ruptures in the membrane. Substances can now cross into and out of the cytoplasm, practically abolishing the membrane functions, thus quickly causing the death of the organism. It is interesting to note that polymyxin acts as a disinfectant, and affects by simple contact a main organ of the bacterium; this accounts for the quick, bactericidal effect of the polymyxins, whether the cell is metabolically active or not. Recent evidence indicates that polymyxin, in addition to its action on the cytoplasmic membrane, affects the outer layer of the cell wall of the gram-negative bacilli.[31]

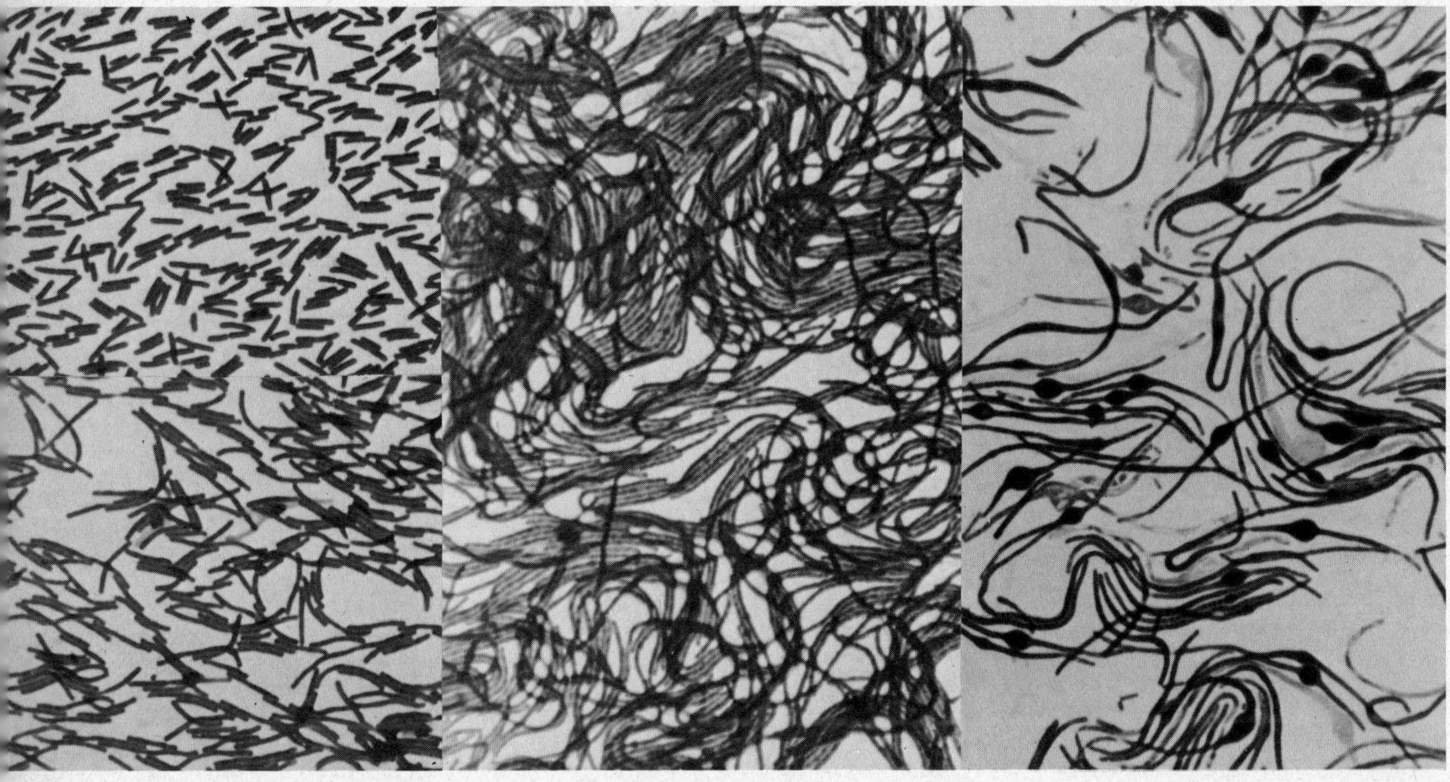

Fig 6.—Morphological changes produced by penicillin on gram-negative bacilli. Upper left, *Normal bacilli;* lower left, *elongated bacilli;* center, *filamentous forms;* right, *globular forms.*

Fig 7.—The mechanism of protein synthesis.

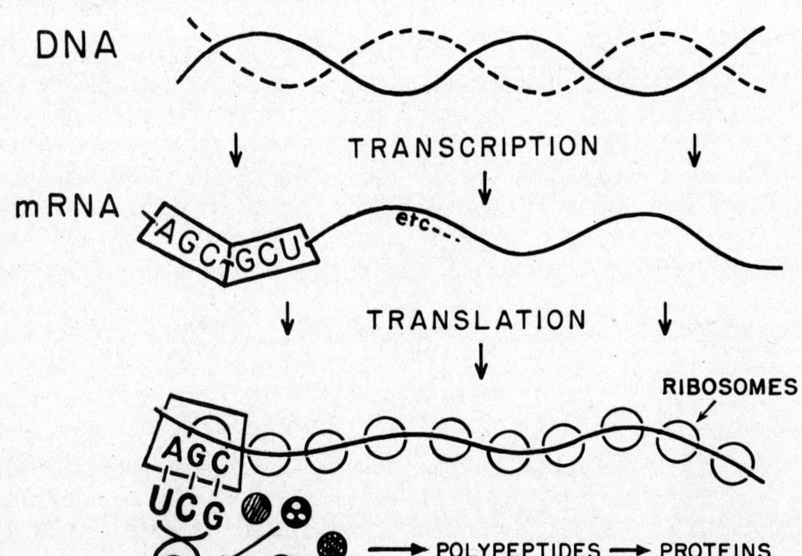

For all practical purposes, the polymyxins are inactive against gram-positive bacteria, as already mentioned, they are unable to cross the magnesium ribonucleate coating of the cell wall.[32] Their efficiency against gram-negative organisms is due to the fact that they can affect the outer layer of their cell wall and then penetrate to the cytoplasmic membrane without other opposition.

The resistance of some gram-negative bacilli to polymyxin is probably due, as demonstrated for *Proteus mirabilis*, to the exclusion of the antibiotic from the susceptible membranes.[33]

Nalidixic acid blocks DNA synthesis.[34] It has been demonstrated that it inhibits thymine incorporation into DNA with only negligible effects on the incorporation of protein or RNA precursors. But the precise

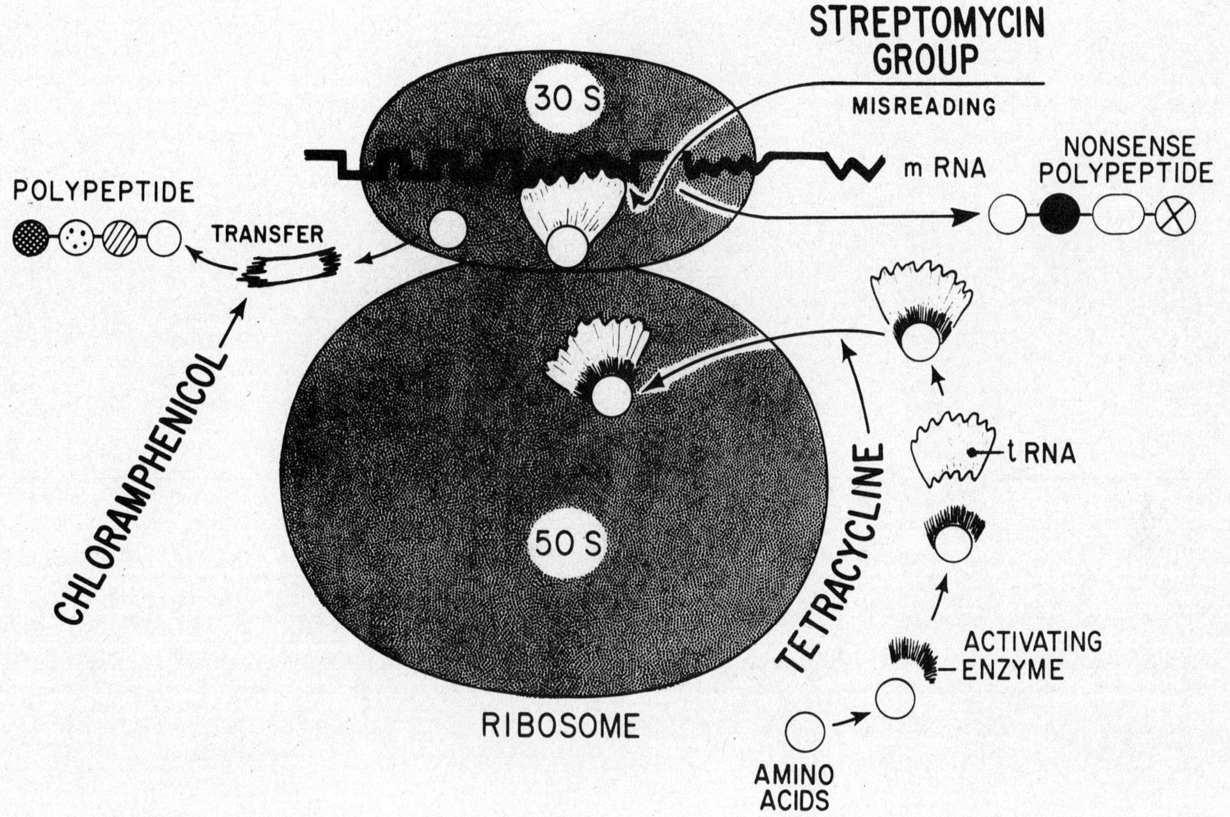

Fig 8.—The effect of chloramphenicol, tetracycline, and streptomycin on protein synthesis at the ribosome level.

mechanism is still unclear.

Rifampin and related derivatives prevent bacterial multiplication by blocking the synthesis of RNA.[35] Scientists in Israel and Scotland recently reported rifampin to be active against certain viruses as well as against bacteria, but the antiviral activity does not seem to be related to the effect on RNA.

Several practical implications result from the mode of action of antibiotics on gram-negative bacilli. As mentioned before, antibiotics, in order to act, have to penetrate the microorganism. One mechanism of bacterial resistance to antibiotics already exemplified is a change in permeability.[36]

Some of the synergistic and antagonistic effects of various antibiotic combinations can also be explained and predicted through their mechanism of action. Penicillin is expected to be antagonized by all drugs stopping protein synthesis (Fig 10). If the cytoplasm cannot grow, inhibition of the cell wall synthesis remains without effect. The cell will not increase its volume, the autolytic enzymes which are proteins will not act, and, therefore, the cell will not lyse. Streptomycin is synergistic with penicillin because it does not stop protein synthesis; it just alters it, producing nonfunctional proteins and enzymes (Fig 10). At the same time, penicillin, which damages the cell wall, facilitates the penetration of streptomycin into the cell (Fig 11, at left). It has been shown that microorganisms treated with penicillin bind significantly more streptomycin than nontreated organisms.[37]

By varying the concentrations of some antibiotics, the primary sites of action can be changed and, consequently, the effect of the cell is different. Cycloserine, at low concentrations, inhibits cell wall synthesis and is bactericidal. At high concentrations, it inhibits transaminases, resulting in an inhibition of protein synthesis; in this case, cycloserine is only bacteriostatic.[38]

Figure 6 shows the filamentous and the globular forms produced by gram-

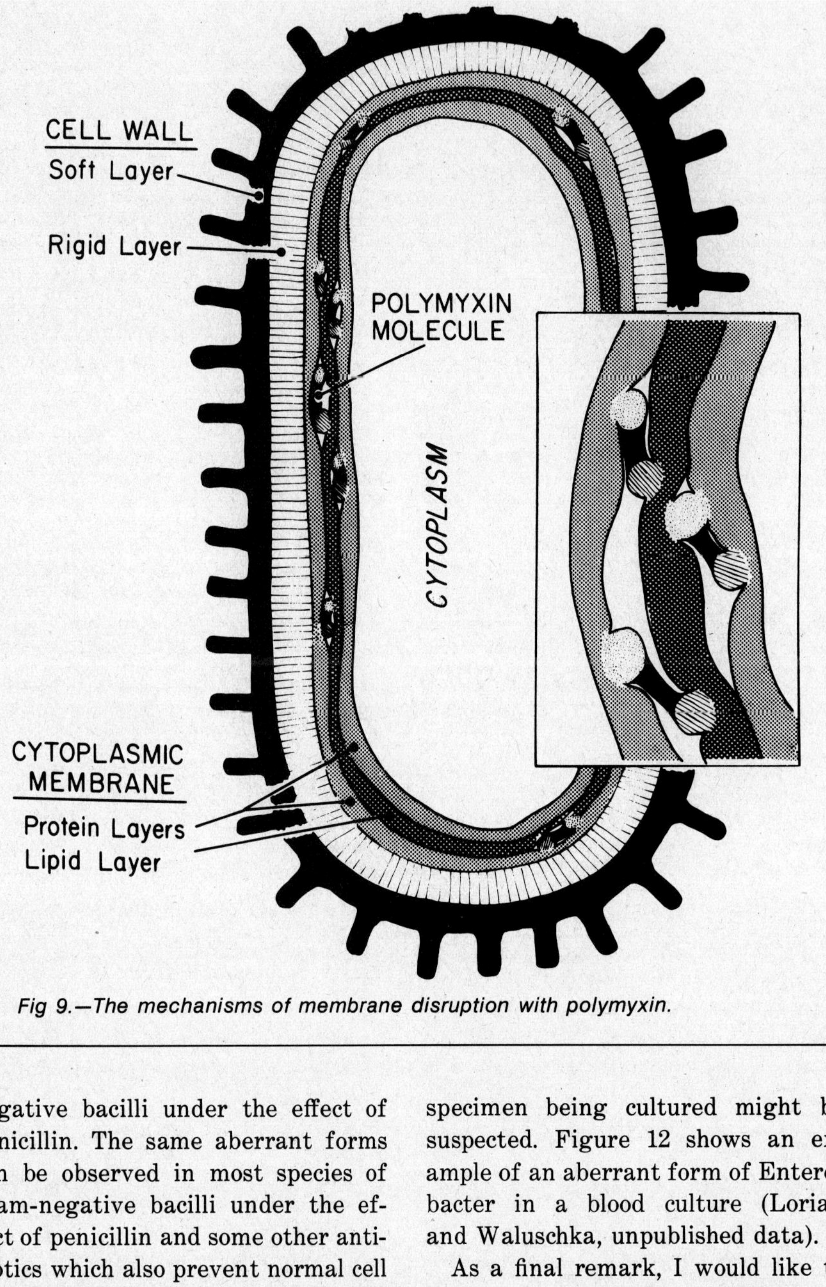

Fig 9.—The mechanisms of membrane disruption with polymyxin.

negative bacilli under the effect of penicillin. The same aberrant forms can be observed in most species of gram-negative bacilli under the effect of penicillin and some other antibiotics which also prevent normal cell wall formation. Such a peculiar bacillary morphology can be observed not only in vitro, but also sometimes in smears from different parts of the body, eg, urine and sometimes even in blood cultures. In those cases, previous antibiotic therapy or the presence of traces of antibiotics in the specimen being cultured might be suspected. Figure 12 shows an example of an aberrant form of Enterobacter in a blood culture (Lorian and Waluschka, unpublished data).

As a final remark, I would like to comment on those disk sensitivity tests which are made for different compounds of the same antibiotic.

The various compounds of a given antibiotic differ mostly as to their pharmacologic properties. The antibacterial spectrum is usually very similar to the antibiotic base and certainly their mode of action is the same. Consequently, a disk sensitivity test of one compound is sufficient to indicate the sensitivity of a bacterial strain to any of the other compounds. This is the case with the tetracyclines, the polymyxins, and the cephalosporins, among others.

Summary

The mode of action of any antibiotic is essentially the same whether it is against gram-positive or gram-negative microorganisms. The gram-positive organisms have a thick cell wall which contains a rigid layer of mucopeptides representing about 60% or more of the cell wall. The gram-negative bacilli have a very thin layer of this rigid component—10% or less. The osmotic pressure is about 20 atmospheres in the gram-positives with only about 5 atmospheres in the gram-negative organisms. These are essential differences and a cause of different behavior in the presence of antibacterial agents. The antibiotics can be divided into four groups according to the mechanism of action as related each to a different anatomical part of the bacteria.

1. The first group consists of those antibiotics which affect the cell wall synthesis. They can be subdivided into three subgroups: cycloserine which deprives the bacteria of the elements necessary for synthesis of the complete cell wall, vancomycin, ristocetin and bacitracin which inhibit the second stage of the mucopeptide synthesis, and the penicillins and the cephalosporins which stop the cross-linking of the linear peptide strands that are so important to confer the rigidity of the cell wall.

2. Another group of antibiotics among which we can find most of the large spectrum agents like chloramphenicol and tetracycline, inhibit the

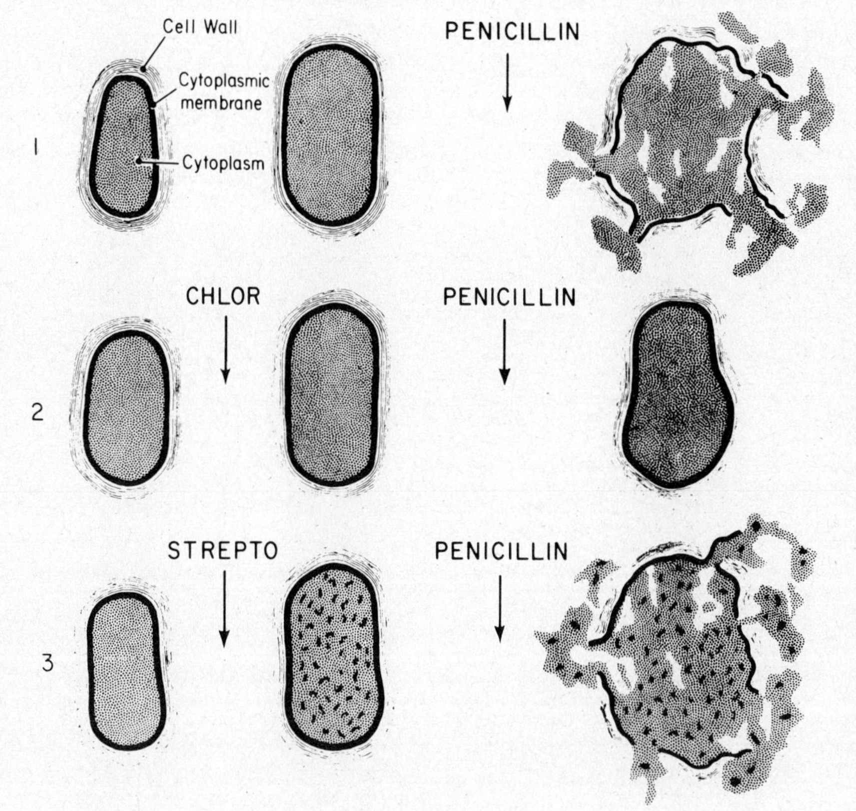

Fig 10.—Antagonism and synergism produced by chloramphenicol (CHLOR) and streptomycin (STREPTO) with penicillin.

Fig 11.—Left, *Synergism.* Right, *Autoantagonism.*

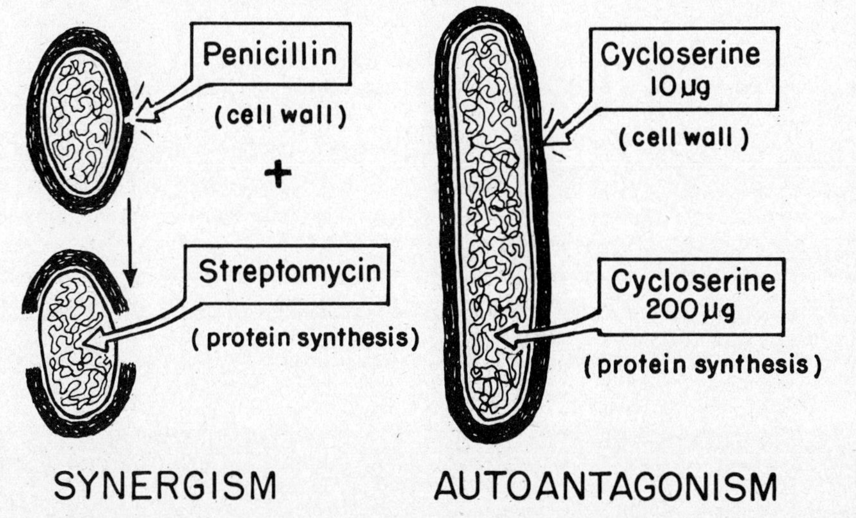

protein synthesis. Tetracycline blocks the binding of the transfer RNA amino acid complex to the ribosome and, therefore, the polypeptide synthesis is stopped. Chloramphenicol blocks the transfer of the amino acids onto the amino acid chain. The streptomycin group of antibiotics interfere with the function of the messenger RNA. These antibiotics produce misreading and although they do not stop the protein synthesis, they produce nonfunctional polypeptides which finally produce a faulty protein.

3. Another group is represented by the polymyxins which act on the cytoplasmic membrane. They disrupt it by direct physical-chemical effect and this accounts for their quick bactericidal action regardless if the cells are metabolically active or not.

4. Finally, nalidixic acid blocks DNA synthesis and rifampin and related derivatives prevent bacterial multiplication by blocking the RNA synthesis.

Some practical applications result from the knowledge of the mode of action of antibiotics. The synergistic and antagonistic effects of various combinations can be predicted and explained. Penicillin is expected to be antagonized by all drugs stopping

Fig 12.—Aberrant forms of Klebsiella *in a blood culture.*

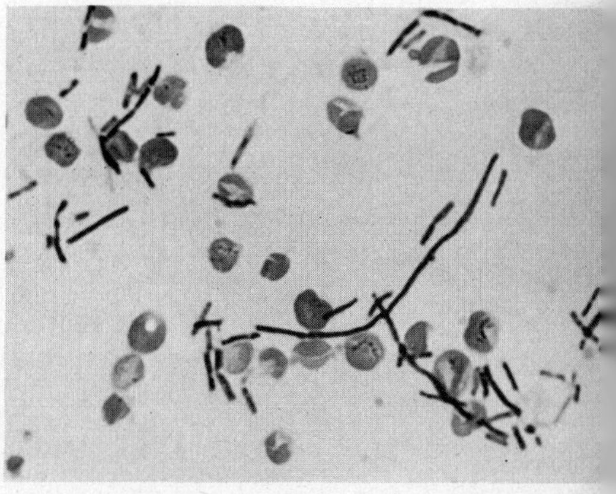

protein synthesis. It is synergistic with streptomycin because penicillin, by damaging the cell wall, allows streptomycin to penetrate better and in larger quantities at its site of action.

Gram-negative bacilli can be seen in filamentous forms in urine or blood. They are gram-negative bacilli which change to filamentous form under the effect of penicillin-type antibiotics.

The various compounds of a given agent differ mostly as to their pharmacologic properties, but antibacterial spectrum and mode of action are similar. Consequently an in vitro sensitivity test for one compound is sufficient to indicate the sensitivity of a strain to any of the compounds.

Nonproprietary and Trade Names of Drugs

Cycloserine—*Seromycin, Oxamycin.*
Rifampin—*Rifadin.*

References

1. Feingold DS: Antimicrobial chemotherapeutic agents: The nature of their action and selective toxicity. *New Eng J Med* **269**:900-906, 1963.
2. Feingold DS: Antimicrobial chemotherapeutic agents: The nature of their action and selective toxicity. *New Eng J Med* **269**:957-964, 1964.
3. Hayflick L: The mycoplasmatales and the L-phase of bacteria, in Hijmans W, van Boven C, and Glasener H: *Fundamental Biology at the L-Phase of Bacteria*, New York, Appleton-Century-Crofts Inc, 1969, p 71.
4. Depetris S: Ultrastructure of the cell wall of *Escherichia coli* and chemical nature of its constituent layers. *Ultrastructure Res* **19**:45-83, 1967.
5. Mitchell P, Moyle J: Osmotic function and structure in bacteria in *Symposium of the Society for General Microbiology*. Cambridge, England, Cambridge University Press, 1956, vol 6, pp 150-180.
6. Few AV, Schulman JH: Absorption of polymyxin by bacteria. *Nature* **171**:644-645, 1953.
7. Few AV, Schulman JH: The absorption of polymyxin E by bacteria and bacterial cell walls and its bactericidal action. *J Gen Microbiol* **9**:454-466, 1953.
8. Dunnick JK, O'Leary WM: Correlation of bacterial lipid composition with antibiotic resistance. *J Bact* **101**:892-900, 1970.
9. Ghuyson JM: Use of bacteriolytic enzymes in determination of wall structure and their role in cell metabolism. *Bact Rev* **32**:425, 1968.
10. Higgins ML, Schockman GD: Model for cell wall growth of *Streptococcus faecalis*. *J Bact* **101**:643-648, 1970.
11. Mitchell P, Moyle J: Autolytic release and osmotic properties of "protoplasts" from *Staphylococcus aureus*. *J Gen Microbiol* **16**:184-194, 1957.
12. Park JT: Discussion of mode of action of penicillins in deReuck AUS, Cameron MP: *Resistance of Bacteria to the Penicillins: Ciba Foundation Study Group No. 13*. Boston, Little Brown & Co, 1962, p 43.
13. Petit JF, Munoz E, Ghuyson JM: Peptide cross-links in bacterial cell wall peptidoglycans studied with specific endopeptidases from *Streptomyces albus* G. *Biochemistry* **5**:2764-2776, 1966.
14. Tipper DJ, Strominger JL: Biosynthesis of the peptidoglycan of bacterial cell walls: Inhibition of crosslinking by penicillins and cephalosporins: Studies in *Staphylococcus aureus* in vivo. *J Biol Chem* **243**:3169-3179, 1968.
15. Strominger JL, Izaki K: Peptidoglycan transpeptidase and D-alanine carboxypeptidase: Penicillin-sensitive enzymatic reactions. *Fed Proc* **26**:9-22, 1967.
16. Strominger JL, Izaki K: Biosynthesis of the peptidoglycan of bacterial cell walls: Peptidoglycan transpeptidase and D-alanine carboxypeptidase: Penicillin-sensitive enzymatic reaction in strains of *Escherichia coli*. *J Biol Chem* **243**:3180-3192, 1968.
17. Butler K, English AR, Ray VA, et al: Carbenicillin: Chemistry and mode of action. *J Infect Dis* **122**:S1-S8, 1970.
18. Truco RE, Pardee AB: Synthesis of *Escherichia coli* cell walls in the presence of penicillin. *J Biol Chem* **320**:435, 1958.
19. Gardner AD: Morphological effects of penicillin on bacteria. *Nature* **146**:837, 1940.
20. Steed P, Murray RGE: The cell wall and cell division of gram-negative bacteria. *Canad J Microbiol* **12**:263-271, 1965.
21. Goldberg IH: Drugs affecting nucleic acid and protein synthesis. *Amer J Med* **39**:722, 1965.
22. Davis BD, Dulbecco R, Eisen HN, et al: *Microbiology*. New York, Harper & Row Publishers Inc, 1967, p 229.
23. Gottlieb D, Shaw PD: Antibiotics, mechanism of action, in Laskin AI: *Tetracyclines*. New York, Springer-Verlag, 1967, p 347.
24. Nathans D, Lipman F: Amino acid transfer from aminoacylribounucleic acid to protein on ribosomes of *Escherichia coli*. *Proc Nat Acad Sci USA* **47**:497, 1961.
25. Nirenberg MW, Matthaei JH: Dependence of cell-free protein synthesis in *Escherichia coli* upon naturally occurring or synthetic polyribonucleotides. *Proc Nat Acad Sci USA* **47**:1588-1602, 1961.
26. Schnitzer RJ, Hawking F: *Experimental Chemotherapy*. New York, Academic Press Inc, 1964, vol 2, p 39.
27. Milanesi G, Ciferri O: Studies on the mechanism of action of gentamicin. Effect on protein synthesis in cell-free extracts of *Escherichia coli*. *Biochemistry* **5**:3926-3935, 1966.
28. Sarre SG, Hahn FE: Mode of action of gentamicin. *Trans NY Acad Sci* **39**:575-578, 1967.
29. Mandelstam J, McQuillen K: *Biochemistry of Bacterial Growth*. New York, John Wiley & Sons Inc, 1963.
30. Gottlieb D, Shaw PD: Antibiotics, mechanism of action, in Sebek OK: *Polymyxins and Circulin*. New York, Springer-Verlag, 1967, p 148.
31. Koike M, Iida K, Matsuo T: Electron microscopic studies on mode of action of polymyxin. *J Bact* **97**:448-452, 1969.
32. Rhodes RE, Vila OA, Ferlanto RJ: The nature of polymyxin activity against a gram-positive organism. *Antibiot Chemother* **3**:509, 1953.
33. Sud TJ, Feingold DS: Mechanism of polymyxin B resistance in *Proteus mirabilis*. *J Bact* **104**:289-294, 1970.
34. Goss WA, Deitz WH, Cook TM: Mechanism of action of nalidixic acid on *Escherichia* coli. *J Bact* **88**:1112-1118, 1964.
35. Rifampicin, news. *J Infect Dis* **121**:461, 1970.
36. Okamato S, Mizuno D: Mechanism of chloramphenicol and tetracycline resistance in *Escherichia coli*. *J Gen Microbiol* **35**:125, 1964.
37. Weinberg AN: A new look in the mechanism of penicillin-streptomycin synergism. Read before the sixth annual meeting of the Canadian Society of Chemotherapy, Quebec, 1970.
38. Curtis R, Charamella LJ, Berg CM, et al: Kinetic and genetic analyses of D-cycloserine inhibition and resistance in *Escherichia coli*. *J Bact* **90**:1238, 1965.

ECG Analysis No. 3

Premature A-V Junctional Contractions

Douglas P. Zipes, MD, and Charles Fisch, MD, Indianapolis

The term "A-V junctional" has replaced "A-V nodal" in recent years, owing to sound arguments voiced by many researchers. A brief review of recent anatomic and electrophysiologic data is necessary to explain this change, since the substitution transcends a simple semantic decree.[1]

The A-V node lies at the base of the interatrial septum between the coronary sinus and the medial tricuspid valve leaflet. It connects to the sinus node by three distinct anatomic pathways which may provide a functional route for rapid transmission of the sinus impulse through the atria to the A-V node.[2] In addition to these internodal pathways, anatomically distinct pathways bypassing all or part of the A-V node have been implicated in the interpretation of a number of electrocardiographic phenomena,[3] and will be discussed in the future.

Past teaching has indicated that the site of the pacemaker focus during nodal beats lay within the A-V node, and could be recognized by the relationship of P to QRS. Thus, a retrograde P wave occurring before ("upper nodal"), during ("mid nodal"), or after ("lower nodal") the QRS complex indicated the level of origin of the impulse within the A-V node (Fig 1). P waves which were small and inverted (negative) in leads II, III aV_F and V_6, and usually upright (positive) in leads I, aV_L, aV_R and V_1 were considered due to retrograde atrial activation; the accepted P-R interval for "upper nodal" beats is 0.12 seconds or less while the R-P interval for "lower nodal" beats is 0.2 seconds or less. In addition to these classifications a normal P-R interval with retrograde P wave contour described a "coronary sinus rhythm," while a short P-R interval with normal P waves indicated a "coronary nodal rhythm." The following data suggest that such precise localization of the site of impulse origin is unwarranted from surface electrocardiography.

Figure 2 demonstrates that antegrade and retrograde conduction times, in addition to the site of impulse origin, determine the P-QRS relationship. It must be remembered that the P-R or R-P interval of beats arising in the A-V nodal area represents the *difference* between the antegrade and retrograde conduction times. Thus, varying conduction velocity in either direction may alter the P-R or R-P interval even in the same patient (Fig 3).[4]

Supraventricular ectopic impulses can originate in other parts of both atria, at the junction of the A-V node and His bundle (NH region), and in the His bundle as well. Ironically, the midportion of the A-V node, called the N region, lacks the electrophysiologic properties necessary for automatic pacemaker activity, and cannot generate ectopic beating. The advent of His bundle recordings in patients has demonstrated that many A-V nodal rhythms begin with a His potential, which suggests that the escape focus lies in the His bundle.

Many studies indicate that stimulating the atria in a retrograde direction does not necessarily produce the typical retrograde P wave contour.[5] The most likely explanation for this observation suggests that rapid transmission of the retrograde impulse occurs over the specialized internodal tracts, to the region of the S-A node, and establishes depolarization of a significant portion of the atria in a normal direction. This would result in P waves with a normal or almost normal contour.

In summary, the following facts ar-

Received for publication July 27, 1971; accepted July 27.

From the Indiana University Medical Center, Krannert Institute of Cardiology, Indianapolis.

Reprint requests to 1100 W Michigan St, Indianapolis 46202 (Dr. Zipes).

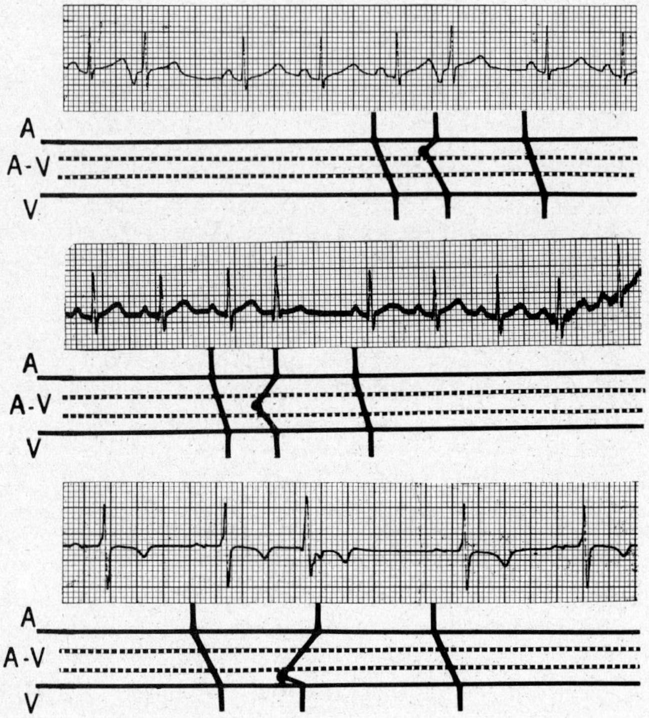

Fig 1.—Premature junctional contractions (PJC). Top, center, and bottom *Demonstrate the P and QRS relationships for PJCs formerly called upper, mid, and lower premature nodal contractions, respectively. Ladder diagram below each recording indicates site in A-V node where impulse was thought to originate.*

Fig 2.—Premature junctional contractions. Diagram indicates that a pacemaker maintaining a constant site of origin may achieve the P and QRS relationships recorded in Fig 1 simply by varying conduction time, in this case, to the atrium.

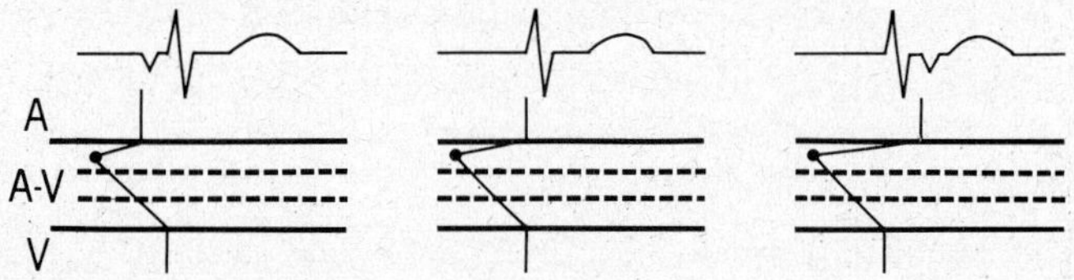

Fig 3.—Junctional tachycardia. In the top tracing, rhythm is regular except for second, seventh, and last beats which occur prematurely. P waves are not visible, which suggests the diagnosis of a junctional tachycardia (discussed in later sessions) with premature junctional contractions. Two days later (lower tracing) the rate of junctional tachycardia has increased to 100 beats per minute; R-R interval now equals coupling interval of the PJCs in the top tracing. Retrograde conduction to the atria has lengthened so that P wave now follows the QRS complex. Thus, in the same patient, increased discharge rate apparently delayed retrograde conduction from example in Fig 2, to right center.

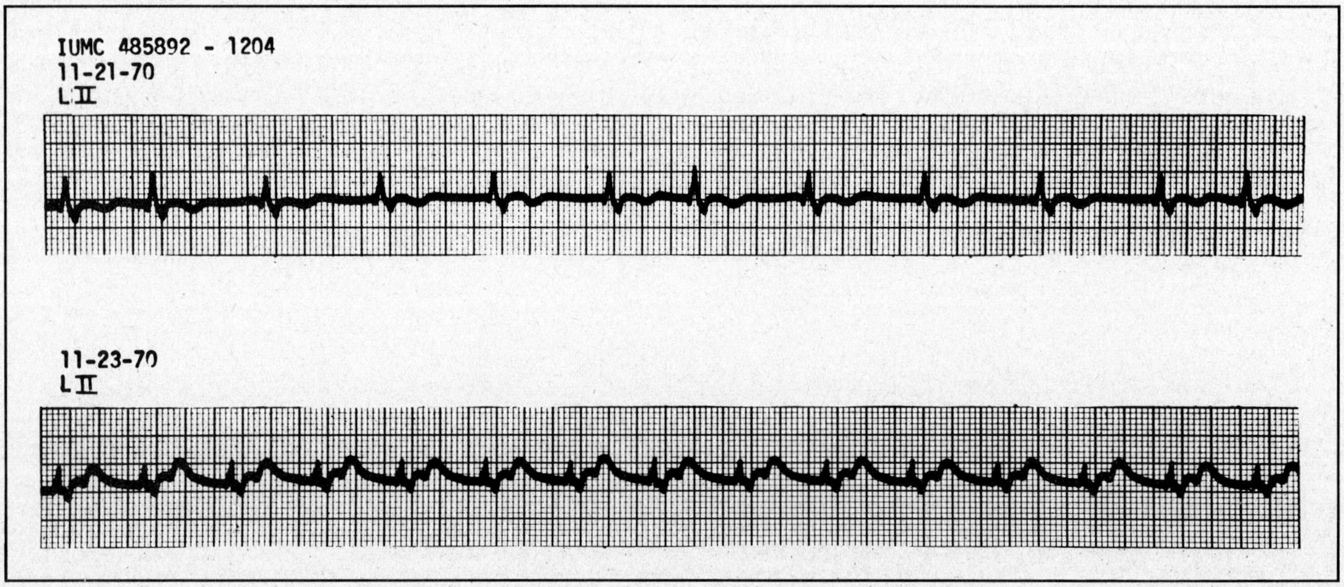

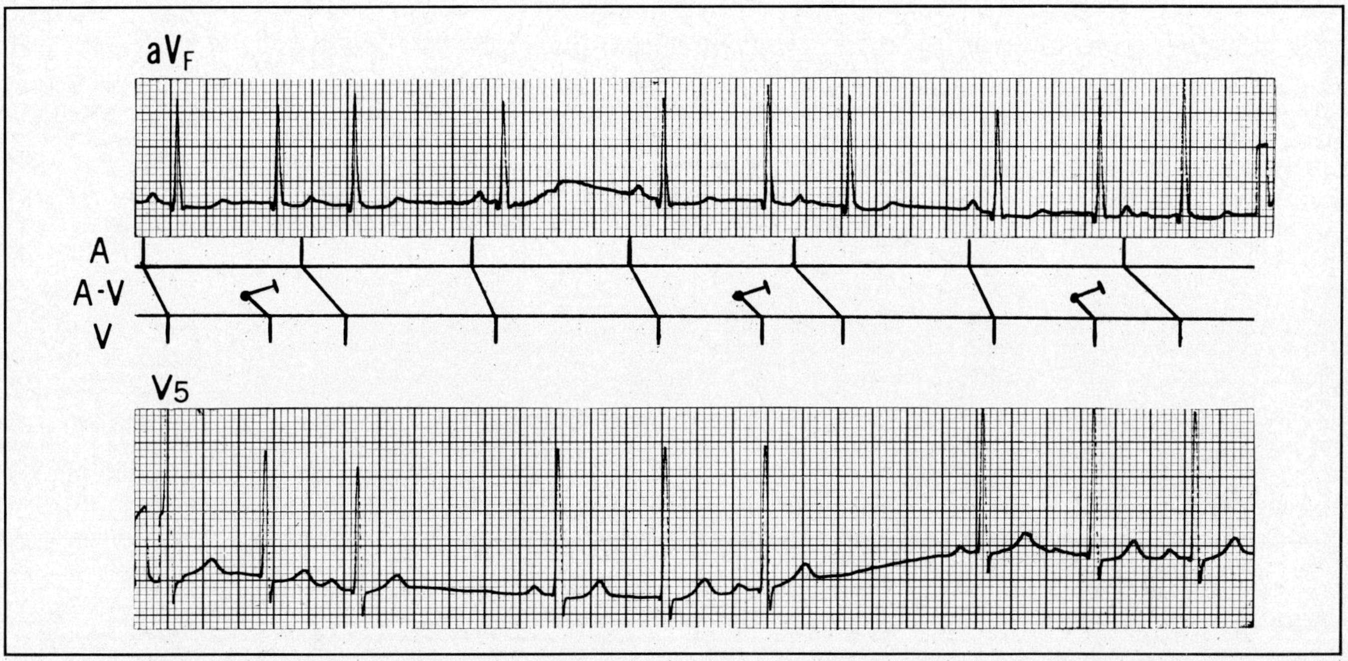

Fig 4.—Interpolated premature junctional contractions. Retrograde conduction from premature junctional contractions does not reach atria to cause deplorization. The next sinus-initiated P wave arrives on time and conducts to the ventricles with some A-V delay, because of partial retrograde penetration from PJC. Slight variation in sinus discharge rate is present.

gue that the terms upper, mid, and lower nodal, coronary sinus and coronary nodal imply a precision in impulse localization not found in the surface electrocardiogram, and that the less precise term A-V junctional be substituted: (1) Variations in A-V and V-A conduction, in addition to the site of impulse formation, affect the relationship of P to QRS. From the surface ECG, it is difficult if not impossible, to differentiate impulses originating in or near the coronary sinus, A-V node proper, and the bundle of His. For example, a coronary sinus rhythm with its normal P-R interval cannot be differentiated from an impulse arising in the A-V node with depression of antegrade conduction. (2) The N region of the A-V node lacks the property for automatic pacemaker discharge, while other sites in the atria, NH portion of the A-V node, and His bundle may initiate ectopic beating. (3) Retrograde atrial depolarization may result in P waves which have vectors and contours similar to those found during normal antegrade activation.

All of the phenomena we described at length which may occur following premature ventricular or atrial contractions may also succeed premature junctional contractions. These include both compensatory and noncompensatory pauses, echo beats, interpolated beats, and so forth. Figure 4 illustrates an example of interpolated premature junctional contractions.

References

1. Pick A, Langendorf R: Recent advances in the differential diagnosis of A-V junctional arrhythmias. *Amer Heart* **76**:553-575, 1968.
2. James TN: The connecting pathways between the sinus node and the A-V node, and between the right and left atrium in the human heart. *Amer Heart J* **66**:498-508, 1963.
3. Ferrer MI: New concepts relating to the pre-excitation syndrome. *JAMA* **201**:1038-1039, 1967.
4. Goldreyer BN, Bigger JT Jr: Site of re-entry in paroxysmal supraventricular tachycardia in man. *Circulation* **43**:15-26, 1971.
5. Waldo AL, Vitikainen KJ, Kaiser GA, et al: The P wave and P-R interval: Effects of the site of origin of atrial depolarization. *Circulation* **42**:653-671, 1970.

Societal Health and Medical Services

Caustic commentaries on the state of American Medicine continue to be pronounced at a high rate. Hearings conducted before Senator Edward Kennedy's senate subcommittee on the state of health care in the nation are frequently punctuated by testimony from disaffected patients and distressed community workers. These hearings, though well-publicized in the press, are not easy to obtain in the form of proceedings. Another set of interviews, however, is available, and this collection proves to be an extraordinarily trenchant record of unhappy experiences with American health care facilities and personnel. Presented in the form of a pamphlet, entitled *Heal Your Self*, this monograph is a most important publication. It emanates from the universities of California and North Carolina and is the official and final report of a special study group that was organized by these two universities. The group was constituted as the Citizens Board of Inquiry into Health Services for Americans, developing out of a joint project established at both universities, and supported by grant funds raised from private foundations. What the Citizens Board did was to travel throughout the nation on a series of field trips and site visits to hospitals, clinics, and offices of all types and conduct a large number of tape-recorded interviews with patients, patients' families, clinic workers, hospital administrators, physicians, nurses, insurance agents, and any other representative health worker in the field. These interviews were then edited, summarized, and a series of conclusions and recommendations was drawn. The final report is the monograph now available; it is well-written, presented in a format that engages the eye, and demands a careful assessment from the medical profession. For the purposes of this discussion it may be permissible to offer the following abbreviated summary of the conclusions and recommendations:

1. Continual, immediate, daily access to medical care should be available for everyone. This is not the case now.
2. Health care should not be expensive, unnecessarily time-consuming, impersonal, noneducative, uncoordinated, discriminatory, nor nonassessable by the patient. It has all of these qualities for many Americans now.
3. The public, as the consumer, must have the directing role in the design and execution of the health care delivery system for the nation. It has little role in the process now.
4. The federal government must look after the health care needs of the public and when there are deficiencies and inadequacies it must act with dispatch. Sufficient legislative permission for such involvement is not now established. The public should work for such legislation immediately.

The interviews that constitute this report are well-drawn and are presented in such a manner as to provide an almost unending indictment of the health care that is available for the socially and economically disadvantaged individuals in our nation. Vignette after vignette focuses on the anger and fury of disappointed patients and their families. Repeatedly, people could not get a physician, or had to wait too long, or were forced to pay too much, or were led to believe that their insurance would pay more than it actually did, or were sent to the wrong office, or never got to see anyone at all, and on and on. There is no sense of relief in this tale of unfortunate experiences. Most, but not all, of these experiences relate to people in the lower income groups of our society. When one finishes this monograph there is a sense of despair and depression.

There is, however, a most interesting addition to the report: the dissenting opinion of one of its members, Gerald Besson, MD. He is a practicing physician in Sunnyvale, Calif, and he participated fully in all the work of the Board. He makes several important points:

1. Though he acknowledges the inadequacy of health care services for many Americans he insists that the inadequacy be viewed as part of the total milieu in which these individuals live and work. Medical health is but one part of an individual's total social health;
2. The participation of consumers in the administration of health care services should lead to a reflective and equitable participation with professionals, not a preemptive bid for power and control that exceeds equity;
3. The locus for administrative decision-making should be as proximate to the point where the decisions are going to have an effect as is possible; health care delivery by distant, remote control is likely to depersonalize further the services to the patients.

He closes his dissent eloquently: "... ultimately our problems revolve around our choice of national priorities. Human needs and the quality of our lives must be our focus. Our affluent society cannot tolerate the gross social inequities that this report documents. In the necessities of life, a basic minimum for all is economically feasible, just and timely."

Here then is one of the sharpest joining of the issues that confront American medicine: in the midst of affluence, medical care for many is inadequate; in the midst of affluence, many live in poverty. If we are to repair the deficiencies of the medical care system we must first and foremost repair the larger and more pervasive insufficiencies of housing, clothing, food, and the opportunity for a full and rich life. When medical care delivery is poor, it means that all of the social functions of that area are poor. The reason so many Americans are receiving inadequate health care is because the cultural subsets in which they live are impoverished, disorganized, disassembled. How can we provide first-rate medical care for the inner cities of our nation when those inner cities are architecturally necrotic, socially destructive, and emotionally erosive? What comes first: medical care or total human social care? And if the medical care is far from ideal, is the repair of the health services an item for priority concern before the reconstitution of a decent society for the disadvantaged people? Besson maintains that the report tends to miss the underlying importance of these primary issues, focusing instead on the glaring inadequacy of health care.

His statement is a cogent and persuasive dissent. There are two societies in America—the advantaged and the disadvantaged, the wage earners and the unemployed, the well-housed and the tenement and shack dwellers, the educated and the unschooled, the hopeful and the hopeless. When we discuss the inequities and insufficiencies of health care services we must take into account the central social and economic issues that burden our nation; the medical profession may wish to do all that it can to institute the changes recommended by the Citizens Board, but it cannot rebuild inner cities with multiphasic screening nor modernize the rural backlands with comprehensive personal health services. This position is not to deny the issue that major reforms in the health system (or nonsystem as critics prefer to remark) are necessary. But it is to say what the first-order problem really is, and for the health care system difficulties to be viewed in a different and more comprehensive perspective.

Many critics, including the Citizens Board, suggest that American medicine has dealt with the problem of insufficient numbers and of a maldistribution of services with an air of arrogant unconcern. It may also be said, however, that the American community has faced the larger issues of social distress with an even greater degree of arrogance. For haven't we all—industry, unions, government, professions, artists—placed the growth and development of our own spheres and arenas somewhat before the successful and complete rehabilitation of our disadvantaged? If we are to do a better job in caring for the health of our citizens, must not we first care for the total social and economic health of society? *Heal Your Self* may well be the banner phrase for the nation as a whole as well as for the medical profession. Such a call for action need not be considered solely as a condemnatory comment, as some critics wish to imply, but rather as a command for community committment to make major changes in the total social milieu of our nation. In light of Besson's articulate addendum to the Citizens Board report, it is fair to hope that physicians and their colleagues will help to demonstrate how to accomplish that goal.

M.D.B.

Members of the Citizens Board of Inquiry into Health Services for Americans are as follows:

Chairman of the Board
Lester Breslow, MD
Chairman
Department of Preventive and Social Medicine
School of Medicine
University of California
Los Angeles

Chairman, Executive Committee
C. Arden Miller, MD
Vice Chancellor
Health Sciences
University of North Carolina
Chapel Hill, NC

Members
David Bazelon
Chief Judge
US Court of Appeals
Washington, DC

Stephen Becker
Author
Katonah, NY

The Hon. Joe Bernal
State Senator
San Antonio, Tex

Roberta Bessette
Supervisor
Combined Nursing Services of Minneapolis
Minneapolis

Gerald Besson, MD
Sunnyvale, Calif

Julian Bond
Georgia State House of Representatives
Atlanta

George F. Burket, Jr., MD
Kingman, Kan

Victoria DeLee
Ridgeville, SC

Dorothy DiMascio
Anchorage, Alaska

Marian Wright Edelman
Attorney
Washington Research Project
Washington, DC

Rashi Fein, PhD
Professor of the Economics of Medicine
Harvard University
Boston

Richard Fitzsimons
Minnesota State Legislature
Warren, Minn

H. Jack Geiger, MD
Department of Community Health and Social Medicine
School of Medicine
Tufts University
Boston

Robert Haggerty, MD
Professor and Chairman
Department of Pediatrics
School of Medicine and Dentistry
University of Rochester
Rochester, NY

Harry Huge
Attorney
Arnold and Porter
Washington, DC

Bertha Johnson
Detroit

Sanford Kravitz, PhD
Dean
School of Social Welfare
State University of New York
Stony Brook, Long Island, NY

Harry Lipscomb, MD
Xerox Center for Health Care Research
Baylor College of Medicine
Houston

C. Clement Lucas, Jr., MD
Special Assistant to the Administrator for Youth Affairs
Health Services and Mental Health Administration
Department of Health, Education and Welfare
Rockville, Md

Peter McColough
President
Xerox Corporation
Stamford, Conn

Einar Mohn
International Director
Western Conference of Teamsters
Burlingame, Calif

Rodney Powell, MD
Department of Pediatrics
School of Medicine
University of Minnesota
Minneapolis

John D. Rockefeller IV
Secretary of State
Charleston, WV

Bayard Rustin
Executive Director
A. Philip Randolph Institute
New York

Lisbeth Bamberger Schorr
Washington, DC

Milton Senn, MD
Professor of Pediatrics
School of Medicine
Yale University
New Haven, Conn

Nathan Stark
Vice President
Hallmark Cards
Kansas City, Mo

George Wiley, PhD
Director
National Welfare Rights Organization
Washington, DC

Jerry Wurf
President
American Federation of State, County and Municipal Employees
Washington, DC

Letter to the Editor

Treatment of *Candida* Infection

To the Editor.—The review of Toala et al on the lack of significance of 371 *Candida* isolates from specimens submitted for bacteriological examination presents the clinician's dilemma but few clues to its resolution. Although *Candida* from any specimen should not be ignored, the organism is so ubiquitous that the recovery of the fungus from sputum, stool, vagina, cervix, and umbilicus is of little significance. The recovery of *Candida* from a noncatheterized or midstream urine is not pathognomonic. Patients with indwelling catheters frequently have *Candida* in the urine. The recovery of *Candida* from a local abscess or wound infection rarely warrants systemic treatment. However, Toala et al reported eight isolates from the blood, and nine from intravenous catheters. These 17 isolates out of the 371 are the ones that should give the greatest concern.

The lumping of isolates of unequal significance leads to more befuddlement of the clinician. In differentiating between *Candida* as a comparatively harmless commensal, and as an agent of infection, it is important to consider the patient's clinical and serological reactions to the organism.

We have studied 33 high risk patients that came to autopsy. Histopathologic evidence of systemic candidal infection was correlated in a blind study with the titers of *Candida*-agglutinating and the presence or absence of *Candida*-precipitating antibodies during life. Both serodiagnostic tests showed high correlation of diagnostic accuracy for both positive and negative cases. In patients with postmortem evidence of systemic candidal infection, the agglutinin titer were significantly raised (>160), and precipitins were present. No false positive precipitin reactions were noted. However, both serological reactions may be minimal to negative in cases of terminal or disease-induced anergy. In serologically competent patients, moreover, hypergammaglobulinemia is a nonspecific concomitant of systemic candidiasis.

This is not to say that systemic antifungal therapy should be instituted immediately upon establishing the diagnosis of systemic candidiasis. On the other hand, one should not wait for a rapidly deteriorating clinical condition and masses of yeast appearing in the urine. One should begin by removing iatrogenic factors favoring systemic dissemination of the organism, discontinuation of antibiotics and steroids if the patient's condition permits, replacement of plastic catheters with scalp vein needles, and reevaluation of the necessity for Foley catheters. Systemic antifungal therapy should be considered if these measures fail to improve the patient's clinical condition, if cultures remain positive, if agglutinating and precipitating antibodies persist or show increase in titers or if hypergammaglobulinemia continues. Prompt therapy is especially important in the presence of an underlying disease that impairs the immune mechanism, since immunologically incompetent patients are unable to neutralize the infection on their own.

If these measure are followed, harmless colonization can be distinguished in most instances from infection and a more judicious choice will be made of patients for systemic antifungal therapy.

PHILIP J. KOZINN, MD
GEORGE DEGENSHEIN, MD
Brooklyn, NY

Reference

1. Toala P, Schroeder SA, Daly AK, et al: *Candida* at Boston City Hospital: Clinical and epidemiological characteristics and susceptibility to eight antimicrobial agents. *Arch Intern Med* **126**:983-989, 1970.

Books

Signs and Symptoms, ed 5. By Cyril M Mac-Bryde, MD, Robert S Blacklow, MD. Price, not given. Pp 1,025, with 241 figures and 4 color plates. JB Lippincott Co, 227-231 S Sixth St, Philadelphia, 1970.

It is always curious to reflect upon the episodes in one's life—often quite inconsequential at the moment of their happening—that modify the subsequent course of events. Most often, it is the impact of one or several people, either from personal contact or through their words, eg, as written in a book.

As a House Officer there were perhaps two or three physicians and an equal number of books that played significant roles in my selection of a career pattern and life style. And one of the books that influenced me greatly was MacBryde, the third edition.

I recall the book with pleasure. It was like reading a good novel. Here were all the answers to the mysteries—the explanation for the curious constellations of signs and symptoms I was encountering each day on the wards. It provided the link between the classic texts of physiology, whose fare was often parched and laborious, and the books of physical diagnosis where the going was easier, but too many questions were unresolved.

MacBryde was beautiful: the language was clear; the syntax was orderly; there was no clutter—no confusion. If the mechanism was unknown, it was so stated. There was no mumbo-jumbo or escape into fuzzy physiology. I reread it the month before my internal medicine boards; it was an old friend revisited.

The present (fifth) edition is a bit more than a chip off the old block; it is a grandly contemporary revision. The coauthor list has expanded to 37 (15 new faces) in addition to editors MacBryde and Blacklow.

The same painstaking effort to present the facts as to why things are happening has been preserved in each edition, and this one is no exception. Five new sections have beeen added: "Loss of Vision: Eye Pain" by Reinecke of Albany; "Problems of Communication, Speech and Hearing: Ear Pain" by Catlin of Baltimore; "Urinary Tract Pain, Hematuria and Pyuria" by Perlmutter and Blacklow of Boston; "Anemia, Weakness, and Palor" by Reinhard of St. Louis; and "Conversion Symptoms" by Engel of Rochester.

The other chapters range from MacBryde and Blacklow's classic on "Study of Symptoms" to my favorite, "Pigmentation of the Skin," by my old chief Harold Jeghers and Edelstein. There are outstanding contributions by medical celebrities such as Eugene A. Stead, Jr., Henry A. Schroeder, Leon Schiff, John A. Pierce, Harold G. Wolff; and Richard W. Vilter. Other chapters have equally distinguished authors, and all offer the same meaty, no nonsense content. Diagrams, photographs, and roentgenographic reproductions are scattered throughout the text in strategic profusion.

It is altogether a splendid book. It was like meeting an old friend, who has now become famous and even more replete in wisdom with the passage of years. Every physician—regardless of age or discipline—will be a little better doctor for having read, savored, and digested his new MacBryde and Blacklow.

ROBERT H. MOSER, MD
Haiku, Maui

Medicine: Essentials of Clinical Practice. Edited by Chester S Keefer, MD, Robert W Wilkins, MD. Price, $11.50. Pp 1,053, with 103 illustrations. Little Brown & Co, 34 Beacon St, Boston 02106, 1970.

This is a fine textbook of internal medicine that will surely be accepted with enthusiasm by the student and the seasoned clinician, a safe prediction for many reasons. When the student buys such a book he hopes it will give him everything his instructors expect him to know, in painless prose and in an inexpensive, lightweight form.

The resident wants a lot of hard information, easily locatable, with a minimum of medical philosophy. He certainly doesn't want to lug around in his bag instructions on how to take a history or do a physical examination. The older clinician wants to be able quickly to find and read about specific points, such as what kind of bone changes his current sarcoid patient might have or what's good for meningococcemia these days. And, whether student or professor, at some time the medical text buyer will want to make a quick survey of some large (but uncommon) subject, such as the porphyrias, so they won't nail his ears to the post at Grand Rounds tomorrow morning.

All of our heroes will find what they want to Keefer and Wilkins, 1970. The organization of the material is

Communications to this Department may be sent directly to Robert H. Moser, MD, the Maui Medical Group, 99 Market St, Wailuku, Maui, Hawaii 96793, or to the Chief Editor for transmittal to him.

particularly good for straight reading. There is a most satisfying continuity (the new Harrison is chopped up into 401 chapters; there are 46 here). At the same time, the index is so well done that spot information can be picked out quickly.

This is, as intended, strictly a down-to-earth book and one directed squarely at the practicing clinician. It is good to be reassured in discussion after discussion that internal medicine is still being presented to the student as a classical art, and that the experts still admit there is no substitute for the history and physical examination for understanding the patient.

There are many highlights; eg, it would be hard to find a more satisfactory discussion of diabetes. Fluid and electrolyte balance are explained so that ordinary mortals can understand. To this noncardiologist, the whole matter of valvular heart disease seems better dealt with here than it has been in the other standard textbooks of medicine (I have just read through the new Harrison and discovered that no where are there instructions on how one should digitalize a patient). Superb tables, eg, the ones on the antihypertensive drugs, are appreciated by tyro and expert alike, and there might have been more of them. It was good to see a chapter entitled "Psychosomatic Medicine," although the discussion doesn't seem to be about psychosomatic medicine.

This is clearly an excellent book for the third and fourth year medical student and for the house-staffer. I recommend that every gray and wrinkled, exhausted-minded internist who has been out doing it for 30 years read it through from start to finish, for an especially pleasant and profitable experience.

EDDY D. PALMER, MD
Schooley's Mountain, NJ

Handwriting: Revelation of Self: A Source Book of Psychographology. By Harry O Teltscher, PhD. Price, $6.95. Pp 338. Hawthorn Books Inc, 70 Fifth Ave, New York, 1971.

It would be remarkable, indeed, if handwriting held no message about the function of the brain, whose product it indubitably is. It is as Freud said about impulses in dreams: they cannot be dealt with if they are inspired by alien spirits and considered as foreign to one's own being.

I have long had a passing interest in handwriting. As Lincoln said, "I can never think except with my fingers." It is likely that this state of affairs partly arose because of the overwhelming attention devoted to handwriting in elementary school when I was a boy. A good deal of emotion was stirred up by the rewards and punishments awarded for writing. This was followed in a few years by complete relaxation of any care with it at all, which appears to be the case today. This has given me a modicum of distress as a teacher. In high school I experienced further surveillance of handwriting when I entered a commercial course. Our instructor was one of those remarkable experts in penmanship, who could produce the most lovely forms, birds for instance, with a few strokes of his pen or chalk.

Later in my occupational endeavor I worked as a mail clerk in a large general hospital and came to pride myself on the relatively unique ability—in that institution at least—to decipher any and all scribbles, and identify most of them without other hints about who the perpetrator might have been. A career in medicine has led me to further survey some of the most execrable script.

Observing the signatures of acquaintances and friends over the years, I developed a facetious formula that success must somehow be correlated with illegibility. But legibility doesn't carry much weight in psychographology. The very awkwardness of a child's script may be indication of his trying to think for himself; the process of identification has all sorts of determinants.

In this country, the business of graphology has been so hedged round by quackery that most of the scientifically inclined paid little or no attention to it. It is usually consigned a role akin to that of spiritualism and fortune-telling, although neurologists have long recognized the signature of certain diseases such as Parkinson's disease, where writing becomes smaller as the sentence proceeds.

Teltscher's current volume is a completely revised edition of a book that appeared first in 1942. The author was born in Vienna and is a practicing psychologist in New York City with memberships in the Society for Clinical and Experimental Hypnosis, American Psychological Association, and the American Sociological Association.

Teltscher takes up the technique of analyzing handwriting. More than 300 specimens illustrate the book. The chapters on children's writings, vocational skills, personnel selection, progress in psychotherapy, criminology, famous personalities, and the growth and decline of personality are among those of particular interest for the professional as well as nonprofessional. Chapter 8, "The Applications of Grapho-diagnosis in Medicine and Psychology," concerns diagnosis, prognosis, and evaluation of treatment. Among other findings of interest, the handwriting of patients with carcinoma showed changes in writing on an average of two to five years before the disease was otherwise detected. Other diseases, physical and mental, reflect themselves in handwriting, and these are considered anecdotally. The only statistical consideration is that dealing with carcinoma.

A study of the writing of the last six presidents and many other successful people is included. Several pages are devoted to the writing of Franklin D. Roosevelt, which required months of study in the archives of the Hyde Park Library. Evidence suggested brain changes as early as 1940, five years prior to death. Every sample of Roosevelt's handwriting after 1944 showed unmistakable change that could have alerted the country before the Yalta Conference of March and April 1945.

Teltscher does not advocate the lifting of handwriting out of context to make an evaluation, except for research purposes. It is merely another means among many, heretofore neglected, in the evaluation of potential, skill, ambition, stamina, capacity, growth, and liabilities. It seems that handwriting specimens might become part of the physical examination. They could be useful diagnostically, and in the progress of treatment.

This interesting book raises many ideas. Forgery comes to mind. I would like to know an expert's opinion of forgery. Is it possible to exactly duplicate handwriting so that even a person as psychologically competent as Teltscher cannot tell the difference? The brain is a fantastic organ, and it would seem likely that this were possible.

What about the influence of practice and of identification on handwriting? I recall adopting one or another rather profound alteration in script after working for a time with another person who had something rather unique in his own writing.

It would be interesting to know the author's thoughts on handedness and if they accord with Blau's views (Blau A: *The Master Hand: A Study of the Origin and Meaning of Right Hand and Left Sidedness and its Relation to Personality and Language.* New York. American Orthopsychiatric Association Inc, 1946, Pp 206.) that sinistrality is a developmental anomaly of preferred laterality, a mishap to the normal development of dextrality, probably most often a relic of emotional negativism.

Most left-handed people have to exert considerably more effort in writing than do right-handers and their script usually reflects it. According to Blau's thesis, they would seem to be contending with something. I have known only a few persons who appear to write entirely comfortably with the left hand.

Since the author has competence in hypnosis, he could, if he liked, settle one facet of the problem of hypnotic regression, ie, its effect on handwriting. Will this technique temporarily bring back the script of yesteryears?

But this is the usual reviewer's wanting something from an author that he had no intention of doing, and has little to do with psychographology. While I don't pose as anything but an interested amateur, it appears to me that Teltscher has done what he intended to do—write a source book of psychographology. For anyone interested in it and wanting to inform himself in this area, this straightforward, easily readable text is the book for him. This book contains nothing technical that cannot be understood by the layman as well as the professional. A bibliography, an index of handwriting specimens by notables, and a general index comprising the final 22 pages are most helpful.

Charles D. Aring, MD
Cincinnati

Coronary Atheroma: A Diary of Discovery. By Norman GB McLetchie, MB, ChB, MD. Price, $10. Pp 114. Charles C Thomas Publisher, 301-327 E Lawrence Ave, Springfield, Ill 62703, 1970.

This small book reports the work and thinking of McLetchie concerning the origin and morphologic development of the coronary atheroma. The major theme of this work is that the atheroma is a "thrombogenic evil" and results from the normal reaction to the laying down of fibrin. This material is incorporated into the intima and, under conditions of rapid sequential deposition, there is hypoxia, granular disintegration, and finally, progressive fatty metamorphosis deep in the intima. The phagocytic disposal of this fibrin results in the formulation of foam cells which in turn, invite more fibrin deposition. The conclusion is that "the growth of an atheroma is a proper reaction to a surfeit of fibrinous deposit." What appears to be pathological "is the failure of the physiologic mechanisms to . . . completely return fibrin to the circulation." The theory is not new but echoes the thinking of Rokitansky and, later, Duguid.

McLetchie brings to this theory a descriptive, thoughtful analysis, extending over about a quarter of a century, of the morphological pattern of atheromata as seen in a series of 22 young subjects, victims of sudden death, each without previous disease such as severe hypertension or diabetes. The basis for his observation is a special staining technique developed by him, which allows the identification of fibrin and its degradation and transformation products. The book is a series of descriptions of atheromata accompanied by color plates of histologic sections; some are very poorly reproduced.

There are also detailed line drawings interpreting these histologic sections. As is the case with most pathology treatises, the ordinary clinician must accept the interpretations on faith. The verbal descriptions have the tendency to run to the fanciful and to develop a cant which requires a glossary for the uninitiated. "A sunburst diving through a weave may sometimes be seen to end as a zareba of mesenchymal cells which choir around a melt pattern" (!) is a typical example of the florid descriptive style.

McLetchie writes that his work truly belongs to the classic age of pathology, depending only on the methods used in that age and requiring not the teamwork of a scientific taskforce but only the dedicated, painstaking work and thinking of one man.

The book is the monument to this work and will be of interest to those scientists and physicians interested in the genesis of the coronary atheroma.

COL MELVIN D. CHEITLIN, MC, USA
San Francisco

Biology of the Immune Response. By Peter Abramoff, PhD, Mariano F La Via, MD. Price, $12.95. Pp 492. McGraw-Hill Book Co, 330 W 42nd St, New York 10036, 1970.

In this present day era of "clinical immunology" there has been a deluge of books and symposia dealing with varied aspects of hypersensitivity and autoimmunity. *Biology of the Immune Response* must stand out as a most notable achievement. Fundamental aspects of immunology, approached from a biological basis, are covered in a thorough and generally lucid presentation. Appropriate clinical references are made without attempting to present medical diagnoses or therapy.

The range of topics is most complete and presented in a well integrated manner. Included are discussions of antigens, antibodies, immunoglobulins, immunity, hypersensitivity, immunoenchancement, immunosuppression, and transplantation. Eleven contributing authors of international reknown are responsible for the excellent overall quality, eg, Kimishige Ishizaka, Richard Farr, Henry Claman, and David Talmage. Superb illustrations and references are found throughout the book.

This book should serve as an excellent reference for clinicians perplexed by the ever-expanding concepts of immunity, hypersensitivity, and clinical immunology and as a highly recommended core text for serious students of allergy and immunology.

ROBERT E. REISMAN, MD
Buffalo, NY

Differential Diagnosis: The Interpretation of Clinical Evidence. By A McGehee Harvey, MD, J Bordley III, MD. Price, $29.50. Pp not given. WB Saunders Co, 218 W Washington Sq, Philadelphia 19105, 1970.

This is a very large book which tries to encompass a very large subject with moderate success. I am not sure what I expected to find when I read it, but I was left with an ill defined sense of disappointment.

This text could be conveniently divided into three separate publications. The first would be a short paper introducing the work: a lucid exposition of the basic principles and elements of differential diagnosis. However, this information is available elsewhere in greater detail and in at least as good form.

The second publication would be a textbook containing descriptions of disease entities. This has been done better, with more detail and better organization, in standard texts, although the large "Tables of Differential Diagnosis" are among the best I have seen anywhere.

The third text would be a compilation of illustrative case records, most of them previously published, which demonstrate the thought processes of various outstanding clinicians as they develop the differential diagnosis and arrive at a well reasoned final diagnosis. This, too, has been done very well in the Case Records of the Massachusetts General Hospital. Although this largest portion of the book is interesting, reading the many case records is somewhat analogous to a police detective watching reruns of Perry Mason mysteries on television!

For some reason, the "Illustrative Cases" are not always representative of the topics. For example, the chapter on "Sudden Death" states that diseases of the coronary arteries are the most important causes of sudden death, yet the two case records in that chapter are concerned with pulmonary emboli and primary pulmonary hypertension. Too, the case records are oriented to rare diseases. When is the last time you saw a patient with a left atrial myxoma (two cases), amyloidosis (five cases) or "Malignant Myelosclerosis With Nodular Atypical Reticulum Cell Hyperclasia of the Bone Marrow, Spleen, Lymph Nodes and Liver"? However, *Show and Tell*, even the sophisticated medical variety, is much more exciting when the subject is exotic!

There is no apparent organization to the book by order of topics, and little effort was made to write discussions of topics by their relative importance or by the frequency of their occurrence. Inexplicably, "Aortic Insufficiency" is accorded a separate chapter whereas most of the other subjects are under broad headings like "Circulatory Failure," or "Pain in the Chest and Abdomen."

I did enjoy the book, but I am obliged to submit that an important part of the differential diagnostic process is the judicious selection of diagnostic maneuvers at rational points in time rather than only discussion of data retrospectively. This aspect is largely neglected in favor of the stereotyped clinicopathology conference and therein lies my vague feeling of discontent.

Differential Diagnosis is recommended for purchase by medical libraries and by physicians who are intrigued by CPC-manship. But for most of us, borrowing would seem to be a satisfactory and reasonable alternative.

DAVID J. CROSBY, MD
Tuscon, Ariz

McGraw-Hill Encyclopedia of Science and Technology, ed 3. Fifteen volumes. Price, $360. McGraw-Hill Book Co, 320 W 42nd St, New York 10036.

This third edition of the most complete and authoritative science reference ever published demands recognition by every physician. More than 2,500 experts, including many Nobel prize winners, contributed to the 15 excellently bound, highly readable volumes which are kept up-to-date by a series of yearbooks. The borders of modern medicine are limitless: molecular biology is now upon us and many articles refer to subjects ranging from high temperature physics to ecology. It is a pleasure to use this encyclopedia to obtain clearly written information outside of one's field of specialization. With over 12,000 photographs and an entire index volume, this work is very easy to utilize. Many articles bear directly on medicine and closely related subjects. It is both a vocation and an avocation to read this work. For example, there are over 110 articles on modern meteorology, over 90 on solid state physics, over 250 on organic chemistry, and nearly 200 on paleontology.

One may read such experts as Christian DeDuve on "Lysosome," Fernandez-Moran on "Myelin," L. S. B. Leaky on *"Australopithecus,"* Suess on "Cosmic Abundance of Elements," B. H. Billings on "Polarized Light," V. McKusick on "Human Genetics," and Glenn Seaborg on "Transuranium Elements." Space technology is covered in detail, as are the modern disciplines of oceanography, computers, comparative physiology, and biophysics.

I know of no more facile way a physician can become up-to-date on such subjects as atomic and nuclear physics, interstellar matter, elementary particles, nova, pulsar, or quasar. Genetics, experimental embryology, and nuclear engineering are covered in detail. By using this work, the clinician will see the artificiality of dividing biology into just botany and zoology.

I can recommend this work without qualification. The articles proceed from elementary to more advanced discussion of a subject so that even in complex topics, the reader is always able to pick up useful information. In many cases the articles are written by the actual scientist who made the discovery. Any physician will broaden his professional knowledge and greatly increase his general scientific scope by frequent use of this work. This third edition, with nearly 1 million additional words of text, is a major contribution to the scientific literature of 1971.

THOMAS AUERBACH, MD
Chicago

Ulcerative Colitis. By JC Goligher ChM, FRCS; FT de Dombal, MS, MB, FRCP; J McK Watts, MB, FRACS; G Watkinson, MD, FRCP; and BC Morson, DM, MCPath. Price, $16.75. Pp 365, with 114 figures and 69 tables. Williams & Wilkins Co, 428 E Preston St, Baltimore 21202, 1968.

Ulcerative colitis is, as the authors point out, a most imprecise disease. Its etiology is now known, and various methods of treatment are rather empirical. In addition, other inflammatory conditions of the large and small bowel must be excluded in order to make accurate diagnosis and evaluations of the results of medical and surgical treatment. The authors have made an exhaustive, clearly written, and reasonable attempt to clarify diagnosis and treatment. Their considerable experience in managing ulcerative colitis is presented in a particularly enlightening fashion. Analysis of the pertinent literature, as well as their own results, is objective and well conceived. Details of all aspects of ulcerative colitis are examined minutely and carefully, and conclusions are set forth clearly and statistically.

These conclusions are heavily in favor of operative intervention in all patients 60 years of age and older and those with total involvement of the large bowel. The operation of choice is total proctocolectomy and ileostomy. The rationale of surgical as compared to medical therapy in these groups of patients seems well substantiated on the basis of their figures and literature review. The medical treatment and indications for surgical intervention in younger patients and more restricted bowel involvement are also evaluated statistically and thoroughly. Again, one can hardly quarrel with the conclusions drawn, at least in their experience in analyzing this group of patients as compared to other published series.

The practitioner inexperienced in ulcerative colitis may well feel, on reading this book, that treatment has become largely surgical. Approximately one third of the volume is taken up with the various indications, surgical procedures, and follow-up care of surgical patients. For the internists, these may seem rather repetitively, even if appropriately expressed. As the authors point out, their experience with ulcerative colitis is in considerable contrast with at least one other large patient group treated medically in the United States. It is left for the reader to decide whether he should accept the authors' point of view in regard to early surgical intervention, or to continue medical treatment in patients with severe and diffuse disease of the colon. At the present stage of knowledge, one must admit the authors make a strong case, and their conclusions coincide with that of many gastroenterologists in the United States.

The volume is distinctly British in flavor and personal in tone. It is written pleasantly and clearly throughout, and though several authors have collaborated, there is little overlap in style. A slight bias for the British form of medicine may be imputed from the statement that patients in Britain can obtain ileostomy appliances on the National Health Scheme (page 285) which apparently infers that this makes it easier to have severe ulcerative colitis and surgery in Great Britain. In the present stage of the British economy, it is to be hoped that there will be no rush from other countries to obtain this "free" service, but the nature of the operation probably renders this unlikely.

The book is highly recommended to all physicians interested in ulcerative colitis. It represents an excellent statement of the present status of the disease, both medically and surgically, and all the opinions are presented in a most objective manner. It may be particularly recommended to the American physicians as perhaps the best overall review of ulcerative colitis in British medicine in recent years.

ROBERT S. NELSON, MD
Houston

Radiation Biology of the Fetal and Juvenile Mammal. Edited by Melvin R Sikov, MD, D Dennis Mahlum, MD. Price, $3. Pp 1,026, with many illustrations. US Atomic Energy Commission, Division of Technical Information Extension, PO Box 62, Oak Ridge, Tenn 37830, 1969.

No diminished interest in the biological effects of irradiation has occurred since Muller demonstrated the mutagenic potentialities of x-rays. This volume is a collection of papers presented at the Ninth Annual Hanford Biology Symposium, Radiation Biology of the Fetal and Juvenile Mammal, cosponsored by Battelle Memorial Institute-Pacific Northwest Laboratories and the US Atomic Energy Commission.

Because there are nearly 90 reports in just over 1,000 pages, excluding remarks of the chairmen, the reports are generally brief. This necessity for brevity may be responsible for the uneven character of the papers. More extensive development of papers could well have made many more informative.

As a mutagen, ionizing radiation has a multiple potential for disease production: by solitary gene-effects it may simulate hereditary disorders; or, by another mechanism, affect karyokinesis and produce cytogenetic abnormalities. Effects on genes during development implies the potential for diverting differentiation; also, there are the oncogenic aspects, another face of the mutational impact. An attempt to cover the field is made here, but with uneasy success.

In one report, "Analysis of the Morbidity and Mortality of Children Irradiated in Fetal Life (II)" by M. L. Griem et al, the authors are sufficiently self-critical to limit additional comment. In this study of 1,008 offspring of mothers subjected to pelvimetry during pregnancy, no increase in leukemia or congenital anomalies was detected. However, as the authors state, changes due to irradiation are dependent in part upon the developmental stage. Inspection of Table 4 shows that most of the women in the study were x-rayed during the second and third trimesters, not critical periods for low radiation doses. They further state, "It should be noted that the number of cases studied is insufficient to reliably detect any but fairly large differences between the groups in the incidence of abnormalities".

While many papers may have been marred by ambiguity, Hardy et al in "Comparative Utilization of Dietary Radium 226 and Other Alkaline Earths by Pigs and Sheep" were decisive. Their investigations showed that there were marked species differences in the utilization of alkaline earths. Less than 50% of the radium burden was in the skeleton of the pig, while 97% was in the skeleton of the sheep. Such differences in species emphasizes the need for exercising care in the extrapolation of animal data to humans.

Other examples of informative reports in this volume occur, of course. But, it is difficult to envision the reading audience that would be attracted to this volume. The hidden and obvious inadequacies remove it from recommendation to the novice. And, certainly, the radiation expert would be discouraged. Nevertheless, it does possess an orientation that is not present in any other single volume. On this basis it may have use in biomedical libraries as a reference volume.

RAYMOND L. TEPLITZ, MD
Pasadena, Calif

Progress in Clinical Pathology, vol 3. By Mario Stefanini, MD. Price, $19.75. Pp 426, with many illustrations. Grune & Stratton Inc, 757 Third Ave, New York 10017, 1970.

The major current thrusts in clinical pathology are (1) management, (2) patient-focused activities, (3) quality assurance, (4) automation, (5) data handling, and (6) the biology of disease. *Progress in Clinical Pathology*, vol 3 presents a mixed bag of 12 chapters of variable nature and quality touching upon three of these areas. The difference between "Clinical Chemical Analyses via an Automated System" and "Tumor Embolization in Man" emphasizes the wide range of subjects.

One wonders at the value of the proliferation of the "Review of," "Yearbooks of," "Progress in," "Advances," etc, etc, which appear at frequent intervals. Apparently, the philosophic purpose of a book like this is to bridge the gap between journals and textbooks. Most such books simply summarize existing literature, rather than present original material.

In point of fact, the active clinical laboratory worker generally derives new information about his own area of interest from professional meetings (papers, panels, and exhibits), journal publications, instrument and reagent manufacturing companies, and conversations and visits with peers. If he is to enter a subject outside his own major area of expertise, he uses textbooks, workshops, short courses, journals, and visits to exemplary laboratories.

These actual approaches to acquisition of working knowledge leave a book such as this out in the cold, with a very limited group of readers. Most fields dealt with in this book are advancing so rapidly that once it was published, it was substantially out of date and of little but historical interest. In addition, the treatment of most subjects is so brief and superficial as to leave the reader wanting for in-depth information. For example, the chapter entitled "Advances in Electrophoretic and Chromatographic Technics" deals with the entire subject of "Gas Chromatography" in less than one page—and its vital application to toxicology in one sentence!

Potential readers may include the early resident in pathology, the student of medical technology, and the clinician interested in an overview of some limited area of laboratory medicine.

GEORGE D. LUNDBERG, MD
Los Angeles

Control of Gastrointestinal Function. By Frank P Brooks, MD, ScD (Med). Price, $7.95. Pp 222. Macmillan Co, 866 Third Ave, New York 10022, 1970.

The author has aptly described his work as a concise summary of gastrointestinal physiology. There is not a wasted word. Long segments seem to have a reference after each sentence, ie, denoting separate scientific observations. There is little interpretive formulation, or clarification by discussion or analysis. However, the book is well documented so that further reading can be directed properly.

There are several chapters on secretion and motility with one each on digestion and absorption. This division is partly organizational since each segment of the alimentary tract participates as a motile or secretory organ. The very short chapter on digestion is sufficient, since it follows the chapters on gastric, pancreatic, and biliary secretion. In the same theme as the text, illustrations are almost all reproduced from original scientific papers.

This is a physiology book, not a text on clinical medicine. However, at the end of each chapter or sometimes following topics within chapters, there is a short paragraph entitled "Pathophysiology." This paragraph relates to specific disease states.

This book would be an excellent text for a course for medical students in gastrointestinal physiology. It could serve as well for postgraduate training in gastroenterology. It is not a book for casual reading, or at least casual reading would not do justice to the tremendous amount of information present. More elaborate discussions would certainly be helpful, but then, the work is intended to be a concise summary.

This book can be recommended to anyone at any level of training who wishes to learn more about gastrointestinal physiology. Abundant information is present, but one may have to refer to the original references or review monographs to gain full understanding of the topic.

ERL DORDAL, MD
Chicago

Fifth Symposium on Advanced Medicine. Edited by Roger Williams, MD, FRCP. Price, $10.50. Pp 380, with few illustrations. Williams & Wilkins Co, 428 E Preston St, Baltimore 21202, 1969.

This paperback book covers main sessions presented at a conference of the Royal College of Physicians of London on "Advanced Medicine" and purports to cover "recent advances in various fields." There are eight major sections, including gastroenterology, endocrinology, lung disease and thromboembolism, treatment of malignant disease, calcium metabolism and bone disease, biochemical screening, neurology, and drug addiction. Each of the sections has much to recommend it. In some instances, however, the material presented is more a review of standard material rather than a summary of recent advances. This is especially true in the sections on gastroenterology, and lung disease and thromboembolism, although both are well written. The cautious optimism expressed for ancrod (Arvin [Britain; no comparable US product]) in the treatment of thrombosis and thromboembolism will be of interest to American readers who have less experience with this agent than our British Colleagues.

Although most of the articles are written in a crisp, terse manner this pithy style occasionally is a drawback to lucid presentation of some material. For example, there is a one-sentence paragraph in the discussion of "Pre-malignant Disease of the Gut" which states that "Sideropenia, oesophageal web and upper oesophageal carcinoma are well known associations: prevention by an adequate iron intake needs no justification." While sideropenia, per se, and sideropenia in association with the other two entities can certainly be prevented by adequate iron, there is no justification for the implication that adequate iron will also prevent oesophageal carcinoma! Likewise, in the excellent discussion on urinary tract stone disease, the use of allopurinol (Zyloprim) in treating uric acid stones is dismissed cursorily with the comment, "Allopurinol, a xanthine oxidase inhibitor, has also been recommended."

In general, the articles are timely commentaries on newly developed concepts. Especially valuable are the essays on "The Immunoassay of Peptide Hormones" and "Insulin Secretion in Man", even though proinsulin receives no mention. Neatly tucked away at the end of the section on lung disease is an absolute gem entitled "The Pleura and Its Effusions." "Immunity and Malignant Disease in Experimental Animals" is also well presented and should provide a concise and clear picture of this complicated subject to those who lack a sophisticated background in this area.

The presentations on radiotherapy and chemotherapy are far too brief to represent anything but generalizations in areas which deserve detailed presentations. Furthermore the author, in his introduction to "Radiotherapeutic Achievements," seems overly defensive and somewhat testy about his topic as he protests "radiotherapy is a much maligned specialty and its potentialities and achievements rarely appreciated." Of all the sections, "Calcium Metabolism and Bone Disease" was the most enjoyable and informative to me. Each of the four chapters has new data, clearly presented in a most pragmatic fashion. That dealing with "Urinary Tract Stone Disease" deserves special kudos.

The book makes for worthwhile reading on topics of practical interest, and because of the brevity of the articles is especially convenient for reading in "quick snatches."

COL O'NEILL BARRETT JR., MC, USA
Honolulu

Electronic Measurement Techniques in Anaesthesia and Surgery. By DW Hill, PhD, FIEE. Price, $13.50. Pp not given. Appleton-Century-Crofts Inc, 35 W 32nd St, New York 1970.

This excellent monograph is well organized for the purpose of orienting and educating the surgeon and anesthesiologist to electronic equipment in the areas of monitoring, measuring, and scanning. This book contains (A) "Recording Systems and Signals," (B) "Pressure Transducers and Myograph," (C) "Measurement of Respiratory Function," (D) "Measurement of Blood Flow," (E) "Electrodes," (F) "Gas and Vapor Analysis," (G) "Electrode Systems for pH, P_{CO_2}, P_{O_2}," (H) "Cardiac Output," (I) "Defibrillators," (J) "Pacemakers," (K) "Diathermy and Electrical Safety," (L) "Temperature," and (M) "Isotopes." *Electronic Measurement Techniques in Anaesthesia and Surgery* is based on the author's lecture series. The references are largely British and equipment as well, but most of the common or popular American equipment is covered adequately.

There are up-to-date references at the end of each chapter and a good index at the end of the book, clear line drawings to illustrate the principles involved in most of the chapters, and many mathematical formulas to explain principles involved in instrumentation. To many physicians not used to this technique, this may be a difficult area, but it is necessary for the student who wishes to understand the instruments.

This book is definitely of value to people who are interested in monitoring in the coronary care unit, intensive care unit, surgical monitoring, and operating room monitoring. It should be available in the libraries of hospitals having these facilities.

MAX S. SADOVE, MD
Chicago

Gastrointestinal X-Ray Diagnosis. By DH Cummack, MB, ChB, DMR. Price, $24.50. Pp 55. Williams & Wilkins Co, 428 E Preston St, Baltimore 21202, 1970.

By definition, an atlas is a compilation of plates, charts, or tables illustrating any subject; the word derives from Atlas, who carried the world on his shoulders. It is indeed a heavy burden that D. H. Cummack bears, that of collecting in one book the roentgenographic manifestations of disorders of the gastrointestinal and biliary tracts, and the liver. To accomplish this goal, Cummack presents more than 1,000 high quality reproductions of appropriate roentgenographs. A book of this sort is autobiographical: it tells of the author's encounters with the common and the uncommon; of landmarks he has learned to recognize as significant of disturbances—or not; of shortcuts or newly discovered roads he has taken to find the enemy—despite nature's camouflage and the limitations of the method.

The author possesses a rare talent—brevity. His illustrations are explained by terse captions containing relevant clinical and roentgenographic data, their succinctness refreshing when compared to the wandering, prolix captions fashionable in certain roentgenographic publications, in which the space allocated for them exceeds the area of the accompanying reproductions.

Pearls abound, a not unexpected windfall in this material which comes from the Gastrointestinal Unit of the University of Edinburgh. I find very little to carp at: a few interpretations with which I disagree, and a mild feeling of frustration induced by the failure to find references to such esoterica as "Stammer's Hernia" and the "*Formation de Moutier*."

With this atlas, I can relax in a comfortable chair, read at my own pace, return for a second look, and, perhaps, even think a little. I cannot react this way when I am exposed to the conventional method of studying gastrointestinal disorders—the review course, in which a speeding (and droning) pedagogue flies through 200 slides in 50 minutes, while I drift off into a state of eyelid-drooping, head-swaying semiconsciousness.

A good descriptive atlas—such as this one—is an effective educational tool, equally valuable to the eager young student and the crusty old practitioner.

MARCUS J. SMITH, MD
Santa Fe, NM

Encyclopedia of Medical Radiology, vol 17. **Radiation Therapy of Benign Diseases.** Edited by A Zuppinger, E Ruckensteiner. Price, $50.10. Pp 584, with 76 figures, Springer-Verlag, 1 Berlin 33, Heidelberger Platz 3, 1970.

This volume is the latest in a comprehensive series of German reference works on diagnostic and therapeutic radiology which have been published since 1963. The editors state that "in non-malignant diseases radiotherapy has fallen into neglect" and that this book ". . . should help to ensure the wider use of this form of treatment." The relatively impartial reader can glean reasons for the former statement from the text, but not for the latter. The 15 contributors present the subject matter without relation to its contemporary importance and only occasionally concede the obsoleteness of the information.

The undoubtedly definitive presentation of the use of x-ray therapy for angina pectoris(!) occupies 26 pages. Various methods are recommended, from irradiation of the stellate ganglia to irradiation of what is hoped to be the adrenal medullas. One is more chagrined by the absence of controlled evaluations of therapy than enlightened by the impartially recorded disputes. One author (p 283) concludes that "Oliguria or anuria which develops during the course of acute glomerulonephritis or nephrosis can with great probability be alleviated by x-irradiation of the kidneys," while another informs us (p 319) that it is "difficult" to influence renal function by x-ray therapy and that there is danger of damaging the renal tubules. This internist also was surprised to learn, for instance, that asthma has been treated roentgenologically—by irradiation of the lungs alone or together with the spleen. While these and other obsolete topics are presented in detail, x-ray therapy of ankylosing spondylitis, which is still widely practiced in Europe, receives only one page. Technical aspects of therapy are presented adequately.

There is an excellent chapter on the use of ^{131}I in thyroid diseases, an adequate presentation of the use of ^{32}P in polycythemia vera, but little about the newer uses of other isotopes.

The quality of the illustrations is excellent, as is the total manufacture of the volume. Each chapter has a voluminous bibliography, and there is an index in German and English. This is a fine source for a student of the history of radiation therapy, but it can not be recommended as a contemporary reference.

THOMAS G. BENEDEK, MD
Pittsburgh

Involuntary Movement Disorders. By Irving Spencer Cooper, MD. Price, $29.50. Pp 432, with 521 illustrations. Harper & Row Publishers Inc, 48 E 33rd St, New York 10016, 1969.

This most recent volume by Irving S. Cooper is a magnificent book from the point of view of medical artistry and photography. It is filled with photographs of patients and drawings based on the photographs. Anatomic tracts, pathologic material, and illustrations of surgical technique occupy a good part of the book.

The volume is divided into six sections: (1) "Hypertonus and Hyperkinesis of Parkinson's Disease," (2) "Bilateral Thalamic Surgery in Parkinson's Disease," (3) "Intention Tremor," (4) "Dystonia," (5) "Hemiballismus and Hemichorea," and (6) Surgical Treatment of the Dyskinesias."

Cooper has been a pioneer in concert with A. E. Walker, R. Myers, and P. C. Bucy in the field of surgery for Parkinson's disease and other dyskinesias. He has without doubt the most experience of all with basal ganglia and thalamic surgery. He has also operated upon patients with intention tremor of an hereditofamilial nature, Wilson's disease, and multiple sclerosis. The section on dystonia is devoted to discussion and surgical treatment of dystonia musculorum deformans. Torticollis is looked upon by Cooper as a dystonic variant and has been treated by a lesion placed in the contralateral ventrolateral nucleus of the thalamus. On the other hand, athetosis has not responded well to thalamic surgery. Finally, a discussion of hemiballism and hemichorea, as well as the surgical management of this condition, concludes the specific disease entities reviewed in the book. The volume is closed by a section on the surgical treatment of the dyskinesias with particular emphasis on surgical technique and placement of the lesion.

The book is overwhelming in surgical detail, case presentation, and in an undertow of enthusiasm for the surgical attack on the involuntary movement disorders. There is absolutely no doubt that Cooper has contributed significantly to our knowledge of basic physiologic and anatomic mechanisms as well as clinical insights concerning the involuntary movement disorders. He has played an innovating role with consummate flair and bravery.

Yet, despite all this, it would seem to this reviewer that both the public and the profession have been oversold on the surgical procedures outlined in this book. The enthusiasm and reported early results were, to some extent, premature and misplaced. There isn't a neurologist in practice who has not seen poor or indifferent results from the procedure. But few of us have seen enough postoperative patients so that we can make an independent judgment on the operation. Neither the public nor the profession were made fully aware of the highly selective type of patient Cooper insisted upon. Finally, the law of "thirds" in therapy often catches up with the dyskinetic patient treated either with surgery or L-DOPA (levodopa); ie, a third do well, a third so indifferently, and a third do poorly. Thalamic surgery for the diskinetic patient has suffered from the same unabashed enthusiasm and malhandling by the Delilahs of the press in the past as has L-DOPA recently. Both methods of therapy are of help in a limited percentage of patients. However, their influence may be far reaching as a stimulus to further research, and I feel certain that Cooper's book will take its place in the history of medicine as a stepping stone in this regard.

DAVID GREEN, MB, BS
Albany, NY

Art Interpretation and Art Therapy. Edited by Irene Jakab. Price, $15.60. Pp 258, with 161 illustrations. S Karger AG (American agent, Albert J Phiebig, PO Box 352, White Plains, NY), 1969.

This is a rather small book (22 original communications and summaries of others) for a rather large sum of money with primary appeal to a rather elite group of specialists. It represents the legible products of the Fifth International Colloquium on Psychopathology of Expression, a 1968 meeting in Los Angeles that also included films, psychodrama, hypnosis, a panel on hippiedom, and a live stage demonstration of expressive movements!

Most of the communications present a narrow focus, such as discussion of the ceramic productions of a schizophrenic patient during a span of 13 years, artistic evidence in support of Jungian archetypes, and suggestion that the sexual molestation of young female children is perhaps psychologically more traumatic than some recent literature might imply. Physician readers will almost certainly be attracted by Fischer's essay entitled "On Creative, Psychotic and Ecstatic States" in which he postulates a continuum of arousal phenomena (presumably related to reticular function), a cybernetic model of data input and data processing, and correlation with experiential states such as relaxation, anxiety, catatonia, and mystical rapture.

Quite apart from the issue of specialization, however, perhaps the very printed words themselves illustrate the more general truth that whole segments of human experience can be expressed best through the nonverbal arts. Very appropriately, I think, two authors quote Archibald MacLeish as follows: "What is wrong is not, of course, the great discoveries of science—information is always better than ignorance, no matter what information or what ignorance. What is wrong is the belief behind the information, the belief that information alone will change the world. It won't. Information without human understanding is like an answer without its question—meaningless. And human understanding is only possible through the Arts."

GEORGE BOLIAN, MD
Honolulu

Atomic Absorption Spectroscopy: Applications in Agriculture, Biology, and Medicine. By Gary D Christian, Frederic J Feldman. Price, not given. Pp 490. Wiley-Interscience, Division of John Wiley & Sons Inc, 440 Fourth Ave, New York, 1970.

The role of trace elements in biological systems has become prominent in clinical medicine during the past few years as reliable analytical methods suited to the clinical laboratory have been developed. The beginning of modern trace element analysis was the introduction of the flame photometer in the 1940's. This instrument is severely limited in its range; sodium, potassium, lithium, and to a lesser extent, calcium, barium, and magnesium are the only elements that can be quantitated readily by this technique. The availability of the much more versatile atomic absorption spectrophotometer in the early 1960's lead to the development of methods which allowed clinical laboratories to measure a large number of trace elements with relative ease.

Still, the lack of readily available literature on biological applications of atomic absorption spectrophotometry hindered its acceptance by the clinical laboratory. It was not until 1967 that slim volumes of biomedical orientation began to appear. They were primarily concerned with basic principles; the clinical chemist was left to search the reference lists for specific details.

The present text, in contrast, not only covers principles and theory, but gives detailed directions on collecting and storing of biological specimens, wet and dry ashing procedures, preconcentration of elements, calibration of instruments, and specific instructions on the analysis of each of 77 elements.

Although not immediately apparent, this book is an excellent source of information on physiological effects of the trace elements considered. For example, a capsule summary of Wilson's disease appears in the section describing copper analysis. Mechanisms of toxicity and procedures for the treatment of poisoning produced by most elements are presented.

The detailed description of several commercially available instruments spanning a price range from $3,000 to $10,000 will be most helpful to clinical laboratories contemplating the purchase of an atomic absorption spectrophotometer.

The authors may be accused of being overdiligent in stating what atomic absorption techniques cannot do in specific instances, but low sensitivities, interferences by other substances present or by scattered light, and other sources of error can quickly lead to erroneous results if they are not taken into consideration. An appendix listing atomic absorption detection limits reinforces these cautions.

In short, this volume is the most comprehensive contribution to the use of atomic absorption spectroscopy in biomedical applications published to date.

LTC WALTER J. DECKER, MSC
El Paso, Tex

Electrophoresis and Immunoelectrophoresis. By Leo P Cawley, MD. Price, $15. Pp 360. Little Brown & Co, 34 Beacon St, Boston, 1969.

This book explains the basic principles of electrophoresis and immunoelectrophoresis, discusses specific applications of these techniques in the clinical laboratory, and is appended with technical details of each of the methods considered.

The advantages of this text are numerous. It fills a need to assemble information of this type in a concise format. Liberal use is made of well-planned and amply explained illustrations. The excellent drawings and fundamental exposition of basic principles in chapter 1 represent one of the stronger areas of the book, providing a firm foundation for the remaining chapters. Chapter 12 ("Analytical Methods") is particularly strong in relation to the author's stated purpose of a unified approach to laboratory diagnosis. Chapter 15, a compendium of methodology with brief summaries of interpretation, significance, theoretical principles, technical steps, and suggestions is perhaps the most practical part of the book. The addition of an appendix of technical details such as buffer composition is wise; it prevents such necessary information from cluttering the discussions. In general, this is a solid, thoughtful approach to the subject; such aspects as the prozone phenomenon (page 254) are properly emphasized; the table of immunoglobulin structural fragments (page 50) is noteworthy; chapter 14 ("CPK") is an excellent example of a clinically oriented, straightforward approach. The index is adequate, the size of the book not forbidding, and such material features as binding and paper quality are reasonable. The price is not immodest, nor is it excessive.

Certain disadvantages, though detracting little from the overall usefulness of the book, appear as dilutional factors. While the format of separating the discussions of specific electrophoretic and immunoelectrophoretic applications from the technical details is sound, the arrangement and organization of the chapters preceding the technical compendium are open to question, since the subjects appear in seemingly random order. While the author's concept of the "disease-oriented" laboratory is of highest merit, his use of a separate language in this connection ("bioware," "hardware," "software," "on-line advice lines," orchestration," etc) appears somewhat contrived. No correlation of the causes of pseudo-M protein spikes, practical information needed for proper interpretation, is attempted in the discussions of monoclonal spikes, although scattered references to such misleading patterns appear. More clearcut guidelines for moving from qualitative screening procedures to specific quantitation or in-depth studies would be desirable. Admittedly, the length required to explain a given topic is often inversely proportional to the concrete knowledge of that topic, since brevity often reflects certainty. Nonetheless, there appears some discrepancy between the volume of material presented on the proven clinically useful tool of hemoglobin electrophoresis (chapter 10) and the nonhemoglobin proteins of erythrocytes.

Future editions would probably benefit from the inclusion of a chart of hemoglobin electrophoretic mobilities, a table of abnormal hemoglobins, and certain clinical guidelines. Additional minor points are noted. For example, chapter 5 ("Urine") leaves the impression that concentration of urine is always necessary for examination of urinary protein, and on the discussion of "Continuous Particle Electrophoresis," one could argue about the author's conclusions.

Typographical errors, unavoidable in a first edition of this length, are aggravating rather than misleading: reference 50 on page 60 should read "Houston" rather than "Honston," the legend to Fig 3-7 should refer to a monoclonal peak in the beta-globulin region rather than gamma, page 167 should describe EM examination of albumin as revealing a ring structure with a central hole, not "control," and "lycine" (page 337) is of course "lysine."

The overall impression of this book is favorable, and the criticism should not detract from its usefulness. It is highly recommended for anyone faced with establishing and maintaining a laboratory with electrophoretic and immunoelectrophoretic techniques. Most technicians, the experienced as well as the beginner, will be greatly comforted to have Cawley's book at hand.

WILLIAM C. LEVIN, MD
Galveston, Tex

Radionuclide Applications in Neurology and Neurosurgery. Edited by Yen Wang, MD, DSC Pietro Paoletti, MD. Price, $27.50. Pp 367, with many illustrations, Charles C Thomas Publisher, 310-327 E Lawrence Ave, Springfield, Ill 62703, 1970.

In all probability, most practicing physicians are familiar with the scintillation brain scan for the detection of intracranial disease. It is equally safe to assume that radionuclide cisternography, radioactive xenon (^{133}Xe) cerebral blood flow, and neutron capture therapy are techniques of which few can claim expertise, yet these procedures are in routine clinical use in a number of hospitals throughout this country. This book deals with the theory and application of these and other radioisotopic methods in neurological disease.

The chapters on diagnostic procedures include sections on pathophysiology, methodology, and clinical application. The portions devoted to therapy include material on interstitial applications, stereotactic implantation, and heavy particle irradiation. Each chapter is written authoritatively in review style, but details (especially mathematical) are rare. The interested reader must of necessity go to the original communications on each subject. Extensive bibliographies follow each chapter.

It would be a mistake to assume that this volume is suited only to the neurologist or neurosurgeon; such is not the case at all. The diagnosis of normal pressure hydrocephalus or cerebrospinal fluid rhinorrhea by radionuclide cisternography, "luxury perfusion" (loss of vasomotor autoregulation) detection with ^{133}Xc gas, or the treatment of diabetic retinopathy with alpha particles from a cyclotron are topics of interest to internists, generalists, and specialists in neurological disease alike. The book is well suited to the hospital library where it can serve as a reference work for the specialist in neurosensory disorders, but it would repay any physician interested in keeping abreast of current trends in medical practice to peruse its contents.

N. DAVID CHARKES, MD
Philadelphia

So You Have Glaucoma. By Everett R Veirs, MD. Price, $5.75. Pp 84. Grune & Stratton Inc, 757 Third Ave, New York 10017, 1970.

The purpose of the second edition of *So You Have Glaucoma* is to present information to the patient with glaucoma that will give him a better understanding of his condition and enable him to take better care of himself. It is not the intent of the authors to suggest the best forms of treatment in a specific case of glaucoma, a complex disease which manifests itself in varying types and varying degrees of severity.

The author stresses the necessity of the patient following the advice of his or her own ophthalmologist. There is repeated warning throughout the text that damage resulting from carelessness is cumulative and can make the difference between useful vision and blindness. It also stresses the fact that the diagnosis is not a verdict of future blindness. There are only a few patients who do not keep useful vision as long as they live in spite of the fact that most patients with glaucoma cannot be dismissed as cured. There is a definite amount of repetition from chapter to chapter, but the author feels that the patient will benefit by this repetition.

There is no doubt that a patient who reads this understandable text may find out more about glaucoma than he needs to know. There are a few points which might be questioned. The author does feel that any patient who maintains a constant intraocular pressure in the high twenty's unequivocally has glaucoma and in time will experience permanent damage.

There are many equally qualified ophthalmolgists who feel that there is a condition which may be called ocular hypertension. These individuals have pressures running in the high twenty's but fail to show any visual field loss, optic nerve changes or visual dysfunction that is due to the high pressures. Many of these individuals do not seem to show any evidence of glaucoma over two or more decades of observation. Such individuals do not require therapy. Often these patients have been diagnosed as having glaucoma and instructed carefully on the use and importance of regular, repeated instillation of drops of topical therapy. This has been stressed so many times to them by their own ophthalmologist, and again in this text that they would be quite fearful of stopping the drugs for even a trial period.

Many questions that the patients ask are not answered in this text. Although the author talks about avoiding excess intake of fluid at any time, he does not discuss the imbibition of alcoholic beverages. Many patients are concerned about the role of exercise and sex. These are not discussed. However, it is a short text in large print with several helpful illustrations and figures. It is true that the author suggests that the patient consult his ophthalmologist about the use of drugs, sun glasses or any other questions that he may have. So he, too, recognizes that this small text does not answer all questions.

IRVING H. LEOPOLD, MD
New York

Abdominal Trauma. By Meyer O Cantor, MD. Price, $9.50. Pp 212. Charles C Thomas Publisher, 301 E Lawrence Ave, Springfield, Ill 62703, 1970.

This book which is devoted to abdominal trauma has 38 chapters and an index within its 212 pages. Several chapters are only one page in length, and some of them are short as one half page. These would have better been included as paragraphs in other chapters but have apparently been included as a means of increasing the size of the volume. Even the longer chapters are written in a rather casual manner with little indication that the book contains anything other than personal opinion in spite of the fact that there is a rather extensive bibliography. There is no indication that the bibliography is pertinent to the text itself except for rare reference contained within the pages of the volume.

The principles set forth in the various chapters are in general sound, but there is little in these pages to instruct the uninitiated about how these principles are derived and the basis for diagnosis and therapy. To the experienced surgeon there is nothing here worthy of more than casual perusal and indeed it is difficult to maintain any sustained interest.

JOHN A. MONCRIEF, MD
Charleston, SC

Advances in Microcirculation. Edited by Hamburg H Harders. Price, $13.50. Pp 158 with 62 figures and five tables. S Karger Ag, Arnold Böcklinstrasse 25, Basel (American agent, Albert J Phiebig, PO Box 352, White Plains, NY), 1970.

This volume is the third in a series publishing selected important research work presented at the European Conference on Microcirculation. This group is extremely active and capable in this field which cuts across many fields including anatomy, physiology, clinical medicine, pharmacology, biophysics, rheology, immunology, transplantation, coagulation, and other fields. It is a book of broad interest. Certainly knowledge of contemporary events in microcirculation progress is essential for the understanding of disease. The present volume has an extremely comprehensive chapter on the influence of intravenous fat emulsions on the microcirculation; another on the evaluation of infrared thermography; methods of examining the microcirculation in nerves, cochlea, and nucleus pulposus; and last on the influence of smoking on the microcirculation.

With the development of sophisticated methods of observing the microcirculation in various disease states, it is possible for the first time to understand some of the events which transpire in tissue. Certainly this volume will be of interest to most academic minded physicians.

BG ROBERT M. HARDAWAY, MC, USA
El Paso, Tex

Psychedelic Drugs. Edited by RE Hicks, PJ Fink, VO Hammett. Price, not given. Pp 249. Grune & Stratton Inc, 381 Fourth Ave, New York, 1969.

Psychedelics. Edited by Bernard Aaron and Humphrey Osmond. Price, $2.45. Pp 512. Doubleday & Co Inc, 277 Park Ave, New York 10017, 1970.

The first of these two recent books on a related subject is a collection of communications read at a Hahnemann Symposium in November 1968. Hahnemann symposia are wonders of organization. First a large number of authorities in a particular field are assembled in one place to deliver prepared communications. Then, as soon after as possible, these are published in book form. Numerous volumes have already appeared, although few are as elegant as this one. The limited scope of the subject, which in effect is concerned solely with lysergic acid diethylamide (LSD), has led to a relatively few communications. These have been logically divided into those dealing with research, hazards associated with nonmedical use, legal issues, social use, and clinical use.

As is often the case, quality of the presentations varies considerably, and much has been published elsewhere. Still, a sampling of such communications under a single cover may provide an impression of the state of the art of LSD. After two decades of clinical use, and one of widespread social use, it is appalling how little we know about LSD and related drugs. Do psychedelic (mind-revealing) drugs really live up to their name? Can they be used to alter the mind in some directed way? Do they add to spiritual growth? Do they aid traditional analytically oriented psychotherapy? Are they specifically useful for treating alcoholics or terminal cancer patients? What is the risk of adverse psychiatric effects, whose types are well documented? Are genetic disturbances real and of clinical importance? Do legal restrictions impede proper scientific research or impair the personal freedom of people to use these drugs in a nonmedical way?

Many of these questions have partial answers, such as provided by mounting experimental evidence that LSD offers nothing specially beneficial for alcoholics. The group gathered together for this symposium tends on the whole to be favorably inclined to the expanded medical and social use of this drug. Unfortunately, the drug scene is highly volatile. Concerns about LSD have been superseded by those about whether marihuana should be admitted to the company of social drugs or whether we are witnessing the first wave of a pandemic of heroin abuse which may destroy a large portion of our youth. LSD may be temporarily in eclipse, but its brief and turbulent history suggests that it will not be for long. For those who maintain a special interest in this topic, the book will be a useful reference; it is not a book for general reading.

Even the psychedelic drug movement has its hips and squares. The hippiest of those in the movement have prepared the series of communications edited by Aaronson and Osmund. The emphasis is on experimental, anthropological, and sociological aspects of the use of mind-altering drugs. Besides LSD, mescaline, psilocybin, and marihuana are mentioned. The questions mentioned above trouble this group far less, and they produce answers such as one might expect from strong proponents of these drugs. Still, for all the evident biases, the book provides a lot of information at very little cost. If the lack of scientific objectivity does not offend, then this modest paperback may provide a rather broad view of such drugs.

LEO E. HOLLISTER, MD
Palo Alto, Calif

Fundamentals of Tuberculosis Today. By William A. Stead, MD. Price, not given. Marquette University Press, 1131 W Wisconsin Ave, Milwaukee 53233, 1971.

William A. Stead is worried that physicians and nurses have forgotten about tuberculosis. He has written a pleasant little booklet reviewing the pertinent data on pathophysiology, clinical manifestations and contemporary treatment. He has ornamented his modest booklet with cunning diagrams of rotund body cells being defended by devilish–INH (isoniazid) against alligatorish AFB (acid fast bacilli) (from his handbook *Understanding Tuberculosis Today*). One might carp that some of the lingo and diagrams are frivolous for a dour physician audience, but they make their point, and painlessly.

ROBERT H. MOSER, MD
Haiku, Hawaii

Rapid Interpretation of EKG's. By Dale Dubin, MD. Price, $9.50. Pp 265, with 236 illustrations. Cover Publishing Co, PO Box 1092, Tampa, Fla, 1970.

As an introduction to electrocardiography, this paperbacked "programmed" course will probably appeal most to paramedical and coronary care unit personnel. The approach is elemental and overly simplistic; the serious student will desire more depth and detail. There is minimal written text, the major portion of the book being comprised of large half tone, predominantly schematic illustrations, supplemented by brief legends and "fill-in-the-blank," programmed statements.

Simplification results in taking considerable liberty with fundamental electrophysiologic concepts and in the incorporation of errors. These include the derivation of the augmented limb leads, the genesis of Q waves in infarction and bundle block, and incorrect identification of 4:1 AV block as 3:1, to mention a few. To most physicians desiring an introduction to electrocardiography, this book will prove far too elemental and cannot be recommended. It may serve some advantage in instructing nursing and monitoring personnel, although many better texts are available which illustrate and discuss disorders of rhythm with greater clarity and detail.

ROBERT J. HALL, MD
Houston

BRIEF REVIEWS

Biographical History of Medicine. By John H Talbott, MD. Price, $60. Pp 1,211. Grune & Stratton Inc, 757 Third Ave, New York 10017, 1970.

John H. Talbott, distinguished investigator and recently retired editor of *JAMA*, has performed a unique service to medicine. His most recent contribution is this remarkable series of biographical sketches in which the history of medicine is traced through the lives of great physicians (from Hammurabi, 2250 BC to Banting, 1891-1941). These are expanded versions of essays which the author wrote for *JAMA* over the years of his editorship. They are remarkable examples of fine medical-reportorial style (the author says that some underwent five to ten revisions). They reflect the background, historical sensitivity, and broad knowledge of the biographer.

Line drawings by Gabriel Bako adorn much of the book; quotations from original articles citing key contributions by the biographees, and a few of the cardinal contributions to the literature of each of the individuals add great flavor to the presentations.

The skein of each life is woven into the grand tapestry of the history of our art. This is a worthy tome and should find its place in every medical library. There is no doubt that some future medical historian will include John Talbott in a similar book of medical heroes.

Oxford Medicine. Edited by Kenneth Dewhurst. Price, not given. Pp 212. Sandford Publications, Manor House, Sandford-upon-Thames, City of Oxford, 1970.

This is a collection of essays edited and gathered by medical historian-clinician Kenneth Dewhurst to commemorate the bicentenary of the Radcliff Infirmary at Oxford. It offers remarkable insight into the evolution of clinical medicine at that noble institution. It is written by 24 eminent contributors, and is noteworthy for its literary style as well as historical interest.

Modern Treatment, vol 7, No. 3. **Treatment of The Systemic Mycosis: Treatment of Calcium Disorders.** By John P Utz, MD, Gilbert S Gordan, MD, PhD. Price, $20 (per year). Pp 712. Harper & Row Publishers Inc, 49 E 33rd St, New York 10016, 1970.

This is another in the splendid *Modern Treatment* series. The first section is edited by John P. Utz of Richmond who, with nine collaborators, tackles the vexing area of systemic mycoses. As is customary in this series, there is heavy stress on diagnosis and therapy. The articles are frank in their discussion of the many problems and frustrations in the diagnosis and management of systemic mycoses. However, the overall flavor is optimistic.

The sharing symposium is on disorders of calcium metabolism edited by Gilbert S. Gordan of San Francisco with eight co-authors. Individual essays span the entire subject, including diseases of the parathyroids, renal contributions to calcium perturbations, and intestinal malabsorption problems. This is a most current review of the management of calcium metabolic difficulties. As is typical of all books in this series, the discussions are crisp, pertinent, and current.

BOOKS RECEIVED

Forensic Medicine. By Keith Simpson, MA, MD, FRCP. Price, $10.75. Pp 36, with few illustrations. Williams & Wilkins Co, 428 E Preston St, Baltimore 21202, 1969.

Cerebral Blood Flow. Edited by M Brock, C Fiechi, DH Ingvar, NA Lassen, K Schurmann. Price, $16. Pp 291, with 113 figures. Springer-Verlag New York Inc, 195 Fifth Ave, New York 10010, 1969.

The Anatomy of the Developing Lung. Edited by John Emery. Price, $7. Pp 223, with many illustrations. Grune & Stratton Inc, 381 Park Ave S, New York 10016, 1969.

A Manual of Antimicrobial Therapy. By George A Pankey, MD. Price, $5.50. Pp 149, with no illustrations. Charles C Thomas Publisher, 301-327, E Lawrence Ave, Springfield, Ill 62703, 1969.

Guide to Clinical Laboratory Diagnosis. By John A Koepke, MD. Price, $6.75. Pp 310, with few illustrations. Appleton-Century-Crofts Inc, 440 Park Ave S, New York 10016, 1969.

Radioiodinated Rose Bengal and Colloidal Radiogold in the Diagnosis of Hepatobiliary Disease. By Leonard Rosenthal, MS, MD. Price, $7.50. Pp 88, with many illustrations. Warren H Green Inc, 10 S Brentwood Blvd, St. Louis 63105, 1969.

Clinical Nuclear Medicine. By Douglas Maynard, MD. Price, $12.50. Pp 280, with 354 illustrations. Lee & Febiger, 600 Washington Sq, Philadelphia 19106, 1969.

Lymphography in Cancer. By WA Fuchs, MD; JW Davidson, MD; HW Fischer, MD. Price, $21. Pp 294, with 189 illustrations. Springer-Verlag New York Inc, 175 Fifth Ave, New York 10010, 1969.

Virology Monographs: Polyoma Virus and Rubella Virus. By Bernice E Eddy, MD, E Norby, MD. Price, $17.60. Pp 174, with 20 illustrations. Springer-Verlag New York Inc, 175 Fifth Ave, New York, 10010, 1969.

Mental Retardation: Approaches to Institutional Change. By Charles Carr Cleland, PhD; Jon David Swartz, PhD. Price, $12.50. Pp 270, with no illustrations. Grune & Stratton Inc, 381 Park Ave S, New York 10016, 1969.

Fundamentals of Visual Science. By Mevlin L Rubin, MS, MD, Gordon L Wall, ScD. Price, $17.50. Pp 435, with no illustrations. Charles C Thomas Publisher, 301-327 E Lawrence Ave, Springfield, Ill 62703, 1969.

The Thyroid and the Blood. By GR Tudhope, MD, MRCP, FRCP. Price, $4.50. Pp 102, with few tables. Charles C Thomas Publisher, 301-327 E Lawrence Ave, Springfield, Ill 62703, 1969.

Progress in Surgery, vol 8. Edited by M Allgower, SE Bergents, RY Calne, WF Gruber. Price, $13.20. Pp 146, with 41 figures and 10 tables. S Karger AG, Basel, PO Box 352, White Plains, NY, 1970.

Hormonal Contraception. By Jurgen Haller, MD. Price, $12. Pp 288, with many tables and few illustrations. Geron-X Inc, Box 1108, Los Altos, Calif 94022, 1969.

Advances in Internal Medicine. By Gene H Stollerman, MD. Price, $15. Pp 494, with few figures. Year Book Medical Publishers Inc, 35 E Wacker Dr, Chicago 60601, 1969.

Manual of Clinical Microbiology. Edited by John E Blair, PhD; Edwin H Lennette, MD; Joseph Truant, PhD. Price, $12. Pp 727, with many illustrations. Williams & Wilkins Co, 428 E Preston St, Baltimore 21202, 1970.

ERRATUM

In the Original Article entitled "Evaluation of Equilin-3-Monosulfate and Other Estrogens: Comparison by Study of Urinary Gonadotropins in Women" by R. Palmer Howard, MD, and E. Corinne Keaty, PhD, which appeared in the August issue of the ARCHIVES (**128**:229-234, 1971), the following errors appeared: On page 232, Table 3, the second footnote should read †X signifies **no** test conducted at a lower amount but the amount shown was adequate for maintenance. The third footnote should read ‡Y signifies **no** test conducted at a higher amount, but the amount shown was inadequate for maintenance. Also on page 232, in the third column of the text, the sixth line from the bottom should read 17β-estradiol.

Internal medicine at large

Drug laboratory

An Anonymous Drug Analysis Laboratory, possibly the first in the nation with government sanction, is being set up by the School of Pharmacy at the University of Maryland in Baltimore.

Maryland's new Drug Abuse Administration is providing a $30,000 grant. The DAA officials, pharmacy dean William J. Kinnard, Jr., PhD, and S. Edward Krikorian, Jr., PhD, head of the new laboratory, now face the task of collecting drug samples while assuring the anonymity and legal immunity of those who submit them.

Dr. Krikorian believes the samples probably will come from worried parents, treatment centers seeking an antidote, users who experienced an unusual reaction, and police officials who encounter drugs which defy analysis in their more limited laboratories.

One complication: mailing drugs is unlawful and many drug users might fear a police stake-out at any collection box or other delivery point.

It is generally agreed by those involved that the laboratory can only be successful if those who operate it are trusted fully by those who turn to it. This of course would include addicts but, on the other hand, requires precautions against pushers who might regard the laboratory as a means of checking on the quality of their wares.

Drug analysis is enough of a problem in itself, Dr. Krikorian admits, "if only because of the sheer numbers of drugs in use and small size of the sample ordinarily available."

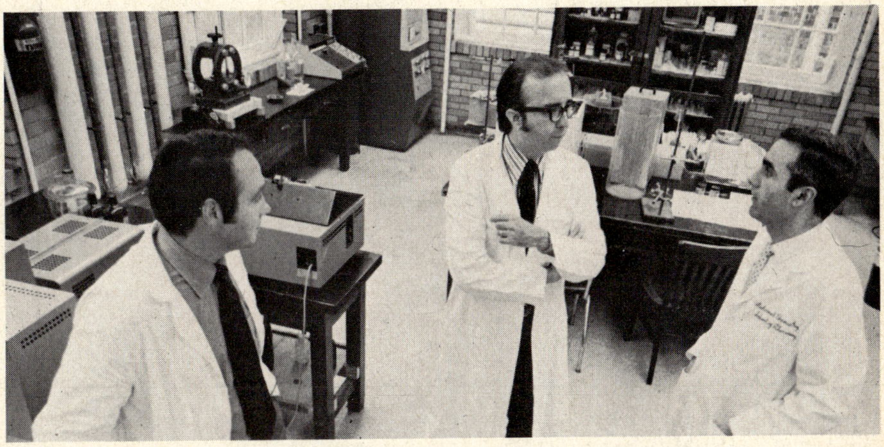

Drs. Blake, Kinnard and Krikorian (left to right) in the new laboratory.

Another faculty member who will be participating in the effort, David A. Blake, PhD, believes that exposing deceit among drug traffickers may prove an added benefit.

"Most kids experimenting with drugs don't take our warnings seriously," he says, "because they don't get the effects that we predict."

The reason, Dr. Blake believes, is because there is little correlation between controlled experiments with pure drugs in the laboratory "and the kids' experience with adulterated street drugs. We can gain a lot of credibility by supplying accurate information about the actual drugs

continued

Highlights of the Month

Boston researchers say much of the blood used in transfusions is too old to deliver oxygen properly . . . page 692.

Members of the Select Society of Seeking Scientists, Saints and Sinners devote their time to help with research on aging . . . page 693.

Developer of automated test for sickle cell hemoglobin believes that the physician's obligation does not stop with telling a person he has the condition . . . page 695.

Internists in the news . . . pages 699, 702.

Internal medicine at large

Drug analysis continued

which these youngsters are using."

Dean Kinnard says analysis will be just one function of the new facility. Other goals are "to develop better methods to identify drugs, better antidotes, and better educational programs. Then, when we have established procedures, we will train people who can set up their own laboratories. That is the function of a university."

Old blood and frozen blood

Three-fourths of all blood transfused in the United States is more than 12 days old, say two Boston researchers whose animal studies suggest that much transfused blood is too old to deliver oxygen effectively.

The best approach, they said at the Society for Cryobiology meeting in Washington, DC, is to freeze blood a day or so after collection. One investigator, Charles E. Huggins, MD, calculates that present practices lead to the annual waste of 1.2 million units, worth about $25 apiece, or a total of $30 million.

Dr. Huggins, associate professor of surgery at Harvard Medical School and clinical director of the Blood Bank and Transfusion Service at Massachusetts General Hospital, said fresh or freshly-frozen blood was far superior to blood stored for 10 to 20 days in sustaining rats which have undergone 16 exchange transfusions.

He and Hiroshi Suzuki, MD, worked with rats and mice, perhaps the only laboratory animals with no specific antibodies to human group 0 blood cells.

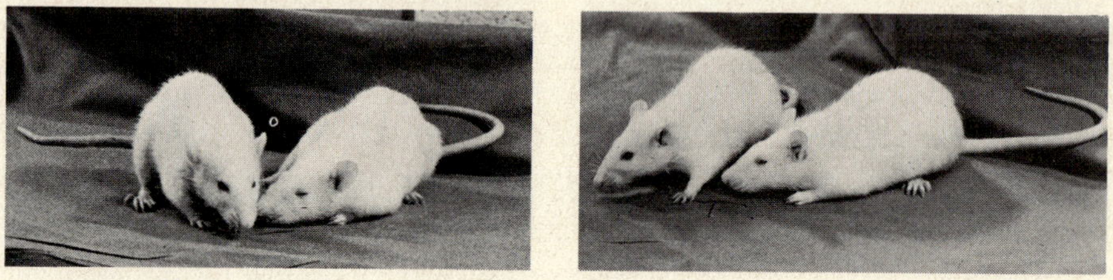

The healthy, inquisitive rat (left) received blood that had been frozen 24 hours after collection and stored for 2 months. He explores his surroundings, while another animal that was given blood stored at 4 C for 14 days remains motionless.

Some 97% of the animals' red blood cells (the most that can be removed without killing the animal) were taken, and a saline-low molecular weight dextran solution was substituted. Human red blood cells in 20% to 60% concentration were added to the solution.

The investigators reported these results:

- Three of 13 rats survived when given transfusions containing a 20% concentration of blood stored at 4 C for 20 days (normally considered acceptable for human use).
- Seven of 26 survived with 10-day-old blood.
- Five of 18 animals survived with blood stored for three or four days.
- Thirteen of 16 survived with blood stored for 24 hours.
- Ten of 10 survived with blood stored for six hours.
- Ten of 13 survived with blood frozen within 24 hours of collection and stored at -85 C for one week to two years.

According to the investigators, their results—and those obtained at other laboratories—indicate that "some major effort is needed to change blood bank practices and equipment."

Giant cell arteritis

The patient is over 50. The symptoms are nonspecific and the physical examination unremarkable.

Now what? Well, says a Seattle researcher, "when older people begin to fail, giant cell arteritis is one of the first diseases that should be considered."

This condition can respond dramatically to steroids if treated in time, says Kenneth R. Wilske, MD, chief of the section of immunology and rheumatic diseases at the Mason Clinic. Otherwise, it may lead to stroke, myocardial infarction, and blindness.

Dr. Wilske, who also is clinical associate professor at the University of Washington School of Medicine, and Louis Healey, MD, reported on 92 giant cell arteritis patients seen at the Mason Clinic between 1965 and 1969. The disease often is characterized by a high sedimentation rate, they said, and may be associated with symptoms ranging from headache to strokes, personality changes, and myocardial infarctions. Local expressions of the disease include polymyalgia rheumatica and temporal arteritis.

Research on aging

The Select Society of Seeking Scientists, Saints, and Sinners (total membership about 650) has two scheduled meetings this week at the Baltimore City Hospitals complex. Less than 1% of the members will attend either session.

But that is the way the Six S's want it. There were two meetings last week, and there will be two more next week. In fact, the Six S's have been meeting almost every week for more than a decade, with never more than six members on hand at any one time.

The society consists of male volunteers who are participating in longitudinal studies on aging at the federal Gerontology Research Center. The center's $7.5 million research facility, dedicated three years ago in Baltimore, is about 50 miles from the parent National Institute of Child Health and Human Development in Bethesda, Md.

Even as the longitudinal studies continue, a decade's worth of data has been stored electronically for rapid computer retrieval by investigators interested in various aspects of aging. That should be a lot of information, Center chief Nathan W. Shock, PhD, says, "and it is, but it's only a fraction of a 70-year lifespan."

Indications from cross-sectional data to date include:

• Aging proceeds at different rates in different individuals. Some 90-year-old men, for instance, have renal blood flow as high as 70-year-old average subjects.

• Age doesn't affect all human organ systems the same way. While there is no assurance that an individual will follow organ system age curves developed so far from test averages, the basal metabolic rate, for example, (in terms of surface area) seems to decline about 20% between the ages of 30 and 90. At the same time, renal blood flow and maximum breathing capacity are apparently halved.

• Aging is accompanied by reduction in reserve capacities. This involves gradual loss of functioning cells from many organs and tissues. The amount of work that most 80-year-old men tested could do, and still have their heartbeat return to normal within two minutes, is 60% less than that for most 20-year-old men tested. These octogenarians also require about twice as long as 20-year-olds to clear the bloodstream of injected sugar.

• Aging appears to have less effect on decision-making processes than on motor control. In tests that involve rapid tapping of a pencil between targets on a sheet of paper, older men had relatively little difficulty making decisions for "homing in" on the targets, but showed age-related decreases in sense of position and motor control.

Testing a Six S's member requires 2½ days. He travels to Baltimore, at his own expense and often from many states away, approximately ev-

continued

Investigators at the Gerontology Research Center have found that age-related changes in conduction velocity in normal subjects contribute little to the slowing of reflex and reaction time in older persons.

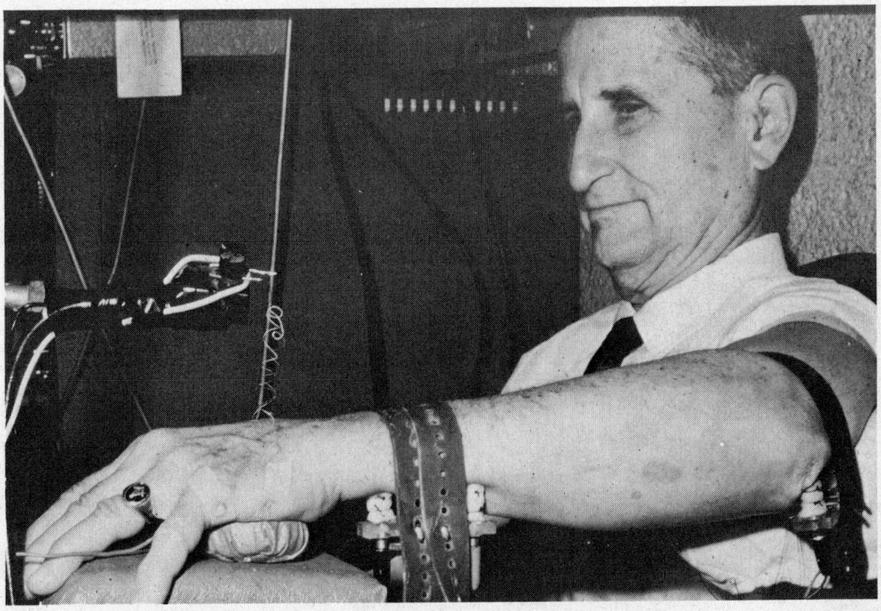

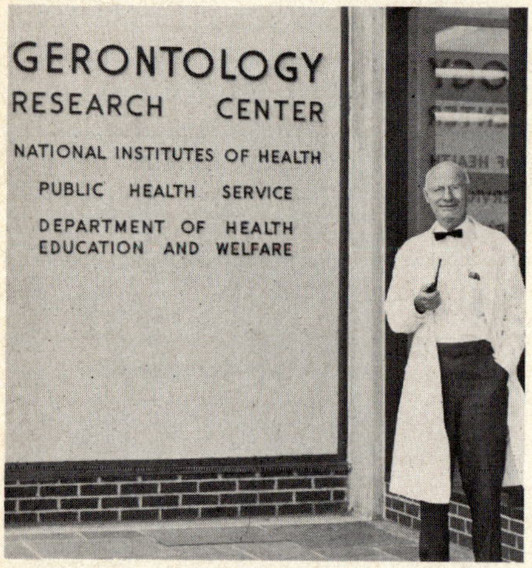

Dr. Shock, who will be 65 on Christmas Day, is starting his fourth decade as head of the center. The grip strength test (center) records age-related changes in muscle performance; tonography (bottom) can detect glaucoma in the volunteers.

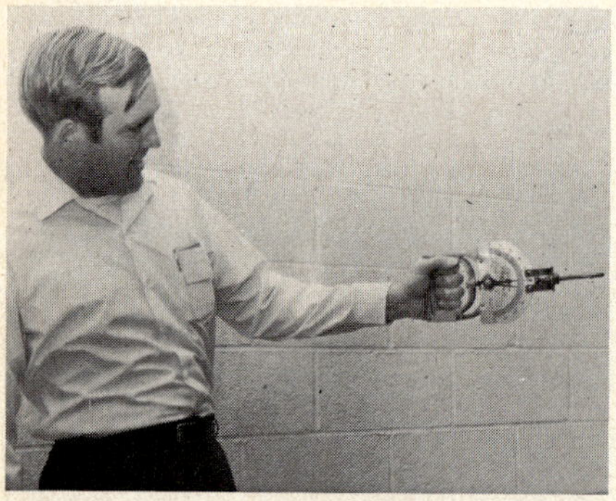

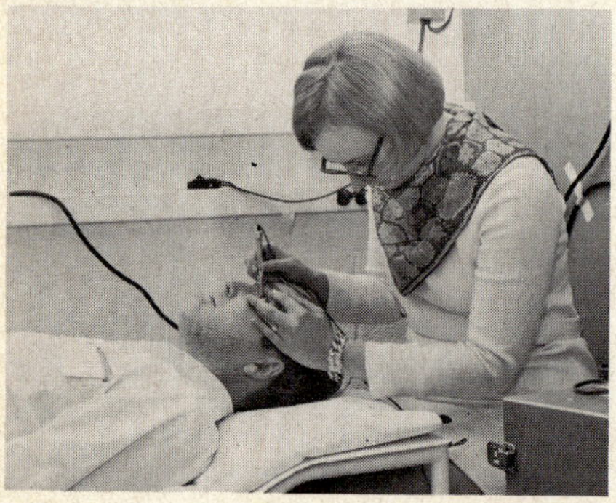

Aging

continued

ery 18 months. Those over 70 are asked to come once a year.

These volunteers have been described as "some of the nation's most distinguished guinea pigs." It's also been noted that "these are not health nuts or hypochondriacs, but business and professional men who are helping scientists in Baltimore to find out how and why people grow old."

Some 85% of the volunteers have at least a bachelor's degree, about 25% hold a master's degree, and around 15% have earned doctorates. Former Vice President Henry Wallace used to participate. The volunteers also include nearly 100 father-son pairs.

The oldest man to participate so far (now dead) was 103 years old, and the oldest volunteer at present is 96. The youngest to enter was 18, the son of another participant. The Center likes participants to be at least 20, not for any lack of interest in younger people but, as Human Performance Section head Arthur H. Norris, MS, explains: "We're concentrating here on physiology and other aspects characteristic of the adult."

There's a reason why the Six S's, and not that traditional subject, the medical student, are involved in these studies.

The society stems from a conversation in October 1957 between Dr. Shock and the late William Wesley Peter, MD, whose career included missionary health personnel recruiting in China, the Indian Health Service, and teaching.

Dr. Shock felt that comparing the test results of medical students and elderly, usually indigent, patients, in which most of the differences were attributed to aging, left something to be desired.

But the problem was to find non-institutionalized subjects in a cross-section of ages who would return regularly. There also was the matter of cost.

Dr. Peter came to the rescue. He would be the first volunteer, he said, and on February 2, 1958, he received the first physical examination and began the first tests of the longitudinal studies.

Further, Dr. Peter promised, he would recruit others. By the end of the first year (and Dr. Peter died shortly thereafter on March 31, 1959) there were 60 volunteers. By the end of the second year, 100 men were involved, thanks to Dr. Peter's idea of having each participant recruit a friend or associate. By the close of the third year, the total had reached 150.

All in all, more than 900 men have been tested. The dropout rate since 1958 for reasons other than death is about 18%, and the investigators know the reasons for most of these cases.

"If we're going to lose a man," Mr. Norris says, "it probably will be between his first visit and scheduled third visit. After that, except for severe health reasons or death, the probability of dropout declines to near zero."

About 90 of the participants have died.

There is such an abundance of would-be participants that no applications presently are being accepted from 40 to 70-year-olds. Those under 40 usually have to wait for about five years. This is partly due to present budgetary and personnel restrictions, although Center officials are encouraged by the President's recent emphasis on problems of the aging.

Some epidemiologists have suggested that the longitudinal study, is too heavily oriented toward business and professional men. This may be due in part to Dr. Peter's original recruiting pitch, which went something like this:

"There is a reason why people like us should volunteer. We are not receiving custodial care and we are not living institutionalized lives.

"Nor are we medically indigent. Such research material, if preponderant, distorts the picture. Many persons being cared for in old people's homes have been buffeted by the storms of life for so many years that they present more than the average number of abnormal findings, both physical and psychological.

"More persons are needed from the outside; persons who live normal lives in their communities."

Dr. Peter was also responsible for the name of the Six S's: "Select, because each member is selected by another participant. Seeking, because all want to know more about aging. Scientists, to include the investigators. Saints and Sinners, because this will include everyone."

There is one more S which Dr. Peter hoped to see added to the alliterative society—Sisters. So far, budgetary and personnel restrictions have prevented adding women to the studies. But when Center officials receive the green light, they know who their first woman volunteer will be—Eleanor E. Whipple Peter, MD, physician-widow of the man whom Dr. Shock credits with "putting into action the dreams of the gerontologist."

12 groups of tests

There are essentially 12 groups of tests and procedures in the Gerontology Research Center's longitudinal studies.

Some are performed each time the volunteer comes to Baltimore. Others may be done as infrequently as every fourth visit.

There is a medical summary (history, physical examination, x-rays, and other studies). Next come tests of each individual's hearing and vision, carbohydrate metabolism, nutrition, genetics, biochemistry, psychology, exercise and neurosmuscular function, renal function, pulmonary function, and body composition.

Results are reported to the volunteer's personal physician.

One drawback, Center officials admit, is that the volunteers who drop out for health reasons usually are lost to follow-up. Also, there is no formal provision for autopsies. Some volunteers have arranged for their own autopsies, with data being sent to the Center.

"For the present," says Arthur H. Norris, MS, head of the Human Performance Section, "about all we can do is ask the man's physician to advise us of cause of death, and the results if an autopsy was done locally."

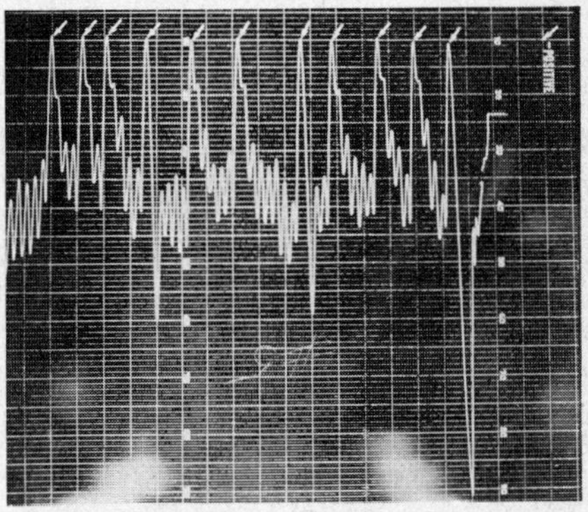

The "peaks" on the AutoAnalyzer indicate the presence of hemoglobin S in 10 of 11 subjects; the test was negative in the 11th individual ("valley" at extreme right).

Sickle cell anemia

Merely detecting sickle cell disease is not enough, says a researcher connected with an automated procedure for revealing the presence of hemoglobin S.

"It's immoral to go into a person's mind and tell him that he has a disease without doing more than just disclosing the fact," says Robert M. Nalbandian, MD.

"If you're going to do mass screening, it carries with it the moral obligation of treatment and genetic counseling."

Dr. Nalbandian, associate pathologist at Blodgett Memorial Hospital, East Grand Rapids, Mich, told the American Association of Blood Banks' annual meeting in Chicago that the automated procedure for detecting sickle cell hemoglobin is ready for use in urban and military screening programs.

continued

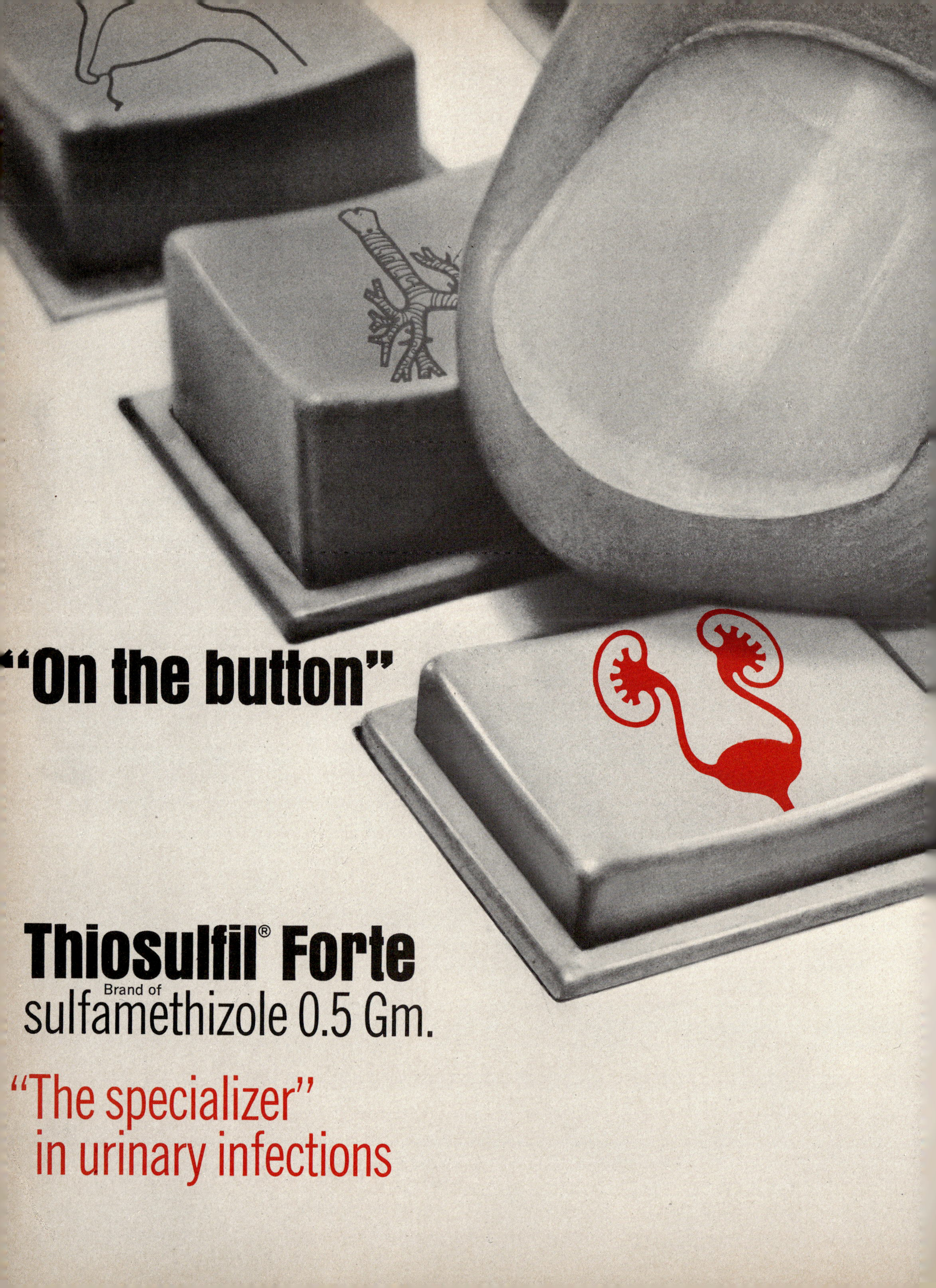
"On the button"
Thiosulfil® Forte
Brand of
sulfamethizole 0.5 Gm.
"The specializer"
in urinary infections

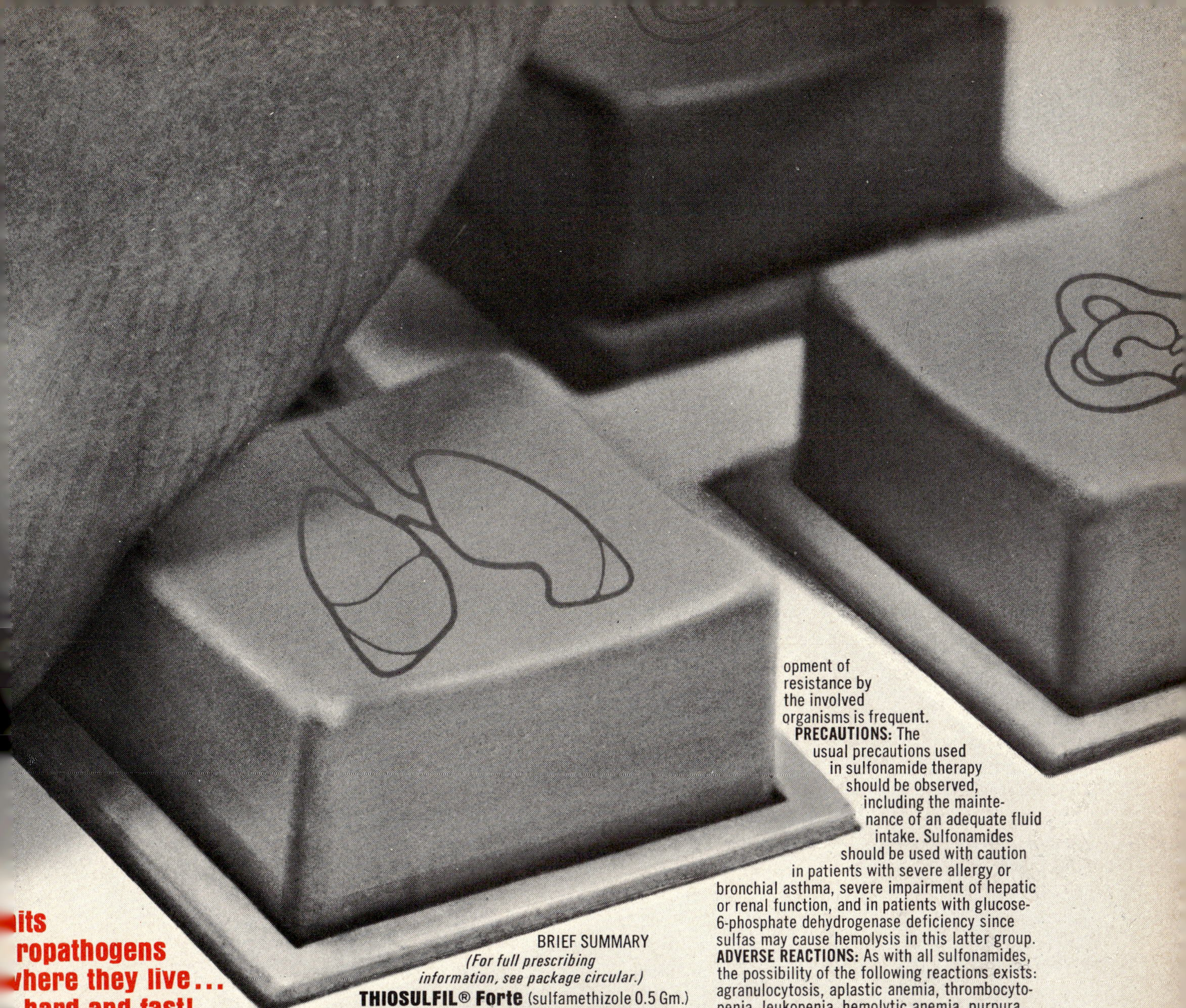

its
ropathogens
vhere they live...
hard and fast!

A *true specific* in cystitis... a *true specific* in pyelitis. In fact, THIOSULFIL Forte sulfamethizole 0.5 Gm.) accumu-ates so *little* in the respiratory ract and other tissues that it has nly *one* indication—urinary ract infections due to susceptible rganisms.

Rapidly absorbed and excreted, HIOSULFIL Forte delivers its otent antibacterial action *locally*. Vithin eight hours, about 80 er cent of the drug is in the rinary tract in free, active form—) fight the infection where it is.

The patient on THIOSULFIL orte uses less sulfonamide... ets more action for his money. nd there's no need for excessive ading or priming doses.

BRIEF SUMMARY
(For full prescribing information, see package circular.)

THIOSULFIL® Forte (sulfamethizole 0.5 Gm.)
Bacteriostatic agent for use in Urinary Tract Infection (due to susceptible organisms)

INDICATIONS: THIOSULFIL is indicated in the treatment of acute and chronic urinary tract infections—cystitis, urethritis, prostatitis, pyelonephritis, and pyelitis—caused by susceptible bacteria, normally *Escherichia coli, Klebsiella aerobacter, Staphylococcus aureus, Proteus mirabilis,* and less frequently, *Proteus vulgaris.* As with most antibiotics and all antimicrobials, THIOSULFIL is most effective in acute, uncomplicated urinary tract infections. **CONTRAINDICATIONS:** Sulfonamides should not be used in patients hypersensitive to sulfa drugs. They should not be used in infants less than two months of age, in pregnancy at term, and during the nursing period because sulfonamides pass the placenta and are excreted in the milk and may cause kernicterus. **WARNINGS:** Sulfonamides should not be used to treat group A streptococci infections or their sequelae. The occurrence of sore throat, fever, pallor, purpura, or jaundice during sulfonamide administration may be an early indication of serious blood dyscrasias. Frequent blood counts and renal function tests should be carried out during sulfonamide treatment, especially during prolonged administration. Microscopic urinalyses should be done once a week when a patient is treated for longer than two weeks. Urine cultures should be made to confirm eradication of bacteriuria. (Para-aminobenzoic acid must be added to the culture media while the patient is on sulfonamide.) Because sulfonamides are bacteriostatic, development of resistance by the involved organisms is frequent. **PRECAUTIONS:** The usual precautions used in sulfonamide therapy should be observed, including the maintenance of an adequate fluid intake. Sulfonamides should be used with caution in patients with severe allergy or bronchial asthma, severe impairment of hepatic or renal function, and in patients with glucose-6-phosphate dehydrogenase deficiency since sulfas may cause hemolysis in this latter group. **ADVERSE REACTIONS:** As with all sulfonamides, the possibility of the following reactions exists: agranulocytosis, aplastic anemia, thrombocytopenia, leukopenia, hemolytic anemia, purpura, hypoprothrombinemia, methemoglobinemia, erythema multiforme (Stevens-Johnson Syndrome), generalized skin eruptions, exfoliative dermatitis, anaphylactoid reactions, periorbital edema, conjunctival and scleral injection, photosensitization, arthralgia, allergic myocarditis, drug fever, chills, toxic nephrosis with oliguria and anuria, periarteritis nodosum, L. E. phenomenon, hepatitis, pancreatitis, stomatitis, nausea, emesis, abdominal pains, diarrhea, anorexia, headache, peripheral neuritis, mental depression, convulsions, ataxia, hallucinations, tinnitus, vertigo, and insomnia. The sulfonamides bear certain chemical similarities to some goitrogens, diuretics (acetazolamide and the thiazides), and oral hypoglycemic agents. Goiter production, diuresis, and hypoglycemia have occurred rarely in patients receiving sulfonamides and cross-sensitivity may exist with these agents. However, the incidence of severe reactions following the use of THIOSULFIL (sulfamethizole) has been very low. **HOW SUPPLIED:** THIOSULFIL Forte—No. 786—Each tablet contains sulfamethizole 0.5 Gm. (scored), in bottles of 100 and 1,000. Also in unit dose package of 100. THIOSULFIL—No. 785—*Tablets*—Each tablet contains sulfamethizole 0.25 Gm. (scored), in bottles of 100 and 1,000. No. 914—*Suspension*—Each 5 cc. (teaspoonful) contains sulfamethizole 0.25 Gm., in bottles of 16 fluidounces.

Ayerst. AYERST LABORATORIES
New York, N.Y. 10017

7128

Sickle cell continued

Developed by Dr. Nalbandian in 1970, the test—based on the theories of Makio Murayama, PhD, National Institutes of Health, and work by Nobel laureate Linus Pauling, PhD, and Harvey Itano, MD, PhD—makes it possible to screen 120 samples per hour.

Potassium, phosphate, sodium dithionite, and saponin are the reagents. Upon exposure, the hemoglobin S red cells lyse, the hemoglobin deoxygenates, and a threadlike liquid crystal system is formed, interfering with the passage of light.

All this is reflected in the distinctive curve obtained with an AutoAnalyzer.

The test however does pick up other sickling hemoglobins that do not signify sickle cell disease—such as hemoglobin C (Harlem)—and electrophoresis is necessary for differential diagnosis.

Hemoglobin S was detected in 309 of 5,192 black school children tested in Grand Rapids, where the total cost per test was 83 cents (2 cents for reagents, 81 cents for personnel, equipment, and other expenses), and the cost of each positive finding came to $13.85. The cost of screening 20,000 troops was 17 cents per test, and $19.03 per positive finding.

In Grand Rapids, the alternatives that are offered to persons with a positive test (and their families) include no action, advice from a physician of the patient's choice, help from a physician who treats sickle cell disease with urea therapy, visiting the sickle cell anemia clinic at Blodgett, or obtaining genetic counseling.

Dr. Nalbandian is an adjunct associate professor of physiology and pharmacology at Wayne State University School of Medicine in Detroit and consultant to the Army Medical Research Laboratory, Fort Knox, Ky. His colleagues in developing the test are Blodgett chemist Bruce M. Nichols, BS; Lt Col Frank R. Camp, Jr., BA, of the AMRL blood transfusion division; Raymond L. Henry, PhD, and Jeanne M. Lusher, MD, of Wayne State; and Paul L. Wolf, MD, of Stanford University Medical Center.

Granulocytes

Granulocyte collection and transfusion have been made easier and more practical by using a steroid and a starch in combination.

Giving normal donors etiocholanolone (a natural steroid hormone which can cause granulocytosis) up to 12 hours before leukapheresis has increased the median number of collected cells by nearly 60%, while the granulocyte total goes up threefold.

According to Kenneth B. McCredie, MB, ChB, there is a way to increase the harvest even more. He said the addition of hydroxyethyl starch—used to facilitate the separation of erythrocytes and granulocytes—has resulted in an eightfold increase in the number of obtained granulocytes. When the starch was used in conjunction with etiocholanolone, the increase was tenfold.

Dr. McCredie, a investigator at the M.D. Anderson Hospital and Tumor Institute, Houston, told the American Association for Cancer Research meeting in Chicago that the procedure will make it possible to make more use of normal donors. They can now give therapeutic amounts of granulocytes without harmful effects, he said.

Most of the donors have been chronic myelogenous leukemia patients who have large numbers of circulating leukocytes.

Syphilis vaccine

A syphilis vaccine that has been tested successfully in rabbits may mean another step forward in man's battle with venereal disease.

Inactivated *Treponema pallidum* organisms from rabbit testicular tissue produced "an apparent complete immunity," reported James N. Miller, MD, of the UCLA School of Medicine, Los Angeles, during the First International Congress of Immunology in Washington, DC. Intravenous administration of the material was carried out over a 37-week period to give the animals a total of 3.7×10^9 organisms.

Mieczyslaw Metzger, MD, of the Polish Academy of Science, reported similar results with penicillin and time-inactivated treponemes—administered intravenously or intramuscularly—over a seven-week period. His test animals received 8 to 12 $\times 10^9$ organisms. The vaccines produced complete symptomatic protection, but only partial protection against asymptomatic infection was observed.

Attempts to cultivate *T pallidum* in vitro have so far been unsuccessful.

The recipients of the six 1971 **Gairdner Foundation Awards** are being honored for their contributions to the field of insulin research. The awards were presented October 29 at the University of Toronto to **Solomon A. Berson,** MD, of Mt. Sinai School of Medicine, New York; **Charles H. Best,** MD, of the University of Toronto-**Rachmiel Levine,** MD, of the City of Hope Medical Center, Duarte, Calif; **Frederick Sanger,** MD, of Cambridge University; **Donald F. Steiner,** MD, of the University of Chicago, and **Rosalind F. Yalow,** PhD, of Mt. Sinai School of Medicine. The awards consist of $5,000 each.

William C. Roberts, MD, medical officer of the cardiology branch of National Heart Institute, has been named professor and chairman of the Department of Pathology at Baylor College of Medicine.

Susan C. Dees, MD, professor of pediatrics at Duke University School of Medicine, has received the 1971 **Bret Ratner Award** of the American Academy of Pediatrics for her contributions in the field of pediatric allergy.

Vernon W. Lippard, MD, former dean of Yale Medical School, has succeeded **Robert A. Moore,** MD, as medical director of the National Fund for Medical Education. Dr. Moore will continue as a consultant to the Fund and Dr. Lippard will remain a consultant to the Josiah Macy, Jr., Foundation.

Leonard P. Eliel, MD, has been appointed executive vice president for medical affairs at the University of Oklahoma. He had held the position on an interim basis since the death of **John P. Colmore,** MD, last November.

Luther L. Terry, MD, former Surgeon General of the US Public Health Service, has resigned as vice president for medical affairs of the University of Pennsylvania to devote full time to teaching as professor of community medicine and medicine. **Robert D. Dripps,** MD, professor and chairman of the Department of Anesthesiology, was named the university's acting vice president for medical affairs.

Charles U. Lowe, MD, scientific director of the National Institute of Child Health and Human Development, is the recipient of the 1971 **Clifford G. Grulee** Award of the American Academy of Pediatrics for service to the academy.

Richard C. Reynolds, MD, professor of medicine at the University of Florida College of Medicine, has been appointed first chairman of the university's Department of Community Health and Family Medicine. Dr. Reynolds joined the Florida faculty in 1968.

The new president of the American Association of Medical Clinics is **Walter I. Buchert,** MD, medical director of the Geisinger Medical Center, Danville, Pa.

The recipients of the 1971 **E. Mead Johnson Awards** for outstanding research in pediatrics are **Paul G. Quie,** MD, and **Fred S. Rosen,** MD. Both men are noted immunologists and received the awards at the annual meeting of the American Academy of Pediatrics in Chicago. Dr. Rosen is associate professor of pediatrics at Harvard Medical School and Dr. Quie is professor of pediatrics and laboratory medicine at the University of Minnesota. Each award consists of $3,000, a scroll, and a certificate.

Fred Gorstein, MD, has been promoted to professor of pathology at New York University School of Medicine.

Tsung O. Cheng, MD, associate professor of medicine at George Washington University School of Medicine, has been appointed chief of cardiology at the District of Columbia General Hospital.

Recent appointments at the Chicago Medical School include those of two professors of pathology—**Parker R. Beamer,** MD, and **William Thomas, Jr,** MD.

Recent promotions at the Albany Medical College include those of **Edward Attarian,** MD; **C. Maynard Guest,** MD; **George W. Hemstead,** MD; **Anthony Nardacci,** MD; **Robert H. Randles,** MD; **Robert W. Raymond,** MD; **Robert Rosenthal,** MD, and **Danica K. Vedder,** MD. All eight were promoted to the rank of associate professor of medicine.

Internal Medicine at large

Alfred S. Ketcham, MD, is the new clinical director of the National Cancer Institute.

Harold Brody, MD, PhD, professor of anatomy at the State University of New York at Buffalo, has been named chairman of the department. He succeeds **O.P. Jones**, MD, PhD, who retired August 31 and remains on the faculty as professor of anatomy.

Charles D. May, MD, former professor of pediatrics at New York University School of Medicine, has been named professor of pediatrics at the University of Colorado School of Medicine. Dr. May came to Denver earlier this year to join the staff of National Jewish Hospital.

The new president of the American Association of Blood Banks is **William G. Battaille**, MD, pathologist at Sibley Memorial Hospital, Washington, DC. **Robert D. Langdell**, MD, professor of pathology at the University of North Carolina School of Medicine, was chosen president-elect of the organization.

Robert H. Felix, MD, dean of the St. Louis University School of Medicine, has been appointed chairman of the Special Medical Advisory Group of the Veterans Administration. The group's purpose is to ensure the maximum mutual support between the VA system and other elements of the health care system.

Buris R. Bushell, MD, the Ruth Lawson Hanson Professor of Medicine in Diabetes and Metabolism at the University of Alabama School of Medicine, has been appointed director of the university's newly-formed Division of Diabetes, Endocrinology and Metabolism.

The new president of the American Dietetic Association is Col **Katharine E. Manchester**, chief of the Food Service Division at Walter Reed General Hospital, Washington, DC. She was the first Regular Army member of the Army Medical Specialist Corps to be promoted to the permanent rank of colonel.

Edward C. Heath, PhD, professor of physiological chemistry at Johns Hopkins University School of Medicine, has been appointed the William S. McEllroy Professor and chairman of the Department of Biochemistry at the University of Pittsburgh School of Medicine.

Nevin S. Scrimshaw, MD, PhD, DPS, professor and head of the Department of Nutrition and Food Science at Massachusetts Institute of Technology, has been named a honorary member of the American Dietetic Association.

Jerome Beloff, MD, has joined the University of Miami School of Medicine faculty as associate professor of family medicine and pediatrics.

Daisuke Nakada, PhD, has been promoted to professor of biochemistry at the University of Pittsburgh School of Medicine.

Herbert J. Kaufmann, MD, has been appointed professor of pediatric radiology at the University of Pennsylvania School of Medicine. Dr. Kaufmann was formerly professor of radiology on the medical faculty of the University of Basel, Switzerland.

The new president of the American Academy of Family Physicians is **J. Jerome Wildgen**, MD, of Kalispell, Mont. **James L. Grobe**, MD, of Phoenix, Ariz, was named president-elect of the organization of 31,000 family physicians. The organization was formerly called the American Academy of General Practice.

LeRoy A. Pesch, MD, is leaving his post as dean and director of University Hospitals, State University of New York at Buffalo, to become the first full-time president of the Michael Reese Hospital and Medical Center in Chicago.

Gustave J. Dammin, MD, the Elsie T. Friedman Professor of Pathology at Harvard Medical School, has been awarded the **Walter Reed Medallion** presented to individuals who have made substantial contributions to the Army Medical Department and to distinguished foreign military and civilian leaders.

Volume 128, Number 5, November 1971

Archives of Internal Medicine

Original Articles

Prophylactic Gamma Globulin for Prevention of Endemic Hepatitis

Effects of US Gamma Globulin Upon the Incidence of Viral Hepatitis and Other Infectious Diseases in US Soldiers Abroad

A Cooperative Study

A prospective double-blind study was performed in 107,803 US soldiers assigned to Korea to determine if prophylactic injections of US-derived human serum gamma globulin prevented icteric endemic viral hepatitis abroad. Each soldier received an intramuscular injection containing either 2, 5, or 10 ml of gamma globulin or a placebo solution upon arrival in Korea and 65% received a second injection of the same material five to seven months later. Gamma globulin prophylaxis significantly decreased the incidence of hepatitis and provided passive protection for about six months. The 5-ml dosage produced maximal protection. Similar protection occurred in patients with both Australia antigen (HAA)-positive and HAA-negative endemic hepatitis. The severity of illness was slightly diminished in the gamma globulin-protected group. Prophylactic injections of gamma globulin did not significantly alter the incidence of other commonplace infectious diseases.

In 1945, Stokes and Neefe reported that the parenteral administration of human serum gamma globulin prevented or attenuated epidemic icteric hepatitis.[1] Subsequently, many investigators have provided evidence which attests to the efficacy of injections of gamma globulin in the prevention of epidemic and endemic hepatitis.[1-52] Various dosages and schedules of administration of gamma globulin have been recommended for the protection of individuals who have been exposed or may become exposed to the disease. Some of these programs are reported to have prevented hepatitis whereas others provided partial protection. In most studies, nationally obtained gamma globulin was used to protect citizens. In a few studies, international protection seemed to be derived from the prophylactic use of gamma globulin.[3,21,35,45,48,49] Experimental studies have indicated that gamma globulin prophylaxis reduced the incidence of icteric hepatitis, but did not decrease the occurrence of anicteric liver disease.[17,18,51]

For many years, gamma globulin prophylaxis was believed to reduce the incidence of serum hepatitis.[53-56] Other studies have indicated that gamma globulin administration has no significant effect upon the incidence of transfusional hepatitis and experimental studies provided support of these data.[51,57-60] Observations showing that many patients with endemic hepatitis have Australia antigen (HAA) in their serum and that HAA-positive hepatitis can be transmitted by the oral route makes the problem of serum hepatitis more important than was previously realized.[51,61]

Reports of the efficacy of gamma globulin to prevent hepatitis have led physicians to use this biologic mate-

Received for publication March 12, 1971; accepted April 14.

From the Division of Medicine, Walter Reed Army Institute of Research, Washington, DC.

This cooperative study was conducted by Walter Reed Army Institute of Research, US Army Medical Research and Development Command.

This material has been reviewed by US Army Medical Research and Development Command and there is no objection to its publication. The opinions or assertions contained herein are the private views of the author and are not to be construed as official or as reflecting the views of the Department of the Army or the Department of Defense.

Reprint requests to Division of Medicine, Walter Reed Army Institute of Research, Washington, DC 20012 (COL Marcel E. Conrad, MC, USA).

rial during epidemics of hepatitis, for the protection of transfused patients, and for the prevention of disease among contacts of patients with hepatitis. Military usage of gamma globulin was extended further; gamma globulin injections were utilized prophylactically to reduce the incidence of hepatitis in soldiers in certain overseas areas. This prophylactic use of gamma globulin was based upon the assumptions that the intramuscular administration of gamma globulin is innocuous, anicteric hepatitis may be less noxious than icteric hepatitis, and nationally obtained gamma globulin provides worldwide protection and in a similar dosage.

During 1964 a program was initiated to protect all military personnel stationed in Asia from hepatitis. A 16% solution of human immune serum gamma globulin was used which was prepared from blood donated in the United States. Soldiers were injected with 0.05 ml/lb of body weight of the gamma globulin solution upon arrival overseas and again five months later.[62] Preliminary observations seemed to indicate that this program was effective. During 1964 and 1965, the incidence of hepatitis among US soldiers stationed in Korea was three to four cases per thousand per year; whereas in previous years the incidence was 0.7%.[63] However, scrutiny of the monthly hepatitis rates showed that the decrease began four months before the gamma globulin inoculations were initiated (Fig 1). Similarly, in Vietnam, gamma globulin prophylaxis was initiated during a period when the incidence of hepatitis was decreasing rapidly. During 1965 the number of military personnel assigned in Asia markedly increased because of the escalation of the conflict in Vietnam.[64] This significantly depleted available stockpiles of gamma globulin and made reassessment of the prophylactic program necessary. It was decided that only persons with a high risk of exposure to infectious hepatitis would receive inoculations of gamma globulin. An incidence greater than five cases per thousand soldiers per year in a geographic area was recommended as the guideline for a high-risk group. In addition, the dose of gamma globulin administered to soldiers was reduced to 5 ml of a 16% solution upon arrival overseas and again five months later. This policy markedly reduced the usage of gamma globulin but did not cause a perceptible increase in the incidence of hepatitis among soldiers stationed in Korea or Vietnam during the next year. These data made it impossible to ascertain whether the administration of gamma globulin from the United States had a significant effect upon the incidence of hepatitis among troops stationed in Asia.

During May 1967 a prospective study was initiated to evaluate the effectiveness of prophylactic injections of gamma globulin obtained from the United States in the prevention of clinical hepatitis among US soldiers stationed in Korea. Korea was selected because it is an Asian country where about 50,000 US soldiers are assigned each year for a one-year tour of military duty, all soldiers arrive in Korea through a single aerial port of debarkation, all patients with hepatitis are hospitalized at one of two military hospitals, and peacetime operations in this country permitted greater medical and logistical support and control of the study than was possible in South Vietnam.[65]

This article reports the results of observations in 107,803 US soldiers who arrived in Korea between May 15, 1967, and Aug 1, 1969. Upon arrival in Korea each soldier received either an injection containing one of three doses of gamma globulin or a placebo solution. Sixty-five percent of these soldiers received a similar injection five to seven months later (Fig 2). The incidence of icteric hepatitis and other commonplace diseases in these soldiers is the subject of this report.

Subjects, Methods, and Procedures

The subjects of this study were 107,803 US male soldiers who arrived in Korea for military assignment between May 15, 1967, and Aug 1, 1969. The military rank and age distribution of this population and their length of military service are shown in Fig 3 and 4 and Table 1.

During May 1967 an immunization station was established at Kimpo Air Force Base, the aerial port of debarkation for all US Army personnel reporting to Korea for assignment. This facility was operated by a team from Walter Reed Army Institute of Research. Each incoming aircraft was met to assure that arriving personnel were informed of the study, records were initiated, and injections were received. Each subject of the study received an intramuscular injection of 10 ml which contained either one of three doses of gamma globulin or placebo solution. The dose was divided such that half was injected into each buttock. A special record was initiated which included the name, military rank, army service number, age, body weight, previous history of hepatitis, the identification number on the vial used for injection, the date of injection, and the proposed date for a second inoculation. A duplicate card with instructions for receipt of a second injection five months later was affixed to each soldier's Health Record and forwarded to his assigned military unit. The second injection was administered at inoculation centers established at the principal medical facility for each large population of troops. Each soldier reporting to the secondary inoculation centers received the contents of a vial labeled with the same identification number as at the time of initial injection. These centers entered the date of the second injection and the identification number of the vial used on the duplicate special record card and mailed it to the immunization team at Kimpo Air Force Base. If a completed duplicate card was not received for a soldier during the sixth month after his initial injection, his military unit was notified and requested to send him to a designated immunization facility.

During the performance of this study the only adverse reaction observed or reported following an injection of gamma globulin or placebo solution was syncope. This was more common during the summer months. It was usually transitory and recovery was prompt.

During the period from May 15, 1967, until May 15, 1970, all soldiers who developed clinical or laboratory evidence of infectious hepatitis were hospitalized at the 121st Evacuation Hospital or the 11th Evacuation Hospital. Diagnosis and hospital care was performed by board-certified or qualified internists who had been assigned to Korea for their military service. The diagnosis of viral hepatitis was established in patients with a medical history and physical findings suspicious for this disease by laboratory studies which included an abnormal serum bilirubin concentration (>1.5 mg/100 ml), abnormal serum glutamic oxaloacetic and serum glutamic pyruvic transaminase determinations (SGOT or SGPT, or both, > 200 units), and lack of evidence of infectious mononucleosis by either the infectious mononucleosis spot test or heterophil agglutination studies including absorption with guinea pig kidney or both. Only icteric cases of hepatitis were included in this report. Anicteric hepatitis is rarely a cause of hospitalization among US soldiers; symptomatic patients hospitalized without icterus usually are found to have or develop an abnormal total serum bilirubin concentration with an increased direct-reacting fraction. A liver biopsy was performed in all patients who volunteered for the procedure (82% of patients). The liver biopsy specimens were examined by the pathologist assigned to the 121st Evacuation Hospital. In addition, the specimens were reexamined by H. F. Smetana, MD, without knowledge of either clinical history or laboratory data.

Patients with viral hepatitis were detected by surveillance of the admission diagnoses of all soldiers to each hospital in Korea and a review of all hospital records made during the period of study. This was performed by both the registrar of each hospital and members of the study team, respectively. The incidence of other infectious diseases which occurred among subjects of this study who required hospitalization was quantified by examination of all hospital records in US Army hospitals from May 15, 1967, to May 15, 1970. The study team recorded the occurrence of infectious diseases in nonhospitalized subjects of this study by maintaining daily surveillance of soldiers reporting to the 548th General Dispensary for monthly intervals during October 1968, January 1969, and April 1969. The maintenance of individual inoculation records at the aerial port of debarkation permitted confirmation that each patient reported in this study received gamma globulin or a placebo injection and provided the dates of inoculations.

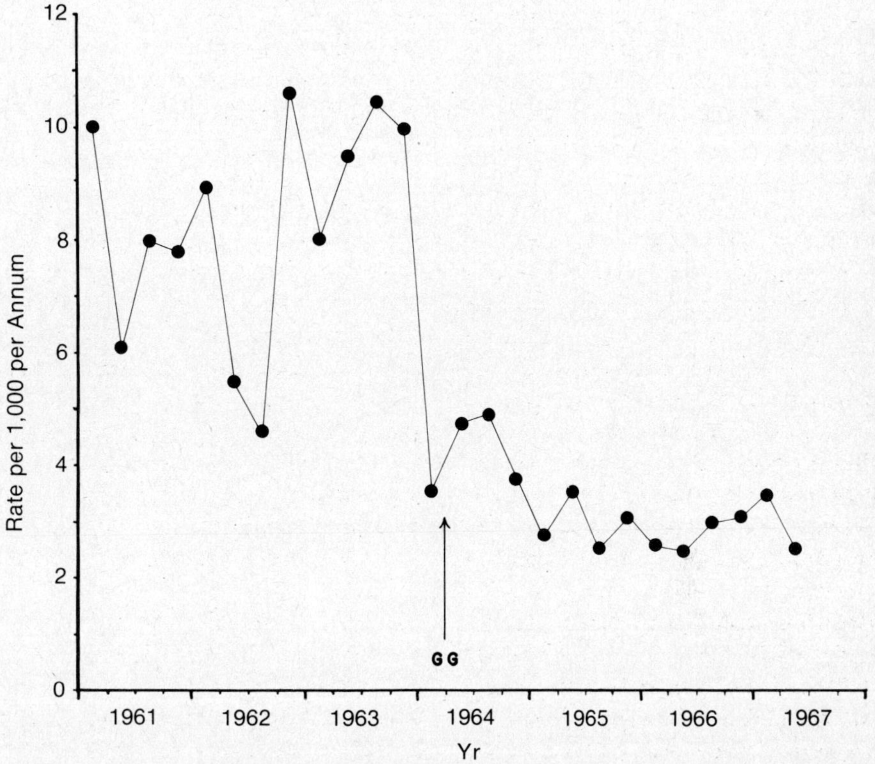

Fig 1.—A significantly greater incidence of viral hepatitis was observed among soldiers assigned to Korea before 1964 than afterwards. This change could not be attributed to the use of gamma globulin because the decrease in incidence occurred several months before the prophylactic program was initiated (GG).[63]

A survey form was mailed to each patient who developed hepatitis requesting his place of birth; years of education; the geographic location of his elementary school, high school, and college; areas travelled outside the United States; previous personal and family history of hepatitis, jaundice, gallstones, anemia, liver disease, cirrhosis, and malaria; a personal history of blood transfusion and immunizations; and history of blood donation, drug ingestion, and dental work during the six months before hospitalization for hepatitis. A response was obtained from 96% of the patients. A similar survey form was completed by 4,000 soldiers who did not develop viral hepatitis. They were selected by requesting all soldiers on certain aircraft arriving in Korea to complete the questionnaire. The survey form was placed on various aircraft in a random manner at intervals during the study.

Serum was obtained during the first week of hospitalization from 211 patients with viral hepatitis for Australia antigen (HAA) studies. These specimens were obtained from all patients hospitalized with hepatitis at the 121st Evacuation Hospital from September 1969 to March 1970. The serum was examined by both the agar gel precipitin test and a quantitative complement fixation test for HAA.[66-68] Examination of serial serum specimens obtained at weekly intervals for one month from several patients with and without HAA as determined by the complement fixation test showed changes in titer but would not

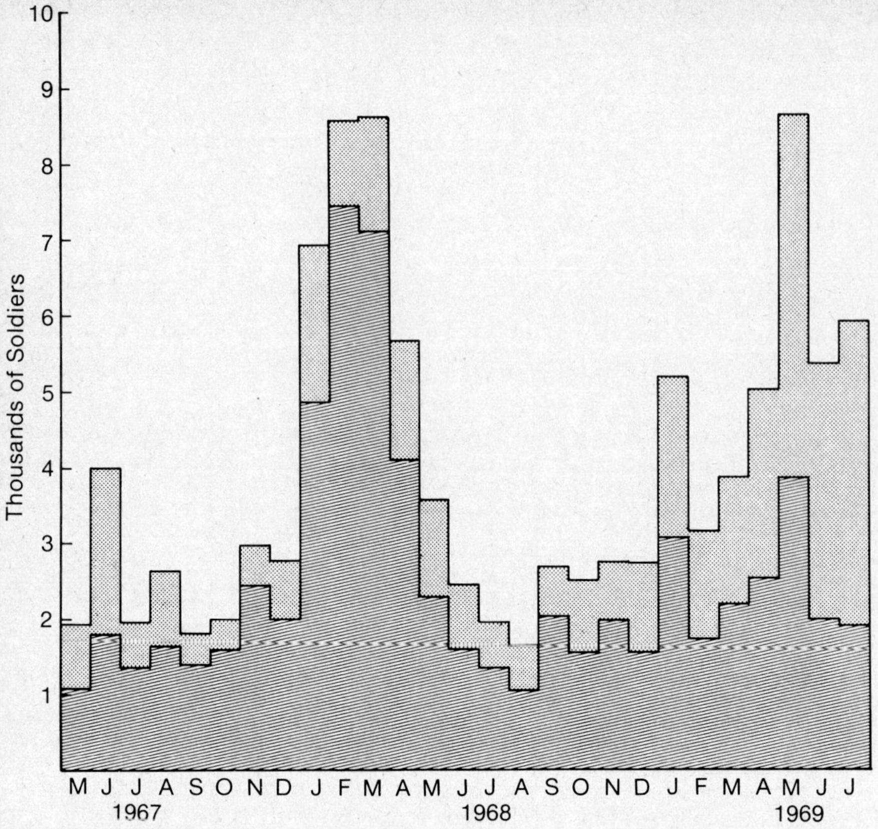

Fig 2.—The dotted bars show the number of US soldiers arriving in Korea during each month of the study. The crosshatched bars show the number of these soldiers who received a second injection of gamma globulin five to seven months later. The uneven assignment of soldiers to Korea was a military response to political events.

Fig 3.—The percentage of soldiers in various age groups who developed hepatitis (solid bars) *in comparison to the age distribution of normal soldiers* (crosshatched bars). *Viral hepatitis was more prevalent than expected between the ages of 20 to 29 years and less prevalent among both younger and older soldiers.*

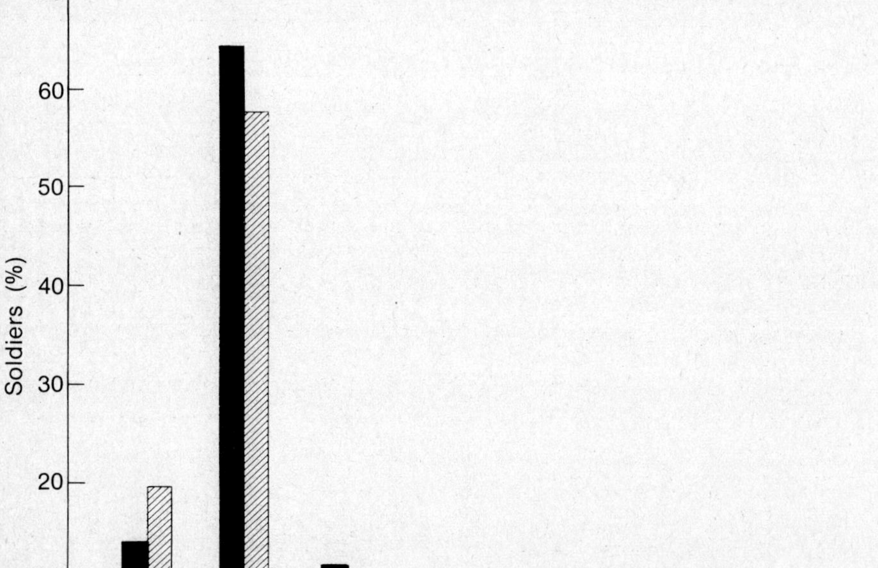

have altered their inclusion in either the HAA-positive or HAA-negative groups.

Materials

The solutions used for injection in this study were purchased (Hyland Division, Travenol Laboratories, Los Angeles) in sterile stoppered labeled glass bottles. Each bottle contained a sufficient volume so that 10 ml could be withdrawn with a hypodermic needle and syringe. The solutions contained either (1) 10 ml of human serum gamma globulin (16%), (2) 10 ml of a sucrose potassium glutamate solution containing 2.5% human serum albumin, (3) 5 ml of 16% gamma globulin and 5 ml of the control solution, or (4) 2 ml of gamma globulin and 8 ml of the albumin control solution. The various solutions used for injection were bottled in containers labeled with a single-digit identification number. An equal number of bottles were labeled with each integer, 0 through 9. Bottles containing various quantities of gamma globulin were assigned one of two integers and the control solutions were labeled with one of the remaining four integers. Bottles were packaged in cartons containing an equal number of bottles labeled with each of the ten possible integers. This permitted random utilization of the coded solutions. Each subject of the study was injected with contents of a vial labeled with a number identical to the last integer of his army service number. The code was unknown to all participants and subjects of the study and was not decoded until all data had undergone statistical analysis.

All solutions and materials utilized in this study were obtained, produced, and packaged in accordance with the US Pharmacopoeia (USP) requirements for sterile and pyrogen-free solutions prepared for parenteral injection into humans. The gamma globulin and albumin were obtained, prepared and tested in accordance with the standards and regulations of the Division of Biologic Standards, Public Health Service for immune human serum gamma globulin and human serum albumin. The albumin sucrose potassium glutamate solution used in this study was prepared to contain sucrose, USP, 74.6 gm/liter; KH_2PO_4, analytical reagent (AR), 0.51 gm/liter; K_2HPO_4, AR, 1.22 gm/liter; and potassium glutamate, 0.72 gm/liter. The pH of the aqueous solution was adjusted to 7.0 with KOH, AR. To each 900 ml of the sucrose potassium glutamate solution, 100 ml of a 25% solution of human serum albumin was added. The gamma globulin was prepared from plasma which was recently bled from paid donors in various geographic areas of the US and anticoagulated in either acid citrate dextrose solution or citrate. Gamma globulin was prepared by Cohn ethanol fractionation.

Four separate lots of material were manufactured for use in this study. They were prepared and shipped at six-month intervals to avoid the use of aged biologic materials in the performance of the study. Each lot was dated and the cartons marked with a different colored label to insure that older lots were used first. Each lot was air transported in single shipments. These shipments were made during the spring and fall to avoid freezing or overheating. Other than the day of shipment, the biologic materials were refrigerated at 4 C until they were used for injection.

Certain characterizations of the four lots of human serum gamma globulin used in this study are shown in Table 2. These studies were performed because of accumulating evidence that some gamma globulin preparations may be less effective than others in preventing hepatitis due to factors such as source of the plasma, age of the plasma, fragmentation of gamma globulin, and antibody levels.[69] The total protein concentration was measured by the biuret method. The IgG, IgA, IgM, and albumin concentrations were quantified by the radial diffusion method of Feinberg as modified by Mancini et al.[70] Fragmentation of the gamma globulin was quantified by both the trichloroacetic acid precipitation method and by estimation of the molecular size of the protein in solution using a Sephadex G 100 column as previously described.[71,72] Diphtheria antitoxin was measured by toxin neutralization tests in rabbits and is reported in international units with comparison to National Institutes of Health (NIH) standard antitoxin lot A25. Measles and poliovirus type 2 antibodies were measured by viral neutralization tests in tissue culture. Results are reported as a potency ratio in which the reciprocal of the 50% end point dilution of the gamma globulin solution in viral neutralization studies were compared to NIH lot 1 using lot MV5 virus pool and NIH lot 174 using PV TC4 virus pool, respectively. Studies of this gamma globulin for Australia antibody were performed by radioimmune assay and showed a reciprocal dilution titer greater than 1,280; this titer was tenfold greater than that observed with three commercially available lots of gamma globulin from other sources.

The albumin-sucrose potassium gluta-

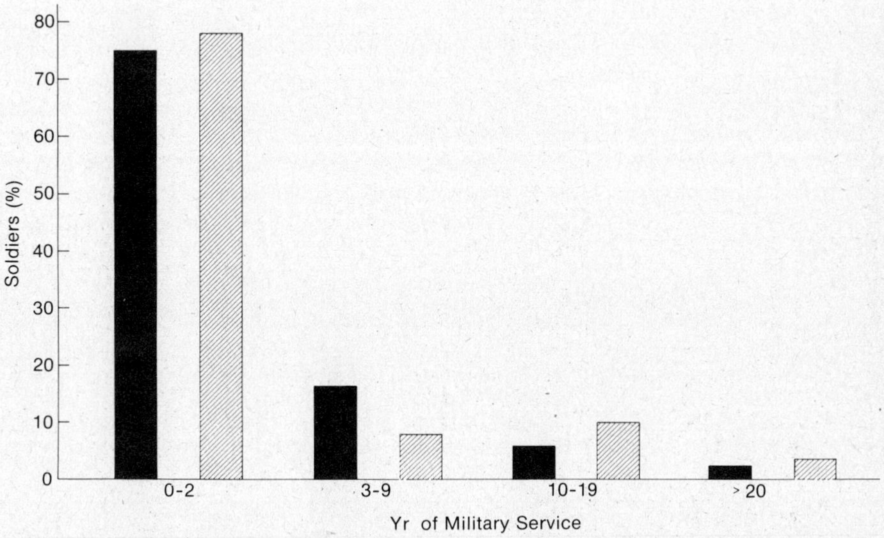

Fig 4.—The percentage of soldiers with various periods of military service who developed hepatitis (solid bars) *and the duration of military service among normal soldiers* (crosshatched bars). *A greater per capita incidence of hepatitis was observed in soldiers with three to nine years of military service.*

Table 1.—Distribution of Hepatitis Patients and Normal Soldiers by Military Rank*

	Hepatitis Patients (%)	Normal Subjects (%)
E1-E5	83.95	80.94
E6-E7	11.50	9.55
E8-E9	1.10	1.49
Warrant officers	0.22	0.96
01-03	3.23	5.59
04-06	0	1.47

* Private, E1 and E2; Private First Class, E3; Corporal, E4; Sergeant, E5; Staff Sergeant, E6; Sergeant First Class, E7; Master Sergeant, E8; and Sergeant Major, E9. Second Lieutenant 01; First Lieutenant, 02; Captain, 03; Major, 04; Lieutenant Colonel, 05, and Colonel, 06.

Table 2.—Certain Characteristics of the Serum Gamma Globulin Used in This Study

		Protein Composition					Percentage Fragmentation of Globulin		Antibody Content		
Lot	Date of Manufacture	Total Protein (gm/100 ml)	γG (gm/100 ml)	γA (mg/100 ml)	γM (mg/100 ml)	Albumin (mg/100 ml)	Trichloroacetic Acid Method	Sephadex G 100	Measles*	Polio II†	Diphtheria‡
1	April 1967	17.0	16.2	113	131	23	3.6	2.7	0.52	1.8	4
2	September 1967	16.8	15.8	82	109	16	3.0	2.8	0.88	1.1	5
3	April 1968	17.1	16.6	95	120	8	4.8	3.5	0.56	1.0	5
4	October 1968	17.3	16.4	110	85	12	3.5	2.9	0.64	1.2	5

* Potency ratio by neutralization testing compared with National Institutes of Health lot 1 with the use of lot MV5 virus pool.
† Potency ratio by neutralization testing compared with National Institutes of Health lot 174 with the use of PV II TC4 virus pool.
‡ Reported in international units and compared to National Institutes of Health standard antitoxin lot A25.

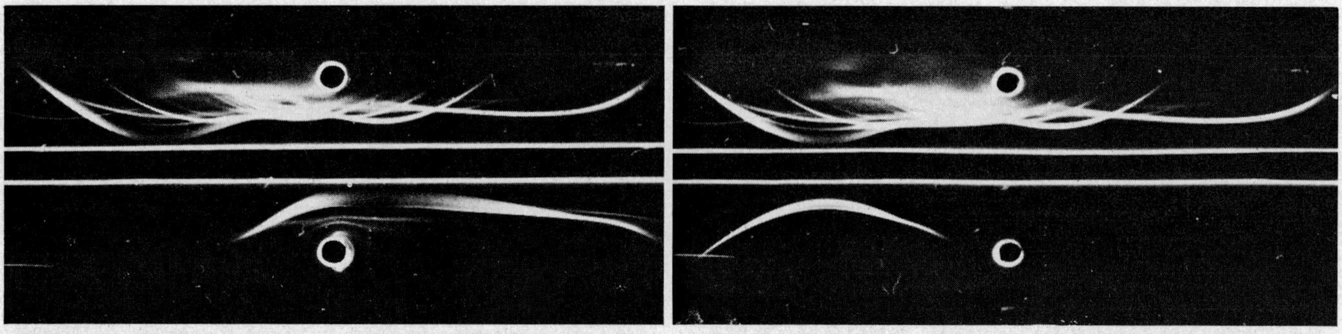

Fig 5.—Left *and* right, *Immunoelectrophoresis of normal human sera* (above) *and either gamma globulin* (left, below) or albumin placebo solution (right, below). *Longitudinal troughs contained horse antiserum to whole human sera. Circular reservoirs contained human sera* (left *and* right, above) *and either gamma globulin* (left, below) *or placebo solution* (right, below). *The anode was to the left. No gamma globulin was detected in the placebo solution. The gamma globulin contained mostly IgG and small amounts of IgA and IgM. Similar findings were observed with all four lots of material (Table 2).*

Table 3.—Distribution of Hepatitis Patients and Normal Subjects by Race

	Hepatitis Patients (%)	Normal Subjects (%)
White	75.22	69.94
Black	23.45	25.59
Mongolian	1.33	3.57
Other	0	0.90

Table 4.—Population of Geographic Locations Where Normal Soldiers and Soldiers With Hepatitis Lived at Various Stages of Life—Percentage of Group

	Birth		Elementary School		High School	
Population	Hepatitis Patients	Normal Soldiers	Hepatitis Patients	Normal Soldiers	Hepatitis Patients	Normal Soldiers
<2,500	21.6	20.9	31.6	27.5	28.3	24.4
2,500 to 25,000	28.7	27.6	29.3	28.7	30.0	30.5
25,000 to 250,000	24.5	24.7	19.9	24.2	22.0	25.7
>250,000	25.2	26.8	19.2	19.6	19.7	19.4

mate solution used as a placebo in this study contained no detectable IgG, IgA, or IgM. Immunoelectrophoresis of the control solution against horse antiwhole human serum showed only an albumin arc (Fig 5).

Results

Icteric Hepatitis in a Military Population.—A comparison was made between patients admitted to the hospital with hepatitis and the normal subjects of this study. The incidence of icteric hepatitis was significantly greater among soldiers between the ages of 20 and 30 years who had three to ten years of military service than was expected from enumeration of the normal subjects in these groups (Fig 3 and 4). A greater than anticipated incidence of hepatitis was observed among enlisted men of lower military rank (E1 to E7) than in officers or senior enlisted men (Table 1). A greater per capita incidence of hepatitis was observed in white soldiers than black soldiers (Table 3). There was no significant difference in the size of the city of birth of hepatitis patients than normal subjects. However, more hepatitis patients spent their childhood and adolescence in rural communities, small cities, and suburbs than was found in the normal population (Table 4). The hepatitis patients had completed more years of education than the control population (Table 5).

A lifetime history of hospitalizations and of hospitalizations within the previous six months was more frequent in normal subjects than hepatitis patients. A family history of hepatitis was twice as frequent among the normal subjects as among the hepatitis patients. Slightly more hepatitis patients donated blood within the previous six months than normal subjects. However, more normal subjects had received a blood transfusion than hepatitis patients. A history of dental work, immunizations, and use of medications was similar in both groups of subjects (Table 6). Only three of the hepatitis patients in this study were believed to have used habituating drugs intravenously; one received 10 ml of gamma globulin, another 2 ml of gamma globulin, and the third patient had received placebo solution.

Six of the 467 patients who developed hepatitis in this study stated that they had developed hepatitis previously (1.28%), whereas 2,091 of 107,803 soldiers indicated that they had been treated for hepatitis before arrival in Korea (1.94%). Among the hepatitis patients, the previous diagnosis had been established within two years in two patients and might represent a relapse—one patient who received placebo solution had hepatitis nine months before arrival in Korea; the other patient who received 2 ml of serum gamma globulin upon arrival in Korea had developed hepatitis four months after a blood transfusion 18 months previously. A relapse of hepatitis seemed less likely in the remaining four patients because the previous diagnosis was established more than three years before their arrival in Korea and there was no intervening history of recurrence.

Occurrence of Icteric Hepatitis Among Soldiers at Intervals Following Assignment to Korea.—A soldier is usually assigned to this geographic area for one year. During the period of this study approximately 2% of soldiers had a shorter military assignment and about 5% requested and obtained an extension of the Korean tour. Figure 6 shows a graphic representation of the month of the Korean tour during which 467 patients of this study developed hepatitis. Similar to previously reported studies,[73,74] there was a low incidence of hepatitis among soldiers during the first few months of assignment to Korea with the majority of cases occurring 7 to 11 months after arrival overseas. Likewise, soldiers remaining in Korea for more than one year continued to develop icteric hepatitis. That the reduced incidence of hepatitis during the initial months of assignment overseas was not solely caused by the administration of gamma globulin upon debarkation is shown by examination of the monthly incidence among soldiers receiving injections of the placebo solution.

Effect of Gamma Globulin Upon the Incidence of Icteric Hepatitis.—The incidence of icteric hepatitis among the 107,803 soldiers who received either gamma globulin or a placebo injection was 0.433% (Fig 7, Table 7). The number of soldiers was similar in the groups which received either 2 ml, 5 ml, or 10 ml of gamma globulin or were included in one of the two control groups both upon arrival in Korea (19.87% to 20.21%) and five to seven

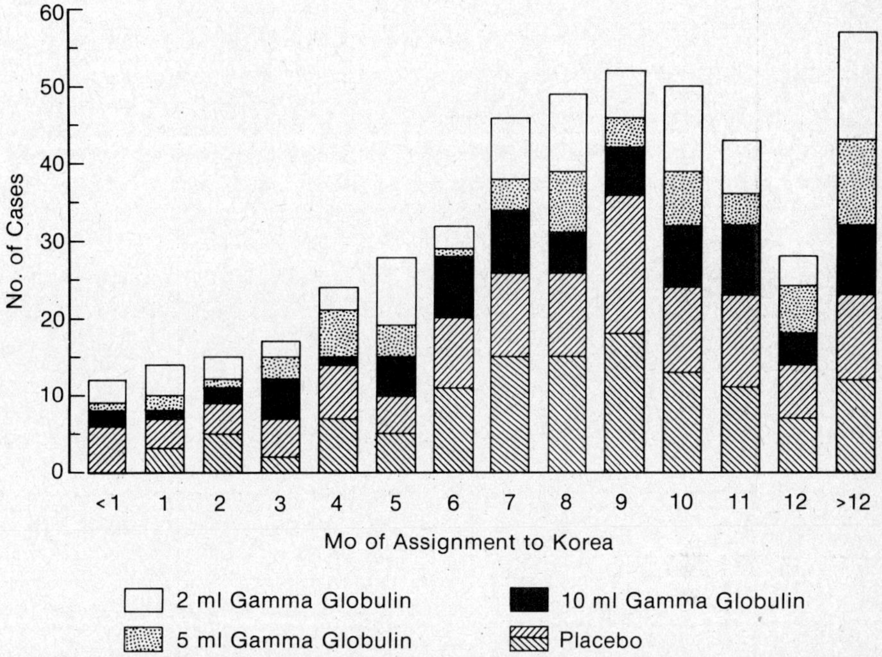

Fig 6.—Graphic representation of the month following assignment to Korea during which soldiers developed icteric hepatitis. Each bar is divided to show whether soldiers received one of three doses of gamma globulin or placebo solution. All groups had a lower incidence of hepatitis during the first months of assignment.

months later (12.80% to 13.20%). A clinical diagnosis of hepatitis was established in each of the 467 soldiers in this group of patients. Each patient had bilirubinemia and abnormal serum transaminase determinations. An adequate liver biopsy specimen was obtained from 352 of these patients and showed abnormalities consistent with diagnosis of viral hepatitis.

There were 121 and 123 cases of hepatitis from the two groups of soldiers injected with placebo solutions, respectively. Among soldiers receiving various amounts of gamma globulin; 87 cases were observed in the group that received 2 ml of gamma globulin, 62 cases occurred in soldiers who were injected with 5 ml of gamma globulin, and 74 cases were observed in the subjects who received 10 ml of gamma globulin. Statistical analysis of these data by χ^2 analyses showed no significant difference between the two placebo groups or between groups of soldiers receiving 5 and 10 ml of gamma globulin. On the contrary, a comparison between the placebo groups and soldiers receiving either 5 or 10 ml of gamma globulin showed a significant difference ($P<.001$). The 2-ml dose of gamma globulin provided some protection ($P<.01$) but less than that observed among soldiers receiving larger dosages of gamma globulin ($P<.05$).

Table 5.—Grade in School Completed by Hepatitis Patients and Normal Soldiers

Grade Completed (yr)	Hepatitis Patients (%)	Normal Subjects (%)
Less than 8	6.92	11.81
9 to 12	69.78	75.94
Greater than 12	23.30	12.25

Figure 7 shows the interval between an injection of various doses of gamma globulin and the occurrence of clinically apparent icteric hepatitis in each member of this study. Signifi-

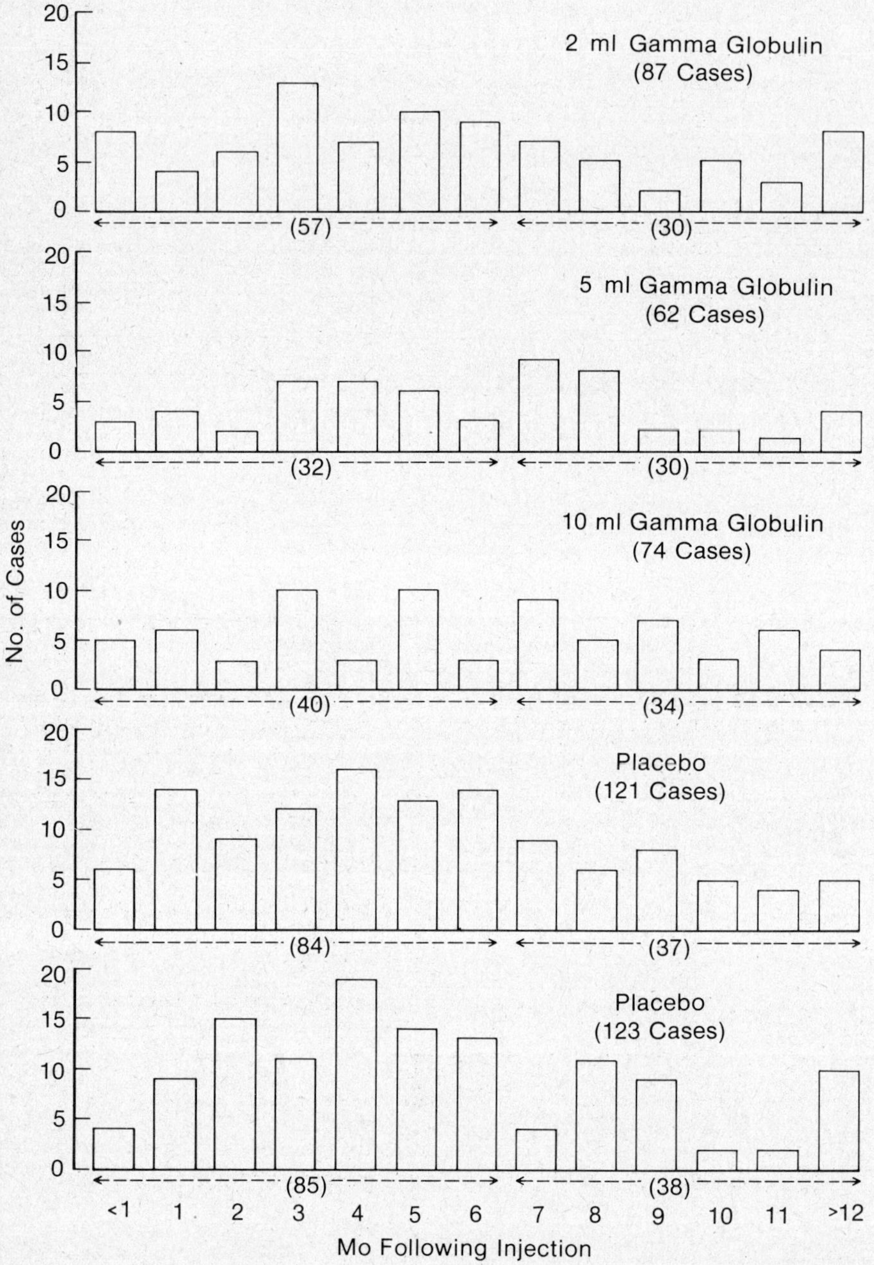

Fig 7.—A lower incidence of hepatitis was observed in soldiers who received gamma globulin. Protection lasted six months. Soldiers who received 5- or 10-ml doses of gamma globulin had less than half the incidence of hepatitis during the six months following injection when compared to control subjects. Two-milliliter doses of gamma globulin provided less protection than larger doses.

cant differences were observed between groups of soldiers who had received either placebo or gamma globulin within six months of the time the diagnosis of hepatitis was established. The protection afforded by gamma globulin during the six months after inoculation with various doses of gamma globulin seemed to be generalized and could not be temporarily related to the dose of gamma globulin. Contrariwise, no significant difference was observed in the incidence of hepatitis among groups of soldiers who had not received an injection for six months; this suggested the gamma globulin provides only passive protection and not passive-active immunity.[4]

A similar mean body weight was observed in soldiers with icteric hepatitis whether they received various doses of gamma globulin or placebo injections; this suggested that the administration of a weight-calculated dose of gamma globulin was relatively unimportant in a military population (Table 9).

Australia Antigen Among Soldiers Developing Icteric Hepatitis in Korea.— A blood specimen was obtained from 211 consecutive admissions with icteric hepatitis to the 121st Evacuation Hospital. The blood was drawn within one week of the onset of icterus and was tested for HAA by both agar gel immunoprecipitation and complement fixation methods. Twenty-five patients (11.8%) were found to have HAA in their serum by a complement fixation technique; ten of these specimens showed a positive reaction by an immunoprecipitation method. Two patients with HAA had received blood transfusions during the previous six months in Vietnam and developed hepatitis two months after assignment to Korea. Among patients without detectable HAA, one developed hepatitis within six months after blood transfusion and became icteric during his third month of assignment to Korea. Among soldiers with and without detectable HAA in their serum, the incidence of hepatitis was significantly less during their first months of assignment overseas than later during their military tour (Fig 8). The effect of the administration of gamma globulin upon the incidence of HAA-positive and HAA-negative icteric hepatitis is shown in Fig 9. Patients who had received either a 5-ml or 10-ml dose of gamma globulin were compared with soldiers who had received injections of the placebo solution. Among 148 patients without demonstrable HAA, the incidence of icteric hepatitis was significantly less in those who had received gamma globulin (52 patients) than among those who had received the albumin solution (96 patients) ($P<.001$). Among the 20 soldiers who developed HAA-positive icteric hepatitis, 4 had received gamma globulin and 16 had received placebo injections. This difference is statistically significant by χ^2 analysis using Yates' correction for continuity ($P=.02$). The only patient with HAA-positive hepatitis who became ill within six months after an injection of gamma globulin had been transfused in Vietnam five months before the onset of jaundice.

Effect of Gamma Globulin Upon Clinical Course of Hepatitis.—The use of a standardized medical history form which included the common symptoms of hepatitis on a checklist permitted a comparison of the frequency of these symptoms in groups of patients who received either various doses of gamma globulin or placebo (Table 8). Comparison of data from patients who received the placebo solution and either 5 ml or 10 ml of gamma globulin showed that a history of chills ($P<.05$), fever ($P<.01$) and yellow skin ($P<.05$) were more frequent complaints of the control subjects than among the soldiers who received gamma globulin. Similarly, albuminuria was more frequent among patients who had received placebo injections ($P<.01$). There was no significant difference in the incidence of other symptoms and physical findings between groups.

Comparison of quantitative data obtained during hospitalization of soldiers of this study for icteric hepa-

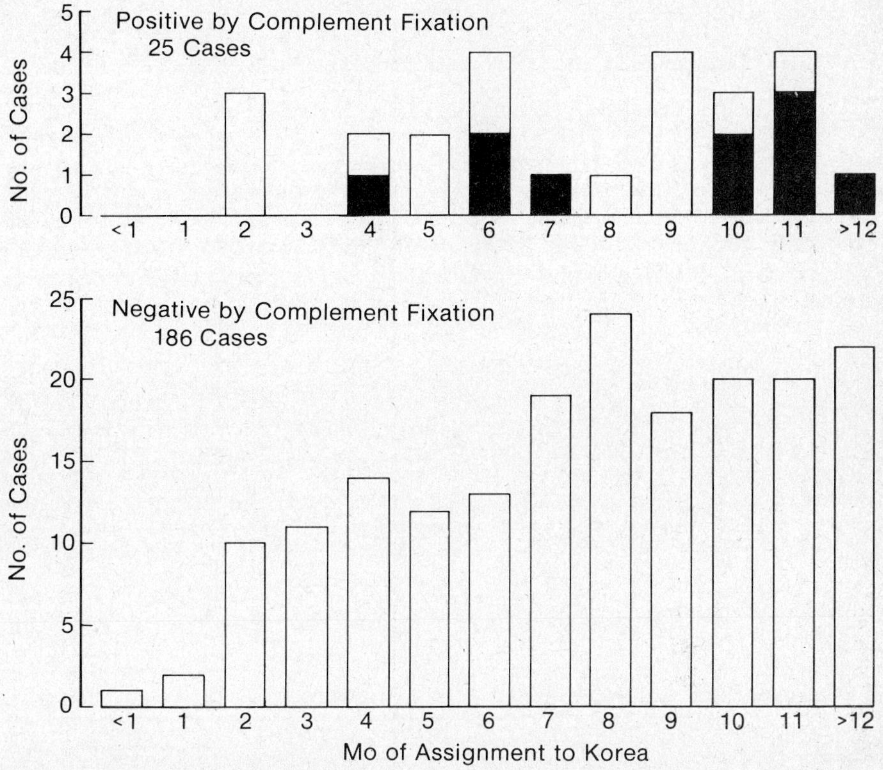

Fig 8.—Sera obtained during the first week of illness from 211 patients with viral hepatitis were tested for Australia antigen (HAA). A complement fixation test was positive for HAA in 12% of patients and 40% of these specimens were positive by the immunodiffusion method (solid portion of bars). *The majority of both HAA-positive and HAA-negative cases of hepatitis occurred after soldiers were assigned to Korea for several months.*

Fig 9.—Comparison of the prevalence of HAA-positive and HAA-negative hepatitis among soldiers who received either 5-ml or 10-ml doses of gamma globulin or placebo solution at intervals following injection. Solid portion of bars show patients positive for HAA by both complement fixation and immunodiffusion methods.

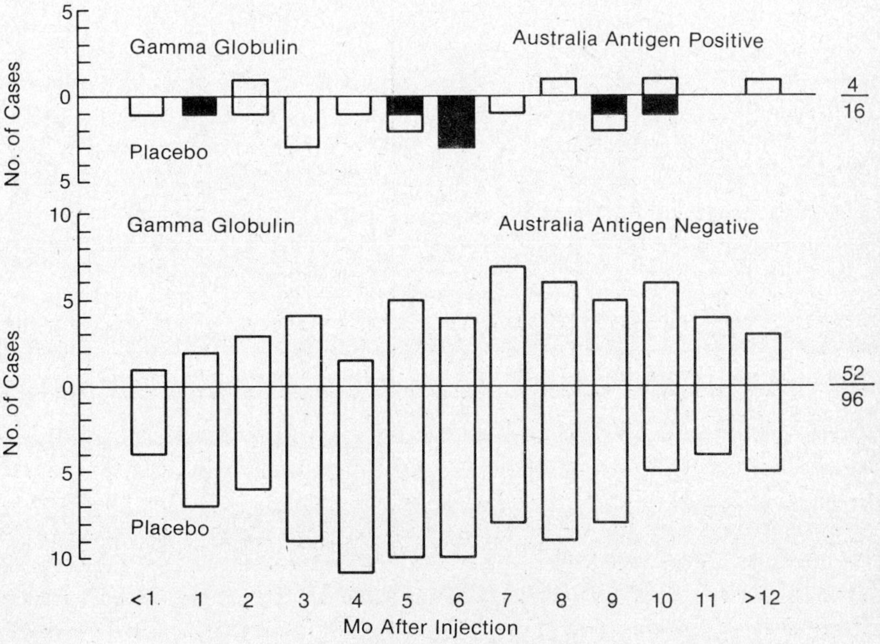

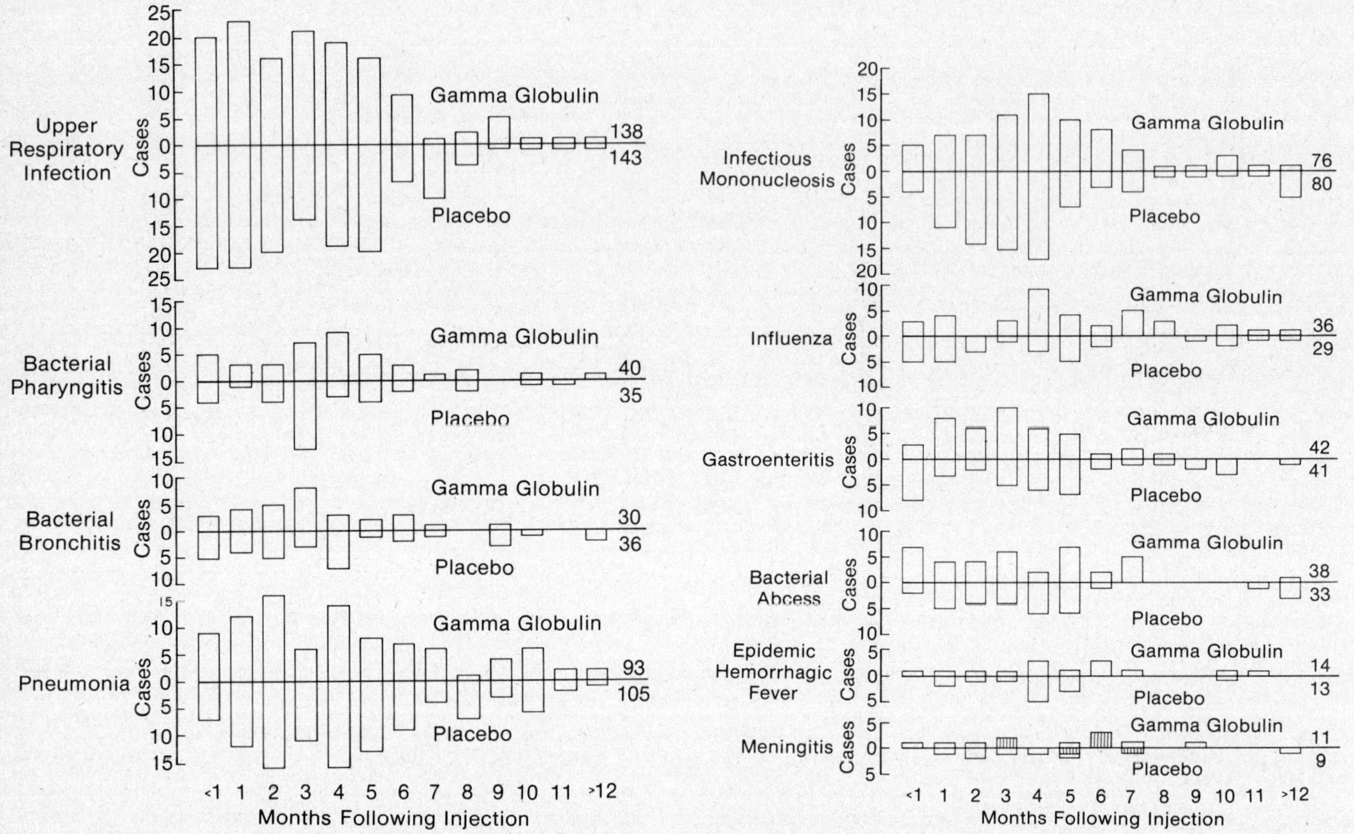

Fig 10.—Left *and* right, *Graphic representation of patients admitted to the hospital with an infectious disease at intervals after receiving either 5 or 10 ml of gamma globulin* (above horizontal line) *or placebo solution* (below). *No significant protection was afforded by gamma globulin prophylaxis. Among meningitis patients, the crosshatched bars show bacterial infections and the remainder are aseptic meningitis.*

titis showed no significant difference between groups injected with placebo solution and either 5 ml or 10 ml of gamma globulin with reference to the length of hospitalization, the duration of symptoms before hospitalization, and the maximal increase in the serum alkaline phosphatase and in hematologic measurements made at the time of admission to the hospital (Table 9). There was a slight but statistically significant increase in the maximal total bilirubin and one-minute direct bilirubin serum measurements in subjects who received placebo injections ($P<.01$). Although mean maximal serum transaminase values were similar in both groups, a statistical comparison could not be made because serum measurements greater than 2,000 units were not quantified and the values were not normally distributed.

Effect of Gamma Globulin Administration Upon the Incidence of Diseases Commonly Encountered in Soldiers.—During the period of this study, the medical records of each military hospital in Korea were periodically examined to detect hospitalized soldiers who had received an injection of the placebo and either 5 or 10 ml of gamma globulin. Figure 10, *left* and *right,* provides a comparison of the incidence of various infectious diseases which occurred in the subjects of this study. Gamma globulin did not significantly reduce the incidence of upper respiratory infections, bacterial pharyngitis, bacterial bronchitis, pneumonia, infectious mononucleosis, influenza, gastroenteritis, bacterial abscess, epidemic hemorrhagic fever, or meningitis. Likewise, there did not seem to be an interval following gamma globulin administration when protection occurred.

Figure 11, *left* and *right,* shows the results of a survey conducted to determine if gamma globulin reduced the incidence of infectious diseases which were treated in outpatient facilities. The clinical diagnosis established at the time the patient was examined was used for these data. The survey included all soldiers examined at the 548th Medical Dispensary during October 1968, February 1969, and April 1969. A comparison was made between soldiers who had received

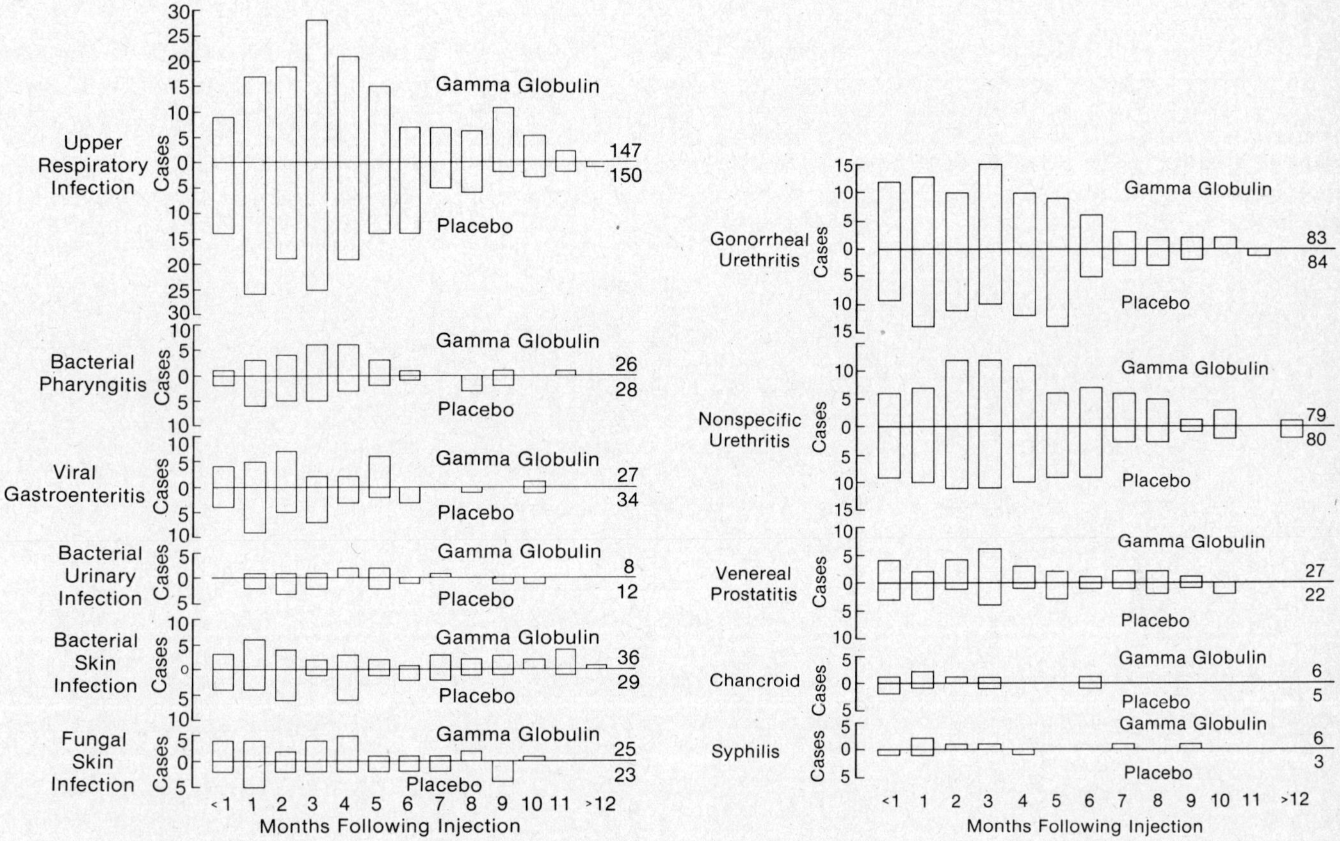

Fig 11.—Left *and* right, *Graphic representation of patients seen on an outpatient basis with various infectious diseases at intervals after receiving either 5 or 10 ml of gamma globulin* (above horizontal line) *or placebo solution* (below horizontal line). *No significant protection was observed for any disease.*

the placebo solution and those who had received either 5 or 10 ml of gamma globulin. Gamma globulin did not significantly reduce the incidence of upper respiratory tract infections, bacterial pharyngitis, nonbacterial gastroenteritis, bacterial urinary tract infections, bacterial or fungal skin infections, and venereal diseases.

Comment

Clinical studies of viral hepatitis contracted by US soldiers stationed in Korea have shown that it is a relatively mild disease.[73,74] Usually, symptoms persist for about two weeks and laboratory studies become normal within one month after the onset of jaundice. Since the Korean war, the mortality from hepatitis has been one death in 4,000 cases. Despite the seemingly benign course of illness among soldiers with viral hepatitis in Korea, clinically recognized cases of anicteric hepatitis (serum bilirubin value < 1.5 mg/100 ml) are uncommon and constitute less than 1% of patients. In part, the low mortality and morbidity of hepatitis in this geographic area may be attributed to the occurrence of this disease in a young, healthy, and well nourished male population. However, a more prolonged illness with a greater mortality has been observed among US soldiers with hepatitis in other geographic areas of the world.

Most US soldiers who are assigned to Korea remain in that geographic location for 13 months and are garrisoned in military compounds where there is careful surveillance and control of their food and water supply. Among these soldiers the incidence of viral hepatitis has varied from three to ten cases per 1,000 per annum during the past ten years.[63] Clinical hepatitis was a relatively uncommon disease among soldiers newly assigned to Korea. We believe that sanitation was responsible for the low incidence of hepatitis during the first four to five months of a soldier's military assignment to Korea and the marked increase in incidence of disease among soldiers who were in Korea for longer intervals was caused by voluntary increased exposure to the local environment during the later portion of a military tour. The relatively

Table 6.—Medical History From Normal Soldiers and Those Who Developed Hepatitis

	Hepatitis Patients (%)	Normal Soldiers (%)
Previous hospitalization	38.69	52.57
Previous hospitalization within six months	1.09	3.17
Blood donor within six months	32.63	25.47
Transfused previously	0.43	1.06
Dental work within six months	44.16	54.26
Immunizations within six months	64.87	76.83
Medications and drugs within six months	24.29	28.46
Previous hepatitis	1.28	1.94

Table 7.—Prophylactic Use of Gamma Globulin in Soldiers Dose of Gamma Globulin and Distribution and Cases of Hepatitis

Human serum gamma globulin (16%) (ml)	10	5	2	0	0
Albumin sucrose potassium glutamate (ml)	0	5	8	10	10
No. of soldiers First injection	21,788	21,392	21,558	21,287	21,778
No. of soldiers Second injection	14,233	13,799	13,921	13,826	14,176
No. of cases of icteric hepatitis	74	62	87	121	123

greater incidence of hepatitis among enlisted men than officers, and junior noncommissioned officers than master sergeants, probably reflects a greater exposure to the local native environment. However, this explanation could not be used to explain the relatively decreased incidence of hepatitis among soldiers who were either black, reared in a large city, or had completed fewer years of schooling because each of these groups had a greater incidence of venereal disease during their military tour in Korea. A plausible explanation is that these groups contained more immune subjects because of greater exposure to hepatitis during childhood. Acceptance of this hypothesis would suggest that there was antigenic similarity between some strains of hepatitis in Korea and the United States.

The clinical symptoms, physical findings, and laboratory studies observed in the patients of this study were qualitatively similar to those reported elsewhere.[73,74] In previously reported studies of US soldiers who developed viral hepatitis in Korea, we observed a greater incidence of splenomegaly, albuminuria, and relapses. These differences were probably caused by dissimilar goals and different methods of performance of each study. The older studies were reports of prospective investigations to document the clinical course and complications of hepatitis in small groups of patients in which the investigators scrutinized each patient for a prolonged interval. On the contrary, the present study was designed primarily to establish the diagnosis of viral hepatitis in a large number of subjects and clinical observations were made by many physicians who were assigned to Korea.

In this study, we believe most of the patients were infected by the oral route. Only a few patients had received blood transfusions during the six months before the development of icterus and there was little evidence by history or physical examination of the parenteral use of narcotics or habituating drugs among the hospitalized soldiers. It seemed unlikely that immunizations or dental work contributed significantly to the prevalence of hepatitis. Disposable hypodermic needles and syringes and pressure sterilization have been used in all military medical facilities during recent years. Surveillance is maintained over shipments of vaccine so that outbreaks of disease could be rapidly traced to their source. Further, in this study there was a similar history of dental work, immunizations, and use of medications among patients with hepatitis and soldiers who did not develop this disease. The finding of HAA in only 12% of serum specimens from patients during the acute stage of disease is significantly less than has been observed in studies of patients with hepatitis in the United States. That this was not caused by the use of less sensitive laboratory methods to detect HAA antigen was shown by our detection of the same number of HAA-positive specimens from aliquots distributed in a national cooperative study that included many of the laboratories which had reported a greater prevalence of HAA-positive hepatitis in their studies of patients. Probably, the number of HAA-positive cases in our studies would have increased if multiple serial serum specimens were obtained from each patient. However, it has been shown that the majority of HAA-positive patients will be detected by examination of a serum specimen obtained during the first few days following the onset of icterus. The detection of HAA-positive sera in 12% of patients in whom a 2% incidence of serum hepatitis was expected based upon the history of recent blood transfusions or parénteral use of drugs is probably due to the oral transmission of the virus which causes the HAA-positive type of hepatitis. In human experimental studies, Krugman and Giles showed that sera containing MS2 agent which produces HAA-positive hepatitis after a long incubation period can be transmitted by the oral administration of infective sera.[51]

The primary goal of the reported study was to determine if commercially produced gamma globulin made from blood donated in the United States protected US soldiers who were stationed abroad from hepatitis. Although previous clinical and experimental studies indicated that the injection of human serum gamma globulin reduced the incidence of hepatitis among recipients, implementation of a widespread program of prophylactic administration of gamma globulin to US soldiers during 1964 in South Vietnam and Korea failed to produce an apparent decrease in the prevalence of hepatitis. Explanations which were considered were that (1) changes in the prevalence of hepatitis among soldiers in these geographic areas disguised protection afforded by gamma globulin and (2) lack of protection by US serum gamma globulin was caused by the existence of antigenically different strains of hepatitis in Asia. Support for the existence of different strains of hepatitis virus include (1) differences in the incubation period of *serum* and *epidemic* hepatitis and the demonstration of HAA antigen in serum from most patients with *serum* hepatitis and few patients with *epidemic* hepatitis,[51] (2) the occasional recurrence of hepatitis in patients who previously had the disease, and (3) demonstration of a variation in the hepatic pathology in different epidemics of infectious hepatitis.[75-77]

Table 8.—Percentage of Patients With Viral Hepatitis in Various Experimental Groups With Symptoms, Physical Findings, and Laboratory Abnormalities That Frequently Occur in Patients With This Disease*

	Gamma Globulin (10 ml)	Gamma Globulin (5 ml)	Gamma Globulin (2 ml)	Placebo	Placebo
Symptoms					
Chills†	15.3	17.0	17.8	24.6	25.4
Fever‡	27.8	17.0	26.2	36.8	39.3
Malaise	82.1	86.6	78.5	87.1	80.5
Anorexia	75.0	93.3	82.2	86.0	82.0
Nausea	59.8	67.8	67.8	68.5	58.3
Vomiting	37.5	42.4	33.4	47.4	37.7
Diarrhea	23.6	20.3	15.5	20.2	14.7
Tobacco distaste	31.9	40.7	36.9	43.8	30.2
Dark urine	93.3	96.8	94.0	94.6	92.6
Light-colored stools	25.0	18.7	23.8	21.0	21.3
Yellow skin†	18.2	18.7	19.1	24.61	30.4
Scleral icterus	65.4	59.4	71.5	79.3	73.0
Physical findings					
Jaundice	96.0	93.8	96.5	96.5	97.5
Hepatomegaly	79.2	78.0	77.5	82.5	74.5
Splenomegaly	5.6	11.8	9.5	5.2	6.5
Lymphadenopathy	1.4	1.7	5.1	3.5	4.1
Laboratory data					
Biluria	98.6	91.6	92.6	94.5	98.5
Albuminuria‡	8.3	10.1	15.5	21.9	16.4

* Data from patients who received the placebo solution was compared with that obtained from patients who received either 5 ml or 10 ml of gamma globulin by χ^2 analysis. Data showing a significant difference is indicated by a single or double dagger.
† $P<.05$.
‡ $P<.01$.

Our study showed that prophylactic injections of serum gamma globulin derived from US-donated blood significantly reduced the incidence of icteric hepatitis in US soldiers stationed in Korea. Intramuscular administration of 2 ml of a 16% solution of human serum gamma globulin at six-month intervals provided significant protection but less than was observed with a 5-ml injection. The use of a larger dose of gamma globulin (10 ml) did not cause a greater reduction in the incidence of icteric viral hepatitis. Prophylactic injection of gamma globulin provided partial protection for about six months. No definite periods of protection were observed during this interval which could be related to the dose of gamma globulin. The marked reduction in the incidence of icteric hepatitis among US soldiers in Korea suggests that certain strains of hepatitis encountered in this geographic area are antigenically similar to those which exist in the United States. On the contrary, the failure to protect 40% of patients during the six months following an injection of 5 or 10 ml of gamma globulin may indicate that strains of hepatitis exist in Korea which are antigenically dissimilar from those which occur in the United States. Alternative hypotheses are that gamma globulin either increases the dose of virus which may be tolerated or it lessens the severity of illness so that many cases are undetected. Data from experimental studies of Krugman favor the latter

Table 9.—Icteric Hepatitis in US Soldiers; Quantitative Data (Mean ± Standard Error)

	10 ml of Gamma Globulin	5 ml of Gamma Globulin	2 ml of Gamma Globulin	Placebo	Placebo
Body weight (lb)	166 ± 3.2	165 ± 2.7	167 ± 2.4	164 ± 2.1	166 ± 2.0
Hospitalization (days)	31.5 ± 1.82	34.0 ± 2.54	35.0 ± 1.80	31.3 ± 1.78	34.4 ± 1.81
Prodrome (days)	6.0 ± 0.55	6.8 ± 0.51	6.5 ± 0.35	6.3 ± 0.35	6.3 ± 0.38
Maximal transaminase value (units)	997 ± 49	949 ± 55	1007 ± 43	1018 ± 37	1001 ± 38
Maximal total bilirubin value (mg/100 ml)	6.4 ± 0.39	6.2 ± 0.44	6.9 ± 0.47	7.4 ± 0.38	6.5 ± 0.32
Maximal direct bilirubin value (mg/100 ml)	3.4 ± 0.24	3.3 ± 0.25	3.6 ± 0.25	4.0 ± 0.22	3.6 ± 0.19
Alkaline phosphatase value (Sigma units)	3.8 ± 0.22	4.5 ± 0.72	4.3 ± 0.37	4.2 ± 0.22	4.0 ± 0.19
White blood cell count (10^3 cells/mm)	6.2 ± 0.21	6.1 ± 0.23	6.2 ± 0.24	5.7 ± 0.15	5.9 ± 0.20
Polymorphonuclear granulocytes (%)	48.9 ± 1.30	51.4 ± 1.09	50.5 ± 1.11	47.3 ± 0.94	49.5 ± 0.90
Lymphocytes (%)	42.1 ± 1.35	41.0 ± 1.15	40.1 ± 1.14	43.4 ± 0.96	41.8 ± 0.94
Hematocrit (%)	46.3 ± 0.37	46.2 ± 0.30	46.2 ± 0.30	46.4 ± 0.25	46.4 ± 0.26

possibility because injections of gamma globulin diminished the incidence of icteric hepatitis but increased the number of cases of anicteric hepatitis in children exposed to hepatitis.[16-18] This possibility was considered during the planning of our study and could have been solved by determination of the incidence of anicteric hepatitis among soldiers who received either gamma globulin or placebo solution. It was not performed because (1) anicteric hepatitis causes little identifiable morbidity among soldiers overseas, (2) biweekly blood analyses from 10,000 soldiers for one year would be necessary to obtain significant data from a population with an incidence of hepatitis of 3 to 5 per 1,000 per year, and (3) these additional studies would triple the cost of the investigation. However, some information can be obtained from scrutiny of the morbidity of hepatitis patients who received either gamma globulin or placebo solution and developed icteric hepatitis. If the administration of serum gamma globulin only diminished the severity of illness without affecting the incidence of anicteric plus icteric hepatitis, a decrease in the morbidity of icteric hepatitis should be observed.

A slight but significant decrease in the occurrence and severity of certain clinical and laboratory findings was observed among patients who received gamma globulin and developed icteric hepatitis when compared to patients who were injected with placebo solution. This suggests that gamma globulin diminishes the morbidity of hepatitis. We believe the lack of magnitude of these differences continues to make the other speculations worthy of continued consideration.

Although relatively few patients with HAA-positive hepatitis were found in this study, statistical analysis indicated that prophylactic administration of gamma globulin provided similar protection to this group of patients as was observed among those with HAA-negative hepatitis. On the contrary, most recent studies of transfusional hepatitis have shown that gamma globulin did not prevent the disease and hepatitis occurred in children who received parenteral doses of MS2 infective sera mixed with gamma globulin but not in experimental subjects given mixtures of MS1 sera and gamma globulin.[51,58-60] An explanation of these seemingly diverse observations is that the protection afforded by gamma globulin is dose related.[56] Prophylactic injections of gamma globulin may reduce the incidence of clinically apparent hepatitis following small oral doses of HAA-positive virus but fail to diminish icteric hepatitis among patients who receive large parenteral infusions. Whereas gamma globulin may not significantly protect patients receiving transfusions of HAA-positive blood, it may be useful in the prevention of hepatitis among close contacts of patients who develop transfusion-induced HAA-positive disease. Another possibility is that the source and quality of the gamma globulin may be an important factor in providing protection. Our gamma globulin was made from blood let from a paid donor population; it was prepared from recently obtained plasma and carefully refrigerated until it was used. Further, it had a high titer for Australia antibody in comparison to other commercial lots of gamma globulin.

Last, the development of a large population in which individuals received either gamma globulin or placebo by random selection permitted an evaluation of the effect of prophylactic injections of gamma globulin upon the prevalence of commonplace infectious diseases. Scrutiny of the hospitalizations of all soldiers included in this study and periodic surveys of outpatient visits showed no diminution in the prevalence of these diseases. This suggests that human serum gamma globulin is not a prophylactic panacea for all infectious diseases and should be reserved for the prevention of specific diseases in which it has been shown to be useful and for replacement therapy in patients with the antibody deficiency syndromes.[78]

This investigation was supported by US Army Medical Research and Development Command with the collaboration of the personnel of the Eighth US Army and the Fifth US Air Force: Project Director: COL Marcel E. Conrad, MC, USA; Immunization Center Director: MSG Allen A. Young; Coordinator with Eighth US Army: LTC Richard L. Park, MC, USA. Members of the Immunization Team were as follows: SSG John Dinger, SP5 Alan R. Gerling, SP5 James M. Bickley, SP5 Robert A. Boykins, SFC Roger L. Tidwell, SFC Thomas L. Petty, SP5 Donald H. Knowles, and SFC Otha L. Dupree. The Australia antigen studies were performed by MAJ William H. Bancroft, MC, USA, and the gamma globulin was characterized by LTC George M. Bernier, MC, USA. Liver biopsy specimens were examined independently by Hans F. Smetana, MD. The Liver Advisory Board to the US Army Medical Research and Development Command provided both advice and support in the planning of this study. The investigations were made possible by the professional and logistical support of the Office of the Surgeon of the Eighth US Army, 121st Evacuation Hospital, 11th Evacuation Hospital, 65th Military Airlift Group, 38th Replacement Battalion, and Sixth Medical Depot. Collation of the data was performed by Sophia W. Tate and Patricia H. Conrad. Studies of gamma globulin for Australia antibody were performed by Lacy R. Overby, PhD.

References

1. Stokes J Jr, Neefe JR: Prevention and attenuation of infectious hepatitis by gamma globulin. *JAMA* **127**:144-145, 1945.
2. Havens WP Jr, Paul JR: Prevention of infectious hepatitis with gamma globulin. *JAMA* **129**:270-272, 1945.
3. Gellis SS, Stokes J Jr, Brother GM, et al: Use of human immune serum globulin (gamma globulin) in infectious (epidemic) hepatitis in Mediterranean Theater of Operations: I. Studies on prophylaxis in two epidemics of infectious hepatitis. *JAMA* **128**:1062-1063, 1945.
4. Stokes J Jr, Farquhar JA, Drake ME, et al: Infectious hepatitis: Length of protection by immune serum globulin (gamma globulin) during epidemics. *JAMA* **147**:714-719, 1951.
5. Capps RB, Bennett AM, Stokes J Jr: Endemic infectious hepatitis in infants' orphanage: I. Epidemiologic studies in student nurses. *Arch Intern Med* **89**:6-23, 1952.
6. Brooks BF, Hsia DY-Y, Gellis S: Family outbreaks of infectious hepatitis: Prophylactic use of gamma globulin. *New Eng J Med* **249**:58-61, 1953.
7. Drake ME, Ming C: Gamma globulin in epidemic hepatitis: Comparative value of two dosage levels, apparently near the minimal effective level. *JAMA* **155**:1302-1305, 1954.
8. Ashley A: Gamma globulin: Effect on secondary attack rates in infectious hepatitis. *New Eng J Med* **250**:412-417, 1954.
9. Hsia DY, Lonsway M Jr, Gellis SS: Gamma globulin in prevention of infectious hepatitis: Studies on use of small doses in family outbreaks. *New Eng J Med* **250**:417-419, 1954.
10. Barondess JA, Drake ME, Bashe WV Jr, et al: Epidemic of infectious hepatitis: Some notes on delineation of high risk groups and protection of exposed susceptibles by gamma globulin. *Arch Intern Med* **95**:633-645, 1955.
11. Krasna V, Radkovsky J, Klouckova A: An evaluation of the efficacy of gamma globulin in the prophylaxis of infectious hepatitis in Prague, 1953-1956. *J Hyg Epidem* **1**:413-422, 1957.
12. Tarantaev TM, Tokar CKH, Kuvshinnikov SM, et al: Seroprophylaxis of infective hepatitis. *Zh Mikrobiol* **30**:9-14, 1959.
13. Fadeeva TL: Serum prophylaxis of infective hepatitis in children's establishments in Rostov on Don. *Zh Mikrobiol* **29**:515-519, 1958.
14. Losonczy GY: Beiträge zur Prävention der epidemischen Hepatitis mittels Gammaglobulins. *Ann Immunol Hungaricae* **3**:134-137, 1960.
15. Stoll K: Epidemiologische Beobachtungen bei Hepatitisfällen in Budapester Kindergemeinschaften mit Hinblick auf die Wirksamkeit des Gamma-globulins. *Ann Immunol Hungaricae* **3**:138-148, 1960.
16. Krugman S, Ward R, Giles JP, et al: Infectious hepatitis: Studies on the effect of gamma globulin and on the incidence of inapparent infection. *JAMA* **174**:823-830, 1960.
17. Krugman S, Ward R: Infectious hepatitis: Current status of prevention with gamma globulin. *Yale J Biol Med* **34**:329-339, 1961-1962.
18. Krugman S: Clinical use of gamma globulin. *New Eng J Med* **269**:195-201, 1963.
19. Cervenka J: Gamma globulin in the prevention of infectious hepatitis, in *European Symposium on Hepatitis*. Geneva, 1963, pp 96-111.
20. Paktoris EA: Aktul'nye voprosy epidemiologii i profilaktiki bolezni Botkina. *Vestn Akad Med Nauk SSSR* **18**:55-66, 1963.
21. Kluge T: Gamma-globulin in the prevention of viral hepatitis, Hoonah, Alaska, 1961. *Amer J Pub Health* **53**:1623-1629, 1963.
22. Aach RD, Elsea WR, Lyerly J, et al: Efficacy of varied doses of gamma globulin during an epidemic of infectious hepatitis, Hoonah, Alaska, 1961. *Amer J Pub Health* **53**:1623-1629, 1963.
23. Paktoris EA, Podsedlovskii TS: Opyt massovoi profilaktiki γ-globulinom epidemicheskogo gepatita v Litovski SSR: I. Diitel' nost' profilakticheskoi aktivnosti γ-globulina pri epidemicheskom gepatite. *Zh Mikrobiol* **4**:112-116, 1964.
24. Szmuness W: Bewertungsversuch der Wirksamkeit einzelner, bei der Bekaempfung der Hepatitis epidemica angewendeten Massnahmen. *Zbl Bakt (Orig)* **194**:161-182, 1964.
25. Szmuness W: Skuetecznosc globuliny gamma w zwalczaniu wirusowego zapalenia watroby. *Tyg Lek* **19**:1734-1736, 1964.
26. Yarrow A: Infective hepatitis in a rural school: The use of gamma globulin. *Lancet* **1**:485-487, 1964.
27. Zak MR, Sheinbergas MM, Moteyunas LI, et al: O vyyavlenii subklinicheskikh form epidemicheskogo gepatita (bolezn' Botkina) v ochage pri profilaktike gamma-globulinom. *Zh Mikrobiol* **41**:31-34, 1964.
28. Noble HB, Peterson DR: Evaluation of immune serum globulin for control of infectious hepatitis. *Public Health Rep* **80**:172-177, 1964.
29. Fiabane L, Targon A: La profilassi dell' epatite viral con gamma-globuline in una comunita infantile. *Ann Sclavo* **7**:440-444, 1965.
30. Podsedlovskii TS, Paktoris EA: Opyt massovoi profilaktiki γ-globulinom epidemicheskogo gepatita v Litovskoi SSR: II. Sravnitel' nye dannye po effektivnosti razlichnykh doz i metodov profilaktiki γ-globulinom epidemicheskogo gepatita. *Zh Mikrobiol* **42**:61-66, 1965.

31. Zibitsker DE, Kieselev AV: Provedenie planovoi profilaktiki bolezni Botkina γ-globulinom s uchetom prodoizhitel' nosti sozdavaemogo immuniteta. *Zh Mikrobiol* **43**:116-122, 1965.

32. Zikitsker DE: Oprofilaktike γ-globulinom bolezni Botkina i drugikh infektsionnykh zabolevanii (V poryadke obsuzhdeniya). *Zh Mikrobiol* **43**:57-61, 1965.

33. Keen TEB: Prophylactic use of gamma globulin infectious hepatitis: A survey in general practice in Victoria. *Med J Aust* **52**:135-139, 1965.

34. Fiabane L, Targon A: La profilassi dell' epatite viral con gamma-globuline in una comunita infantile. *Ann Sclavo* **7**:440-444, 1965.

35. Borg LG: Immune gamma globulin as a control for infectious hepatitis in Bolivia (man). *Milt Med* **130**:389-392, 1965.

36. Klots VI, Babayants RA, Sultanov AS, et al: Opyt profilaktiki epidemicheskogo gepatita gamma-globulinom u detei v vozraste 5 mesyatev—7 let. (Po materialam Andizhanskoi oblasti). *Med Zh Uzb* **5**:69-70, 1966.

37. Spotarenko SS, Paktoris EA: Itogi opytov po ratsional' nomu ispol' zovaniyu γ-globulina v profilaktike infetsionnogo gepatita. *Zh Mikrobiol* **43**:52-56, 1966.

38. Estrin BM, Nikolaevskaya AD, Tverdokhlebova VA, et al: Opyt profilaktiki infektsionnogo gepatita gamma-globulinom. *Vrach Delo* **8**:143-144, 1967.

39. Khramova LP: Opyt massovoi profilaktiki gammaglobulinom epidemicheskogo gepatita. *Zh Mikrobiol* **44**:127-129, 1967.

40. Burlai VV: Gamma-globulinoprofilaktika infektsionnogo gepatita. *Vrach Delo* **7**:128-129, 1967.

41. Spotarenko SS: Otdalennye rezul' taty massovogo primeneniya gamma-globulina kak metoda profilaktiki epidemicheskogo gepatita. *Zh Mikrobiol* **44**:58-62, 1967.

42. Shteinbakh AE, Lapin NN, Shevchenko EM, et al: K otsenke effektivnosti protivoepidemicheskikh i profilakticheskikh meropriyatii pri bolezni Botknia. *Zh Mikrobiol* **45**:7-11, 1968.

43. Pollock TM, Reid D: Assessment of British gammaglobulin in preventing infectious hepatitis: A report of the Director of the Public Health Laboratory Service. *Brit Med J* **3**:451-454, 1968.

44. Spotarenko SS, Karon BI: O deistvii γ-globulina pri infektsionnom gepatite. *Zh Mikrobiol* **45**:66-69, 1968.

45. Mosley JW, Reisler DM, Brachott D, et al: Comparison of two lots of immune serum globulin for prophylaxis of infectious hepatitis. *Amer J Epidemiol* **87**:539-550, 1968.

46. Pille ER, Spotarenko SS, Itselis FG, et al: Epidemiologicheskaya effektivnost' malkyh doz gamma-globulina pri infektsionnom gepatite. *Zh Mikrobiol* **45**:35-41, 1968.

47. Masar I, Pucekova G, Stukovsky R: Rodinny vyskyt infekonej hepatitidy v podraienkach profylaxie gamaglobulinom. *Cesk Epidemiol* **17**:257-269, 1968.

48. Woodson RD, Clinton JJ: Hepatitis prophylaxis abroad: Effectiveness of immune serum globulin in protecting Peace Corps volunteers. *JAMA* **209**:1053-1058, 1969.

49. Pollock TM, Reid D: Immunoglobulin for the prevention of infectious hepatitis in persons working overseas. *Lancet* **1**:281-283, 1969.

50. Masar I, Pucekova G, Stukovsky L: Analyza gamaglobulinovej profylaxie v ohniskach infekcnej hepatitidy. *Cesk Epidemiol* **18**:325-336, 1969.

51. Krugman S, Giles JP: Viral hepatitis: New light on an old disease. *JAMA* **212**:1019-1029, 1970.

52. Silverberg M, Neumann PZ: Infectious hepatitis: Gamma-globulin prophylaxis in a community outbreak. *Amer J Dis Child* **119**:117-121, 1970.

53. Grossman EB, Stewart SC, Stokes J: Post-transfusion hepatitis in battle casualties and study of its prophylaxis by means of human immune serum globulin. *JAMA* **129**:991-994, 1945.

54. Duncan GG, Christian HA, Stokes J Jr, et al: An evaluation of immune serum globulin as a prophylactic agent against homologous serum hepatitis. *Amer J Med Sci* **213**:53-57, 1947.

55. Mirick GS, Ward R, McCollum RW: Modification of post-transfusion hepatitis by gamma globulin. *New Eng J Med* **273**:59-65, 1965.

56. Kawakami K: Clinical study on prevention of serum hepatitis gamma-globulin administration in large amount. *Bull Kobe Med Coll* **28**:66-77, 1966.

57. Drake ME, Barondess JA, Bashe WJ Jr, et al: Failure of convalescent gamma globulin to protect against homologous serum hepatitis. *JAMA* **152**:690-693, 1953.

58. Holland PV, Rubinson RM, Morrow AG, et al: γ-Globulin in the prophylaxis of posttransfusion hepatitis. *JAMA* **196**:471-474, 1966.

59. Elblom L, Olsson P, Aberg T: The effect of gammaglobulin in prevention of fibrinogen transmitted hepatitis. *Acta Chir Scand* **133**:351-354, 1967.

60. A Cooperative Study: Prevention of posttransfusion hepatitis by γ-globulin: Preliminary report. *JAMA* **214**:140-142, 1970.

61. Shulman NR, Hirschman RJ, Barker LF: Viral hepatitis. *Ann Intern Med* **72**:257-269, 1970.

62. *Infectious Hepatitis Control,* circular 40-l. Department of the Army, 1964.

63. *Health of the Army,* 1950 to 1968. Department of the Army, vol 5 to 23.

64. *Infectious Hepatitis Control,* circular 40-31. Department of the Army, 1966.

65. Conrad ME: Infectious hepatitis in military populations: Problems encountered with gamma globulin prophylaxis. *Bull NY Acad Med* **45**:167-180, 1969.

66. Blumberg BS, Sutnick AI, London WT: Hepatitis and leukemia: Their relation to Australia antigen. *Bull NY Acad Med* **44**:1566-1586, 1968.

67. Prince AM: An antigen detected in the blood during the incubation period of serum hepatitis. *Proc Nat Acad Sci* **60**:814-821, 1968.

68. Purcell RH, Holland PV, Walsh JH, et al: A complement-fixation test for measuring Australia antigen and antibody. *J Infect Dis* **120**:383-386, 1969.

69. Mosley JW, Brachott D: Variations in effectiveness of gamma globulin preparations for prophylaxis against infectious hepatitis, in Merler E (ed): *Immunoglobulins: Biologic Aspects and Clinical Uses.* National Academy of Science, 1970, pp 234-243.

70. Mancini G, Vaerman PP, Carbonara AO, et al: A single radial-diffusion method for the immunological quantification of proteins: Protides of the biological fluids, in Peeters H (ed): *Proceedings of the 12th Colloquium.* Amsterdam, Elsevier, 1964, pp 370-373.

71. Sgouris JT: Stability of immunoglobulin G preparation. *Fed Proc* **25**:726, 1966.

72. Connell GE, Painter RH: Fragmentation of immunoglobulin during storage. *Canad J Biochem* **44**:371-379, 1966.

73. Conrad ME, Schwartz FD, Young AA: Infectious hepatitis: A generalized disease: A study of renal gastrointestinal and hematologic abnormalities. *Amer J Med* **37**:789-801, 1964.

74. Conrad ME, Weintraub LR, Schwartz FD, et al: Viral hepatitis in Korea: Clinical observations and studies performed during prospective studies to obtain specimens for virologic culture, in Popper H, Schaffner F (ed): *Progress in Liver Diseases.* New York, Grune & Stratton, 1965, vol 2, pp 395-415.

75. Smetana HF: Pathology of hepatitis, in Schiff L (ed): *Diseases of the Liver,* ed 2. Philadelphia, JB Lippincott Co, 1963, pp 369-424.

76. Gupta DN, Smetana HF: The histopathology of viral hepatitis as seen in the Dehli epidemic (1955-56). *Indian J Med Res* **45**(suppl):101-113, 1957.

77. Dubin IN, Sullivan BH Jr, Legolvan PC, et al: The cholestatic form of viral hepatitis: Experiences with viral hepatitis at Brooke Army Hospital during the years 1951 to 1953. *Amer J Med* **29**:55-72, 1960.

78. Janeway CA, Rosen FS, Merler E, et al: *The Gamma Globulins.* Boston, Little Brown & Co, 1967, pp 97-113.

Granulomatous Bowel (Crohn's) Disease

A Retrospective Study of the Course and Treatment

Hans Fromm, MD; Frederick A. Wilson, MD;
John B. Rodgers, Jr., MD; and
John A. Balint, MB, MRCP, Albany, NY

Ninety-two patients had regional enteritis or granulomatous colitis, or both. The variable nature of this disease and the difficulty of evaluating therapy are illustrated by patient summaries. Site and extent of bowel involvement at the time of diagnosis did not influence prognosis. Mortality, operation rate, and number of complications were similar in steroid and nonsteroid treated patients when they were matched retrospectively by age, sex, site, and extent of disease. An actuarial analysis of results of surgical therapy suggested a higher risk of recurrence and consequent further resection after each additional major operation. Presence of Crohn's disease indicated need for supportive medical care. If this fails steroid therapy should be given a trial. Surgical intervention should be reserved for patients with mandatory surgical indication and those with incapacitating symptoms which have failed to respond to medical therapy.

In 1932 Crohn et al[1] first described the clinical and pathological picture of "regional ileitis" as a distinct entity. Since then, many studies of this disease have appeared in the medical literature.[2,3] However, our knowledge about the etiology of this disorder remains speculative.[4,5] The treatment of regional enteritis is still empirical and symptomatic; opinions as to the effectiveness of various treatments differ widely.[6,10] The purpose of this paper is to examine the results and complications of medical and surgical treatment in a group of patients with regional enteritis. The variable nature of the disease and the difficulty of evaluating treatment is stressed, and illustrative case reports are presented.

Methods

All of the 92 patients seen at the Albany Medical Center Hospital between January 1960 and December 1968 whose studies met established histologic, radiologic, or surgical criteria[5,11] for the diagnosis of regional enteritis are included in this evaluation. The diagnosis of granulomatous bowel disease was made in 62 patients from histological sections of resected bowel. Of these the complete histological picture with noncaseating granulomata containing epitheloid, mononuclear, and Langhans giant cells was found in 29 cases. In 33 patients the histological diagnosis was based on the findings of transmural inflammation with lymphocytes and monocytes in association with deep fissures and fistula formation but without granulomata being observed. Skip areas of normal intervening mucosa between areas of diseased bowel were also generally noted in these cases. In 14 of the remaining cases, regional enteritis was diagnosed on the basis of finding an inflamed, edematous, and thickened segment of bowel during an exploratory laparotomy. Thirteen cases were diagnosed on the basis of typical clinical and radiological features of this disease.[2-11] Three cases included in this series fulfilling the criteria for granulomatous colitis[12,13] were found after reviewing the medical records of all 165 patients with a diagnosis of ulcerative colitis treated at the Albany Medical Center Hospital during this same period.

Eighty patients (87%) were followed from the time of diagnosis to the end of 1968. Seventy-two patients were followed by sending questionnaires to them and to their physicians in 1967 and again in 1968. Questionnaires completed by the patients provided information about their latest physical condition, working ability, and present treatment, whereas questionnaires completed by the physicians gave additional information about new radiologic findings and laboratory data. Completed questionnaires on 41 patients were obtained from their physicians, 19 more from the patients, and 12 more from both the patients and their physicians. Eight patients are still being followed by the authors. The average patient follow-up was 6.6 years (range, one month to 41 years) since the time of diagnosis and 17 years (range, 1 to 42 years) since the onset of symptoms. The anatomical site and extent of granulomatous bowel involvement at the time of diagnosis were correlated with mortality and incidence of major bowel operations per 100 person-years of observation. Extent of regional enteritis was graded by the number of bowel segments involved as evident by roentgenogram or surgical exploration, or both. Jejunum, ileum, ascending colon, transverse colon, descending colon, and rectosigmoid were each counted as one segment. There were only two patients in whom the duodenum was involved as well as the jejunum and ileum, and in one of these the stomach was affected in addition to the other segments of small bowel. These two were evaluated as patients with two segments involved.

An evaluation of steroid treatment was attempted by retrospective matching of steroid-treated patients with a group of patients who did not receive steroids. The patients were matched by age, sex, and site and extent of disease at the time of diagnosis. Patients who had one major bowel operation (intestinal resection, bypass, or change of bowel continuity) before steroid treatment were matched with nonsteroid-treated patients who had at least one major operation. The matched groups were examined for the incidence of deaths, major operations (after starting steroid therapy), and complications during the entire time of follow-up per 100 person years of observation. Incidences of the following

Received for publication June 21, 1971; accepted Aug 6.

From the Department of Medicine, Division of Gastroenterology, Albany Medical College, Albany, NY.

Reprint requests to Department of Medicine, Division of Gastroenterology, Albany Medical College, Albany, NY 12208 (Dr. Balint).

complications were determined: fistula and abscess formation, perforation, peritonitis, infections, and peptic ulcer.

In addition to evaluating steroid therapy, an effort was made to assess the success of surgery. This was done by determining the risk a patient faced of requiring another major surgical procedure following an attempt at surgical management of this disease. The risk of having another major surgical procedure after each major operation was examined by an actuarial analysis. To make maximum use of the operative experience of this study, a cohort approach using person years at risk was employed. The probability of surviving successive years without an additional operation was estimated by relating the number of "new" operations to the number of person years at risk. For this analysis the first, second, and third major operation of all patients were used which were performed between 1960 and 1968.

Results

The site and extent of regional enteritis in the 92 subjects were estimated by radiologic examination and from operative findings. Fifty-five patients had barium contrast studies, both of the upper intestine (including the small bowel) and of the large intestine. In 44 of these, radiologic findings were confirmed by a laparotomy. Twenty-three additional patients had one radiologic study of either the upper intestine (small bowel) or large bowel. In 21 of these, the radiologic diagnosis was confirmed by laparotomy. The anatomical bowel involvement of the remaining 14 patients who had no serial x-rays of the upper gastrointestinal tract was determined by exploratory laparotomy. Sigmoidoscopy was performed in 51 of the 92 patients during their stay in the hospital. In 19 of these, the rectum was reported to show an inflamed, granular, edematous, and friable mucosa which was apparently difficult to distinguish from idiopathic ulcerative colitis. In five patients a rectal biopsy was obtained and showed nonspecific inflammation in four cases and granuloma formation in one.

In 40 patients evidence of granulomatous disease was confined to the small bowel, with ileal involvement alone in 32 and disease in ileum and jejunum in 6. Two other patients showed in addition disease of the duodenum with apparent gastric lesions in one of these (Table 1). Forty-seven patients had evidence of both small and large bowel disease. In three of these patients, the large bowel disease was at first confined to the rectum but involved the colon after resection of diseased ileum and ileotransverscolostomy had been performed for ileitis. In five patients the granulomatous changes appeared to be limited to the colon. In four of these, the diagnosis was based on the barium contrast studies of the colon and on histological examination of surgically resected specimens. During surgical exploration no evidence of small bowel involvement was found in these four patients. No evidence of recurrent disease was found in these four patients at follow-up two to nine years later.

The age of onset of the first symptoms of regional enteritis in 89 patients ranged from 3 to 68 years, with a mean of 30.7 years. In three patients the age of onset of the disease was unknown. The figure demonstrates the interval between onset of symptoms and time of diagnosis of regional enteritis. In almost a quarter of the patients, unexplained gastrointestinal symptoms were present for more than five years before the diagnosis of regional enteritis was established.

Table 2 shows the clinical findings in this group of patients. Abdominal pain and diarrhea were the most frequent symptoms, followed by weight loss, anemia, nausea, vomiting, fever and gastrointestinal bleeding. Splenomegaly was found in three patients. The incidence of these symptoms was similar in patients whose disease was apparently limited to the small bowel and in those with documented disease of both large and small bowel.

Sixty-six patients suffered 130 local and systemic complications (Table 3). The remaining 26 patients escaped such additional problems. The incidence of the different complications was similar in patients with small bowel disease only and those with both the small and large bowel involved, except for iritis which occurred only in patients with involvement of the colon. One patient developed a polypoid adenocarcinoma at the site of the enterocolostomy. Two patients with granulomatous colitis developed toxic megacolon.

Of the total of 92 patients, 81 underwent at least one surgical procedure (see below). Only 11 patients were managed by medical means alone. Medical therapy consisted of various combinations of rest, bland diet, replacement of fluids, electrolytes, blood and albumin as indicated, antidiarrheal and spasmolytic agents, nonabsorbable sulfonamides, systemic antibiotics, and supplementation with iron and cyanocobalamin. Steroid therapy used in 40 patients was usually started with administration of prednisone at a dose of 60 to 80 mg orally per day and later tapered to approximately 10 to 15 mg per day and discontinued after six to eight weeks. Because evaluation of steroid treatment in a retrospective study is difficult due to lack of good control data, an attempt was made to match steroid-treated patients with ones who did not receive steroids. Twenty-one of 40 steroid-treated patients of whom 13 had no major operation before the start of steroid therapy and 8 who had had one major operation prior to the start of steroid treatment were matched restrospectively with 21 comparable nonsteroid-treated patients. The total duration of steroid treatment in these 21 patients was one to six months in 12 patients and more than one year (range, one to seven years) in 9 patients. Table 4 summarizes the calculated prognosis of the matched patient groups in terms of mortality, incidence of major operations, and complications per 100 person years of follow-up. No significant differences were found in respect to any of these indexes between the two groups of patients.

The following patient summaries further document spontaneous fluctuations in the course of Crohn's disease and emphasize the difficulty in evaluating the results of steroid therapy in a retrospective study:

Patient 1 was a white woman with Sjorgren's syndrome and erythema nodosum who presented with fever, diarrhea, and severe crampy, abdominal pain. Radiographs revealed marked narrowing of the terminal ileum. She was treated with 60 mg of prednisone per day orally. The patient responded well symptomatically and steroids were gradually tapered and then stopped after six months' therapy. Despite symptomatic improvement progression of segmental involvement to various parts of the colon was demonstrated radiologically. Because the patient was clinically well despite radiographic evidence of advancing disease, steroids were not resumed and the patient continued to be essentially asymptomatic. Fifteen months after discontinuance of prednisone, radiologic studies of the small intestine showed no further significant changes. However, another barium enema showed remarkable improvement of the colon with disappearance

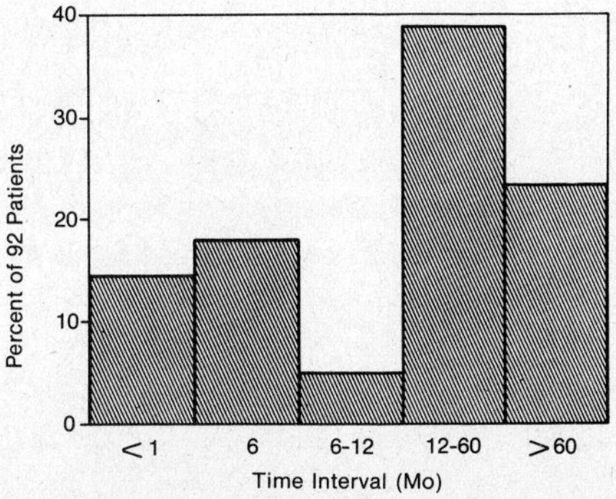

Time interval between onset of symptoms and diagnosis of granulomatous bowel disease in 92 patients.

of all evidence of disease. The terminal ileum still appeared to be narrowed, and changes diagnostic of regional ileitis were still present two years later when the patient had an elective hysterectomy for an unrelated problem. In summary this patient improved symptomatically on steroid treatment although x-ray examination revealed evidence of further progression of bowel disease. After discontinuation of steroids the patient remained asymptomatic and later x-ray studies demonstrated greatly diminished involvement of the large bowel by this disease process.

Patient 2 was a 47-year-old white woman who underwent an exploratory laparotomy for abdominal pain five years after roentgenograms had shown changes consistent with Crohn's disease of the terminal ileum. Exploration revealed inflammatory involvement of the entire small bowel. No resection was performed. A mesenteric lymph node biopsy showed a single foreign body type granuloma. After six years of medical treatment without steroids, the patient underwent a subtotal gastrectomy and gastrojejunostomy for a bleeding gastric ulcer. During this operation there was no small bowel disease detectable, except for the inflammation of the terminal ileum. Following this procedure the patient remained symptomatic and at the age of 61 years, 14 years after the initial laparotomy, she had a right ileocolectomy for partial small bowel obstruction and fistula formation to the anterior abdominal wall. The resected ileum and ascending colon exhibited extensive chronic and acute ulcerating enteritis. Three months later the patient died in septic shock following a protracted course of increasing diarrhea and right lower quadrant abdominal pain. The autopsy revealed 4,500 cc of fibropurulent fluid in the peritoneal cavity and a 1.0 × 0.5 cm, dome-shaped, polypoid, well differentiated mucin-producing adenocarcinoma, 1 cm distal to the enterocolostomy. No metastases were found. The microscopic sections of the enterocolostomy, gastrojejunostomy, and mesenteric lymph nodes showed foreign body type granulomata. Here again evidence of spontaneous fluctuation of the extent of granulomatous bowel disease is demonstrated.

Patient 3 was a 31-year-old white man who entered the hospital with evidence of intestinal obstruction, carpopedal spasm, and positive Trousseau's and Chvostek's signs. The patient had a five-year history of intermittent, mild abdominal pain and diarrhea. One year prior to admission an x-ray examination revealed marked changes consistent with regional enteritis of the entire small bowel including the duodenum. On admission, three positional films of the abdomen revealed multiple loops of distended small bowel with air-fluid levels. On sigmoidoscopic examination the rectal mucosa appeared beefy red, granular, and friable. A perirectal fistula was present. Barium enema demonstrated abnormalities of the terminal ileum consistent with regional enteritis.

The laboratory values obtained were as follows: serum potassium, 2.9 mEq/liter; serum calcium, 2.8 mEq/liter; serum magnesium, 0.77 mEq/liter; total serum protein, 6.9 gm/100 ml; and serum albumin, 3.1 gm/100 ml. After intravenous replacement of fluids, potassium, calcium, and magnesium, the patient recovered dramatically with a return of normal bowel function, and no further tetany was observed. The patient has since done well over a follow-up period of 18 months with a 40-lb weight gain and the ability to work full-time. Treatment has consisted of only parenterally administered vitamin D and cyanocobalamin and a low-fat (50-gm) diet. Roentgenograms one year after discharge from the hospital showed evidence of improvement of the jejunum and ileum and a normal appearing duodenum. This patient is presented as another example of spontaneous improvement of granulomatous bowel disease while receiving very conservative medical treatment without steroid therapy. Symptoms and signs of intestinal obstruction were successfully treated by correction of electrolyte and fluid depletion.

Review of the medical records of the surgically treated patients in this series show that the indications for operations were as follows in order of frequency: intractable abdominal pain and diarrhea, intestinal obstruction, abdominal mass, abscess of fistula, perirectal disease, and severe abdominal pain of unknown origin; possible intestinal carcinoma and gastrointestinal bleeding were also indications for surgery in a few cases.

Only 11 patients had no operations, whereas 81 patients underwent a total of 193 major and minor operations. Twenty-nine patients had more than one major operation. Of the 193 surgical procedures, 115 represented major operations with bowel resection, colostomy, ileostomy, or bypass of the diseased bowel. The remaining 78 operations were either for incision and drainage of abscess or fistulae or exploratory laparotomies without intestinal resection or bypass. The chance of not having another operation after each major operation was examined by actuarial analysis. The chance of surviving five years without another major operation was 17% lower after two operations than after one (Table 5). This difference between the two groups (one and two operations at the start, respectively) approximately met the criteria for independence but was not significant at the 5% level. These findings suggested that there may exist a patient group with a high risk of having repeated operations. Features of the disease in its presurgical stages which might correlate with the number of surgical procedures in the subsequent course of the disease were therefore sought. We examined the following features occurring before the first operation in patients who had one, two, or three operations: sex; age at time of first operation; duration of symptoms before the first operation; extent of disease; presence of anemia, hypoalbuminemia, or both; systemic manifestations; weight loss; treatment with corticosteroids; and completeness of follow-up. No statistically significant differences were found in the occurrence of these features among the patients with one, two, or three operations. However, the average age at time of the first operation and the duration of symptoms before the first operation showed a tendency to increase with the number of operations. Patients who had three operations were an average of seven years older and had symptoms for two years longer at the time of their first operation than patients who had only one operation. Further studies may clarify these differences.

Table 1.—Anatomical Involvement

No. of Patients	Site of Involvement
32	Ileum
6	Ileum + jejunum
1	Ileum + jejunum + duodenum
1	Ileum + jejunum + duodenum + stomach
5	Colon
47	Small intestine + colon

Table 2.—Incidence of Symptoms and Signs in 92 Patients With Regional Enteritis

	In 40 Patients With Small Bowel Disease (%)	In 47 Patients With Small and Large Bowel Disease (%)	In 5 Patients With Large Bowel Disease Only (%)
Abdominal pain	88	81	100
Diarrhea	75	81	100
Weight loss	55	64	40
Anemia	38	49	40
Nausea, vomiting	50	38	20
Fever	35	42	60
Minor gastrointestinal bleeding	28	25	80
Major gastrointestinal bleeding	3	14	20
Abdominal mass	20	10	20
Constipation	15	14	20
Anorexia	15	12	0
Hepatomegaly	10	4	0
Fatigue	8	8	0
Splenomegaly	8	0	0

Of the 64 patients who were treated by at least one major abdominal operation, four went on to repeated bowel resections causing a short bowel syndrome. The remaining small bowel length in these four patients ranged between 41 and 228 cm, and the large bowel length varied from 5 to 25 cm. Three patients with a short bowel syndrome are still alive and doing well. One patient with a short bowel syndrome died at the age of 47 years in septic shock.[14] Four patients died shortly after operation: two at the age of 36 and 62 years, respectively, from bronchopneumonia, one at the age of 61 years from a subphrenic abscess, and one at the age of 58 following a severe wound infection. Three other patients died more than 90 days after surgery. One of these died at the age of 42 years from a cerebrovascular accident following severe dehydration; another died at the age of 61 of sepsis and was incidentally found to have an adenocarcinoma of the colon, and the third patient died from a metastatic ovarian carcinoma at the age of 52. Thus, a total of eight patients in this series died after an attempt at surgical therapy.

The site and extent of the disease was correlated with the incidence of major bowel operations and mortality per 100 person years of observation since the time of diagnosis. As Table 6 depicts, the prognosis in terms of operation rate and mortality was similar in patients who had only small bowel disease and in those who had both small and large bowel involvement. Also, the number of bowel segments involved at the time of diagnosis did not seem to influence significantly the prognosis for the patient. The average number of operations was about 20 and the average mortality between 1 and 2 per 100 person years irrespective of site and extent of the disease at the time of diagnosis.

Table 3.—Main Local and Systemic Complications Found in 66 Out of 92 Patients With Regional Enteritis

	% of 92 Patients
Local	
Fistulae	
Total	34.8
Anal and perirectal	17.4
Enterocutaneous	10.9
Internal	9.8
Rectovaginal	4.3
Enterovaginal	3.3
Abscesses	
Total	29.3
Anal and perirectal	14.1
Abdominal wall	6.5
Mesentery	6.5
Pelvic	5.4
Hip	2.1
Stricture of rectum	2.2
Toxic dilatation of colon	2.2
Systemic	
Total	42.4
Arthritis	25.0
Malabsorption	25.0
Erythema nodosum	4.3
Iritis	2.2

Table 4.—Retrospective Comparison of Prognosis of Matched* Patients Treated With and Without Steroids

	Steroids Given Before a Major Operation†	No Steroids Given Before a Major Operation	Steroids Given After One Major Operation‡	No Steroids Given After One Major Operation
No. of patients	13	13	8	8
Average length of patient follow-up§ (yr)	4.5	9.2	9.0	9.9
No. of deaths‖	0	0	0	1.3
Incidence of major operations	18.9‖	13.4‖	2.8¶	2.5¶
Incidence of complications during time of follow-up	15.5	10.9	4.2	3.8

* Matched by age at time of diagnosis, sex, site, and extent of disease at time of diagnosis.
† Nine patients received steroids for one to six months and four for more than one year (range, one to six years).
‡ Three patients received steroids for one to six months and five for more than one year (range one to seven years).
§ Refers to length of follow-up since the time of diagnosis.
‖ Numbers refer to incidence per 100 person-years of follow-up as described in the text.
¶ Refers to incidence of major operations per 100 person-years after first major operation.

Table 5.—Chance of Surviving Five Years Without Another Operation in Relation to Number of Previous Operations

No. of previous operations at start of analysis*	1	2	3
No. of patients at start of analysis	47	24	12
Number of operations during next five years	13	10	5
Percent chance of surviving five years without another operation	63	46	41

* Refers to all first, second, and third major operations of this series performed in the time period between 1960 and 1968.

Table 6.—Anatomical Involvement and Prognosis of Patients

	Site of Involvement						
	Small Bowel		Large Bowel	Small and Large Bowel			
Extent of Involvement	1*	2	4	2	3	4	5
No. of patients	32	8	5	24	9	8	6
No. of person-years followed since diagnosis	124	82	18	220	54	58	54
No. of operations per 100 person-years	21.0	19.5	22.0	12.7	25.9	24.1	25.9
No. of deaths per 100 person-years	1.6	2.4	0	0.5	1.9	3.5	0

* Numbers refer to number of bowel segments involved.

† One patient had in addition to ileum and jejunum the duodenum involved and one other patient additional involvement of the stomach.

‡ All five patients with disease confined to the large bowel had all segments of the large bowel involved.

Comment

This group of 92 patients appears to be similar to other series of patients with Crohn's disease in terms of clinical, radiological, and pathological features.[2,11] Frequent local and systemic complications were characteristic also for this series. In particular, the high incidence of internal and perirectal fistulae found in this study has been reported by other investigators.[2,12]

Three patients in this series had distinct splenomegaly. No other reports were found in the literature of the incidence of splenomegaly in regional enteritis. One patient in the present study was found at autopsy to have a colon carcinoma. This patient had died after a 19-year course of regional enteritis. The occurrence of colonic cancer in patients with granulomatous ileocolitis appears to be rare. Only 17 cases have been reported in the world literature prior to November 1969.[10,15]

The patients reported here were treated by several physicians without a uniform approach. Interpretation of the results and complications of treatment must, therefore, be limited. Forty of 92 patients were treated with steroids at some time during the course of the disease. Twenty-one of these 40 could be matched retrospectively with patients who did not receive steroid treatment. The mortality rate and incidence of major operations and complications in steroid- and nonsteroid-treated patients of this study appeared to be similar. Therefore, it is impossible to make a firm judgement concerning the possible beneficial or harmful effect of steroid treatment in regional enteritis. The patient summaries presented in this paper further document the difficulty in evaluating an apparent "treatment effect" and illustrate the variable course of this disease. The first case presented illustrates the dilemma of steroid treatment in a patient who improved symptomatically upon steroid administration but whose disease, as judged radiographically, progressed markedly at the same time. After discontinuance of steroids this patient continued to be asymptomatic, and almost all of the bowel disease disappeared without specific treatment. Similar spontaneous fluctuations of the granulomatous bowel involvement were documented by surgical exploration in the second case. The third patient summary demonstrated radiological evidence of regression of the disease with nonspecific measures alone. Studies by other authors[10,16,17] leave the question as to the effectiveness of steroid treatment in Crohn's disease unsettled. Sparberg and Kirsner[16] concluded from their study that long-term steroid treatment might decrease the incidence of operations in patients with regional enteritis. However, the authors also emphasized the unpredictable response to steroids, the infrequency of radiographically evident improvement after steroid administration, and the frequency of recurrent symptoms after reduction of the steroid dose or its discontinuance. Jones and Lennard-Jones[17] observed a good initial symptomatic response in the majority of their patients. However, their long-term results were reported to be less encouraging. Brill and associates[10] were unable to determine from their retrospective study the long-term efficacy or potential harmful effects of steroids. They found an increase of bowel perforations and mortality with steroid treatment. These authors, therefore, advise withholding steroids whenever possible. The obvious diversity of opinion as to the effectiveness of corticosteroids in Crohn's disease can only be resolved by a controlled prospective study, which has yet to be done.

The failure of medical treatment led to surgical intervention in 81 of the 92 patients with a total of 115 major and 78 minor operations. Review of other studies[2,3,7,18] reveals that most patients with Crohn's disease are finally treated by surgery. Earlier studies[7,18] were optimistic about the outcome of patients treated with resection of diseased intestine. In the series of Colcock and Vansant,[7] 76.3% of the patients had no evidence of recurrent regional enteritis after one or even more bowel resections. Barber et al[18] reported similar results. More recent papers, however,[9,10] emphasize the high rate of recurrence of the disease after bowel resection. In this study it was found that the risk of having further major operations was higher after the second or third operation than after the first. Lennard-Jones and Stalder,[9] found the probability of having another operation increased in patients who had two operations in comparison to those who had only one operation. Analysis of a larger series of patients could perhaps confirm this observation since in the present study the operation rate showed a tendency to increase after each additional operation, though this trend did not reach statistical significance. Age, sex, and duration of the disease did not affect the prognosis of the patients in the series of Lennard-Jones and Stalder,[9] an observation confirmed by this study.

There appeared to be no correlation between site and extent of regional enteritis at the time of diagnosis and the incidence of major operations and mortality per 100 person years of follow-up since the time of diagnosis in this series. The mortality and operation rates were similar in patients who had one, two or more bowel segments involved. The lack of correlation between the prognosis of the disease and site or extent of anatomical involvement at the time of diagnosis could perhaps be explained by the fluctuating nature of the bowel disease, which has been documented by case reports in this study.

The average mortality rate in this series ranged between 1 and 2 per 100 person years, and the average incidence of major operations was approximately 20 per 100 person years of follow-up since the time of diagnosis. Prior et al[19] followed 295 patients for an average of 13.8 years since the time of onset of symptoms and found a mortality of 18% which was reported to be twice as high as that expected in the general population. In the present series the mortality was 9% of 92 patients who were followed for an average of 17 years from the onset of symptoms.

The case histories presented here show that patients with Crohn's disease may show remarkable improvement on supportive care, with careful attention to maintenance of nutritional, fluid, and electrolyte balance without other "specific" therapy. Our studies do not indicate that steroid therapy is definitely beneficial or harmful. However, patients not responding to very conservative therapy should probably have a trial of steroids prior to being considered for surgical management, as this approach is often not curative, is associated with a high recurrence rate, and may add to the morbidity of Crohn's disease.

This investigation was supported in part by Public Health Service training grant TO1 AM 05507.

References

1. Crohn BB, Ginzburg L, Oppenheimer GD: Regional ileitis: Pathologic and clinical entity. *JAMA* **99**:1323-1329, 1932.

2. Van Patter WN, Bargen JA, Dockerty MB, et al: Regional enteritis. *Gastroenterology* **26**:347, 1954.

3. Banks BM, Zetsel L, Richter HS: Morbidity and mortality in regional enteritis: Report of 168 cases. *Amer J Dig Dis* **14**:369-379, 1969.

4. Golde DW, McGall LM: Aetiology of regional enteritis. *Lancet* **1**:1144-1145, 1968.

5. Morson BC: Histopathology of Crohn's disease. *Proc Roy Soc Med* **61**:79-81, 1968.

6. Lennard-Jones JE: Medical aspects of Crohn's disease. *Proc Roy Soc Med* **61**:81-83, 1968.

7. Colcock BP, Vansant JH: Surgical treatment of regional enteritis. *New Eng J Med* **262**:435-439, 1960.

8. Brooke BN, Hoffmann DC, Swarbrick ET: Azathioprine for Crohn's disease. *Lancet* **2**:612-614, 1969.

9. Lennard-Jones JE, Stalder GA: Prognosis after resection of chronic regional ileitis. *Gut* **8**:332-336, 1967.

10. Brill CB, Klein SF, Kark AE: Regional enteritis and enterocolitis: A study of 74 patients over 15 years. *Ann Surg* **170**:766-774, 1969.

11. Marshak RH, Wolf BS: Roentgen findings in regional enteritis. *Amer J Roentgen* **74**:1000-1014, 1955.

12. Marshak RH, Lindner AE, Jannowitz HD: Granulomatous ileocolitis. *Gut* **7**:258-264, 1966.

13. Lockhart-Mummery HE, Morson BC: Crohn's disease of the large intestine and its distinction from ulcerative colitis. *Gut* **1**:87-105, 1960.

14. Bochenek W, Rodgers JB, Balint JA: Effects of changes in dietary lipids on intestinal fluid loss in the short bowel syndrome. *Ann Intern Med* **72**:205-213, 1970.

15. Jones HJ: Colonic cancer and Crohn's disease. *Gut* **10**:651-654, 1969.

16. Sparberg M, Kirsner JB: Long-term corticosteroid therapy for regional enteritis: An analysis of 58 courses in 54 patients. *Amer J Dig Dis* **11**:865-880, 1966.

17. Jones JH, Lennard-Jones JE: Corticosteroids and corticotrophin in the treatment of Crohn's disease. *Gut* **7**:181-187, 1966.

18. Barber KW, Waugh JM, Sauer WG: Surgical treatment of complications of regional enteritis: A ten-year follow-up. *Arch Surg* **86**:442-444, 1963.

19. Prior P, Fielding JF, Waterhouse JA, et al: Mortality in Crohn's disease. *Lancet* **1**:1135-1137, 1970.

Gastric Secretory and Serologic Studies on Patients With Neoplastic and Immunologic Disorders

Two-hour gastric acid and intrinsic factor (IF) secretory capacity determinations after betazole hydrochloride stimulation were performed on 21 patients with multiple myeloma, 10 each with lymphoproliferative disorders, rheumatoid arthritis, extragastric cancer, and 40 controls, all less than 65 years old. One patient with multiple myeloma had pernicious anemia (PA); four patients with multiple myeloma had close relatives with PA, gastric carcinoma, or thyroid disease. Two other elderly patients had myeloma and atrophic gastritis. Two patients with lymphoproliferative disorders had severely impaired gastric secretion. Parietal cell, IF, and thyroid autoantibodies were not detected in serum from any of the patients.

Jeremiah J. Twomey, MB; Arline H. Laughter, MSc;
Nelda D. Villanueva, MD; Yuan S. Kao, MD;
Martin D. Lidsky, MD; and Paul H. Jordan, Jr., MD, Houston

Patients with atrophic gastritis and pernicious anemia (PA) have an increased prevalence of gastric carcinoma,[1] thyroid disease,[2,3] and idiopathic delayed onset immunoglobulin (Ig) deficiency.[4,5] Reports from Scandinavia suggest that the prevalence of PA is also increased among patients with multiple myeloma. Larsson found three definite and two probable cases of PA among 69 patients with multiple myeloma[6] and Nordenson mentioned three cases of PA in a review of 310 patients with multiple myeloma.[7] One definite and another probable case of PA were found among 72 other patients with multiple myeloma.[8,9] Reduced serum vitamin B_{12} levels were reported more frequently than PA among patients with multiple myeloma.[9,10]

There is little known about gastric function in patients with other immunologic diseases. We are aware of only two case reports of coexistent Hodgkin's disease and PA.[11,12] In one survey of 432 patients with rheumatoid arthritis, 18.5% had histamine-fast achlorhydria.[13] However, parietal cell autoantibodies have not been detected with excessive frequency in serum from patients with rheumatoid arthritis[14,15]; parietal cell antibodies have been found with excessive frequency in serum from females with Sjögren's syndrome.[16]

The purpose of this study was to evaluate gastric secretion by patients with lymphoproliferative disorders and rheumatoid arthritis and to search for a coincidental relationship between these diseases and PA.

Material and Methods

Twenty-one patients with multiple myeloma, ten with rheumatoid arthritis, and ten with other lymphoproliferative disorders (four with chronic lymphocytic leukemia, three with Hodgkin's disease, two with lymphosarcoma, and one with reticulum cell sarcoma) were studied. All were less than 60 years of age. None of the patients was acutely ill when studied or had received abdominal irradiation, adrenocorticosteroids, or chemotherapy during the preceding four weeks. The diagnosis of multiple myeloma was based upon the presence of at least 20% plasma cells in bone marrow aspirates or 10% plasma cells plus osteolytic lesions, together with an IgG or IgA monoclonal gammopathy or Bence Jones proteinuria. Lymphoma and Hodgkin's disease were diagnosed histologically from biopsy specimens. Patients with chronic lymphocytic leukemia had $>$50,000 mature lymphocytes/cu mm of blood and generalized lymphadenopathy. The diagnosis of definite rheumatoid arthritis was based upon the criteria of the American Rheumatism Association.[17]

Control studies were performed on 40 hospitalized men without known gastric disease or history of excessive alcohol intake. Ten were from each age decade between the ages of 20 and 60 years. We also studied gastric secretion by 10 patients with histologically proved extragastric disseminated carcinoma whose ages ranged from 45 to 60 years.

Gastric secretions were collected for two hours using constant suction after an overnight fast and after stimulation with 1.7 mg/kg of betazole hydrochloride given subcutaneously. In almost all instances, the nasogastric tube was positioned under fluoroscopic control. The hydrochloric acid content of each sample of gastric juice was calculated after the pH was titered to 7.3 using 0.1N sodium hydroxide. (Studies performed in this laboratory have shown that

Received for publication March 8, 1971; accepted July 13.

From the departments of medicine and surgery, Veterans Administration Hospital and Baylor College of Medicine, Houston.

Reprint requests to Veterans Administration Hospital, 2002 Holcombe Blvd, Houston 77031 (Dr. Twomey).

Table 1.—Results of Two-Hour Betazole Hydrochloride Stimulated Gastric Secretory Studies*	Volume (ml)		HCl (mEq)		IF ($\mu g\ B_{12}$ bc)	
Normal controls (40)	463 ± 141		47.5 ± 18.9		19.4 ± 8.4	
Multiple myeloma (21)	301 ± 120	$P<.001$†	30.1 ± 16.7	$P<.001$	8.7 ± 4.6	$P<.001$
Lympho-proliferative disorders (10)	292 ± 117	$P<.001$	30.4 ± 15.3	$P<.005$	9.6 ± 6.1	$P<.001$
Carcinoma (10)	293 ± 120	$P<.001$	24.6 ± 13.2	$P<.001$	8.5 ± 4.7	$P<.001$
Rheumatoid arthritis (10)	344 ± 155	$P<.05$	31.0 ± 22.3	$P<.05$	10.8 ± 5.1	$P<.005$

* Mean ± SD.
† Student's *t* test: patient vs control groups.

two-hour collections of gastric juice following stimulation with subcutaneously administered betazole encompass the response to this stimulus and yield results comparable to those reported by others on one-hour collections following stimulation with histamine.[18,19]) Aliquots were depepsinized[20] and stored at pH 7 and −70 C for IF assay. Multiple biopsy specimens of proximal gastric mucosa were obtained under fluoroscopic supervision using Brandborg and Rubin's suction biopsy apparatus. Vitamin B_{12} absorption was studied using the isotopic method described by Schilling.[21]

Intrinsic factor, IF-vitamin B_{12} blocking antibody, and serum vitamin B_{12} were assayed by radioimmunologic methods using albumin-coated charcoal.[22,23] Intrinsic factor quantitation was expressed as its capacity to bind vitamin B_{12}(B_{12} bc). Serum folic acid levels were assayed by a microbiologic method using *Lactobacillus casei*.[24] The presence of parietal cell autoantibody in serum was sought with the use of an immunofluorescence technique. Thyroid hemagglutinating antibodies in serum were assayed using commercial kits.[25] IgG, IgA, and IgM were quantitated by a radial immunodiffusion method using rabbit antiserum specific for human Ig heavy-chain determinants.[26]

Results

Gastric Secretory Capacity.—Total volume, HCl, and IF content in two-hour gastric aspirates from each group of patients was significantly less than in aspirates from control subjects (Table 1). Secretory capacity was least reduced in patients with rheumatoid arthritis. The volume of gastric juice collected from two patients with multiple myeloma, one with chronic lymphocytic leukemia, and one with malignant melanoma was more than 2 standard deviations less than the mean control value. Aspirates from two patients with multiple myeloma, two patients with cancer, two patients with rheumatoid arthritis, and one patient with chronic lymphocytic leukemia contained less HCl than 2 standard deviations below the mean control output. Only one patient with multiple myeloma had $< 2.1 \mu g$ of vitamin B_{12} bc of IF in two-hour collections which is 2 standard deviations less than the mean control value.

Patients With Gastric Dysfunction.—Secretory studies were repeated on the patients whose total two-hour HCl or IF secretion was at least 2 standard deviations below mean control values. Three of these patients had additional evidence of gastric dysfunction (Table 2): (1) A 52-year-old man with multiple myeloma and an IgG monoclonal gammopathy, diagnosed 17 months earlier, had betazole-fast achlorhydria with minimal IF secretion on two occasions and histologic evidence of atrophic gastritis. (2) A 48-year-old man with chronic lymphocytic leukemia, diagnosed 19 months prior to study, had impaired ability to secrete HCl and IF. A second-stage Schilling test determination was also suggestive of IF secretory failure. Biopsies showed a pleomorphic inflammatory infiltrate and shortened glands in the gastric mucosa; numerous parietal cells were seen. (3) Results of gastric secretory studies and Schilling tests on a 50-year-old man with lymphocytic lymphosarcoma involving the spleen and axillary lymph nodes for at least 28 months prior to study were suggestive of impaired IF secretion. Gastric biopsy specimens were normal. The gastric biopsies from these patients did not demonstrate mucosal infiltration with their underlying lymphoproliferative diseases. Their serum vitamin B_{12} levels were not reduced.

Autoantibody Studies.—Parietal cell, IF-vitamin B_{12} blocking, and antinuclear antibodies were not detected in serum from any of the patients. Three patients with rheumatoid arthritis had significant serum titers of thyroid hemagglutinating antibody; one of these patients had hypothyroidism.

Serum from two patients not included in the survey was also studied for autoantibody. One was a 77-year old man with multiple myeloma, an IgA monoclonal gammopathy, achlorhydria, IF secretory failure, and atrophic gastritis. The second patient was an 89-year-old man with multiple myeloma, an IgG monoclonal gammopathy, polyposis, atrophic gastritis, and adenocarcinoma of the stomach. Neither had detectable parietal cell, IF-vitamin B_{12} blocking, or thyroid hemagglutinating antibodies.

Serum Vitamin B_{12} and Folic Acid Levels.—None of the patients had reduced serum levels of vitamin B_{12} (normal range: 200 to 1,000 pg/ml). Two patients with multiple myeloma had reduced serum folic acid levels (3.7 pg/ml each) (normal range: 7 to 15.9 ng/ml). These patients had not been treated with either vitamin B_{12} or folic acid.

Family History.—Four patients with multiple myeloma gave family histories pertinent to the diagnosis of PA: (1) The mother of a 57-year-old woman physician had PA and hypothyroidism; her father died from carcinoma of the stomach. (2) A maternal aunt of a 58-year-old man died from gastric carcinoma. Both of these patients had light-chain gammopathies. (3) A 64-year-old lady reported a maternal aunt had PA and a sister was under treatment for hypothyroidism. (4) A 59-year-old woman had a sister with well-documented hyperthyroidism. The latter two patients had IgG monoclonal gammopathies. It was not possible to substantiate this information. Family histories from the other patients were noncontributory.

Table 2.—Findings on Three Patients With Evidence of Gastric Dysfunction

	Patient 1	Patient 2	Patient 3
Diagnosis	Myeloma	CLL*	LSA†
HCl (mEq/2 hr)	0	8.5	19.9
	0	8.8	26.8
IF (μg B_{12} bc 2 hr)	1.2	3.9	1.2
	1.0	2.7	3.5
Schilling test (%/48 hr)‡			
Stage 1	2.8	4.3	4.9
			5.5
Stage 2	13.4	9.6	10.8
Gastric biopsy	Atrophic	Abnormal§	Normal
Serum vitamin B_{12} (pg/ml)	1057	760	796

* CLL = chronic lymphocytic leukemia.
† LSA = lymphosarcoma.
‡ Normal value is >8%.
§ Pleomorphic infiltrate and shortening of mucosal glands.

Comment

1. This survey indicates that gastric juice volume, HCl, and IF secretory capacity by groups of patients with multiple myeloma, lymphoproliferative disorders, metastatic cancer, and rheumatoid arthritis were significantly less than by a group of patients without known gastric disease who were hospitalized for minor surgery. This reduction of gastric secretion may be specifically related to the underlying diseases or may be a nonspecific consequence of chronic illness. Gastric irritation caused by salicylate ingestion may have affected gastric secretion by the patients with rheumatoid arthritis.

2. Measurement of the IF content in stimulated collections of gastric juice has been found useful in detecting PA in its early stages.[27] Three patients from this survey (one with multiple myeloma, one with chronic lymphocytic leukemia, and one with lymphosarcoma) had impairment of IF secretion to a degree where vitamin B_{12} absorption was reduced. The first two had histologic evidence of gastric atrophy.

Eight definite and three probable cases of PA have been diagnosed among surveys totaling 440 patients with multiple myeloma.[6-9] This prevalence is considerably higher than the 0.2% prevalence of PA among an unselected adult hospital population in the United States.[28] The frequent family histories of PA, gastric carcinoma, and thyroid disease elicited from our patients with multiple myeloma adds indirect evidence of a coincidental relationship between PA and multiple myeloma. Familial multiple myeloma affecting two brothers whose mother had PA has been previously reported.[29] Our survey suggests a need for a more extensive search for a coincidental relationship between other lymphoproliferative disorders and PA.

3. Studies on 12 Ig-deficient patients with a PA-like syndrome failed to demonstrate serum parietal cell or IF antibodies.[4,5] We have also failed to detect parietal cell, IF, or thyroid hemagglutinating antibody in serum from two patients with coexistent multiple myeloma and PA and a third patient with polyposis and adenocarcinoma of the stomach. Polyposis of the stomach is usually associated with gastric atrophy and hyposecretion.[30] Substantiation of this limited experience would provide further evidence that detectable serum levels of gastric autoantibodies are not essential to the pathogenesis of atrophic gastritis. An increased incidence of thyroid autoantibodies in serum from patients with rheumatoid arthritis has been reported.[31] Three of the ten patients we surveyed with rheumatoid arthritis had elevated serum titers of thyroid hemaggluti-

nating antibodies.

4. Results of serum vitamin B_{12} and folic acid assays in this survey contrast with previous reports of reduced serum vitamin B_{12} and folic acid levels in many patients with multiple myeloma.[9,10]

Patients with idiopathic delayed onset Ig deficiency and multiple myeloma have in common defective humoral immune mechanisms and an increased incidence of a PA-like disorder. However, the patterns of their gastric disease differ: (1) We have found a PA-like disorder in five out of ten unselected adult patients with idiopathic delayed onset Ig deficiency.[5] This suggests that atrophic gastritis occurs more frequently in patients with delayed onset Ig deficiency than with multiple myeloma. (2) The PA-like disorder is recognized at an unusually young age in most patients with coexistent Ig deficiency (mean age for 12 patients: 30 years[4,5]). In patients with multiple myeloma, the plasma cell dyscrasia and gastric disease are recognized at a later age as in Addisonian PA. (3) This study suggests that IF secretion declines with prolonged survival with multiple myeloma. In contrast, there tended to be a close relationship between the onset of idiopathic delayed onset Ig deficiency and coexistent PA. In this study, such a relationship was not evidenced between duration of multiple myeloma and gastric secretory capacity. Atrophic gastritis is a consequence of gastric disease. It may well be a consequence of a number of pathophysiologic mechanisms.

This investigation was supported in part by Veterans Administration research funds.

Raymond Alexanian, MD, Robert Hettig, MD, Thomas Jarrold, MD, and Charles Douglass, MD, permitted the study of their patients. Franz Leidler, MD, provided some histologic information.

References

1. Harris JW: *The Red Cell.* Cambridge, Mass, Harvard University Press, 1963, p 153.
2. Soborg M, Halberg P: Cellular hypersensitivity in Hashimoto's thyroiditis. *Acta Med Scand* **183**:101-105, 1968.
3. Nakamara RM, Weigle WO: Transfer of experimental autoimmune thyroiditis by serum from thyroidectomized donors. *J Exp Med* **130**:263-285, 1969.
4. Twomey JJ, Jordan PH Jr, Jarrold T, et al: The syndrome of immunoglobulin deficiency and pernicious anemia. *Amer J Med* **47**:340-350, 1969.
5. Twomey JJ, Jordan PH Jr, Laughter AH, et al: The gastric disorder that occurs in immunoglobulin deficient patients. *Ann Intern Med* **72**:499-504, 1970.
6. Larsson SO: Myeloma and pernicious anemia. *Acta Med Scand* **172**:195-205, 1962.
7. Nordenson NG: Myelomatosis: A clinical review of 310 cases. *Acta Med Scand* **179**(suppl 445):178-186, 1966.
8. Fraser KJ: Multiple myeloma and pernicious anemia. *Med J Aust* **1**:298-299, 1969.
9. Hoffbrand AV, Hobbs JR, Kremenchusky S, et al: Incidence and pathogenesis of megaloblastic erythropoiesis in multiple myeloma. *J Clin Path* **20**:699-705, 1967.
10. Killander A, Larsson SO: Serum B_{12} concentration in multiple myeloma and other forms of hypergammaglobulinemia, in *Proceedings of the 8th Congress of the European Society of Haematology, Vienna, 1961.* Basel, Switzerland, S Karger AG, 1962.
11. Steinbrinck W: Über besondere Verlaufsformen der Biermerschen Anämie und ihre Begleitsymptome. *Z Klin Med* **139**:67-88, 1941.
12. Cieza Rodriguez LF, Tau R: Enfermedad de Hodgkin asociada con una anemia perniciosa. *Día Méd* **15**:1322-1323, 1943.
13. Edström G: Magensekretion und Grundumsatz bei den chronischen rheumatischen Arthritiden. *Acta Med Scand* **99**:228-256, 1939.
14. Roitt IM, Doniach D, Shapland C: Autoimmunity in pernicious anemia and atrophic gastritis. *Ann NY Acad Sci* **124**:644-656, 1965.
15. Armstrong EM: An investigation of the prevalence and significance of gastric parietal-cell autoantibody in rheumatoid arthritis. *Ann Rheum Dis* **26**:499-505, 1967.
16. Goudie RB, Buchanan WW: Autoimmunity in rheumatoid arthritis. *Scot Med J* **12**:87-95, 1967.
17. Ropes MW, Bennett GA, Cobb S, et al: 1958 Revision of diagnostic criteria for rheumatoid arthritis. *Bull Rheum Dis* **9**:175-176, 1958.
18. Ardeman S, Chanarin I, Doylé JC: Studies on secretion of gastric intrinsic factor in man. *Brit Med J* **2**:600-603, 1964.
19. Rødbro P, Christiansen PM, Schwartz M: Intrinsicfactor secretion in stomach diseases. *Lancet* **2**:1200-1203, 1965.
20. Sullivan LW, Herbert V, Castle WB: In vitro assay for human intrinsic factor. *J Clin Invest* **42**:1443-1458, 1963.
21. Schilling RF: Intrinsic factor studies: Effect of gastric juice on urinary excretion of radioactivity after oral administration of radioactive vitamin B_{12}. *J Lab Clin Med* **42**:860-866, 1953.
22. Gottlieb C, Lau K-S, Wasserman LR, et al: Rapid charcoal assay for intrinsic factor (I.F.), gastric juice unsaturated B_{12} binding capacity, antibody to I.F. and serum unsaturated B_{12} binding capacity. *Blood* **25**:875-884, 1965.
23. Lau K-S, Gottlieb C, Wasserman LR, et al: Measurement of serum vitamin B_{12} level using radioisotope dilution and coated charcoal. *Blood* **26**:202-214, 1965.
24. Herbert V: The assay and nature of folic acid activity in human serum. *J Clin Invest* **40**:81-91, 1961.
25. Stavitsky AB: Micromethods for study of proteins and antibodies. II: Specific application of hemagglutination and hemagglutination-inhibition reactions with tannic acid and protein-treated red blood cells. *J Immun* **72**:368-375, 1954.
26. Fahey JL, McKelvey EM: Quantitative determination of serum immunoglobulins in antibody-agar plates. *J Immun* **94**:84-90, 1965.
27. Irvine WJ, Davies SH, Haynes RC: Secretion of intrinsic factor in response to histamine and to gastrin in the diagnosis of Addisonian pernicious anemia. *Lancet* **2**:397-401, 1965.
28. Schwartz SO, Gore M: Pernicious anemia in Negroes. *Arch Intern Med* **72**:782-785, 1943.
29. Herrell WE, Ruff JD, Bayrd ED: Multiple myeloma in siblings. *JAMA* **167**:1485-1487, 1958.
30. Stout AP: Tumors of the stomach, in *Atlas of Tumor Pathology,* section VI, fascicle 21. Armed Forces Institute of Pathology, 1953.
31. Rose NR, Witebsky E: Thyroid autoantibodies in thyroid disease. *Advances Metab Dis* **3**:231-277, 1968.

Patients undergoing surgery for fibroid tumors of the uterus had significantly higher blood pressures (140.3/89.6 mm Hg) than those undergoing other gynecological procedures (129.5/83.5 mm Hg) in this institution. Though the fibroid patients were significantly older, heavier, and had fewer children, stratification on these variables failed to remove the blood pressure disparities. The incidence of cardiomegaly and of abnormalities found on intravenous pyelograms (IVP) was greater in the fibroid patients. The blood pressure difference between the groups persists after operation. The triad of obesity, fibromyomata uteri, and hypertension appears to constitute a syndrome.

Hypertension, Obesity, and Fibromyomata Uteri, as a Syndrome

William E. Summers, MD; Robert L. Watson, DVM; William H. Wooldridge, MD; and Herbert G. Langford, MD, Jackson, Miss

In recent years primary aldosteronism and renovascular hypertension have emerged as distinct entities and have, therefore, been split off from the larger category of essential or idiopathic hypertension. We have obtained evidence to suggest that the triad of hypertension, obesity, and fibromyomata uteri may also represent such a syndrome.

Reports of an association between fibroid tumors of the uterus and hypertension appeared in the late 1800's, and numerous reports appeared during the period 1900 to 1942 with the papers of Castaño,[1] Kretschmer and Kanter,[2] Moehlig,[3] and Everett and Scott[4] typical of the period. Little was reported for the next 20 years, though short statements regarding the association were made in standard textbooks, such as that by Te Linde[5]: "One of the commonest clinical pictures we encounter, especially in colored wards, is an obese, middle-aged woman with a large symptomatic fibroid, considerable hypertension, and evidence of beginning myocardial failure." In 1966, Lovell et al[6] reinvestigated the relationship in a predominately Negro Jamaican population admitted for fibroid surgery and in those admitted for other gynecological operations. They found that the blood pressures were significantly higher in the patients with fibroids than in patients in their comparison groups, and that the disparities could not be explained by age, parity, or weight differences between the groups. Clinch and Sweetnam,[7] however, failed to find such an association in an English white population. We have investigated the question in a population more closely resembling Lovell's.

Received for publication June 3, 1970; accepted March 8, 1971.

From the departments of medicine and preventive medicine (Dr. Watson), and medicine and physiology (Dr. Langford), University of Mississippi Medical Center, Jackson.

Reprint requests to Department of Medicine, University of Mississippi Medical Center, Jackson, Miss 39216 (Dr. Langford). Dr. Summers is now with the Department of Pediatrics, University of Mississippi Hospital, Jackson. Dr. Wooldridge is now with the Department of Pediatrics, Children's Memorial Hospital, Oklahoma City.

Methods

The study groups consisted of all Negro women admitted to the University of Mississippi Medical Center in 1965 and 1966, with a diagnosis of carcinoma in situ of the cervix; or who were scheduled for either uterine leiomyoma (fibroid) removal, repair of the anterior (cystocele), posterior (rectocele), or anterior and posterior vaginal wall; vaginal hysterectomy; or complete or partial salpingectomy as well as ligation or transection of the fallopian tube. The charts of these patients were abstracted for diagnosis and procedures carried out, marital status, parity, age, place of residence, blood pressure upon admission, laboratory test results, surgical and pathological reports, and presence or absence of conditions or therapy which might affect blood pressure. The blood pressure measurement used for the analysis, recorded by the lowest ranking member of the medical team examining each subject (ie, student > intern > resident), was usually selected as being the closest to admission and least likely to be influenced by previous measurements.

All coding was carried out by two of us (W.E.S. and W.H.W.) and upon initial completion of the record review, a random sample of 25 charts was reviewed by the opposite coder. All of the charts were then reviewed and jointly coded for those items in which systematic discrepancies were noted: bacteriuria, heart enlargement, and results of intravenous pyelograms. In addition, if questions of inclusion or exclusion arose, charts were reviewed jointly by all four investigators. Finally, a frequency distribution was obtained for each variable by each observer and no systematic differences in coding were noted.

Those subjects in all groups of the original study still residing in the three counties closest to the Medical Center were contacted during the summer of 1968 (18 to 42 months after the index hospitalization) for follow-up observations. Each subject was interviewed and blood pressure (two readings), arm circumference, and pulse rate were measured in the subject's home. The blood pressure measurements were obtained after five minutes of rest in a sitting position. All interviews and measurements were obtained after a period of laboratory standardization. Satisfactory agreement in recorded pressures was achieved between the two doctors, with staff personnel, and with a standard training film before field interviews were initiated.

Results

The final study groups were smaller than expected because there were duplications in the diagnosis and operation file listings, and because of exclusion for the lack of confirming evidence of fibroids in subjects listed with that diagnosis. Of the 264 fibroid listings there were 206 subjects, and of these, a fibroid was removed surgically in 172 patients. In another 34 patients a fibroid was noted on pelvic examination or incidental to surgical procedure but was not removed, and confirming evidence was therefore lacking. These 34 patients have been omitted from the analyses. Of the 226 listings for conditions considered in our comparison group, there were 132 subjects, of whom 36 were also included in the fibroid listings. In 17 of these 36, the fibroids were clinically diagnosed before operation and these subjects have been transferred to the confirmed fibroid group. In the other 19 subjects, fibroids incidentally found during surgery for a control procedure were removed and confirmed by a pathologist. We considered this group separately from the confirmed fibroid groups, as the fibroids were not clinically diagnosed and may, therefore, have been smaller. We thus arrived at three separate study groups: (*a*) 189 subjects in whom fibroids were clinically diagnosed, removed, and confirmed by a pathologist (confirmed fibroid group); (*b*) 96 subjects who were admitted only for nonfibroid operations (control group); and (*c*) 19 subjects who were admitted for nonfibroid operations but had a fibroid which was found incidentally to the performed surgical operation (incidental fibroid group).

The mean age, weight, parity, gravidity, interval since last pregnancy, and systolic and diastolic blood pressure for each of the groups are shown in Table 1. The means obtained among the confirmed fibroid group differed from the means of the control group at $P < .05$ for all the

Table 1.—Comparison of Patients With Clinically Diagnosed and Removed Fibroids and Three Control Groups*

	Comparison Group With Control Procedures Only		Comparison Group With Incidental Fibroids		Fibroids Diagnosed and Removed With Pathological Confirmation	
Variables	No.	Mean and SD	No.	Mean and SD	No.	Mean and SD
Age	96	38.27† ± 14.1	19	43.47 ± 9.5	189	44.74† ± 10.0
Weight	90	149.49† ± 36.0	18	161.22 ± 28.3	169	167.20† ± 39.9
Parity	96	5.96† ± 3.5	19	5.05† ± 4.0	186	2.74† ± 2.9
Gravidity	96	6.65† ± 3.9	19	5.89 ± 4.0	186	3.48† ± 3.5
Years since last pregnancy	80	8.26† ± 11.9	13	10.00 ± 9.2	131	15.56† ± 11.2
Systolic blood pressure	96	129.52† ± 22.9	19	133.21 ± 27.6	189	143.70† ± 29.7
Diastolic blood pressure	96	83.53† ± 16.3	19	80.21 ± 9.7	189	90.16† ± 16.4

* The fibroid patients are significantly higher in all variables than the comparison group with control procedures only.
† $P \leq .05$.

Table 2.—Blood Pressure of Patients With Clinically Diagnosed and Removed Fibroids and Three Control Groups*

		Comparison Group With Control Procedures Only					Fibroids Diagnosed and Removed With Pathological Confirmation				
			Systolic Pressure		Diastolic Pressure			Systolic Pressure		Diastolic Pressure	
Variables		No.	Mean	SD	Mean	SD	No.	Mean	SD	Mean	SD
Age	≤ 35	50	122.08	20.909	80.64	17.924	26	120.15	13.229	78.12	12.166
	36-50	27	129.89†	20.872	83.96†	13.016	123	146.20†	30.294	92.46†	16.519
	> 50	19	148.58	20.120	90.53	14.327	40	151.30	28.871	90.95	15.392
Weight	≤ 139	43	125.19†	22.784	78.95	17.171	51	137.18†	29.340	85.10	13.543
	140-179	31	132.19	23.644	87.03	12.742	59	138.88	26.596	86.36	14.842
	≥ 180	16	139.94	22.242	90.38	17.576	59	154.49	32.670	96.47	18.670
	Unknown	6	127.00	18.363	80.00†	15.492	20	142.30	22.471	95.70†	13.350
Parity	0	4	119.50	15.524	79.00	12.275	44	141.23	26.910	87.70	16.378
	1-4	34	132.18†	27.349	86.03	17.492	97	144.46†	31.654	91.20	14.298
	≥ 5	58	128.48†	20.523	82.38†	15.824	45	144.36†	29.283	93.52†	17.966
	Unknown	0					3	145.33	21.572	90.06	17.217

* The blood pressure of the patients with fibroids is significantly higher (systolic and diastolic), as well as for the 36 to 50 year age range, for ≤63.0 kg (139 lb) (systolic), and for one to four and ≥ five parity (systolic and diastolic).
† $P \leq .05$.

Table 3.—Fibroid: Control Differences Among All Subjects

		Regression Statistics					
	Variable	Mean	SD	Regression Coefficient	Standard Error of Regression Coefficient	Computed *t* Value	Partial Correlation Coefficient
Systolic pressure	F:C*	2.30	0.96	2.74	1.75	1.57	0.10
	Age	42.60	11.92	0.87	0.14	6.37	0.37
	Weight	161.37	39.79	0.18	0.04	4.51	0.27
Diastolic pressure	F:C*	2.30	0.96	0.92	1.07	0.85	0.05
	Age	42.60	11.92	0.25	0.084	3.00	0.19
	Weight	161.37	39.79	0.13	0.025	5.17	0.31

* F:C signifies Fibroid:control, the former being assigned the value three and the latter one. These values are chosen arbitrarily, but the choice does not affect the results. The variable may be thought of as a linear function or "composite" of fibroid; control differences with respect to blood pressure-related variables, other than age and weight.

Table 4.—Comparison of Fibroid and Control Study Groups

Variable	Fibroid-Control Differences: Fibroid	Control	Δ (F-C)
F:C*	3	1	2
Age	44.74	38.54	6.20
Weight	167.60	149.64	17.96
Systolic blood pressure	143.86	129.69	14.17
Diastolic blood pressure	89.51	83.77	5.74

* See Table 3, footnote for explanation.

Table 5.—Variable of Blood Pressure Disparities

	Variable	Contributions of Variables to Blood Pressure Differences: (1) Observed Contribution to Blood Pressure (mm/unit)	(2) Observed F:C Difference (units)	(1) × (2) Estimate of Contribution to Difference (mm)
Systolic	F:C	2.74	2.	5.48
	Age	.87	6.20	5.39
	Weight	.18	17.96	3.23
	Total			14.10*
Diastolic	F:C	.92	2	1.84
	Age	.25	6.20	1.55
	Weight	.13	17.96	2.33
	Total			5.72*

*Slight discrepancies (14.17 − 14.10 = 0.07 and 5.74 − 5.72 = 0.02) are attributable to rounding error.

Table 6.—Hospital Blood Pressures and Home Blood Pressures of Subjects Reexamined Three to Four Years After Operation*

	Comparison Group With Control Procedures Only					Fibroids Diagnosed and Removed With Pathological Confirmation				
		Systolic Pressure		Diastolic Pressure			Systolic Pressure		Diastolic Pressure	
	No.	Mean	SD	Mean	SD	No.	Mean	SD	Mean	SD
Hospital pressure	24	124.58	14.664	83.38	14.400	37	130.81	18.532	87.35	12.781
Average home pressure	24	123.23†	18.746	83.75†	12.973	37	135.07†	23.373	92.64†	16.152

* Although the hospital pressures were not significantly different in this subset, systolic and diastolic pressures of patients with clinically diagnosed and removed fibroids were significantly higher at follow-up than the pressures of the control group.

† $P \leq .05$.

listed variables. The means of the incidental fibroid group occupied an intermediate position between the means of the control group and the confirmed fibroid group for all but one variable. The means for age and weight of this group closely resembled the confirmed fibroid group, while parity, gravidity, interval since last pregnancy, and systolic and diastolic blood pressure were more similar to those of the control group.

Since the group of patients with confirmed fibroids were older, heavier, and had fewer children than the comparison group, the higher blood pressures observed in that group could be a reflection of those differences. To examine this, we partitioned by age, weight, and parity (Table 2).

A rise in blood pressure with age was observed in both groups. The comparison subjects < 35 years of age had slightly higher systolic and diastolic pressures than their counterparts with fibroids, and those > 50 years of age had slightly lower pressures than those of the same age with fibroids. Both the mean systolic and diastolic blood pressures were significantly ($P < .05$) higher in those 36 to 49 years of age in the confirmed fibroid group than in the control subjects of the same age range, ie, 146.2 vs 129.9 and 92.5 vs 84.0 mm Hg, respectively. To further evaluate the influence of the observed age differences between the groups we used scores as described by Hamilton et al[8] to adjust the blood pressure in each group to age 60. The mean score for systolic pressures was significantly higher in the fibroid group than in the control group, +8.15 ± 2.62 vs - 1.61 ± 3.74, (t = 2.15, P = .04). The mean diastolic score was higher in the fibroid group also, though the differences were not statistically significant, 9.13 ± 1.40 vs 5.57 ± 2.43 (t = 1.35, P = .12).

To evaluate age, weight, and blood pressure at one time, the regression of the Hamilton-Pickering systolic scores on weight[8] was determined. The correlation of the fibroid patients scores with weight (r = .34) was significantly different from 0 ($P \leq .05$) and from the correlation of the control patients (r = .05). The latter correlation did not differ significantly from 0.

Systolic and diastolic blood pressures were higher in the heavier weight groups. The confirmed fibroid group had higher systolic pressures at each weight level and higher diastolic pressures in two of the three weight levels (Table 2). The disparities were consistent, ie, higher in five of six cells, but not statistically significant.

It has been shown in several studies that blood pressure levels decrease with increasing parity[9,10]; however, after partitioning on parity a distinct blood pressure-parity relationship was not detectable in either group. The mean blood pressures, both systolic and diastolic, were consistently higher among subjects with confirmed fibroids than among comparison subjects. The differences, though only statistically significant ($P < .05$) for systolic pressures in two of three parity levels and for diastolic pressures at one of the three levels, were relatively large: 21.7, 12.3, and 15.9 mm Hg, respectively, for systolic pressures; and 8.7, 5.2, and 11.2 mm Hg, respectively, for diastolic pressures. It seems unlikely that parity can explain the blood pressure differences between the two groups (Table 2).

Multiple regression studies were performed for the 90 control and 169 fibroid cases for which records were complete with respect to systolic and diastolic blood pressure, age, weight, and parity. The contribution of parity to the blood pressure differences between the fibroid and control groups was found to be < .50 mm Hg and of no statistical significance. The analysis was repeated, omitting parity as a variable (Tables 3, 4, and 5).

As shown in Table 3 the contribution fibroid: control ratio (F:C), loosely ascribed to the blood pressure associated with the presence of fibroid tumors, is not significantly different from zero at the sample sizes used ($P > .10$ systolic; $P > .20$ diastolic). Age and weight differences between the study groups, however, do contribute to the blood pressure differences ($P < .01$).

Table 5 shows that despite a lack of statistical significance, the contributions ascribed to the tumors are sizable and, if real, are of clinical importance. Of the 14 mm Hg systolic disparity between the two groups, less than 9 mm can be attributed to age and weight differences, while 5 to 6 mm can be attributed to other influences. Of the 6 mm difference in diastolic pressure, about 2 mm can be attributed to these other influences.

Two other disparities were noted between the two major groups. The diagnosis of cardiac enlargement by a radiologist was made more frequently in the confirmed fibroid group, 59 of 182 (32%, 7 not done) than in the control subjects were 16 of 89 (18%, 7 not done) had roentgenographic evidence of cardiac enlargement ($\chi^2 = 6.3$ $P < .05$). Cardiac enlargement was defined as a cardiac-thoracic ratio of ≥ 50%. The presence of abnormalities of IVP was more frequently noted in the confirmed fibroid patients (53 of 76, 69.7%) than in the control patients (6/17, 35%, $\chi^2 = 7.1$). Since IVPs were not ordered for 60% of those with fibroids and 82% of control subjects, however, the opportunities for selective biases to operate were many. The abnormalities noted were of several types including hydroureter, hydronephritis, and extrinsic pressure on the bladder.

There were no significant differences noted between the groups with respect to place of residence, marital status, hospital service status, past diagnosis of toxemia of pregnancy; pyelonephritis; blood urea nitrogen (BUN), serum creatinine, serum potassium, or hemoglobin levels; hematocrit reading; urine specific gravity; or frequency of bacteriuria or proteinuria. Of the subjects in the control group, 12 of 96 (12.5%) had taken medication to reduce blood pressure in the past, as opposed to 31 of 189 (16%) in the confirmed fibroid group. This difference was not significant ($P > .25$), however. All medication had been discontinued prior to surgery and should not have affected the admitting blood pressure levels.

Blood pressure measurements were obtained on 70 subjects in their homes as part of the follow-up study by two of us (W.E.S. and W.H.W.). Included were 24 of 37 (64.8%) of control subjects and 37 of 57 (65%) of fibroid patients residing in the immediate three-county area. These pressures were obtained 18 to 42 months after surgery. The mean systolic and diastolic pressures recorded in the hospital and obtained at home in these groups are shown in Table 6. There was remarkably little difference between the pressures taken at the two different times, ie, mean systolic difference of 1.69 and 4.26 mm Hg, respectively, for the control group and fibroid group when examined as matched pairs. Though the subsets sampled did not have significantly different hospital pressures, at follow-up the differences were significant: $\bar{x} = 123.23$ vs $\bar{x} = 135.07$ mm Hg systolic, $P < .05$; and 83.75 vs 92.64 mm Hg, $P < .02$ for diastolic pressures, respectively, in the control and fibroid groups.

Comment

In any case-comparison study based on hospital charts the possibility of selective bias in the admission of patients with the combination of conditions under study must be considered. Such a bias could have operated in this study if (*a*) patients with fibroids and hypertension were more likely to bleed than patients with lower pressures, and (*b*) if hypertension did not affect the hospitalization rate for the comparison conditions. There was, however, no difference in the hemoglobin levels or hematocrit readings between the fibroid and control groups, and few of the fibroid patients were seen for problems relating to vaginal bleeding. The lack of differences between the fibroid and comparison groups with respect to blood and urine laboratory values and medical histories would suggest that major biases were not operating.

Our data are in agreement with the findings of Lovell et al,[6] but in apparent conflict with the report of Clinch and Sweetnam.[7] The association between blood pressure and the presence of fibroids might, therefore, be a peculiarity of Negroes. We are reluctant to accept this explanation at the moment, for both of the other reports[6,7] and the present one share the weakness of lack of data on fibroid size. If there is a relationship between fibroid size and blood pressure, as is suggested by the intermediate position of our incidental fibroid group, it is quite possible that smaller fibroids were removed from Clinch and Sweetnam's patients in Wales than from Jamaican and Mississippi Negroes. Also, all studies were based on data from hospital charts, which probably accounts for the large blood pressure variances.

Two salient points emerge: patients with fibroid tumors of the uterus have higher blood pressures and are heavier than patients admitted to the same institution for other gynecological surgery. In at least two other studies weight differences do not completely explain the blood pressure disparities. Intuitively, one gets the impression that the presence of a fibroid may be equivalent to about 6 years of age or 30 lb of weight (Table 5).

If the higher blood pressure of the fibroid patients is merely the effect of obesity, the important association is between fibroid tumors and obesity and the blood pressure association is secondary. To examine this question, we partitioned on weight. The blood pressure disparity between controls and patients with fibroids remained. Partitioning failed to answer the question completely, because the fibroid patients were older, and blood pressure increases with age. To assess the contribution of age and weight together, the regression of the blood pressure score of Hamilton, et al[8] on weight was calculated for the fibroid patients and the controls. The use of these scores, by adjusting each patient to age 60, takes into account the influence of age.

The fibroid patients' blood pressures were significantly correlated with weight; the controls were not; and the correlations were significantly different from each other. Multiple regression techniques showed that age and weight, though making significant contributions to the blood pressure disparities, do not account for the entire blood pressure difference. At leas one third, must be ascribed to the presence of the fibroid or associated factors or both.

The much stronger relationship between weight and Pickering blood pressure score[8] in the fibroid patients suggests to us that both variables represent a reaction to a third factor, which we presume may be the same factor that made the fibroids grow. The best candidate for this unknown factor which we postulate increases obesity, blood pressure, and fibroid growth is increased secretion of, or reaction to, estrogenic hormones resembling the "blend" found in oral contraceptives. Oral contraceptives have been shown to cause weight gain, fibroid growth,[11] and hypertension.[12] Modifications of this explanation for the coincidence of these findings would include (*a*) estrogenic activity causes fibroid growth, fibroids secrete renin (present in normal uterus), and the renin causes the hypertension; and (*b*) estrogens cause the weight gain while the estrogen-induced fibroid growth produces pressure on the urinary tract and this results in elevated blood pressure levels.

Hysterectomy failed to remove the blood pressure difference between the fibroid patients and the controls; in fact, the blood pressure disparities became more distinct when blood pressure was remeasured 18 to 42 months after surgery. The persistence of the blood pressure disparity argues against a continuing response to a humoral agent from the uterus, such as renin, as the cause of the blood pressure findings. Also, the failure of the blood pressure to fall after hysterectomy makes unlikely the possibility that mild hydronephrosis produced by the fibroids had interfered with renal function, for some improvement in renal function should occur after operation.

"One of the paths of progress in medicine is to define, and refine, 'syndromes' among the undifferentiated mass of clinical data—by discovering that apparently unrelated phenomena have the same cause."[13] The evidence cited here suggests to us that hypertension, obesity, and fibroids are interrelated and, thus, constitute a syndrome, and that the triad represent a reaction to some common cause.

This study was supported by Public Health Service grant HE-10721 from the National Heart Institute and Public Health Service general research support grant FR-5386.

Suggestions and encouragement were offered by William Miall, MD. Paul Woosley provided assistance with statistical computations.

References

1. Castaño CA: The kidney's role in uterine fibroids. *Prensa Med Argent* **6**:147, 1919.
2. Kretschmer HL, Kanter AE: Effect of certain gynecologic lesions on the upper urinary tract: A pyelographic study *JAMA* **109**:1097-1101, 1937.
3. Moehlig RC: Association of uterine fibromyomas with other clinical conditions. *J Clin Endocr* **2**:219-222, 1942.
4. Everett HS, Scott RB: The possible etiologic role of gynecologic lesions in the production of hypertension. *Amer J Obstet Gynec* **44**:1010-1025, 1942.
5. Te Linde RW: *Operative Gynecology*, ed 3. Philadelphia, JB Lippincott Co, 1962.
6. Lovell HG, Miall WE, Stewart DB: Arterial blood pressure in Jamaican women with and without uterine fibroids. *W Indian Med J* **15**:45-51, 1966.
7. Clinch J, Sweetnam PJ: Fibroids and hypertension. *J Obstet Gynaec Brit Comm* **75**:1052-1053, 1966.
8. Hamilton M, Pickering GW, Roberts JAF, et al: The aetiology of essential hypertension: IV. The role of inheritance. *Clin Sci* **13**:37-49, 1954.
9. Humerfelt S, Wedervang F: Study of the influence upon blood pressure of marital status, number of children and occupation. *Acta Med Scand* **159**:489-497, 1957.
10. Miall WE, Oldham PD: Factors influencing arterial blood pressure in the general population. *Clin Sci* **17**:409-444, 1958.
11. Evaluation of oral contraceptives: COUNCIL ON DRUGS, *JAMA* **199**:650-653, 1967.
12. Laragh JE, Sealey JE, Ledingham JGG, et al: Oral contraceptives: Renin, aldosterone, and high blood pressure. *JAMA* **201**:918-922, 1967.
13. Morris JN: *Uses of Epidemiology*, ed 2. Baltimore, Williams & Wilkins Co, 1964, p 141.

Some Epidemiological Clues in Thyroid Cancer

Tonsillectomy, Acne, Allergy, Ethnicity

Irwin D. J. Bross, PhD; Katsutaro Shimaoka, MD; and John Tidings, Buffalo, NY

A computerized procedure for screening of etiological factors over cancer sites has revealed some interesting differences between patients with thyroid cancer and those with other types of cancer or with nonneoplastic diseases. This screening procedure utilized approximately 22,000 epidemiological interviews on patients admitted to Roswell Park Memorial Institute from 1957 to 1965. Patients with thyroid cancer reported seven of 15 specific complaints or pathologic conditions, as well as tonsillectomies, more frequently than did patients in the comparison series. An excess of Jewish patients occurred in the thyroid cancer group, and the sex ratio of these patients differed from that of non-Jewish patients. Statistical analysis of these differences indicates that they are significant and suggests that further medical investigation be carried out.

In the usual epidemiological study of cancer, the first step is to choose a site (or group of sites) which will be the focus of the study. The next step, ordinarily, is to consider the various etiological hypotheses that have been suggested for cancers at the given site and to select those items of information reported in the data which would allow a test of the hypotheses. The investigator then looks for differences between cancer and control series (or between cancer sites) which would either support or contradict the hypotheses about the genesis of the cancer. In a sense, the screening approach employed here turns the usual procedure inside out. Instead of starting with a focus on a given site of cancer, the screening procedure, if successful, ends with a focus on some site. The starting point for the screen is a given item of information from the interview question schedule. The investigator then looks for patterns in the data for this item which are unusual—patterns at a particular cancer site which are different from the usual patterns for other cancers or for the controls. Because three unusual patterns occurred for thyroid

Received for publication July 29, 1970; accepted Feb 2, 1971.

From the departments of biostatistics (Dr. Bross), medicine (Dr. Shimaoka), and epidemiology (Mr. Tidings), Roswell Park Memorial Institute, Buffalo, NY.

Reprint requests to Biostatistics Department, Roswell Park Memorial Institute, 666 Elm St, Buffalo, NY 14203 (Dr. Bross).

cancer, we made it our focus of attention.

The procedure for screening over sites is not new but is rarely used, mainly because special circumstances are needed for success. If the estimates at the rarer sites are to be reliable, subdivision of a series over sites necessitates a very large initial sample. This series started from a data base of approximately 25,000 interviews. Even though coding has not been completed for all items in the interview, at least 22,389 interviews were available for analysis of the items. Another practical limitation of this "inverted" approach is the size of the clerical task that is required. Until recently, the amount of clerical work was almost prohibitive. Now, however, with the advent of modern electronic computers and special programs for preprocessing of data, this approach has become more feasible. The screening approach is a useful adjunct to the more conventional approaches to the analysis of epidemiological data, rather than a rival or replacement for these approaches. It is primarily useful in discovering unexpected relationships, the further investigation of which would ordinarily follow the traditional lines.

One useful method for screening over sites is illustrated by the Figure. This graph shows the percentage of hospital patients reporting tonsillectomy by site of cancer (or by the diagnoses of the patients with nonneoplastic disease). In this particular graph there is no subdivision by sex or age, but in much of our actual screening, six age:sex categories were routinely used.

It can be seen from the Figure that the proportion of patients reporting tonsillectomies is higher in the controls than at most of the sites of cancer. There are, however, two cancer sites which stand out when the data is viewed in this way: thyroid cancer and Hodgkins disease. These series appear to have a high proportion of tonsillectomies, even when compared to the controls. Thus, the Figure shows that 22.0% of the thyroid cancer patients reported this surgery, as compared to 10.4% in the overall cancer series and 16.6% in the controls.

Screening results of this type do not ordinarily establish a scientific finding. Rather, they suggest a possible starting point for the further analysis which may establish a finding. It was known, for instance, that the ages of the cancer and control patients were different and that the proportion of patients reporting tonsillectomies tended to diminish with increasing age. Hence, it requires further analysis to rule out the possibility that the differentials seen in the Figure are merely due to age differences. In general, then, screening results are suggestive rather than definitive, and they have to be followed-up by additional analysis to establish any definite conclusions.

In the secondary screening, the series were separated into three age categories (1-50, 51-65, 66-98 years) with roughly equal numbers in each category. By making comparisons within categories, it was possible to reduce the risk of spurious differences arising from gross differences between age distributions at different sites. By making comparisons between these categories, it was possible to avoid the masking effects of recall problems (mainly in the group over 65) and to look at possible etiological differences between cancers occurring early (under 50) and those occurring in the traditional "cancer ages."

Tonsillectomies and Thyroid Cancer.—Our screening process picked out three of the 12 areas of the interview schedule in which the patterns for the thyroid cancer differed from the patterns for most of the other cancer sites. The first area of the schedule concerned the patient's hospitalizations prior to admission to Roswell Park Memorial Institute (RPMI). In this area the screen singled out the tonsillectomy hospitalizations. The second area concerned the patient's report of 15 specific diseases or pathologic conditions; here, allergic and skin responses were singled out. The third area was religious and ethnic background; here, the focus was on Jewish patients. The findings for tonsillectomy will be discussed in this section and the other screening results will be dealt with in later sections.

Our first concern with the tonsillectomy differences between cancers and controls was whether they would disappear when the age and sex of the patients were taken into account. However, the differences between cancer and control patients continue to be apparent even within these categories (Table 1). While the number varies in the different categories, roughly 40% more tonsillectomies are reported by the controls. Since there is a fairly consistent effect over the sites of cancer—apart from the thyroid and Hodgkins disease cases—this result suggests the peculiar hypothesis that removal of the tonsils in some way affords protection against cancer. An alternative hypothesis would be that some factor associated with tonsillectomies, eg, availability of better childhood health care, was responsible for the relationship.

The overall pattern of Table 1 is in line with what would be expected from the history of surgery in the United States in the present century. The younger patients have a far higher proportion of tonsillectomies than the older ones. About 20% of the cancer patients under 40, for instance, have tonsillectomies; the percentages are similar for males and females. Among the cancer patients 40 to 59 years of age, the percentage with tonsillectomies is about halved and it is halved again for the patients over 60. In interpreting these results, it might be noted that in the older series two factors are likely to be involved: the real changes in surgical practice in the first half of the 20th century, and the artifactual "recall effect" that is often found in survey data when elderly persons are questioned about events in the distant past. The size of the "recall effect" cannot be easily estimated. However, it may in part account for the smaller differences between cancer and control patients at the older ages.

In judging the compatability of these findings for tonsillectomies and the history of this operation, it might be noted that these interviews were made during the period 1957 to 1966. Thus, for example, a patient in the 40 to 59 age group was growing up in the period just before or just after World War I when there were rapid changes in the practice of surgery.

A further question which arises here concerns the age of the patient at the time of tonsillectomy. The distribution of cases and controls by age at surgery and at interview is shown in Table 2. This table combines data over sexes in view of the similarity in rates in Table 1. The corresponding

Table 1.—Proportion of Hospital Patients Reporting Tonsillectomies, by Age and Sex

Age at Interview, Yr	Males: Cancers	Males: Controls	Females: Cancers	Females: Controls
1-19	18.6	29.9	19.7	27.8
20-39	21.0	25.8	18.9	26.0
40-59	11.7	16.5	13.7	20.6
60+	2.8	4.9	7.4	8.1

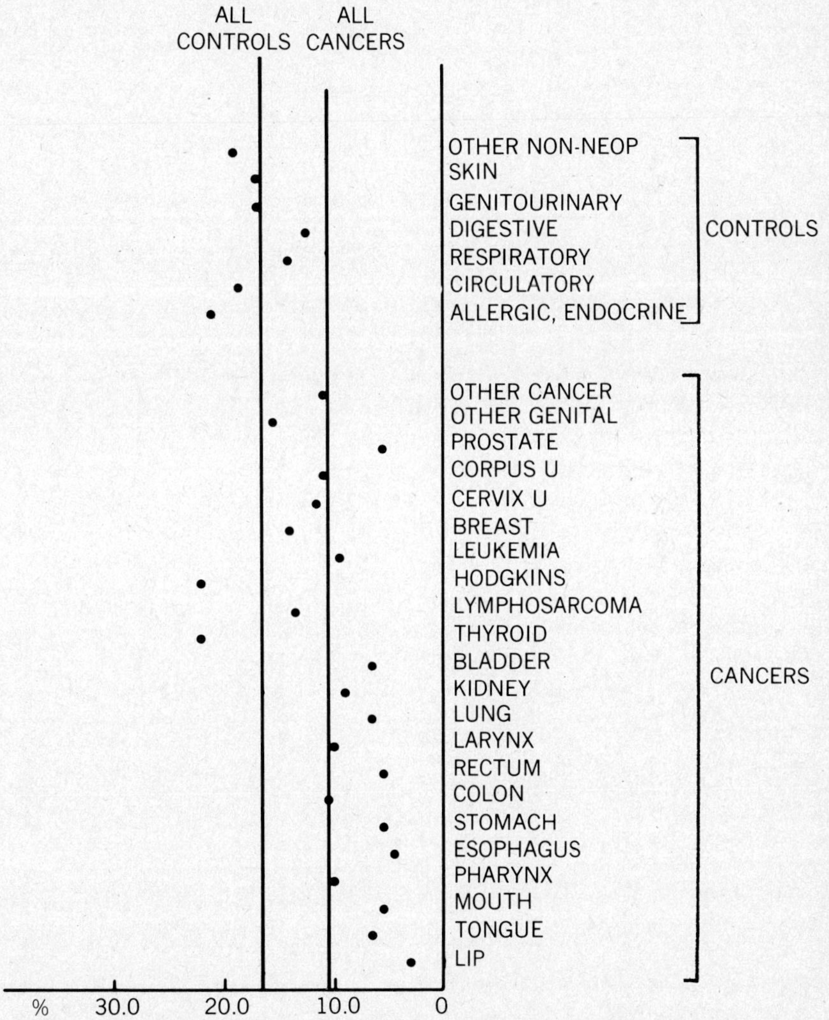

Percentage of hospital patients reporting tonsillectomy. The X axis represents the diagnosis groups; the Y axis, the percentage of patients in diagnosis groups reporting tonsillectomy. Solid lines marked "All Cancers" or "All Controls" represent the mean percentage point for all patients.

percentages by age at surgery and at interview are shown in Table 3. The percentages of tonsillectomies in Table 3 suggest that the differential between cancer cases and controls occurs even in those patients whose tonsillectomy came later in life. It may be noted that most of the patients in the over 60 series, both cases and controls, have had their tonsillectomies after they were adults. In the younger series the tonsillectomies tend to occur before the age of 20.

Since the pattern for tonsillectomies persists even when the age:sex factors are controlled, the next question is whether the differences between thyroid cancer and other cancers also persist when these other factors are taken into account. Table 4 shows the observed and expected number of tonsillectomies in the thyroid cancer patients. The expected numbers are calculated in two ways: on the basis of the rates for the cancer cases (A), and on the basis of the rates for the controls (B). There is an excess number of male thyroid cancer cases with tonsillectomies by either calculation. The females show a similar excess, although it is not very large in the comparison with the controls. An approximate chi-square test gives statistically significant differences between the thyroid cases and the other cancers for both males (at 1%) and females (at 5%) and for the combination of both (at 1%) sexes. However, the differences from the controls do not reach statistical significance at the 5% level. From these results it follows that the difference in percentage of tonsillectomies between thyroid cases and other cancers is clearly demonstrable, but there is some question whether or not the thyroid cancer patients are also different

Table 2.—Distribution of Hospital Patients by Age at Interview and Age at Tonsillectomy—Numerical Distribution

Age at Interview, yr	No. of Cancer Patients	No. of Control Patients	No. of Patients With Tonsillectomy by Age at Tonsillectomy, yr: 1-19 Cancer	1-19 Cont	20-39 Cancer	20-39 Cont	40+ Cancer	40+ Cont	Total Cancer	Total Cont
1-19	268	301	53	87					53	87
20-39	851	1,013	138	198	28	65			166	263
40-59	3,695	2,237	244	196	202	198	32	28	478	422
60+	5,237	2,243	24	8	158	79	83	57	265	144
Totals	10,051	5,794	459	489	388	342	115	85	962	916

Table 3.—Distribution of Hospital Patients by Age at Interview and Age at Tonsillectomy—Percentage Distribution

Age at Interview	% of Patients With Tonsillectomy, Age at Tonsillectomy: 1-19 Cancer	1-19 Cont	20-39 Cancer	20-39 Cont	40+ Cancer	40+ Cont
1-19	19.8	28.9				
20-39	16.2	19.5	3.3	6.4		
40-59	6.6	8.8	5.5	8.8	0.9	1.2
60+	0.4	0.3	3.0	3.5	1.6	2.5

Table 4.—Observed and Expected Numbers of Tonsillectomies in Thyroid Cancer Patients

Sex	Age	No. of Patients	No. of Patients With Tonsillectomy: Observed	Expected (A)*	Expected (B)
Male	1-19	0	0	0	0
	20-39	7	4	1.5	1.8
	40-59	14	4	1.6	2.3
	60+	12	1	0.4	0.6
	Total	33	9	3.6	4.9
Female	1-19	8	2	1.6	2.2
	20-39	19	8	3.6	4.9
	40-59	27	3	3.7	5.6
	60+	34	6	2.5	2.7
	Total	88	19	11.9	16.1
X^2	Male			8.10	3.43
	Female			4.24	0.52
	Combined			10.08	2.33

* Expectations in (A) are calculated from cancer rates and in (B) are calculated from control rates (Table 1).

Table 5.—Hospital Patients With Asthma, Hay Fever, Hives, Eczema, Neurodermatitis, Contact Dermatitis, Acne

			No. of Complaints							
			None		One		More than One		Total	
Sex	Age, yr	Diagnosis	No.	%	No.	%	No.	%	No.	%
M	1-50	Thyroid cancer	7	50.0	4	28.6	3	21.4	14	100
		All cancer	1,162	83.0	196	14.0	43	3.0	1,401	100
		Controls	759	83.1	133	14.6	21	2.3	913	100
M	51-65	Thyroid cancer	10	90.9	1	9.1	0	0	11	100
		All cancer	2,145	84.3	349	13.7	50	2.0	2,544	100
		Controls	673	81.4	123	14.9	31	3.7	827	100
M	66-98	Thyroid cancer	8	100.0	0	0	0	0	8	100
		All cancer	2,452	88.5	280	10.1	40	1.4	2,772	100
		Controls	747	86.5	106	12.3	11	1.2	864	100
F	1-50	Thyroid cancer	29	70.8	6	14.6	6	14.6	41	100
		All cancer	1,917	81.6	356	15.2	75	3.2	2,348	100
		Controls	1,289	79.1	265	16.3	75	4.6	1,629	100
F	51-65	Thyroid cancer	19	86.4	3	13.6	0	0	22	100
		All cancer	1,961	80.9	381	15.7	83	3.4	2,425	100
		Controls	725	79.5	146	16.0	41	4.5	912	100
F	66-98	Thyroid cancer	19	76.0	4	16.0	2	8.0	25	100
		All cancer	2,072	85.5	302	12.5	48	2.0	2,422	100
		Controls	624	85.0	96	13.1	14	1.9	734	100

Table 6.—Thyroid Cancer and Religion

Sex	Age, yr	No. of Cases	No. of Jewish	% Jewish
Males	1-50	14	4	28.6
	51-65	11	0	0
	66+	8	1	12.5
Females	1-50	41	1	2.4
	51-65	22	2	9.1
	66+	25	1	4.0
	Total	121	9	7.4

from the controls.

It might be noted that there is a preponderance of female patients in the thyroid series—almost 3:1—and that the female patients are often relatively young. The age:sex distribution for the thyroid cancer series is, therefore, quite different from the usual age:sex distribution at a nonreproductive site.

The proximity of the tonsils and the thyroid gland raised the possibility that there might be some connection between surgery and the locations. Most of the thyroid cancer patients reported that they had had neck surgery for the thyroid condition prior to their admission at RPMI. However, a case history review showed that in only two cases was tonsillectomy performed within a year of the surgery for the thyroid problems.

Allergies and Skin Complaints.—A second area of the interview schedule where our screening procedures picked up distinctive patterns for thyroid cancer was in the patient's re-

Table 7.—Patients With Cancer of the Thyroid

	Males		Females	
	Jewish	Non-Jewish	Jewish	Non-Jewish
Histology				
Papillary and mixed cancer	4	12	4	45
(with psammoma bodies)	3	2	3	14
Follicular cancer		5		13
(with psammoma bodies)		2		1
Hurthle cell cancer		2		4
Cancer unspecified		2		6
Anaplastic cancer	1	7		16
Involvement				
Limited to thyroid		5	1	28
Neck	4	21	3	51
Distant metastases	1	14	1	31
Treatment				
Less than subtotal				
Thyroidectomy	2	11	2	34
Total thyroidectomy	3	14	2	46
Right dissection	3	6	1	19
Left dissection	3	8	1	12
Bilateral dissection	3	2		6
Postoperative radiation	1	6	1	21
Radioiodine	1	6	1	17
Suppression	3	11	2	39
Sequelae				
No evidence of disease	2	10	0	35
Living, with disease	0	3	1	6
Died	1	12	2	39
No follow-up	2	3	1	4
Total	5	28	4	84

port of 15 specific diseases or pathologic conditions (Table 5). These were goiter, diabetes, allergy, asthma, hay fever, hives, eczema, psoriasis, neurodermatitis, contact dermatitis, acne, heart disease, pneumonia, influenza, and chronic bronchitis. When the individual complaints were considered, the differences were, at best, only faintly visible in the screening results. Of the 15 conditions, seven showed some suggestion of a relationship in the initial analysis. These were asthma, hay fever, eczema, neurodermatitis, contact dermatitis, and acne—a somewhat heterogeneous group.

When, as here, the initial screening results are inconclusive for individual conditions, it is sometimes possible to clarify the situation by considering the persons who report more than one of the seven suspect conditions. A report of two or more conditions is rare among the control patients and also among cancer patients as a whole. There is some variation by age and sex, but only about 3% of the controls and cancer patients report more than one of the seven complaints.

Multiple reports are somewhat more frequent among the thyroid cancer patients. In those over 50 there is no sign that multiple reports are more frequent than in the controls, but in the younger patients—young males in particular—there appears to be an excess of multiple reports. The numbers are small—three males in 13 report two or more complaints—but it is very unlikely (at the 1% level) that this result would occur by sampling variation alone.

Religion and Other Factors.—In the hospital patient population surveyed here, less than 2% of the population were Jewish. In the cancer series, 221 out of 13,916 patients were Jewish, as well as 61 out of 5,036 controls. The proportion of Jewish patients was similar in all of the age and sex categories. Of the 33 males in the thyroid cancer series five were Jewish (15%). Of the 88 females in the series four were Jewish (4%). The effect becomes more noticeable when the age of the patients is taken into account (Table 6). Four of the 14 younger males are Jewish. The excess of Jewish patients in the thyroid cancer series is statistically significant at the 1% level by a chi-square test.

A case history review (Table 7) of the Jewish patients in the thyroid cancer series disclosed some differences between the Jewish patients and the non-Jewish patients. The sex ratio for this series is 3:1 in favor of females, as it is in most other studies. For Jewish patients in this series the sex ratio is 1:1.

None of the Jewish patients had follicular type cancer. Jewish patients had notably more psammoma bodies than did non-Jewish patients. Jewish patients tended to have more kinds of treatment for their conditions than did non-Jewish patients.

Since thyroid cancer is the only diagnosis category in our hospital population which shows these differences, there is probably a strong selective factor operating for Jewish patients with this malignancy. These results are included here because of the differences previously noted. The reader is cautioned, however, that the numbers involved (nine Jewish patients) are too small to draw any definite conclusions.

Conclusions

A procedure used at RPMI for screening epidemiological data over a site has revealed several interesting differences between the patients with thyroid cancer and the patients with other cancers or with nonneoplastic disease. These differences tend to become more rather than less noticeable when the age and sex distribution of the thyroid cancer patients is taken into account. The screening technique operated from a population base of over 22,000 hospital patients, of which 125 had cancer of the thyroid gland. The distinguishing features of the thyroid cancer patients were as follows:

1. They reported more tonsillectomies than the other cancer patients (with the possible exception of patients with Hodgkins disease). They also reported more tonsillectomies than the nonneoplastic controls, but the differences are not statistically significant. Although there was some variation by age and sex, the RPMI controls reported about 40% more tonsillectomies than the corresponding cancer patients.

2. They had a greater chance of reporting more than one complaint on a list of seven allergy and skin complaints. The effect seemed more pronounced in the younger patients but is of borderline statistical significance.

3. They were more likely to be Jewish than the controls or the other cancer cases. In the thyroid patients 7% were Jewish compared to less than 2% of the patients in either the cancer or the control series.

4. These findings should be viewed as leads for possible future investigations and probably should not be taken at face value. For this reason, no attempt to provide any detailed explanation of these findings has been made.

Screening for Adrenocortical Insufficiency With Cosyntropin (Synthetic ACTH)

Paul F. Speckart, MD; John T. Nicoloff, MD; and John E. Bethune, MD, Los Angeles

A screening procedure for adrenocortical insufficiency, utilizing (synthetic α 1-24 adrenocorticotropic hormone [ACTH] and a cortisol-binding globulin technique for serum cortisol, has been evaluated in normal subjects and in patients with primary and secondary adrenal insufficiency. Cosyntropin is injected by vein, and a serum cortisol concentration 60 minutes later is compared with a sample removed just prior to the cosyntropin administration. A clear separation of normal subjects from those with adrenal insufficiency is achieved.

It is generally accepted that a single plasma cortisol or urinary steroid determination may not distinguish adrenal insufficiency from normal adrenal function. Therefore, corticotropin stimulation is required to differentiate one from the other. A standard corticotropin stimulation test requires either a prolonged intravenous infusion or repeated intramuscular injections of corticotropin, along with frequent venipunctures or 24-hour urinary collections. This type of testing is time consuming and may necessitate hospitalization in order to obtain accurate results. A more rapid screening procedure for the detection of adrenal insufficiency which may be employed in either hospital or office is needed. The recent availability of a commercial form of synthetic adrenocorticotropic hormone (ACTH), combined with improved methods for determining plasma cortisol levels, has provided an opportunity for the development of an accurate, rapid, simple, and safe testing procedure for the detection of adrenocortical insufficiency.

Shorter procedures for testing adrenal reserve have been recently developed and widely used in Europe.[1-3] These methods have employed cosyntropin (synthetic α 1-24 ACTH) intramuscularly and have measured adrenocortical response by the use of a fluorometric cortisol determination. A similar procedure utilizing the plasma fluorescent cortisol response to the rapid intravenous administration of a commercial corticotropin extract has also been reported.[4] Cosyntropin possesses low antigenic potency and can usually be employed safely in patients known to have allergies to ACTH extract.

We describe a testing procedure which can be used for the assessment of adrenocortical response, employing a single intravenously administered dose of cosyntropin. Plasma cortisol has been measured by a competitive protein-binding assay method utilizing cortisol-binding globulins (CBG).[5] This method, in our experience, is superior to the standard fluorometric cortisol technique in that it possesses greater sensitivity and reliability.[6-8] It appears that a single intravenous dose of cosyntropin, when employed with the CBG method, fulfills the clinical requirements for a rapid, accurate, and simple screening test for the detection of adrenocortical insufficiency.

Received for publication July 31, 1970; accepted Dec 22, 1970.

From the Department of Medicine, University of Southern California School of Medicine and the Los Angeles County-University of Southern California Medical Center, Los Angeles.

Reprint requests to University of Southern California School of Medicine, 2025 Zonal Ave, Los Angeles 90033 (Dr. Bethune).

Materials and Methods

The adult study subjects were selected from the wards and clinics of the Los Angeles County-University of Southern California Medical Center. Nine patients formed the control group. A deliberate effort was made to select patients with moderate to severe nonendocrine illnesses for use as control subjects; this type of patient is most frequently evaluated for adrenal cortical insufficiency. Seven patients with proven Addison's disease and five patients with known panhypopituitarism were studied. An additional three patients receiving long-term glucocorticoid therapy for collagen disease were also examined.

Baseline blood samples from all patients were collected between 8 and 9AM. Patients receiving steroid therapy were instructed to take their last medication 24 hours before testing. A 10 ml blood sample was collected in evacuated tubes at "0" time. After the initial blood samples were drawn, 0.25 mg of cosyntropin in 1 ml of normal saline was injected intravenously as a single dose. Blood samples were then collected after intervals of 30, 60, 120, and 180 minutes. The blood was allowed to clot, and the serum was separated and frozen until cortisol was measured.

Serum cortisol determinations were performed by the method of Nugent and Mayes.[5] The only deviation from the described procedure was that the assay incubations were all carried out at 4 C, thus eliminating the variations caused by changes in ambient temperature and improving the sensitivity of the CBG assay system. The maximum quantity of serum required for single cortisol determinations was 1 ml.

Results

The mean plasma cortisol response to the intravenous administration of

0.25 mg of cosyntropin in each patient group is shown in the Figure. Individual values which were obtained are given in the Table. The baseline serum cortisol concentration in patients with no known adrenal abnormality showed considerable variation. The mean baseline value was 16.7μg/100 ml with a range of 11μg/100 ml to 25μg/100 ml. In seven of the nine control subjects tested, the absolute increase in cortisol concentration at 60 minutes was greater than 7μg/100 ml. In one patient, the 30 minute value was somewhat higher than the 60 minute value. Another patient had only a modest rise of 4.2μg/100 ml at 60 minutes. All values, however, equalled or exceeded 18μg/100 ml at the 60 minute interval. In contrast, all patients with Addison's disease had low baseline cortisol concentrations and none demonstrated an increase in serum concentration after the administration of a single intravenous dose of cosyntropin.

Patients with either panhypopituitarism or adrenocortical suppression due to long-term exogenous steroid therapy demonstrated a definite but blunted serum cortisol response to a single intravenous injection of cosyntropin. The mean baseline cortisol value for this group was 3.9μg/100 ml and was not statistically different from that of patients with Addison's disease. All patients with secondary adrenocortical insufficiency demonstrated a serum cortisol response to cosyntropin of at least 1.6μg/100 ml or greater at the 60 minute period. As a group, these values differed statistically from those of patients with primary adrenal failure. However, in any individual patient, the response up to three hours following a single dose of cosyntropin did not always distinguish primary from secondary adrenal insufficiency.

Examination of the baseline cortisol values and those 60 minutes after corticotropin stimulation permitted a clear separation of any patients studied into one of two categories: those with normal adrenal function and those with either primary or secondary adrenal insufficiency.

Serum Cortisol Response to a Rapid Bolus of 0.25 mg Cosyntropin in Three Groups of Patients

Patient	Corticotropin Concentration, μg/100 ml: 0 min	30 min	60 min	120 min	180 min
			Without Adrenal Disease		
1	12.2	26.6	30.0	37.0	35.0
2	11.0	13.4	18.0	15.0	19.0
3	11.4	16.0	20.0	...	19.0
4	17.4	38.0	38.0	39.0	24.5
5	19.6	24.6	27.0	29.6	19.2
6	24.6	33.4	34.8	36.6	37.2
7	11.6	15.6	25.6	29.8	29.8
8	25.0	36.4	30.6	35.0	31.6
9	17.3	...	21.5	17.8	15.9
Mean ± SD	16.7 ±5.6	25.5 ±9.8	27.3 ±6.8	30.0 ±9.0	25.7 ±7.7
			Primary Adrenal Insufficiency		
1	0	3.0	2.9	2.2	2.9
2	ND*	ND	ND	ND	ND
3	0.9	0.8	0.6	0	0
4	2.0	0.3	0	0	0
5	...	2.7	2.3	2.0	0
6	6.4	3.0	3.1	2.9	2.7
7	2.7	0	0	0	0
Mean ± SD	2.1 ±2.2	1.8 ±1.3	1.6 ±1.4	1.4 ±1.3	1.2 ±1.4
			Secondary Adrenal Insufficiency		
1	9.2	8.5	11.1	13.0	11.6
2	2.8	10.8	9.6	15.5	15.0
3	1.3	9.7	11.0	11.6	8.0
4	5.5	8.2	8.8	12.7	12.6
5	0.8	1.2	2.4	0.8	0
6†	9.8	12.2	10.7	11.8	9.4
7†	0	1.3	2.2	2.3	1.3
8†	1.8	3.4	...	3.4	2.8
Mean ± SD	3.9 ±3.8	6.9 ±4.3	8.0 ±4.0	8.9 ±5.7	7.6 ±5.6

* ND signifies not done.
† Patient on long-term steroid therapy.

Comment

The testing procedure proposed in this study has several important assets. Cosyntropin is a material of low antigenicity with predictable hormonal effects.[9] It can be used in patient populations with a high potential for allergic reactions, such as those receiving steroids for asthma. Therefore, it is considerably safer to employ for office use than ACTH extracts, although an occasional allergic reaction has been reported.[10,11] The CBG method for serum cortisol determination was found to be accurate and reproducible, particularly in the lower ranges such as are found in patients with Addison's disease. The CBG method is relatively specific for cortisol with the exception of exogenously administered cortisone.[6] It has an advantage over the routine

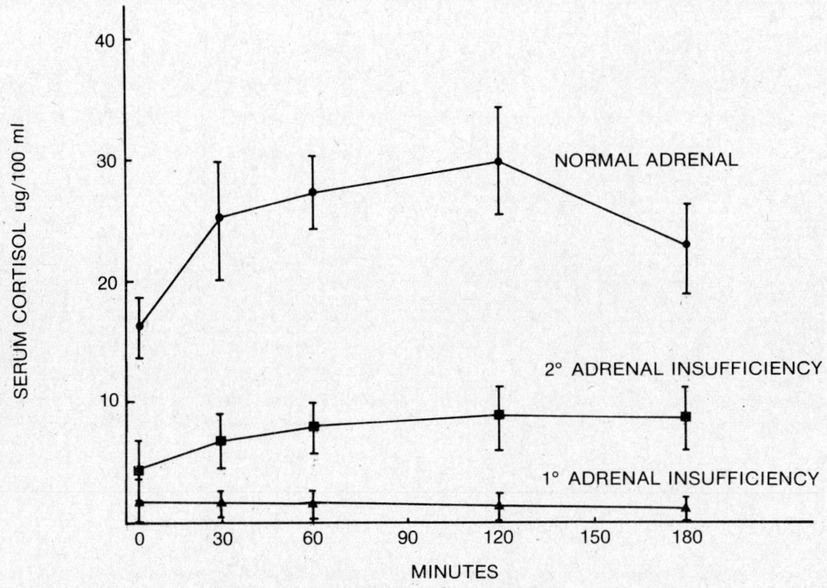

Serum cortisol response to 0.25 mg of cosyntropin in normal subjects (n = 9), hypopituitarism (n = 8), and Addison's disease (n = 7). P < .01 between all means except zero times in primary and secondary adrenal insufficiency.

fluorometric methods employed for measuring serum cortisol in that the values are more reproducible and extraneous compounds, such as spironolactone, will not interfere with the determination. In addition, this method requires only 1 ml or less of serum for one determination, a distinct advantage over other methods such as the Porter-Silber technique. The CBG method is highly specific for the cortisol molecule. The only likely interference would be in pregnancy in which case the very high circulating level of progesterone, which binds slightly to CBG, would cause a modest elevation in plasma cortisol concentration.

The results suggest that as a screening procedure for adrenocortical insufficiency, a baseline sample followed by one 60 minutes after stimulation by intravenously administered cosyntropin is capable of detecting insufficient adrenal function. To prove that the adrenal insufficiency is primary or secondary to pituitary insufficiency or adrenal suppression would require, in most instances, a more prolonged period of ACTH stimulation.[12] However, this testing technique does meet the major clinical requirement of indicating whether a sick patient suspected of having Addison's disease does or does not possess adequate adrenocortical reserve. If the response to this simple procedure is normal, adrenal function can be considered normal. If the response is abnormal, a prolonged period of corticotropin stimulation by standard procedures would be indicated.

This investigation was supported in part by Public Health Service research grant RR-43, from the General Clinical Research Centers, and training grant AM-05176 from the National Institute of Arthritis and Metabolic Diseases.

Nonproprietary and Trade Names of Drug

Cosyntropin—*Cortrosyn.*

References

1. Wood JB, Frankland AW, James VHT, et al: A rapid test of adrenocortical function. *Lancet* **1**:243-245, 1965.
2. Greig WR, Browning MCK, Boyle JA, et al: Effect of the synthetic polypeptide β 1-24 (Synacthen) on adrenocortical function. *J Endocr* **34**:411-412, 1966.
3. Hicklin JA, Wills MR: Plasma "cortisol" response to synacthen in patients on long-term small-dose prednisone therapy. *Ann Rheum Dis* **27**:33-37, 1968.
4. Musa BU, Dowling J: Rapid intravenous administration of corticotropin as a test of adrenocortical insufficiency. *JAMA* **201**:633-635, 1967.
5. Nugent CA, Mayes DM: Plasma corticosteroids determined by use of corticosteroid-binding globulin and dextran-coated charcoal. *J Clin Endocr* **26**:1116-1122, 1966.
6. Bowman RE, DeLuna RF: Assessment of a protein-binding method for cortisol determination. *Anal Biochem* **26**:465-469, 1969.
7. Kraicer J, Conrad RG, Bicknese MB: Abnormally high plasma corticosterone values using the acid fluorescence method. *Clin Chim Acta* **23**:512-513, 1969.
8. Kendall JW, Egans ML, Stott AK: Fluorometric determination of corticosteroids: An interfering substance in impure dichloromethane which fluoresces with benzyl alcohol preservative in heparin. *J Clin Endocr* **28**:1373-1376, 1968.
9. Danowski TS, Hofmann K, Weigand FA, et al: Steroid responses to ACTH-like polypeptides. *J Clin Endocr* **28**:1120-1126, 1968.
10. Charpin J, Zafiropoulo A, Aubert J, et al: Donnees actuelles concernant l'allergie a l'ACTH. *Presse Med* **72**:3025-3028, 1964.
11. Zarate O, Quinteros H: Preliminary report on the therapeutic use of a synthetic corticotrophin. *J Allerg* **38**:51-55, 1966.
12. Christy NP, Wallace EZ, Jailer JW: The effect of intravenously-administered ACTH on plasma 17, 21-dihydroxy-20-ketosteroids in normal individuals and in patients with disorders of the adrenal cortex. *J Clin Invest* **34**:899-906, 1955.

Rheumatoid Pleurisy With Effusion

Glen A. Lillington, MD, Palo Alto, Calif; and David T. Carr, MD, and John G. Mayne, MD, Rochester, Minn

Rheumatoid pleuritis characteristically occurs in middle-aged male rheumatoid patients and may antedate the arthritis. The pleural fluid is an exudate, frequently turbid, and may be milky. The glucose content of the fluid is less than 30 mg/100 ml in 70% to 80% of effusions. A low glucose level in pleural fluid that is nonpurulent, negative for bacteria on smear and culture, and negative for malignant cells on cytologic examination almost invariably indicates that the effusion is due to rheumatoid pleuritis unless pleural biopsy reveals tuberculosis.

Various pleuropulmonary disorders may occur in association with rheumatoid arthritis, the most common being pleurisy or pleural effusion.[1,2] It is now generally agreed that rheumatoid pleuritis is a specific entity which can be diagnosed clinically if certain characteristic manifestations are present.

In some patients with rheumatoid arthritis and pleural effusion, histologic examination of the pleural membranes at thoracotomy or autopsy has revealed granulomatous inflammation, the features of which are identical with, or similar to, the characteristic microscopic changes found in the subcutaneous nodules of rheumatoid arthritis and in the rheumatoid nodules of the lung.[3-13] In many instances, however, only nonspecific pleuritis, pleural fibrosis, and pleural adhesions have been demonstrated.[1,14,15]

Needle biopsy of the parietal pleura has demonstrated characteristic rheumatoid tissue in some instances,[16-21] but in most cases, needle biopsy has revealed only nonspecific chronic pleuritis.[22-29] Needle biopsy and even open thoracotomy with biopsy of the pleura may fail to provide a specific histologic diagnosis in rheumatoid pleuritis.

The possibility that examination of the pleural fluid might prove useful in the diagnosis of rheumatoid pleuritis was first suggested by the demonstration by Carr and Power[30] of low glucose levels in the pleural fluid of three rheumatoid patients. Subsequently, Carr and Mayne[23] noted low concentrations of glucose in ten of 11 rheumatoid pleural effusions. A total of 27 pleural effusions were aspirated from 25 patients with rheumatoid arthritis in this series, but the glucose concentrations of the pleural fluid were measured in only 11 instances. Other features that have been reported to occur in at least some rheumatoid pleural effusions include positive latex fixation titers (rheumatoid factor),[21] elevated lipid levels,[23,28,31] elevated lactic dehydrogenase levels,[10,20,21,28,32] and the presence of rheumatoid arthritis (RA) cells[21,32,33] (phagocytic leukocytes containing inclusion bodies).

The purposes of this paper are as follows: (1) to review all reported cases of rheumatoid effusions in which the pleural fluid glucose was measured, (2) to report the characteristics of the rheumatoid pleural effusions in patients studied at the Mayo Clinic in the decade 1960 through 1969, and (3) to assess the diagnostic

Received for publication Dec 1, 1970; accepted May 6, 1971.

From the Department of Medicine, Palo Alto Clinic, Palo Alto, Calif (Dr. Lillington) and the Department of Internal Medicine, Mayo Clinic and Mayo Foundation, Rochester, Minn (Drs. Carr and Mayne).

Reprint requests to Section of Publications, Mayo Clinic, Rochester, Minn 55901.

value of other pleural fluid characteristics in rheumatoid patients.

Materials and Methods

A search of the records of the Mayo Clinic revealed that 18 pleural effusions were aspirated from 17 patients who had RA (one patient had bilateral effusions) in the decade 1960 through 1969. Rheumatoid patients in whom there was reasonable evidence that the pleurisy was due to some other disease were excluded from this series. All patients except one (patient 13, Tables 1 and 2) satisfied the criteria of the American Rheumatism Association for "classic" RA. This patient had recurring episodic attacks of polyarthritis which occurred between visits to the Mayo Clinic; the serologic test for rheumatoid factor was positive. The anatomic staging and functional classification were done according to Steinbrocker's method.[34]

In some instances, the effusions were recurrent or persistent, and several aspirations were carried out on a single effusion. Tests performed included determination of protein, fat, and glucose concentrations; cultures for fungi, acid-fast bacilli, and common pyogens; and microscopic examination for malignant cells. Not all of these tests were performed on every effusion. Needle biopsy of the pleura was done in five patients, and surgical biopsy (thoracotomy) in two others. Glucose levels in pleural fluid and blood were determined by automated analysis (AutoAnalyzer method)[35]—a method that gives values approximating those for "true" glucose. Serologic tests for "rheumatoid factor" (RF) were performed in all patients, and studies of peripheral blood for lupus erythematosus (LE) cells were done in 15 of the 17 patients.

Table 1.—Selected Clinical Data in Patients With Rheumatoid Arthritis and Pleural Effusion

		Characteristics of Arthritis					
Patient No.	Sex and Age (yr)	Year of Onset	Stage	Functional Class	Year of Thoracentesis	Side	Pulmonary Lesions
1	M, 67	1957	III	2*	1966	Left	None
2	M, 62	1955	III	3	1965	Right	Bilateral nodules
3	F, 43	1962	II	2	1967	Right Right	Nodule, right lung
4	M, 62	1961	III	3	1967	Left	None
5	M, 62	1961	III	2*	1968	Left	None
6	M, 44	1956	II	2*	1965	Left Left Left	Bilateral nodules
7	M, 55	1961	I	1	1961	Left Left Left	None
8	M, 54	1950	III	2*	1960	Right	None
9	M, 39	1949	III	3	1969	Left	None
10	M, 57	1958	I	3	1966	Right	None
11	M, 44	1963	I	1*	1965	Right Right	None
12	M, 39	1956	III	2	1961	Right	None
13	M, 39	1957	I	1	1962	Right	None
14	M, 47	1967	II	3	1967 1968	Left Right	Nodules, left lung
15	M, 60	1964	III	2	1967	Left	None
16	F, 77	1960	II	3	1964	Left	None
17	F, 45	1950	III	3	1967	Right	None

* Degree of disability due to the arthritis. Each had additional disability due to the pleuropulmonary disease.

Results

The data are shown in Tables 1 and 2. Fourteen of the 17 patients were men, and no patient was younger than 39 years of age at the time of onset of the effusion. Nine patients were more than 50 years of age. This age and sex incidence has been noted previously.[23] The blood test for rheumatoid factor was positive in 16 patients, and negative (twice) in 1 patient (case 17). Blood tests for LE cells were negative in 11 patients. A questionably positive response was noted in one patient (case 8), and one or more positive reactions for LE cells were obtained in three patients (cases 11, 16, and 17).

The gross appearance of the aspirated pleural fluid was turbid or opaque in 12 of the 18 effusions and was usually yellow-green; in 3 of these effusions, a chyliform (milky) appearance was noted.

The concentration of glucose in the pleural fluid was 37 mg or less per 100 ml on at least one occasion in 15 of the 18 effusions; in 11 of these, the glucose level was less than 20 mg. The patients with high levels of pleural fluid glucose (cases 15, 16, and 17) had certain special clinical characteristics and will be discussed later.

The protein concentration of pleural fluid was greater than 3.0 gm/100 ml in 17 effusions. Smears and cultures were done for acid-fast organisms (17 of 18 effusions), other bacteria (14 of 18 effusions), and fungi (12 of 18 effusions) and were invariably negative. Cytologic examination for malignant cells was carried out in 16 effusions and findings were negative in each case.

Needle biopsy of the parietal pleura was carried out in five patients (cases 5, 10, 12, 13, and 16). In each instance, histologic examination showed nonspecific chronic inflammation of the pleura. One patient (case 14) had bi-

Table 2.—Selected Laboratory Data in Patients With Rheumatoid Arthritis and Pleural Effusion

	Pleural Effusion					
Case	Volume (ml)	Gross Appearance	Protein (gm/100 ml)	Glucose (mg/100 ml)	Fat (mg/100 ml)	Blood Glucose (mg/100 ml)
1	500	Creamy	4.9	18	2,100	100
2	110	Yellow	3.2	37	. . .	116
3	1,000	Dark green	4.7	0	289	. . .
	25	Milky	5.3	34	208	. . .
4	75	Amber	4.1	17	. . .	82
5	100	Straw	3.9	36	. . .	78
6	800	Milky	4.8	5	1,350	93
	50	. . .	5.1	5	336	. . .
	1,600	Milky	3.6	20	1,006	. . .
7	325	Amber	5.0	83	. . .	. . .
	. . .	Cloudy brown	. . .	22	226	. . .
	. . .	. . .	5.7	11	. . .	. . .
8	400	Milky	7.5	26	1,023	. . .
9	120	Cloudy green	7.3	<10	1,180	92
10	500	Cloudy	5.5	0	. . .	85
11	500	Yellow	4.3	18	. . .	79
	1,600	Amber	4.5	10	. . .	. . .
12	100	Turbid green	6.8	0	. . .	75
13	1,300	Cloudy green	5.2	0	. . .	95
14	300	Cloudy green	4.5	10	289	79
	550	Cloudy green	5.7	26	. . .	. . .
15	20	Straw	2.6	81	. . .	. . .
16	200	Yellow	4.7	118	. . .	84
17	150	Cloudy	6.9	98	. . .	77

lateral effusions; bilateral thoracotomies were performed, and histologic examination of the pleura showed typical changes of rheumatoid pleuritis[23]; autopsy revealed pericarditis.

Concentrations of fat in the pleural fluid were measured in six effusions and were significantly elevated in four, with fat levels between 1,023 mg/100 ml and 2,100 mg/100 ml. Three of these four effusions were milky white (chyliform), and one was cloudy green. In three of these four patients (cases 1, 6, and 8), the effusion was known to have been present 1½ to 2 years. In the fourth patient (case 9), the duration of the effusion was unknown.

Three patients (cases 15 through 17) merit special comment. Although each patient had the typical joint manifestations of RA, there was evidence that some other disease process might have caused the pleural effusions. This was not definite enough, however, to exclude these from the series. All three patients had clinical features suggestive of systemic lupus erythematosus (SLE), and this diagnosis was, in fact, made in each case by at least one of the various consultants who examined the patients. Our studies[36] of pleural effusions in patients with SLE have indicated that the pleural fluid glucose content is normal in this disease. If patients 15 through 17 were excluded from this series, then all of the remaining 15 rheumatoid pleural effusions in the series had glucose levels of 37 mg or lower per 100 ml.

Diagnostic Significance of Pleural Fluid Glucose

The diagnostic value of a symptom or sign as an index of the presence of a given disease process depends upon its incidence (that is, how commonly the sign occurs in the disease) and its specificity (that is, how rarely the sign occurs in other diseases). To obtain an approximate value for the incidence of a low glucose level in the pleural fluid of patients with RA, we have reviewed all reported cases of rheumatoid pleural effusions in which the glucose content of the fluid was recorded.[10,17,19-21,23,26-33,37-43] The total number of cases collected may not be correct, because in some instances a given patient has been reported in two or more separate publications, and we are not certain whether we have detected all such "overlaps." In addition, the specific values for pleural fluid glucose were reported in different ways by different authors, and some ambiguity remains.

The results are shown in Table 3. Values for pleural fluid glucose were reported for 76 effusions in rheumatoid patients (including the 17 patients reported in this paper). The glucose content was greater than 50 mg/100 ml in 13 cases (17.1%) and was less than 30 mg/100 ml in 59 cases (77.6%). The true incidence of low glucose probably is even greater, as some of the pleural effusions with normal glucose concentrations may be due to a cause other than the rheumatoid disease.

Low levels of pleural fluid glucose occur in empyemas (bacterial, fungal, or tuberculous)[44-46] and in some neoplastic pleural effusions.[38,44,47,48] Clark-

Table 3.—Pleural Fluid Glucose in Rheumatoid Pleural Effusion*

Glucose Concentration (mg/100 ml of Pleural Fluid)	No. of Cases	% of Total
0-9	32	42.1
10-19	16	21.1
20-29	11	14.4
30-50	4	5.3
>50	13	17.1
Total	76	100.0

* Data from literature plus from present report.

son[44] noted a glucose content of less than 60 mg/100 ml in 25% of patients with neoplastic pleural or peritoneal effusions; in almost all instances, the glucose content was less than 25 mg/100 ml, and the effusions were usually bloody and contained large numbers of tumor cells. Because the true nature of purulent or neoplastic effusions is usually indicated promptly by smears, cultures, and cytologic studies, the low glucose level in pleural fluid in these cases rarely leads to diagnostic confusion.

The glucose level in pleural fluid may be significantly reduced in nonpurulent tuberculous effusions.[47,49] The values are usually below 60 mg/100 ml and often are less than 30 mg/100 ml, particularly when the effusion yields tubercle bacilli on smear or culture.[46]

Nonpurulent and nonmalignant effusions due to diseases other than tuberculosis or RA almost invariably have glucose levels greater than 70 mg/100 ml.

Specific Characteristics of Rheumatoid Pleural Effusions

Glucose.—In most pleural transudates and exudates, the glucose content is approximately equal to that in the blood. An abnormally low concentration of glucose in pleural fluid (in a normoglycemic patient) can result from (1) abnormalities in the pleural membrane reducing transfer of glucose, or (2) excess glycolysis in the fluid. Increased glycolysis due to large numbers of inflammatory or neoplastic cells in the pleural fluid seems to be the explanation for the low glucose levels noted in some neoplastic pleural effusions and in many purulent pleural effusions. A decreased glucose level is commonly found in tuberculous pleural effusions, even if nonpurulent[46,47,49,50]; while the cause of this is not clear, it is probably not due to increased glycolysis because the cell counts in many tuberculous pleural effusions are not inordinately high.

The low levels of glucose in rheumatoid pleural effusions are apparently due to impaired transport of glucose from the blood to the pleural fluid across the inflamed pleural membrane.[29,37]

Lipids.—High concentrations of total lipids[23,28,31] and of cholesterol[28,29,39] have been noted in some rheumatoid pleural effusions. The fluid may be chyliform or may have the "opalescent sheen" noted in some chronic cholesterol effusions that have cholesterol crystal formation. Four of the 18 effusions in our series contained high levels of lipids. The effusions were known to be chronic or recurrent in three patients, and no specific information on the duration of the effusion was available in the fourth. Chronicity and high cellularity are probably necessary for the development of a high lipid or cholesterol content in a pleural effusion unless it is a true chylothorax.

Rheumatoid Factor.—The presence of RF in high titers in rheumatoid pleural effusions was first noted by Berger and Seckler.[21] However, RF may be found by some techniques in a significant percentage of pleural effusions secondary to bacterial pneumonia, carcinoma, and tuberculosis.[51] These patients did not have RA; and, in many instances, the serum levels of RF were low despite high levels in the pleural fluid. This test was not performed on the pleural effusions of our patients.

Lactic Dehydrogenase.—High levels of lactic dehydrogenase (LDH) have been reported in rheumatoid pleural effusions[10,20,21,28,32] and, in most instances, the level of LDH in the pleural fluid has exceeded that in the serum. Elevations of LDH are commonly found in chronic pleural effusions due to other causes[2] and the test is of little value in the identification of rheumatoid effusions.

Cytology.—In most reported cases, cytologic examination of rheumatoid pleural effusions has not been particularly helpful in the differential diagnosis. Recently, there have been several reports[21,32,33] of the identification of RA cells in rheumatoid pleural effusions. The RA cell or "ragocyte" is a polymorphonuclear leukocyte that contains characteristic cytoplasmic inclusion bodies thought to represent phagocytosed RF complex. These cells are freuquently found in synovial fluid from rheumatoid joints. Typical RA cells were noted in the pleural fluid in patient 1 of the current series.

Nosanchuk and Naylor[41] have described "a unique cytologic picture" in five of ten pleural effusions in patients with rheumatoid arthritis. The glucose concentrations in pleural fluid ranged from 0.0 to 25.0 mg/100 ml in these five patients. The cytologic findings comprised three "characteristic" elements: large elongated cells, multinucleated giant cells, and a background of orange (Papanicolaou stain) or red (hematoxylin-eosin stain) granular material. They did not describe RA cells in their cases.

References

1. Baggenstoss AH, Rosenberg EF: Visceral lesions associated with chronic infectious (rheumatoid) arthritis. *Arch Path* **35**:503-516, 1943.
2. Turner-Warwick ME: Rheumatoid arthritis, rheumatoid factors and lung disease. *Brit J Hosp Med* **2**:507, 1969.
3. Bennett GA, Zeller JW, Bauer W: Subcutaneous nodules of rheumatoid arthritis and rheumatic fever: Pathologic study. *Arch Path* **30**:70-89, 1940.
4. Gruenwald P: Visceral lesions in a case of rheumatoid arthritis. *Arch Path* **46**:59-67, 1948.
5. Bevans M, Nadell J, Demartini F, et al: The systemic lesions of malignant rheumatoid arthritis. *Amer J Med* **16**:197-211, 1954.
6. Lee PR, Sox HC, North FS, et al: Pleurisy with effusion in rheumatoid arthritis. *Arch Intern Med* **104**:634-639, 1959.
7. Raven RW, Weber FP, Price LW: The necrobiotic nodules of rheumatoid arthritis: Case in which the scalp, abdominal wall (involving striped muscle), larynx, pericardium (involving myocardium), pleurae (involving lungs), and peritoneum were affected. *Ann Rheum Dis* **7**:63-75, 1948.
8. Ellman P, Cudkowicz L, Elwood JS: Widespread serous membrane involvement by rheumatoid nodules. *J Clin Path* **7**:239-244, 1954.
9. Robertson JL, Brinkman GL: Nodular rheumatoid lung disease. *Amer J Med* **31**:483-487, 1961.
10. Basten A, Camens I, Schwartz CJ: Rheumatoid lung disease with report of a case. *Aust Ann Med* **15**:175-181, 1966.
11. Rubin EH, Gordon M, Thelmo WL: Nodular pleuropulmonary rheumatoid disease: Report of two cases and review of literature. *Amer J Med* **42**:567-581, 1967.
12. Horler AR, Thompson M: The pleural and pulmonary complications of rheumatoid arthritis. *Ann Intern Med* **51**:1179-1203, 1959.
13. Brunk JR, Drash EC, Swineford O: Rheumatoid pleuritis successfully treated with decortication: Report of a case and review of the literature. *Amer J Med Sci* **251**:545-551, 1966.
14. Fingerman DL, Andrus FC: Visceral lesions associated with rheumatoid arthritis. *Ann Rheum Dis* **3**:168-181, 1943.
15. Sinclair RJG, Cruickshank B: Clinical and pathological study of 16 cases of rheumatoid arthritis with extensive visceral involvement ("rheumatoid disease"). *Quart J Med* **25**:313-332, 1956.
16. Heller P, Kellow WF, Chomet B: Needle biopsy of the parietal pleura. *New Eng J Med* **255**:684-690, 1956.
17. Schools GS, Mikkelsen WM: Rheumatoid pleuritis. *Arthritis Rheum* **5**:369-377, 1962.
18. Lassiter GS, Tassy FT: Malignant rheumatoid disease with aortic stenosis. *Arch Intern Med* **116**:930-936, 1965.
19. Portner MM, Gracie WA Jr: Rheumatoid lung disease with cavitary nodules, pneumothorax and eosinophilia. *New Eng J Med* **275**:697-700, 1968.
20. Campbell GD, Ferrington E: Rheumatoid pleuritis with effusion. *Chest* **53**:521-527, 1968.
21. Berger HW, Seckler SG: Pleural and pericardial effusions in rheumatoid disease. *Ann Intern Med* **64**:1291-1297, 1966.
22. Ward R: Pleural effusion and rheumatoid disease. *Lancet* **2**:1336-1338, 1961.
23. Carr DT, Mayne JG: Pleurisy with effusion in rheumatoid arthritis, with reference to the low concentration of glucose in pleural fluid. *Amer Rev Resp Dis* **85**:345-350, 1962.
24. Mattingly S: The lungs and rheumatoid arthritis. *Ann Phys Med* **7**:185-202, 1964.
25. Poppius H, Tani P: Non-tuberculous pleurisy. *Acta Tuberc Scand* **44**:310-315, 1964.
26. Walker WC, Wright V: Rheumatoid pleuritis. *Ann Rheum Dis* **26**:467-474, 1967.
27. Martel W, Abell MR, Mikkelsen WM, et al: Pulmonary and pleural lesions in rheumatoid disease. *Radiology* **90**:641-653, 1968.
28. Stengel BF, Watson RR, Darling RJ: Pulmonary rheumatoid nodule with cavitation and chronic lipid effusion. *JAMA* **198**:1263-1266, 1966.
29. Dodson WH, Hollingsworth JW: Pleural effusion in rheumatoid arthritis: Impaired transport of glucose. *New Eng J Med* **275**:1337-1342, 1966.
30. Carr DT, Power MH: Pleural fluid glucose with special reference to its concentration in rheumatoid pleurisy with effusion. *Chest* **37**:321-324, 1960.
31. Bower GC: Chyliform pleural effusion in rheumatoid arthritis. *Amer Rev Resp Dis* **97**:455-459, 1968.
32. Mandl MAJ, Watson JI, Henderson JAM, et al: Pleural fluid in rheumatoid arthritis. *Arch Intern Med* **124**:373-376, 1969.
33. Carmichael DS, Golding DN: Rheumatoid pleural effusion with "R.A. cells" in the pleural fluid. *Brit Med J* **2**:814, 1967.
34. Steinbrocker O, Traeger CH, Batterman RC: Therapeutic criteria in rheumatoid arthritis. *JAMA* **140**:659-662, 1949.
35. McGuckin WF, Power MH: Determination of blood sugar by an automatic method, abstracted. *Clin Chem* **4**:541, 1958.
36. Carr DT, Lillington GA, Mayne JG: Pleural-fluid glucose in systemic lupus erythematosus. *Mayo Clin Proc* **45**:409-412, 1970.
37. Carr DT, McGuckin WF: Pleural fluid glucose: Serial observation of its concentration following oral administration of glucose to patients with rheumatoid pleural effusions and malignant effusions. *Amer Rev Resp Dis* **97**:302-305, 1968.
38. Carr DT, McGuckin WF: Chemistry of pleural effusions. *Biochem Clin* **4**:283-286, 1963.
39. Ferguson GC: Cholesterol pleural effusion in rheumatoid lung disease. *Thorax* **21**:577-582, 1966.
40. Petty TL, Wilkins M: The five manifestations of rheumatoid lung. *Chest* **49**:75-82, 1966.
41. Nosanchuk JS, Naylor B: A unique cytologic picture in pleural fluid from patients with rheumatoid arthritis. *Amer J Clin Path* **50**:330-335, 1968.
42. Champion GD, Robertson MR, Robinson RG: Rheumatoid pleurisy and pericarditis. *Ann Rheum Dis* **27**:521-530, 1968.
43. Sulavik S, Katz S: *Pleural Effusion: Some Infrequently Emphasized Causes.* Springfield, Ill, Charles C Thomas Publisher, 1963, pp 18-25.
44. Clarkson B: Relationship between cell type, glucose concentration, and response to treatment in neoplastic effusions. *Cancer* **17**:914-928, 1964.
45. Peterson JE: Quantitative sugar estimations in pleural fluid—An aid to diagnosis. *Med Arts Sci* **2**:124-128, 1948.
46. Barber LM, Mazzadi L, Deakins DD, et al: Glucose level in pleural fluid as a diagnostic aid. *Chest* **31**:680-687, 1957.
47. Glenert J: Sugar levels in pleural effusions of different etiologies. *Acta Tuberc Scand* **42**:222-227, 1962.
48. Durieu H: Mécanismes de la régulation du taux du glucose dans les épanchements pleuraux. *Acta Tuberc Belg* **45**:205-238, 1954.
49. Gelenger SM, Wiggers RF: Relationship of the pleural fluid sugar to pulmonary tuberculosis. *Chest* **15**:325-328, 1949.
50. Calnan WL, Winfield, BJO, Crowley MF, et al: Diagnostic value of the glucose content of serous pleural effusions. *Brit Med J* **1**:1239-1240, 1951.
51. Levine H, Szanto M, Grieble HG, et al: Rheumatoid factor in nonrheumatoid pleural effusions. *Ann Intern Med* **69**:487-492, 1968.

Factors Affecting Plasma Calcium Concentration During Hemodialysis

Harry S. Tamm; Karl D. Nolph, MD; and John F. Maher, MD, Columbia, Mo

Plasma concentrations of calcium often increase during hemodialysis. To evaluate the mechanisms involved, total (Ca) and ionized (Ca^{++}) calcium, protein, pH, P_{CO_2}, and sodium (Na^+) were measured in plasma (P) at the beginning and end of 17 six-hour coil dialyses using bath with 5.27 ± 0.04 mg/100 ml of Ca^{++}. Simultaneously, ultrafiltrates (UF) collected directly from coils (after isolating and draining the cannister) were analyzed for Ca, Ca^{++}, and Na^+. Increases in plasma Ca reflected mainly increases in protein-bound calcium (secondary to bath hemoconcentration of protein and increased binding per gram of protein) without an increase in plasma Ca^{++} or complexed Ca. With increases in plasma pH and protein concentration, $(UF/P\ Na^+)^2$ decreased only slightly suggesting minimal changes in net protein anionic concentration and Gibbs-Donnan effects.

Plasma calcium concentration usually increases acutely during hemodialysis with the use of dialysis bath prepared from commercially available concentrates. Several explanations for this phenomenon have been proposed:

1. diffusion of calcium to blood from dialysate higher in calcium concentration than plasma, which causes a rise in plasma ionized calcium concentration[1,2];

2. increased calcium binding per gram of protein subsequent to a rise in plasma pH, with simultaneous influx of ionized calcium from the bath, which prevents a detectable decrease in plasma ionized calcium concentration[3]; and

3. increased net negative charge per gram of protein secondary to an increase in blood pH, which results in greater Gibbs-Donnan effects.[4] The latter would favor diffusion of ionized calcium from bath to blood, even in the absence of a concentration gradient.

Another mechanism not previously proposed might involve the following:

4. proportional increases in the concentrations of plasma proteins and protein bound calcium secondary to the ultrafiltration (and subsequent hemoconcentration) which often accompanies dialysis.

Recent reports suggest that the calcium balance or changes in plasma calcium concentration during dialysis, or both, may have long-term effects on parathyroid function and calcium homeostasis in patients undergoing chronic hemodialysis.[5] Further evaluation of the factors affecting plasma calcium during hemodialysis is required.

In this paper, analyses of changes in plasma calcium concentration during hemodialysis are reported. The results demonstrate that protein hemoconcentration and increased protein calcium binding (mechanisms 2 and 4) can alone account for increases in plasma calcium concentration observed during routine hemodialysis.

Study Design

Studies were performed during 17 six-hour routine hemodialyses in six patients. Five patients had end-stage chronic renal disease and one had postsurgical acute renal failure. Commercially available cellophane coils were perfused in the usual manner with the use of a standard blood pump and coil dialysis apparatus. Dialysis bath containing sodium, 130 mEq/liter; chloride, 101 mEq/liter; acetate, 35 mEq/liter; potassium, 2 mEq/liter; magnesium, 1.5 mEq/liter, calcium, 2.5 mEq/liter; and 200 mg/100 ml of dextrose prepared from a concentrate and deionized tap water was used in all studies. Bath flow rate into the recirculating reservoir was 350 ml/mm. Blood flow rate varied from study to study (approximately 75 to 200 ml/min). Outlet pressure was varied as

Received for publication March 22, 1971; accepted Aug 3.

From the Department of Medicine, Division of Nephrology, University of Missouri Medical Center, Columbia.

Reprint requests to Department of Medicine, Division of Nephrology, University of Missouri Medical Center, Columbia, Mo 65201 (Dr. Nolph).

determined by the clinical need for ultrafiltration.

Samples of heparinized arterial blood were collected during the first and last half hour of every dialysis. Early samples were drawn at least 15 minutes after the initiation of dialysis and, thus, any hemodilution from the approximate 700 ml of saline prime had already occurred. Ultrafiltrates (UFs) of blood were collected directly from the dialysis coil during the same early and late periods of dialysis. In order to accomplish this, the coil and its cannister were removed from the dialysis bath, drained by gravity, and placed directly over a graduate cylinder. Ultrafiltrate was collected for ten minutes (50 to 100 ml) and discarded. The next 10 ml of UF following discard were collected directly into 20-ml containers fitted tightly to the cannister outlet to minimize evaporation.

Concentrations of total calcium, ionized calcium, sodium, and protein were determined in arterial plasma and UF samples. Arterial pH and P_{CO_2} were determined in 17 and 11 studies, respectively. Total calcium concentration was also measured in selected bath samples.

Chemical Determinations

Protein concentrations were measured by automatic analysis (Technicon Auto-Analyzer) with the use of a modification of the Biuret reaction.[6] Sodium and total calcium concentrations were also determined by automatic analysis.[7,8] The pH and P_{CO_2} were determined on an analyzer (Corning, model 16 pH/P_{CO_2}). Ionized calcium was determined by a flow through electrode method.[9]

Calculations

All total calcium, ionized calcium, and sodium concentrations in plasma were corrected to and are reported as their approximate concentrations in plasma water using the relationship: Plasma water concentration (P) = (measured plasma concentration) $\frac{100}{(98.6 - 0.73\ \text{Pr})}$, where Pr equals the concentration of protein in grams per 100 ml.[10]

According to the Gibbs-Donnan formulae,[11-13] at diffusion equilibrium:

1. $(P_{Na^+})\ (P_{Cl^-}) = (UF_{Na^+})\ (UF_{Cl^-})$

or

2. $$\frac{(P_{Cl^-})}{(UF_{Cl^-})} = \frac{(UF_{Na^+})}{(P_{Na^+})}$$

(Neglecting correction to ion activities which should be nearly the same for the numerator and demoninator of respective ratios.)

Similarly,

3. $(P_{Ca^{++}})\ (P_{Cl^-})^2 = (UF_{Ca^{++}})\ (UF_{Cl^-})^2$ or

4. $$\frac{(P_{Cl^-})^2}{(UF_{Cl^-})^2} = \frac{(UF_{Ca^{++}})}{(P_{Ca^{++}})}.$$

Squaring equation 2 and substituting into equation 4:

5. $$\frac{(UF_{Na^+})^2}{P_{(Na^+)}^2} = \frac{(UF_{Ca^{++}})^2}{(P_{Ca^{++}})^2} = (UF/P\ Na^+)^2.$$

Calculation of $(UF/P\ Na^+)^2$ during early and late dialysis in each study permitted quantitative assessment of changes in net protein charge and changes in potential Gibbs-Donnan effects on diffusion equilibrium of ionized calcium.

The concentration of mean plasma water complexed calcium was calculated as (mean UF total calcium concentration) − (mean UF ionized calcium concentration). This calculation neglects Gibbs-Donnan effects on the ionic components of complexed calcium and probably underestimates true plasma water complexed calcium concentration. It also neglects any net conversion of ionized to complexed or vice-versa in ultrafiltrate samples. It should be closer to true value than the usual formula of UF calcium − plasma ionized calcium.

Mean plasma protein-bound calcium concentration was calculated as (mean P total calcium) − (mean P ionized calcium + mean P complexed calcium).

Results

Although any or all of the proposed mechanisms might effect plasma calcium concentration during a single hemodialysis, analysis of changes in mean calcium values in a number of dialyses should detect any common predominant mechanism. Table 1 shows the mean arterial plasma measurements during early and late dialysis. Plasma total calcium concentration increased in 12 of 17 studies with a mean increase of 0.7 mg/100 ml in late dialysis. No change in mean plasma ionized calcium concentration was detected. Total protein concentration increased in 16 of 17 studies and the late mean value was higher by 0.6 gm/100 ml. Patients invariably lost weight and mean weight loss was 1.6 ± 0.6 kg. Arterial blood pH increased in all studies. Mean arterial P_{CO_2} decreased slightly from early to late dialysis.

During these studies, mean measured bath calcium concentration prior to circulation was 5.27 ± 0.04 mg/100 ml (greater than both plasma ionized and ultrafiltrable calcium).

Table 2 shows mean UF/P total calcium, UF/P ionized calcium, and $(UF/P\ Na^+)^2$ values at the beginning and end of dialysis. Minimal changes in mean values during dialysis were observed. In both early and late arterial samples, the mean ratio of UF/P total calcium was well below that of $(UF/P\ Na^+)^2$ and UF/P ionized calcium. Mean UF/P ionized calcium and $(UF/P\ Na^+)^2$ were similar in both early and late arterial plasma samples.

The Figure shows the mean plasma composition in early and late dialysis calculated from the mean data shown in Tables 1 and 2. Note that only calculated protein-bound calcium increased during dialysis. The ratio of late over early mean protein-bound calcium concentration was 1.22. The ratio of late over early mean plasma concentration was 1.10.

Comment

Diffusion of Ionized Calcium From Bath to Blood.—In these studies, mean

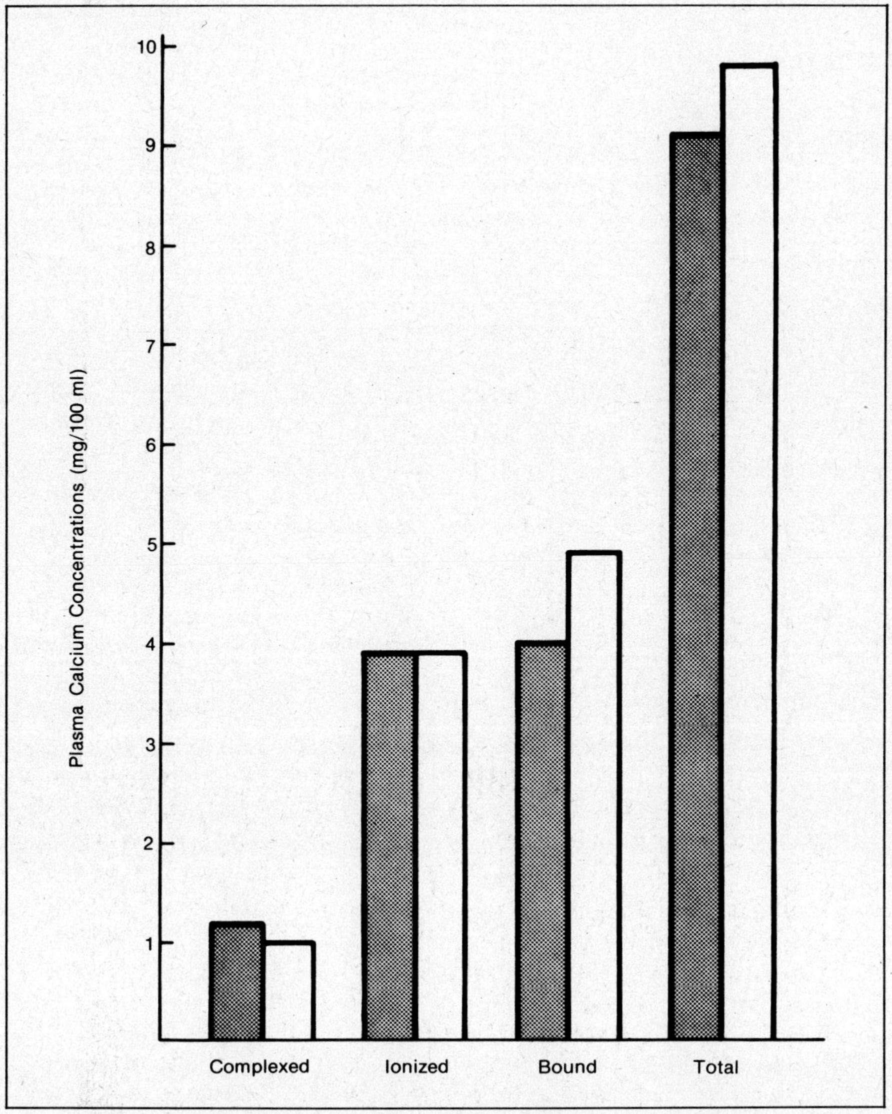

The mean concentrations (vertical axis) *of plasma complexed, ionized, bound, and total calcium during early* (shaded vertical bars) *and late* (clear vertical bars) *hemodialysis. The values for total and ionized concentrations are the means of measured concentrations as in Table 1. The values for complexed and bound concentrations are calculated from mean data shown in Tables 1 and 2 (see text). Only the mean concentration of protein-bound calcium increased during dialysis.*

ionized plasma calcium concentration did not increase in spite of the fact that the bath calcium (presumably mostly ionized) was 1.37 mg/100 ml greater than mean plasma ionized calcium concentration at the beginning of dialysis. Furszyfer et al[5] reported a mean calcium uptake of 0.31 mg/min with the use of a bath of similar calcium concentration to that used in this study (5 to 6 mg/100 ml). They also demonstrated greater calcium absorption from bath containing 7 to 8 mg/100 ml of calcium. Certainly the use of progressively higher levels of dialysate calcium might eventually cause absorption rapid enough to increase serum ionized calcium. In our studies, however, significant increases in plasma total calcium occurred that did not reflect increases in plasma ionized calcium concentration, which demonstrates the pitfalls of assuming that changes in total plasma calcium reflect changes in plasma ionized calcium concentration.

Furszyfer et al[5] have further proposed that the maintenance of normal or slightly elevated ionized calcium concentration in dialysis patients, or prevention of its reduction during dialysis, may avoid repeated parathormone stimulation and prevent or delay the onset of secondary hyperparathyroidism. They also proposed that net calcium transfer depends primarily upon the concentration gradient between dialysate calcium and plasma ultrafiltrable calcium. Ultrafiltrable calcium consists of both ionized and complexed calcium, however, and the concentration gradient for the transfer of complexed calcium should be considered independently in order to accurately predict net calcium movement. Variations in ultrafiltration rate might also effect net solute transport. Further evaluation is needed to identify the best way to predict the net transfer of calcium during dialysis.

During the present studies, the concentration of calcium in the bath relative to plasma ionized calcium favors a net uptake of calcium from dialysate. Due to the use of a large volume of dialysate in our system, the calcium uptake could not be accurately determined from minor changes in bath calcium concentration. Bath calcium postcoil concentration, however, was always slightly less than precoil bath concentration where measured, which suggests that calcium is absorbed from this standard dialysis solution. Mean ionized calcium concentration did not change, however, from early to late dialysis.

Wing[2] also found that the increase

in plasma ultrafiltrable calcium during dialysis was less than anticipated by the measured amount of calcium absorbed. It was assumed that this discrepancy either represented a simultaneous negative calcium balance secondary to metabolic body losses or rapid mobilization of calcium into the noncirculation pools. Measured calcium binding to cellophane was insufficient to explain differences between observed total plasma calcium and that predicted from estimated calcium absorption. This agrees with the work of Freeman et al,[14] who reported negligible adherence of calcium to cellophane when in contact with blood.

Ogden and Holmes also demonstrated an increase in ultrafiltrable plasma calcium when dialysate calcium level was high. At a dialysate calcium level of 7.5 mg/100 ml, ultrafiltrable calcium did not change appreciably, but total calcium level increased by 1.8 mg/100 ml.[1]

Another factor which potentially could affect plasma ionized calcium concentration is a sudden decrease in plasma inorganic phosphate concentration with dialysis.[15] Since ionized calcium concentration did not change, this factor did not seem to affect our studies.

Effects of Increased Net Negative Charge Per Gram of Protein.—The absence of a significant rise in plasma ionized calcium level in these studies suggests that increases in net negative protein charge and Gibbs-Donnan effects on ionized plasma calcium did not play a major role. Arterial plasma pH did increase, however, in every study, which implies that the net negative charge per gram of protein might have increased. Assuming that the ionic activity of sodium remained constant, that sodium is not bound to protein, and assuming that a Gibbs-Donnan-like phenomenon occurs during ultrafiltration,[16] changes in $(UF/P\ Na^+)^2$ and $UF_{Ca^{++}}/P_{Ca^{++}}$ should reflect changes in the net negative charge effect of protein on the concentration of these ions in the UFs. Mean ratios changed only slightly from the beginning to the end of dialysis, which suggests that any increase in net negative protein charge subsequent to an increase in plasma arterial pH from 7.4 to 7.6 was of minor significance. The lower mean $(UF/P\ Na^+)^2$ in late dialysis, however, is in the direction expected with increasing arterial pH.

Table 1.—Mean (± SD) Arterial Plasma Concentrations During Hemodialysis

	Total Calcium (mg/100 ml)	Ionized Calcium (mg/100 ml)	Total Protein (gm/100 ml)	pH	P_{CO_2} (mm Hg)
Early dialysis	9.1 ± 1.0	3.9 ± 0.4	6.0 ± 0.5	7.45 ± 0.04	37 ± 7
Late dialysis	9.8 ± 1.0	3.9 ± 0.8	6.6 ± 0.7	7.54 ± 0.03	34 ± 6

Table 2.—Mean (± SD) UF/P Values During Hemodialysis

	US/P Total Calcium	US/P Ionized Calcium	$(UF/P\ Na^+)^2$
Early dialysis	0.52 ± 0.10	0.90 ± 0.11	0.89 ± 0.05
Late dialysis	0.46 ± 0.12	0.90 ± 0.07	0.84 ± 0.05

The fact that UF total calcium level/P total calcium level was always well below $(UF/P\ Na^+)^2$ suggests that a Gibbs-Donnan-like phenomenon alone does not explain the marked difference between plasma ultrafiltrable and total calcium levels and is compatible with the hypothesis that calcium is bound to protein by coordinate covalent binding. The net negative protein charge influenced ultrafiltrate ionized calcium concentration, however, to the degree predicted by the $(UF/P\ Na^+)$.[2] Similar effects on cationic complexed calcium might be expected.

Increases in Protein Bound Calcium.—Protein concentration increased during every study, reflecting the ultrafiltration loss of plasma fluid during hemodialysis. An increase in mean protein-bound calcium proportional to the increase in mean plasma protein concentration could only account for a rise from 4.0 to 4.4 mg/100 ml (early protein-bound calcium concentration × late/early plasma protein concentration = 4.0 mg/100 ml × 1.1). Since mean protein bound calcium concentration actually increased to 4.9 mg/100 ml, hemoconcentration of plasma proteins alone can only account for 0.4/0.9 or 44.5% of the observed increase. This suggests that increased binding of calcium per gram of plasma protein may occur in addition to protein hemoconcentration compatible with the third mechanism.

The in vitro diffusion equilibrium study of Danesh et al similarly suggested increases in protein binding sites per gram of protein associated with a rise in blood pH.[3] Their study differed markedly from the clinical situation. Blood pH changes were greater than in our study. Ionized calcium concentrations, protein concentrations, or estimates of changes in net protein charge were not reported. A dialysis coil was perfused from a reservoir containing citrated blood which was not in equilibrium with a large extravascular calcium pool and was not under the influence of endocrine regulation of calcium homeostasis as is the case in clinical dialysis. Our results, nevertheless, lend support to their findings and also suggest that plasma protein hemoconcentration during clinical dialysis can explain an almost equal portion of the increase in total plasma calcium concentration.

General Comments.—Our findings suggest that with the use of a standard dialysis bath total plasma calcium concentration usually increases. This does not represent a significant increase in ionized calcium concentration, but mainly a rise in protein bound calcium. This increment was proportionally greater than that of plasma protein concentration, which suggests an increase in protein binding sites. Since the latter may reflect an effect of pH change, the increase in plasma calcium cannot be predicted from ultrafiltration rate and protein hemoconcentration alone. Accordingly, neither weight loss nor change in hematocrit value can be used to predict postdialysis plasma calcium concentration. Little or no change in net protein charge occurred during routine dialysis in spite of an invariable rise in pH.

Although ionized calcium flux into bath could have been enhanced by solvent drag with ultrafiltration,[16] net uptake more likely occurs. Some net removal of complexed calcium seems likely, but the slight decrease in plasma complexed calcium concentration suggests either low dialysis clearance or rapid reformation. As estimated, any increase in the mean number of protein calcium binding sites per gram of protein accommodated only 0.5 mg of calcium per 100 ml of plasma water or 20 mg of calcium per 4 liters of plasma. Thus, any net movement of ionized calcium from bath to plasma in excess of 20 mg must have been associated with simultaneous net movement of calcium from plasma to other body pools. Since mean plasma ionized calcium concentration did not change and since any change in net protein charge was slight, it can be assumed that mean extravascular extracellular fluid ionized calcium concentration remained essentially constant. Thus, movement of absorbed dialysate calcium to cellular, excreted, or crystalline calcium pools would have to be invoked.

All patients were normocalcemic or hypocalcemic prior to dialysis and had no evidence for secondary hyperparathyroidism. The presence of hyperparathyroidism associated with greater rates of bone calcium mobilization might alter the above findings.

Greater changes in blood pH than seen in our studies might cause changes in net protein charge or greater increases in calcium binding sites per gram of protein, or both. Similarly, the use of dialysis bath with higher calcium concentrations would be expected to increase plasma ionized calcium. Nevertheless, our studies show that during routine hemodialysis with a standard bath, hemoconcentration of protein-bound calcium can also contribute significantly to increases in total plasma calcium level. Just as changes in total plasma calcium cannot be assumed to reflect changes in ionized calcium concentrations, changes in protein-bound calcium cannot be assumed to reflect only changes in binding sites per gram of protein. Variations in ultrafiltration and protein hemoconcentration may account in part for discrepant findings between different laboratories. All attempts to analyze plasma calcium homeostasis during dialysis must account for changes in protein-bound calcium concentration associated with ultrafiltration and plasma volume contraction.

This investigation was supported in part by the Missouri Regional Medical Program-Renal Disease and Clinical Research Center grant RR-00287-04.

References

1. Ogden DA, Holmes JH: Changes in total and ultrafiltrable plasma calcium and magnesium during hemodialysis. *Trans Amer Soc Artif Intern Organs* **12**:200-202, 1966.

2. Wing AJ: Optimum calcium concentration of dialysis fluid for maintenance of hemodialysis. *Brit Med J* **4**:145-149, 1968.

3. Danesh BZ, Walker CM, Mathers NP: The relation of post dialysis plasma calcium and magnesium to the dialysate levels and to changes in blood pH. *New Eng J Med* **282**:771-775, 1970.

4. Hattner RS, Jacobs J, Bernstein DS: Letter to the editor. *New Eng J Med* **283**:155, 1970.

5. Furszyfer J, Goldsmith RS, Johnson WJ, et al: Control of secondary hyperparathyroidism during long term hemodialysis. *Proc Cen Soc Clin Res* **43**:119, 1970.

6. Failing JF, Brickley MW, Zak B: Automatic determination of serum protein. *Amer J Clin Path* **33**:83-88, 1960.

7. Mabry CC, Geredon RE, Roekel IE: Automated submicro chemistries: A system of rapid sub-microchemical analysis for the measurement of sodium, potassium, chloride, carbon dioxide, sugar, urea, nitrogen total and direct reacting bilirubin and total protein. *Amer J Clin Path* **46**:265-281, 1966.

8. Manston R: Simultaneous autoanalysis of calcium and phosphorus. *Anal Biochem* **16**:65-69, 1966.

9. Hattner RS, Johnson JW, Bernstein DS: Electrochemical determination of apparent ionized serum calcium using a calcium selective electrode: The method and values in normal humans and a comparison to total serum calcium. *Clin Chim Acta* **28**:67-75, 1970.

10. Waugh WH: Utility of expressing serum sodium per unit of water in assessing hyponatremia. *Metabolism* **18**:706-712, 1969.

11. Donnan FG: The theory of membrane equilibrium. *Chem Rev* **1**:73-90, 1924-1925.

12. Mannery JF: Water and electrolyte metabolsim. *Physiol Rev* **34**:334-417, 1954.

13. Fulton JF: *Howell's Textbook of Physiology*, ed 15. Philadelphia, WB Saunders Co, 1946, pp 570-573.

14. Freeman RB, Maher JF, Schreiner GE: The affinity of synthetic membranes for calcium. *Trans Amer Soc Artif Intern Organs* **11**:99-103, 1965.

15. Bricker NS, Ogden DA, Schreiner GE: Invited discussion. *Arch Intern Med* **124**:292-301, 1969.

16. Nolph KD, Stoltz ML, Carter CB, et al: Factors affecting the composition of ultrafiltrate from hemodialysis coils. *Trans Amer Soc Artif Intern Organs* **16**:495-501, 1970.

Changes in the Diagnostic Process During 40 Years of Clinicopathologic Conferences

Alvan R. Feinstein, MD, and Jennifer R. Niebyl, MD, New Haven, Conn

The topics and diagnostic discussions have been analyzed for the clinicopathologic conferences of the Massachusetts General Hospital, which were published during 1922, 1942, and 1962. The general distribution of topics has remained similar through the years, and the diseases under survey have remained almost exclusively entities of morbid anatomy, with "answers" provided by morphologic evidence. The general accuracy of pre-mortem diagnosis has declined during the 40-year period, probably because increasingly difficult cases have been selected for the conferences, although a misplaced confidence in para-clinical tests may be a contributing factor. In the diagnosis of cardiovascular-respiratory problems, almost half of the errors were due to "inaccurate focus." Other types of diagnostic errors were due to omission, inappropriate exclusion, and extraneous addition.

Making a medical diagnosis is one of the oldest forms of reasoning. Every organized human society has contained members who were adept at contemplating medical ailments and at classifying them according to some ordered system of diagnostic nomenclature. Throughout recorded civilization, many different methods have been used for these contemplations and classifications of disease. In different societies and at different times, diagnostic nomenclature has described either causes, manifestations, or prognosis of disease, and diagnostic procedures have been performed by individuals or groups, with or without examination of the sick person, by logical deduction or mystical revelation, by human thought alone or with the aid of natural, supernatural, or artificial devices.

In medicine today, a new artificial device—the digital computer—has become available for application in diagnostic activities. The ability of this device to store massive amounts of data, to expedite complex calculations, and to operate in a logical sequence has brought optimistic hopes about the contributions computers might make in diagnosis. This potential role of computers has led to several recent appraisals of diagnostic reasoning.[1-6] In some of these appraisals, the diagnostic process has been viewed as an exercise mainly in mathematical logic; in others, the process has been relegated to a series of calculations based on statistical theories of probability; in yet others, the process has been deemed too complex and artful to be delineated and catalogued in a scientific manner.

The existence of these different beliefs about diagnosis is not surprising, since diagnostic reasoning—as a discrete intellectual activity—is seldom discussed in textbooks or taught in medical schools. The procedure has no oral or written rules, tactics, or logic; and physicians usually learn it in a laissez faire manner by observing diverse performances by teachers and colleagues. Without specific guidelines having been established, the activity of diagnostic reasoning is easily susceptible to various interpretations when clinicians and nonclinicians attempt to contemplate it with modern mathematical rigor and computational skills.

Even without the incentive provided by these new technologic adjuncts of the intellect, however, diagnostic reasoning would still warrant formal intensive analysis, if only to enlighten the students and practitioners now contending with all the rational challenges of traditional diagnosis, while simultaneously deciding how to apply the many new ancillary tests used in a diagnostic "work-up." For clinical effectiveness the analysis should be directed not at the abstract theories and models of mathematical logic or of computation but at the actual components of the diagnostic reasoning performed by clinicians. The goal is to discern the distinctive forms of clinical logic and strategy that are contained in the daily realities of medical practice and that are detectable only from examination of those realities.

A useful way to begin such analytic activities is by contemplating a teaching exercise that has been used traditionally to illustrate diagnostic reasoning and that has often been recorded in detail so that its proceedings can be reviewed: the clinicopathologic conference (CPC). Ever since such conferences were suggested by Walter Cannon[7] and initiated by Richard Cabot,[8] the CPC has

Received for publication Oct 19, 1970; accepted Feb 1.

From the Eastern Research Support Center and the Department of Medicine, West Haven Veterans Administration Hospital, and the Departments of Medicine and Epidemiology, Yale University School of Medicine, New Haven, Conn. Dr. Niebyl is now with Johns Hopkins Hospital, Baltimore.

Reprint requests to Department of Internal Medicine, Yale University School of Medicine, 333 Cedar St, New Haven, Conn 06510 (Dr. Feinstein).

been a useful and often entertaining educational activity. In the customary conference, the clinician who acts as discusser receives a summary of what was known during the life of the patient; after reviewing this summary, the discusser presents his diagnostic formulation; when he has finished, the pathologist describes the actual findings noted in surgical specimens or at necropsy.[9]

Published transcriptions of such conferences offer a unique opportunity to study the diagnostic process. The discusser at a CPC cannot rely on probability alone, since uncommon disorders may be selected more frequently than common ones. To attain pedagogic and competitive "success," he must delineate his ideas, specify his reasoning, and justify his conclusions; and the accuracy of those conclusions is promptly established by the pathologist's report. The published records of CPCs are not fully satisfactory for studying diagnostic reasoning: the discusser usually knows that the patient has died or has had surgery; the selected cases are not typical representatives of the range of human ailments, and the reported details represent summaries of data rather than the original evidence. Nevertheless, the CPC has become a standard method for teaching diagnosis, and besides, it is the only diagnostic activity whose verbatim accounts are regularly preserved and made available for analysis.

The classical records of such conferences are from the Massachusetts General Hospital. From 1919 to 1923 these records were printed separately as *Case Records* of that hospital; later they were incorporated into the *Boston Medical and Surgical Journal*, with which they transferred to their current weekly appearances in the *New England Journal of Medicine*. By exploring these records at three different times in a span of four decades, we could evaluate not only the different diagnostic tactics used in each of these eras of medicine but also the changes that had occurred in different eras. We had initially hoped that the published discussions would be specific enough to enable us to construct a "flow-chart" of the logic followed in each diagnostic session. This hope could not be fulfilled because the discussions pursued too many different pathways and because a specific pattern of logic could not always be discerned. Instead, we concentrated on analyzing the characteristics of the patients, the accuracy of diagnosis, and the sources and types of diagnostic errors that had occurred in the conferences.

Although disagreements between clinical and necropsy diagnoses have been noted in several previous investigations,[8,10-12] the patients in those reports were catalogued according to necropsy findings rather than clinical modes of presentation; moreover, the causes of errors in diagnosis were not explored by evaluating the physician's account of his diagnostic reasoning. We hoped that our clinical classification of cases and analysis of diagnostic errors would provide a useful starting point for the more general discussions of diagnostic reasoning that will be presented in a subsequent series of papers.

Materials and Methods

The reviewed material consisted of all the clinicopathological conferences of the Massachusetts General Hospital published in the years 1922, 1942, and 1962. The clinicopathological conferences presented in 1922 were published separately as the *Case Records of the Massachusetts General Hospital;* and the clinicopathological conferences of 1942 and 1962 were published in the *New England Journal of Medicine.*

General Classification of Cases.—Each case was classified according to (1) main clinical topic, (2) source of pathological data, (3) presence or absence of an anatomical lesion, and (4) accuracy of diagnosis.

Main Clinical Topic.—The clinical classification of cases depended on the patient's chief complaint at the time of his last admission. If no chief complaint was evident, the case was categorized according to the major diagnosis stated by the discusser. The categories of clinical topics were as follows: *Cardiovascular-Respiratory, Gastroenterological, Genitourinary, Neurological, Hematological-Lymphatic, Gynecological, Dermatological, Orthopedic, Metabolic,* and *Multisystemic.*

Source of Pathological Data.—The source of pathological data for each case was classified as *Necropsy,* if the discusser knew that the patient had died and as *Surgical Pathology* if the case history ended with the statement that an operation was performed or that a diagnostic procedure was undertaken. For the few instances in which the patient died during or after surgery without the death being revealed until the pathologist's discussion, the category of *Surgical Pathology* was used even if the necropsy findings were presented.

Presence or Absence of an Anatomical Lesion.—When the "disease" was demonstrated as a morphologic lesion, the case was classified as *Anatomical.* When no primary lesion was demonstrated by gross anatomic or microscopic examination (as in some cases of diabetes mellitus or hyperthyroidism), the case was classified as *Nonanatomical.*

Accuracy of Diagnosis.—The ratings of *correct, partly correct,* or *incorrect* were used for the discusser's major diagnosis (or diagnoses). The rating was *Correct* if all the discusser's major diagnoses were correct. The rating was *Partly Correct* if one of two major diagnoses, or a part of more than two major diagnoses, were correct. If a major diagnosis had two components, such as the site and nature of the disease process, and only one component was diagnosed correctly, the rating was also *Partly Correct.* If all the major diagnoses were incorrect, the rating was *Incorrect.*

Separate Analysis of Cardiovascular-Respiratory Cases.—In addition to the above classifications, which were given to all of the cases studied, a further analysis was made of all the cases in the *Cardio-*

vascular-Respiratory group. Each such case was classified as *Clinical* or *Para-Clinical* according to whether the discusser relied mainly upon evidence obtained by a routine history and physical examination or whether the critical information was obtained by some para-clinical procedure, such as a roentgenogram or laboratory test.

In those cases for which the diagnosis was *Incorrect* or *Partly Correct*, the type of error was analyzed. The errors were classified as follows:

1. *Errors of Omission* occurred when the discusser failed to mention the correct diagnosis anywhere in his discussion.

In one case the patient had a firm thyroid nodule and rapid progression of cough, dyspnea, and cyanosis. Patchy confluent densities and a superimposed reticular pattern were seen on roentgenogram. The clinician diagnosed lymphangitic spread of thyroid carcinoma, and his discussion of the diagnostic possibilities completely omitted the correct diagnosis, which was idiopathic interstitial fibrosis of the lungs.[13]

2. *Errors of Inaccurate Focus* occurred when the discusser listed the correct diagnosis among the possibilities but then considered it less likely than his final choice. This label was also used for errors in which the discusser listed only one of two diagnoses, both of which accounted for the symptoms and signs.

The first type of error is illustrated by the case of a patient with dyspnea and bone pain, for whom the clinician, after stating that he could not rule out metastatic lung cancer (which was the correct diagnosis), decided upon multiple myeloma as the most likely explanation.[14] The second type of error is illustrated by the necropsy finding of both lobar pneumonia and congestive heart failure in a patient whose dyspnea had been attributed only to the congestive heart failure.[15]

3. *Errors of Inappropriate Exclusion* occurred when the discusser felt that the correct diagnosis was incompatible with the findings, and definitely ruled it out.

For example, in the discussion of a febrile patient with laborious respirations, diffuse crepitations, and dullness over the right chest, the discusser ruled out tuberculosis on the basis of "repeatedly negative Pirquets and intradermal tests." The patient was found to have widespread tuberculosis in the lungs, intestines, liver, and spleen.[16]

4. *Errors of Addition* occurred when the discusser made the correct diagnosis but felt obliged to add an extra incorrect diagnosis to explain the findings.

For example, in a patient with cardiac murmurs and congestive heart failure, the discusser diagnosed syphilitic aortitis with aortic insufficiency and congenital heart disease with a septal defect. The anatomical diagnosis was syphilitic aortitis with aortic insufficiency, but no congenital abnormality was found.[17]

Results

General Classification of Cases.—The data cited in the sections that follow are summarized in the Figure. Certain additional details, reported in the text, are not contained in that illustration.

Number of Cases.—In 1922, about three cases were published each week, so that 154 clinicopathologic conferences were reported. Five other cases, excluded from tabulation here, were presented for clinical discussion only, without pathologic correlation. The number of weekly cases dropped to about 2 per week in 1942, and 1 to 2 in 1962, so that a total of 105 cases were reported in 1942 and 86 in 1962.

Distribution of Clinical Topics.—Cardiorespiratory and gastroenterological cases occurred most frequently, the combination accounting for more than half of the total cases each year. The proportion of cases in each topic remained essentially unchanged throughout the three time periods. Next most commonly presented were genitourinary and neurologic cases; each of these topics accounted for about 10% of the total in all three years.

Among the small number of cases in the *Miscellaneous* category, dermatologic topics appeared only in 1922 (four cases); metabolic cases decreased from eight in 1922 to two in each of 1942 and 1962 (reflecting mainly a decrease in cases with a major diagnosis of diabetes mellitus); orthopedic cases declined from nine in 1922 to one in each of 1942 and 1962. The proportion of multisystemic cases rose from 3% in 1922 and 1942 to 7% in 1962. Much of the increase was associated with "collagen-vascular" diseases.

Accuracy of Diagnosis.—The percentage of *incorrect* diagnoses in the total cases each year rose sharply from 12% in 1922 to 41% in 1942 and then fell slightly to 31% in 1962. The percentage of *correct* diagnoses began at 71% in 1922 and dropped to 41% in 1942 and 42% in 1962. The percentages of *partly correct* diagnoses were 16%, 18%, and 27%, respectively, in those three annual periods.

Within each of the individual groups of clinical topics, the percentage of incorrect diagnoses was higher in 1962 than in 1922. In the cardiorespiratory and genitourinary categories, the *incorrect* percentage rose at each time period, whereas in other categories the curve was "tent-shaped," with a fall from 1942 to 1962 after a sharper rise from 1922 to 1942. The pattern of percentages of *correct* diagnoses was essentially a mirror image of the *incorrect* pattern.

The greatest consistency of *correct* diagnoses throughout the years was in the *miscellaneous* category where the *correct* percentages were, respectively, 67%, 56%, and 50%. Among the constituent groups of this category, the best performances over the three-year totals were found in Metabolic topics (10/12 correct; 83%), Gynecologic topics (8/12 correct; 75%), and in Orthopedic topics (6/10; 60%).

Only one of seven hematolymphatic cases was *correct,* although four others were partly correct.

Sources of Case Material.—Despite changing techniques of diagnosis, and an increasing modern use of chemical and other functional methods for detecting disease, the diagnostic "endpoint" of the CPC has remained mainly morphologic. The percentage of *anatomical* cases was 96%, 99%, and 98% for the three time periods under survey.

The source of morphologic material has gradually been changing, however, so that the operating room has begun to provide as many cases as the morgue. The percentage of *necropsy* cases in the total group fell from 97% in 1922 to 48% in 1942 and 41% in 1962. This progressive fall was also reflected in each of the main clinical subgroups, except for the neurologic and miscellaneous categories, in which the percentage of necropsy cases rose slightly between 1942 and 1962.

The proportion of Surgical Pathology cases has thus risen from 3% in 1922, to 52% in 1942, and 59% in 1962. In the last two time periods, the proportions of such cases have been particularly high (higher than for the total group) in the gastroenterological and in certain miscellaneous categories.

Source of Material, and Accuracy of Diagnosis.—In 1922, all four surgical pathology cases received correct diagnoses, whereas 71% of the necropsy cases were correct. In 1942, 35% of the surgical pathology and 48% of the necropsy cases were diagnosed correctly; and in 1962, 43% of the surgical pathology and 40% of necropsy cases were correct. Thus, the general declining trends in overall accuracy of diagnosis seemed unaffected by the source of morphologic material, although a slight improvement occurred between 1942 and 1962 for surgical pathology cases.

Within the individual clinical categories, the most striking disparities occurred in the genitourinary and neurological groups, where surgical pathology material in recent years was diagnosed correctly much more often then necropsy material. The other categories showed only minor variations on the main trends already noted.

Analysis of Diagnostic Errors.—The results of the special analyses of

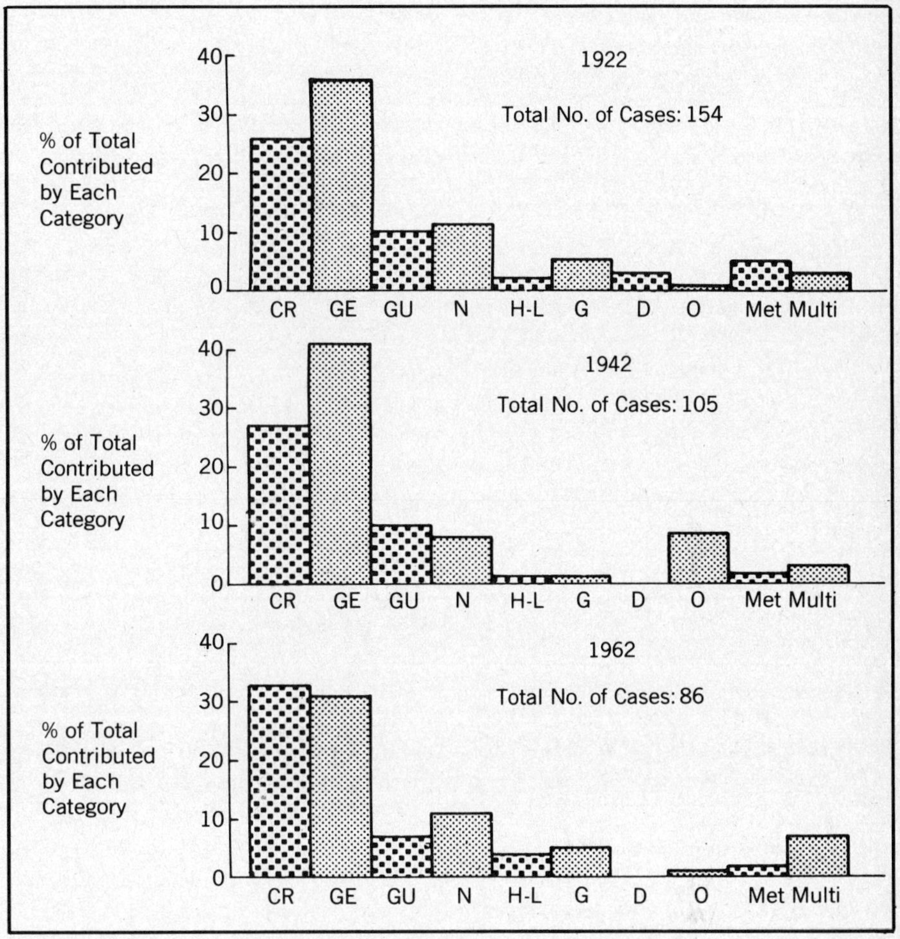

Incidence of types of clinical cases in clinicopathologic conferences. CR = cardiovascular-respiratory, GE = gastroenterological, GU = genitourinary, N = neurological, H-L = hematologic-lymphatic, G = gynecological, D = dermatological, O = orthopedic, Met = metabolic, and Multi = multisystemic.

diagnostic error in the cardiorespiratory category are shown in Table 1. A total of 97 such CPC cases were presented—41 in 1922 and 28 in each of 1942 and 1962.

Principle Source of Evidence.—The discusser placed main diagnostic reliance on para-clinical rather than clinical evidence in 10% of cases in 1922, 39% of cases in 1942, and 43% in 1962. As the reliance on para-clinical cal data increased, however, the percentage of correct diagnoses decreased, from 63% in 1922, to 43% in 1942, and 36% in 1962. The percentage of correct diagnoses was considerably higher in the "clinical reliance" cases than in the "para-clinical reliance" cases in both 1922 and 1962, but was slightly lower in 1942.

Types of Errors.—Of the 97 cardiorespiratory cases in the total group, 49 had been associated with the various types of error shown in Table 2.

The most common type of error was one of inaccurate focus, which occurred in 22 instances, and which was individually most frequent among the errors of 1922 and 1962. Next most common were errors of omission, which occurred in 14 cases. Errors of inappropriate exclusion were individually most frequent in 1942 but third most frequent in the other years and in the total. Errors of addition were uncommon, having occurred in only three cases.

Other Characteristics.—During these four decades, the CPC has changed in several other features that cannot be easily expressed in numbers.

One such feature is the intellectual atmosphere and apparent purpose of the conferences. At many institutions today the CPC has become an exercise in which the pathologist has both the first and the last word. He is usually responsible for choosing the cases to be discussed, and his statements are generally regarded as the solution to the "whodunit" mystery of diagnosis, regardless of whether the clinician's proposals agree or disagree with the morphologic findings. In the CPCs of 1922, however, the cases were selected by clinicians rather than by pathologists, and the atmosphere was one of common concern over the cause of the patient's death. The discussion contained a mutual interchange between clinician and pathologist, rather than a final answer provided by the pathologist, and on several occasions the pathologist could not provide a diagnostic explanation. In one case, the clinician refused to accept the pathologist's findings as an explanation for the clinical problem.[18] The sequence of the discussion in 1922 was also somewhat different from that of 1942 and 1962. In many cases of 1922, the operative findings and subsequent course of the patient were revealed after the initial discussion, and the clinician then continued with further discussion before the necropsy results were presented. In some instances, the clinician was asked specifically to correlate the necropsy findings with the clinical manifestations.

Table 1.—Accuracy of Diagnosis and Major Diagnostic Reliance in Cardiovascular-Respiratory Cases

Year	1922	1942	1962
Total No. of cases	41	28	28
No. and (percentage) of cases diagnosed correctly	26 (63)	12 (43)	10 (36)
No. and (percentage) of cases with major diagnostic reliance on			
Para-clinical data	4 (10)	11 (39)	12 (43)
Clinical data	37 (90)	17 (61)	16 (57)
No. and (percentage) of cases diagnosed correctly when major diagnostic reliance was on			
Para-clinical data	2/4 (50)	5/11 (45)	2/12 (17)
Clinical data	24/37 (65)	7/17 (41)	8/16 (50)

Table 2.—Types of Error in Cardiovascular-Respiratory Cases

Year	1922	1942	1962
Total No. of errors	15	16	18
No. and (percentage) of errors that were due to			
Omission	5 (33)	5 (31)	4 (22)
Inaccurate focus	8 (53)	5 (31)	9 (50)
Inappropriate exclusion	8 (7)	6 (38)	3 (17)
Addition	1 (7)	0 (0)	2 (11)

This early atmosphere, in which the clinician was regarded as a scholarly collaborator rather than as the object of a "test," may have existed because most cases in 1922 were discussed by one of three physicians: Richard C. Cabot, Hugh Cabot, and Edward L. Young, Jr. In 1942 and 1962, however, each case was assigned to a different physician, and the same person rarely appeared as discusser for more than several cases per year.

The earlier conferences also contained therapeutic as well as diagnostic challenges. Three of the cases in 1922 were presented for a discussion of management only, and no pathology report was given. In another case (a neurologic problem), the pathologist was unable to provide an answer because the brain had not been examined. In yet another instance, the "final answer" was provided by a roentgenogram rather than by a pathologist's examination of tissue. (These events occurred in the five 1922 cases excluded from numerical analyses in this report.)

The types of patient and data have also changed in the CPCs of these different eras. In 1922 the patients were generally younger than the types of patient chosen in more recent years, and many deaths due to infectious diseases in 1922 might have been prevented by modern antibiotics. Many of the clinical diagnostic challenges in 1922 would be labelled "straightforward" today, as exemplified by cases with "arteriosclerosis" as the major diagnosis and main cause of death. The available descriptive information in 1922 contained more detailed accounts of history and physical examination than appeared in 1942 and 1962, but the para-clinical data of 1922 were much more limited. Electrocardiography and radiography were rarely used, and laboratory data consisted mainly of findings of urinalysis, white blood cell count, hemoglobin and blood glucose determinations, Wasserman and Widal tests, and bacteriologic cultures.

Comment

Errors in Diagnosis.—Perhaps the most remarkable finding in this survey was that modern clinicians, although aided by the technologic advances of para-clinical tests, were less accurate in CPC diagnoses than were the doctors who worked more than 40 years ago. Moreover, in the cardiorespiratory cases of recent years, discussers relying on adjunctive para-clinical data were diagnostically correct less often than when their main reliance was placed on the conventional data of clinical examination.

The routine diagnostic importance of conventional clinical data was noted by Gruver and Freis during analysis of a consecutive series of premortem and postmortem diagnoses.[11] For patients who had been unable to give a history during life, the rate of diagnostic error was much higher than when such histories were available. In discussing diagnostic reasoning for a CPC presented in 1963, Field[19] found that the patient's record contained "35 positive findings, of which 40% are derived from signs found on physical examination and 30% from the history. Of the nine bits of negative information provided, 85% came from the laboratory determinations. From these figures one can conclude that in the practice of medicine the history and physical examination are still rewarding efforts, and that the laboratory examination can add considerable confusion to the pictures."

Although the decreased attention to clinical phenomena is a tempting explanation for the declining rate of correct diagnoses at CPC, a more likely cause is the type of case selected for the conferences. Because the conference is a special occasion, the cases are often chosen for the challenges they present to the clinician, and a correct diagnosis is usually much more difficult to achieve than in the activities of routine medical practice. For example, in two groups of patients who received routine hospital management during 1952 and 1957, and whose diagnoses were checked at necropsy,[11,12] the rates of correct diagnosis were *higher* than those found in this survey for patients of the 1942 and 1962 CPC cases, where an expert clinician had considerable time for intensive analysis of the data. Moreover, because of the increasing diagnostic accuracy provided by technologic tests, and because the CPC is sometimes regarded as an effort to "stump the clinician," a pathologist today may be particularly likely to select cases for their diagnostic difficulty.[9] In some instances, the cases may even be chosen deliberately to lead the clinician astray if he relies on para-clinical diagnostic procedures. For all these reasons, the clinician's decreasing rate of "success" at CPC seems attributable not so much to diagnostic ineptitude as to a change in the orientation of the conferences and to increasingly difficult case challenges—although a misplaced confidence in para-clinical tests is obviously a contributing factor.

The CPC as a Teaching Exercise.—The teaching value of the CPC in its current format has been questioned elsewhere,[20] and the doubts are not dispelled by the results of the current survey. In an era in which so many diseases occur as functional, biochemical, immunologic or other nonmorphologic disorders, the persistent anatomic "endpoint" of CPCs tends to provide students with a restricted sampling of the spectrum of human ailments. Moreover, since so many morphologic diagnoses can be attained or approximated with the aid of roentgenography, endoscopy, biopsy, and cytology, the number of cases left for a morphologic "revelation" at surgery or necropsy has progressively dwindled, so that the pathologist who relies on anatomic material has fewer and fewer "interesting" cases available to choose for a CPC.

Another issue in the pedagogic value of CPCs is the desirability of showing students so many instances in which thoughtful clinicians, after an intensive appraisal of the data, arrive at wrong diagnoses more often than doctors harriedly working in the routine activities of a large municipal hospital.[11,12] Although a well-analyzed diagnostic error can always be instructive, the published records of contemporary CPCs seldom contain such analyses. Aside from a few brief questions about the pathologic findings, the clinician whose error has just been revealed usually remains silent and generally does not attempt a retrospective assessment of the flaws in his reasoning. In denying this enlightenment to students and himself, the clinician may perhaps be reluctant to pursue his error to its sources, or perhaps time (and publication space) do not permit such a discussion; but another possible explanation is that the clinician believes his reasoning was correct, despite its erroneous conclusions, and that proper clinical logic would compel him to arrive at the same diagnosis were he to repeat his analysis of the same data. In such an instance, the patient may have been a poor choice for CPC, representing a diagnosis that the clinician could get "right" only by thinking "wrong."[9]

Finally, in the emphasis placed mainly on a correct statement of diagnosis, the contemporary CPC may divert attention from two scientific clinical challenges that are of prime importance to clinicians today: the choice of tests in a diagnostic "work-up" and the choice of therapeutic agents.[20] When the CPC was evolving into its current format more than 40 years ago, these challenges were of minor importance because few technologic tests were available, and treatment was frequently ineffective. During the past four decades, however, technology has spawned an enormous array of paraclinical tests and therapeutic agents that require careful scientific appraisal. These new challenges are generally omitted in current CPCs, whose format seems still aimed at the old clinical problems in diagnosis, with no major adaptations having been made for the newer scientific problems in "work-up" and in therapy.

The Potential Contribution of Computers in Diagnosis.—The types of errors noted in these demonstrations of diagnostic reasoning can help indicate the potential role of computers in diagnosis.

Errors of omission had the second highest frequency of the four types of error catalogued in this survey and occurred when the discusser had overlooked the correct diagnosis in preparing his list of diseases for differential consideration. Such errors might be avoided if the computer, with all diagnostic possibilities stored within its bank of data, could be used as a reminder of all the candidate diseases that required consideration in each clinical situation. Such reminders might be particularly useful for doctors who lack convenient access to textbooks[21,22] that contain such listings or who prefer to use a computer rather than a textbook. On the other hand, the mere use of the computer as a mnemonic aid would not affect the many errors due to inaccurate focus or inappropriate exclusion. Besides, by augmenting the list of possibilities to be considered, the computer might actually increase the number of errors of "addition."

Consequently, to provide significant help in the diagnostic process, a computer must act as more than a mere memory bank, containing deposits of "input" symptoms and "output" diseases. For a computer to give important aid in the course of the reasoning, the stored information must be assembled and classified on the basis of an intellectual strategy suitable for the sequential logic and judgmental decisions of diagnosis. A series of subsequent papers (by A.R.F.) will be concerned with identifying and specifying the inherently clinical modes of reasoning that constitute the diagnostic process. The computer can be helpful in this activity, not because of the calculations it can do with its "hardware," but because its "software" methods provide a new type of diagram—the "flow chart"—that can help illustrate the intellectual strategies and sequential paths of the reasoning.

This investigation was supported in part by Public Health Service grant 00408, from the National Center for Health Services Research and Development.

References

1. Ledley RS, Lusted LB: Reasoning foundations of medical diagnosis. *Science* **130**:9-21, 1959.
2. Lipkin M, Engle RL, Zworkin VK: Digital computers as an aid to differential diagnosis. *Arch Intern Med* **108**:56-72, 1961.
3. Warner HR, Toronto AR, Veasy LG, et al: A mathematical approach to medical diagnosis. *JAMA* **177**:177-183, 1961.
4. Engle RL, Davis BJ: Medical diagnosis: Past, present and future: I. Present concepts of the meaning and limitations of medical diagnosis. *Arch Intern Med* **112**:512-519, 1963.
5. Lipkin M: The likelihood concept in differential diagnosis. *Perspect Biol Med* **7**:485-497, 1964.
6. Jacquez JA (ed): *The Diagnostic Process.* Ann Arbor, Mich, Malloy Lithographing Inc, 1964.
7. Cannon WB: The case system in medicine. *Boston Med Surg J* **142**:563, 1900.
8. Hunter WA: A study of diagnostic errors in clinicopathological conferences at the Massachusetts General Hospital during a 25-year period. *Permanente Found Med Bull* **10**:306, 1952.
9. Harvey AM, Bordley J: *Differential Diagnosis: The Interpretation of Clinical Evidence*, ed 2. Philadelphia, WB Saunders Co, 1970.
10. Munck W: Autopsy findings and clinical diagnosis: A comparative study of 1,000 cases. *Acta Med Scand* **266** (suppl):775, 1952.
11. Gruver RH, Freis ED: A study of diagnostic errors. *Ann Intern Med* **47**:108-120, 1957.
12. Prutting J: Lack of correlation between antemortem and postmortem diagnoses. *New York J Med* **67**:2081-2084, 1967.
13. Case 2-1962, case records of the Massachusetts General Hospital. *New Eng J Med* **266**:90-95, 1962.
14. Case 59-1962, case records of the Massachusetts General Hospital. *New Eng J Med* **267**:508-514, 1962.
15. Case 8433, *Case Records of the Massachusetts General Hospital.* **8** (pt 3, No. 43):1-4, 1922.
16. Case 8402, *Case Records of the Massachusetts General Hospital.* **8** (pt 2, No. 40):1-5, 1922.
17. Case 13-1962, case records of the Massachusetts General Hospital. *New Eng J Med* **266**:407-414, 1962.
18. Case 8512, *Case Records of the Massachusetts General Hospital.* **8** (pt 2, No. 51):1-4, 1922.
19. Field R: Case 67-1963, case records of the Massachusetts General Hospital. *New Eng J Med* **269**:919, 1963.
20. Feinstein AR: *Clinical Judgment.* Baltimore, Williams & Wilkins Co, 1967.
21. Douthwaite AH (ed): *French's Index of Differential Diagnosis.* Baltimore, Williams & Wilkins Co, 1967.
22. Matousek WC: *Differential Diagnosis*, ed 2. Chicago, Year Book Medical Publishers Inc, 1967.

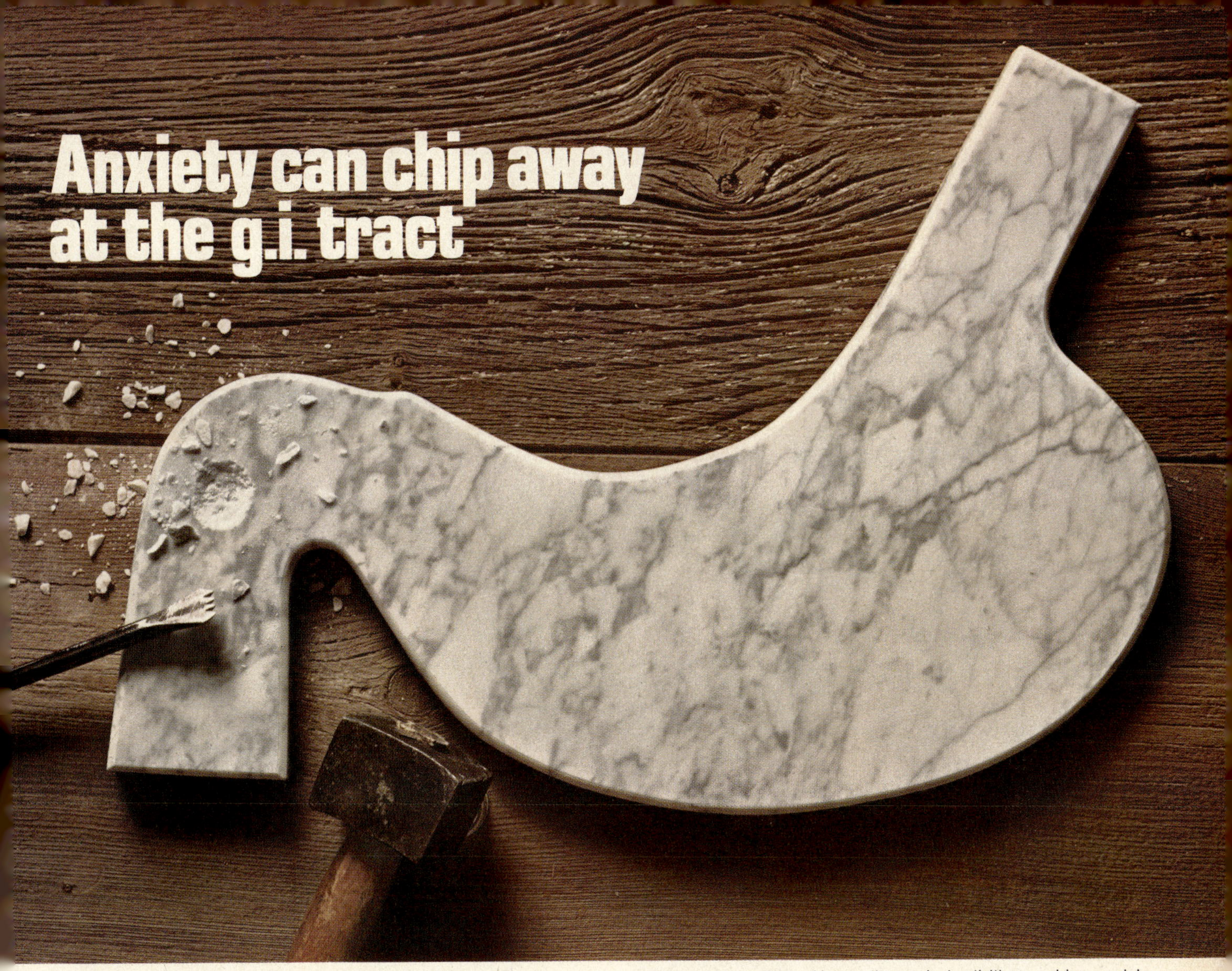

Probably no bodily system is as vulnerable to the relentless pounding of excess anxiety as the g.i. tract. Patients unable to cope with emotional pressures often show such stress physically, as ulcer or other g.i. disorders. 'Combid' can help control the patient's anxiety as well as spasm and excess secretion—round-the-clock with just b.i.d. dosage.

Combid®

Trademark

Each capsule contains: Compazine® (brand of prochlorperazine) 10 mg., as the maleate; Darbid® (brand of isopropamide) 5 mg., as the iodide.

Spansule®

brand of sustained release capsules

Before prescribing, see complete prescribing information, including symptoms and treatment of overdosage, in SK&F literature or *PDR*.

Indications: For adjunctive therapy in peptic ulcer.

Contraindications: Patients with known hypersensitivity to prochlorperazine or isopropamide, existing drug-induced C.N.S. depression, glaucoma, pyloric obstruction, prostatic hypertrophy, bladder neck obstruction, obstructive intestinal lesions and/or ileus, jaundice, hepatic disease, blood dyscrasias, or bone marrow depression. Nausea and vomiting associated with intestinal obstruction or brain tumor. Children under 12 years of age.

Warnings: Use with caution in patients with a past history of jaundice, hepatic abnormality, or blood dyscrasias. Caution patients about concomitant use of alcohol and other C.N.S. depressants because of possible additive effects. Also caution against activities requiring mental alertness (driving, operating machinery). Use in pregnancy, nursing mothers, and in women of childbearing age only when necessary. An inhibiting effect on lactation may occur.

Precautions: Patients sensitive to other drugs may be more liable to have a reaction to prochlorperazine. Use with caution in elderly patients. Discontinue one week prior to I^{131} uptake and PBI tests, as the iodine in isopropamide iodide may alter results.

Adverse Reactions: Drowsiness, dry mouth, blurred vision, urinary retention, dilated pupils, photophobia, constipation and tachycardia. Less frequently, palpitation, nausea, dysphagia, fever, and nasal congestion. Rarely, hypotension, agranulocytosis, cholestatic jaundice, leukopenia, extrapyramidal symptoms (parkinsonism-like symptoms, spasticity, painful constriction of skeletal muscles, or dystonias, chiefly of head, neck and shoulders, oculogyric crises, carpopedal spasms) have occurred with prochlorperazine.

Other Adverse Effects reported with one or more phenothiazines: Some adverse effects are dose-related, others involve patient sensitivity, some occur more frequently in patients with special medical problems, for example, mitral insufficiency or pheochromocytoma. Opisthotonos, hyperreflexia, akathisia, dyskinesia, sometimes lasting months or years; *grand mal* convulsions; altered cerebrospinal fluid proteins; cerebral edema, potentiation of C.N.S. depressants (opiates, analgesics, antihistamines, barbiturates, alcohol) and atropine, heat and phosphorus insecticides; headache, adynamic ileus, inhibition of ejaculation; reactivation of psychotic processes, catatonic-like states; hypotension (sometimes fatal; cardiac arrest); pancytopenia, thrombocytopenic purpura, eosinophilia; lactation, galactorrhea, gynecomastia, menstrual irregularities, false positive pregnancy tests; photosensitivity, itching, erythema, urticaria, eczema, exfoliative dermatitis; asthma, laryngeal edema, angioneurotic edema, anaphylactoid reactions; peripheral edema; reversed epinephrine effect; hyperpyrexia; pigmentary retinopathy; with prolonged administration of substantial doses, skin pigmentation, epithelial keratopathy, and lenticular and corneal deposits. EKG changes—particularly nonspecific, usually reversible Q and T wave distortions—have been reported, but relationship to myocardial damage is not confirmed. Sudden discontinuance in long-term patients may cause temporary nausea, vomiting, dizziness, tremulousness.

NOTE: Sudden death has been reported, though a relationship to phenothiazine administration has not been determined. In some cases the cause appeared to be asphyxia due to failure of the cough reflex; in others, no cause could be determined.

Supplied: Bottles of 50 capsules.

SK&F Smith Kline & French Laboratories

Clinical Notes

Schönlein-Henoch Syndrome Associated With Exposure to Cold

MAJ Philip W. Rogers, MC; MAJ S. M. Bunn Jr., MC;
LTC N.A. Kurtzman, MC; and MAJ M.G. White, MC, Fort Sam Houston, Tex

The terms Schönlein-Henoch syndrome or anaphylactoid purpura have been applied to a specific acquired hemorrhagic disorder without abnormalities of the clotting mechanism or evidence of thrombocytopenia. This syndrome is characterized by a generalized vasculitis involving multiple organ systems.[1] The etiology and pathogenesis of this syndrome are unknown, though rare cases are associated with food allergy and drugs,[2,3] or insect bite.[4] The demonstration of granular and nodular deposits of IgG and β_1C globulin located primarily in the mesangium and to a lesser degree on the basement membrane of glomeruli of patients with this syndrome[5] suggests an immune pathogenesis. Histologic and ultrastructural features of the glomerular lesions, including prominent deposition of platelets and fibrin in the capillary lumen[5] do not specifically distinguish anaphylactoid purpura from other forms of immune renal disease such as acute poststreptococcal glomerulonephritis, systemic lupus erythematosus, and Goodpasture's syndrome[8]; however, normal serum complement levels[6,7] help to distinguish anaphylactoid purpura from these entities.

The following case is presented because of the unusual association of anaphylactoid purpura with apparent hypersensitivity to a physical factor—cold. In 1941, Peters and Horton[9] reported a case of "allergic purpura" produced on exposure to cold; their patient did not have clinical renal disease, gastrointestinal symptoms, or arthralgia.

Received for publication July 29, 1970; accepted Sept 14.

From the departments of medicine and pathology, Brooke General Hospital and the Metabolic Branch, US Army Institute of Surgical Research, Brooke Army Medical Center, Fort Sam Houston, Tex.

Reprint requests to US Army Institute of Surgical Research, Fort Sam Houston, Tex 78234 (Dr. Kurtzman).

Patient Summary

The patient, a 23-year-old, Korean woman, enjoyed good health until November 1968 when, while in Germany with her husband, she began to note painless, purpuric lesions on her lower extremities on exposure to cold. The lesions would persist for several days and then gradually disappear during the following week. They appeared only on exposure to cold and were associated with generalized arthralgia and abdominal pain without evidence of gastrointestinal bleeding. She was hospitalized in February 1969.

Physical examination revealed the patient was alert and well-developed and in no acute distress. The only pertinent findings were the scattered purpuric, erythematous, 0.5- to 1.0-cm lesions over both lower extremities and buttocks. The results of the remainder of the physical examination were unremarkable.

Complete blood cell count was normal, platelet count was 264,000/sq mm, and erythrocyte sedimentation rate was 6 mm/hr. Results of a tourniquet test were negative, clotting time was six minutes, and bleeding time was four minutes. The prothrombin time and serum fibrinogen level were normal. Examination of the peripheral blood smear revealed occasional target cells and mild anisocytosis. The following tests were negative: cryoglobulin, cryofibrinogen, direct and indirect Coombs' tests, rheumatoid arthritis latex fixation, antinuclear antibody, acid hemolysins, cold hemolysins, and lupus preparation. Results of serum protein electrophoresis and immunodiffusion studies were normal. Serum uric acid, calcium, and glucose tolerance test results were also normal.

Twenty-four hour measurement of urine protein excretion was 0.79 to 1.08 gm; creatinine clearances ranged from 82 to 115 ml/min/1.73 sq m. Examination of the urinary sediment revealed occasional white blood cells, numerous red blood cells, and occasional granular casts.

A skin biopsy through a purpuric lesion showed an "acute nonspecific vasculitis." Results of a gastrocnemius muscle biopsy were "normal." A percutaneous renal biopsy specimen containing 28 glomeruli was interpreted as showing "diffuse glomerular disease with hypercellularity due to increased numbers of epithelial or endothelial cells, or both, focal basement membrane thickening, and numerous synechiae." Several small arteries appeared "normal."

The patient was placed on a regimen of prednisone, 40 mg, daily for 30 days, with no change in occurrence of purpura or renal function. She was transferred to Brooke General Hospital in May 1969 because of persistent purpura on exposure to cold. Evaluation again revealed no abnormality other than albuminuria and abnormal urinary sediment as previously described.

The patient remained asymptomatic until Jan 15, 1970, when the temperature in San Antonio, Tex, dropped to 35 F and she again developed arthralgia and small petechial lesions of both lower extremities and her right buttock. There were also several 1 × 1 cm, bright red purpuric areas around the knees. Several pruritic, somewhat painful erythematous, slightly elevated wheals were noted on the plantar surface of the left foot and right knee. The petechiae persisted for approximately three days and disappeared, while the larger lesions became darker in color and finally disappeared in approximately one week. Creatinine clearance was 115 ml/min/1.73 sq m and urinary protein excretion, 0.62 gm/24 hr. Urinary sediment showed two to three white blood cells and three to ten red blood cells per high power field.

She developed similar lesions during two more cold periods in February 1970 when the temperature ranged from 19 to 35 F. The patient did not have central heating in her home. No demonstrable change in renal function was documented during or after each exacerbation. Urinary sediment, however, did show more red blood cells during an exacerbation. Cryofibrinogen and cryoglobulin tests, antinuclear antibody test, direct Coombs' test, cold agglutinins, and antistreptolysin O (ASO) titer were all negative before, during, and after periods of purpura. Complete blood cell count remained normal with erythrocyte sedimentation rate ranging 5 to 6 mm/hr. Prothrombin time and fibrinogen also remained normal. Serum complement level ranged from 105 to 130 mg/100 ml (normal, 123 to 167 mg/100 ml).

She was again hospitalized at Brooke General Hospital on Feb 10, 1970 and extensive evaluation failed to reveal any other cause for her purpuric lesions or renal disease. A percutaneous renal biopsy was performed, and the specimen was examined by both light and electron microscopy.

Biopsy Findings

Light Microscopy.—Glomerular changes consisted of hypercellularity, mesangial prominence, and moderate lobular accentuation, all of these changes being rather diffuse and generalized, though localized portions of some loops appeared relatively uninvolved. The increase in cellularity was mesangial and endothelial. Local and focal nodular sclerosis and capsular synechiae were present (Fig 1). There was local and focal karyorrhexis, but hematoxylin bodies were not appreciated. Many lobules showed increased capillary wall thickness, and not infrequently these thickened loops merged locally with increased mesangial matrix resulting in marked narrowing to virtual complete obliteration of the capillary lumens of some of the tufts. Occasional polymorphonuclear leukocytes were noted within the capillary lumina and mesangium. Minimal focal tubular atrophy and interstitial fibrosis were present without significant inflammation. No significant vascular changes were noted.

Electron Microscopy.—The number of diseased capillary loops was appreciable. The markedly thickened capillary loops displayed the multilayered appearance described by Urizar and Herdman,[10] Kobayashi,[11] and others in anaphylactoid purpura (Fig 2). Changes which seem inseparable from those given the classification of membranoproliferative glomerulonephritis by Hamburger were also noted. These consisted of numerous floccular-nodular subendothelial electron-dense deposits with fusion of the overlying epithelial foot processes and proliferation of mesangial matrix material along the luminal surfaces of the capillary loops. The lobular stalks showed an increase in both mesangial cells and matrix, and electron-dense deposits were frequently observed in this location as well. The lumina of the capillary loops of more than occasional lobules were completely obliterated as the end result of the process described above. A dense deposit within the elastica of an efferent arteriole is a finding not noted in the electron microscopic descriptions of previously reported cases (Fig 3).

Comment

The term "anaphylactoid purpura" was introduced by Frank in 1915 although Osler, in a series of articles between 1895 and 1914, characterized it as a disease entity with variable symptoms, all of which he felt were the result of anaphylaxis. Heberden[12] and Willan[13] in 1808 first described patients with peculiar visceral crises associated with purpura and edema of the hands and feet. Schönlein[14] described the arthritic component of the disease in 1837, and Henoch[15] called attention to the associated renal involvement in 1874. Since then numerous reports[16-20] have documented the association of nephritis with anaphylactoid purpura.

Anaphylactoid purpura of Schönlein-Henoch syndrome is characterized by four main groups of symptoms: first, the pleomorphic and purpuric lesions of the skin; second, gastrointestinal symptoms including vomiting, gastrointestinal bleeding,

Fig 1.—Typical glomerulus showing a diffuse increase in mesangial and endothelial cells associated with nodular accumulations of mesangial matrix. Localized capillary wall thickening is present (small arrows) *as are early synechiae* (large arrows) *(hematoxylin-eosin stain, ×500).*

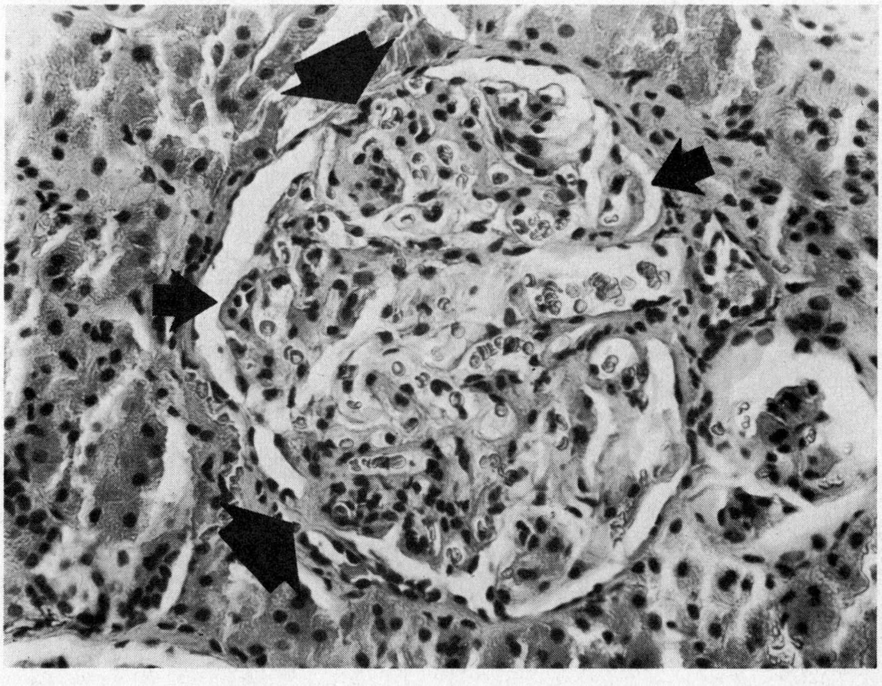

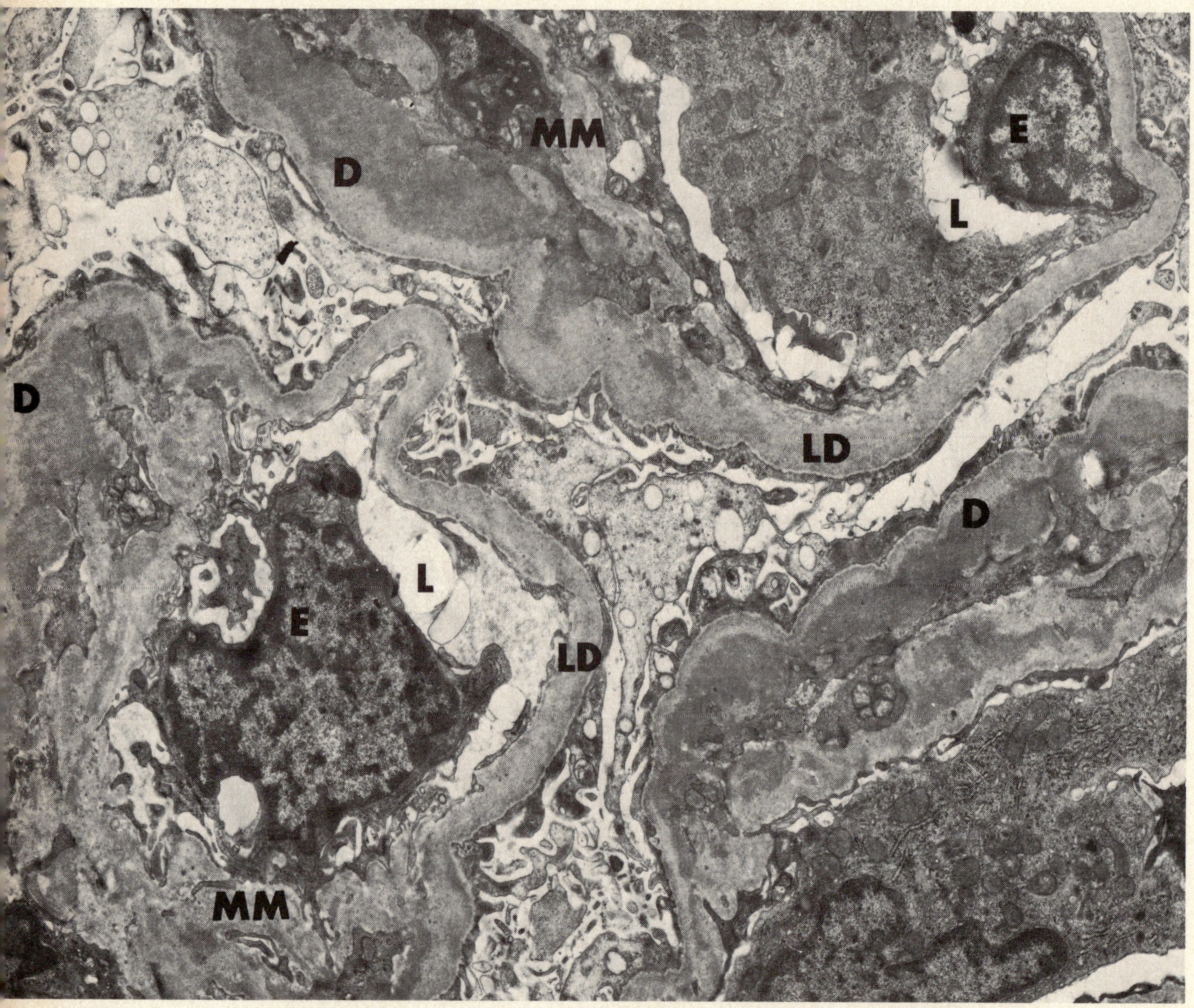

Fig 2.—Portions of three capillary loops in which segments of the capillary walls are markedly thickened by large subendothelial dense deposits and mesangial matrix proliferation (basement membrane "splitting"). Epithelial foot process fusion is marked (×12, 270). Abbreviations are as follows: D = dense deposits; E = endothelial cell; L = capillary lumen; LD = lamina densa; and MM = mesangial matrix.

and abdominal pain; third, arthralgia or true arthritis; and last, glomerulonephritis.

Most patients with anaphylactoid purpura are less than 16 years old, with a median age of about four years.[1] Younger children tend to exhibit transient edema more frequently than older children who are more prone to gastrointestinal symptoms and persistent renal abnormalities.

Most series have shown a preponderance of males—approximately 1.6:1. There is presently no explanation for this higher incidence in males.

The average duration of symptoms has ranged from three days to two years with a mean of approximately four weeks.[1] The average duration of the illness with acute renal involvement is usually somewhat longer—approximately five weeks.[1] Recurrences appear to be more frequent in those patients with renal involvement.

Glomerulonephritis.—The renal manifestations of the Schönlein-Henoch syndrome include microscopic hematuria and albuminuria with normal or reduced renal function. The findings may be present in up to 62% of cases.[19] The percentage of individuals who eventually develop progressive renal failure has varied between 6% and 36%.[1] The renal manifestations may not become evident until several months after the onset of the characteristic syndrome.

Histologic changes seen in the glomeruli in renal biopsy studies of patients with anaphylactoid purpura have frequently been described as local and focal in nature. However, the degree of hypercellularity, attributed to endocapillary proliferation, may vary from a localized process associated with small accumulations of PAS positive material to a more diffuse process in which many segments of the glomerular tufts are involved. Necrotizing changes are not uncommonly seen, and the histologic picture of active lupus glomerulonephritis may be simulated, though karyorrhexis is said to be less frequent, wire loops less common, and hematoxylin bodies *absent*. More chronic glomerular changes of a diffuse and generalized nature have also been described[11] along with accompanying tubular degeneration. Renal vascular changes are usually reported as *absent*.

Renal ultrastructural changes in cases of anaphylactoid purpura include endothelial cell proliferation with focal thickening and splitting of the basement membranes. There is also endothelial or mesangial cell proliferation extending from the axial regions to the periphery of the capillary loops, accompanied by increased mesangial matrix. Kobayashi et al[11] first described nodular subendothelial dense deposits in this syndrome, a finding present in our case. To our knowledge, no other case reports have documented dense deposits in the juxtaglomerular vasculature, as were seen in an efferent arteriole in our case.

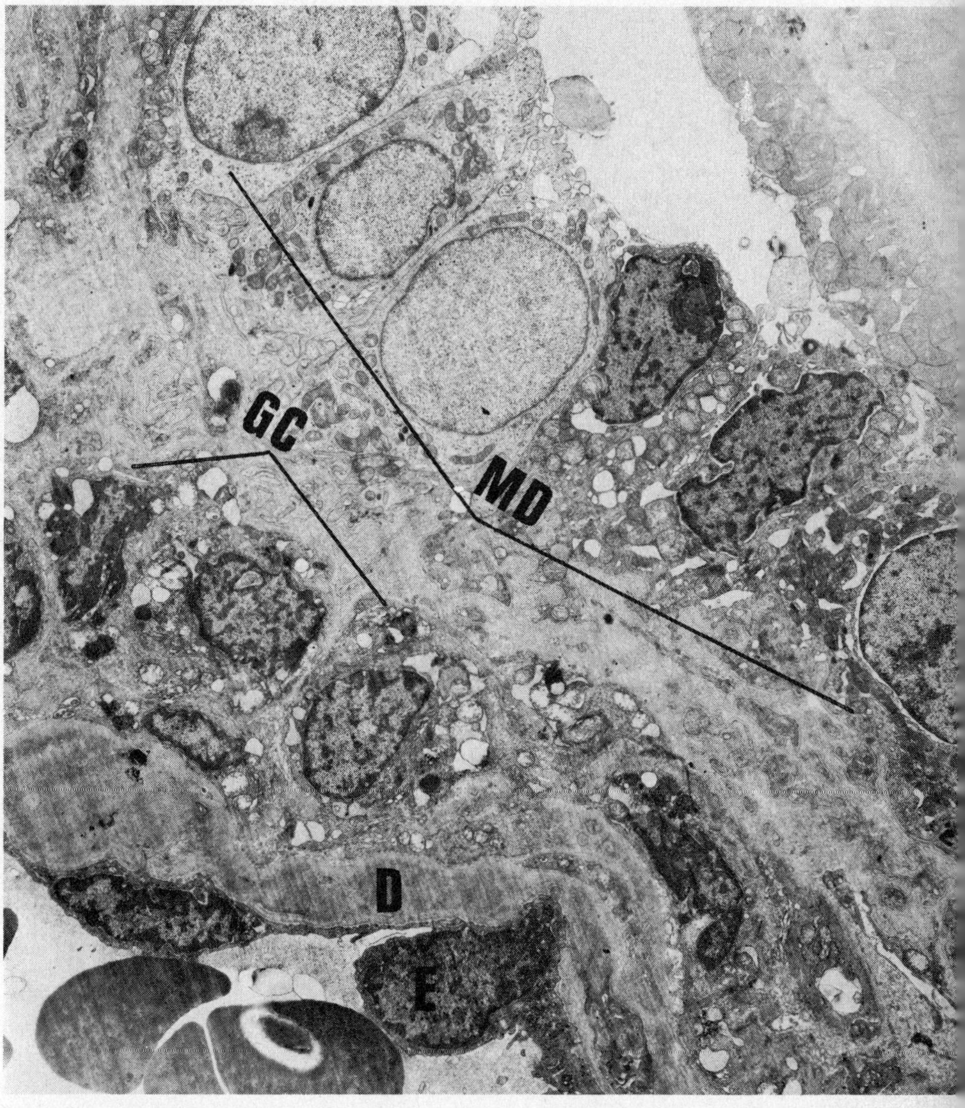

Fig 3.—The macula densa and nearby granular cells of the juxtaglomerular apparatus with dense deposits within the subendothelial elastica of the efferent arteriole (× 6,000). Abbreviations are as follows: D = dense deposits; E = endothelial cell; GC = granular cells; and MD = macula densa.

Skin Rash.—The characteristic skin rash described by Gairdner[21] is frequently urticarial at the onset, then fades to be replaced by red macular or maculopapular lesions. The lesions may remain small and discrete or may enlarge to become blotchy and at times confluent. The initial color of the lesions is red with progression to a brownish discoloration. Petechial and purpuric lesions are also seen. These lesions are usually confined to the area below the waist and are found most commonly on the legs, feet, about the knees, and over the buttocks. They may occasionally be found on the arms, hands, elbows, and face, but are rarely found on the trunk.

Joint Involvement.—Periarticular pain, tenderness, or swelling is a very common finding. The joints most frequently involved are the ankles, knees, wrists, and fingers. Examination reveals mild periarticular edema with no change in the actual joint space. Joint involvement, when present, is usually transient, rarely migratory, and leaves no residual deformity.

Soft Tissue Edema.—Localized swelling of the dorsum of the hands and feet and occasionally the scalp, ears, and periorbital region may be noted.

Gastrointestinal Symptoms.—Colicky abdominal pain is the most common of all symptoms and may precede the purpuric rash. Vomiting, melena, and hematemesis are also frequent symptoms. Massive gastrointestinal bleeding and intussusception are frequent.

Other less frequent manifestations of the Schönlein-Henoch syndrome include hepatomegaly,[1] localized swelling and hemorrhage of the testes,[1] convulsions,[22] intracerebral subarachnoid hemorrhage,[22] myocardial necrosis,[23] and optic neuritis.[22]

Our patient had intermittent abdominal pain, arthralgia, characteristic skin lesions, and renal disease. What makes this patient unique is that all her episodes of purpura have been associated with exposure to cold. The hematuria is more pronounced with exacerbation; however, she showed no decrease in creatinine clearance during an exacerbation as was described by Gary et al.[24]

Anaphylactoid purpura has usually been considered an allergic disorder as implied by the name. In our case, a physical factor, cold, has been implicated as initiating an antigen antibody reaction, which may well be an important pathogenetic factor. The demonstration of immune complexes on the basement membranes of glomeruli in patients with the Schönlein-Henoch syndrome is similar to polyarteritis,[25] systemic lupus erythematosis,[26] the Arthus phenomenon,[19] and Schwartzman reaction.[19] The serum complement in patients with the Schönlein-Henoch syndrome, however, is normal. Urizar and Herdman[10] suggest that the presence of intravascular coagulation may also have a pathogenetic role since patients with early or minimal lesions did not have such immune complexes. Whether cold, or any of the other documented allergens is really the cause of anaphylactoid purpura or just associated with the syndrome still remains unclear. Further, experimental and clinical investigation must be done to clarify the exact role of allergy in the pathogenesis of the Schönlein-Henoch syndrome.

Summary

Anaphylactoid purpura is characterized by a generalized vasculitis, the etiology and pathogenesis of which remain unknown. Immunofluorescent and electron microscopy suggest an immune pathogenesis with the deposition of antigen antibody complexes on the basement membranes of peripheral capillary loops of the glomerulus.

An unusual patient with Schönlein-Henoch syndrome had purpura which was exclusively associated with exposure to cold. Electron micrographs of the renal biopsy reveal numerous floccular-nodular subendothelial electron dense deposits along the basement membranes of the peripheral capillary loops as well as within the elastica of an efferent arteriole.

This syndrome is usually considered an allergic disorder as implied by the name, anaphylactoid purpura; however, our case implicates a physical factor, cold, as initiating the antigen antibody reaction.

Steven W. Miller assisted in the preparation of material for electron microscopy.

References

1. Allen D, Diamond LK, Nowell DA: Anaphylactoid purpura in children (Schönlein-Henoch syndrome). *Amer J Dis Child* **99**:833-854, 1960.

2. Ackroyd JF: Allergic purpura, including purpura due to foods, drugs, and infections. *Amer J Med* **14**:605-632, 1953.

3. Jensen B: Schönlein-Henoch's purpura: Three cases with fish or penicillin as antigen. *Acta Med Scand* **152**:61-70, 1955.

4. Burke DM, Jellinek HL: Nearly fatal case of Schönlein-Henoch syndrome following insect bite. *Amer J Dis Child* **88**:772-774, 1954.

5. Urizar RE, Michael AF, Sisson S, et al: Anaphylactoid purpura: II. Immunofluorescent and electron microscopic studies of the glomerular lesions. *Lab Invest* **19**:437-450, 1968.

6. Wedgwood RJP, Janeway CA: Serum complement in children with "collagen diseases." *Pediatrics* **11**:569-581, 1953.

7. West CD, Northway JD, Davis NC: Serum levels of beta-1-C, a complement component in the nephritides, lipoid nephrosis and other conditions. *J Clin Invest* **43**:1507-1517, 1964.

8. Urizar RE, Schwartz A, Vernier RL: Immunofluorescence microscopy and ultrastructural changes of kidney in experimental anaphylactoid purpura. *Lab Invest* **21**:77-84, 1969.

9. Peters GA, Horton BT: Allergic purpura with special reference to hypersensitivitness to cold. *Mayo Clin Proc* **16**:631-636, 1941.

10. Urizar RE, Herdman RC: Anaphylactoid purpura: III. Early morphologic glomerular changes. *Amer J Clin Path* **53**:258-266, 1970.

11. Kobayashi O, Wada H, Kifurre S: Needle renal biopsy of the nephritis of anaphylactoid purpura in children. *Acta Med Biol* **9**:175-187, 1961.

12. Heberden W, cited by Rook A: William Heberden's cases of anaphylactoid purpura. *Arch Dis Child* **33**:271, 1958.

13. Willan R: *On Cutaneous Diseases*. London, J Johnson, 1808.

14. Schönlein JL: *Allgemeine und Specielle Pathologie und Therapie*, ed 3. Herisau, Switzerland, Lit-Compt, 1837, vol 2, p 48.

15. Henoch E: Über eine eigentümbliche Form von Purpura. *Berlin Klin Wschr* **11**:641-643, 1874.

16. Wedgwood RJP, Klaus MH: Anaphylactoid purpura: A long-term follow-up study with special reference to renal involvement. *Pediatrics* **16**:196-205, 1955.

17. Oliver TK Jr, Barnett HL: Incidence and prognosis of nephritis associated with anaphylactoid (Schönlein-Henoch) purpura in children. *Amer J Dis Child* **90**:544-547, 1955.

18. Derham RJ, Rogerson MM: The Schönlein-Henoch syndrome with particular reference to renal sequelae. *Arch Dis Child* **31**:364-368, 1956.

19. Vernier RL, Worthen HG, Peterson RD, et al: Anaphylactoid purpura: I. Pathology of the skin and kidney and frequency of streptococcal infection. *Pediatrics* **27**:181-193, 1961.

20. Sterky G, Thilen A: A study on the onset and prognosis of acute vascular purpura (the Schönlein-Henoch syndrome) in children. *Acta Paediat* **49**:217-229, 1960.

21. Gairdner D: The Schönlein-Henoch syndrome (Anaphylactoid Purpura). *Quart J Med* **17**:95-122, 1948.

22. Lewis IC, Philpott MG: Neurological complications in the Schönlein-Henoch syndrome. *Arch Dis Child* **31**:369-371, 1956.

23. Lecutier MA: Case of the Schönlein-Henoch syndrome with myocardial necrosis. *J Clin Path* **5**:336-338, 1952.

24. Gary NE, Mazzara JT, Holfelder L: The Schönlein-Henoch syndrome. *Ann Intern Med* **72**:229-234, 1970.

25. Norkin S, Wiener J: Henoch-Schönlein syndrome: Review of pathology and report of two cases. *Amer J Clin Path* **33**:55-65, 1960.

26. Faith GC, Trump BF: The glomerular capillary wall in human kidney disease: Acute glomerulonephritis, systemic lupus erythematosis, and pre-eclampsia: Comparative electron microscopic observations and a review. *Lab Invest* **15**:1682-1719, 1966.

Detection of a Left Atrial Myxoma by Echocardiography

William H. Spencer, III, MD;
Robert H. Peter, MD; and
Edward S. Orgain, MD, Durham, NC

Left atrial myxoma is a rare entity with protean manifestations.[1] In the past, diagnosis has proved difficult partly because of the necessarily elaborate techniques required to establish the presence of the tumor.[2,3] Recently, cardiac echograms have proven successful in the preoperative diagnosis of both right and left atrial myxomas.[4-8] We have recently encountered a dramatic example of the successful preoperative diagnosis of a myxoma which emphasizes the value of ultrasound in the detection of these tumors.

Received for publication May 14, 1971; accepted July 15.

From the Cardiovascular Division, Department of Medicine, Duke University Medical Center, Durham, NC.

Reprint requests to Department of Medicine, Division of Cardiovascular Disease, Duke University Medical Center, Durham, NC 27710 (Dr. Orgain).

Patient Summary

The patient (JO 3777) was a 35-year-old housewife referred for evaluation of pulmonary infiltrates. She was well until late April 1970 when she developed persistent cough, dyspnea on exertion, and a low-grade fever. A brief hospitalization and treatment with several antibiotics produced some subjective improvement. During the next 2½ months the patient had frequent, but mild, afternoon temperature elevations and mild dyspnea. In late July 1970 the patient experienced a return of fever to 104 F (40 C), cough, and shortness of breath. A chest roentgenogram revealed bilateral alveolar infiltrates. She was again hospitalized and treated with antibiotics with some improvement. When, two weeks after discharge, the cough and low-grade fever recurred, she was referred to Duke University Medical Center for further evaluation.

There was no past history of rheumatic fever. Findings of the review of systems were unremarkable.

Physical examination revealed an alert woman not obviously ill. The blood pressure was 104/70 mm Hg; the pulse rate was 108 beats per minute. There were no conjunctival petechiae or splinter hemorrhages. The fundi were normal. Prominent *a* waves were noted in the jugular venous pulse. The chest was clear to percussion and auscultation. The heart was not enlarged. The first sound was loud and appeared doubled. The second heart sound was normal. A third sound with the timing of an opening snap was present. A grade 2/6 holosystolic, blowing murmur was present at the left sternal border and at the cardiac apex. No diastolic murmurs were audible. Findings of the remainder of the physical examination were normal.

Admission laboratory data revealed a normal hemogram, sedimentation rate, urine, quantitative serum protein value, and blood chemistry values, save for a slightly elevated alkaline phosphatase level. The electrocardiogram displayed left atrial enlargement. A chest roentgenogram on admission was interpreted as normal; however, a review of previous

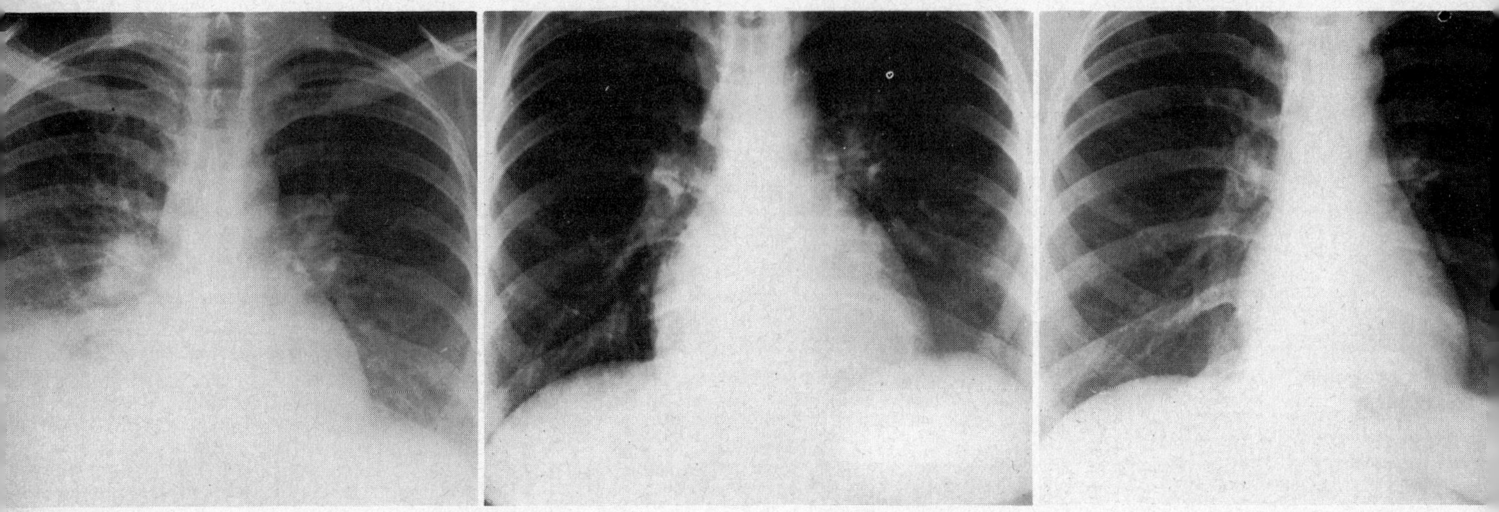

Fig 1.—Three chest roentgenograms performed at appropriate intervals during the patient's course. Left, *Cardiac enlargement and bilateral pulmonary edema during a symptomatic period.* Center, *Preoperative cardiac enlargement.* Right, *Dramatic decrease in heart size six months postoperatively.*

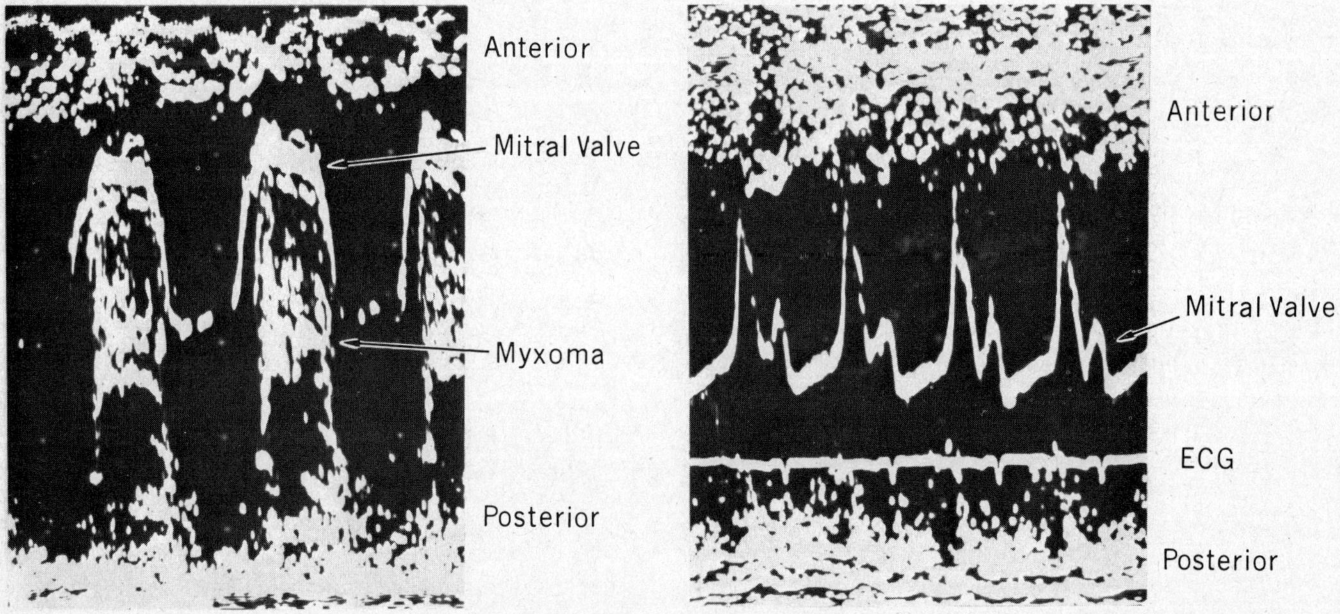

Fig 2.—Preoperative (left) and postoperative (right) *views.* Left, *Echocardiograms showing tumor mass present posterior to the anterior leaflet of the mitral valve.* Right, *Echocardiogram taken five days postoperatively reveals a normal pattern with the area of the mitral orifice free of echoes.*

roentgenograms recorded in May and in July 1970 disclosed the typical pattern of bilateral pulmonary edema (Fig 1, *left*).

An echocardiogram (Fig 2, *left*) revealed the dramatic, unequivocal pattern of a mass occupying the orifice of the mitral valve during diastole. The echo pattern of the anterior leaflet of the mitral valve is seen above the mass in Fig 2, *left*; behind this echo is the mitral orifice. In the normal pattern as seen in Fig 2, *right*, the area behind the anterior leaflet echo is free of echoes. The myxoma, then, occupies the mitral orifice in Fig 2, *left*.

Right-sided cardiac catheterization was performed, and during the levophase of a pulmonary angiogram a 6- by 3-cm mass was observed to occupy the left atrium during ventricular systole (Fig 3, *top*) and to move vigorously into the mitral orifice, partially obstructing it during diastole (Fig 3, *bottom*). Right-sided pressures were elevated with a pulmonary wedge pressure of 32 mm Hg.

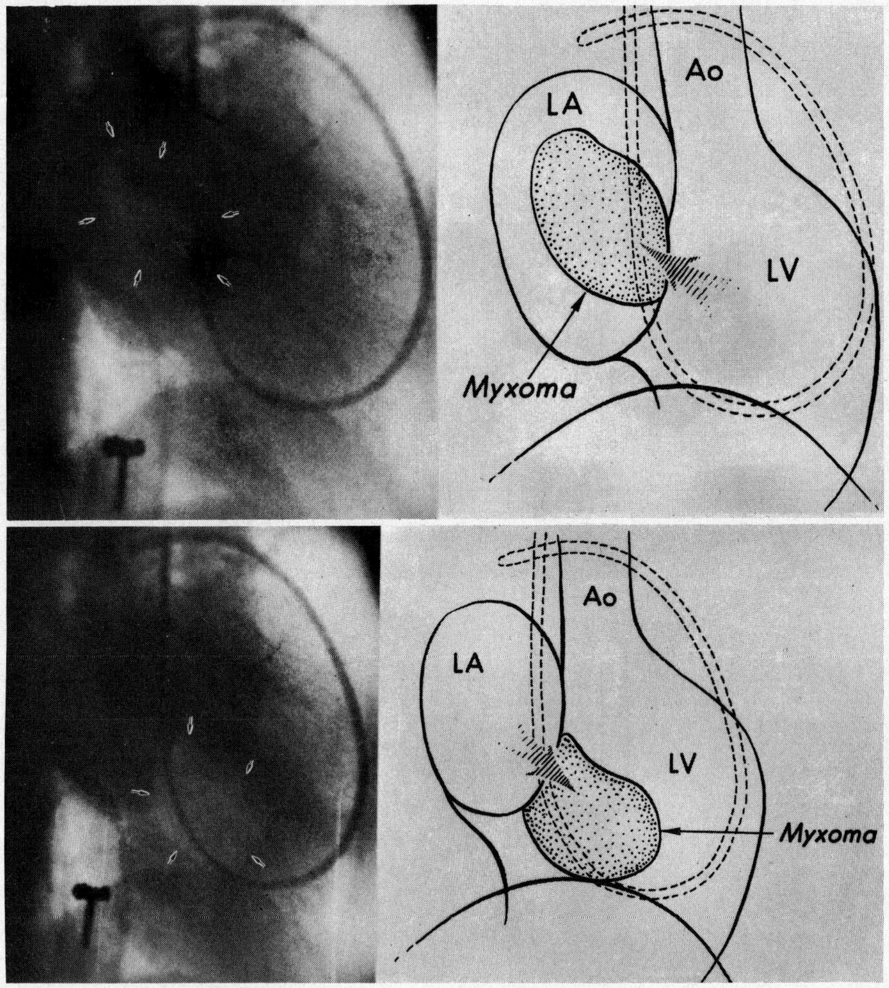

Fig 3.—Frames from cineangiograms during systole (top) *and diastole* (bottom). *The myxoma is seen in the left atrium (LA)* (top). Bottom, *The myxoma is seen after its diastolic descent into the mitral orifice. LV = left ventricle and Ao = aorta.*

Immediately following angiography, surgery was performed utilizing complete cardiopulmonary bypass. A histologically typical left atrial myxoma attached to the interatrial septum by a 1-cm pedicle was excised without difficulty.

A follow-up echocardiogram (Fig 2, *right*) performed four days postoperatively exhibits a perfectly normal pattern in striking contrast to the preoperative echo.

The patient, rechecked in detail six months postoperatively, was found to be completely asymptomatic with a normal heart size and sounds. The change in heart size observable on the chest roentgenogram (Fig 1, *left*, *center*, and *right*) is quite dramatic.

Comment

Because atrial myxomas represent benign tumors which may cause disabling morbidity or rapid mortality if unrecognized, a simple screening technique to establish their presence is a most welcome addition to the diagnostic armamentarium. Previous reviews have stressed the use of angiocardiograms as a means of establishing the diagnosis[1,2]; however, the intricacy of this procedure prohibits its use as a widespread screening maneuver and limits its use to cases where the clinical suspicion is strong. Since most of these tumors, 90% in one series,[3] descend into the mitral valve orifice during diastole, detection by ultrasound techniques is possible, but the accuracy of this technique for this purpose is not known. The present case represents a vivid example of the capacity to recognize such tumors with the simple, noninvasive technique of ultrasound cardiography. We would urge the widespread use of ultrasound to exclude atrial myxoma in patients with unexplained dyspnea, peripheral emboli, atypical murmurs, syncope, or unusual postural effects on symptoms or signs.

This investigation was supported in part by Public Health Service training grant HE 05736.

References

1. Greenwood WF: Profile of atrial myxoma. *Amer J Cardiol* **21**:367-375, 1968.
2. Hair TE, Orgain ES, Sealy WC, et al: Myxoma of the left atrium: Observations on two cases with successful removal and review of diagnostic methods. *Amer J Med* **32**:560-571, 1962.
3. Godwin JF: Diagnosis of left atrial myxoma. *Lancet* **1**:464-467, 1963.
4. Schattenberg TT: Echocardiographic diagnosis of left atrial myxoma. *Mayo Clin Proc* **43**:620-627, 1968.
5. Wolfe SB, Popp RL, Feigenbaum H: Diagnosis of atrial tumors by ultrasound. *Circulation* **39**:615-622, 1969.
6. Popp RL, Harrison DC: Ultrasound for the diagnosis of atrial tumor. *Ann Intern Med* **71**:785-787, 1969.
7. Finegan RE, Harrison DC: Diagnosis of left atrial myxoma by echocardiography. *New Eng J Med* **282**:1022-1023, 1970.
8. Kostis JB, Moghadam AN: Echocardiographic diagnosis of left atrial myxoma. *Chest* **58**:550-552, 1970.

Mechanism of *Aspergillus*-Induced Microangiopathic Hemolytic Anemia

Stanley J. Robboy, MD; Kent Salisbury, MD;
Bruce Ragsdale, MD; Lewis M. Bobroff, MD;
Bernard M. Jacobson, MD; and Robert W. Colman, MD, Boston

Florid microangiopathic hemolytic anemia (MHA) is encountered in few disease states. The most common are thrombotic thrombocytopenic purpura (TTP), hemolytic uremic syndrome of infancy, and disseminated intravascular coagulation (DIC). Red blood cell (RBC) fragmentation may occur clinically in the latter secondary to carcinoma[1] or septicemia and in the laboratory following intravenous injections of thrombin or endotoxin into animals.[2] Less frequently, fragmentation is seen with malignant hypertension, severe preeclampsia or eclampsia, or acute necrotizing glomerulonephritis.[2]

Received for publication Dec 18, 1970; accepted Jan 21, 1971.

From the departments of pathology and medicine, Harvard Medical School, and the James Homer Wright Pathology Laboratories and the Departments of Medicine, Massachusetts General Hospital, Boston. Dr. Robboy is now with US Ireland Army Hospital, Fort Knox, Kentucky.

Reprint requests to Laboratory Service, US Ireland Army Hospital, Fort Knox, Kentucky 40121 (Dr. Robboy).

Recently, we encountered a patient who developed MHA and DIC while he was receiving steroids and antibiotics. Subsequently we encountered a second patient who developed leukoerythroblastosis and DIC, suggestive of MHA, while she too was receiving steroids.[3] Two additional cases[4,5] (Table) suggested that this peculiar combination of findings was not coincidental. These microangiopathic changes appear to be in vivo manifestations of the in vitro models of Bull et al[6] in which RBC moving at high speeds fragmented as they passed through a meshwork of fibrin strands. The current report also illustrates the beneficial clinical and hematological responses to heparin therapy, which was given three times during the hospital course.

Patient Summary

The patient (MGH 1607583) was a 66-year-old man who entered the hospital with bruises and jaundice of 11 days' duration. He had been in Spain two weeks before admission when fever appeared. Influenza had been suspected and chloramphenicol, tetracycline, erythromycin, and prednisolone were prescribed. Although the fever abated, the cough and malaise persisted. Subsequently, large ecchymoses spontaneously appeared on the arms and legs. He returned to the United States and was brought to the Massachusetts General Hospital, Boston.

The past medical history was not suggestive of any bleeding disorder, nor of exposures to any obvious respiratory tract pathogens. For years he smoked one to two packs of cigarettes daily and had a chronic cough productive of 1 cup of sputum each day. X-ray films taken during the preceding ten years disclosed mild emphysema.

On admission, he was slightly icteric and cachectic. The respiratory rate was 28 per minute; the other vital signs were normal. Petechiae covered the arms, legs, and trunk, and nontender ecchymoses, 2 to 4 cm in size, covered the forearms, right pectoral region, and legs. Focal rales were audible. The liver was palpable 6 cm below the right costal margin. Findings from the remainder of the examination were within normal limits.

The hematocrit reading was 23%, and the white blood cell count (WBC) was 9,600/cu mm, with 70% neutrophils, 22%

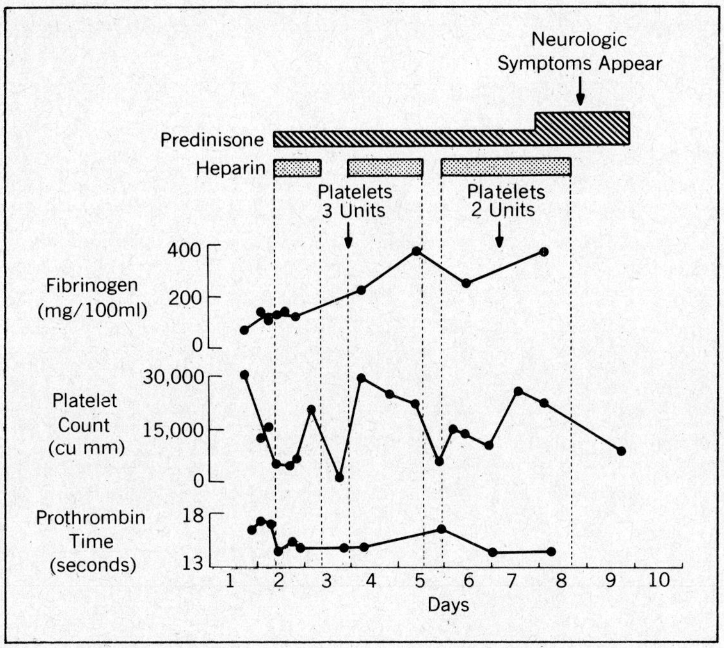

Fig 1.—Clinical and laboratory changes during hospitalization.

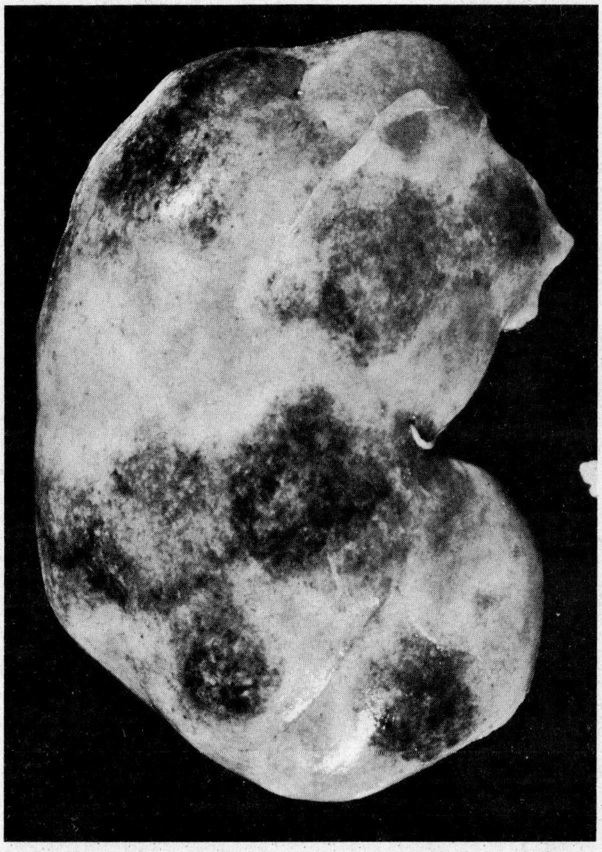

Fig 2.—Surface of renal cortex with focal hemorrhage.

banded neutrophils, 5% metamyelocytes, and 3% myelocytes. In addition there were 32 normoblasts per 100 WBC. The peripheral blood smear disclosed an extraordinary number of schistocytes. A bone marrow aspirate revealed marked erythroid hyperplasia and adequate number of normal megakaryocytes. The prothrombin time was 15.9 seconds (control, 12.1 seconds); platelet count, 32,000/cu mm; fibrinogen value, 70 mg/100 ml; thrombin time, 31.9 seconds (control, 21 seconds); and fibrinogen degradation products (Fi test), 1:32 (normal titer, < 1:8). Cryofibrinogen was present. The reticulocyte count was 9.4%, serum hemoglobin level was 23.2 mg/100 ml (normal, 2 to 3 mg/100 ml), and direct and indirect Coombs tests were negative. The stool was guaiac positive (4 +).

Other laboratory studies included the following values: blood urea nitrogen (BUN), 126 mg/100 ml; creatinine, 3.1 mg/100 ml; calcium, 7.8 mg/100 ml; phosphorus, 6.3 mg/100 ml; and bilirubin, 1.0 mg/100 ml direct and 2.6 mg/100 ml total. The lactic acid dehydrogenase (LDH) level was 720 units, and alkaline phosphatase level was 3.3 Bodansky units. The creatinine clearance was 40 liters/day. The urine sediment contained eight to ten RBC per high-power field (HPF), two to four WBC per HPF, and many coarsely granular pigmented casts. Multiple cultures of sputum, urine, blood, and cerebrospinal fluid were negative. An x-ray film of the chest disclosed bilateral apical pleural scars and upward hilar retraction, but no infiltrates.

On admission (Fig 1), several venipunctures were performed. Within two hours, large ecchymoses developed at the multiple venipuncture sites and substantial oozing occurred about the venous catheter. Purpura now covered the thighs and arms. Whole blood and packed RBC were given. On the morning of the second day, the stools were maroon and the urine slightly bloody. A nasal excoriation oozed blood. Therapy with heparin sodium (50 mg intravenously every four hours) and prednisone (20 mg orally every eight hours) was begun. By the next day the prothrombin time and the platelet count showed modest improvement and the heparin therapy was discontinued. When the platelet count suddenly fell, heparin therapy was reinstituted, 3 units of platelet concentrates were given, and during the next two days the platelet count and fibrinogen level improved. Because of the persistent epistaxis, liquid maroon stools, and hematuria, the heparin was again discontinued. Within six hours the platelet count and fibrinogen level fell, and the prothrombin time became prolonged. Heparin sodium therapy was reinstituted at a constant infusion rate of 10 mg intravenously per hour.

During the sixth through the eighth days (while the patient was receiving heparin) results of the tests of hemostasis improved. The number of transfusions needed to maintain a hematocrit reading of at least 20% dropped from 6 units per day during the early hospital days to 3 each day. The serum hemoglobin level fell to 10 mg/100 ml, and the number of schistocytes in the peripheral smears decreased markedly. Epistaxis and bleeding from the gastrointestinal tract and venipuncture sites continued, but at diminished rates. Confluent ecchymoses and large subcutaneous hematomas were present on the forearms and hands.

By the seventh day, the renal function was improved with a BUN level of 50 mg/100 ml and creatinine level of 1.5 mg/100 ml. Once rehydration was begun, the urine output averaged 2 to 3 liters per day. Repeated gram stains of the urine were negative. On the eighth day, in preparation for splenectomy the dosage of prednisone was increased (to 40 mg orally every six hours) and the heparin therapy discontinued. At about this time, slight ptosis of the right eyelid and anisocoria were noted. By the morning of the tenth day the patient was obtunded, the gaze was disconjugate, flaccid paralysis developed in the left arm and leg, and death occurred.

At autopsy, *Aspergillus fumigatus* was identified in lung, kidneys, brain, heart, thyroid, and spleen. The lungs weighed 2,700 gm combined. Throughout both lungs, but especially in the lower lobe of the left lung, there were tiny, soft, necrotic foci filled with characteristic hyphae that were 3μ to 5μ in diameter, septate, and dichotomously branched.

The kidneys weighed 610 gm combined. The cortices bulged with numerous hemorrhages, 1 to 3 cm in size (Fig 2), that corresponded largely to thrombosed arcuate arteries (Fig 3). Microscopically, each thrombosed artery contained an intricate mesh of intertwined hyphae, some of which were anchored in the muscular wall (Fig 4). Filling the interstices of the hyphal trellis were amorphous fibrin-leukocyte-platelet thrombi, entrapped RBC, and numerous fibrin strands less than 1μ in diameter.

The heart weighed 450 gm and contained four foci of *A fumigatus*, each 1 to 4 mm in diameter. Three were buried within the myocardium; one broke through the endocardial surface of the left atrium, was flat, and did not appear to have interfered with the flow of blood. The fresh brain weighed 1,650 gm and had one large focus, and at least eight foci of cerebral hemorrhages that were 1 to 5 mm in size. Each contained *A fumigatus* hyphae in arteries. In addition, a thrombus with *A fumigatus* obstructed the right internal carotid artery just prior to the origin of the anterior cerebral artery. The spleen and the thyroid both contained foci of hemorrhage, 0.5 to 3.0 cm in size; *A fumigatus* hyphae involved large arteries. Other findings at autopsy included (1) an acute bleeding duodenal ulcer, (2) healed rheumatic mitral valvulitis, (3) erythroid hyperplasia of vertebral and iliac marrow, fatty femoral marrow, and normal lymph nodes, (4) rare fibrin thrombin in heart, pancreas, renal glomerular capillaries.

Comment

In 1962, Brain et al[1] introduced the term "microangiopathic hemolytic anemia" to describe a type of hemolytic anemia in which schistocytes were produced as normal RBC passed through pathological small blood vessels. Recently this group proposed several mechanisms to explain the steps by which the RBC fragment.[6] The injection of thrombin into blood flowing in a closed in vitro circulatory system caused clots of fibrin (up to 11 mm in size) to form; the pressure of the system rose and schistocytes and hemoglobinemia appeared. Such a model may explain in vivo production of schistocytes in two cases of DIC where fibrin thrombin formed about large hyphal tangles of *Aspergillus* organisms in a cardiac chamber[4,5] (Table).

A second in vitro model of Bull et al,[6] and the one applicable to this case and one other,[3] explains how RBC fragment as they are forcibly passed at high speeds through a fine mesh composed of thin fibers. The two essential facets were (1) rapid blood flow, greater than 10 cm/sec, and (2) obstructing fibers 1μ or less in diameter. The composition of the fiber was immaterial; fibrin, glass, metal, or nylon were equally effective. The present case is presented as an in vivo example of this model. *Aspergillus* organisms because of their ability freely to invade blood vessel walls[7] anchored into arterial walls and formed a trellis of interweaving hyphae in the lumina of the renal arteries (Fig 3,4). As fibrin-leukocyte-platelet thrombi formed about the organisms,[7] the two criteria for the model of Bull et al[6] became fulfilled. It is proposed that as the normal RBC were forced through the porous meshwork, they impinged upon thin fibrin strands and eventually fragmented.[8] That *Aspergillus* organisms themselves

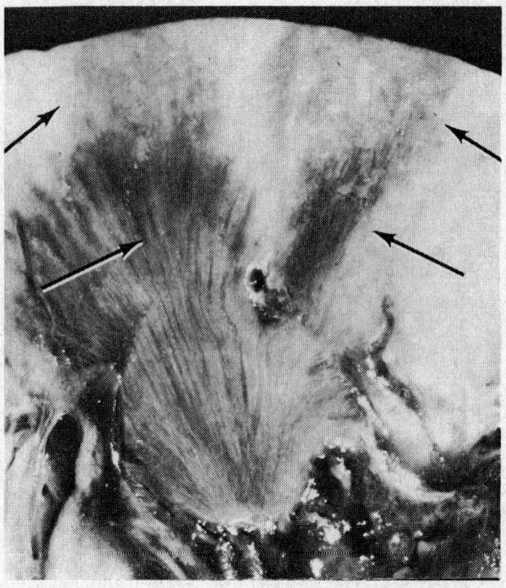

Fig 3.—Cut surface showing thrombosed arcuate artery and cortical hemorrhage (arrows).

Fig 4.—Aspergillus *hyphae appear as black strands in thrombus in lumen and wall of arcuate artery of kidney (methenamine silver, ×170).*

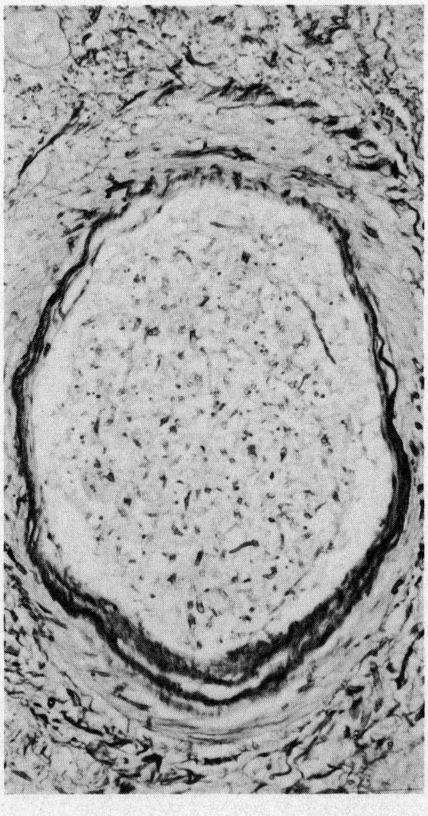

Findings in *Aspergillus*-Induced MHA and DIC*

Patient	Prothrombin Time, Patient/Control (sec)	Fibrinogen (mg/100ml)	Fibrinogen Degradation Products	Schistocytes	Normoblasts (per 100 WBC)	Reticulocytes (%)	Location of Aspergillus
Case record[3]	23.0/12.1	110	Present	"Bizarre" cells	2		Renal arteries
Doughten[4]	28.7/12.2	20	Absent	Numerous	10	6.1	Heart atria
Luke[5]				Present			Kidneys Heart ventricles
Robboy	15.9/12.1	70	Present	Florid	32	9.4	Renal arteries

* MHA signifies microangiopathic hemolytic anemia; DIC, disseminated intravascular coagulation.

neither cause hemolysis nor elaborate a thromboplastic activity into serum has been documented in vitro.[4]

It has been suggested that DIC and microangiopathic hemolytic anemia may be intimately related.[9] This patient had active DIC with secondary fibrinolysis evident both clinically and by laboratory tests. In this case a vicious cycle of DIC and microangiopathy apparently developed. As RBC fragmented, they released procoagulant phospholipids,[10] sustained the DIC, and perpetuated the formation of fibrin which was undergoing continual dissolution by the activated fibrinolytic process. In turn the new fibrin thrombi assured the presence of thin fibrin thrombi upon which RBC could fragment. On three occasions, heparin, a drug useful in abolishing DIC and secondary fibrinolysis,[11,12] was administered. Each time, the prothrombin time, platelet count, and fibrinogen returned towards normal levels (Fig 1). This suggests that the DIC was partially controlled and might account for the improving clinical picture. Unfortunately, heparin does not remove the precipitating cause of DIC. As we have observed previously, the discontinuation of heparin therapy often results in the prompt exacerbation of DIC. During life, the clinical diagnosis was TTP; *A fumigatus* was not suspected. Presumably the steroids given prior to and during hospitalization nurtured the growth of the fungus.[13] Possibly the organism had been present for some period in an asymptomatic focus in the lung.

An *Aspergillus* infection should be considered when signs of MHA, leukoerythroblastosis, and DIC appear in patients who are receiving steroids or antibiotics.

Summary

Florid microangiopathic hemolytic anemia and disseminated intravascular coagulation occurred in a previously healthy man. At autopsy the arcuate arteries of the kidneys were thrombosed and contained an intricate network of intertwined hyphae bridged by fibrin strands. The microangiopathic changes appear to be an in vivo manifestation of an in vitro model in which RBC moving at high speeds fragmented as they passed through a meshwork of thin fibrin strands. It is proposed that the intravascular hemolysis caused the release of procoagulant phospholipids, and a vicious cycle was sustained by further deposition of fibrin. Heparin, administered on three occasions, appeared to ameliorate both the hemolysis and the intravascular coagulation.

References

1. Brain MC, Dacie JV, Hourihane DO: Microangiopathic haemolytic anaemia: The possible role of vascular lesions in pathogenesis. *Brit J Haemat* **8**:358-374, 1962.
2. Brain MC, Microangiopathic hemolytic anemia. *New Eng J Med* **281**:833-835, 1959.
3. Case records of the Massachusetts General Hospital (case 44-1970). *New Eng J Med* **283**:919-927, 1970.
4. Doughten RM, Pearson HA: Disseminated intravascular coagulation associated with *Aspergillus* endocarditis. *J Pediat* **73**:576-582, 1968.
5. Luke JL, Bolande RP, Gross S: Generalized aspergillosis and *Aspergillus* endocarditis in infancy. *Pediatrics* **31**:115-122, 1963.
6. Bull BS, Rubenberg ML, Dacie JV, et al: Microangiopathic haemolytic anaemia: Mechanisms of red-cell fragmentation: In vitro studies. *Brit J Haemat* **14**:643-652, 1968.
7. Case records of the Massachusetts General Hospital (case 23-1970). *New Eng J Med* **282**:1256-1264, 1970.
8. Bull BS, Kuhn IN: The production of schistocytes by fibrin strands (a scanning electron microscopic study). *Blood* **35**:104-111, 1970.
9. Rubenberg ML, Regoeczi E, Bull BS, et al: Microangiopathic haemolytic anaemia: The experimental production of haemolysis and red-cell fragmentation by defibrination in vivo. *Brit J Haemat* **14**:627-642, 1968.
10. Marcus AJ: The role of lipids in blood coagulation. *Advances Lipid Res* **4**:1-37, 1966.
11. Robboy SJ, Minna JD, Colman RW: Resolution of pathological fibrinolysis with heparin. *Clin Res* **18**:414, 1970.
12. Straub P, Riedler G, Frick P: Hypofibrinogenaemia in metastatic carcinoma of prostate: Suppression of systemic fibrinolysis by heparin. *J Clin Path* **20**:152-157, 1967.
13. Zidransky H, Friedman L: The effect of cortisone and antibiotic agents on experimental pulmonary aspergillosis. *Amer J Path* **35**:169-183, 1959.

Osteomalacia Induced by Laxative (Phenolphthalein) Ingestion

Boy Frame, MD; Hernan L. Guiang, MD; Harold M. Frost, MD; and William A. Reynolds, MD, Detroit

A 51-year-old woman developed skeletal symptoms due to histologically proved osteomalacia. The etiology could not be determined until a history of factitial diarrhea due to long-term phenolphthalein (Ex-Lax) ingestion was finally elicited. Normal bowel habits returned after the use of phenolphthalein was discontinued and the osteomalacia showed signs of healing. Surreptitious ingestion of cathartics should be considered as a causal factor in patients with unexplained osteomalacia.

The overuse of phenolphthalein (Ex-Lax) may cause diarrhea and result in a variety of metabolic disturbances. Hypocalcemia has been observed in such cases, but to our knowledge osteomalacia has not previously been recorded. The purpose of this communication is to cite the occurrence of biopsy proved severe osteomalacia in a patient with factitial diarrhea due to phenolphthalein.

Received for publication Sept 8, 1970; accepted Nov 2.

From the departments of medicine (Drs. Frame and Guiang), orthopedic surgery (Dr. Frost), and radiology (Dr. Reynolds), Henry Ford Hospital, Detroit.

Reprint requests to 2799 W Grand Blvd, Detroit 48202 (Dr. Frame).

Patient Summary

A 51-year-old white obese woman was seen in the orthopedic clinic with back and hip pain of six months' duration. She was hostile, combative, and a poor historian. To one observer the patient admitted to having three to four loose stools daily, but later denied this. Her history and family history were otherwise unremarkable. On physical examination, there was moderate obesity, skeletal tenderness over the spine and hips, and emotional lability.

Laboratory results were as follows: hemoglobin, 15.5 gm/100 ml; white blood cell count, 8,000/cu mm; and negative results of venereal disease research laboratory test for syphilis (VDRL). The serum creatinine level was 1.2 mg/100 ml. Serum electrolyte values were sodium, 135 mEq/liter; potassium, 3.1 mEq/liter; chloride, 98 mEq/liter; and carbon dioxide combining power, 24 mEq/liter. Values for the serum calcium were 7.7, 7.8, and 8.0 mg/100 ml and for serum inorganic phosphate 3.1, 3.1, and 3.0 mg/100 ml. Serum alkaline phosphatase levels were 13.1 and 12.0 Bodansky units/100 ml. Serum protein electrophoresis determination showed an albumin value of 3.4 gm/100 ml and normal levels of globulin. A 24-hour urine sample contained 105 mg of calcium in a volume of 2,100 ml. The serum carotene level was 56μg/100 ml and the serum magnesium level was 1.9 mEq/liter. Results of a 25-gm four-hour xylose absorption test on three occasions averaged 1.8 gm. Skeletal roentgenograms demonstrated essentially normal bone density, but pseudofractures of both femoral necks were noted (Fig 1, *left*).

A left 11th rib specimen was removed for study following the administration of a double bone-label with demeclocycline hydrochloride (Declomycin). A review of the histologic changes and bone remodeling data in the removed bone specimen demonstrated changes of florid osteomalacia (Fig 2). Osteoid seam numbers were markedly increased and the mineral appositional rate was decreased (Table).

The etiology of the osteomalacia was

not certain at this stage of our investigation, but the repeatedly impaired absorption of xylose suggested the presence of a malabsorption syndrome. Roentgenograms of the upper-gastrointestinal tract, including the small bowel, were normal. A jejunal biopsy was contemplated but refused by the patient. The patient was discharged on a regimen of a gluten free diet, 15 ml of calcium glubionate (Neo-calglucon) four times daily, and vitamin D, 50,000 units/day.

A return clinic visit a month later was most revealing. The patient was interviewed in the presence of her daughter. When asked again about bowel habits, the patient hesitated, but the daughter than stated that the patient had a long history of frequent watery, black, and foul-smelling stools associated with abdominal cramping. It turned out that the patient had prevailed upon various family members to keep her supplied with phenolphthalein. Further investigation uncovered a 20-year history of taking 15 to 20 phenolphthalein tablets daily. It was estimated that more than $5,000 had been spent on this laxative habit. Apparently the phenolphthalein had produced small watery stools and abdominal cramping. The patient interpreted this as incomplete emptying of the colon and her solution was to take more phenolphthalein.

Dietary history was reviewed with the patient and the family and there appeared to be adequate dietary intake of dairy products and meat. A dietary deficiency of vitamin D was therefore not felt likely.

With the cooperation of the family, many boxes of hidden phenolphthalein tablets were discarded and the patient was watched carefully. She was placed on a regular diet and the use of vitamin D and calcium supplements were discontinued. Bowel habits soon returned to normal. A month later skeletal discomfort was considerably improved as was her mental status. Values for serum potassium, calcium, and phosphorus were now normal. Results of a repeat xylose absorption test were now normal at 3.5 gm in four hours. Value for serum alkaline phosphatase, which may continue elevated for many months during the healing of osteomalacia, remained high at 12 Bodansky units. Repeat skeletal x-ray films showed healing of the femoral neck pseudofractures (Fig 1, *right*).

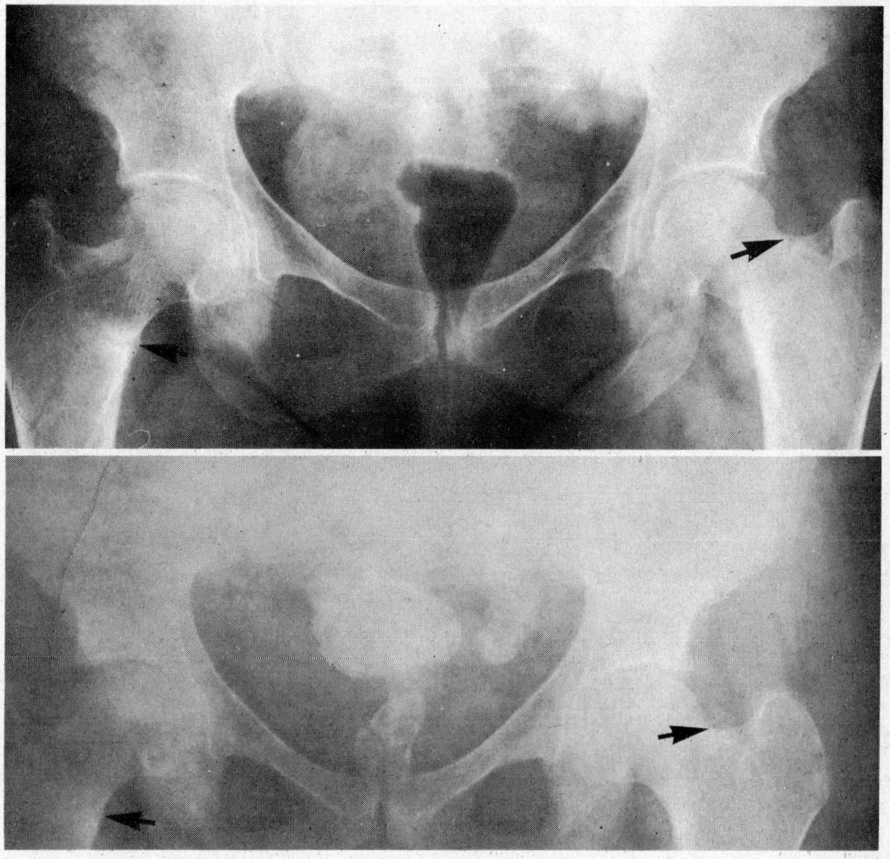

Fig 1.—Top, X-ray film showing pseudofractures about femoral necks. Bottom, *Progress x-ray films showing healed pseudofractures three months after discontinuance of phenolphthalein with vitamin D and calcium.*

Fig 2.—Photomicrograph of rib showing increased numbers of osteoid seams (arrows).

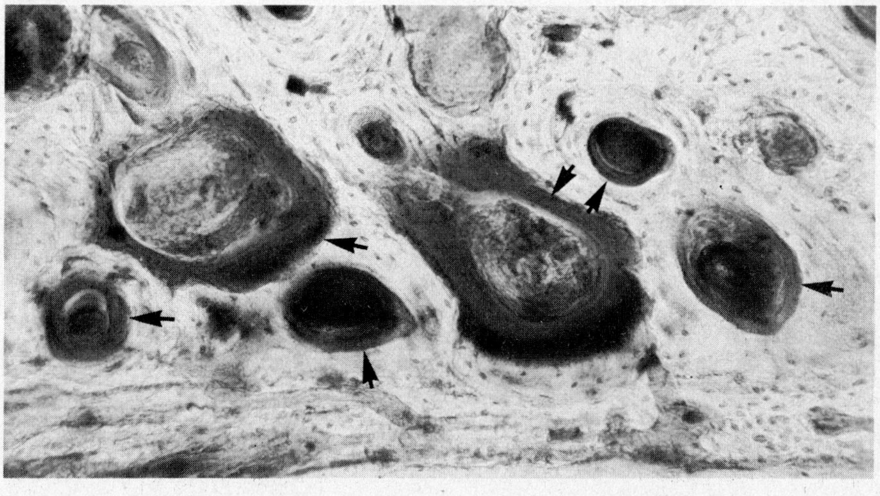

Bone Remodeling Data (11th Rib)

Mean	Patient's Measured Value	Age Comparable Normal, Measured Value
No. of osteoid seams per cu mm	12.5	0.39 ± 0.27
Appositional rate, μ/day	0.28	0.93 ± 0.32
Osteon formation time, yr	2.2	0.23 ± 0.10

Comment

The clinical symptoms and laboratory results in this patient were typical of osteomalacia. Values for serum calcium and inorganic phosphorus were both decreased and the serum alkaline phosphatase level increased. The pseudofractures in the femoral neck regions were considered practically pathognomonic of osteomalacia. Furthermore, the histologic appearance and bone remodeling data obtained from study of the 11th rib specimen confirmed the diagnosis. The number of osteoid seams was increased to 12.5, a 30-fold increase over a comparable normal value of 0.39 ± 0.27/cu mm. Of added significance was decreased mineral appositional rate of 0.28μ/day, compared to a normal value of 0.93 ± 0.32. Both an increase in seam numbers and impaired osteoid mineralization are prerequisites for the histologic diagnosis of dynamic osteomalacia.[1]

The cause of the osteomalacia was not apparent until the delayed history of phenolphthalein overuse was obtained. This had led to frequent watery stools which undoubtedly caused impaired absorption of vitamin D and calcium. The observed hypokalemia was also a result of the chronic diarrhea. Discontinuance of the use of phenolphthalein led quickly to normal bowel habits and healing of the osteomalacia. The vitamin D and calcium supplements given before the history of phenolphthalein ingestion was obtained were of added benefit in therapy.

Several complications of long-term laxative abuse have been emphasized. Potassium depletion due to diarrhea was the first mentioned by Schwartz and Relman in 1953.[2] More recently sodium and potassium deficit in such cases has been reported to result in hyperaldosteronism and to simulate Bartter's syndrome.[3] Protein-losing gastroenteropathy and malabsorption of xylose has also been noted.[4] Although hypocalcemia has been observed as a result of chronic purgation,[5] the patient reported in this communication is thought to be the first reported example of osteomalacia due to the surreptitious ingestion of phenolphthalein.

Phenolphthalein is an irritative cathartic with its greatest effect on the colon and least on the peristaltic activity of the small intestine.[6] The mechanism of action is not definitely known but it is thought to stimulate smooth muscle of the colon and to cause mucosal irritation. Malabsorption arises due to the rapid intestinal transient time as a result of increased peristalsis. In addition, subtle changes in the intestinal mucosal cells may affect further the absorptive capability of the small and large intestine.

Once again the altered psyche of patients subject to long-term laxative habit is noteworthy. Most are women. For various reasons they attempt to hide their ingestion and concerted detective work may be required to uncover the habit. Rarely patients may receive a vicarious pleasure from having frequent bowel movements. In some cases the bowel is purged so completely that the next spontaneous bowel movement may be unduly delayed. The patient then interprets this as constipation which he thinks requires another dose of laxative. Others, as in our patient, interpret the small watery bowel movements and abdominal cramping as incomplete emptying of the colon which required additional purging.

An ether extraction of urine that is treated with 0.1 normal sodium hydroxide indicates the presence of phenolphthalein and its conjugates and may be of aid when patients attempt to conceal the ingestion of phenolphthalein.[7]

References

1. Arnstein AR, Frame B, Frost HM: Recent progress in osteomalacia and rickets. *Ann Intern Med* **67**:1296-1330, 1967.

2. Schwartz WB, Relman AS: Metabolic and renal studies in chronic potassium depletion resulting from overuse of laxatives. *J Clin Invest* **32**:258-271, 1953.

3. Fleischer N, Brown H, Graham DY, et al: Chronic laxative-induced hyperaldosteronism and hypokalemia simulating Bartter's syndrome. *Ann Intern Med* **70**:791-798, 1969.

4. Heizer WD, Warshaw AL, Waldmann TA, et al: Protein-losing gastroenteropathy and malabsorption associated with factitious diarrhea. *Ann Intern Med* **68**:839-852, 1968.

5. Staffurth JS, Allott EN: Paralysis and tetany due to simultaneous hypokalemia and hypocalcemia, with other metabolic changes. *Amer J Med* **33**:800-806, 1962.

6. Abramowitz EW: Phenolphthalein today: A critical review. *Amer J Dig Dis* **17**:79-82, 1950.

7. Fantus B, Dyniewicz JM: Phenophthalein studies: Elimination of phenophthalein. *JAMA* **110**:796-799, 1938.

Coronary Artery Occlusion Due to Neoplasm

A Rare Cause of Acute Myocardial Infarction

Joseph A. Franciosa, MD, and Walter Lawrinson, MD, Washington, DC

Coronary atherosclerosis accounts for virtually all cases of myocardial infarction. On rare occasions other processes may involve the coronary arteries. Anomalous origin, aneurysm, and arteriovenous fistula occur in these vessels.[1-3] Embolization due to bacterial endocarditis, mural thrombi, or during cardiac surgery are well-known phenomena, and thrombosis may occur in patients with hematologic disorders such as polycythemia and sickle-cell anemia. Aortic dissection, infection, collagen-vascular disease, rheumatic fever, amyloidosis, gout, and Buerger's disease have also been reported to involve the coronary arteries.[4-7]

Neoplastic disease also involves the heart; when coronary vessels are affected, ischemia or infarction may result. While this possibility is well recognized in theory, actual cases are apparently exceedingly rare. At Washington Hospital Center from 1958 through 1968, 892 cases of myocardial infarction have come to autopsy. Three of these had the combination of epicardial or myocardial metastases or both and recent infarctions associated with coronary atherosclerosis. In none of these three was there evidence of vascular compromise due to neoplasm.

A search of the literature confirms the rarity of the occurence. The clinical and pathological aspects of a case of acute myocardial infarction due to neoplastic coronary arterial occlusion are reported.

Received for publication Oct 6, 1970; accepted Jan 19, 1971.

From the departments of medicine and pathology, Washington Hospital Center, Washington, DC. Dr. Franciosa is now with the Veterans Administration Hospital, Washington.

Reprint requests to Veterans Administration Hospital, 50 Irving St NW, Washington, DC 20422 (Dr. Franciosa).

Patient Summary

A 52-year-old Negro woman was admitted to the Washington Hospital Center on Nov 1, 1968, complaining of pain in the back and left shoulder.

One year earlier she had undergone a right maxillectomy for squamous cell carcinoma of the maxillary sinus. She did well postoperatively until two months before admission when she began to experience pain in the left scapular region. Six weeks later she noted a weight loss of 10 kg (22 lb) along with nausea, anorexia, dyspnea, and cough with blood-streaked sputum. Her history included total hysterectomy at the age of 36 years and gastric wedge resection of a benign ulcer at the age of 48. At the time of this latter operation, hypertension was noted but not treated.

Physical examination revealed a chronically ill, cachectic, dehydrated woman. The pulse was 80 beats per minute and regular. Blood pressure was 110/80 mm Hg; temperature, 99 F (37.2); and respirations, 20 per minute. There was periorbital edema of the right eye; fundoscopic examination showed arteriolar narrowing and tortuosity without hemorrhages, exudates, or papilledema. In the mouth there was a prosthesis covering a large cavity produced by previous right maxillectomy. No evidence of any new lesions was seen in this region. The lungs were clear to percussion, but there were decreased breath sounds in the left scapular region. A left ventricular apical impulse of normal quality was palpated in the fifth left intercostal space at the mid-clavicular line. Heart sounds were normal,

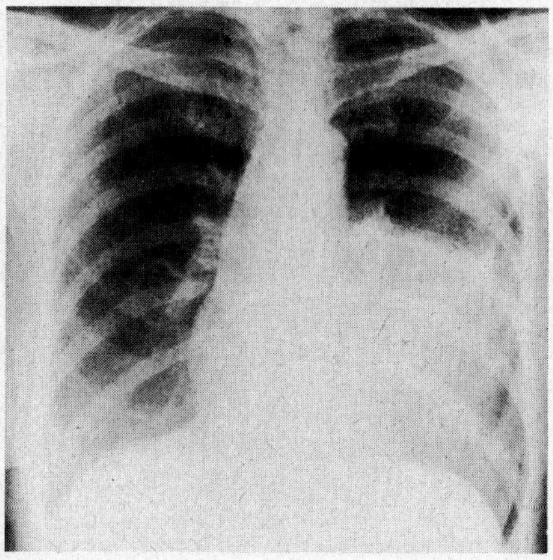

Fig 1.—Admission chest x-ray film. Note left upper lobe consolidation.

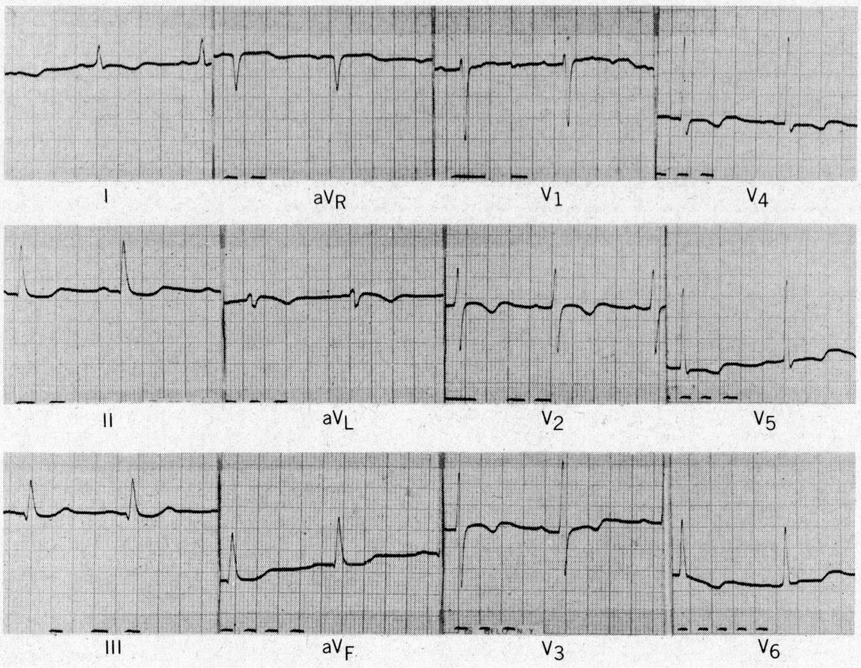

Fig 2.—Admission ECG showing T-wave inversion, with normal R-wave progression across precordium.

Fig 3.—Electrocardiogram on eighth hospital day which shows left bundle branch block.

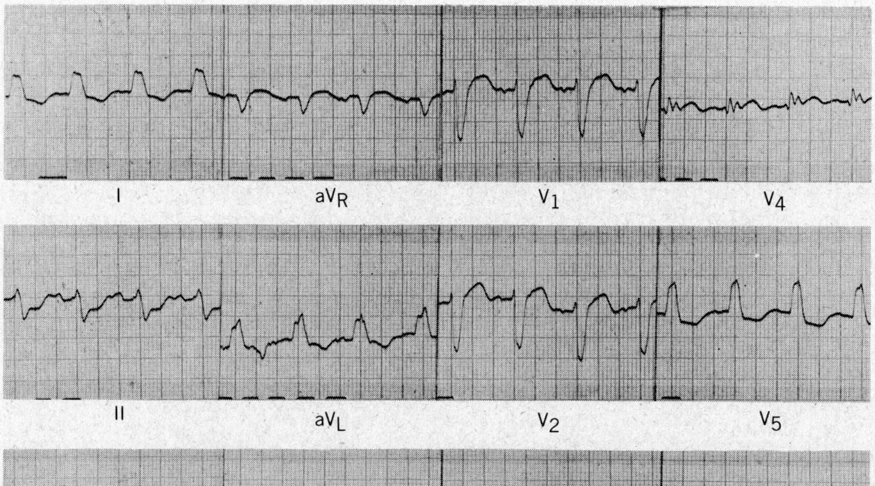

and there were no murmurs, rub, or gallops. The remainder of the findings of physical examination were within normal limits.

Urine, blood urea nitrogen (BUN) value, and electrolytes were normal. Hematocrit value was 33%; hemoglobin value, 10 gm/100 ml; and the leukocyte count, 14,300/cu mm with 86% neutrophils, 8% lymphocytes, 5% monocytes, and 1% eosinophils. The serum alkaline phosphatase level was 2.8 units/100 ml (Bodansky method); serum glutamic oxaloacetic transaminase (SGOT) value, 10 units/ml; and total serum bilirubin, 0.3 mg/100 ml. A chest roentgenogram (Fig 1) showed consolidation of the lingula of the left upper lobe, and an electrocardiogram (Fig 2) showed normal axis, sinus rhythm, and inverted T waves in I, αV_L, V_2, V_3, and V_4. Sputum cytological examination showed class IV cells consistent with epidermoid carcinoma.

General supportive therapy was instituted, and her condition improved gradually until the eighth hospital day when she complained of sudden precordial chest pain and breathing difficulty. She was dyspneic with a pulse rate of 100 beats per minute; blood pressure, 90/60 mm Hg; and temperature, 100 F (37.8 C). There were physical findings consistent with acute biventricular heart failure. An electrocardiogram (Fig 3) revealed left bundle-branch block and a chest roentgenogram showed increase in the left lung consolidation, bilateral pleural effusion, passive vascular congestion, and a mediastinal shift to the right. The next day the

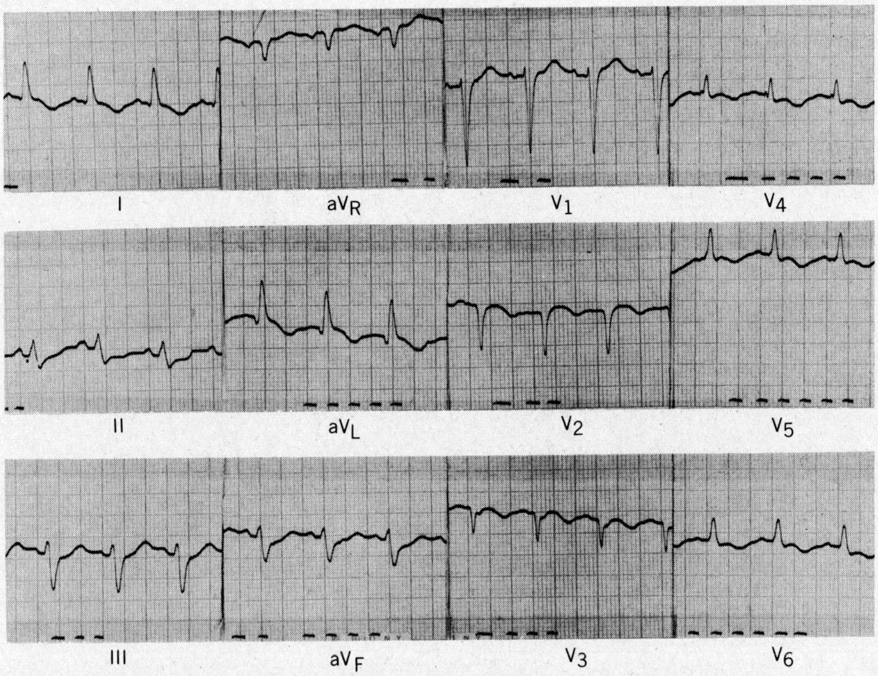

Fig 4.—Electrocardiogram on tenth hospital day which shows Q waves in I, aV_L, V_2, and V_3 consistent with anterolateral myocardial infarction.

Fig 5.—Large pulmonary neoplasm invading the left atrioventricular sulcus and encircling the left coronary artery.

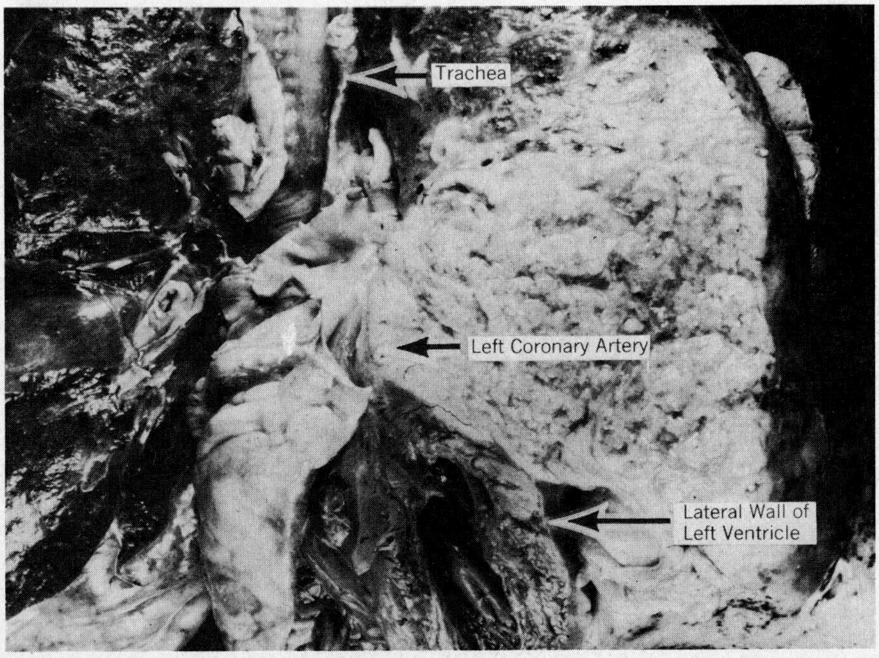

SGOT value was 69 units/ml, and the creatine phosphokinase (CPK) value, 27 mg/100 ml; on the tenth hospital day the lactic dehydrogenase (LDH) value was 1,100 units/ml with a total bilirubin value of 0.5 mg/100 ml. That same day an ECG (Fig 4) showed reversion to normal conduction with Q waves in I, αV_L, V_2, and V_3. On the 13th hospital day, she developed an arrhythmia, which by means of an intraatrial ECG, was interpreted as parasystolic, with an atrioventricular (AV) junctional parasystolic focus at a rate of 80 beats per minute, and a sinus rate of 75 beats per minute. Antiarrhythmic drugs and "overdrive" pacing from the right atrium were unsuccessful in restoring sinus rhythm, and her condition steadily worsened with progressive cardiorespiratory failure and persistent arrhythmia. On the 22nd hospital day she became comatose and died two days later.

Autopsy Report

The heart and lungs together weighed 2,700 gm. Cut sections of the left lung revealed an 8 × 6 × 5 cm tumor mass originating in the left mainstem bronchus and diffusely infiltrating the left upper lobe of the lung, hilum, and adjacent pericardium. There were numerous metastatic nodules scattered throughout both lungs and in the peribronchial and paratracheal lymph nodes.

The heart showed left ventricular hypertrophy and was displaced to the right by the adherent left hilar mass. The anterolateral and posterior walls of the left ventricle showed diffuse grayish pink discoloration and softening. Sections through the left ventricle revealed large areas of softening in a circumferential, transmural distribution. The left atrioventricular sulcus was diffusely infiltrated by tumor which was contiguous with the left hilar mass (Fig 5). The tumor tissue infiltrated the adjacent myocardium, encircling and constricting the origin of the anterior descending left coronary artery and a major portion of the left circumflex coronary artery.

Histologically, the large pulmonary neoplasm showed the typical picture of poorly differentiated squamous carcinoma with areas of focal necrosis. The tumor cells diffusely infiltrated the myocardium of the left ventricle and encircled and compressed the major and minor branches of the left coronary arteries (Fig 6). The lumens were correspondingly narrowed. Several small arterioles were filled with amorphous debris and scattered tumor cells (Fig 7). In addition, the coronary arteries showed a slight degree of atherosclerosis. The myocardium showed massive fresh infarction in the areas corresponding to the changes noted on gross examination.

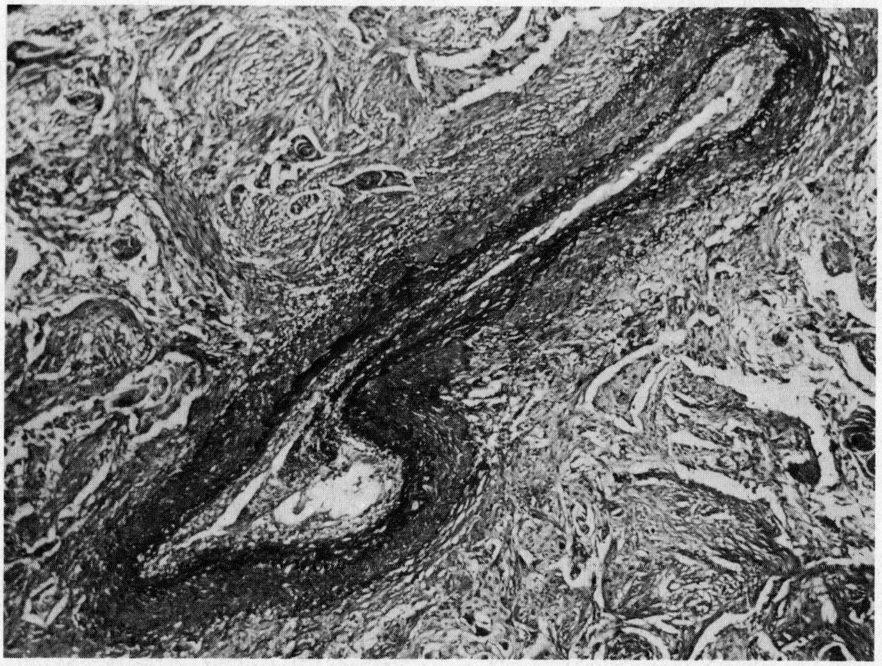

Fig 6.—Medium sized coronary artery showing compression deformity due to extrinsic squamous carcinoma (Verhoeffs elastica stain, ×100).

Comment

Metastatic tumors are much more common than primary neoplasms in the heart. The overall incidence of cardiac involvement in patients dying of cancer is about 5%,[8] with the most common primary lesions being bronchogenic carcinoma, breast carcinoma, malignant melanoma, lymphoma, and leukemia. These tumors reach the heart by hematogenous and lymphatic spread or by direct invasion. The cardiac lesions are diffusely infiltrative or nodular and can involve any part of the heart.

There is no typical symptomatology, but clinical pictures consistent with pericarditis, myocardial disease, and angina are described. Refractory congestive heart failure, conduction disturbances, and uncontrollable arrhythmias are commonly seen. Any of these manifestations in a patient known to have cancer should alert one of the possibility of cardiac metastases.

Fig 7.—Small coronary artery and vein showing occlusion by nests of tumor cells (hematoxylin-eosin stain, ×450).

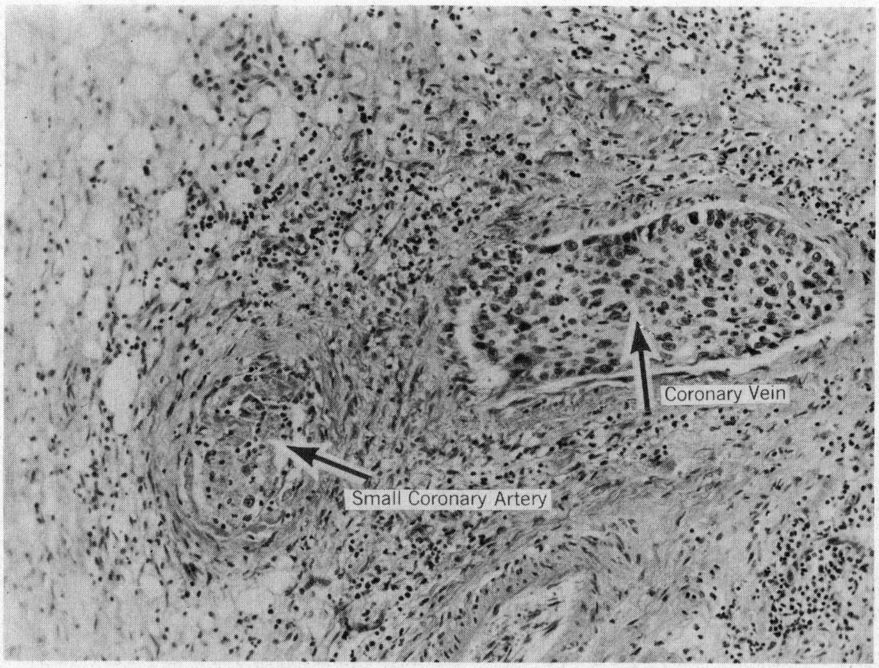

Electrocardiographic patterns are not typical either. Berge and Sievers[9] found 37 abnormal ECGs among 122 cases of metastatic heart disease; arrhythmias, heart block, and S-T, T changes were most commonly observed. Harris et al[10] reported a case with persistent current of injury which did not evolve as a typical myocardial infarct; at autopsy there was myocardial necrosis due to direct tumor invasion without coronary artery involvement.

Very few cases of coronary artery involvement by tumor can be found in the literature. In 1930, Fishberg[11] reported a case of lymphoma which surrounded the left circumflex artery. Frolich et al[12] reported the case of a woman with retroperitoneal fibrosarcoma and cardiac metastases which had surrounded, infiltrated, and occluded a coronary artery; clinically she had had chest pain, arrhythmias, and electrocardiographic changes. Hanfling had a very similar case in his series.

A review of 53 cases of metastatic heart tumors by Javier et al[13] described a 51-year-old man with Hodgkin's disease who suddenly developed atrial fibrillation, syncope, and electrocardiographic evidence of acute diaphragmatic wall damage. Postmortem examination revealed a metastatic nodule occluding the left circumflex artery.

Cancer may produce myocardial infarction without metastatic involvement of the heart. Lisa et al[14] have described a case of bronchogenic carcinoma with multiple miliary type myocardial infarctions due to occlusion of the smaller coronary artery branches by carcinomatous emboli. Cera[15] reported a case of bronchogenic carcinoma with tumor emboli which occluded the left coronary artery and resulted in fatal acute myocardial infarction. Recently, Motte and co-workers[16] reported a case of hypernephroma with secondary polycythemia which resulted in acute coronary thrombosis.

Thus, the case reported here again documents the occurrence of coronary arterial occlusion due to tumor. Our patient presented a clinical picture quite typical of acute myocardial infarction. When this occurs in a patient known to have neoplastic disease, the possibility of tumor involvement of the coronary arteries should be considered, especially in view of the recent advances in surgical treatment of coronary artery disease.

Summary

A 52-year-old woman entered the hospital because of suspected carcinoma of the lung. On the eighth hospital day she had an episode clinically consistent with acute myocardial infarction and died two weeks later. At autopsy she was found to have tumor involving the left coronary artery with resultant myocardial infarction. While recognizing the entity of acute myocardial infarction without demonstrable coronary artery occlusion, it is felt that the lack of significant atherosclerosis in this patient makes it reasonable to assume a direct cause and effect relationship between the cardiac lesions found.

References

1. Keith JD: The anomalous origin of the left coronary artery from the pulmonary artery. *Brit Heart J* **21**:149-161, 1959.

2. Scott DH: Aneurysm of the coronary arteries. *Amer Heart J* **36**:403-421, 1948.

3. Upshaw CB: Congenital coronary arteriovenous fistula: Report of a case with an analysis of 73 reported cases. *Amer Heart J* **63**:399-404, 1962.

4. Hurst JW, Logue RB: *The Heart*. New York, McGraw-Hill Book Co Inc, 1966, pp 733-742.

5. Barnett RN, Zimmerman SL: Coronary arteritis with fatal thrombosis due to salmonella choleraesuis variety Kunzendorf. *Amer Heart J* **34**:441-446, 1947.

6. Traut EF, et al: Specific vascular changes in gout. *JAMA* **156**:591-593, 1954.

7. Saphir O: Thromboangiitis obliterans of the coronary arteries and its relation to arteriosclerosis. *Amer Heart J* **12**:521-535, 1936.

8. Hanfling S: Metastatic cancer to the heart. Review of the literature and report of 127 cases. *Circulation* **22**:474-483, 1960.

9. Berge T, Sievers J: Myocardial metastases: A pathologic and electrocardiographic study. *Brit Heart J* **30**:383-390, 1968.

10. Harris T, Copeland G, Brody D: Progressive injury current with metastatic tumor of the heart. *Amer Heart J* **69**:392-400, 1965.

11. Fishberg A: Auricular fibrillation and flutter in metastatic growths of the right auricle. *Amer J Med Sci* **180**:629-634, 1930.

12. Frolich E, Shnider B, Leonard J: Antemortem diagnosis of metastatic sarcoma to the heart: A case report. *Amer Heart J* **57**:623-629, 1959.

13. Javier B, et al: Cardiac metastases in lymphoma and leukemia. *Dis Chest* **52**:481-484, 1967.

14. Lisa J, et al: Tumors of the heart: Report of four cases and review of the literature. *Arch Intern Med* **67**:91-113, 1941.

15. Cera L, Karlinsky W, Rodin A: Tumor embolism of the left coronary artery. *Amer Heart J* **53**:472-478, 1957.

16. Motte G, et al: Thrombose coronariènne avec troubles due rhythme mortels compliquant une polyglobulie secondaire à un cancer du rein. *Presse Med* **76**:719-722, 1968.

Acute Myelogenous Leukemia Following Localized Radiotherapy

James L. Poth, MD; Ralph P. George, Jr., MD;
William P. Creger, MD; and Stanley L. Schrier, MD, Stanford, Calif

Recent reports have described the occurrence of acute myelogenous leukemia in patients with Hodgkin's disease.[1-3] This occurrence was believed to relate to therapy rather than to a transitional stage in Hodgkin's disease. The development of acute myelogenous leukemia in patients with lymphocytic lymphoma is distinctly unusual,[4] although the termination of reticulum cell sarcoma as acute myeloid leukemia has been reported,[5,6] in which case it usually occurs within 12 months of the diagnosis of reticulum cell sarcoma has generally not been associated with radiotherapy. The incidence of acute myelogenous leukemia in patients with solid tumors is not significantly increased over expected figures, although a higher than expected coincidence has been reported by some observers between chronic lymphocytic leukemia and solid tumors.[7,8]

The increasing use of high dose radiotherapy, particularly in patients with lymphoma, prompts us to report two patients with lymphocytic lymphoma, one patient with laryngeal carcinoma, and one with lymphoepithelioma, in whom acute myelogenous leukemia developed after a temporally remote course of high-dose irradiation.

Received for publication Oct 6, 1970; accepted Dec 15.

From the Division of Hematology, Stanford University School of Medicine, Stanford, Calif.

Reprint requests to Division of Hematology, Stanford University School of Medicine, Stanford, Calif 94304 (Dr. Poth).

Patient Summaries

Patient 1.—The patient was a 43-year-old man who developed bilateral inguinal adenopathy in December 1963. Biopsy showed lymphosarcoma, small cell type. The patient was classified as clinical stage IIa. The complete blood count and bone marrow biopsy findings were normal. From Dec 26, 1963, to Jan 24, 1964, the patient received 4,000 rads tumor dose to periaortic, bilateral iliac, and inguinal nodes. His adenopathy regressed, and he returned to work. Excepting one episode of diarrhea believed to be related to radiation-induced enterocolitis, he was entirely asymptomatic.

In September 1969 inguinal adenopathy reappeared and adenopathy was also noted in the left cervical and supraclavicular regions, the right axilla, and the left iliac fossa. Biopsy of a left supraclavicular node showed replacement of nodal architecture with primitive myeloid cells. Bone marrow aspirate showed nearly complete replacement with primitive cells which demonstrated some differentiation toward bizarre promyelocytes on the one hand and bizarre megaloblasts on the other. The hematocrit value was 46%; white blood cell count (WBC), 7,800/cu mm with 70% polymorphonuclear cells (PMNs), 23% lymphocytes, 1% monocytes, 2% eosinophils, 1% myelocytes, and 3% blast forms. The platelet count was

90,000/cu mm.

During the next month adenopathy progressed rapidly. The WBC in October 1969 was 13,600/cu mm with 20% myeloblasts. The hematocrit value was 27% and the platelet count, 12,000/cu mm. The patient had a partial remission after administration of 180 mg of daunomycin. He was maintained on a regimen of mercaptopurine and methotrexate but relapsed after 56 days. Therapy with cytarabine (cytosine arabinoside) and thioguanine was begun; however, the patient succumbed to overwhelming staphylococcal sepsis.

At postmortem examination there was no evidence of lymphoma, but leukemic infiltration of the bone marrow and spleen was found along with staphylococcal bronchopneumonia.

Patient 2.—The patient was a 48-year-old man who had been in good health until December 1966. At that time a laryngeal biopsy revealed well differentiated, papillary, squamous cell carcinoma of the larynx with involvement of the left true and false cords and the posterior aspect of the epiglottis. Subsequently, a left hemilaryngectomy was performed. No local metastases were present. Following surgery, he received radiotherapy with 7,000 rads tumor dose to the larynx from Jan 3, 1967, to Feb 18, 1967. Upon completion of radiotherapy, he felt entirely well and returned to work. In October 1969 he developed fever, chills, night sweats, and gingival bleeding.

Physical examination showed an acutely ill man with temperature of 102.2 F (39 C), conjunctival hemorrhages, and several areas of ecchymosis in the skin. The hematocrit value was 28%; WBC, 600/cu mm with 32% PMN's, 58% lymphocytes, and 10% myeloblasts; platelet count, 10,000/cu mm; and the reticulocyte count, 1.1%. Bone marrow aspirate showed acute myelogenous leukemia. The patient was treated with 600 mg of daunomycin, but died from fulminant sepsis during the period of drug-induced bone marrow hypoplasia.

At postmortem examination there was no evidence of the original laryngeal carcinoma or of leukemic infiltrate. The bone marrow was hypoplastic to a degree consistent with recent chemotherapy. Numerous yeast colonies *(Candida albicans)* were found throughout the renal and pulmonary parenchyma and the upper gastrointestinal tract.

Patient 3.—The patient was a 66-year-old white man who in 1964 was found to have a lymphoepithelioma involving the base of the tongue with extension to the left lateral pharyngeal wall and epiglottis. No adenopathy was noted. From June 23, 1964, to Aug 7, 1964, he received 6,150 rads tumor dose to opposing lateral face fields and 5,950 rads to anterior-posterior tangential neck fields. Eighteen hundred milligrams of methotrexate were delivered via bilateral carotid artery perfusion from June 22, 1964, to July 30, 1964. Complete blood cell counts were normal prior to therapy. The patient did well until Aug 29, 1969, at which time he developed grossly bloody diarrhea, accompanied by chills and fever. Significant physical findings included palatal and lower extremity petechiae; a spleen palpable 4 cm below the left costal margin; hepatomegaly with an overall breadth of 16 cm; cervical, axillary, and inguinal adenopathy with an average node diameter of 3 cm; and grossly bloody stool on rectal examination. The WBC was 99,000/cu mm with 11% PMNs and 81% myeloblasts; hematocrit value, 24%; and platelet count, 40,000/cu mm. Bone marrow examination disclosed acute myelogenous leukemia. Liver function studies and coagulation measurements were within normal limits. X-ray examination of the upper gastrointestinal tract revealed submucosal infiltrate involving the distal jejunum and ileum; no gastric or duodenal pathology was demonstrated. Sigmoidoscopy revealed no bleeding site.

The patient continued to bleed massively per rectum and, despite blood and platelet transfusion, died 36 hours after admission.

Postmortem examination revealed only fibrous tissue at the site of his original tumor. Generalized organ infiltration with early myeloid cells was present. The jejunum, ileum, and cecum demonstrated dense leukemic infiltration with overlying mucosal necrosis and hemorrhage.

Patient 4.—The patient was a 53-year-old white man who from July 20, 1959, to Sept 1, 1959, received 2,900 rads tumor dose to bilateral inguinal and iliac areas after biopsy of a right inguinal node yielded a diagnosis of lymphosarcoma (Fig 1). From May 20, 1960, to June 3, 1960, an additional 2,400 rads tumor dose was administered to the left supraclavicular area for recurrent disease. The patient did well until 1966 when systemic symptoms accompanied by hepatosplenomegaly prompted treatment with vincristine sulfate and chlorambucil. Further radiotherapy included 2,500 rads tumor dose to a 4 × 4 cm lesion at the base of the tongue which was administered from Jan 10, 1967, to Feb 24, 1967. At the completion of the third course of radiotherapy, the WBC was 2,350/cu mm with 56% PMNs, 40% lymphocytes, and 4% eosinophils. He did well on chlorambucil therapy, 4 mg per day, until June 1969 when systemic symptoms and left upper abdominal quadrant pain occurred. He received 2,687 rads tumor dose to the left upper retroperitoneal area and an additional 1,800 rads to the entire retroperitoneal area between June 9, 1969, and Oct 15, 1969. Symptomatic relief was obtained, but in November 1969 epistaxis and gingival bleeding developed for which he was admitted to Stanford University Hospital for the first time on Dec 13, 1969.

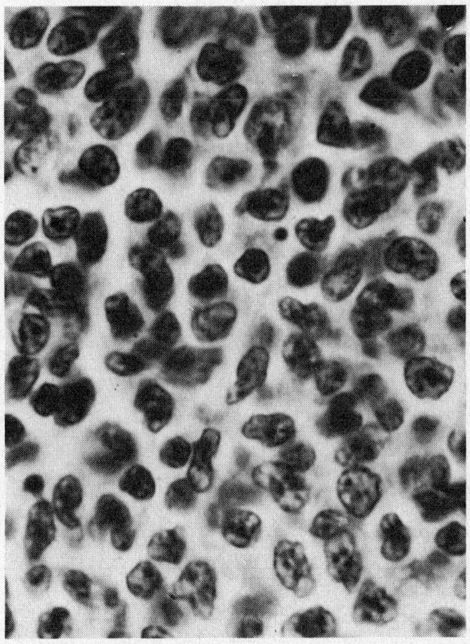

Fig 1.—Patient 4: Right inguinal node biopsy demonstrating poorly differentiated lymphocytic lymphoma (hematoxylin-eosin stain, ×800).

Significant physical findings on admission included a spleen palpable 6 cm below the left costal margin, absence of adenopathy or hepatomegaly, petechiae over the lower extremities, and oozing of blood from the gums. Laboratory data included the following: WBC, 1,000/cu mm with 50% PMNs (many bilobed), 44% lympho-

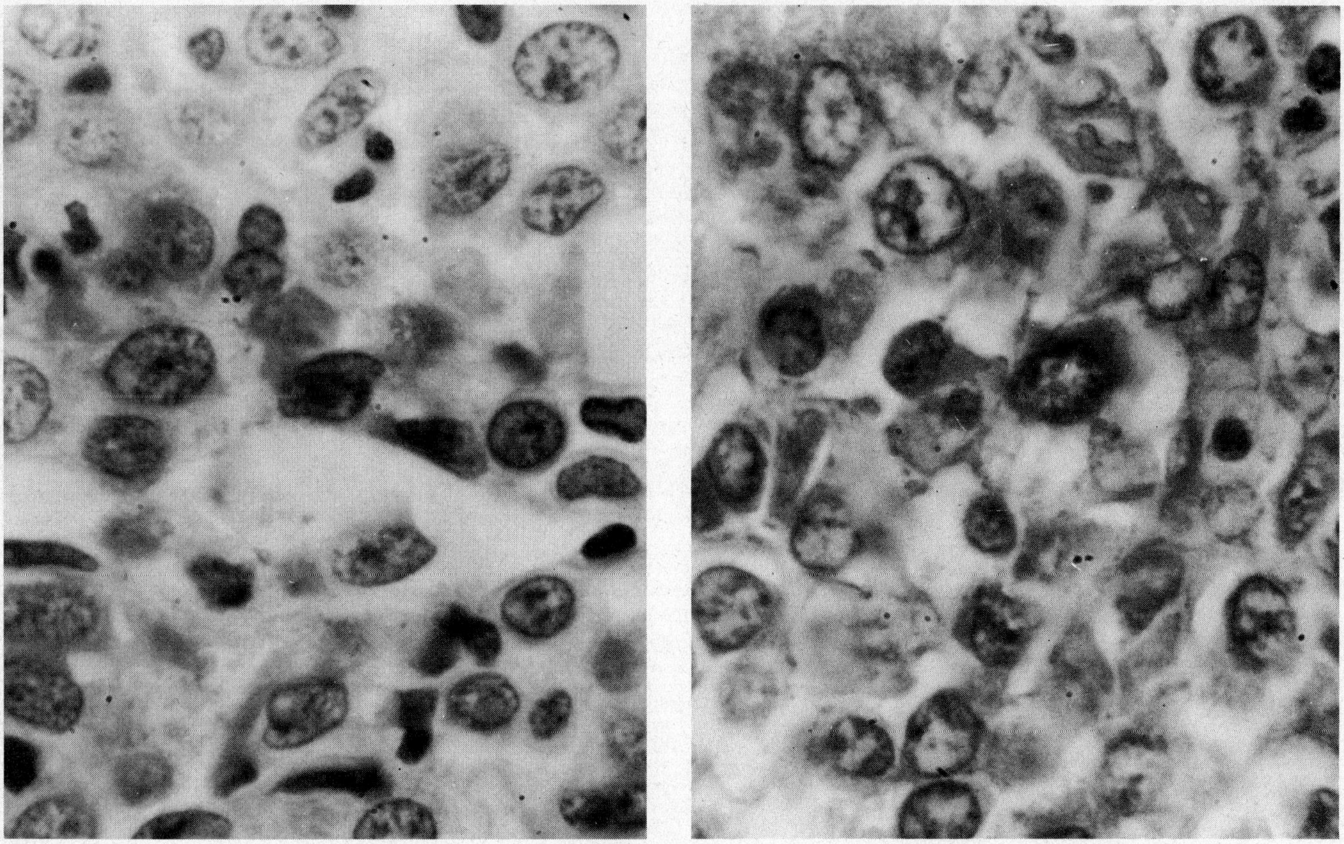

Fig 2.—Patient 4: Representative areas from bone marrow biopsy (left) *and spleen* (right) *which show infiltration with primitive myeloid cells (hematoxylin-eosin stain, ×800).*

cytes, 6% primitive blast cells, and rare nucleated red blood cells; platelet count, 12,000/cu mm; hematocrit value, 29.5%; and reticulocyte count, 0%. Liver function test results and coagulation measurements were normal. Bone marrow biopsy demonstrated infiltration with early myeloid cells; megakaryocytes and red blood cell precursors were distinctly reduced (Fig 2, *left*).

Splenectomy was performed on Dec 18, 1969, in an attempt to alleviate uncontrollable thrombocytopenic bleeding. At surgery, there was no evidence of retroperitoneal lymphoma. The spleen weighed 880 gm; microscopic sections revealed infiltration with primitive myeloid cells (Fig 2, *right*), some of which were esterase positive. Following splenectomy the patient achieved transient improvement in platelet count but within three weeks required intermittent platelet transfusion for protracted gingival bleeding, and he died Feb 3, 1970, from a presumed central nervous system hemorrhage. Postmortem examination was not performed.

Comment

In each of the four patients described herein, acute myelogenous leukemia developed 32 months to ten years following a minimum of 2,900 rads localized radiotherapy. This time lapse corresponds to the reported appearance time of radiation-induced leukemia which has ranged from 3 to 15 years following exposure.[9-11] In the three of our patients who were autopsied, no trace of the primary tumor was found.

The overall annual prevalence of acute myelogenous leukemia in the general population has been estimated at 1.5 per 100,000.[12] Between 1960 and 1965, approximately 7,200 patients were treated at this institution with 3,000 or more rads to single, as well as multiple, fields. Thus far, two instances of acute myeloid leukemia have developed in this group (patients 2 and 4 were treated elsewhere). The significance of the incidence of leukemia in this group of irradiated patients is open to question. The numbers are small and the two cases of leukemia could obviously be coincidental. Alternatively, our cases could reflect an underlying oncogenic predisposition in the leukemic patients. This situation was suggested by Carey et al[13] who reported four women with acute myelocytic leukemia developing within 1 to 11 months following diagnosis of carcinoma of the breast. No radiotherapy was involved. The coincidence of the two entities was 30 times more frequent than would have been expected on the basis of individual occurrence rates applicable to the general population. Recently, acute myelomonocytic leukemia following prolonged melphalan therapy for multiple myeloma was reported.[14] None of our patients received melphalan and only one (patient 4) received alkylator therapy.

Finally our data could indicate a real relationship between prior radiotherapy and the subsequent development of myeloid leukemia. Evidence for the association of leukemia with limited, as well as generalized, irradiation is available. Court-Brown[15] noted a 4 per 1,000 incidence of leukemia, predominately myeloid, in 14,554 patients treated with irradiation to the spine and pelvis for ankylosing spondylitis. Doll[16] reported five myeloid leukemic deaths (three acute and two chronic) in 2,068 patients who, in the course of ovarian irradiation for induction of menopause, received an average of 136 rads to the pelvic marrow. Contrary data are provided by Hutchison,[17] however, who was unable to find an increased incidence of myeloid leukemia in over 20,000 patients followed for a total of 60,000 patient-years after irradiation for cervical cancer. However, the mean interval follow-up of three years in that study is short in comparison to the 3 to 15 year appearance time of radiation-induced leukemia.[9-11] The increased incidence of leukemia following generalized irradiation has been most vividly seen in atomic blast survivors[9,10] and in patients with polycythemia vera treated with x-ray, radioactive phosphorus (^{32}P), or both.[11]

These four cases, added to the recent reports of radiation-associated leukemia in Hodgkin's disease, suggest that an increased frequency of leukemia may be found in patients given high-dose radiation for various neoplasms. The ultimate possible risk of future leukemia will probably be an acceptable one for the complete control of a potentially fatal malignancy. However, interim follow-up of all irradiated patients is crucial in determining the approximate leukemogenic risk of this form of therapy.

Summary

Four patients developed acute myelogenous leukemia 32 months to ten years following a minimum of 2,900 rads localized radiotherapy for neoplastic disease. The underlying malignancies comprised two cases of lymphocytic lymphoma and single cases of lymphoepithelioma and laryngeal squamous cell carcinoma. In three of the patients no evidence of the original tumor was found at postmortem examination.

This investigation was supported in part by Public Health Service training grant T1-AM5239.

Ronald F. Dorfman, MD, interpreted the biopsy material from two patients.

Nonproprietary and Trade Names of Drug

Melphalan—*Alkeran*.

References

1. Ezdinli EZ, Sokal JE, Aungst CW, et al: Myeloid leukemia in Hodgkin's disease. *Ann Intern Med* **71**:1097-1104, 1969.
2. Newman DR, Maldonado JE, Harrison EG, et al: Myelomonocytic leukemia in Hodgkin's disease. *Cancer* **25**:128-134, 1970.
3. Steinberg, MG, Geary CG, Crosby WH: Acute granulocytic leukemia complicating Hodgkin's disease. *Arch Intern Med* **125**:496-498, 1970.
4. Rosenberg SA, Diamond HD, Jaslowitz B, et al: Lymphosarcoma: A review of 1,296 cases. *Medicine* **40**:31-84, 1961.
5. Laszlo J, Grode HE: Granulocytic leukemia and reticulum cell sarcoma. *Cancer* **20**:545-551, 1967.
6. Zeffren JL, Ultmann JE: Reticulum cell sarcoma terminating in acute leukemia. *Blood* **15**:277-284, 1960.
7. Bousser J, Mathé G: Association du cancer épithélial et de lymphomatose (leucosique ou non). *Sem Hôp Paris* **30**:821-837, 1954.
8. Gunz F, Angus HB: Leukemia and cancer in the same patient. *Cancer* **18**:145-152, 1965.
9. Bizzozero OJ Jr, Johnson KG, Ciocco A: Radiation-related leukemia in Hiroshima and Nagasaki, 1946-1964: I. Distribution, incidence and appearance time. *New Eng J Med* **274**:1095-1101, 1966.
10. Bizzozero OJ Jr, Johnson KG, Ciocco A, et al: Radiation-related leukemia in Hiroshima and Nagasaki, 1946-1964: II. Observations on type specific leukemia survivorship and clinical behavior. *Ann Intern Med* **66**:522-530, 1967.
11. Modan B, Lilienfeld AM: Polycythemia vera and leukemia—The role of radiation treatment: A study of 1,222 patients. *Medicine* **44**:305-344, 1965.
12. Crosby WH: Acute granulocytic leukemia: A complication of therapy in Hodgkin's disease, abstracted. *Clin Res* **17**:463, 1969.
13. Carey RW, Holland JF, Sheebe PR, et al: Association of cancer of the breast and acute myelocytic leukemia. *Cancer* **20**:1080-1088, 1967.
14. Kyle RA, Pierre RV, Bayrd ED: Multiple myeloma and acute myelomonocytic leukemia. *New Eng J Med* **283**:1121-1125, 1970.
15. Court-Brown WM, Doll R: Mortality from cancer and other causes after radiotherapy for ankylosing spondylisis. *Brit Med J* **2**:1327-1332, 1965.
16. Doll R, Smith PG: The long-term effects of irradiation in patients treated for metropathia haemorrhagica. *Brit J Radiol* **41**:362-368, 1968.
17. Hutchison GB: Leukemia in patients with cancer of the cervix uteri treated with radiation: A report covering the first five years of an international study. *J Nat Cancer Inst* **40**:951-982, 1968.

Cardiac Syncope Due to Glossopharyngeal Neuralgia

Treatment With a Transvenous Pacemaker

Basheer A. Khero, MD, and Charles B. Mullins, MD, Dallas

Glossopharyngeal neuralgia associated with bradycardia and syncope is a rare syndrome. The pain is paroxysmal and intense, felt in the ear, throat, posterior part of the tongue, soft palate, and lower lateral and posterior parts of the pharynx. The pain is accompanied by bradycardia or asystole and, at times, syncope with associated convulsions.[1-5]

This report describes the clinical picture and hospital course of a patient with this syndrome whose syncopal attacks were prevented by a cardiac pacemaker. A 14-day trial of diphenylhydantoin (Dilantin) was used in an attempt to control the paroxysms of pain but was unsuccessful, necessitating surgical resection of the glossopharyngeal nerve.

Patient Summary

A 46-year-old woman was admitted to Parkland Memorial Hospital for the first time in February 1969. She had been seen as an outpatient at another hospital seven years previously when she complained of paroxysms of severe pain below the right ear radiating down to the neck and up into the face, lasting no more than a minute. A diagnosis was not made and the symptoms disappeared spontaneously within a few days.

She remained symptom free for a year. The pain then began to recur at irregular intervals, lasting for one to two weeks with remissions varying from four to six months. Three years after the onset of her pain symptoms, her tonsils and upper right teeth were removed because of chronic infection which was thought to be the cause of the pain, but no relief of her paroxysms of pain was noted.

In January 1969 the patient developed severe pain which was precipitated by swallowing of either solid or liquid foods, especially cold liquids. The symptoms became progressively more severe and in the 15 days prior to admission, paroxysms of pain appeared six to eight times a day, lasting one to two minutes. For the first time, the paroxysms of pain were associated with an occasional loss of consciousness, but no convulsions occurred. The syncopal attacks occurred several times, always following severe episodes of pain, and were unassociated with other neurological manifestations.

While in the emergency room waiting to be examined, the patient had an attack of pain which resulted in loss of consciousness. An electrocardiogram recorded sinus arrest and sinus bradycardia (Fig 1, *top*). She was given atropine 0.4 mg intravenously and responded with a sinus rate of 100 beats per minute. Massage of the carotid sinus did not cause bradycardia, but when pain was produced by touching the right tonsillar fossa, sinus bradycardia developed. A diagnosis of glossopharyngeal neuralgia was made.

Other findings of physical examination were within normal limits. The white blood cell count, and levels of fasting blood glucose, blood urea nitrogen, and serum electrolytes, were normal; findings of serologic study and urinalysis were normal.

A temporary transvenous demand pacemaker was inserted via the subclavian vein percutaneously to the right ventricular apex for use as a standby pacemaker in the event of paroxysms of pain and bradycardia. She was placed on a continuous cardiac monitor and started on diphenylhydantoin 100 mg three times daily. During this period, the patient continued to have spontaneous attacks of neuralgia associated with bradycardia, but syncopal attacks were prevented by demand pacing (Fig 1, *bottom*). After two weeks of ineffective medical therapy with dosage of diphenylhydantoin up to 500 mg daily, right occipital craniotomy and resection of the right glossopharyngeal nerve were performed without complications. She has had no further attacks following the resection and has remained symptom free for 12 months without medication.

Comment

Glossopharyngeal neuralgia is uncommon, compared to trigeminal neuralgia. The condition was first described by Weisenburg[6] in 1910 in a patient with a tumor of the cerebel-

Received for publication Oct 22, 1970; accepted Jan 13, 1971.

From the Pauline and Adolph Weinberger Laboratory for Cardiopulmonary Research, Department of Internal Medicine, University of Texas (Southwestern) Medical School at Dallas; and Parkland Memorial Hospital, Dallas.

Reprint requests to Cardiopulmonary-D-710, 5323 Harry Hines Blvd, Dallas 75235 (Dr. Mullins).

lopontine angle, whereas Harris[7] was the first to describe it in a patient with no underlying pathology. Riley and associates in 1942[1] were the first to report cardiac arrest associated with the neuralgia. Subsequently, several cases of this syndrome have been reported.

Although in most cases glossopharyngeal neuralgia occurs as an isolated condition, it may be associated with trigeminal neuralgia, vagal neuralgia,[8] cardiac arrhythmias, syncope, and seizures,[1-5] hypersection from the parotid gland on the affected side,[3] and convulsions and unconsciousness in the presence of a normal heart rate and blood pressure.[2]

In most of the cases the cause of the neuralgia is unknown. Occasionally, cerebellopontine tumors[4] or an elongated styloid process and calcified stylohyoid ligament[9] may be the etiological factor. It has been suggested that the abnormally long styloid process or calcified stylohyoid ligament may cause chronic compression of nerves during swallowing, and Graf[9] reported cases which were benefited by surgical extirpation of the anomalous process.

Paroxysms of pain are precipitated by mechanical touch or swallowing of foods, particularly cold, salty, bitter, or acid.[3-5,10] The most common trigger zone is the tonsillar fossa on the affected side. In the present case, as in other reported cases,[2-5] bradycardia, hypotension, and syncope followed severe paroxysms of pain, while massage of the carotid sinuses did not reproduce the symptoms. Sinus arrest, sinus bradycardia, and wandering atrial pacemaker are the most common arrhythmias reported in the syndrome. The cause of the arrhythmias is not completely understood, but it is likely that vagal reflexes initiated by the pain are involved.

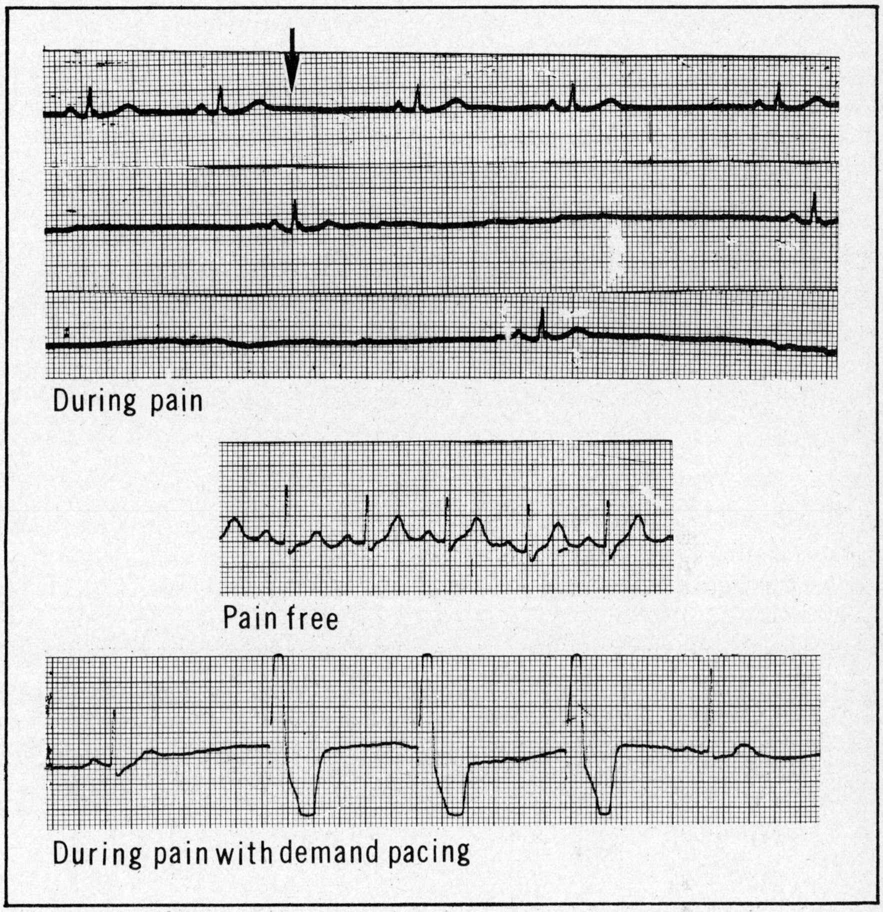

Patient's electrocardiogram. Top, *Taken during an attack of pain showing sinus bradycardia and sinus arrest;* center, *when free of pain;* bottom, *during pain after insertion of a pacemaker. Arrow* (top) *indicates time of onset of pain.*

The intimate relationship of the ninth and tenth cranial nerves, particularly in reference to sensory function, has been implicated as a possible reason for reflex arrhythmias in association with the neuralgia.[10] Sensory fibers arise from cells in the superior and inferior ganglia of the glossopharyngeal nerve. Those from the cells of superior ganglion mediate sensation of touch, pain, and heat from the posterior third of the tongue, posterior pharynx, and posterior part of the mouth. The fibers from the inferior ganglion supply the taste buds of the posterior third of the tongue. The central fibers from the superior ganglion terminate in the solitary tract, and its nucleus in the medulla oblongata which communicates with the dorsal nucleus of the vagus through collateral fibers. The dorsal nucleus of the vagus is the principal autonomic nucleus supplying parasympathetic fibers to the heart, bronchi, and abdominal viscera. The carotid sinus nerve is another important afferent branch of the glossopharyngeal nerve; it conducts impulses from the carotid body and carotid sinus to the medulla oblongata, and plays a role in the regulation of the heart rate, respiratory rate, and blood pressure. It has been suggested that intense impulses arriving from the irritative lesion in the peripheral course of the glossopharyngeal nerve may reach the solitary tract and then be relayed to the dorsal nucleus of the vagus through collaterals; or, less likely, there may be functional spillover of the impulses into the carotid sinus nerve as it travels with the glossopharyngeal nerve.[3-5]

The treatment of glossopharyngeal neuralgia is directed toward control of pain and abolition of the reflex bradycardia and syncope. Atropine sulfate and isoproterenol (Isuprel) hydrochloride are used as temporary emergency measures to abolish the bradycardia, but have no effect on the pain and cannot be used for long-term therapy. Spraying of the pharyngeal and oral mucosa with local anesthetics or nerve block are of temporary benefit.[5] Anticonvulsant therapy has been suggested as a treatment of trigeminal neuralgia and results have sometimes been satisfactory. Diphenylhydantoin has been advocated since, in addition to its central action, it also stabilizes the peripheral nerve fibers against hyperexcitability. The effect of the drug is noted after 24 hours of administration orally, but intravenous use offers a more rapid method of obtaining relief from pain.[11] However, the response of glossopharyngeal neuralgia to diphenylhydantoin has been variable.[3,7,11,12] In the present case, diphenylhydantoin was ineffective with doses up to 500 mg per day despite plasma levels of 0.9 mg/100 ml, which are within advocated therapeutic levels. Kong and associates[5] suggest that blood levels of 1 mg/100 ml of diphenylhydantoin are the best therapeutic levels and that level can be reached with daily doses of 5 to 6 mg/kg of body weight.

This is the first report of the use of a temporary pacemaker to prevent the sinus bradycardia and syncope associated with trigeminal neuralgia. The advantage of a standby temporary demand pacemaker during the institution of drug therapy is that it can maintain a reasonable heart rate at any moment when bradycardia ensues due to paroxysms of pain. The side effects and delay in administration of atropine and isoproterenol as short-term treatment are avoided.

Surgical resection of the glossopharyngeal nerve is the most effective permanent form of treatment. There are no recurrences, particularly when the upper two rootlets of the vagus nerve are also sectioned.[3,4,8,10] The only postoperative complication may be mild sensory depression of the areas supplied by afferent fibers,[3,4,8] a problem that did not occur in our case. Until definitive treatment with nerve resection can be accomplished, life-threatening attacks of cardiac syncope can be prevented by the use of a temporary transvenous cardiac demand pacemaker.

Summary

Glossopharyngeal neuralgia manifested by paroxysms of pain in the right ear, neck, jaw, and tonsillar area associated with episodes of sinus arrest and bradycardia resulted in syncope in a 48-year-old woman. A temporary transvenous cardiac demand pacemaker was used to prevent the syncopal attacks during an unsuccessful trial of diphenylhydantoin therapy. Surgical resection of the glossopharyngeal nerve was accomplished without complications and with a complete remission of symptoms.

This study was supported in part by Public Health Service grant HE-06296 to Dr. Khero. Dr. Mullins is a Teaching Scholar of the American Heart Association.

References

1. Riley HA, German WJ, Wortis H, et al: Glossopharyngeal neuralgia initiating or associated with cardiac arrest. *Trans Amer Neurol Assoc* **68**:28-29, 1942.
2. Thomson JL: Glossopharyngeal neuralgia accompanied by unconsciousness. *J Neurosurg* **11**:511-513, 1954.
3. Kjellin K, Müller R, Widén L: Glossopharyngeal neuralgia associated with cardiac arrest and hypersecretion from the ipsilateral parotid gland. *Neurology* **9**:527-531, 1959.
4. Garretson HD, Elvidge AR: Glossopharyngeal neuralgia with asystole and seizure. *Arch Neurol* **8**:26-31, 1963.
5. Kong Y, Heyman A, Entman ML, et al: Glossopharyngeal neuralgia associated with bradycardia, syncope, and seizures. *Circulation* **30**:109-113, 1964.
6. Weisenburg TH: Cerebello-pontile tumor diagnosed for six years as tic douloreux: The symptoms of irritation of the ninth and twelfth cranial nerves. *JAMA* **54**:1600-1604, 1910.
7. Harris W: Persistent pain in lesions of the peripheral and central nervous system. *Brit Med J* **2**:896-900, 1921.
8. Chawla JC, Falconer MA; Glossopharyngeal and vagal neuralgia. *Brit Med J* **2**:529-531, 1967.
9. Graf CJ: Glossopharyngeal neuralgia and ossification of the stylohyoid ligament. *J Neurosurg* **16**:448-453, 1959.
10. Karnosh LJ, Gardner WJ, Stowell A: Glossopharyngeal neuralgia: Physiologic considerations of role of the ninth and tenth cranial nerves: Report of cases. *Trans Amer Neurol Assoc* **72**:205-207, 1947.
11. Iannone A, Baker AB, Morrell F: Dilantin in the treatment of trigeminal neuralgia. *Neurology* **8**:126-128, 1958.
12. Kersley JA: A case of glossopharyngeal neuralgia. *J Laryng* **79**:734-737, 1965.

Calcium Free Peritoneal Dialysis

Treatment of Vitamin D Intoxication

Karl D. Nolph, MD; Michael Stoltz, MD; and John F. Maher, MD, Columbia, Mo

Peritoneal dialysis with calcium free dialysis solution has been reported to lower effectively total serum calcium concentration in hypercalcemic patients.[1,2] Lack of availability of calcium free solutions most likely explains infrequent reports of use of this form of therapy in spite of frequent need to treat hypercalcemia in the presence of impaired renal function and in spite of the relative safety and technical simplicity of the procedure.

Commercially available dialysis solutions contain ionized calcium concentrations higher than those in normal serum and do not provide a maximum concentration gradient for diffusion of calcium from peritoneal capillary blood. In fact, calcium absorption usually occurs from such solutions during dialysis in patients with chronic renal disease and low serum calcium concentrations.[3]

This study describes a patient with vitamin D intoxication and severely impaired renal function who underwent repeated peritoneal dialyses with calcium free peritoneal dialysis solutions. Changes in serum total and ionized calcium per total amount of calcium removed, total and ionized peritoneal calcium clearances relative to the clearances of other solutes, and analyses of factors affecting calcium removal rate during calcium free peritoneal dialyses are reported for the first time.

Received for publication Dec 18, 1970; accepted March 25, 1971.

From the Department of Medicine, Division of Nephrology, University of Missouri Medical Center, Columbia.

Reprint requests to Department of Medicine, Division of Nephrology, University of Missouri Medical Center, Columbia, Mo 65201 (Dr. Nolph).

Patient Summary

A 38-year-old white woman was admitted for the eighth time in two years to the University of Missouri Medical Center, Columbia, on April 29, 1970, because of chest pain, diffuse pruritus, nausea and vomiting, dyspnea, dysuria, and increasing weakness during the previous week. She had been a well controlled insulin-dependent diabetic for eight years until July 1968 when she first entered this hospital complaining of decreased vision in the left eye. Examination at that time revealed severe diabetic retinopathy, hematuria, proteinuria, blood urea nitrogen level of 40 mg/100 ml and a creatinine clearance of 18.2 ml/min. Her subsequent six hospitalizations were related to problems of decreasing renal function, hypertension, congestive heart-failure, and severe retinopathy.

Sixteen weeks before her eighth admission, the patient had been admitted with symptoms attributed to congestive heart-failure. Creatinine clearance was 5 to 6.5 ml/min, serum calcium value was repeatedly between 6 and 7 mg/100 ml and inorganic phosphorus level was 7.7 mg/100 ml. Daily protein excretion was 4.6 gm and serum albumin value was 1.9 gm/100 ml with a total protein level of 6.1 gm/100 ml. Discharge medications included ergocalciferol (vitamin D_2), 500,000 units daily, and aluminum hydroxide gel, 15 ml three times daily. During the next 5 weeks, the serum calcium level increased to 10 mg/100 ml as shown in Fig 1 and the ergocalciferol dosage was reduced to 300,000 units/day. During a routine visit to the ophthalmology clinic, slit-lamp examination showed no evidence of calcium deposition in the cornea. By ten weeks from the start of ergocalciferol therapy, the serum calcium level had increased to 11.8 mg/100 ml. After 12 weeks on ergocalciferol therapy, the serum calcium value was 8.1 mg/100 ml; ergocalciferol dosage of 500,000 units/day was reinstituted. By the 16th week, the serum calcium value had increased to 12.2 mg/100 ml and the patient presented with the symptoms described. On physical examination, blood pressure was 200/100 mm Hg; temperature 101.8 F (38.8 C); pulse rate, 100 beats per minute; and respirations, 26 per minute and labored. Her skin was covered with numerous factitial infected wounds. Fundoscopic examination revealed hemorrhages, exudates, microaneurysms, A-V nicking, and arteriolar narrowing. In addition to findings of congestive heart-failure, a loud pericardial friction rub was present. Bilateral costovertebral angle tenderness was noted. Peripheral pulses in the lower extremities

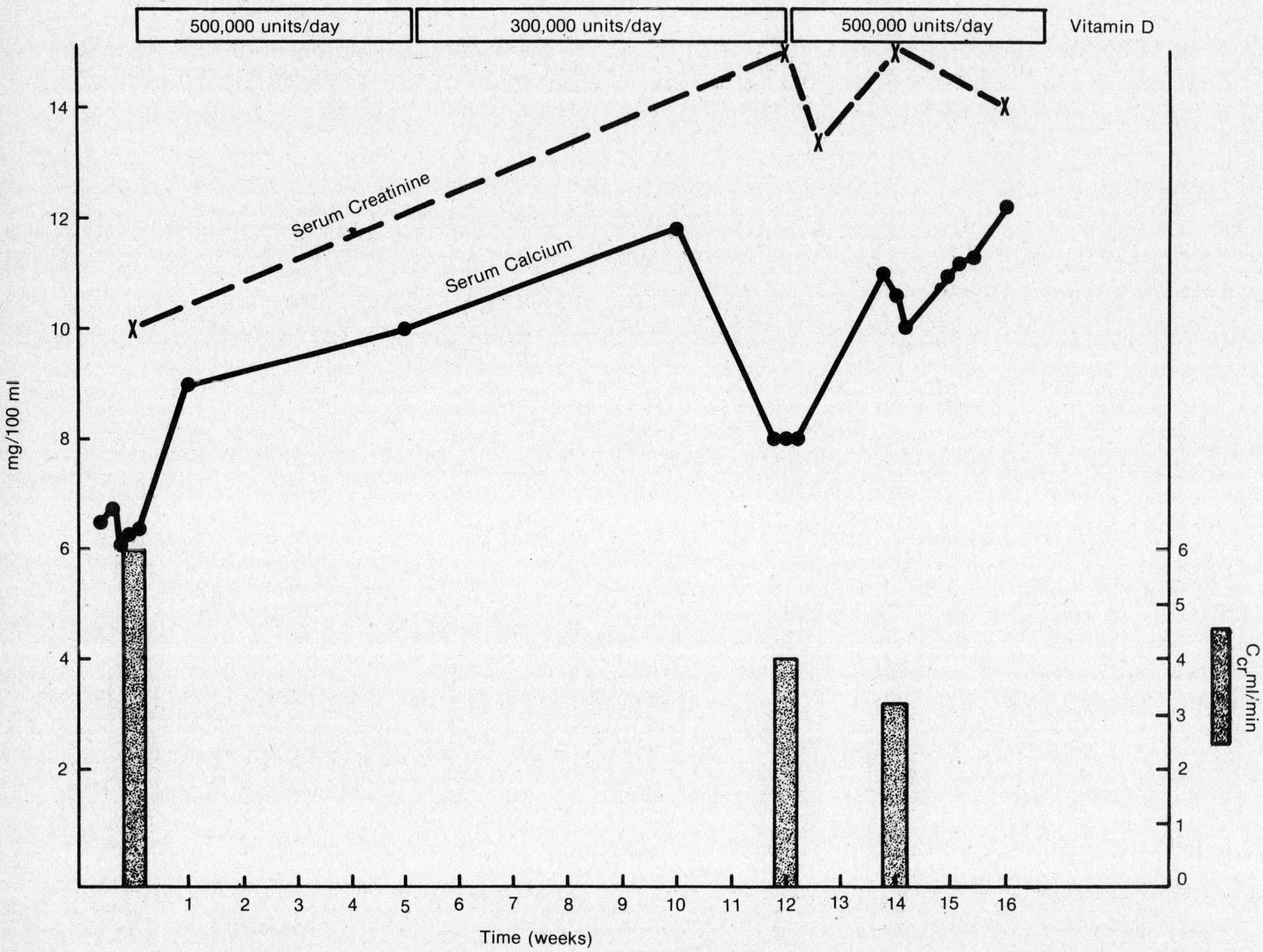

Fig 1.—Serum concentrations of total calcium and creatinine levels (vertical axis, left) *and creatinine clearance* (vertical axis, right) *are related to time* (horizontal axis) *during four-month period preceding dialysis.*

were diminished. The patient was obtunded and weak. Urinalysis showed an albumin value of 300 mg/100 ml, trace of glucose, 7 to 8 red blood cells per high powered field, numerous white blood cells, and hyaline and coarse granular casts. Hematocrit reading was 18% and white blood cell count was 19,000/cu mm. Serum electrolyte values were sodium, 135 mEq/liter; potassium, 7.3 mEq/liter; chloride, 95 mEq/liter; bicarbonate, 14 mEq/liter. Serum creatinine was 15.6 mg/100 ml. Serum calcium values ranged from 11.2 to 12.3 mg/100 ml. Other pertinent serum chemical values were serum inorganic phosphorus, 10.3 mg/100 ml; serum urea nitrogen (SUN), 165 mg/100 ml; and fasting serum glucose, 109 mg/100 ml. Serum albumin values ranged from 2.2 to 2.6 gm/100 ml and total serum protein levels were 5.9 to 6.5 gm/100 ml. Culture of the nasopharynx showed a heavy growth of *Diplococcus pneumoniae*. Slit-lamp examination now demonstrated deposits in the limbic area of the cornea and x-ray films of the hands disclosed calcifications of radial and ulnar arteries. Serum alkaline phosphatase value was normal. Blood cultures and urine repeatedly showed no bacterial growth. Therapy included insulin injection, digoxin, antibiotics, diuretics, aluminum hydroxide gel, packed blood cell transfusions, and other supportive measures. Creatinine clearance ranged from 3 to 4 ml/min. Since multiple infections were suspected prednisone therapy for hypercalcemia was not initiated immediately. Because of possible reversible contributions of hypercalcemia to the patient's deterioration, calcium free peritoneal dialysis was begun on April 30, May 12, May 26, and June 9 in an effort to keep the serum ionized calcium level below 5 mg/100 ml. Dialyses consisted of 39, 42, 31, and 46 hourly exchanges, respectively. The changes in serum total calcium and ionized calcium and inorganic phosphorus levels throughout this period are shown in Fig 2.

Following the first dialysis, symptoms attributable to hypercalcemia or uremia or both diminished. The white blood cell count returned to normal. Fever, pyuria, pericardial friction rub, and congestive heart-failure resolved. On May 9, prior to the second dialysis as shown in Fig 2, prednisone therapy was initiated. This did not prevent, however, a rapid rise in serum calcium to values in excess of 14 mg/100 ml by May 12. Throughout the course, prednisone, 30 to 60 mg/day, had no obvious effect on the serum calcium level. The rapid rise in the serum calcium level before the second dialysis was associated with a rapid reduction of serum inorganic phosphorus value. Following the fourth peritoneal dialysis, serum calcium returned to levels below normal and the patient was discharged on June 13, 1970, with a serum total calcium value of 10 mg/100 ml and serum ionized calcium value of 4.2 mg/100 ml. The patient was readmitted on June 24, 1970, for problems related to hyperglycemia, acidemia, anemia, and congestive heart-failure. Throughout this admission, total calcium values ranged from 6 to 9 mg/100 ml. Prednisone therapy was tapered and she was discharged on July 8 improved with a SUN level of 132 mg/100 ml, a serum creatinine value of 9.3 mg/100 ml and creatinine clearance of 3.8 ml/min. She was readmitted in congestive heart-failure again on July 15. Total serum calcium values throughout this final admission ranged from 6 to 8 mg/100 ml. On admission the SUN level was 125 mg/100 ml, and the serum creatinine value was 12.5 mg/100 ml. X-ray film of the chest and heart scan showed pleural and pericardial effusions, respectively. She died on July 19, following aspiration.

Postmortem examination revealed hyalinization and thicknening of arteriolar walls in the myocardium, liver, pancreas, spleen, and kidney. Only small focal areas of calcification in arteriolar walls were noted. The kidneys showed nodular glomerulosclerosis compatible with diabetes mellitus. No evidence for significant metastatic calcification or renal parenchymal calcifications was seen in tissues examined. Parathyroid glands were not hyperplastic.

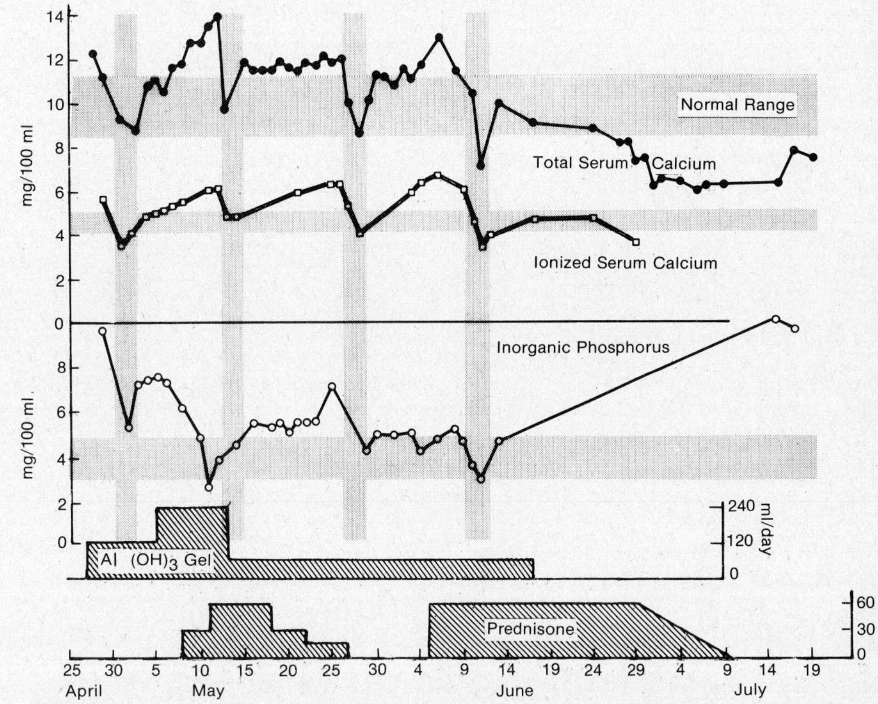

Fig 2.—Serum concentrations of total calcium level (solid circle) and ionized calcium (x) (vertical axis, upper left) *and inorganic phosphorus (open circle)* (vertical axis, lower left) *are related to time* (horizontal axis) *throughout and after dialysis period. Aluminum hydroxide gel and prednisone therapy are indicated as hatched bars below with vertical scales* (lower right). *Vertical shaded bars indicate periods of dialysis. Each horizontal shaded area represents range of normal serum concentration of respective overlapping serum solute plotted.*

Clearance Studies

Peritoneal clearances of urea (C_{urea}), creatinine (C_{cr}), urate (C_{urate}), total calcium (C_{Ca}) and ionized calcium ($C_{Ca^{++}}$) were determined during the multiple exchanges. Two liters of calcium free dialysis solution containing sodium, 140 mEq/liter; chloride, 99.5 mEq/liter; acetate, 45 mEq/liter; magnesium, 1.5 mEq/liter; and potassium, 3 mEq/liter and 1½% dextrose were warmed to body temperature and instilled during a ten-minute period into the peritoneal cavity and allowed to remain thereafter for 30 minutes. As complete drainage as possible was then accomplished by gravity during a 20-minute period. During the clearance measurements, concentrations of the study solutes were determined in serum at the beginning of every other exchange and in dialysate. Clearances were calculated as follows: (the concentration of a respective solute in the dialysate/the concentration in serum at the time of the exchanges) × (the drainage volume in milliliters/the total time of the exchange in 60 minutes). The total calcium removed per dialysis was calculated as the sum of the respective products of the dialysate calcium concentration (milligram per milliliter) and the exchange volume (milliliter) for every exchange. Inulin space was measured as an estimate of extracellular fluid space (ECF) prior to dialyses 1 to 3 as the total amount of inulin (milligrams) administered divided by the serum concentration of inulin (milligrams per liter) two hours after the injection (urinary losses were neglected because of the low glomerular filtra-

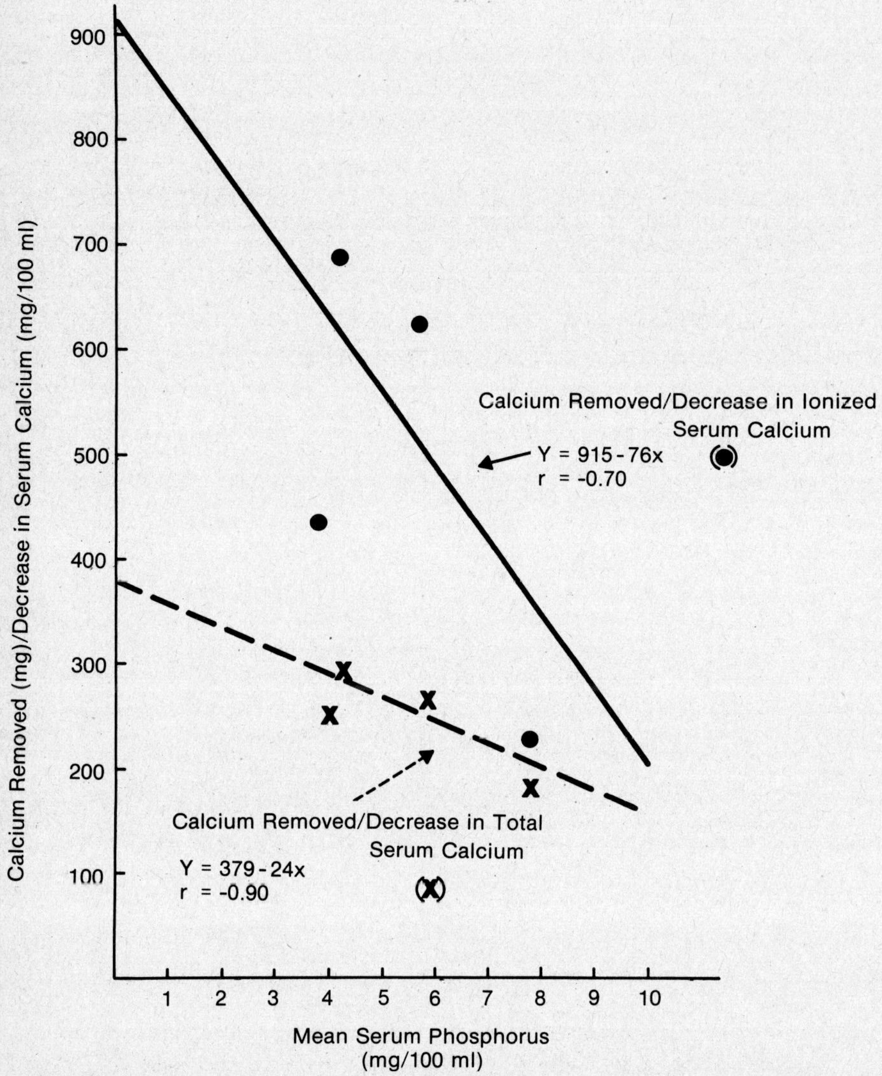

Fig 3.—Ratios of total calcium removed per decrease in total serum calcium concentration (x) (vertical axis) *and per decrease in ionized serum calcium (open circle)* (vertical axis) *are related to mean serum phosphorus* (horizontal axis) *during each dialysis.*

Table 1.—Comparison of Mean* Solute Clearance Values

	C_{Ca}	C_{Ca++}	C_{urea}	C_{cr}:C_{urea}	C_{urate}:C_{urea}
Patient	6.9±1.1	10.7±2.4	14.1±4.1	0.59±0.08	0.53±0.06
No. of Exchanges	11	11	22	22	22
Control Values	9.6±1.0	17.0±2.6	18.9±3.4	0.77±0.03	0.70±0.10
No. of Exchanges	9	3	13	13	13
Significance† of Difference of Means	$P<0.01$	$P<.01$	$P<.01$	$P<.01$	$P<.01$

* ± SD.
† Nonpaired *t* test.

tion rate). The value in this patient was repeatedly near 16 liters (28% of body weight). Maximum ionized calcium (milligrams) in the inulin space at initiation of each dialysis was calculated as the initial ionized serum calcium concentration (milligrams per liter) times the inulin space (16 liters). This is probably an overestimate of ionized calcium in the inulin space since the lower extravascular ionized calcium concentrations secondary to the Gibbs-Donnan phenomenon were neglected. Concentrations of total calcium, urea, creatinine, urate, and inulin levels were measured by reported methods.[4-6] Ionized calcium concentrations in serum and dialysate were measured by a flow-through ion-exchange electrode method.[7]

Peritoneal clearances are shown in Table 1, and compared to values measured similarily in five patients with chronic renal failure (three with chronic glomerulonephritis, two with chronic pyelonephritis and one patient with postpartum acute renal failure) unassociated with systemic vascular disease. All values in our patient were significantly less than control values and showed selectively greater reduction in clearances of larger molecular weight (MW) solutes. This latter point is evident from the significant reduction in the clearances of creatinine (MW, 113) and urate (MW, 168) as compared to urea (MW, 60). Clearance values were persistently below control values with no tendency to increase in the later dialysis.

The total amount of calcium removed for each dialysis and the percent of the initial ionized calcium in the inulin space thereby represented are shown in Table 2. The decreases in total ionized calcium per dialysis and the ratio of the change in serum

Table 2.—Effects of Calcium Free Peritoneal Dialysis on Serum Calcium

Date Dialysis Started	No. of Exchanges	Total Calcium Removed (mg)	ECF* Ionized Calcium Remover (%)	Predialysis Total Serum Calcium (mg/100 ml)	Postdialysis Total Serum Calcium (mg/100 ml)	Predialysis Ionized Serum Calcium	Postdialysis Ionized Serum Calcium	$\frac{\Delta \text{ Ionized}}{\Delta \text{ Total}}$ Serum Calcium
5/1/70	39	650	68	12.3	8.7	6.2	3.4	0.78
5/13/70	42	1,526	159	14.2	9.7	5.7	3.5	0.49
5/26/70	31	882	92	12.0	8.7	6.2	4.8	0.42
6/9/70	46	931	97	11.2	7.7	6.2	4.2	0.57

$$* \left(\frac{\text{mg Calcium Removed}}{[\text{Initial Serum Ionized Calcium (mg/ml)}]\ [\text{Inulin Space (ml)}]}\right) \cdot 100$$

In this approximation the numerator includes some complexed calcium and thus errs high; the denominator also errs high since Gibbs-Donnan corrections were neglected (see text).

ionized to the change in serum total calcium are also shown in Table 2. Note that total serum calcium concentrations always decreased more than ionized calcium concentrations. The mean ratio of the total:ionized calcium concentration in the dialysate was 1.46 ± 0.30. The mean ratio of ionized:total serum calcium was 0.49 ± 0.06 predialysis and 0.46 ± 0.10 postdialysis (not significantly different [$P > .50$]).

During the different peritoneal dialyses, serum inorganic phosphorus varied markedly due to variations in dosage of aluminum hydroxide gel and the effects of the previous dialysis. The ratio of the total calcium removed to the decrease in total serum calcium concentration from beginning to end of each dialysis and the corresponding ratio of calcium removed to the decrease in the serum ionized calcium were calculated. These values correlated inversely with the mean of serum phosphorus concentrations determined before and after each dialysis, as shown in Fig 3.

Comment

The ergocalciferol (vitamin D_2) doses used in our patient were extraordinarily high[8,9] for reasons that are not clear. It is much better to start with smaller doses (25,000 units ergocalciferol per day recommended) and increase cautiously according to the response in serum calcium as necessary.[8,10] Also the low serum albumin level in this patient makes interpretations of the low initial total serum calcium difficult without an ionized calcium measurement. The question can also be raised as to whether the use of vitamin D therapy with its associated risk was indicated in this patient in whom prognosis was poor because of many associated problems.

In this patient, the ionized and total calcium clearance values as well as the clearances of other solutes were significantly less than values measured in patients with renal failure without systemic vascular disease such as diabetes. The selectively greater reduction in clearances of larger molecular weight solutes might reflect altered peritoneal permeability associated with diffuse vascular disease, metastatic calcification or hypercalcemia itself or both.

Since serum total calcium invariably decreased more than serum ionized calcium, dissociation of protein-bound calcium or removal of complexed calcium or both must have occurred. The fact that the ratio of dialysate total: ionized calcium concentration was 1.46 also suggests removal of complexed calcium by this technique; however, formation of calcium complexes in dialysate cannot be excluded. The insignificant change in the ratio of ionized: total serum calcium represents the net effect of changes in total calcium and protein concentration, changes in pH and possible other factors.

To lower ionized calcium concentrations to normal values, a total quantity of calcium representing at least 68% to 159% of the ionized calcium initially in the extracellular fluid space had to be removed. Removal of complexed calcium, dissociation of bound calcium from protein, and mobilization of calcium from pools outside the extracellular space (primarily from bone), may all have prevented larger decreases in ionized calcium concentration per unit total calcium removed. Similarly, Boen considered that bone calcium mobilization explains the relatively small decreases in total serum calcium per unit calcium removed by calcium free peritoneal dialysis in a patient with mammary carcinoma, skeletal metastasis, and hypercalcemia.[1] In contrast, Maxwell et al[2] reported the use of the dialysis technique in a patient with sarcoidosis, calcium carbonate ingestion, and hypercalcemia where decreases in total calcium concentration multiplied by extracellular fluid volume approximated the total calcium removed and suggested little or no net bone calcium mobilization. Lemann and Donatelli[11] reported little effect of calcium free peritoneal dialysis on the serum calcium concentration of a patient with primary hyperparathyroidism. Rapid calcium mobilization from bone and a short dialysis (ten hours) may explain their poor results. The need for greater calcium removal per unit fall in serum calcium at lower serum phosphorus values in Fig 3 suggests an effect of serum phosphorus on calcium pool mobilization, also noted by other investigators.[10]

It has been recommended that the treatment of hypocalcemia associated with chronic renal failure should be an attempt to restore serum calcium and serum phosphate values to normal levels, particularly in the presence of osteomalacia.[8,9] Vitamin D resistance is usually observed in such patients and large doses of vitamin D are often required to increase serum calcium levels. Recent work with animals suggests that the vitamin D resistance in uremia is in part due to the inability to readily convert vitamin D to its most active form, 25 hydroxycholecalciferol, and to the absence of a calcium-binding protein in the small intestine.[12] Secondary malabsorption of calcium and defective vitamin D influence on bond calcium mobilization may then lead to hypocalcemia. Early treatment of hypocalcemia is intended to restore serum concentrations to normal and prevent the later development of osteomalacia or secondary hyperparathyroidism or both with osteitis fibrosa cystica. There is no evidence that secondary hyperparathyroidism played a significant role in our patient. Hyperplastic parathyroid glands were not found at autopsy and serum calcium had returned to normal to low levels. Alternatively hyperplastic glands could have been suppressed by the hypercalcemia.

The studies in this patient thus provide additional evidence that calcium free peritoneal dialysis offers a form of treatment for hypercalcemia in patients with severe impairment of renal function. Furthermore, the studies suggest that the rate of reduction in serum calcium concentration is related inversely to bone calcium mobilization and directly to serum ionized and complexed calcium concentrations, serum inorganic phosphorus concentration, and peritoneal permeability.

Summary

A patient with severe diabetes mellitus, advanced nephropathy, retinopathy, cardiomyopathy, and hypocalcemia was treated with excessive amounts of vitamin D and hypercalcemia developed. Repeated calcium free peritoneal dialyses corrected the hypercalcemia, reduced her degree of azotemia and markedly improved her symptoms. Serum calcium levels eventually returned to values below normal but the patient died later of further complications of her disease. Calcium free peritoneal dialysis offers a form of treatment for hypercalcemia in patients with severe impairment of renal function. Factors which may influence the efficiency of the technique include bone calcium mobilization, serum ionized and complexed calcium concentrations, serum inorganic phosphorus concentration and peritoneal membrane permeability.

This investigation was supported in part by Public Health Service grant RR-00287-04.

Dr. Stoltz performed this investigation while a medical student research fellow supported by the University of Missouri General Research Support Award.

The calcium free dialysis solution used in this investigation was supplied by McGaw Laboratories, Division of American Hospital Supply Corp, Glendale, Calif.

References

1. Boen ST: *Peritoneal Dialysis in Clinical Medicine.* IN Kugelmass (ed), Springfield, Ill, Charles C Thomas Publisher, 1964, p 36-40.
2. Maxwell MH, Rockney RE, Kleeman CR, et al: Peritoneal dialysis: I. Techniques and applications. *JAMA* **170**:917-924, 1959.
3. Garrett JJ, Cuddihee RE: Calcium absorption during peritoneal dialysis. *Trans Amer Soc Artif Intern Organs* **14**:372-375, 1968.
4. Nolph KD, Whitcomb ME, Schrier RW: Mechanisms for inefficient peritoneal dialysis in acute renal failure associated with heat stress and exercise. *Ann Intern Med* **71**:317-326, 1969.
5. Nolph KD, Stoltz ML, Carter CB, et al: Factors affecting the composition of ultrafiltrate from hemodialysis coils. *Trans Amer Soc Artif Intern Organs* **16**:495-501, 1970.
6. Wieme RJ, Van Raetenbusch FR: Automatic determination of calcium in blood and urine using Corinth Ca. *Clin Chim Acta* **7**:883-887, 1962.
7. Moore EW: Ionized calcium in normal serum ultrafiltrates and whole blood determined by ion-exchange electrodes. *J Clin Invest* **49**:318-334, 1970.
8. Kaye M: Concepts of therapy, prevention and management of osteodystrophy in patients with long-term hemodialysis. *Arch Intern Med* **124**:656-662, 1969.
9. Rubini ME, Coburn JW, Massry SG, et al: Renal osteodystrophy. *Arch Intern Med* **124**:663-669, 1969.
10. Bricker NS, Ogden DA, Schreiner GE, et al: Pivalent ion metabolism and osteodystrophy in chronic renal failure: Invited discussion. *Arch Intern Med* **124**:292-301, 1969.
11. Lemann J Jr, Donatelli AA: Calcium intoxication due to primary hyperparathyroidism. *Ann Intern Med* **60**:447-461, 1964.
12. Avioli LV, Birge SJ, Slatopolsky E: The nature of vitamin D resistance of patients with chronic renal disease. *Arch Intern Med* **124**:451-454, 1969.

ECG Analysis No. 4

Ventricular Tachycardia

Douglas P. Zipes, MD, and Charles Fisch, MD, Indianapolis

The diagnosis of ventricular tachycardia (VT) should be considered when there occurs a series of three or more bizarrely shaped premature QRS complexes that are prolonged greater than 0.12 second, with ST-T vector pointing opposite to the major QRS deflection. The rhythm may be quite regular, or it may vary; the ventricular rate is usually between 100 and 250 beats/min. The atria may beat independently to produce A-V dissociation or they may be depolarized by the ventricles in a retrograde fashion, in which case A-V dissociation is *not* present. If ventricular fusion or capture beats are present—the latter demonstrated by the appearance of an early QRS complex with a supraventricular contour occurring in the midst of the VT—they provide weighty evidence in favor of the diagnosis of VT. The ventricular fusion beat indicates simultaneous activation of the ventricles by two separate impulses, inferring that one of the impulses arises in the ventricles. The capture beat signals supraventricular control of the ventricles generally at a rate faster than the VT; this proves that normal ventricular conduction can occur at cycle lengths equal to or shorter than the tachycardia in question, again inferring that the site of origin of the wide QRS complexes lies in the ventricles.

Unfortunately, certain supraventricular tachycardias (SVT) may mimic VTs and satisfy *all* the criteria previously outlined. Because of the overlapping features of SVT and VT, and because many of the criteria established to diagnose VT cannot be met during a given recording of VT, it would appear best to ascribe a certain probability to the diagnosis, depending on how many and how well the criteria are satisfied.

Figure 1 demonstrates the classic features of VT. A bizarre premature QRS complex prolonged greater than 0.12 seconds interrupts the rhythm after the initial two sinus beats, and continues for two more discharges. Since the third P wave occurs on schedule, simultaneously with the third QRS complex, we assume it was not fired retrogradely by the ventricles; therefore, one beat of A-V dissociation exists. The fourth P wave unaccountably is delayed slightly, but the sharp deflection in the T wave of the fourth QRS complex suggests retrograde capture, as indicated in Fig 1; it may be argued that A-V dissociation is still present since the fourth P wave may be of sinus origin, blocked in transit to the ventricles in the same manner as the third P wave. The distinction is of little consequence, merely serving to determine whether or not A-V dissociation continues. The fifth P wave occurs early because of retrograde capture by the fifth QRS complex; this certainly terminates the period of A-V dissociation, although the VT persists. Retrograde conduction delay to the atria permits antegrade return of the impulse to the ventricles (ventricular echo or reciprocal beat) in time to share with the VT in the activation of

Received for publication June 15, 1971; accepted July 29.

From the Indiana University Medical Center, Krannert Institute of Cardiology, Indianapolis.

Reprint requests to 1100 W Michigan St, Indianapolis 46202 (Dr. Zipes).

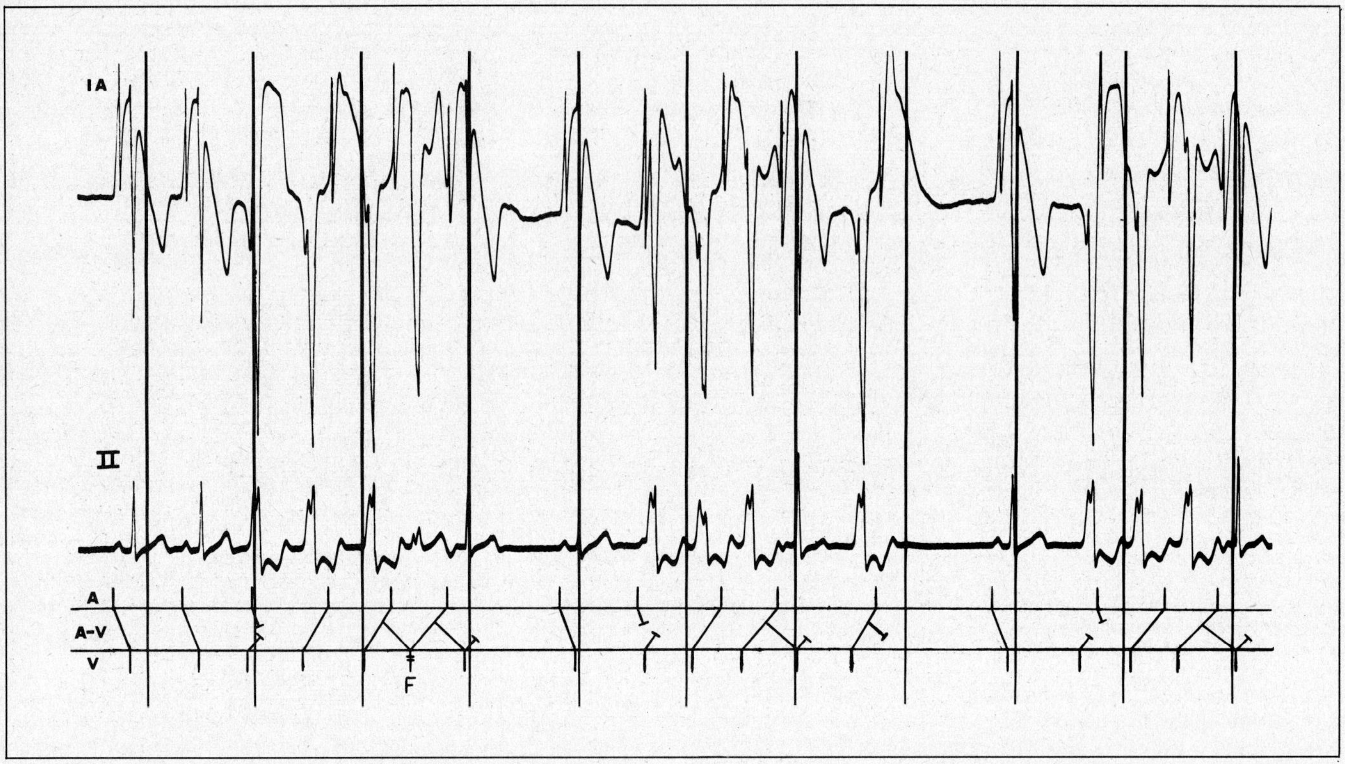

Fig 1.—Ventricular tachycardia. IA indicates intra-atrial recording from the cavity of the right atrium used to identify atrial activity. Lead II is recorded simultaneously. The ladder diagram displays the interpretation of this complex arrhythmia. Because of the position of the intraatrial recording lead, both antegrade and retrograde P waves have very similar contours. The fact that these retrograde P waves, for the most part, occur early and inscribe small negative deflections in lead II substantiates the analysis that they are retrograde captures.

Fig 2.—Repetitive ventricular tachycardia in a 23-year-old woman with syncopal episodes. Sinus beats are interspersed between runs of an ectopic tachycardia, most likely ventricular in origin. The lack of fusion or capture beats and precise determination of atrial activity during the tachycardia prevent an unequivocal diagnosis of ventricular tachycardia from this tracing.

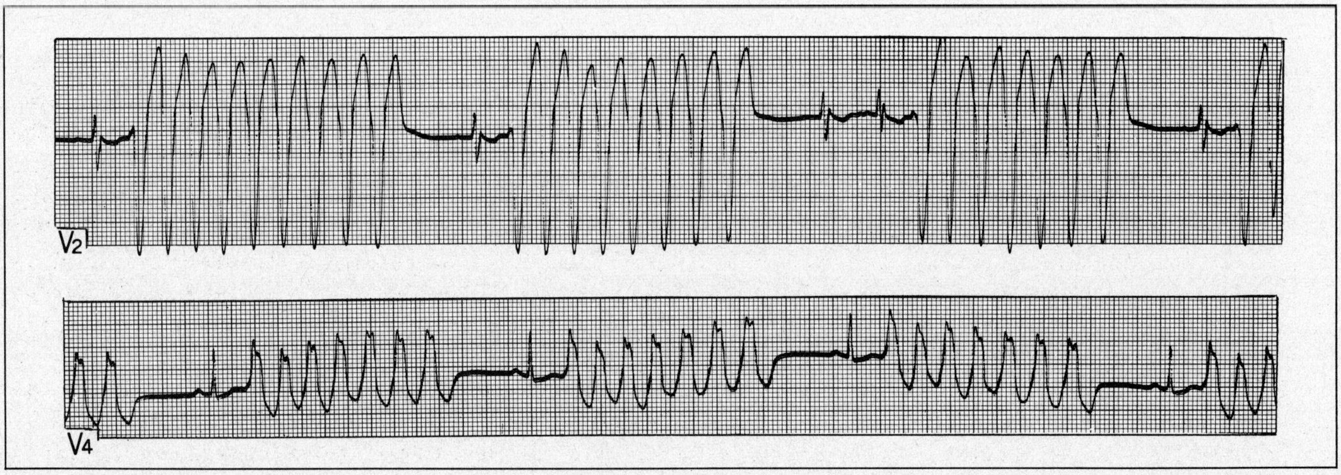

the ventricles. The resulting fusion beat (F) actually represents a supraventricular capture of a part of the ventricles. Retrograde stimulation of the sixth P wave incurs further retrograde delay (retrograde Wenckebach block), and again allows antegrade return of the impulse, this time to solely capture the ventricles. The seventh QRS complex occurs at a rate slightly faster than the VT but maintains a supraventricular contour, thus establishing the ventricular origin of the tachycardia. Retrograde conduction to the atria does not take place after this capture and, following a slight pause, the sequence repeats.

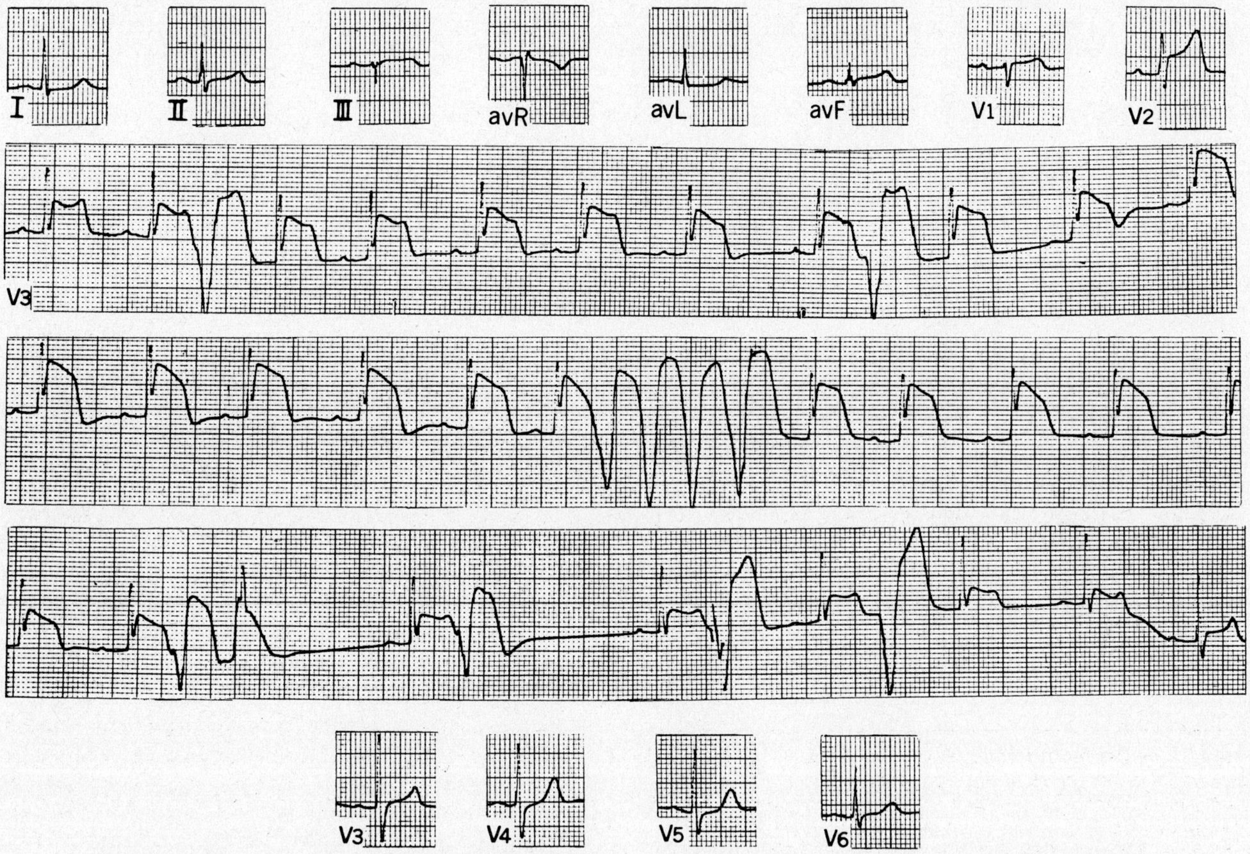

Fig 3.—Ventricular tachycardia during atypical angina pectoris. Transient S-T segment elevation occurs while recording V_2 and V_3. Premature ventricular contractions trigger a short run of ventricular tachycardia. S-T segments return to the baseline as the chest pain abates, and the ectopic ventricular activity ceases.

Fig 4.—Ventricular tachycardia developing into ventricular fibrillation. Irregularly occurring ectopic beats (downward deflections) *increase their discharge rate, and ventricular fibrillation follows, in the midportion of the tracing.*

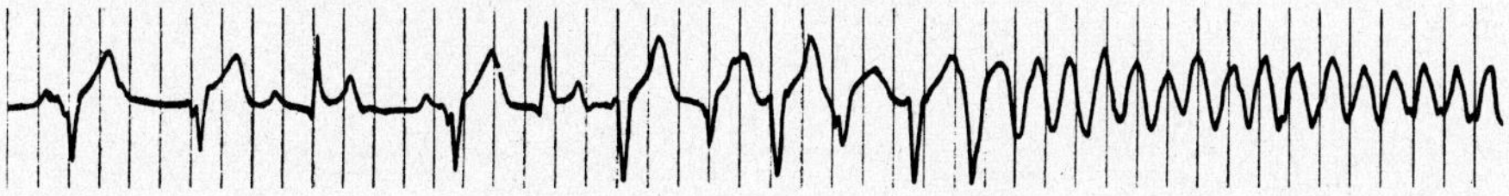

A repetitive type of intermittent VT has been described and is characterized by bursts of ectopic ventricular beating, beginning prematurely and followed by a pause. Single or many sinus beats separate the runs of the VT (Fig 2).

In certain clinical situations, practical considerations of therapy may urge the diagnosis of VT "by the company it keeps," even though many of the criteria graphically analyzed in Fig 1 are lacking. Figure 3 illustrates this problem. During the course of a routine ECG recording, the patient complained of chest pain and the S-T segment elevated as V_2 was recorded. Long samples of V_3 illustrate frequent premature ventricular complexes (PVCs), discharging very close to the preceding T wave, and apparently initiating a run of these wide QRS complexes in the midportion of the second strip. At the end of the third tracing, the S-T segments return to normal and the PVCs cease, confirmed in V_{3-6} (Fig 3, *bottom*). The patient has a variant type of angina described by Prinzmetal et al,[1] during which S-T segments elevate and VT, as well as A-V block, have been demonstrated. Not many would quibble with the diagnosis of VT and the need for therapy, even though distinct fusion and capture beats are absent in this recording. Similarly, when the tachycardia terminates in ventricular fibrillation, VT should be strongly considered (Fig 4).

Reference

1. Prinzmetal M, Ekmekci A, Kennamer R: Variant form of angina pectoris. *JAMA* **174**:1794-1802, 1960.

Special Commentary

The Problem-Oriented Record and the Measurement of Excellence

J. Willis Hurst, MD, Atlanta

The problem-oriented medical record system was introduced by Weed and executed successfully by Bjorn and Cross.[1-5] The system will, in my opinion, serve as a rudder to guide us through the rough but interesting water that lies ahead of our profession in its quest for excellence.

Whereas the problem-oriented medical record solves many practical problems, it also demands that those who use it take their stand for excellence. The purpose of this brief communication is to point out how excellence can be measured when the problem-oriented record is used.

Comment

The following paragraph was written by John Gardner.[6] Examine the last sentence of the paragraph carefully.

> Not only the claims of civility but the realities of individual development call for some measure of self-discipline. Every great artistic performance is the consequence of self-discipline long and faithfully applied. So is every great athletic or intellectual performance. Discipline in that sense—schooling, a conscious adherence to standards, *an effort to bring performance into line with an admired ideal*—is the essence of craftsmanship.[6]

The preceding paragraph indicates how excellence is measured. Gardner's words, as usual, stay with you. Having read them let us now think through how to identify excellence in the context of two specific activities. One activity will be nonmedical and the other activity will be medical.

The Identification of Excellence in a Nonmedical Activity.—The sport called football will serve as the analogue for this discussion. Let us assume for the moment that a group of neighborhood boys finds a football and begins to toss the ball around. Let us also assume they have never heard of the game known as football and, therefore, do not know the rules of the game. Suppose Johnny Unitas appears on the scene and asks if he can play with the neophytes. He does. He catches the ball and runs past all of the boys without being touched. We can not judge the talent of Johnny Unitas based on this performance. The reason we cannot is that he did not perform against any real obstacles. All one could deduce from such action is that Johnny Unitas played better than the boys who are amateurs. Therefore, Unitas' actual ability has not been tested.

The identification of excellence cannot be accomplished unless there are rules. In fact, the rules of the game must be very specific. For example, the real game of football came into being when the agreement was reached that the field would be 360 feet long and 160 feet wide; that the field would be marked off in such a way that a grid would be formed with each line separated by an interval of 30 feet; that there would be eleven players on opposing sides and that each would have certain duties and be called a certain name; that each game would last a certain length of time and be divided into definite time intervals; that several officials would watch the game carefully and that

Received for publication July 28, 1971; accepted Aug 2.

From the Department of Medicine, Emory University School of Medicine, Atlanta. Dr. Hurst is professor and chairman of the Department of Medicine.

Reprint requests to 69 Butler St SE, Atlanta 30303 (Dr. Hurst).

they would fault the players and penalize them if they broke the rules of the game; that the ball itself would be a certain size and weight; and that there were times when other people could go on the field and times when they could not. The sport called football, seen in this light, is a very *rigid* sport. Despite the obvious rigidity of the sport, we rarely hear the fans or the players complain that the sport is too rigid for them. This is because the rules are rigid but do not limit the action. Therefore, the rules of the game do not stifle the imagination of the coaches and players. When Johnny Unitas plays football in the context of such rules, he can be judged. He is not only playing against other players, but he is playing against the obstacles created by the rules of the game. Now he can be judged because all players must, within definable limits, play against the same obstacles. The rules do not prevent creativity. In fact, it is within such a rigid setting that creativity is identifiable. One might conclude that creativity and excellence can only be determined in a system that has identifiable obstacles built into the system. Do not misinterpret my view. I do not believe in rules that limit creativity. Should this happen a football player could be restricted to such an extreme degree that he could not move. I am simply saying that an open field, no rules, situation would produce a nonreproducible, nonteachable activity and that a system that limits the players severely would produce a reproducible, easily taught activity, but it would test the skill of no one. Accordingly, the rules of the game must be set somewhere *between* no rules and rules that inactivate the participants. Rules that evolve in this manner must be carefully defined and must be rigid. It is in this setting that excellence is definable. It is in this context that we all know that Johnny Unitas is excellent.

The Identification of Excellence in a Medical Activity.—Let us now look at the medical record. It is the objective account of the physician's performance. When there are no rules pertaining to the records, the performance of a physician cannot be judged. The physician cannot even judge himself. He cannot define his problems. He cannot improve because there are no identifiable, reproducible obstacles to work against. On the other hand, I am against a set of rules that would cripple the creative thoughts of a physician. No thinking physician would accept a system of accounting medical data that keeps him from thinking. Accordingly, I support the idea that we establish a set of rules pertaining to medical records that are somewhere between no rules and rules that limit thought and creativity. These inbetween rules are absolutely necessary if one is to judge excellence. The guidelines I support are those of Lawrence Weed. He has set forth the rules that we must all adopt. He has suggested that the medical record should reveal an identifiable data base from which a complete problem list should evolve. Each problem is identified by title and number and the problem list is placed at the front of the chart. A numbered and titled initial plan should be developed for each problem. Each medical order should be identified by problem number and title. Numbered and titled progress notes must be written by the physician and nurse. A discharge note must be written that identifies the problems by numbers and titles.[1-6] This record structure must be adhered to rigidly. It will in no way interfere with the thought process of the physician. It simply demands the self-discipline that makes reproducibility possible. It is the framework within which excellence can be achieved and judged.

Conclusions

Excellence in patient care, education, and individual performance cannot be measured in a system without rules. Excellence in patient care, education, and individual performance cannot be measured in a system where the rules are so limiting that no thought or action is possible. Excellence can only be achieved or judged where we impose rules that are in between the extremes just mentioned. The record structure suggested by Weed is such a system. There could be other systems devised that would be acceptable, but, since we must arbitrarily accept only one set of rules for our profession, I suggest we accept the problem-oriented record system devised by Weed as meeting most of the obvious needs.

Excellence in sports, art, science, or medicine cannot be pursued, achieved, or measured without appropriate rules.

References

1. Weed LL: *Medical Records, Medical Education, and Patient Care.* Cleveland, Press of Case Western Reserve University, 1969, pp 1-273.
2. Bjorn JC, Cross HD: *Problem Oriented Practice.* Chicago, Modern Hospital Press, McGraw-Hill Publications, 1970.
3. Hurst JW: Ten reasons why Lawrence Weed is right. *New Eng J Med* **284**:51-52, 1971.
4. Hurst JW: How to implement the Weed system. *Arch Intern Med* **128**:456-462, 1971.
5. Hurst JW: The art and science of presenting a patient's problems. *Arch Intern Med* **128**:463-465, 1971.
6. Gardner JW: *The Recovery of Confidence.* New York, WW Norton & Company Inc, 1970, p 81. Quote reprinted with permission of author and publisher.

Review

Current Studies Regarding Diabetes

Robert H. Williams, MD, and John W. Ensinck, MD, Seattle

The recent pessimistic report by the University Group Diabetes Program[1] regarding the value of tolbutamide in the treatment of diabetes, combined with the continued high frequency of coronary disease, blindness, uremia, neuropathy, and other complications, even in "well treated" diabetes, emphasize the need for detailed analysis of the current status of study in this area. In most diabetics, despite the association of decreased glucose tolerance with decreased insulin secretion, it has not been proved that the primary etiology is in the pancreas. We know relatively little about the exact sequential abnormalities involved in the angiopathies—the concomitants that cause the greatest morbidity and mortality. In spite of the supposed genetic basis for the diabetes in most instances, blood glucose abnormalities are not found in the majority of patients until after the age of 30, even though significant microvascular abnormalities have developed in the interim. Various therapies have been employed without adequate evaluation of their benefits and hazards. Therefore, major new approaches to these diverse problems are sorely needed. We present the current status of some phases of diabetes-related research, examining in particular the factors involved in the synthesis and release of proinsulin, insulin, and glucagon. More basic information in these areas might lead to significant improvement in the management of diabetes. The present status of some of the clinical problems is also discussed briefly; more controversy and less recent progress has occurred in this area.

Received for publication Jan 25, 1971; accepted May 24.

From the Division of Endocrinology and Metabolism, Department of Medicine, SK-30, University of Washington, Seattle.

Read in part as the Ninth Elliott P. Joslin Lecture.

Reprint requests to Department of Medicine, SK-30, University of Washington, Seattle 98105 (Dr. Williams).

Development and Functions of the Fetal Pancreas

Studies of the development and function of the fetal pancreas, especially in humans, might be helpful in ascertaining early manifestations of genetic alteration in diabetes.

The pancreatic islets arise from the gut, and there are many interrelations among hormones produced by the two structures, particularly with respect to the transit, absorption, and assimilation of food. The pancreas evolves as a diverticulum from the duodenum.[2] In rats the islet cells are derived from the primitive gut before day 12 and then from the pancreatic ducts.[3] The endocrine cells coalesce to form islets, with differentiation initially of the alpha cells, followed by beta and D cells, which secrete glucagon, insulin, and gastrin, respectively.[4,5]

Transitional phases in the evolution of rat fetal pancreas include[6] (*a*) the undifferentiated state (fetal age <11 days), with little specific protein production; (*b*) the protodifferentiated state (fetal age, 12 to 14 days), with marked increases in specific proteins; and (*c*) the differentiated state (fetal age >19 days), with the levels of specific proteins modulated by extrinsic stimuli. From fetal age 15 to 19 days, there is a marked increase in the concentration of insulin, other proteins, and enzymes needed in the synthesis and release of insulin and glucagon. The peak concentration of proinsulin per cell occurs at day 12 and decreases rapidly thereafter.[3,6] By day 14, the number of islet cells and the insulin content increase markedly.[7] The initial level of glucagon is higher than that of insulin, but by day 14 the glucagon-insulin ratio equalizes.

Neither glucose nor tolbutamide caused insulin to be released from islets of human fetuses 12 to 16 weeks of age, and glucagon had only a slight effect.[8] Pieces of human fetal pancreas were found to have immunoassayable insulin and glucagon by the 50th day; concentrations and total amounts were higher by the 90th day and markedly increased by the 110th day (L. D. Schaeffer, M. L. Wilder, R. H. Williams, unpublished data) (Fig 1). Neither hormone was found in the pancreas of a fetus aged 25 days. During one-hour incubation of minced pancreas of a 115-day fetus, arginine (5 millimolar) markedly augmented the release of insulin (Fig 2) and glucagon. With glucose (16.7 millimolar), much less insulin was released than with arginine, but glucagon release was the same. In another study,[9] insulin was found in the blood of fetuses, aged 15 to 20 weeks, but the amount did not change after infusion of 50% glucose into the umbilical vein. These and other studies need to be extended to prediabetic subjects. They might reveal anatomic or physiological changes or both in the islet cells that are pertinent to the pathogenesis and progression of the diabetic process.

Synthesis, Release, and Actions of Proinsulin and Insulin

Abnormality of the formation, release, action, or metabolism of pro-

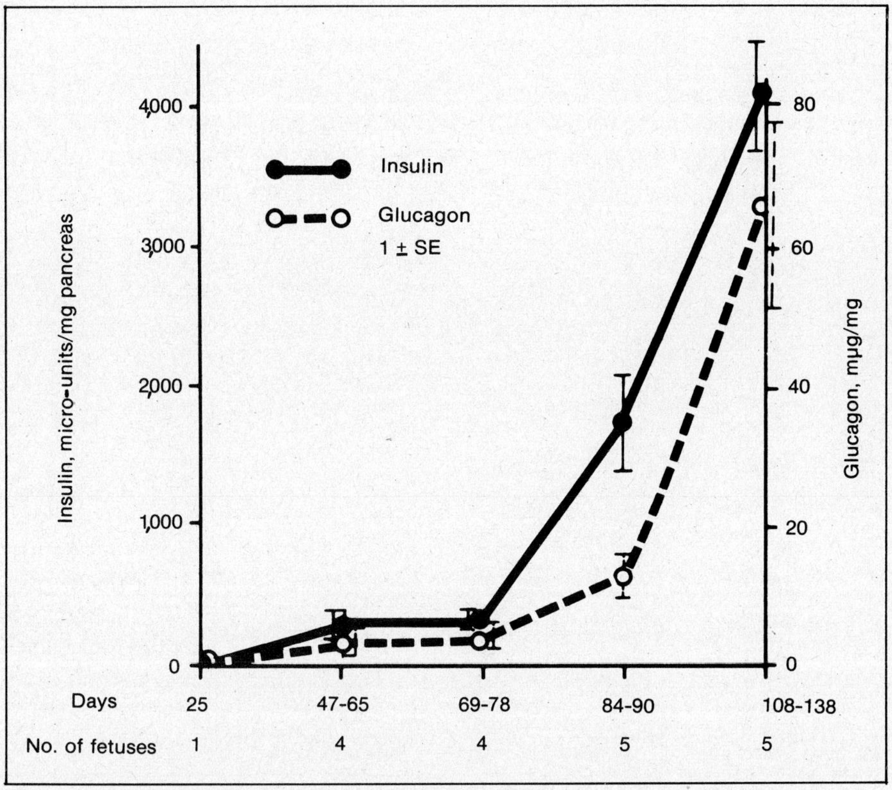

Fig 1.—The results of the hormone assays are averaged for four fetal age ranges. Insulin and glucagon were first found in the pancreas of a human fetus aged about 47 days. The total amounts increased markedly after approximately 80 days of age.

insulin or insulin seems a likely etiology of diabetes. Some recent basic studies[10-26] of these hormones will be described briefly. Steiner and coworkers' discovery of proinsulin and related intermediates[13] has been a strong stimulus to studies in this area. In proinsulin, the single-chain precursor of insulin, the types of amino acids and their sequential arrangement facilitate proper folding of the molecule[12,13]; this folding aids in insulin formation. In human proinsulin, there are 30 amino acids in chain B and 21 in chain A; hydrolysis of proinsulin liberates 31 amino acids in the connecting (C) peptide. In vitro, proinsulin is readily reconstituted oxidatively from the reduced form.[14] The composition of amino acids in the C-peptide differs significantly in various species; one influence of this is upon immunoreactive assays.

Proinsulin is synthesized in the endoplasmic reticulum and is transferred in small granules[4,10] (possibly some nongranulated)[11] to the Golgi complex, where most of it[15,16] is converted to insulin and C-peptide. The latter two compounds are packaged in similar quantities in beta granules and released into the cytoplasm. Apparently about ten minutes are required for transit of the proinsulin from the rough endoplasmic reticulum to the Golgi apparatus, while about one hour is needed for packaging and releasing insulin from the Golgi apparatus. Some beta granules become attached to a microtubular-microfilament system which may aid their rapid extrusion into the extracellular space; calcium stimulates this secretory mechanism, particularly during the initial phase. The part of proinsulin that is not hydrolyzed in the beta cells apparently is secreted as such in nongranular form. During incubation of islets, the ratio of intracellular to extracellular insulin is 8.5:1, while the ratio of intracellular to extracellular proinsulin is 13.8:1.[15] High glucose concentrations increase the amount of proinsulin released into the incubation medium.

The half-life of insulin perfused through rat liver was found to be 17 minutes, but during one hour there was *no change* in the levels of proinsulin or connecting peptide.[17] In animals, almost ten times (by weight) more proinsulin than insulin is required to produce hypoglycemia, and the duration of hypoglycemia is much longer.[18] Proinsulin simulates insulin action on diaphragm and adipose tissue cells, but does not antagonize insulin. Whereas bioassays of insulin show about 25 units/mg, the relative activity of proinsulin is 1.1 units/mg for rat adipose tissue cells and 1.8 units/mg for diaphragm.[19] A significant amount of this activity may occur without the need of conversion to insulin.[20,21] In contrast, the C-peptide does not exert significant action in adipose tissue cells. Reducing the length of the C-peptide attached to insulin increases the insulin-type action upon tissues and reduces the immunoreactivity with proinsulin antibody. However, even with the two arginines (arg_{31}-arg_{32}) attached to the B chain of insulin, Chance found[14] that the biologic activity was only 62% of that of insulin. Some of the amino acids in the C-peptide exert much greater influences than others on the amount of the immunoreactivity. In the assay for proinsulin, attention must be given to the significant species differences in the composition of C-peptide.

In man, some increase in proinsulin occurs after glucose administration, and there is an equal increase in the plasma C-peptide and insulin.[22] Increases in plasma "big insulin" (proinsulin or its products or both) after administration of glucose, tolbutamide, or arginine are slower and more prolonged than are those of insulin[23,24]; the ratio of "big insulin" to insulin increases with time. In obese or acromegalic subjects, glucose causes a hypernormal increment in the ratio of "big insulin" to insulin. Intravenous infusion in swine of various compounds (eg, glucose, glucagon, and arginine) equally increases plasma insulin and C-peptide. A combination of glucose, tolbutamide, and glucagon causes far greater increases in the insulin and C-peptide levels than any of these compounds individually.[25] In diabetic serum, an "abnormal insulin" (possibly proinsulin or related compounds or both) has been reported.[26] It is degraded less rapidly by "insulinase" than is insulin in the serum of normal subjects, and it has subnormal biologic activity. However, abnormal levels of proinsulin in the plasma of diabetics have not been shown.

Despite excellent progress regarding proinsulin-insulin synthesis, metabolism, and actions, much more information is needed to clarify their role in diabetes.

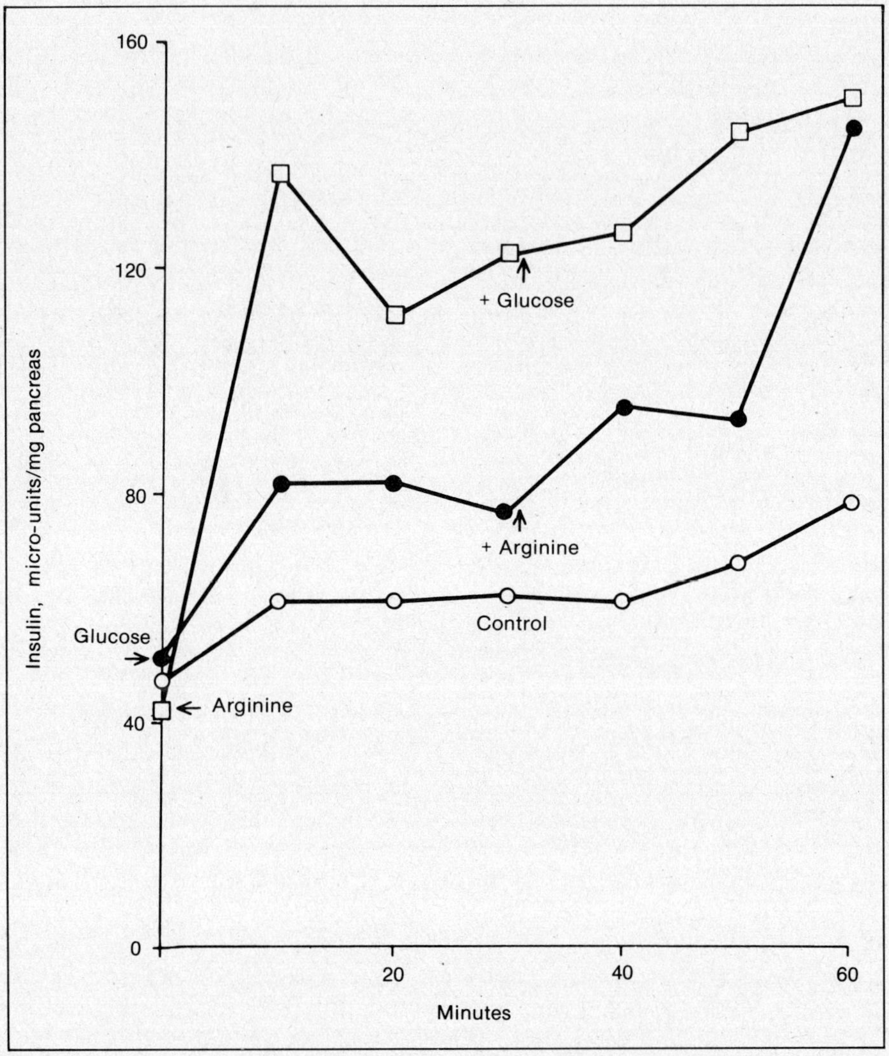

Fig 2.—Arginine caused more insulin secretion than did glucose when they were incubated with minced pancreas of a human fetus aged 115 days.

Factors Affecting Synthesis and Release of Insulin

Effect of Energy Supply.—Glucose-evoked synthesis and release of insulin is an energy-dependent process,[27] depending especially upon oxidative phosphorylation, which in turn is dependent upon glucose metabolism. The following factors are among those that decrease glucose oxidation and/or phosphorylation and insulin release: mannoheptulose, deoxyglucose, glucosamine, anoxia, cyanide, iodoacetate, azide, and oligomycin.[28,29] Insulin release by many compounds (eg, glucose, tolbutamide, glucagon, leucine) is inhibited by agents that inhibit adenosine triphosphate (ATP) formation.[28,30-33] Certain sugars metabolized by the islets (eg, mannose, fructose, ribose) are insulinogenic, but others (eg, galactose, xylose) are not. Beta cells contain glucokinase, hexokinase, and glucose-6-phosphatase, which are important in glucose uptake and utilization. The islets are very active in forming glycogen but store little.[34] Deoxyglucose decreases insulin release produced by glucose and glucagon, but has little effect on the action of tolbutamide and arginine.[35] Tolbutamide, glucagon, theophylline, and almost all other agents that increase insulin release cause an increase in 6-phosphogluconate.[34]

Compounds that increase oxidative phosphorylation increase formation of ATP, which is a high-energy compound. One important function of ATP is to serve as a precursor of cyclic adenylate (c-AMP). An increase in c-AMP in the beta cells increases the release of insulin.[36-38] Methylxanthines increase insulin release, presumably by inhibiting phosphodiesterase action and increasing c-AMP in beta cells.[36,39-41] A number of studies have indicated that an increase in beta adrenergic activity elevates c-AMP levels, whereas an increase in alpha adrenergic activity diminishes c-AMP.[36,38]

Much higher concentrations of glucose are required for release of proinsulin and insulin than for their synthesis.[15] Glucose perfused through rat pancreas for 50 minutes releases insulin very rapidly in the first few minutes, has little effect in the next several minutes, and then progressively increases it. The amount of insulin release over the more prolonged period is larger and depends partially upon new protein synthesis.[42] When a prolonged infusion is followed by glucose restimulation, after a ten-minute rest period, a much faster rate of release occurs than at any other time. Thus, beta cells seem to have two insulin compartments ("pools"), one small and one big.[42-44] The concept of two pools should not be adopted too readily, since several pools could exist. The small compartment responds rapidly and briefly to most agents and is the primary site of insulin secretion.[42] Glucagon and tolbutamide seem to stimulate only the small pool, and for further effect they depend upon glucose metabolism. In man, the release from the small pool depends upon (*a*) the dose of glucose or other stimulant, (*b*) the carbohydrate tolerance, (*c*) the basal insulin level, and (*d*) the size of the pool. The amount of insulin release depends upon the amounts, times, and durations of glucose administration.[44] Ordinarily, the amount of insulin released early is a very small part of that in the beta cell. Also, the amount released by glucose, glucagon, or tolbutamide is much less than that released by their combination.[45] They may act upon the same or different receptors or both.

Effect of Insulin Concentration in Extracellular Fluid.—It has been suggested that levels of insulin surrounding beta cells influence significantly the rate of insulin release. For example, beta cell depletion of insulin is greater in rats injected with anti-insulin serum than in those maintained at a comparable level of hyperglycemia by glucose infusion.[46] Increases in insulin added to incubation fluid containing isolated rat islets proportionately decrease insulin release.[47] It is not known whether such a reaction occurs at physiologic insulin levels in man.

Effect of Electrolytes.—The intracellular levels of calcium, magnesium, zinc, potassium, and sodium ions, play an important role in insulin release. The ratios of some of these compounds, as well as their total intracellular and extracellular concentrations, are important (eg, Na:K). The ions affect electrical potentials, membrane permeability, enzyme activity, and other processes. Calcium ion increases insulin release but not its synthesis[43]; Ca^{++} and Na^{+} increase the release produced by glucose, glucagon, tolbutamide, and leucine.[48] Marked changes in intracellular Ca^{++} may result from changes in intracellular Na^{+}; the uptake of Ca^{++} depends upon intracellular Na^{+}. A high level of Ca^{++} or Mg^{++} inhibits insulin release. Low Ca^{++} concentration decreases insulin release caused by tolbutamide, leucine, and glucagon.[28] The beta cells, especially their granules, have a relatively high zinc concentration, much of which is bound to insulin.[49,50] To what extent primary pancreatic electrolytic changes occur in diabetes and influence its course is not known.

Effect of Amino Acids and Fatty Acids.—Carbohydrate, protein, and fat increase insulin release. The following amino acids stimulate insulin-releasing activity in decreasing order: arginine, lysine, leucine, phenylalanine, valine, and methionine.[51-53] The response to arginine occurs at five minutes, declines by ten minutes, and then gradually rises, suggesting a two-pool system as with glucose. With increasing doses of amino acid, the increments of plasma insulin are larger and longer. Glucose utilization is important in the maximal stimulatory effect of some of the amino acids. Glucose augments insulin release by arginine, but deoxyglucose does not affect it; mannoheptulose blocks it. Glucose plus arginine, leucine, isoleucine, lysine, or protein cause synergistic responses. Leucine is the only one of ten amino acids that stimulates insulin release in vitro in the absence of extracellular glucose.[54] Certain combined amino acids (eg, arginine with leucine or with phenylalanine) act synergistically. Growth hormone increases the insulin-releasing effects of the amino acids.

In dogs, the infusion of oleate complexed with plasma lipoprotein markedly increases plasma insulin levels.[55]

Effect of Catecholamines and Cholinergics.—The autonomic nervous system plays an important role in the secretion and action of insulin, but it has not been shown to have a primary role in the etiology of diabetes. The sympathetic nervous system is activated by absolute or relative hypoglycemia.[56,57] Epinephrine or norepinephrine inhibits insulin release[56] induced by glucose, glucagon, and tolbutamide infusions in man. Decreased alpha adrenergic activity or increased beta adrenergic (eg, isoproterenol) function causes insulin release. Neither secretin- nor arginine-stimulated insulin release is inhibited by epinephrine in man. Acetylcholine or carbamyl choline,[58] or vagal stimulation, increases insulin release from pieces of pancreas. With isolated rat islets, epinephrine or norepinephrine decreases insulin release, but acetylcholine increases it.[59]

Effect of Glucagon.—Glucagon markedly influences, directly or indirectly, net insulin release and action. Alpha cell granules are rich in glucagon. They are formed in the Golgi complex, migrate to the cell membrane, and soon after extrusion (emiocytosis) undergo dissolution.[60] Increases in pancreatic glucose level progressively increase insulin release caused by glucagon.[61] Mannoheptulose and deoxyglucose do not block glucagon-induced insulin release. Glucagon can increase insulin release without increasing the glucose-6-phosphate level.[32] Glucagon decreases the plasma level of amino acids, including essential, nonessential, and glycogenic[62]; it increases the level of fatty acids when there is insulin deficiency. It may increase the release of catecholamines.[63]

Table 1.—Comparisons of Pancreatic Glucagon and Glucagon-Like Immunoreactivity (GLI)*

	Pancreatic Glucagon	Enteric Glucagon-Like Material Gel-Fraction Peak 2	Enteric Glucagon-Like Material Gel-Fraction Peak 1	Net
Molecular weight	3,485	3,500±	7,000+	(2 fractions)
Reaction with specific pancreatic glucagon antibody	+	Very slight	Very slight	Very slight
Reaction with GLI-crossreactive antibody	+	+	+	+
Liver glycogenolysis	++++	+	0	+
Hyperglycemia	++++	+	0	+
Insulin-releasing action	+	? Slight	0	? Slight
Changes after glucose	Decrease	Incomplete	Incomplete	Incomplete
Changes after amino acids	Incomplete	0	0	0
Increased by starvation	+	0	0	0
Increased by pancreozymin	+	0	0	0

* These data are based chiefly on studies in the laboratory of Roger Unger.[67,68]

Table 2.—Some Factors Affecting Insulin Release

	Increase		Decrease	
Sugars and related compounds	Glucose Mannose Fructose Ribose	Xylitol Sorbitol Pyruvate Citrate	Mannoheptulose Deoxyglucose Glucosamine	
Amino acids	Arginine Lysine Leucine	Phenylalanine Valine		
Fat derivatives	Fatty acids Ketones			
Electrolytes	K^+ Ca^{++}	Na^+ Mg^{++}		
Hormones	Glucagon Gastrin Secretin Pancreozymin Acetylcholine Prostaglandins	Somatotropin Placental lactogen ACTH* Glucosteroids Estradiol Progesterone	Epinephrine Norepinephrine Serotonin Insulin	
Other compounds	Sulfonylureas, acutely Methyl xanthines α-adrenergic blockers c-AMP ATP	Methacholine Ouabain Choline	Sulfonylureas, chronically ? Thiazides Biguanides β-adrenergic blockers Hypoxia Cyanide	Azide Iodoacetate Dinitrophenol Oligomycin Proteogenic inhibitors Imidazole

* ACTH signifies adrenocorticotropic hormone.

Glucagon and Gastrointestinal Hormones

Glucagon release is increased by amino acids, theophylline, catecholamines, or hypoglycemia. It is decreased by glucose, fructose, galactose, xylose, xylitol, or ribose,[64] and is not affected by mannoheptulose or deoxyglucose. Cottonseed oil infused into heparinized dogs decrease plasma glucagon.[65] Insulin concentration does not directly affect glucagon release. In vivo, pancreozymin increases the release of insulin and glucagon.[66] Samols et al found that tolbutamide decreases glucagon release in ducks and man,[67,68] Fajans reported that it caused no change in the glucagon levels in man (personal communication, 1971). Diazoxide increases glucagon release in ducks and man, but decreases insulin release.[67]

After an overnight fast, the molar ratio of plasma insulin to glucagon is 2.3:1, but after a carbohydrate meal,

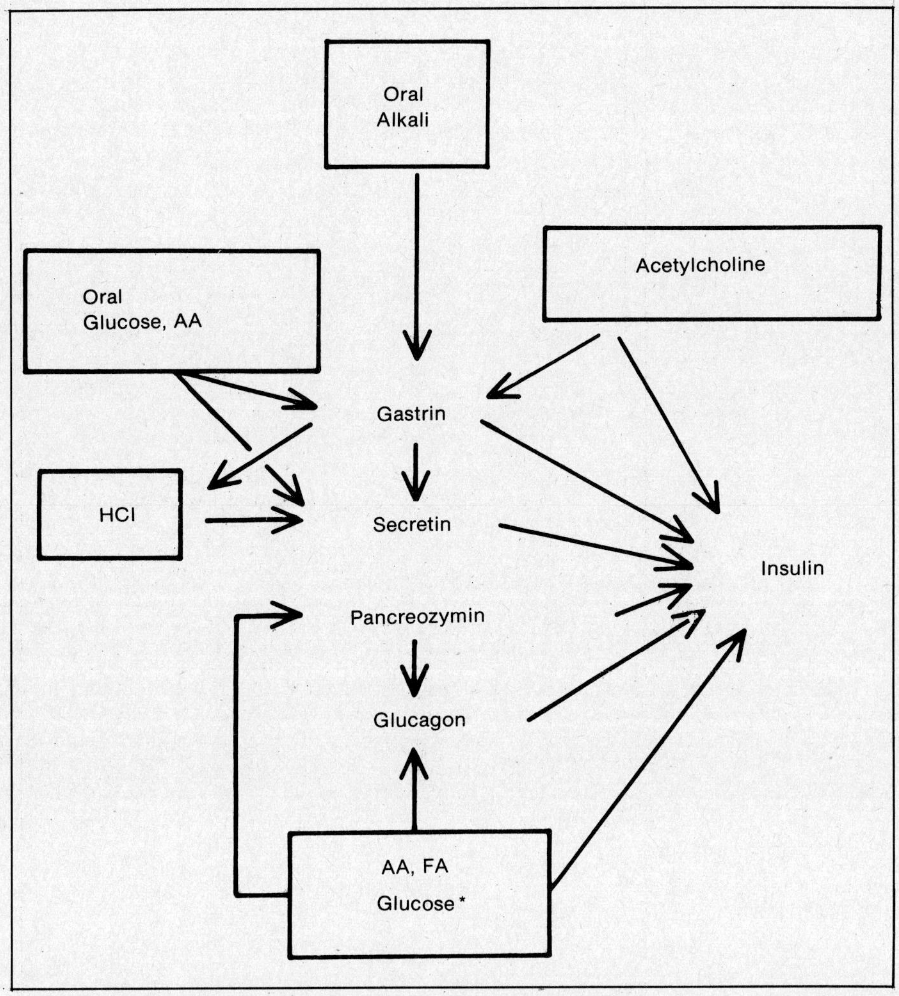

*Fig 3.—Gastrin, secretin, pancreozymin, and glucagon directly or indirectly increase insulin release. The influences of the other compounds are discussed in the text. *Glucose suppresses release of pancreatic glucagon but increases glucagon-like immunoreactivity. AA signifies amino acids; FA, fatty acids.*

it is 36:1.[69] Glucagon is very important in preventing hypoglycemia during fasting.[70] Hypoglycemia is produced by giving antiglucagon antibody to fasting rats.[71]

Many reports of plasma immunoreactive glucagon levels have not indicated correctly the amounts of pancreatic glucagon secretion, because varying amounts of glucagon-like material from the gut have reacted with the antibody used for assay. Recently, this field has been greatly clarified. Extracts of gastrointestinal tissue contain glucagon-like biological activity and glucagon-like immunoreactivity (GLI),[72,73] separable by gel infiltration into two fractions (Table 1). The similar molecular size, glycogenolytic activity, and electrophoretic behavior of peak 2 GLI and pancreatic glucagon indicate that the two substances are closely related, yet peak 2 GLI differs from the pancreatic glucagon with respect to its reactivity with certain antisera, suggesting that its molecular structure differs in some way from that of glucagon. Certain hexoses (eg, fructose, glucose) given intravenously increase GLI but decrease pancreatic glucagon.[72-74] After amino acid infusion, the pancreaticoduodenal vein plasma shows a large peak of immunoreactivity in the glucagon-^{131}I zone and a very small peak in the preinsulin-^{131}I zone. Both peaks were readily measured in the glucagon-specific assay system, indicating their pancreatic origin.

The following hormones are secreted by the gastrointestinal tract and, under one condition or another, promote insulin release[57,66,75-79]: gastrin, secretin, pancreozymin, glucagon, acetylcholine, and serotonin. A given amount of glucose administered orally causes much greater insulin release than an equivalent intravenous dose; indeed, rapid entrance of glucose into the duodenum eventually may cause hypoglycemia, apparently resulting from an excessive insulin-releasing action of gastrointestinal hormones.

Gastrin.—Gastrin is secreted by the gastric mucosa and by the pancreatic D cells.[80] Its release is increased by orally ingested glucose, amino acids, other food, alkali, insulin, and vagal stimulation (acetylcholine), and decreased by secretin, or by hydrochloric acid in the stomach or duodenum. Gastrin, directly or indirectly, rapidly increases insulin release in man and dogs. Tetragastrin briefly increases pancreaticoduodenal vein glucagon in dogs.[81]

Secretin.—Glucose, protein, HCl in the duodenum, and gastrin increase secretin release. In man, secretin increases insulin release,[79,82,83] especially in the presence of glucose. Some reports have shown that it increases insulin secretion in vitro.[84]

Pancreozymin.—Pancreozymin secretion is stimulated by fatty acids, glucose, and essential amino acids,[85] especially phenylalanine, methionine, and valine. Pancreozymin promotes gallbladder contraction and bile flow, pancreatic exocrine flow, and release of insulin and glucagon in vivo.[79,81,86-89] Perfusion of isolated rat pancreas with pancreozymin increases insulin and glucagon release.[90]

Serotonin.—Low doses of serotonin decrease insulin release and high doses increase it. Gastrin, pancreozymin, secretin, and glucagon have close chemical similarities and have several similar targets and actions in the gastrointestinal tract.[91] Pancreozymin has a much greater effect on insulin release than gastrin or secretin, and it is the only one of these three that significantly stimulates glucagon release.

Figure 3 presents the actions of several of the gastrointestinal hormones, and of other factors, on insulin secretion.

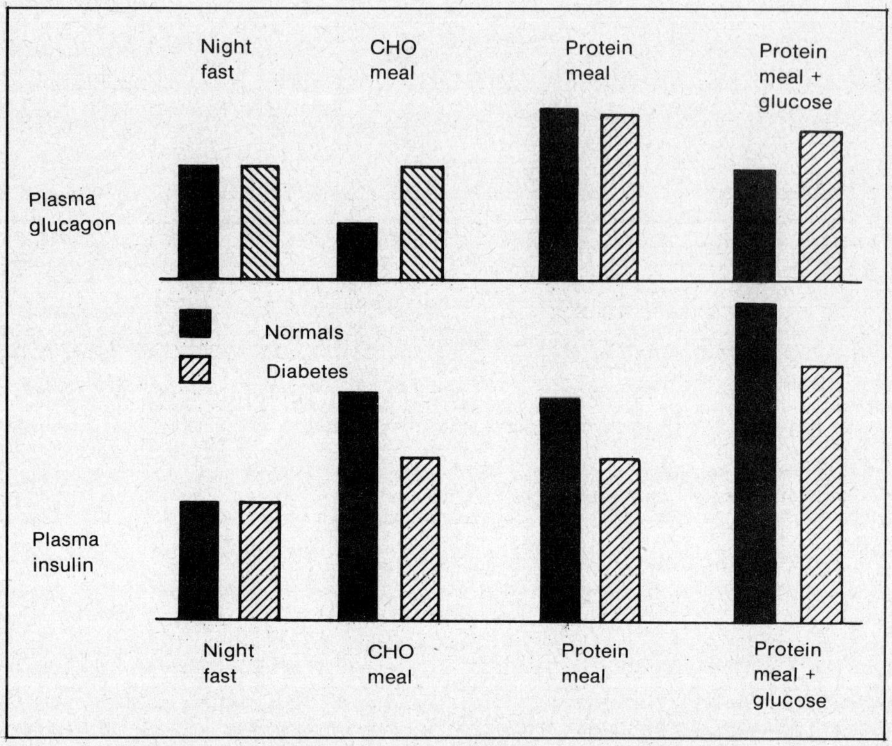

Fig 4.—This figure indicates the relative changes in plasma glucagon and insulin produced by fasting, or carbohydrate or protein meals or both. Detailed assay values are presented by Unger et al.[93] In nondiabetics a high CHO meal decreases plasma glucagon, but in diabetics it has relatively little effect. A protein meal significantly increases plasma glucagon in nondiabetics and in diabetics. Either a carbohydrate meal or a protein meal causes subnormal increases in plasma insulin levels of diabetics.

Major Factors Influencing Synthesis and Release of Insulin

Numerous compounds influence synthesis and release of insulin[58,92] (Table 2). Its secretion is stimulated by the main supplies of energy—carbohydrate, protein, and fat. Glucose, amino acid, fatty acid, glucagon, and some of the gastrointestinal hormones promote rapid insulin release. The detailed mechanism by which the compounds produce these actions is not clear, but effects upon oxidative phosphorylation are important in many ways. One result is the formation of ATP, which engages in numerous reactions, including production of c-AMP. Some compounds (eg, theophylline, glucagon, β-adrenergens) that increase insulin secretion produce an increase in c-AMP in beta cells.

Insulin and Glucagon in Prediabetes and Diabetes

After an overnight fast, the plasma level of immunoreactive (pancreatic) glucagon (IRG) is approximately 100 pg/ml in normal and diabetic people.[93] However, when sufficient glucose is given to nondiabetics to produce plasma glucose levels equal to those of diabetics, the IRG drops to 57 pg/ml (Fig 4). Arginine infusion causes much greater rises in IRG in diabetics than in nondiabetics. Diabetics have a marked increase in IRG after a protein meal, but normal subjects whose blood sugar levels are increased to diabetic levels show relatively little increase in IRG after a protein meal. A carbohydrate meal suppresses IRG in diabetics far less than in nondiabetics. Thus, in normal subjects, the glucagon level falls after ingestion of carbohydrates and rises after protein intake, unless carbohydrate-induced hyperglycemia is present. In diabetics, the glucagon level is not suppressed significantly by carbohydrate, a fact which possibly contributes to many of the metabolic abnormalities in diabetes; for example, in the diabetic state, the excess glucagon causes increased gluconeogenesis, glycogenolysis, blood sugar levels, fatty acids, and ketones. In diabetic ketoacidosis, hypernormal levels of plasma IRG are found. We cannot interpret the full significance of the glucagon changes in diabetes because we do not know to what extent they are subsidiary to, and accompanied by, other changes.

In prediabetics, following oral or intravenous administration of glucose, there often is a decrease and delayed increment in plasma immunoreactive insulin (IRI), but in some instances the response is normal and in a few even hypernormal. Since all prediabetics have normal glucose tolerance tests, those with subnormal insulin levels presumably have increased sensitivity to insulin.[94,95] These people sometimes have a normal insulin secretory response to tolbutamide, even when the response to glucose is decreased.[91,96,97] The delayed and deficient insulin response to glucose in prediabetics may be restored to normal by theophylline,[98] suggesting that c-AMP levels play a role. Healthy subjects given propranolol had delayed insulin response to glucose, simulating prediabetics; this abnormal response was reversed by theophylline.[98] Insulin release caused by tolbutamide was not inhibited by propranolol. Tolbutamide and arginine require normal blood glucose levels in order to exert their insulin-releasing activity.

In maturity-onset diabetics, after orally ingested glucose there is a delay in the initial rise in plasma IRI,[99] but the insulin apogee and the total insulin release may be high. Controversy has existed regarding the significance of the high plasma insulin levels in diabetes. Some state that when the insulin values are related to the glucose level, there is too little insulin,[99] whereas others have suggested that there is resistance to insulin action in diabetes.[100] For example, during the steady-state infusion of glucose over a period of three hours, mildly diabetic persons continue to maintain higher blood sugar levels despite relatively high levels of plasma insulin. Obese diabetics have resistance to insulin action and have high plasma levels of insulin after glucose, amino acids, or glucagon, but the levels are less than in nondiabetics of comparable weight.

The concept that diabetes may result from subnormal action of a given quantity of insulin suggests this question: Does all of the material that registers in the immunoassay have fully normal insulin structure? Based on immunologic, biologic, spectroscopic, and other studies, change in the conformation or composition of insulin or both results in a proportionate decrease of biological activity; indeed, even minor changes can alter its actions.[101]

Microangiopathy in Diabetes

Most of the morbidity and mortality in diabetes result from microangiopathy and atherosclerosis. In diabetics the basement membrane of capillaries tends to be thickened, partially owing to deposit of excess glycoproteins. Although synthesis from glucose of the carbohydrate component of glycoproteins is not directly under the regulation of insulin,[102] increased sugar levels increase glucosyltransferase, which is involved in the manufacture of hydroxylysine-linked carbohydrate units of the basement membrane. Insulin decreases this enzyme activity. The basement membranes of diabetic kidneys have a composition similar to the normal except that there is a decrease in lysine and a reciprocal increase in hydroxylsine.[103] These biochemical changes may be important in the pathogenesis of many of the chronic complications of diabetes.

Siperstein[104,105] found basement membrane thickening (BMT) in midthigh muscle capillaries in 8% of normal subjects, 98% of diabetics, and 74% of prediabetics. Similar lesions were also found in nerves, cerebral cortex, retina, pancreas, skin, and other tissues. He states the following:

BMT is found in most human diabetics. Basement membrane thickening is not affected by the duration or severity of the diabetes, the age, sex, or weight of the subject, or whether diabetes is of juvenile- or adult-onset type.

Within 20 months of implantation of a sponge in muscle, most diabetics show significant BMT in surrounding capillaries.

Most patients with diabetes resulting from chronic pancreatitis or other extensive destructive lesions of the pancreas do not develop significant BMT of the muscle capillaries.

Basement membrane thickening of glomerular capillaries is associated with hyperglycemia of pancreatitis and hemochromatosis and with the duration of such disorders, but the lesions are nonspecific; lesions in the muscle are much more specific.

Animals with spontaneous or induced diabetes do not develop significant BMT in muscle capillaries regardless of the severity or duration of the diabetes.

The associated relative hypoinsulinism in diabetes is a *result* of BMT, involving especially the pancreas.

Basement membrane thickening results from biochemical abnormalities in the synthesis or destruction of basement membrane surrounding the capillaries in most of the tissues of the body.

Others[106,107] have drawn conclusions different from those of Siperstein, particularly concerning the frequency and amount of BMT in the development and course of diabetes. They have emphasized that BMT results from insulin deficiency.

Nondiabetics and diabetics have marked variations in the thickness of the basal laminase (synonymous with basement membrane) within each specimen, between specimens from identical sites of different individuals, and between different anatomical sites in the same individual.[108] In diabetics the capillaries in muscles from the distal abdomen and proximal thigh are not thickened, but there is BMT in the muscles of the midabdomen, chest wall, hand, midthigh, mid lower leg, and foot. The increased BMT in capillaries in diabetics was found to be associated with increased laminations of the basement membrane,[109] which were presumed to result from accelerated cell death. It was suggested that the basal lamina provides a scaffolding for regenerating cells. Other observations suggest premature aging in diabetes.

In considering Siperstein's suggestion that diabetes results from decreased insulin passage through pancreatic vessels,[105] it is of note that insulin I^{131} injected subcutaneously in the thigh of diabetic patients enters the blood stream at a normal rate.[110]

Diagnosis and Treatment

Most diagnostic tests for diabetes are based upon hypernormal blood glucose levels. The oral and the intravenous glucose tolerance tests, the cortisone glucose tolerance test, and the tolbutamide tolerance test have been useful, with the oral glucose test used most.[111] Since "diabetic" angiopathies may develop years before abnormal blood sugar values are found, a very important phase of diabetes presumably progresses before the main criterion for diagnosis is manifested. Therefore, earlier chemical changes must be explored, including abnormalities in the metabolism of proteins, nucleotides, metals, and lipids. Because of problems in the early diagnosis of diabetes, its prevalence has not been determined accurately.

Because diabetes presumably results predominantly from genetic defect(s), its occurrence varies markedly among peoples. It occurs more often in Pima Indians than in any other group (> 50% using standard diagnostic criteria).[112] With oral glucose tolerance tests in the adults, the two-hour blood sugar level was bimodal, with an antimode around 200 mg/100 ml in males and one somewhat higher in females. Even with two-hour values above 200 mg/100 ml in males and 250 in females used as criteria, more than 35% of these people have diabetes. The relatively high prevalence of retinopathy and nephropathy emphasizes the intensity of the diabetes.

Therapies in diabetes have included dietary restrictions, sulfonylureas, biguanides, and insulin, but their effects, beneficial or deleterious, have not been completely evaluated. Knowles[113] indicates that most relevant opinions are based upon personal impressions and observations. Studies commonly fail to provide adequate controls to maintain a given type of experimental design, to acquire complete data, to remove investigator bias, and to take other important objective measures.

The main goal of the University Group Diabetes Program was to ascertain whether control of the blood glucose level helps to prevent or delay vascular disease in diabetics not requiring insulin for antiketoacidosis.[1] The 823 patients were divided into four groups: (*a*) those receiving sufficient insulin to maintain "normal" blood glucose levels; (*b*) those receiving a set amount of insulin, 10 to 16 units per day, depending upon body surface; (*c*) those receiving 1.5 gm per day of tolbutamide; and (*d*) those receiving placebo. All were on prescribed diets with caloric contents adjusted to achieve and maintain normal body weight. Control of the blood glucose level was best in the patients with the adjustable insulin dosage, poorest in the placebo group, and about equal for the tolbutamide and insulin standard groups. The percentage mortality from all causes combined among 181 of the patients after 8.8 years was as follows: 8.8 for the insulin-regulated group, 9.5 for the insulin standard group, 10.2 for the placebo group, and 14.7 for the tolbutamide group. The percentage cardiovascular mortality was 5.9 for the insulin-regulated group, 6.2 for the insulin standard group, 4.9 for the placebo group, and 12.7 for the tolbutamide group. The investigators in this study agreed that "the findings of this study provide no evidence that the combination of diet and tolbutamide therapy used for treatment of mild noninsulin-dependent diabetics is more effective than diet alone, except for lowering blood glucose levels," and that "the findings suggest that tolbutamide and diet may be less effective than diet alone or than diet and insulin, at least insofar as cardiovascular mortality is concerned." These observations have led to recommendations that tolbutamide no longer be used for prolonged therapy, but some other diabetologists indicate that its favorable effects outweigh its disadvantages. More information is required to determine the net status of therapy. There is no justification for concluding that other sulfonylureas have the same long-range adverse effects as tolbutamide.

Certainly, insulin has prolonged the lives of many patients, particularly those with ketoacidosis, but we have insufficient objective data regarding the ultimate advantages and disadvantages of its prolonged usage in mild diabetes. There are times when its actions are excessive but not recognized.

Weight reduction is advantageous in obese patients, but what *type* of diet is most appropriate in obese or normal-weight diabetics is not clear. A low carbohydrate-high fat diet lowers the blood glucose level and improves symptoms in some patients, but it sometimes increases plasma triglyceride. A high carbohydrate-low fat diet increases the blood sugar level in others, but it sometimes improves glucose tolerance. In a prospective ten-year study using unmeasured diet in juvenile-onset diabetics, the prevalence of degenerative complications was similar to that reported with the use of restricted diet, and the general course of the disease was similar.[114]

The gaps in our knowledge of the etiology, pathogenesis, course, diagnosis, and treatment of diabetes, combined with long-time publication of unsubstantiated statements, but physicians in a distressing position. At best, treatment has been poor, permitting frequent blindness, coronary thrombosis, uremia, etc. We are justified in giving insulin daily to those with moderately severe or severe diabetes. Although questions prevail concerning the best treatment for the others, we are compelled to proceed with what *seems* to be the best treatment. Present choices in our clinic are (*a*) *diet*—attempt to attain and maintain a normal body weight. Give somewhat more than average protein and less than average carbohydrate (unmeasured) and relatively little free sugar; (*b*) *exercise*—regular daily exercise; (*c*) *Sulfonylureas and phenformin hydrochloride*—use either chlorpropamide, tolazamide, or acetohexamide in conservative doses, and tolbutamide rarely; (*d*) *insulin*—use when the blood glucose level is not appropriately controlled otherwise. Insulin zinc suspension is used most often, with three intermediate feedings and three meals. However, we repeat that much more data is required for appropriate management. Meanwhile, all drugs should usually be used in moderation.

The University Group Diabetes Program has now reported (*JAMA* **217**:777-784, 1971) that the mortality from all causes, and from cardiovascular causes per se, was higher in the phenformin group than in the other treatment groups, including diet alone.

This study was supported in part by Public Health Service grants AM-05020 and AM-02456 from the National Institute of Arthritis and Metabolic Diseases.

Nonproprietary and Trade Names of Drugs

Tolazamide—*Tolinase*.

References

1. The University Group Diabetes Program: A study of the effects of hypoglycemic agents on vascular complications in patients with adult-onset diabetes: II. Mortality results. *Diabetes* **19**(suppl):789-830, 1970.
2. Pictet RL, Clark WR, Williams RH, et al: Electron microscopic study of the histogenesis and cytodifferentiation of the developing embryonic pancreas. *J Cell Biol*, to be published.
3. Clark WR: *The Synthesis and Accumulation of Insulin in the Rat Embryo During Development*, thesis. University of Washington, Seattle, 1968.
4. Lacy PE: Beta cell secretion: From the standpoint of a pathobiologist. Read before the American Diabetes Association, St. Louis, 1970.
5. Gomez-Acebo J, Parrilla R, R-Candela JL: Fine structure of the A and D cells of the rabbit endocrine pancreas in vivo and incubated in vitro: I. Mechanism of secretion of the A cells. *J Cell Biol* **36**:33-44, 1968.
6. Rutter WJ, Clark WR, Kemp JD, et al: Multiphasic regulation in cytodifferentiation, in Fleischmajer (ed): *Epithelial-Mesenchymal Interactions*. Baltimore, Williams & Wilkins Co, 1968, pp 114-131.
7. Brock LC, Clark WR, Williams RH, et al: Embryonic development of the endocrine pancreas: I. Analysis of hormonal levels. *Diabetes* **18**(suppl): 321, 1969.
8. Espinosa de los Monteros MA, Driscoll SG, Steinke J: Insulin release from isolated human fetal pancreatic islets. *Science* **168**:1111-1112, 1970.
9. Adam PAJ, Teramo K, Raiha N, et al: Human fetal insulin metabolism early in gestation. *Diabetes* **18**:409-416, 1969.
10. Lacy PE: Functional morphology of the islet cells, in Cerasi E, Luft R (eds): *Pathogenesis of Diabetes Mellitus (Nobel Symposium No. 13)*. Stockholm, Almqvist & Wiksell, 1970, pp 109-122.
11. Renold AE: Insulin biosynthesis and secretion: A still unsettled topic. *New Eng J Med* **282**:173-182, 1970.
12. Steiner DF, Clark JL, Nolan C, et al: The biosynthesis of insulin and some speculations regarding the pathogenesis of human diabetes, in Cerasi E, Luft R (eds): *Pathogenesis of Diabetes Mellitus (Nobel Symposium No. 13)*. Stockholm, Almqvist & Wiksell, 1970, pp 57-80.
13. Steiner DF, Oyer P, Cho S, et al: Structural and immunological studies on human proinsulin. Read before the International Diabetes Federation, Buenos Aires, 1970.
14. Chance RE: Chemical, physical, biological, and immunological studies on porcine proinsulin and related polypeptides. Read before the International Diabetes Federation, Buenos Aires, 1970.
15. Tanese T, Lazarus NR, Devrim S, et al: Synthesis and release of proinsulin and insulin by isolated rat islets of Langerhans. *J Clin Invest* **49**:1394-1404, 1970.
16. Rastogi GK, Letarte J, Fraser TR: Proinsulin content of pancreas in human fetuses of healthy mothers. *Lancet* **1**:7-9, 1970.
17. Stoll RW, Touber JL, Menahan LA, et al: Clearance of porcine insulin, proinsulin, and connecting peptide by the isolated rat liver. *Proc Soc Exp Biol Med* **133**:894-896, 1970.
18. Lazarus NR, Penhos JC, Tanese T, et al: (A) Studies on the biological activity of porcine proinsulin. *J Clin Invest* **49**:487-496, 1970.
19. Lavis VR, Ensinck JW, Williams RH: Effects of insulin and proinsulin on isolated fat cells and hemidiaphragms from rats. *Endocrinology* **87**:135-142, 1970.
20. Challoner DR, Yu P: Differential effect of porcine on rat epididymal fat cells and fat pieces. *Diabetes* **19**:289-295, 1970.
21. Kitabchi AE: The biological and immunological properties of pork and beef insulin, proinsulin, and connecting peptides. *J Clin Invest* **49**:979-987, 1970.
22. Melani F, Rubenstein AH, Steiner DF: Human serum proinsulin. *J Clin Invest* **49**:497-507, 1970.
23. Gorden P, Roth J: Circulating insulins. *Arch Intern Med* **123**:237-247, 1969.

24. Gorden P, Roth J: Plasma insulin: Fluctuations in the "big" insulin component in man after glucose and other stimuli. *J Clin Invest* **48**:2225-2234, 1969.

25. Stoll RW, Touber JL, Ensinck JW, et al: Porcine insulin, proinsulin, and connecting peptide response to various stimuli. *J Clin Invest* **49**:93a, 1970.

26. O'Brien D: Evidence for an abnormal insulin in diabetes mellitus, in Camerini-Davalos RA, Cole HS (eds): *Early Diabetes*. New York, Academic Press Inc, 1970, suppl 1, pp 135-140.

27. Aleyassine H: Energy requirements for insulin release from rat pancreas in vitro. *Endocrinology* **87**:84-89, 1970.

28. Randle PJ: Islet metabolism and insulin secretion. Read before the International Diabetes Federation, Buenos Aires, 1970.

29. Milner RDG, Hales CN: The mechanism of insulin secretion studied through the effects of electrolytes and inhibitors, in Camerini-Davalos RA, Cole HS (eds): *Early Diabetes*. New York, Academic Press Inc, 1970, suppl 1, pp 59-69.

30. Grey NJ, Goldring S, Kipnis DM: Evidence for a glucose-inducible glucoreceptor for insulin secretion in the rat, in Cerasi E, Luft R (eds): *Pathogenesis of Diabetes Mellitus (Nobel Symposium No. 13)*. Stockholm, Almqvist & Wiksell, 1970, pp 155-172.

31. Matschinsky FM, Ellerman JE: Metabolism of glucose in the islets of Langerhans. *J Biol Chem* **243**:2730-2736, 1968.

32. Montague W, Taylor KW: Islet-cell metabolism during insulin release. *Biochem J* **115**:257-262, 1969.

33. Hellman B, Idahl L-A. Danielsson A: Adenosine triphosphate levels of mammalian pancreatic B cells after stimulation with glucose and hypoglycemia sulfonylureas. *Diabetes* **18**:509-516, 1969.

34. Taylor KW, Montague W: The synthesis, storage and release of insulin, in Cerasi E, Luft R (eds): *Pathogenesis of Diabetes Mellitus (Nobel Symposium No. 13)*. Stockholm, Almqvist & Wiksell, 1970, pp 123-136.

35. Goldsmith SJ, Yalow RS, Berson SA: Effects of 2-deoxy-D-glucose on insulin-secretory responses to intravenous glucose, glucagon, tolbutamide and arginine in man. *Diabetes* **19**:453-457, 1970.

36. Turtle JR, Kipnis DM: An adrenergic receptor mechanism for the control of cyclic 3′5′ adenosine. *Biochem Biophys Res Commun* **28**:797-802, 1967.

37. Park CR, Sneyd JGT, Corbin JD, et al: Role of cyclic adenylate in the actions of insulin, in Ostman J, Milner RDG (eds): *Diabetes*. Amsterdam, Excerpta Medica Foundation, 1969, pp 5-15.

38. Sutherland EW, Robison GA: The role of cyclic AMP in the control of carbohydrate metabolism. *Diabetes* **18**:797-819, 1969.

39. Ensinck JW, Stoll RW, Gale CC, et al: Effect of aminophylline on the secretion of insulin, glucagon, luteinizing hormone and growth hormone in humans. *J Clin Endocr* **31**:153-161, 1970.

40. Cerasi E, Luft R: Further studies on prediabetes. Read before the International Diabetes Federation, Buenos Aires, 1970.

41. Allan W, Tepperman HM: Stimulation of insulin secretion in the rat by glucagon, secretin and pancreozymin: Effect of aminophylline. *Life Sci* **8**:307-317, 1969.

42. Grodsky G, Landhal H, Curry D, et al: A two-compartmental model for insulin secretion, in Camerini-Davalos RA, Cole HS (eds): *Early Diabetes*. New York, Academic Press Inc, 1970, suppl 1, pp 45-50.

43. Curry DL, Bennett LL, Grodsky GM: Dynamics of insulin secretion by the perfused rat pancreas. *Endocrinology* **83**:572-584, 1968.

44. Porte D, Pupo AA: Insulin responses to glucose: Evidence for a two pool system in man. *J Clin Invest* **48**:2309-2319, 1969.

45. Ryan WG, Nibbe AF, Schwartz TB: Beta-cytotrophic effects of glucose, glucagon, and tolbutamide in man. *Lancet* **1**:1255-1256, 1967.

46. Logothetopoulos J, Davidson JK, Haist RE, et al: Degranulation of beta cells and loss of pancreatic insulin after infusions of insulin antibody of glucose. *Diabetes* **14**:493-500, 1965.

47. Sodoyez J-C, Sodoyez-Goffaux F, Foa PP: Evidence for an insulin-induced inhibition of insulin release by isolated islets of Langerhans. Proc Soc Exp Biol Med **130**:568-571, 1969.

48. Milner RDG, Hales CN: The role of calcium and magnesium in insulin secretion from rabbit pancreas studied in vitro. *Diabetologia* **3**:47-49, 1967.

49. Coore HG, Hellman B, Pihl E, et al: Physiochemical characteristics of insulin secretion granules. *Biochem J* **111**:107-113, 1969.

50. Falkmer S, Havu N, Boquist L: Role of sulfhydryl compounds and heavy metals in the synthesis and storage of insulin, in Falkmer S, Hellman B, Taljedal I-B (eds): *The Structure and Metabolism of the Pancreatic Islets: A Centennial of Paul Langerhan's Discovery*. Oxford, England, Pergamon Press Inc, 1970, pp 203-212.

51. Fajans SS, Floyd JC Jr, Knopf RF, et al: Effects of amino acids on insulin release in vivo. Read before the International Diabetes Federation, Buenos Aires, 1970.

52. Fajans SS, Floyd JC Jr, Knopf RF, et al: Effect of amino acids and proteins on insulin secretion in man. *Recent Progr Hormone Res* **23**:617-662, 1967.

53. Floyd JC Jr, Fajans SS, Pek S, et al: Synergistic effect of essential amino acids and glucose upon insulin secretion in man. *Diabetes* **19**:109-115, 1970.

54. Milner RDG: Stimulation of insulin secretion in vitro by essential amino acids. *Lancet* **1**:1075-1076, 1969.

55. Crespin SR, Greenough WB III, Steinberg D: Stimulation of insulin secretion by infusion on free fatty acids. *J Clin Invest* **48**:1934-1943, 1969.

56. Porte D Jr: Sympathetic regulation of insulin secretion. *Arch Intern Med* **123**:252-260, 1969.

57. Porte D Jr, Bagdade JD: Human insulin secretion: An integrated approach. *Ann Rev Med* **21**:219-240, 1970.

58. Malaisse WJ, Malaisse-Lagae F, Wright PH: Diabetogenesis, in Camerini-Davalos, Cole HS (eds): *Early Diabetes*. New York, Academic Press Inc, 1970, pp 79-85.

59. Vance JE, Buchanan KD, Williams RH: Glucagon and insulin release: Influence of drugs affecting the autonomic nervous system. *Diabetes* **20**:78-82, 1971.

60. Lazarus SS, Shapiro S, Volk BW: Secretory granule formation and release in rabbit pancreatic a-cells. *Diabetes* **17**:152-160, 1968.

61. Curry DL: Glucagon potentiation of insulin secretion by the perfused rat pancreas. *Diabetes* **19**:420-428, 1970.

62. Bromer WW, Chance RE: Zinc glucagon depression of blood amino acids in rabbits. *Diabetes* **18**:748-754, 1969.

63. Lefebvre PJ, Cession-Fossion AM, Luyckx AS, et al: Interrelationships of glucagon-adrenergic system in experimental and clinical conditions. *Arch Inter Pharmacodyn* **172**:393-404, 1968.

64. Foá P: The secretion of glucagon in vitro and vivo. Read before the International Diabetes Federation, Buenos Aires, 1970.

65. Madison LL, Seyffert WA Jr, Unger RH, et al: Effect of plasma free fatty acids on plasma glucagon and serum insulin concentrations. *Metabolism* **17**:301-304, 1968.

66. Buchanan KD, Vance JE, Morgan A: Effect of pancreozymin on insulin and glucagon levels in blood and bile. *Amer J Physiol* **215**:1293-1298, 1968.

67. Samols E, Tyler JM, Kajinuma H: Influence of the sulfonamides on pancreatic humoral secretion and evidence for an insulin-glucagon feedback system. Read before the International Diabetes Federation, Buenos Aires, 1970.

68. Samols E, Tyler JM, Mialhe P: Suppression of pancreatic glucagon release by the hypoglycemic sulphonylureas. *Lancet* **1**:174-176, 1969.

69. Unger RH, Faloona GR: The roles of pancreatic glucagon in health and diabetes mellitus. Read before the International Diabetes Federation, Buenos Aires, 1970.

70. Levy LJ, Spergel G, Bleicher SJ: Glucagon deficient man: Model for the role of glucagon in fasting, in *Proceedings of the 52nd Annual Meeting of the Endocrine Society*, St. Louis, 1970, p 134.

71. Grey N, McGuigan JE, Kipnis DM: Neutralization of endogenous glucagon by high titer glucagon antiserum. *Endocrinology* **86**:1383-1388, 1970.

72. Valverde I, Rigopoulou D, Marco J, et al: Characterization of glucagon-like immunoreactivity (GLI). *Diabetes* **19**:614-623, 1970.

73. Valverde I, Rigopolou D, Marco J, et al: Molecular size of extractable glucagon and glucagon-like immunoreactivity (GLI) in plasma. *Diabetes* **19**:624-629, 1970.

74. Assan R: Study of some factors affecting secretion and catabolism of glucagon. Read before the International Diabetes Federation, Buenos Aires, 1970.

75. Forssmann WG, Orci L, Pictet R, et al: The endocrine cells in the epithelium of the gastrointestinal mucosa of the rat. *J Cell Biol* **40**:692-715, 1969.

76. Orci L, Pictet R, Forssmann WG, et al: Structural evidence of glucagon producing cells in the intestinal mucosa of the rat. *Diabetologia* **4**:56, 1968.

77. Frohman LA: The endocrine function of the pancreas. *Ann Rev Physiol* **31**:353-382, 1969.

78. Levine R: Mechanisms of insulin secretion. *New Eng J Med* **283**:522-526, 1970.

79. Dupre J, Curtis JD, Unger RH, et al: Effects of secretin, pancreozymin, or gastrin on the response of the endocrine pancreas to administration of glucose or arginine in man. *J Clin Invest* **48**:745-757, 1969.

80. Lomsky R, Langr F, Vortel V: Immunohistochemical demonstration of gastrin in mammalian islets of Langerhans. *Nature* **223**:618-619, 1969.

81. Kaneto A, Mizuno Y, Tasaka Y, et al: Stimulation of glucagon secretion by tetragastrin. *Endocrinology* **86**:1175-1180, 1970.

82. Dupré J: Regulation of the secretions of the pancreas. *Ann Rev Med* **21**:299-316, 1970.

83. Chisholm DJ, Young JD, Lazarus L: The gastrointestinal stimulus to insulin release: I. Secretin. *J Clin Invest* **48**:1453-1460, 1969.

84. Kraegen EW, Chisholm DJ, Young JD, et al: The gastrointestinal stimulus to insulin release: II. A dual action of secretin. *J Clin Invest* **49**:524-529, 1970.

85. Go VLW, Hofmann AF, Summerskill WHJ: Pancreozymin bioassay in man based on pancreatic enzyme secretion: Potency of specific amino acids and other digestive products. *J Clin Invest* **49**:1558-1564, 1970.

86. Grossman MI: Gastrin, cholecystokinin, and secretin act on one receptor. *Lancet* **1**:1088-1089, 1970.

87. Lazarus NR, Voyles NR, Devrim S, et al: Extragastrointestinal effects of secretin, gastrin, and pancreozymin. *Lancet* **2**:248-250, 1968.

88. Unger RH, Eisentraut AM: Enteroinsular axis. *Arch Intern Med* **123**:261-266, 1969.

89. Creutzfeldt W, Feurle G, Ketterer H: Effect of gastrointestinal hormones on insulin and glucagon secretion. *New Eng J Med* **282**:1139-1141, 1970.

90. Fussganger RD, Straub K, Goberna R, et al: Primary secretion of insulin and secondary release of glucagon from the isolated perfused rat pancreas following stimulation with pancreozymin. *Horm Metab Res* **1**:224-227, 1969.

91. Grossman MI: Physiological role of gastrin. *Fed Proc* **27**:1312-1313, 1968.

92. Williams RH, Ensinck JW: Secretion, fates and actions of insulin and related products. *Diabetes* **15**:623-654, 1966.

93. Unger RH, Aguilar-Parada E, Muller WA, et al: Studies of pancreatic alpha cell function in normal and diabetic subjects. *J Clin Invest* **49**:837-848, 1970.

94. Kipnis DM: Does diabetes begin with insulin resistance? in Cerasi E, Luft R (eds): *Pathogenesis of Diabetes Mellitus (Nobel Symposium No. 13)*. Stockholm, Almqvist & Wiksell, 1970, pp 45-56.

95. Kipnis DM: Insulin secretion in diabetes mellitus. *Ann Intern Med* **69**:891-901, 1968.

96. Serrano-Rios M, Ramos F, Rodriguez-Miñon JL, et al: Studies in prediabetes: Insulin response to oral glucose, intravenous tolbutamide and rapid intravenous glucose infusion in genetic prodiabetics. *Diabetologia* **6**:392-398, 1970.

97. Rojas L, Soeldner JS, Gleason RE, et al: Offspring of two diabetic parents: Differential serum insulin responses to intravenous glucose and tolbutamide. *J Clin Endocr* **29**:1569-1579, 1969.

98. Cerasi E, Luft R: Diabetes mellitus: A disorder of cellular information transmission? in Cerasi E, Luft R (eds): *Pathogenesis of Diabetes Mellitus (Nobel Symposium No. 13)*. Stockholm, Almqvist & Wiksell, 1970, pp 349-354.

99. Varsano-Aharon N, Echemedia E. Yalow RS, et al: Early insulin responses to glucose and to tolbutamide in maturity-onset diabetes. *Metabolism* **19**:409-417, 1970.

100. Reaven GM, Farquhar JW: Steady state plasma insulin response to continuous glucose infusion in normal and diabetic subjects. *Diabetes* **18**:273-279, 1969.

101. Arquilla ER, Bromer WW, Mercola D: Immunology conformation and biological activity of insulin. *Diabetes* **18**:193-205, 1969.

102. Spiro RG: Glycoproteins: Their biochemistry, biology and role in human disease. *New Eng J Med* **281**:991-1001, 1969.

103. Beisswenger PJ, Spiro RG: Human glomerular basement membrane: Chemical alteration in diabetes mellitus. *Science* **168**:596-598, 1970.

104. Siperstein MD: The relationship of carbohydrate derangements to the microangiopathy of diabetes, in Cerasi E, Luft R (eds): *Pathogenesis of Diabetes Mellitus (Nobel Symposium No. 13)*. Stockholm, Almqvist & Wiksell, 1970, pp 81-102.

105. Siperstein MD: Recent studies on capillary basement membrane of the diabetic. Read before the International Diabetes Federation, Buenos Aires, 1970.

106. Ireland JT: Diagnostic criteria in the assessment of glomerular capillary basement membrane lesions in newly diagnosed juvenile diabetics, in Camerini-Davalos, Cole HS (eds): *Early Diabetes*. New York, Academic Press Inc, 1970, suppl, pp 273-278.

107. Bloodworth JMB Jr, Engerman RL, Camerini-Davalos RA, et al: Variations in capillary basement membrane width produced by aging and diabetes mellitus, in Camerini-Davalos RA, Cole HS (eds): *Early Diabetes*. New York, Academic Press Inc, 1970, suppl, pp 279-295.

108. Vracko R: Skeletal muscle capillaries in diabetes. *Circulation* **41**:271-283, 1970.

109. Vracko R, Benditt EP: Capillary basal lamina thickening: Its relationship to endothelial cell death and replacement. *J Cell Biol* **47**:281-285, 1970.

110. Balodimos MC, Williams RH: Absorption of insulin I^{131} from subcutaneous tissue in diabetic patients. *Amer J Med Sci* **243**:49-56, 1962.

111. Kahn CB, Soeldner JS, Gleason RE, et al: Clinical and chemical diabetes in offspring of diabetic couples. *New Eng J Med* **281**:343-347, 1969.

112. Bennett PH, Burch TA, Miller M: Hyperglycemia in North American (Pima) Indians: Diabetes mellitus or not? Read before the International Diabetes Federation, Buenos Aires, 1970.

113. Knowles, cited by Ricketts HT: The influence of diabetic control on angiopathy, in Leibel BS, Wrenshall GA (eds): *On the Nature and Treatment of Diabetes*. Amsterdam, Excerpta Medical Foundation, 1965, pp 588-600.

114. Knowles HC Jr, Guest GM, Lampe J, et al: The course of juvenile diabetes treated with unmeasured diet. *Diabetes* **14**:239-273, 1965.

Editorial

The Challenge and the Opportunities of the Weed System

There is a refreshing enthusiasm abroad in internal medicine these days, vibrant and challenging. It is the enthusiasm for the Weed system, that manner of approach to the keeping of patient records which Lawrence Weed, MD, has so forcefully expounded. To a certain extent, the enthusiasm has managed to override all the anxieties and concerns occasioned by budgetary cuts and freezes. It has put a theme of purposeful pride into many distant corners and it has stirred young students and old professors alike to think more sharply and to work more precisely. Larry Weed's way has become a professional cause for many thoughtful men.

The story, although familiar to many now, merits retelling. Weed, an established bench scientist in the Department of Microbiology at Western Reserve, maintained his continued concern for clinical training. In the early 1960s he began to catalyze a generation of students at Metropolitan General Hospital by patrolling the wards of Charles Rammelkamp's service and asking that all clinical issues be treated as precisely as any other significant scientific problem. He cajoled, probed, badgered, alerted, and inspired the students and house staff of that department to change their way of record keeping and approach to patients. He pointed out that there is absolutely no way to know what a physician thinks, plans, and does with his patients other than to have it written down in the record. He made it clear that if the physician approaches the patient's problems in a way analogous to the bench scientist—be specific about the problem, record accurately each detail of observation that relates to that problem, state clearly what next steps in the pursuit of the problem are being planned, and indicate when a problem has either been resolved or remains uncertain—then the scientific method will more likely become an integral part of every patient's care. He wrote down some of his thoughts of these matters and they appeared in the *Irish Journal of Medical Sciences*, a much respected but not a widely read publication.[1]

Gradually others took up the

cause. Weed himself began to travel and to demonstrate to the staffs that he visited that patients' charts were woefully imprecise and that most of what physicians do and think is undocumented. He urged that people change their ways, and though many physicians agreed and some made the attempt, it was clearly hard for both the young and the old to learn new techniques. His forum grew, however, and he synthesized and summarized his ideas in a set of articles in *The New England Journal of Medicine*[2] and in a handbook monograph.[3] Two very busy and effective practitioners put his method into action in their office practice, and they described the highly gratifying effects that this approach had on their professional performance.[4] And now a series of medical centers and hospitals are following suit, with Willis Hurst, MD, at Emory, being both a very articulate proponent[5,6] and an organizer of a national teaching conference to demonstrate the educational and quality control value of the Weed system.

Why should there be all this stir about record keeping? How can a method of charting and clinical recording really be so significant? For, after all, will the disordered biology of man that constitutes his diseases and his distresses be any better understood by a new approach to record keeping? Scientific research and advance means the identification of new substantive themes and newly discovered processes. It is unlikely that a good journalist—no matter how accurate—will uncover a find unless he is actually studying the biological processes with biological techniques. Weed's answers to these very questions would be to agree that his method of data recording is nothing more than that—a technique for clinical record keeping. But he would quickly add—as would his adherents—that the first step in ever achieving a successful scientific approach to many clinical problems is to be very sure just what the problem is and to note as detailedly and as accurately as possible just what we are now doing and not doing about these problems. In effect, then, the Weed system provides us with a way in which to organize our thoughts so we can more effectively organize our care and our research pursuits. This seems so common-sensical and patently necessary that there can hardly be any further argument about the scientific value of the Weed system.

Two other very important consequences of the Weed approach to record-keeping also must be emphasized and appreciated. The first is the utility of his method for the computerization of patient information and the development of a truly up-to-date national library of clinical medicine. The second is the ability of the profession to provide a monitoring and auditing of medical care that would permit continuous surveillance of medical practice. The Weed system allows for assessment of the scientific bases for clinical decisions and thereby reexamination and recertification of the practicing physician.

The delineation of specific clinical problems by number and the consistent ordering of observations and assessments in a preset manner make it possible for each patient's experience of care to be placed into a specific file on the computer. Weed's group has designed a program that allows for complete identification of the patient's characteristics both as part of that individual's health record and also as one entry in a comprehensive collection of all the comparable clinical characteristics that many different patients display. Thus, not only is a computer library developed for the life health history of any one individual, but a library of clinical experiences for all patients is arrayed according to process and action. In effect, each patient's course becomes a chapter in the file that can be analyzed according to topic and scientific issue. Only on a computer could such a massive amount of information be stored, and yet be so continuously accessible for analysis. Patient's records, therefore, become actual elements in an up-to-date library of clinical medicine. With the development of this technique, it now becomes possible for the clinical experiences of all physicians to become part of the national experience. The observation of a patient in one area and in one institution can be collated and analyzed with the observations made on patients at any other place and locale, no matter how distant geographically. What is learned about patients in San Francisco can be immediately compared with patient data in New York, Boston, Chicago, Boise, Burlington, etc. Nationwide clinical experiences thus become components in a truly national library. The occurrence of various syndromes, the use of a wide variety of treatments, the consequences of a wide diversity of procedures—all can be subject to on-line assessment and evaluation. What has been accomplished for the airline industry could be comparably accomplished for the health care activities of the nation. This is no pipe dream. The techniques and hardware are available. The commitment and dollar investment are what is needed now. The anatomy of the Weed system has made such a function possible.

As for the ability to audit and monitor medical practice: there is the real power in the Weed method. If a physician records thoroughly what he is thinking and what he is doing about each of his patient's problems, and if he arrays all those formulations in a manner which makes it possible to track his course unmistakably, then it becomes possible to review that record and make an independent assessment or evaluation of that physician's pattern of clinical behavior. The more structured the record, the more critical and precise may be the analysis. The more complete the data base, the more thorough the evaluation. The Weed record allows the physician to be examined by his colleagues in a continuous manner. It makes it possible for each patient's care to be reviewed and compared to a set of standard criteria for the specific problem under management. What it all means, of course, is that the graduate physician's clinical care can be subject to constant assessment, a career-long reexamination and recertification. And thus the day-to-day activities of the physician, throughout his entire life span as a clinician, may become continuously educational.

The consequences of rigorous patient assessment—an audit of what has and is being done about the specific problems in the specific patient—can only be salutary for both the patients and the clinician. We have never had any long-term, continuous, quality control for the practice of internal medicine. Once a man graduates, completes his training and takes his board examinations, he, for all intents and purposes, is finished with critical peer review. True enough, flagrant wayward paths are monitored—but it has been possible for a physician to practice internal medicine and not ever again be reassessed during all of his post-certification years. The use of formalized patient records, the patterning of these records according to the Weed method, the storage of these records on a computer, the ability to cross-check and cross-assess these records with established bench marks—all of this now makes it possible to evaluate the practice of medicine at any point in time. It would mean that we could continue to learn from what we are doing, that we could maintain an intellectual formality and design that is sure to lead to more expert care. It is clear that the Weed method asks much of us in terms of redesigning our methods of data-recording. It also means that it promises ever so much more in the understanding and improvement of patient care. It is because of these opportunities that the Weed approach evokes such an enthusiastic response. As we make new adjustments in the many phases of clinical medicine—in the delivery system, in the organization of the practice community, in the arrangements governing payments—we should also take up the challenge for a uniform and comprehensive system of record-keeping that Larry Weed has placed before us. That means we should institute his technique as widely as possible throughout the nation.

M.D.B.

References

1. Weed LL: Medical records, patient care, and medical education. *Irish J Med Sci* **6**:271-282, 1964.
2. Weed LL: Medical records that guide and teach. *New Eng J Med* **278**:593-600, 652-657, 1968.
3. Weed LL: *Medical Records, Medical Education, and Patient Care: The Problem-Oriented Record as a Basic Tool.* Cleveland, Press of Case Western Reserve University, 1969.
4. Bjorn JC, Cross HD: *Problem Oriented Practice.* Chicago, Modern Hospital Press, McGraw-Hill Publications, 1970.
5. Hurst JW: Ten reasons why Lawrence Weed is right. *New Eng J Med* **284**:51-52, 1971.
6. Hurst JW: How to implement the Weed system. *Arch Intern Med* **128**:456-462, 1971.

Books

Endoscopic Color Atlas of Gastric Diseases. By Shinroku Ashizawa, MD; Tsutomuu Kidokoro, MD. Price, not given. Pp 223. Intercontinental Medical Book Corporation, 381 Park Ave S, New York 10016, 1970.

Living in Hawaii, one becomes impressed by the Japanese. No one would attempt to categorize a race; there are as many variations in individuals as there are people. But over many years of observation one gains an overall impression that is inescapable. And words such as humility, industry, meticulousness, and integrity keep creeping into descriptions.

In recent years the reborn Japanese nation has emerged as a successful international competitor in dozens of industrial enterprises. I have watched with interest the evolution of their medical publications, and I have noted the same ability to learn from others—and then improve upon it—and then make it cheaper—which has been the hallmark of their success in commerce.

This book is a prime example: a remarkable compilation of gastrocamera color photographs, gross pathology photos, and diagrams. The fibre-optic endoscope is a Japanese invention; it has revolutionized gastrointestinal and bronchial endoscopy. In the past the principal resistance to more widespread application of endoscopy was the ordeal endured by the patient due to the rigid instrument, the limitations in what one could see, and the problems of interpreting what often was a fleeting, poorly illuminated glimpse of the area of pathology. The skilled scope-wielder was a prized commodity in the medical community; yet, even he cracked an occasional tooth or perforated a rare Zenker's diverticulum. Only a careless fellow could commit such sins with the fibre-optic instruments. And now one can peer at leisure into all the nooks, crannys, and secret places that were often inaccessible even to the most skillful endoscopist using the older instrument. The addition of the marvelous camera permits one to photograph the questionable area and review the movies or color slides at leisure.

Several modifications of the scope permit direct vision biopsy—another boon. In some sophisticated centers, the view-through-the-scope can be relayed via closed circuit TV and shared with the chief or an entire audience of students. No longer will we have the mad flurry of activity in the darkened room with the patient pinned to the table while an army of residents and fellows take turns peering into his gizzard.

This book demonstrates the versatility of the fibre-optic instrument. The authors have provided detailed instructions on what model instrument to use in different portions of the stomach and how to take the superior photographs. Each of the several hundred gastric camera photographs is provided diagrammatic explanation, and a descriptive commentary which is clear and helpful. The range of pathology is somewhat limited, however. I was surprised not to see lymphomas and infiltrative disease, Mallory-Weiss gastroesophageal tears, erosive gastritis, Menetrier's, and a few other rare birds. However, it is replete with polyps, ulcers, and malignancies.

A complementing feature would have been roentgenographic correlation and microscopic pathology of some ulcers and tumors. The table of contents is adequate, but an index is almost mandatory for hurry-up American readers. I feel sure that future editions will encompass these things. The book is handsomely turned out, sturdily bound, and the color reproduction is superb.

There is little doubt that the flexible scope and its cunning camera have added a new dimension to gastroenterologic diagnosis.

ROBERT H. MOSER, MD
Wailuku, Hawaii

Communications to this Department may be sent directly to Robert H. Moser, MD, the Maui Medical Group, Maui Professional Center, Wailuku, Maui, Hawaii 96793, or to the Chief Editor for transmittal to him.

The Founders of Neurology. Edited by Webb Haymaker MD; Francis Schiller, MD. Price, $18. Pp 616. Charles C Thomas Publisher, 301-327 E Lawrence Ave, Springfield, Ill, 1970.

Some years ago, when writing the biography of a British brain-surgeon, I wrote to ask the late Sir Gordon Holmes if he could help me. In his reply he said that his memory was excellent, he probably had information for me, but he was not prepared to write a long letter. He invited me to visit him. He bade me come on any day except Thursdays which were sacred to golf; he was then 86 years old.

When next in London I set an afternoon aside and took a train to Farnham. After we had disposed of the main purpose of my visit the conversation became more general and to my delight he reminisced about his early years at the National Hospital, Queen Square. At the time Ferrier had a big practice and spent little time at the hospital. Jackson, in retirement, was consulting physician and came there once or twice a week. He would select a case from the house physician's list, sit on the bed, make friends with the patient and bring out points that no one else had noticed. Then, he would say to the house physician: "Write up the case in detail and let me have the notes by tomorrow morning's post."

Holmes thought that Gowers, at his best, was the finest clinician he had ever encountered, better than Erb or Marie. Now and then, Eveleen Gowers came to the hospital to play the violin for the patients. Holmes made a point of escorting her home, but when they were approaching the house she would not let him come further, saying that her father would not approve of her being escorted unchaperoned by a young gentleman.

Despite his great age at the time of my visit, Holmes seemed physically hardly touched by the years; he talked fluently but was somewhat deaf and occasionally unable to remember a name. I still treasure the memory of an afternoon spent with a man who had worked with Edinger and Weigert, who had collaborated in research with Henry Head and had himself contributed fundamentally to knowledge of cerebellar function and introduced into clinical practice the modern technique of neurological examination.

I gather that similar conversations during a conference in Atlantic City, when men recalled their teachers and the past, inspired *The Founders of Neurology*, a splendid collection of brief biographies. I recall how eagerly I awaited the publication of the first edition of this book in 1953 and how avidly I read it. Now I note that Webb Haymaker's co-editor is Francis Schiller who has published a number of erudite papers in recent years in the *Bulletin of the History of Medicine*.

A series of articles by Genevieve Miller appeared in that journal in 1969. Her subject was teaching of medical history in the United States and Canada, and it seems that "indifferent," "mixed," and "politely interested" were commonly encountered faculty attitudes; and one misguided group of students regarded anyone with an historical interest as "bearing the hallmark of someone who is no longer competing." Haymaker and Schiller may be cited in rebuttal of that vapid judgment: whole men, actively "competing" in medical science—as witnessed by their contribution to *Bing's Local Diagnosis in Neurological Diseases*—but aware of the intellectual value of historical insights and susceptible to the pleasure of belles-lettres. Theirs is an achievement that youth might envy rather than misprize.

Under their editorship 89 authors give short accounts of the lives and careers of 145 men and one woman (Cecile Vogt), who have made basic contributions to anatomy, physiology, or nosology. The book is a cornucopia of factual and diverting information. In its pages we encounter familiar figures in new rôles—Babinski the gourmet, Bárány the philanthropist and pacifist—and learn of the tribulations of others; Winterstein the neurochemist who lost his chair in Breslau when a student whom he had failed came to power in the Nazi party, Bielschowsky similarly disposed, General Hammond (who introduced the term *athetosis*) dismissed by a "packed" jury and later vindicated by an act of Congress.

For Osler the master word in medicine was "work," and these men were prodigious workers. Vulpian rose to start his day at 4 AM. Clovis Vincent, the French neurosurgeon, was in the wards by five—he boxed a little every morning to warm up and at one time was Georges Carpentier's sparring partner. Moritz Schiff would appear briefly among his dinner guests at 10:30 PM retiring to his study as soon as he could.

The editors admit that the first edition was criticized for its "somewhat anecdotal treatment" of its subjects but to my mind these anecdotes are interesting and enlivening. We find Dusser de Barenne dozing after a night of insomnia; he dreams of an egg cooking slowly; he jumps from his bed, rushes to the laboratory, and devises the method of laminar thermocoagulation. Similarly, under the influence of a dream, Otto Loewi realized that the vagus works by chemical transmission and saw how to prove it; he woke up, scribbled down the details, fell asleep again, and in the morning could not read his own writing—but on the following morning the idea and how to prove it were clear to him. Freud told his class that all dreams are an expression of desire and invited them to come to see him if they could not explain their dreams; soon he was faced by Bárány who related a dream with no element of desire: "That's simple," said Freud. "You had the desire to contradict me."

Very occasionally one disagrees or senses omission: Hughlings Jackson must surely have been interested in epilepsy long before his wife developed "Jacksonian" convulsions in her fatal illness; Sherrington's *The Assaying of Brabantius* deserved mention; the baronet rather than the baron is next in rank to the knight.

These, of course, are trivial points not detracting in any way from my admiration for a book which I recommend warmly. Because I realize that the editors' selection cannot possibly satisfy everyone, I offer only gentle remonstrance for their elevation of George Huntington to the dignity of a "founder" (he is really rather lucky to have attained eponymous fame). But I am cross with them for not including Sir Gordon Holmes.

J. B. LYONS, MD
Dublin

Principles of Internal Medicine. By Maxwell M Wintrobe, MD; George W Thorn, MD; Raymond D Adams, MD; Ivan L Bennett, Jr, MD; Eugene Braunwald, MD; Kurt J Isselbacher, MD; Robert G Petersdorf, MD. Price: vol 1, $26.50, vol 2, $30.50. Pp 2,094. McGraw-Hill Book Co, 330 W 42nd St, New York 10036, 1970.

The panel of contributors to this sixth edition has grown to 171. Many familiar names from earlier editions are no longer on the list, but they have been replaced by others of equal competence. One cannot fault the information presented by this distinguished faculty.

Thus, any appraisal of this, or a similar textbook purporting to cover the expansive field of internal medicine, must be made on items such as the care in selection from the "dreadful abundance" of available material, the clarity of presentation of the various portions, and the general readability of the volume. This volume follows by four years the fifth edition, and significant updating is evident in many sections. Although the general organization of the textbook remains the same, some logical reorganization of material has occurred which has improved the reader's ability to find things.

There remains a problem with the basic design of the textbook which detracts, somewhat, from its presentation. The material on the subject of neurology may serve as a case in point. If all of the pertinent material were to be extracted and published separately as a small textbook of neurology, it would need only little modification to be superb. This section is well organized, beautifully written, and comprehensive enough for the internist's needs.

Because of the fundamental arrangement of *Principles of Internal Medicine*, which presents cardinal manifestations of disease in one part, and description of various specific disease entities later, one finds in one place an excellent section on "Pain," then equally fine sections on "Alterations in Nervous Function," and, further on, sections of "Disorders of the Nervous System," "Diseases of Striated Muscle" (including material on neuromuscular disorders), "Errors of Metabolism," "Disorders due to Chemical and Physical Agents," and several chapters on infections of the central nervous system. Because of an extensive, carefully prepared index and cross-references in the text, there should be little difficulty in locating the specific information needed on any aspect of neurology. The basic problems, however, are that there is duplication in several of these chapters, and there is just too much material for a textbook of internal medicine.

Similar comments may be made about some other important areas. The section on "Disorders Caused by Biologic Agents" is excellent and generally written well, but it attempts to be a textbook on infectious disease. A chapter on "Intermediary Metabolism of Protein, Fat, and Carbohydrate" is written superbly, as are many other individual "orienting" chapters. But can a contemporary textbook of medicine afford to expand to cover, reasonably, all things? It cannot have enough anatomy, physiology, biochemistry, pharmacology, toxicology, pathology, elements of physical examination, clinical material, philosophy of medicine, or geographic incidence of disease and still remain reasonable in size. This is not a new problem; it was recognized and discussed by the editors of the first edition many years ago.

Many sections are rewritten completely by authors different from those who contributed to the preceding edition. In general, the revisions, reorganization of certain material, and newly written chapters have improved the textbook. One can read entire chapters, however, with feeling of nostalgia, for the same words, emphases, clichés, and references appear in this edition which were present in the fifth, and earlier editions. Of course, some principles, facts, and ideas do not change with the years, and certain portions of earlier works do not require revision if they were clear and well-written. Sad to say, some of the chapters which could have benefited from reorganization, rewriting, and pruning are nearly untouched in this new edition.

The single volume copy of this edition of *Principles of Internal Medicine* runs to 2,007 pages of text, about 5 pages of "Laboratory Values," 7 color plates, and an index of 78 pages. (A volume version is available.) Except for the list of laboratory values, all of these portions are expanded over the entries in the previous edition. The covers are somewhat thinner (although apparently equally strong) and the volume is somewhat heavier than its predecessor. One is led to wonder if such expansion can long continue! It was true some time ago that no man could write an adequate textbook of medicine. It may well be true now that no one textbook can be designed to meet the needs of the medical student, the resident, and the busy practitioner.

On the whole, one must recognize that this is a better, more readable textbook than its predecessor, and it clearly should displace the earlier volume (or volumes) on any internist's desk.

JACQUES L. SHERMAN, MD
Northport, NY

Hepatic Failure. By Henry Brown, MD. Price, $10.50. Pp 137. Charles C Thomas Publisher, 301-327 E Lawrence Ave, Springfield, Ill, 1970.

This is another monograph in *American Lectures In Living Chemistry,* and there is no doubt concerning the author's credentials. There are over two dozen references to his own work and many of the tables and illustrations are from his previous publications.

He writes most interestingly (and exhaustively) when referring to his own work–especially his laboratory techniques–and that is its strength. It is not an easy book for a clinician to read, and it will take an *unusual* clinician to appreciate the author's work. One of its weaknesses for the practicing physician is an *inadequate* number of diagrams (eg, the sections on the metabolism of carbohydrates, fats, and proteins).

I believe I have been unfair to the author: the book was *not* written for the clinician (or, if it was, it did not help me); I think it is a text for someone with a special interest in liver disease–and, primarily, the clinical investigator.

NICHOLAS J. COTSONAS, Jr., MD
Peoria, Ill

Advances in Blood Grouping III. Edited by Alexander S Wiener, MD. Price, $19.75. Pp 658. Grune & Stratton Inc, 757 Third Ave, New York 10017, 1970.

This volume is a collection of reprints compiled, and for the most part written, by A. S. Wiener. It is a testimonial to the tremendous productivity of this unique worker. The reprints are offered exactly as they appeared in their original publication; therefore, they are typeset in different styles. The contributions range from articles in prestigious journals as *Blood*, *The American Journal of Clinical Pathology*, and *Nature* to brief communiques to "house organs," eg, Bulletin Adelphi Hospital; and "medical throwaways," eg, *Medical Opinion and Review*.

The book has a particularly extensive and valuable section on the blood groups in nonhuman primates, but the lack of editorial review, synthesis, and emendation permits unnecessary repetitiveness (one diagram appears four times); this defect reduces it to a mere source book.

The price of $19.75, over 600 large pages of differing print, and the lack of editorial guidance do not add up to an attractive package. If one wished to study the complexity of the ABO system, one would go instead to Prokop and Uhlenbruck's magnificent volume on *Human Blood and Serum Group*, or Race and Sanger's *Blood Groups in Man*.

RALPH O. WALLERSTEIN, MD
San Francisco

The Immunology of Malignant Disease. By Jules E Harris, MD; Joseph G Sinkovics, MD. Price, $15. Pp 251. CV Mosby Co, 3207 Washington Blvd, St. Louis 63103, 1970.

The *Immunology of Malignant Disease* is an admirable book from several aspects. Harris states in the Preface that the intended readers are "physicians concerned with the management of malignant disease." This group will find the book rewarding within the immunological scope offered. Doubtlessly, many physicians will find the many chemotherapeutic applications and their rationale practical and useful. The book, although modest in length, deserves a much wider audience. Immunologists, virologists, and all investigators interested in cancer will find at least one or two chapters, if not the whole text, an excellent comprehensive review of the subject. Because of the lucid and eloquently written introductory first chapter, "Normal Immune Response in Man and Its Reaction to Malignant Disease," the book is recommended unhesitatingly to medical students as well. This chapter has well over 200 references. It is a tribute to the authors and publisher that each of the five chapters is documented extensively. Yet, the text reads smoothly and logically, and the small font reference numbers do not intrude on the reader's consciousness. There are few books offering the myriad well-chosen references. Harris and Sinkovics are to be commended for their scholarly approach.

The authors are well known in the field of cancer immunology; thus, they write with authority. Harris has contributed the introductory chapter as well as "Suppression of Human Immune Response" and "Immune Deficiency States Associated with Human Malignant Disease." The latter one and Sinkovics' on "Immunology of Tumors in Experimental Animals" are models of their kind.

The last chapter, "Tumors of Man," is a collaborative effort, and some readers may find certain tumors accorded only a brief exposition. Multiple myeloma is especially notable for the brevity of the presentation. Indeed, the immunology of myeloma would appear to deserve more attention in a text of this kind. Harris, Sinkovics, CV Mosby Co, or some combination thereof has also achieved another exemplary feat of publication. The text is easily read with clear typography on quality paper, and the change of authors from chapter to chapter is not manifestly apparent. One could quarrel with the need to present more information in certain areas (neoantigens, tolerance), but this will more likely be a reflection of a particular reader's background than an intrinsic fault.

The relatively few charts or tabular presentations are quite good with one exception. Readers new to this field would profit from application of this treatment to more complex information. The one chart that doubtlessly is meant to be helpful clinically is an extensive cataloging of suggested antimicrobial agents and their doses for infections in acute leukemia. This kind of material becomes passe very quickly. Worse, particularly for a number of the *enterobacteriaciae*, it suggests implicitly that accurate in vitro sensitivity testing of these organisms to select the proper antibiotic may not be necessary. Nearly a page of footnotes as caveats to this guide to therapy do not vitiate this criticism. Nonetheless, this is a minor point and does not detract from the overall excellence.

The book is recommended highly to those with an interest in tumor immunology. Biennially revised editions might be indicated for this fascinating and rapidly advancing field.

R. E. RITTS, JR., MD
Rochester, Minn

Handbook of Experimental Pharmacology. Edited by O Eichler; A Farsh; H Herken; AD Welch. Price, $68.20. Pp 768, with 117 figures. Springer-Verlag, 1 Berlin 33, Heidelberger Platz 3, Berlin-West, 1970.

This volume provides an easy access to a review of the complex literature of kinin physiology. Like most multi-author books, the quality is variable. Some chapters are little more than an encyclopedic compilation of the literature. In other chapters, an attempt has been made to evaluate the investigations cited, with a critical eye.

This volume will be of interest to libraries of medical schools and departments of pharmacology, physiology, biochemistry, and other investigative branches of medicine. The cost of $68.20 will make private purchase prohibitive for all except those who have keen interest in the area.

J. W. MEAKIN, MD, FRCP
Toronto

Essentials of Clinical Endocrinology. By Norman G Schneeberg, MD. Price, $22.50. Pp 449, with 210 illustrations and two color plates. CV Mosby Co, 3207 Washington Blvd, St. Louis 63103, 1970.

Schneeberg and his contributors (Banghart, Bendersky, Eskin, Paul, Shaw, Smith, and the Steinbergers) have accomplished exactly what they set out to do in superb fashion: prepare a tight, up-to-date synopsis of clinically relevant endocrinological information. The style is simple and straightforward, and it makes an extraordinary density of information quite readable. A very practical clinical orientation is evident throughout: in discussing the treatment of hyperthyrodism, Schneeberg states:

> Criteria useful in selecting individual treatment are outlined below, but the choice depends to a large extent on the experience of the physician, local surgical skills and isotope facilities, and the convenience, comfort and wishes of the patient.

How refreshingly different from the usual dogmatic recommendations!

In controversial areas, the author treads a very reasonable middle-ground; perhaps the necessity for conciseness made it impossible to indicate in greater detail the range of authoritative opinions. However, the reader is given excellent bibliographic referrals, should he wish to explore some of these questions further.

Criticisms which might be offered are for the most part trivial, and are not intended to detract from the overall excellence of the book.

In discussing radioactive iodine therapy, it is recommended that antithyroid therapy be omitted for three to five days beforehand. However, there is evidence that the effects of antithyroid drugs persist for about two weeks; further, that retreatment should be withheld until the ^{131}I has had a few biological half-lives to do its job. With the availability of reserpine, guanethidine sulfate, and propranolol hydrochloride, this delay is entirely safe and practical, and the maximum thyroid effect for the total body dose is realized. In discussing adrenal steroid biosynthesis, the "progesterone pathway" is illustrated, although it is by now well established that cortisol synthesis proceeds by way of the "pregnenolone pathway."

In dealing with the therapy of polycystic ovarian disease, the author recommends therapy with clomiphene citrate (Clomid) or gonadotropins, although this therapy is of use only in the event that the subject is interested in immediate fertility. No mention is made of maintenance treatment, as with steroid contraceptives, which produce ovarian shrinkage, decrease of androgen production (and, consequently, of ovarian fibrosis), and regulated cycles, pending a time when the more definitive therapy is desired.

The book is well printed on fine coated paper. The line drawings and reproductions of x-ray films are excellent. The color in the two color plates is abominable, and the drawing of estrogen effects on vaginal cytology appears to have been taken from a medical student's sketchbook.

Overall, this is probably the best summarization of current clinical endocrinological information which is available, and it is highly recommended at all levels of clinical readership.

JOSEPH W. GOLDZIEHER, MD
San Antonio, Tex

Pulmonary Edema in Man and Animals. By Aldo A Luisada, MD. Price, $10.50. Pp 154, with illustrations. Warren H Green Inc, 10 S Brentwood Blvd, St. Louis 63105, 1970.

This small volume attempts to present a comprehensive review of the experimental and clinical aspects of pulmonary edema. To me, its chief strengths were its recitation of the names of the various scientists who have studied the problem, (with brief mention of their specific contributions) and summaries of experimental approaches to mechanisms and management.

It is well for the physician to be reminded of the diverse laboratory and clinical situations in which pulmonary edema may be encountered. The chief weaknesses are the incomplete description or lack of documentation of certain clinical states mentioned as causes of pulmonary edema, ie, uremia, bronchial asthma, pleurisy.

The references are adequate in some sections and almost totally lacking in others. Certain of the material presented in earlier chapters is repeated later. The recommended measures for home, emergency room, and hospital treatment would not find universal acceptance and the dose of lanatoside C (Cedilanid) is incorrect on pages 117, 119, and 120. It is a mixed bag.

OGLESBY PAUL, MD
Chicago

Progress in Immunobiological Standardization. Edited by RH Regamey; A De Barbieri; W Hennessen; D Ikic; FT Perkins. Price, $19.20. Pp 707, with 290 figures and 185 tables. S Karger AG Medical and Scientific Publishers, Arnold-Bocklin-Strasse 25, CH- 4000 Basel 11 (Switzerland): S Karger GmbH, Postfach 1027, D-8034 Germering/Munchen (Germany); Academic Press, Berkeley Square House, Berkeley Sq, London, W1X 6BA; and Albert J Phiebig Inc, PO Box 352, White Plains, NY 10602, 1970.

This volume contains approximately 200 abstracts presented at the 11th International Congress for Microbiological Standardization, held in Milan, Italy, Sept 16-19, 1968. It is composed of four sections. Section 1 deals with immunoglobulins, their immunochemistry, molecular biology, preparation, assays, and standardization, antilymphocytic immunoglobulins, and preparation, standardization, and clinical use of anti-D immunoglobulins for the prevention of Rh sensitization. The material on antilymphocytic globulin and anti-D immunoglobulins should be of particular interest to the internist.

Section 2 deals with local immunity and investigations on orally administered vaccines, which hopefully point the way toward greater clinical application in this field.

The third section discusses the immunochemistry of enzymes. Section 4, composed of "free" papers, includes such subjects as antivenom sera, tuberculin, toxoids, bacteriology, and virology.

The book constitutes a good coverage of the subject of immunobiology and its standardization up to a certain period. Unfortunately, the time lag in producing a volume of this sort does not make for up-to-date coverage. The Congress was held in the latter part of 1968, the participating papers were probably committed to the program in 1967, and the material is presented to the reader three or four years later. Perhaps that is why none of the exciting work on IgE, developed particularly by Ishizaka's and

Johansson's group, is included. Since some of it was published in 1967, the deficiency of this type of coverage presented in this volume is obvious.

This book should be useful to bacteriologists, virologists, immunologists, and some other investigators, and some clinicians, providing they realize the limitations it presents.

SAMUEL M. FEINBERG, MD
Winnetka, Ill

In Case of Emergency: What to do Until the Doctor Arrives. By Bry Benjamin, MD; and Annette Francis Benjamin. Price, $5.95. Pp 224. Doubleday & Co, Garden City, NY, 1970.

Physicians in their offices or in hospital emergency rooms are presented a spectrum of medical and surgical problems varying in severity and urgency. It is difficult to estimate, because of geographic differences in availability of care, but perhaps 20% of these problems are of such a minor degree that the opinion of a physician is not needed. Patients often realize this, but they may not have been able to speak to their doctor or they do not have a reference source at hand to allay their apprehensions.

In Case of Emergency attempts to provide such a source of first-aid advice. In most instances it achieves the goal by providing a well-indexed and organized manual for an immediate self-help.

I tried to read this book not as a physician, but as a worried parent of a sick child in the small hours of the morning, or as a witness to an accident on the highway. I recalled situations from personal experience, the stories of neighbors and friends, the telephone calls from patients at all hours, and my experiences as an emergency room physician. I tried to use this book for each of those situations.

For the most part, it was quite helpful. But I was disappointed not to find mention of croup, for this stands out as one of the more common and frightening experiences that young parents face. The section on head injuries might have included the possible delayed effects and the importance of awakening the victim for periodic examinations.

I was a little surprised to read that a doctor should be called for every bee sting, even in a person with no known allergic reaction. Having worked in emergency rooms during summer months, I feel this could lead to chaos.

A running theme in the book is that the doctor will arrive. But there are many conditions which require hospital emergency room or in-patient care. Perhaps this could have been mentioned more frequently rather than "waiting for the doctor." I found this book informative and well organized. With a few reservations I would recommend it to my neighbors and friends.

JOHN LODMELL, MD
Olney, Md

BOOKS RECEIVED

Adam's Rib. By Simon S Levin, MB, MRCP, DCH. Price, $6.95. Pp 180. Geron-X Inc Publishers, Box 1108, Los Altos, Calif 94022, 1970.

Bannerstone House. By Tom R Cavanaugh, Payne EL Thomas. Price, not given. Charles C Thomas Publisher, 301-327 E Lawrence Ave, Springfield, Ill 62703, 1970.

The Biochemistry of Clinical Medicine. By William S Hoffman, MD, PhD. Price, $15.75. Pp 856, with 68 figures. Year Book Medical Publishers Inc, 35 E Wacker Dr, Chicago 60601, 1970.

General Physiology: A Molecular Approach. By Robert M Dowben. Price, $15. Pp 619, with many graphic illustrations. Harper & Row Publishers Inc, 49 E 33rd St, New York 10016, 1969.

Brain Tumor Scanning With Radioisotopes. Edited by Louis Bakay, MD. Price, $19.50. Pp 217, with numerous illustrations. Charles C Thomas Publisher, 301-327 E Lawrence Ave, Springfield, Ill 62703, 1969.

The Medical Report: Theory and Practice. By Robert M Fox, Attorney at Law. Price, $11.50. Pp 260, with few illustrations. Little Brown & Co, 34 Beacon St, Boston 02106, 1969.

Essentials of Pharmacology: A Textbook for Students. Edited by John A Bevan, BSc, MB, BS. Price, $16.50. Pp 722, with 179 illustrations. Hoeber Medical Division, Harper & Row Publisher Inc, 49 E 33 St, New York 10016, 1969.

Current Status of Drugs in Cardiovascular Disease, Edited by Charles K Friedberg, MD. Price, $9.75. Pp 262, with many illustrations. Grune & Stratton Inc, 381 Park Ave S, New York 10016, 1969.

The Hormones: Endocrine Physiology. By Clark T Sawin, MD. Price, $9.75. Pp 308, with few illustrations. Little Brown & Co, 34 Beacon St, Boston 02106, 1969.

Computer: Werkzeug der Medizin. By CTh Ehlers; N Hollberg; A Proppe. Price, $6.10. Pp 258, with 41 illustrations. Springer-Verlag New York Inc, 175 Fifth Ave, New York, 1970.

Your Child and Ileal Conduit Surgery. By Alan D Perlmutter, MD; William M Crowell, MD. Price, $4.25. Pp 99. Charles C Thomas Publisher, 301-327 E Lawrence Ave, Springfield, Ill 62703, 1970.

Carcinoma of the Colon and Antecedent Epithelium. Edited by Walter J Burdette, PhD, MD. Price, $20.50. Pp 375. Charles C Thomas Publisher, 301-327 E Lawrence Ave, Springfield, Ill 62703, 1970.

Ventriculocisternostomy: Long-Term Experiences. By Robert C Cantu, MD; Jost J Michelsen, MD; James C. White, MD; Paul FJ New, MD. Price, $12.25. Pp 138. Charles C Thomas Publisher, 301-327 E Lawrence Ave, Springfield, Ill 62703, 1970.

Anaesthesiology and Resuscitation: Anaesthesiologie und Wiederbelebung: Anesthésiologie et Réanimation. Intensivtherapie Beim Akuten Nierenversagen. By E Buchborn, and O Heidenreich. Price, $6.80. Pp 78, with 31 illustrations. Springer-Verlag, New York, 1970.

Autogenic Therapy. By Wolfgang Luthe, MD. Price, $17.50. Pp 344. Grune & Stratton Inc, 757 Third Ave, New York 10017, 1970.

Tumours of the Testicle. By John P Blandy, DM, MCH, FRCS; HF Hope-Stone, MB, BS, DMRT, FFR; Anthony D Dayan, BSC, MD, MRC (PATH). Price, $7. Pp 199. Grune & Stratton Inc, 757 Third Ave, New York 10017; 23 Bedford Sq, London, WC1, 1970.

Drug Abuse and What We Can Do About It. Edited by James C Bennett, EdD, George D Demos, PhD. Price, $8.50. Pp 138. Charles C Thomas Publisher, 301-327 E Lawrence Ave, Springfield, Ill, 1971.

ERRATUM

In the Clinical Note entitled "Erosive Osteoarthritis and the Main en Lorgnette Deformity: (Opera Glass Hand)" by Robert L. Swezey, MD, and Stanley J. Alexander, MD, which appeared in the August issue of the ARCHIVES (**128**:269-272, 1971), an error appeared on page 271. The second sentence in the second column should read as follows: A characteristic distribution of osteoarthritic joints involving primarily **the DIP joints by Heberden's nodes, the PIP joints by Bouchard's nodes,** and, in addition, the carpal metacarpal joint of the thumb is well recognized.[12]

Alcohol and atherosclerosis

Moderate drinking can hasten the progress of atherosclerosis in some individuals, according to a preliminary study by a group of Pennsylvania investigators.

Alcohol has not been singled out as a specific causal factor in the genesis of atherosclerosis, "but an alcohol-induced augmentation of underlying genetic-metabolic hyperlipoproteinemia appears to play an important role in sustaining a persistent—and perhaps in contributing toward—arterial deterioration," said Peter T. Kuo, MD, at the third annual Western Nutrition Congress in Miami.

The data have not been fully analyzed, Dr. Kuo stressed, but preliminary observations suggest that alcohol restriction is ". . . of prime importance in the successful control of the great majority of atherosclerosis- and arteriosclerosis-prone patients who have elevated serum lipid levels."

Dr. Kuo, professor of medicine at the Hospital of the University of Pennsylvania, based his hypothesis on two related studies that led to strikingly similar results. One study dealt with 125 randomly selected chronic alcoholics; the other, with 120 hyperlipidemic control-study patients.

Forty-eight (or 38.4%) of the 125 chronic alcoholics, tested before and after a six-week restriction on alcohol, had persistent hyperlipidemia. Seventy-seven (or 61.6%) of the alcoholics maintained normal plasma lipid-lipoprotein levels throughout. What caught the attention of the Pennsylvania research team, however, was that, when drinking, 45 of the 48 patients had elevated levels of prebetalipoprotein, either alone or in combination with chylomicron—and yet these triglyceride-bearing fractions "cleared" when the subjects stopped drinking.

Abstinence from alcohol for four to six weeks had little effect on hyperbetalipoproteinemia (hypercholesterolemia). However, the period of abstinence resulted in a significant reduction in the triglyceride-rich plasma prebetalipoprotein and chylomicron fractions in patients with type IV and V hyperlipoproteinemia. Conversely, the investigators noted a rapid rise in prebetalipoprotein and chylomicron concentrations in these patients within two weeks after they started drinking again.

"An increase in plasma prebetalipoprotein concentration with associated hypertriglyceridemia was the predominant feature in (all cases of) the alcoholic hyperlipidemia," said Dr. Kuo. He added that investigators studying post-heparin plasma lipolytic activity—which is a measure of lipoprotein lipase levels—have found that the action of that enzyme is frequently depressed in cases of alcoholic lipemia.

Dr. Kuo's team also discovered 21 cases of the same abnormalities among 98 parents, children and siblings of 29 alcoholic patients who had increases in prebetalipoprotein and chylomicron levels. "Although these data are insufficient to support the thesis of genetic alcoholic lipemia," Dr. Kuo observed, "they tend to suggest increased individual susceptibility to the effect of alcohol on prebeta and chylomicron production and retention."

The results of the controlled study

continued

Highlights This Month

Survey shows that diagnostic x-rays are used with more precision—and more frequently than before . . . page 860

Single, heavy dose of radiation appears to produce temporary improvement in cancer patients with brain metastases . . . page 861

Growing popularity of exotic pets may lead to new health dangers . . . page 865

Internists in the news . . . pages 868, 871.

Internal medicine at large

Atherosclerosis

continued

of 120 hyperlipidemic atherosclerotic patients also supported the hypothesis that prebetalipoproteinemia, with or without accompanying chylomicronemia, can be aggravated and sustained by daily consumption of even moderate amounts of alcohol.

The diet of each patient had been followed for about six months prior to the study. They drank an average of three to five ounces of alcohol a day. Their diets generally consisted of 15% to 20% protein, 40% fat, and 40% to 50% carbohydrates. A complete lipoprotein analysis before the patients stopped drinking daily cocktails showed that a little more than 10% of them had some increase in betalipoprotein or in both prebeta and chylomicron levels.

Other members of his investigative team are Gene F. Myers, MD, Alvan Rosen, MD, and Louise Y. Feng, MD, of the University of Pennsylvania School of Medicine.

X-ray survey

Diagnostic x-rays are being used more—and with more precision—than was the case in the middle 1960's, but there is still plenty of room for improvement.

Public Health Service officials, in discussing preliminary data from the *1970 X-ray Exposure Study,* said the increase seems to reflect a broader application of roentgenographic services rather than the use of larger doses of radiation for each patient.

The study uses data from 1964 as a basis for comparison. The complete

ANNUAL RATE OF MEDICAL ROENTGENOGRAPHIC VISITS (PER 100 POPULATION) BY BODY AREA

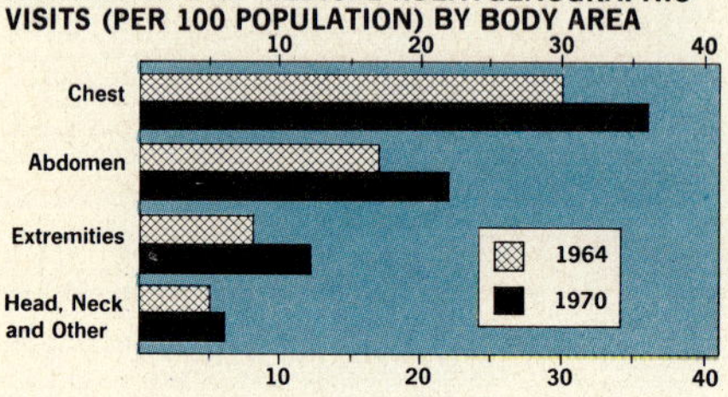

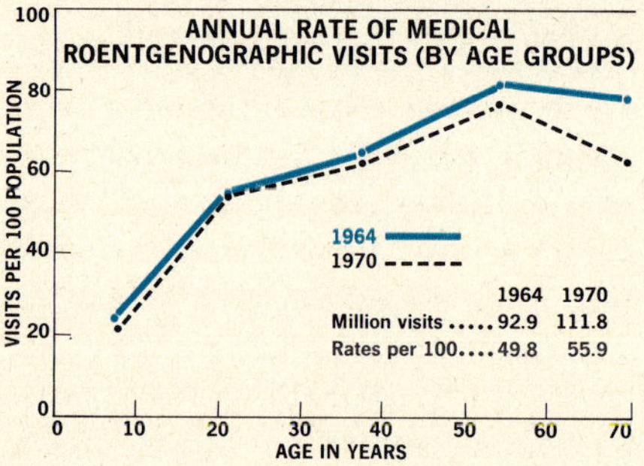

report will be released early next year, but PHS officials disclosed some data during the Boston meeting of the American Roentgen Ray Society:

- The number of patient visits to physicians, dentists and others who use diagnostic x-rays rose from 143 million in 1964 to 179 million in 1970.
- During the same period, the number of x-ray examinations increased from 173 million to 210 million.
- The amount of film used for diagnostic x-rays increased from 506 million sheets to 650 million sheets.
- The 1964 survey showed "adequate collimation" in less than half of all examinations. This proportion rose to two-thirds in 1970, and the PHS officials stressed still more improvement is needed.
- There is little difference in the use of medical x-rays in persons from various income groups, while the use

ESTIMATED DISTRIBUTION OF RADIOGRAPHIC FILMS
BY BEAM AREA VS FILM AREA

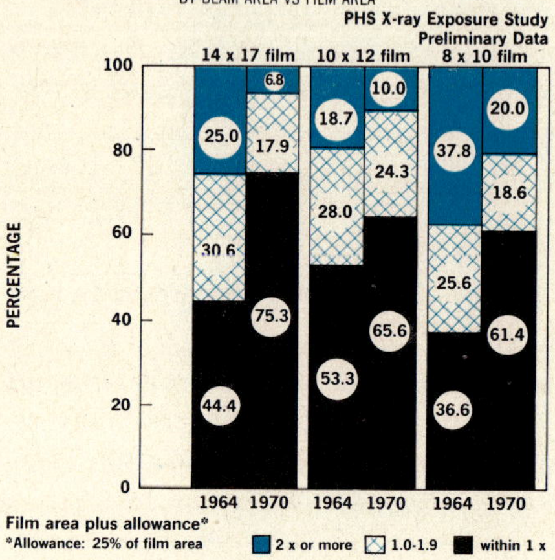

of dental roentgenograms continues to vary according to family income.

The study, based on data from 5,000 x-ray facilities and more than 22,000 households, was sponsored by the Bureau of Radiological Health and National Center for Health Statistics. According to the report, a total of 75.4 million persons had radiographic examinations in 1970 compared with 66.1 million in 1964; 59.2 million persons had dental x-rays, compared with 45.9 million six years earlier, and 8.6 million individuals had fluoroscopic examinations in 1970, compared with 7.8 million in 1964. The proportion of medical roentgenographic examinations performed in hospital x-ray departments rose from 57.6% to 60.3%.

These increases naturally raise some questions, and Reynold F. Brown, MD, chairman of the American College of Radiology's Commission on Radiological Units, Standards and Protection, attempted the following explanation:

"Don't be too quick to assume . . . that while we are doing more radiology, that it is a change in the attitudes and decision-making in the practice of medicine . . . If you increase the access to medical care, such as with the enactment of Medicare, and begin to give medical care to persons who did not have access to it, the total rate (of x-ray use) goes up, but not in the sense (that physicians) are doing anything different in the practice of medicine."

Dr. Brown, who is director of the Office of Environmental Health and Safety of the University of California, San Francisco, noted that older persons accounted for much of the increase.

Young adults are also receiving more roentgenographic examinations—possibly reflecting the increase in accident rates—but the rate of x-ray examinations declined among women between the ages of 15 and 29.

Supervoltage therapy

Patients whose cancer has spread to the brain appear to tolerate, and even show temporary improvement after, single 1,000-rad supervoltage treatments, early data suggest.

If future results support these findings, Frank R. Hendrickson, MD, told the American Society of Therapeutic Radiologists' second annual scientific program in Phoenix, the single treatment could reduce cost, travel, and time away from home for cancer patients with brain metastases.

Dr. Hendrickson is chief of the Department of Therapeutic Radiology at Presbyterian-St. Luke's Hospital, Chicago, and professor of therapeutic radiology at Rush Medical College.

Presbyterian-St. Luke's is among 22 centers studying radiation therapy approaches for the National Cancer Institute in an effort to find the most efficient, economical way to relieve the symptoms of cancer metastizing to the brain.

The centers are working on five different approaches to therapy, ranging from the single treatment to as many as 20 courses of treatment in a four-week period.

Four patients have received the single dose radiation at Presbyterian-St. Luke's during this year of the study, but the Center's over-all experience is 78 patients, dating back three years. In more than half of these patients, the primary cancer was in the lung. About one-third had breast cancer.

Seventy of the 78 have died, he said, but autopsies have not revealed any deleterious changes that could be attributed to the high-dose radiation. The series included four comatose patients who died within 48 hours of treatment, and five others whose condition appeared to be worse after the single dose treatment.

Some patients complain of transient headache after treatment, suggesting there may be edema which so far has escaped postmortem detection. Further, radiation of this magnitude probably would result eventually in thickening of blood vessels in the brain, but the development of this phenomenon would require many more months than cancer allows these patients to live.

Fifty-three of the patients—most of whom were between 50 and 70 years old, some with controlled and some with uncontrolled primary cancer—required hospitalization for serious symptoms at the time of single-dose treatment. Twenty-seven were able to go home improved.

Thirty-two patients were retreated with another single high dose. The mean time between first and second radiation was five months. Half showed improvement again, and 11 were treated a third time. Four patients received a fourth treatment. The longest survival of any patient to date is 18 months.

All of the patients lost hair after the treatment. The loss proved temporary in those who survived for any length of time.

Presbyterian-St. Luke's uses two cobalt 60 units. Dr. Hendrickson said he believes therapy with 600 rads on each of two consecutive days might be better tolerated, although the NCI study presently has no provision for such an approach.

Latest cancer data

Men, especially black men, are more likely to develop cancer now than they were two decades ago—while the incidence of cancer among women is declining, according to a new nationwide survey.

Details of the Third National Cancer Survey will not be available until early next year, but preliminary results released by the National Cancer Institute's Biometry Branch indicate

continued

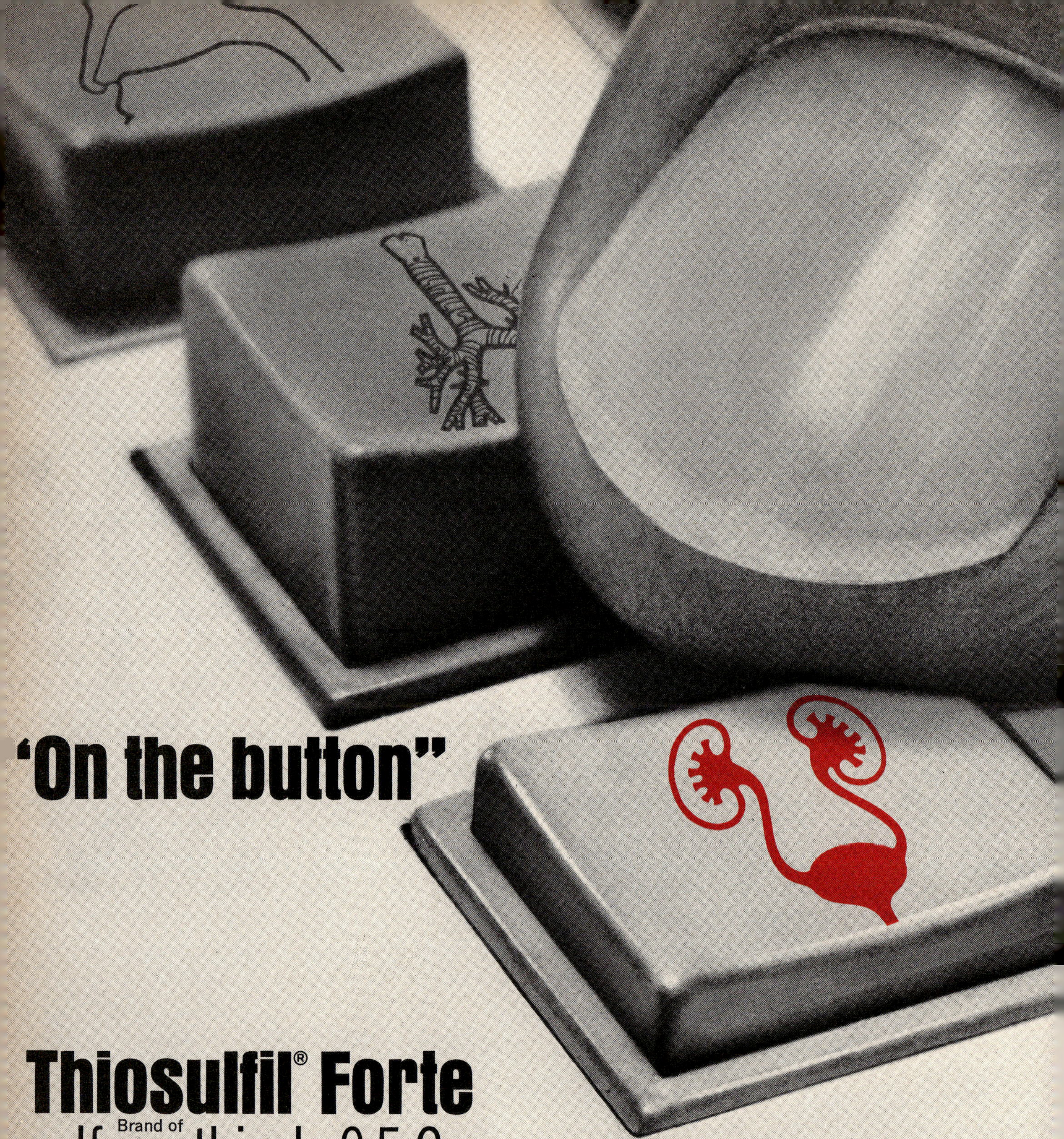

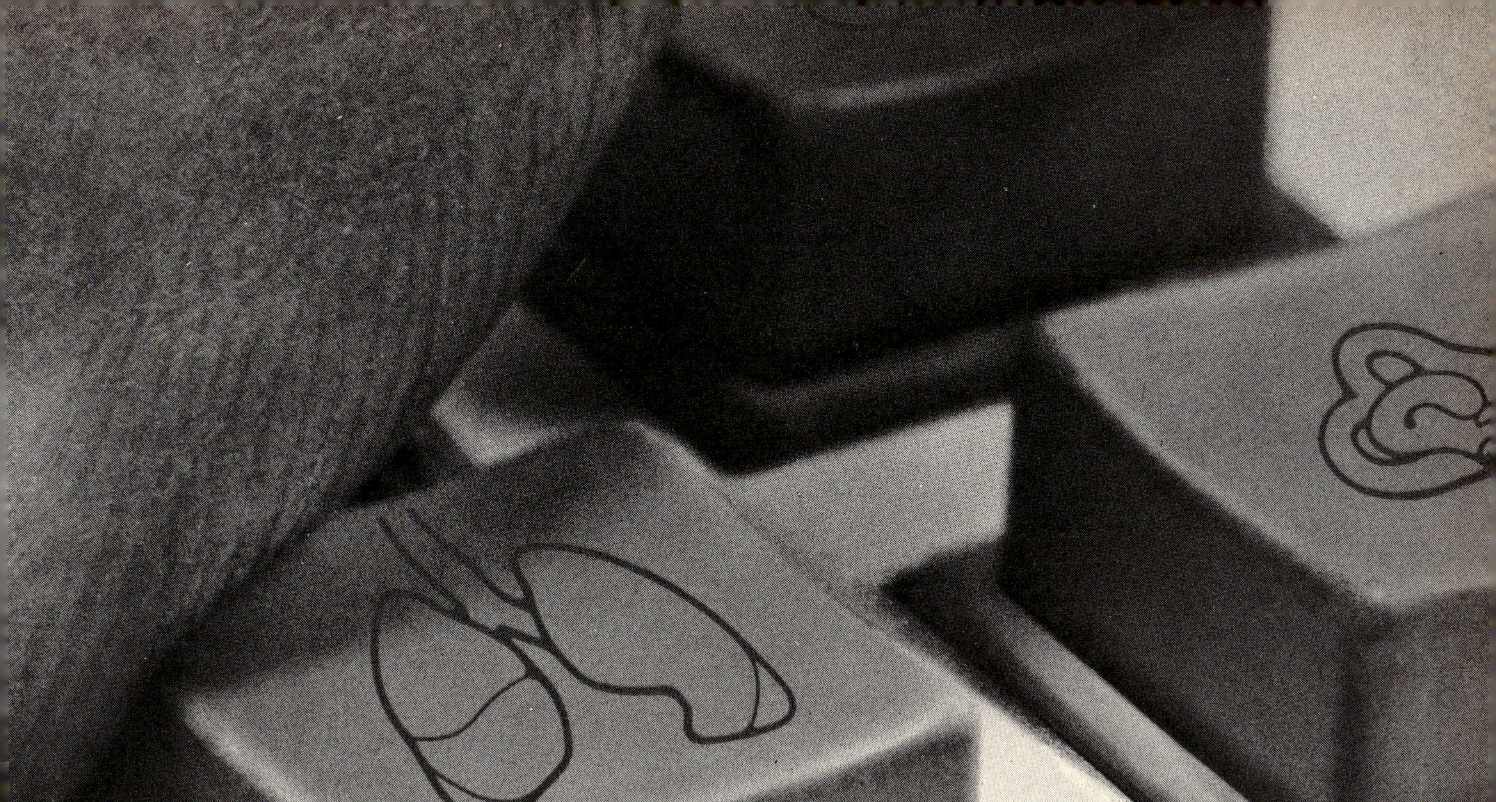

Cancer data

continued

that:

- The incidence of lung cancer has doubled for both men and women.
- The overall incidence of cancer among men rose from 280 cancers per 100,000 population in 1947 to 304 cancers per 100,000 population in 1969. At the same time, the incidence among women declined from 294 to 256 cancers per 100,000 population.
- The incidence of cancer among blacks (especially black men) is substantially higher than among whites. The difference is particularly marked by the higher incidence of cancers of the prostate and esophagus in men.

Most of the increase in the rate of cancer among all men was due to cancers of the prostate and the lungs, and, to a lesser extent, of the colon. The decreased incidence of cancer among women resulted from fewer cancers of the uterine cervix, stomach and rectum.

Biometry Branch statisticians point out that the populations and geometric areas included in the 1947 and 1969 surveys are not exactly the same.

The Third National Cancer Survey is a sequel to the Ten Cities Surveys of 1937 and 1947. These covered ten large cities and surrounding areas. The present study includes data from Iowa, Detroit, Minneapolis-St. Paul, Pittsburgh, Atlanta, Birmingham, Dallas-Fort Worth, Denver and San Francisco-Oakland—nine areas with an estimated population of 20 million, in which 61,409 new cancers were diagnosed during 1969.

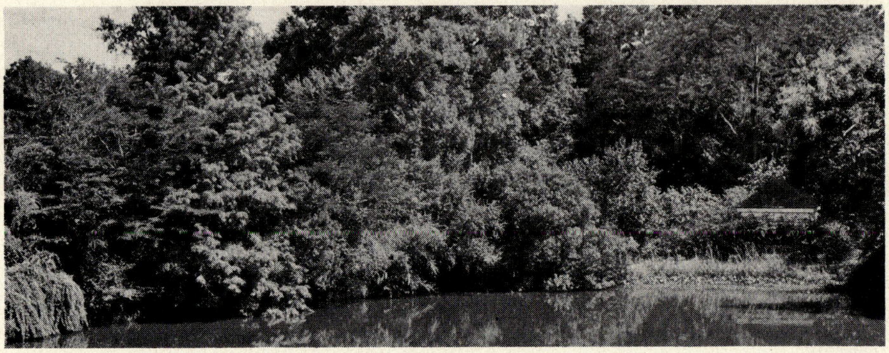

The swamps around New Orleans provide fine growing conditions for ragweed and fungi.

New Orleans asthma

The swamps which virtually surround the city of New Orleans help to create a particularly nasty type of "air pollution" caused by ragweed pollen and spores from dozens of varieties of fungi. The result: New Orleans asthma.

In a discussion of this seasonal disorder, John E. Salvaggio, MD, said that no single source accounts for the disease which is at its worst in September, October and November. It is debatable whether industrial air pollution has much to do with the problem, although he emphasizes that nothing in his work rules out this form of pollution as a contributing source of asthma attacks. What his research does show is a high correlation between natural pollutants and respiratory disease.

Even so, the same atmospheric conditions that make industrial air pollution a major health threat in some cities also worsens the effects of natural irritants. New Orleans asthma "epidemics" are associated with conditions which closely resemble the temperature-inversion phenomena that have trapped pollutants over such cities as Los Angeles. Dispersion of surface pollutants by vertical convection currents is impossible because of the layer of warm air above relatively cool surface air.

Dr. Salvaggio outlined his findings in a telephone interview after publishing a report in the *Journal of Allergy*. He is on the faculty of the Department of Medicine of Louisiana State University School of Medicine.

Drug inventory

The Food and Drug Administration is starting an inventory of all drugs marketed for human use in the United States.

The agency asked the drug industry to voluntarily furnish information on all prescription and non-prescription drugs, vitamins, and antibiotics.

Legislation requiring mandatory registration of all drugs is before Congress. The proposed bill would require the industry to submit inventory information, starting Dec 31, 1972.

Perilous pets?

Exotic animals can be a pain—quite literally. And it is increasingly important for physicians to know something about the associated health hazards because many so-called exotic pets are so easily available—not to mention the busy traffic in laboratory animals.

Luther E. Fredrickson, DVM, MPH, a Tennessee public health official, points out that veterinarians and physicians can provide information that will help people select the right pet for their home and family. "We see too many cases where an appeal to vanity results in the person's obtaining an exotic pet without understanding of its nutritional, environmental, and sexual needs. . . ."

Exotic pets are more likely to injure keepers and to transmit an illness to those who fail to appreciate the special care and handling required, he said. Even zoos are not immune to the health hazards created by—for example—an outbreak of tuberculosis in its monkey colony.

Dr. Fredrickson suggested that smaller zoos with limited funds, facilities, and personnel avoid exotic animals and concentrate on displaying farm animals or small wild creatures native to the region. He spoke in Madison, Wis, at the 13th annual Midwest Interprofessional Seminar on Diseases Common to Animals and Man.

Synthetic tracer

Synthesis of ammonia labeled with nitrogen 13 (^{13}N-ammonia) means that "a new metabolic tracer" may soon be available for dynamic function studies of the heart, brain, kidney, and liver.

Investigators from Memorial Sloan-Kettering Cancer Center described a quick and simple method of synthesizing ^{13}N-ammonia at the Society of Nuclear Medicine meeting in Los Angeles. They said that the short half-life of the new radionuclide results in less than one-third of the radiation dosage of a single chest roentgenogram. ^{13}N-ammonia is a

continued

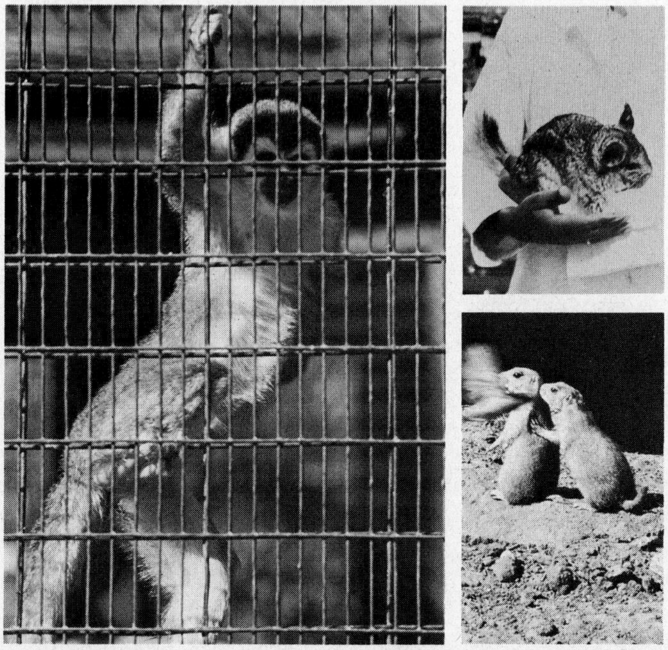

Many pathologic organisms—including *Mycobacterium tuberculosis, Shigella* and *Salmonella*—have been isolated from zoo animals, as well as from household pets and animals used for laboratory research.

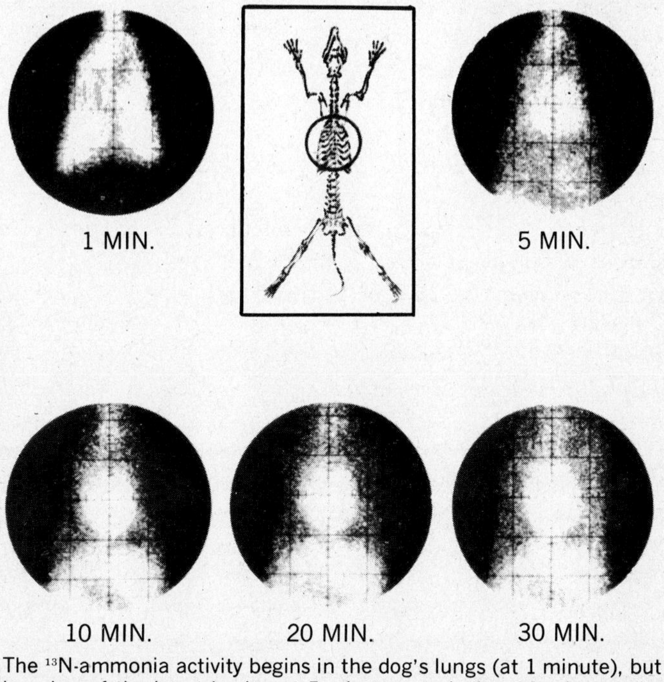

The ^{13}N-ammonia activity begins in the dog's lungs (at 1 minute), but imaging of the heart begins at 5 minutes, and after 10 minutes the heart is shown clearly with some radionuclide activity in the liver.

internal medicine at large

Tracer continued

positron emitter and gives a high count rate per dose with the scintillation camera.

William W. Hunter, Jr., DVM, a visiting investigator at the center, reported that ^{13}N-ammonia should be useful in detecting myocardial infarction and in the evaluation of congestive heart failure. The tracer may also prove useful in scanning tumors, obtaining diagnostic information about the kidneys, and in studying brain function and the actual metabolism of hepatic cells, he said.

Declining fertility rate

The nation's fertility rate declined for the fifth straight month in July, reaching its lowest monthly rate since the late 1930s, according to officials at the National Center for Health Statistics.

The seasonally adjusted fertility rate (the number of births per 1,000 women between the ages of 15 and 44 years) fell from 88.5 in February to 77.5 in July, a decline of about 12%.

An estimated 295,000 babies were born in the United States during July, bringing the total for the first seven months of 1971 to 2,050,000. This is about 2% less than births for the same period of 1970.

According to the Center, there are several possible explanations for the decline.

The increase in the number of abortions during the latter half of 1970 is probably having some impact.

"However, since the declines are fairly general, and are not limited to the states with liberalized abortion laws, there are probably other factors operating," an agency spokesman said. He added that there are not yet enough data to determine the effect of each of the various factors.

How many new TB cases?

No one knows how thorough the tuberculosis case reporting is in the United States. But last year, the actual reports of new cases—of previously unreported, active tuberculosis—totaled 36,137.

The federal Tuberculosis Branch puts the total number of active TB cases on record nationwide for the past year at about 101,000. This includes both known active cases and relapses.

The National Tuberculosis and Respiratory Disease Association estimates that one in four non-hospitalized persons on the active TB registers of health departments is not on chemotherapy. Furthermore, only slightly better than one-third of the contacts of tuberculosis patients receive any prophylactic treatment.

Both the federal TB Branch and NTRDA are working on new approaches, particularly in order to reach patients among minority groups. One of the association's projects is a study of changes in clinic hours to make outpatient treatment more accessible for workers and others whose schedules are limited. NTRDA is also working on informational materials designed for specific cultural groups and seeking to enlist the aid of influential persons in various communities.

NEW ACTIVE TUBERCULOSIS CASES AND DEATHS
UNITED STATES, 1960-1969

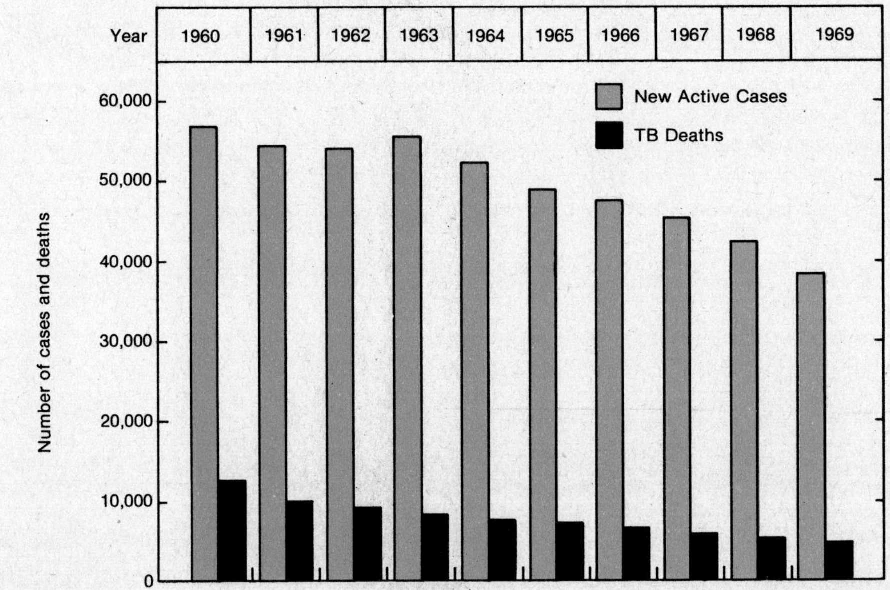

	1960	1961	1962	1963	1964	1965	1966	1967	1968	1969
New Active Cases	55,494	53,726	53,315	54,042	50,874	49,016	47,767	45,647	42,623	39,120
Deaths	10,866	9,938	9,506	9,311	8,303	7,934	7,625	6,901	6,600P	5,340P

P = Provisional

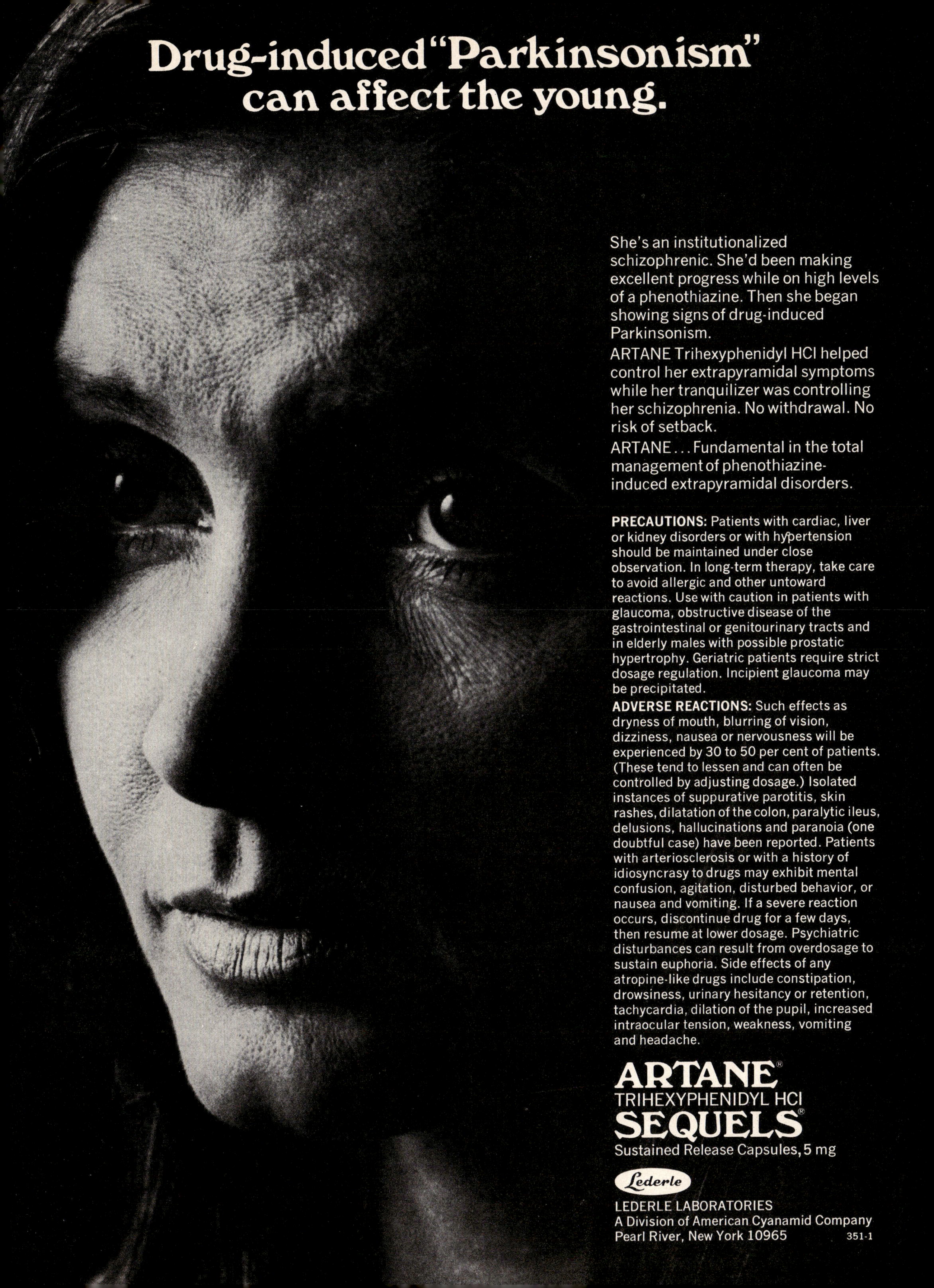
Drug-induced "Parkinsonism" can affect the young.
She's an institutionalized schizophrenic. She'd been making excellent progress while on high levels of a phenothiazine. Then she began showing signs of drug-induced Parkinsonism.
ARTANE Trihexyphenidyl HCl helped control her extrapyramidal symptoms while her tranquilizer was controlling her schizophrenia. No withdrawal. No risk of setback.
ARTANE... Fundamental in the total management of phenothiazine-induced extrapyramidal disorders.
PRECAUTIONS: Patients with cardiac, liver or kidney disorders or with hypertension should be maintained under close observation. In long-term therapy, take care to avoid allergic and other untoward reactions. Use with caution in patients with glaucoma, obstructive disease of the gastrointestinal or genitourinary tracts and in elderly males with possible prostatic hypertrophy. Geriatric patients require strict dosage regulation. Incipient glaucoma may be precipitated.
ADVERSE REACTIONS: Such effects as dryness of mouth, blurring of vision, dizziness, nausea or nervousness will be experienced by 30 to 50 per cent of patients. (These tend to lessen and can often be controlled by adjusting dosage.) Isolated instances of suppurative parotitis, skin rashes, dilatation of the colon, paralytic ileus, delusions, hallucinations and paranoia (one doubtful case) have been reported. Patients with arteriosclerosis or with a history of idiosyncrasy to drugs may exhibit mental confusion, agitation, disturbed behavior, or nausea and vomiting. If a severe reaction occurs, discontinue drug for a few days, then resume at lower dosage. Psychiatric disturbances can result from overdosage to sustain euphoria. Side effects of any atropine-like drugs include constipation, drowsiness, urinary hesitancy or retention, tachycardia, dilation of the pupil, increased intraocular tension, weakness, vomiting and headache.
ARTANE®
TRIHEXYPHENIDYL HCl
SEQUELS®
Sustained Release Capsules, 5 mg
Lederle
LEDERLE LABORATORIES
A Division of American Cyanamid Company
Pearl River, New York 10965
351-1

Internal Medicine at large

The recipient of the 1971 **Bristol Award** of the Infectious Diseases Society of America is **Colin M. MacLeod,** MD, president of the Oklahoma Medical Research Foundation and former president of the Harvey Society and the American Association of Immunologists. Dr. MacLeod received the award for his work in helping to demonstrate the biological activity of DNA.

Herbert J. Kayden, MD, who joined the New York University School of Medicine in 1949, has been promoted to professor of medicine.

Robert D. Conn, MD, has been named professor and first chairman of the Department of Medicine at Southern Illinois University School of Medicine, Springfield. He was formerly associate professor of medicine at the University of Washington, Seattle.

Justus F. Mueller, PhD, professor of microbiology at the State University of New York Upstate Medical Center, Syracuse, is the new president-elect of the American Society of Parasitologists.

Jerome W. Conn, MD, professor of medicine and head of the Division of Endocrinology and Metabolism at the University of Michigan Medical School, has received the 1971 **Heath Memorial Award.** The award was presented in Houston during the 16th Annual Clinical Conference sponsored by The University of Texas M.D. Anderson Hospital and Tumor Institute.

Joseph E. Johnson, MD, who became chancellor of the University of Tennessee Medical Units on an interim basis last December, has been appointed full-time chancellor of the Medical Units as well as vice president for health affairs of the university.

The American Heart Association has presented its 1971 **Louis N. Katz Basic Science Research Prize for Young Investigators** to **Cristobal G. dos Remedios,** PhD. Dr. dos Remedios, acting assistant professor of physiology-anatomy at the University of California in Berkeley, received the award for his work on the molecular basis of muscle contraction.

Robert Messer, MD, has succeeded **Warren Pearse,** MD, as chairman of the Department of Obstetrics and Gynecology at the University of Nebraska Medical Center. Dr. Pearse resigned to become dean of the Medical College of Virginia. Dr. Messer joined the Nebraska faculty in 1963 and became a full professor this fall.

Charles K. Friedberg, MD, clinical professor of medicine at Mount Sinai School of Medicine, has been named a member of the National Heart and Lung Advisory Council of the National Heart and Lung Institute.

Glen E. Tomlinson, MD, has been appointed professor of family medicine and head of the Department of Family Practice at the University of Illinois Abraham Lincoln School of Medicine, Chicago.

Tinsley R. Harrison, MD, a cardiologist who since 1964 has been a Distinguished Professor of the University of Alabama, has won the 1971 **James B. Herrick Award** of the American Heart Association for his work in clinical cardiology. Dr. Harrison is a past president of the association and the author of *Failure of the Circulation* and *Principles of Internal Medicine,* as well as co-author of *Principles and Problems of Ischemic Heart Disease.*

The new president of the American Academy of Pediatrics is **Jay M. Arena,** MD, professor of pediatrics and professor of community health sciences at Duke University School of Medicine. Dr. Arena also heads Duke University Medical Center Poison Control Center and served as president of the American Association of Poison Control Centers from 1968 to 1970.

Carl Eisdorfer, MD, PhD, and **Victor Kassell,** MD, have been named members of the HEW Advisory Committee on Older Americans. Dr. Eisdorfer is director of the Duke University Center for the Study of Aging and Dr. Kassell is a geriatrician in Salt Lake City.

The winners of the 1971 **Bronfman Prizes** for distinguished leadership and achievement in public health are **John H.F. Brotherston,** MD, DPH, chief medical officer of the Scottish Home and Health Department; **Ruth B. Freeman,** RN, EdD, professor emer-

continued

Internal medicine at large

continued

ita of public health administration at Johns Hopkins University, and **James H. Steele**, DVM, MPH, former chief public health veterinarian of US Public Health Service. The awards were presented at the annual convention of the American Public Health Association in Minneapolis.

Robert L. Kroc, PhD, has succeeded **Samuel B. Barker**, PhD, dean of the University of Alabama Graduate School, as president of the American Thyroid Association. Dr. Kroc is president of the Kroc Foundation for the Advancement of Medical Science at Santa Ynez, Calif.

Morton M. Kligerman, MD, chairman of the department of Radiology at Yale University School of Medicine, is leaving to head the new Cancer Research and Treatment Center at the University of New Mexico. Dr. Kligerman was also named chief of the school's Division of Radiation Therapy.

William L. Stewart, MD, former associate professor of medicine at the University of Maryland School of Medicine, has been appointed professor and first chairman of the Department of Family Practice at Southern Illinois University School of Medicine, Springfield.

Giampiero di Mayorca, MD, professor of microbiology at the Eppley Institute of Cancer Research, University of Nebraska, has been named professor of microbiology at the University of Illinois College of Medicine.

Richard E. Marland, PhD, has succeeded **Richard C. Schultz**, MD, as president of the American Association for Automotive Medicine. Dr. Marland is on assignment from the PHS to serve as interim director of Hawaii's Office of Environmental Quality Control. Dr. Schultz is chairman of the Plastic Surgery Department of the University of Illinois College of Medicine, Chicago.

T. Timothy Crocker, MD, has joined the faculty of the University of California Irvine College of Medicine as chairman of the Department of Community and Environmental Medicine. Dr. Crocker was formerly professor of medicine and research physician (oncology) in the Cancer Research Institute of the University of California San Francisco Medical Center.

Jonathan W. Uhr, MD, is succeeding **S. Edward Sulkin**, MD, as chairman of the Department of Microbiology at the University of Texas Southwestern Medical School in Dallas. Dr. Sulkin, who has headed the department since 1945, asked to be relieved of administrative duties to have more time for research. Dr. Uhr, director of the Irvington House Institute for Rheumatic Fever and Allied Diseases at the New York University School of Medicine, was also named professor of internal medicine at Texas, and will assume both positions next fall.

The current president-elect of the American Association of Automotive Medicine is **James L. Weygandt**, MD, a general practitioner from Sheboygan Falls, Wis.

J. Willis Hurst, MD, has been installed as president of the American Heart Association. He is professor and chairman of the Department of Medicine at Emory University School of Medicine. **Paul N. Yu**, MD, Sarah McCort Ward Professor of Medicine and head of the Cardiology Unit at the University of Rochester Medical Center, was chosen president-elect of the association.

Stuart W. Tanenbaum, PhD, has been named program director for biochemistry in the Molecular Biology Section of the Division of Biological and Medical Sciences at the National Science Foundation. He is on leave as professor of microbiology at the Columbia University College of Physicians and Surgeons.

Edward H. Ahrens, Jr., MD, is the first Hilda Altschul Master Professor of Medicine at Cornell University Medical Center. The professorship was endowed in the memory of the late wife of **Arthur M. Master**, MD. Dr. Ahrens will also remain on the Rockefeller University faculty.

Jonathan E. Rhoads, MD, professor and chairman of the Department of Surgery at the University of Pennsylvania School of Medicine, is the new president of the American College of Surgeons. **William P. Longmire, Jr.**, MD, professor and chairman of the UCLA School of Medicine, was chosen president-elect.

The new president of the Flying Physicians Association is **Francis X. Sommer**, MD, of Barbourville, Ky.

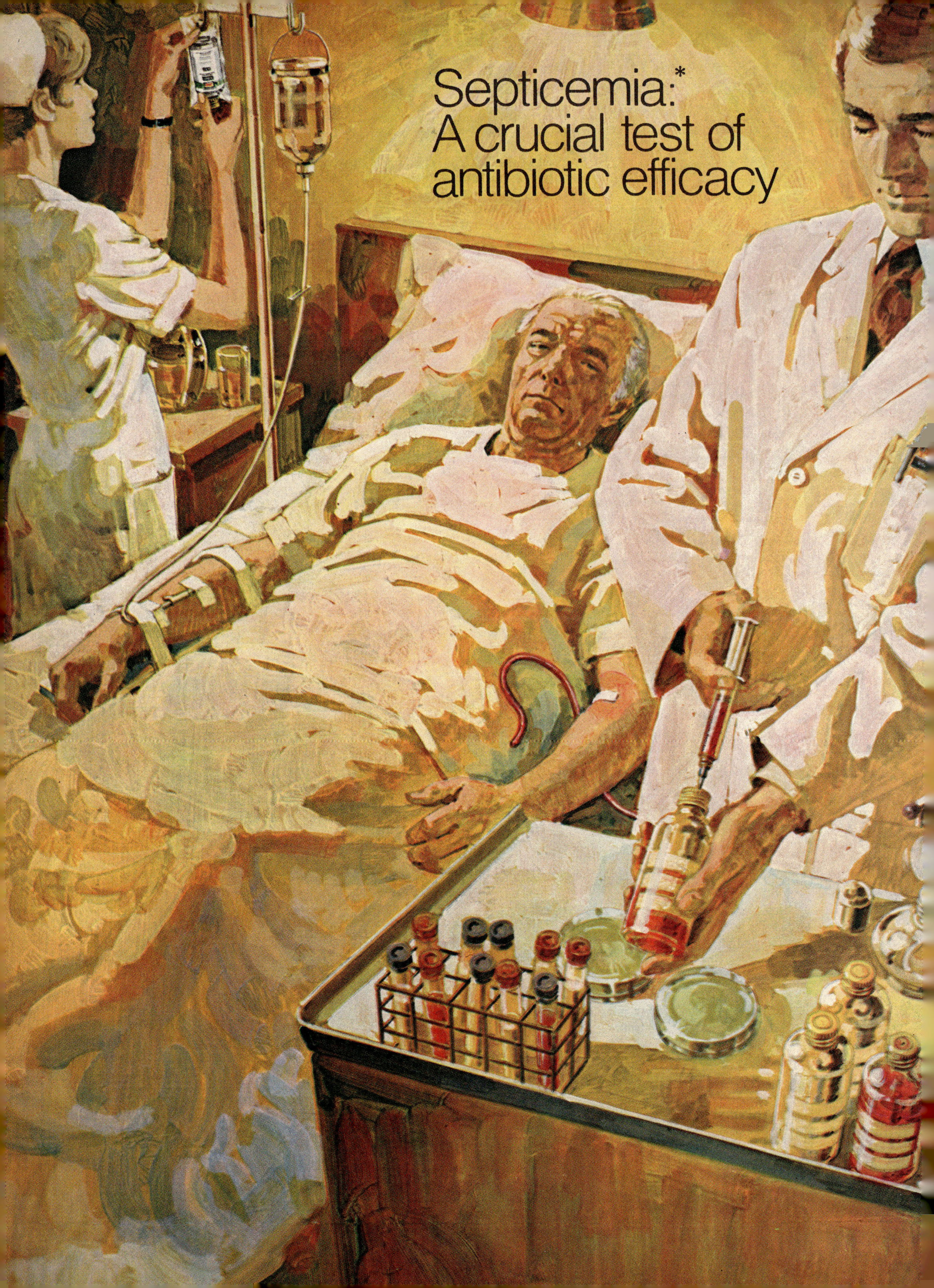
Septicemia:*
A crucial test of
antibiotic efficacy

Volume 128, Number 6, December 1971

Archives of Internal Medicine

Evans County Cardiovascular and Cerebrovascular Epidemiologic Study

Guest Editor: John C. Cassel, MD, MPH

Introduction

Curtis G. Hames, MD, Claxton, Ga

This brief introduction will include a short historical note concerning the development of the Evans County study, a description of the study site, its physical and racial structure, an overview of its accomplishments and hopes for its future.

The Epidemiological Study of Cardiovascular Disease developed in Evans County, Georgia, from the clinical observation that coronary heart disease appeared to occur less frequently among blacks than whites, even though hypertension was obviously more common in blacks and they consumed a higher animal fat diet. In addition there was no difference in coronary mortality by sex in the blacks although such a difference did occur in whites.

The study was, therefore, basically designed to answer two questions: First, were these clinical observations valid? That is, does coronary heart disease really occur more commonly among whites than blacks living in Evans County, and, if so, what was the extent of the differences? Second, presuming a positive answer, what were the reasons for the observed differences?

At about the time these observations were being made in 1956-1967, James Watt, MD, was head of the National Heart Institute. Following a mandate from Congress to expand the base for medical research he envisioned a program to include not only the Institute of Health's own research, the academic and university research, the clinical and laboratory research, facilities of the Veterans Hospitals and other government agencies, industrial and private re-

Received for publication July 25, 1971, accepted Oct 6.

From the Evans County Health Department, Claxton, Ga.

Reprint requests to 2 N Newton St, Claxton, Ga 30417.

search laboratories but also research at the grass roots level where he felt there was a tremendous opportunity for the collection of epidemiological data. Epidemiological research at the community level could provide invaluable information concerning the natural history of many diseases, studies in genetics, delivery of health care systems to name but a few possibilities. In many instances data of these types could not be collected under any other circumstances. He envisioned such a program of research functioning through the local health departments in conjunction with the local practicing physicians. It was at this time, at the suggestion of Jeremiah Stamler, MD, that a small grant had been submitted to the National Institutes of Health for support of such a community study in Evans County.

Dr. Watt became aware of the application and visited this county and its health department as one of several sites for possible pilot study areas. He subsequently was greatly instrumental in nurturing the development of the project; ie, by expanding the concept of its usefulness, providing the administrative machinery for funding and support through the local health department, the assignment of US Public Health Officers for examination of the population and requiring that we seek adequate statistical design and assistance. This was obtained through the support of departments of epidemiology and biostatistics at the University of North Carolina School of Public Health. Dr. Watt had hoped this project might serve as a stimulus for the development of other community based research projects over the entire county; however, the Evans County study is the only black-white epidemiological study in the United States, and it and the Tecumseh study are the only two total community epidemiological studies.

The following brief description of the study site characteristics will give the reader some general feeling for the population under surveillance.

Evans County is located on the coastal plains, about 60 miles inland from the port city of Savannah, Ga. The county is 19 miles at its greatest diameter and consists of flat or slightly rolling terrain of red clay and sandy soil. Much of the county is covered by pine forests which are harvested for pulpwood, turpentine, and lumber. Only small industry is present: fruitcake is manufactured and a local sewing factory employs some 500 people, mostly females. The basic economy continues to be agriculture. However, in recent years there has been a gradual shift to employment at the nearby Fort Stewart under government civil service or to more industrial jobs reached by commuting to Savannah.

The population has been fairly stable as indicated by the fact that the Evans County official population in 1960 was 6,952 and 7,290 in 1970 or a 4.9% increase in ten years. There are approximately 4,847 whites (66.5%) and 2,434 blacks (33.5%.) Only nine persons of other races were enumerated. The black-white ratio has remained almost constant in ten years, showing a surprisingly stable population composition at the time of unusually great black outmigration in other areas of the south. There are 664 children at the age of 5 years, 2,166 ages 5 to 17 years, 3,697 ages 18 to 64, and 763 ages 65 and over. From age 14 and above 3,300 were married, 486 widows, 129 divorced, 1,199 never married. A total of 36.6% are living in incorporated areas while 63.4% are living in a completely rural setting. Households number 2,174, including 324 one person households; in addition, 17 persons are living in group quarters. There are 2,364 housing units in Evans County, 1,348 occupied by owners, 826 occupied by tenants and 190 vacant, mostly for seasonal use by agricultural workers. The proportion of home owners has increased from 49.2% in 1960 to 57% in 1970. In addition to the 2,023 single family units there are now 186 government housing units and 148 trailers or mobile home units. A percentage of occupied units with more than one person per room has decreased from 18.6% in 1960 to 12.6% in 1970. Of all the occupied housing units 1,701 have piped water, toilets, and bath while 473 lack some or all plumbing. The median rent paid by tenants in 1970 was approximately $30 per month.

The original study was launched in this county in 1960 when 100% of all residents over age 40 and a 50% sample of those between 15 and 39 were given a complete physical examination together with a battery of laboratory tests. In addition samples of serum from each individual were frozen and retained for future studies. Since that time the population has been carefully and systematically followed, and survivors reexamined during the period 1967-1969. The results of this follow up and reexamination insofar as cardiovascular and cerebrovascular disease are concerned are reported in the succeeding papers of this issue.

During the period 1960-1970, the availability of a well documented total population under careful surveillance, with frozen serum dating from 1960, has been utilized by numerous academic institutions from various parts of the world as well as by government agencies for a wide variety of research purposes. These studies have extended from molecular biological investigations through clinical research to large scale epidemiological and ecological studies.[1-45] In all such endeavors the principal investigator has served as an interlocutor between the people and the various scientists maintaining rapport and reducing undue confusion or disturbance on the part of the citizens. On numerous occasions it has been demonstrated that such a function is essential for public relations if this delicate balance so vital for the success of any research study in a free living population is to be maintained.

While many of these research projects are not necessarily related to cardiovascular disease, brief comments on a few of them are made here to illustrate the potentialities that can be derived from a close liaison between a practicing physician and academic institutions. The development and supervision of the basic research design by the Department of Epidemiology at the University of North Carolina has made it possible to draw any type of random sample or matched case-control series for purposes of such studies. Further the principal investigator, as a native to the study site, has an unique vantage point, in that he has had direct contact with as many as three to five generations of families and has been able to observe them over time. Such a vantage point displays the potential role of genetics in many diseases in much clearer focus and has lent direction to the research effort. Such effort brought Baruch S. Blumberg MD, PhD, and W. Thomas London, MD, and other geneticists[4,7-9,12,13,23,29,36] to Evans County to utilize the available resources of the study. In a search for the Australian antigen among over 2,000 serum samples from Evans County, Drs. Blumberg and London found a patient with the Australian antigen who also had severe hepatitis. His hepatitis was well documented and served as one of the two original clues to linking the Australian antigen with viral hepatitis. Cardiovascular epidemiology correlates, ie, height, weight, body build, blood pressure, diet, exercise, and social status; levels of triglycerides, cholesterol, γ-globulins, lipoproteins, plasma renin, urinary sodium potassium, carbohydrates, catecholamines; hematocrit value; and numerous clotting factors including platelet stickiness, have been determined in these population groups living side by side where gross differences from coronary heart disease and hypertension exist.[14-22,24-27,30-35,39-44] Studies are also now under way to determine the prevalence of hyperlipoprotemias as classified by Fredrickson along with the correlation of morbidity and mortality with all the various lipid fractions determined in these patients both chemically and by ultracentrifugation. Geneticists from the University of Oslo in Norway and Florence, Italy, are using known genetic markers for possible correlation also with the various same fractions. The computer analysis of electrocardiographic data has been collected to better understand the significance of ST segment elevation in the blacks and its possible relationship to membrane chemistry. A total of 11,000 virus antibody determinations have been made for their possible correlation with congenital heart disease as well as coronary heart disease. The possible relationship of glucose 6-phosphate dehydrogenase deficiency to increased hypertension and decreased CHD as reported by Long and associates,[45] has been determined in the Evans County population. Alpha 2 antitrypsin deficiency was found to occur in about 2% to 3% of the population and its possible relationship to predisposition to develop emphysema has been determined.[12,29] Some 1,400 family aggregations have been characterized in the population. The natural history of transitory ischemic attacks and cerebrovascular accidents are being monitored on a long-term basis. The effects of migration on health is being studied among individuals who have migrated from the study site since 1960. Personality type, incidence of new disease, motivation, social achievement and many other factors are included in the study. No other known southern community has data of this type available for study. The community has also served as a base for training medical students as well as ancillary personnel. The early development of an intensive coronary care unit in the local 42-bed hospital was achieved several years before it became widely utilized even in much larger hospitals.[38]

Our new goals for the future lie not only in the observation of the natural history of disease but also in the area of genetics and ultimately in the utilization of such a well-defined population for preventive intervention studies; ie, with over 1,000 cases of hypertension defined a hypertensive control program could ideally be developed here as a model for use in all parts of the country.

Because of the wealth of data and information that can be obtained from such epidemiological studies other communities should set up similar basic studies where many questions concerning health care and the long-term observation of chronic disease can be answered in the natural environment.

This investigation was supported by Public Health Service research grant HE-03341.

References

1. Hames, CG: An atherogenic profile. *J Med Assoc Georgia* **49**:188-191, 1960.

2. A Report of Selected Characteristic Evans and Bulloch Counties, Ga. 1960, Public Health Service.

3. Hames CG, Greenberg BG: A comparative study of serum cholesterol levels in school children and their possible relation to atherogenesis. *Amer J Public Health* **51**:374-385, 1961.

4. Parker WC, Bearn AG: Haptoglobin and transferrin variation in human and primates: Two new transferrins in Chinese and Japanese populations. *Ann Hum Genet* **25**:227-241, 1961.

5. McDonough JR, Hames CG, Greenberg BG, et al: Observations on serum cholesterol levels in the twin population of Evans County, Georgia. *Circulation* **25**:962-969, 1962.

6. McDonough JR, Hames CG, Stulb SC, et al: Cardiovascular disease field study in Evans County, Ga. *Public Health Rep* **78**:1051-1059, 1963.

7. Robinson JC, Blumberg BS, Pierce JE, et al: Studies on the inherited variants of blood proteins: II. Familial segregation of transferrin $B_{1\text{-}2}B_2$. *J Lab Clin Med* **62**:762-765, 1963.

8. Cooper AJ, Blumberg BS, Workman PL, et al: Biochemical polymorphic traits in a U.S. white and Negro population. *Amer J Hum Genet* **15**:420-428, 1963.

9. Workman PL, Blumberg BS, Cooper AJ: Selection, gene migration and polymorphic stability in a U.S. white and Negro population. *Amer J Hum Genet* **15**:429-437, 1963.

10. McDonough JR, Garrison GE, Hames CG: Blood pressure and hypertensive disease among Negroes and whites: A study in Evans County, Georgia. *Ann Intern Med* **61**:208-228, 1964.

11. Brewer GJ, Gall JC, Honeyman MS, et al: Inheritance of quantitative expression of G-6-PD deficiency in heterozygous Negro females: A twin study. *Clin Res* **13**:265, 1965.

12. Kueppers F, Briscoe WA, Bearn AG: Hereditary deficiency of antitrypsin. *Science* **146**:1678-1679, 1964.

13. Blumberg BS, Workman PL, Hirschfeld J: Gamma globulin, group specific and lipoprotein groups in a U.S. white and Negro population. *Nature* **202**:561-563, 1964.

14. Hames CG, McDonough JR, Elliott JL: Hypertension in identical twins. *Lancet* **2**:585, 1964.

15. McDonough JR, Hames CG, Stulb SC, et al: Coronary heart disease among Negroes and whites in Evans County, Ga. *J Chronic Dis* **18**:443-468, 1965.

16. Lichtman MA, Hames CG, McDonough JR: Serum protein electrophoretic fractions among Negro and white subjects in Evans County, Ga. *Amer J Clin Nutr* **16**:492-508, 1965.

17. Stulb SC, McDonough JR, Greenberg BG, et al: The relationship of nutrient intake and exercise to serum cholesterol levels in white males in Evans County, Ga. *Amer J Clin Nutr* **16**:238-242, 1965.

18. McDonough JR, Hames CG, Garrison GE, et al: The relationship of hematocrit to cardiovascular states of health in the Negro and white population of Evans County, Ga. *J Chronic Dis* **18**:243-257, 1965.

19. Lichtman MA, Hames CG, McDonough JR: Serum gamma globulin levels among Negroes and whites in Evans County, Ga. *Clin Res* **13**:30, 1964.

20. Ibrahim MA, Jenkins CD, Cassel JC, et al: Personality traits and coronary heart disease. *J Chronic Dis* **19**:255-271, 1966.

21. Garrison GE, McDonough JR, Hames CG, et al: Prevalence of chronic congestive heart failure in the population of Evans County, Georgia. *Amer J Epidem* **83**:338-344, 1966.

22. Skinner JC, Benson H, McDonough JR, et al: Social status, physical activity and coronary proneness. *J Chronic Dis* **9**:773-783, 1966.

23. Berg K, Bearn A: An inherited X-linked serum in man: The XM system. *J Exp Med* **123**:379-397, 1966.

24. Hames CG, McDonough JR, Stulb SC: Physical activity and ischemic heart disease among Negroes and whites in Evans County, Ga, in Raab W (ed): *Prevention of Ischemic Heart Disease: Principles and Practice.* Springfield, Ill, Charles C Thomas Publisher, 1966.

25. McDonough JR, Hames CG: Influence of race, sex and occupation on seasonal changes in serum cholesterol. *Amer J Epidem* **83**:356-364, 1967.

26. Lichtman MA, Vaughan JH, Hames CG: The distribution of serum immunoglobins, anti-gamma-G globulins ("rheumatoid factors") and antinuclear antibodies in white and Negro subjects in Evans County, Georgia. *Arthritis Rheum* **10**:204-215, 1967.

27. McDonough JR, Garrison GE, Hames CG: Blood pressure and hypertensive disease among Negroes and whites in Evans County, Ga, in Stamler J (ed): *Epidemiology of Hypertension.* New York, Grune & Stratton Inc, 1967.

28. Brewer GJ, Gall JC, Honeyman M, et al: Inheritance of quantitative expression of erythrocyte glucose-6-phosphate dehydrogenase activity in the Negro: A twin study. *Biochem Genet* **1**:41-53, 1967.

29. Kueppers G, Bearn AG: An inherited A4 antitrypsin variant. *Humangenetik* **4**:217-220, 1967.

30. Lichtman MA, McDonough JR, Hames CG: Serum gamma globulin concentration in related and non-related subjects. *Human Biol* **39**:307-315, 1967.

31. Williams OD, Grizzle JE: Analysis of longitudinal data: An investigation of the relationship among systolic blood pressure, diastolic blood pressure, serum triglyceride, and serum cholesterol, abstracted. *Circulation* **38**(suppl 6):207, 1968.

32. Jenkins CD, Hames CG, Zyzanski SJ, et al: Psychological traits and serum lipids: I. Findings from the California Psychological Inventory. *Psychosom Med* **31**:115-128, 1969.

33. Hames CG: An epidemiological study of platelet stickiness, in Schettler G (ed): *Platelets and the Vessel Wall-Fibrin Deposition: Symposium of the European Atherosclerosis Group.* Stuttgart, Germany, Georg Thieme Verlag, 1970, pp 129-143.

34. Heyden S, Bartel AG, Hames CG, et al: Elevated blood pressure levels in adolescents, Evans County, Georgia: Seven year follow-up of 30 patients and 30 controls. *JAMA* **209**:1683-1689, 1969.

35. Hames CG: Coronary heart disease and smoking: A reducible risk factor. *J Med Assoc Georgia* **58**:440, 1969.

36. Kueppers F: Studies on the Xh antigen in human serum. *Humangenetik* **7**:98-103, 1969.

37. Hames CG: Stress and heart disease. *J Med Assoc Georgia* **59**:194-195, 1970.

38. Bartel AG, Hames CG: Intensive coronary care in a 42-bed rural hospital. *J Med Assoc Georgia* **59**:285-289, 1970.

39. Simpson MT, Hames CG, Olewine DA, et al: Physical activity, catecholamines and platelet stickiness, in *Myocardiology: Recent Advances in Studies on Cardiac Structure and Metabolism.* Baltimore, University Park Press, to be published.

40. Hames CG: The correlation of ischemic heart disease with social class among whites and blacks in a total community epidemiological study. *Lex et Scientia* **7**:53-62, 1970.

41. Heyden S, Bartel AG, Hames CG, et al: Elevated blood pressure levels in adolescents, Evans County, Ga, in Braunwald E (ed): *Year Book of Cardiovascular Medicine and Surgery.* Chicago, Year Book Medical Publishers Inc, 1970.

42. Grim CE, McDonough JR, Dahl LK, et al: On the higher blood pressure of blacks: A study of sodium and potassium intake and excretion in a biracial community, abstracted. *Clin Res* **18**:593, 1970.

43. Grim CE, McDonough JR, Dahl LK, et al: Dietary sodium, potassium, and blood pressure. Three hundred Racial Differences in Evans County, Georgia, abstracted. *Circulation* **62**(suppl 3):85, 1970.

44. Karp H, Heyman A, Heyden S, et al: Incidence and Risk Factors of Stroke Among the Biracial Population in Evans County, Georgia, abstracted. *Circulation* **62**(suppl 3):93, 1970.

45. Long WK, Wilson SW, Frenkel EP: Associations between red cell glucose-6-phosphate dehydrogenase variants and vascular diseases. *Amer J Hum Genet* **19**:35-53, 1967.

Summary of Major Findings of the Evans County Cardiovascular Studies

John C. Cassel, MD, MPH, Chapel Hill, NC

The studies reported in this issue have resulted from an unusual "partnership" between a primary care physician Curtis Hames, MD, and an academic department of epidemiology. The initiative for this collaboration came from Dr. Hames who wished to determine whether certain phenomena he was observing in his practice were occurring throughout the community or were restricted to the types of people who selected him for their physician. To the extent that his practice observations were found to be generalizable, he would then be interested in seeking some explanations. In particular, Hames was impressed with the rarity with which he saw black patients, particularly black men, with any manifestation of coronary heart disease (CHD), despite the fact that levels of blood pressure in many of these patients were markedly elevated. This observation was all the more surprising as coronary disease was a very common manifestation in his white patients. (Evans County, Ga, is situated in the "high coronary belt," the area extending down the Eastern seaboard from Virginia to Georgia which has one of the highest mortality rates from coronary heart disease in the United States.[1])

In an attempt to find answers to these questions it was decided to conduct a study in which every adult resident of the county over the age of 40 years and 50% sample of those between the ages of 15 and 39 years would have a standard medical examination and a battery of laboratory tests. For this purpose a private census of the county was undertaken in 1960, the population divided into ten random subsamples (to avoid the potential problem of examiner variation over time) and over an 18-month period an attempt was made to examine all eligible residents (3,377 in all) by two physicians assigned to this study. Largely due to the excellent rapport between Hames and this population 3,102 (92%) of the residents cooperated and underwent the examinations. The major findings of this study have been published[2,3] and are summarized in this issue.[4] Since that examination the availability of a well categorized defined population has provided the basis for literally dozens of additional studies, conducted by a wide variety of universities.[5] The papers in this issue, however, are restricted to some of the findings in the follow-up study that was conducted between 1967 and 1969 on all those individuals originally examined in 1960 through 1962.

As indicated in this issue[4] the 1960 through 1962 prevalence study documented the fact that all manifestations of coronary heart disease (myocardial infarction and angina) occurred very rarely in black men, their age-adjusted rate being only one half that of white men. Among white men there was a sharp difference in the rate by social class, men in the higher half of the social class scores having a rate of 99 per 1,000, while the rate for those in the lower half was only 40 per 1,000, not very different from the rate for blacks. (There was too little variation in social class among the blacks—as measured by occupation, education, and source of income—to permit any examination for the effect of social class in that group.)

None of the risk factors measured, namely systolic and diastolic blood pressure, serum cholesterol level, cigarette smoking, body weight, or diet could account for either the ethnic or the social class differences in these prevalence rates. Either there

Received for publication May 13, 1971; accepted July 13.

From the Department of Epidemiology, School of Public Health, University of North Carolina, Chapel Hill.

Reprint requests to Department of Epidemiology, School of Public Health, University of North Carolina, Chapel Hill, NC 27514 (Dr. Cassel).

was no difference in the distribution of these risk factors between the various groups (as was the case of diet) or where there were differences (as in the case of blood pressure, cholesterol level, and cigarette smoking) the prevalence rates at comparable levels of these risk factors were always low in black and lower social class whites and high in higher social class whites. Differential rates by occupation groups appeared to offer a clue. These occupational differences suggested that possibly physical activity exerted a protective effect and that variations in the level of physical activity between the various ethnic and social class groups accounted, *at least in part,* for the difference in their rates.

It was recognized at the time of this prevalence study that any conclusions concerning either the difference in occurrence of CHD by ethnic or social class group or the explanation or lack of explanation for such differences provided by the risk factors would have to be made with caution. The problems of selective survival and the possible effects of prior disease affecting risk factor level (rather than vice versa) are common to all cross-sectional prevalence studies and in this case as well may have led to spurious interpretation. For this reason it was recognized that a follow-up incidence study would be required wherein we could determine the fate of all those examined in 1960 through 1962 and found to be free of CHD. Such a follow-up study was conducted between 1967 and 1969, the examining physicians on this occasion using the same criteria for the diagnosis of cases as was used in the initial examinations. Collaboration with the departments of neurology at Duke and Emory Universities made it possible to ascertain all cases of stroke, as well as CHD.[6] All deaths that occurred between the two examinations were identified and all clinical documents and autopsy reports collected so that as accurate an assessment as possible of the cause of death could be made. Strenuous attempts were made to determine the status of all migrants from the county, and as many as possible were visited and examined by study personnel. The health status of those who were not examined was ascertained by mail or through questioning close relatives. The results of these efforts are presented in some detail,[7] but in summary the status of 98.8% of the original cohort was ascertained, 90.9% being examined.

The incidence study revealed, first, that the social class difference in rates originally observed in white men had disappeared.[8] Various analyses indicated that this was most likely a reflection of a changing social class pattern in this disease, particularly affecting younger lower social class men who were beginning to "catch up" if not exceed the higher social class. Such a conclusion received support from the finding that some of the risk factors (particularly systolic and diastolic blood pressure) were increasing in these younger lower social class men to a greater extent than in the higher social class. This phenomenon of a changing social class pattern (which does not seem to be restricted to Evans County) could provide some useful clues in further studies aimed at discovering factors important in the etiology of this disease.

In contrast to the social class findings, the incidence study revealed a persisting difference between blacks and whites with black men having substantially lower rates at each age.[8]

A number of analyses were performed which indicated that it was most unlikely that black cases had been missed or that there had been any systematic under-diagnosing in blacks or overdiagnosing in whites. Further, it was shown that the low rates in blacks could not be accounted for by competing causes of death, particularly death from stroke. Even if all the deaths from stroke in black men were counted as coronary cases (under the extreme assumption if they had lived, they would have developed CHD) and those added to the diagnosed cases of CHD the rates in blacks would still be lower than in whites.

An analysis of various risk factors, systolic and diastolic blood pressure, cholesterol level[9] cigarette smoking, body weight, hematocrit value[10] and ECG abnormalities[11] showed that none of them alone or in combination[12] could account for these differences. At any level of any risk factor or any level of combination of risk factors, black men had comparatively lower rates than did whites.

Examining the relationship between these risk factors and the disease either singly or more importantly in combination (using a multivariate analysis) convinced us that blacks were responding to these factors in a similar fashion to whites but at a much lower level of disease.[12] To put this in other words, most of the factors that increased the risk of CHD in whites also increased the risk of this disease in blacks. Some additional factor or factors had to be present which either potentiated the effect of these risk factors in whites or protected blacks from part of their effect. A clue as to what at least one of these missing factors might be was provided by the finding that the only circumstance in which white men had as low rates as blacks, was when they both were sharecroppers.[13] The only relevant difference between white sharecroppers and all other white men that could be invoked to explain this finding was the high level of physical activity involved in sharecropping. Further, if physical activity is one of the missing factors, making the consequences of the atherosclerotic risk factors less important as far as complications are concerned, it appeared that it only operated above some threshold level. Variations in physical activity among other white occupational groups (ie, nonsharecroppers) surely occur, but these are not reflected in any difference in the rates of CHD.[13]

As a result of these analyses it is now possible to identify three groups of men, two of which, white sharecroppers and all black men, are virtually immune to CHD and the third, all other white men, are as susceptible, (if not more so) as any group in the US. (The incidence rates in white nonfarmers in Evans County are among the highest in the country). Further, these groups could be matched on most, if not all, the currently accepted risk factors allowing an intensive series of studies to be mounted to discover these additional factors which so far have eluded our grasp. As indicated in one of the papers in this series,[14] in addition to the level of physical activity, there is some evidence that psychosocial processes may constitute some of these missing factors. These together with various genetic markers along with some of the postulated pathogenic processes (eg, clotting factors [?]) may be the mediating mechanisms. These possibilities need now to be explored.

Finally, a methodological note: It will be found that tests of statistical significance have been very infrequently used in any of the analyses. This was a deliberate decision on the part of the investigators as it certainly is not clear to us what differences such tests could make to our interpretations in the context of this study. It should be borne in mind that the population over the age of 40 years (no cases occurred under this age) do not constitute a sample of some universe. They are a universe—all the residents of Evans County in the time period 1960 through 1969.

The phenomena we are reporting are those that have been observed to occur in Evans County. Much as we would like to generalize our findings to other men in the United States, we feel that this is not possible without replication. Formal tests of statistical significance would be of little help in this regard as we do not as yet know in what crucial indexes the Evans County population is representative of any other population. We recognize that such tests of significance may serve a useful purpose in quantitating the strength of the relationships found, but we have used other methods to do this. The argument that this represents a sample of a larger time interval, while statistically defensible, is untenable epidemiologically because of the rapid rate of change known to be occurring in Evans County. Nevertheless, recognizing that this is a somewhat unorthodox view, we have included all the data needed so that if he so desires the interested reader can compute these tests himself.

References

1. Sauer HI, Marienfeld CJ, Cartwright RS: *Methods of Mapping Mortality.* Read before the American Public Health Association, Houston, 1970.
2. McDonough JR, Hames CG, Stulb SC, et al: Coronary heart disease among Negroes and whites in Evans County, Georgia. *J Chronic Dis* **18**:443-468, 1965.
3. McDonough JR, Garrison GE, Hames CG: Blood pressure and hypertension disease among Negroes and whites: A study in Evans County, Georgia. *Ann Intern Med* **61**:208-228, 1964.
4. Cassel JC: Review of 1960 through 1962 cardiovascular disease prevalence study. *Arch Intern Med* **128**:890-895, 1971.
5. Hames CG: The Evans County cardiovascular and cerebrovascular epidemiological study: Introduction. *Arch Intern Med* **128**:883-886, 1971.
6. Heyman A, Karp HR, Heyden S, et al: Cerebrovascular disease in the biracial population of Evans County, Georgia. *Arch Intern Med* **128**:949-955, 1971.
7. Cornoni JC, Waller IE, Cassel JC, et al: The incidence study—study design and methods. *Arch Intern Med* **128**:896-900, 1971.
8. Cassel JC, Heyden S, Bartel A, et al: Incidence of coronary heart disease by ethnic group, social class, and sex. *Arch Intern Med* **128**:901-906, 1971.
9. Tyroler HA, Heyden S, Bartel A, et al: Blood pressure and cholesterol as coronary heart disease risk factors. *Arch Intern Med* **128**:907-914, 1971.
10. Heyden S, Cassel JC, Bartel A: Body weight and cigarette smoking as risk factors. *Arch Intern Med* **128**:915-919, 1971.
11. Bartel A, Tyroler HA, Heyden S, et al: Electrocardiographic predictors of coronary heart disease. *Arch Intern Med* **128**:929-937, 1971.
12. Kleinbaum L, Kupper L, Cassel JC, et al: Multivariate analysis of risk of coronary heart disease in Evans County, Georgia. *Arch Intern Med* **128**:943-948, 1971.
13. Cassel JC, Heyden S, Bartel A, et al: Occupation and physical activity and coronary heart disease. *Arch Intern Med* **128**:920-928, 1971.
14. Kaplan BH, Cassel JC, Tyroler HA, et al: Occupational mobility and coronary heart disease. *Arch Intern Med* **128**:938-942, 1971.

Review of 1960 Through 1962 Cardiovascular Disease Prevalence Study

John C. Cassel, MD, MPH, Chapel Hill, NC

The Evans County Cardiovascular Epidemiologic Study was initiated in 1960 in an attempt to confirm the clinical observation that coronary heart disease (CHD) appeared to occur less frequently among blacks than whites.

Following a private census of the county, attempts were made to enroll 100% of those residents over 40 years of age and a 50% random sample of those between 15 and 39 years. Of the 3,371 eligible, 3,102 (92%) cooperated and underwent a complete medical examination, a battery of laboratory tests including a 12-lead electrocardiogram and chest roentgenogram, and for a 10% subsample, a detailed dietary history. The medical examinations were conducted by two physicians, John McDonough, MD, and Glen Garrison, MD, and the dietary history by Sarah Stulb. The results of the prevalence survey, which took approximately 18 months to complete, have been reported in some detail elsewhere.[1,2] What follows here is a brief resume of some of the more important findings which formed the basis for the seven-year follow-up study.

Results

The prevalence of CHD reported by McDonough et al[1] showed that the rates in blacks were lower than in whites, a finding consistent with the clinical impression of one of us (C. G. H.). These rates are shown in Fig 1. The major difference is in men, with black men having markedly lower rates than whites, whereas no such ethnic differences appear in women.

Lower rates in CHD in black men have been reported in the past on numerous occasions in the literature,[3] but the majority of these reports are based upon nonrepresentative samples (usually hospitalized patients where problems of differential utilization patterns and admission policies could have affected the results). Furthermore, until recently many of the studies reporting such differences have been conducted in the South (eg, Blache and Handler,[4] Weiss and Gray,[5] Holman et al,[6] and Groom et al[7]), the few reports from Northern urban centers (eg, Mihaly and Whiteman[8]) reporting no differences. More recently, studies on more representative samples, especially those conducted in the urbanized centers of the country, have tended to confirm, at least as far as mortality from CHD is concerned, that under these circumstances differences between black and white men are minimal.[9]

These findings gain additional support from prevalence data obtained for the country as a whole by the US National Health Survey[10] in which virtually identical rates were found in white and black men.

Thus, to the extent that black-white differences in men do exist, the

Received for publication May 13, 1971; accepted July 10.

From the Department of Epidemiology, School of Public Health, University of North Carolina, Chapel Hill.

Reprint requests to Department of Epidemiology, School of Public Health, University of North Carolina, Chapel Hill, NC 27514 (Dr. Cassel).

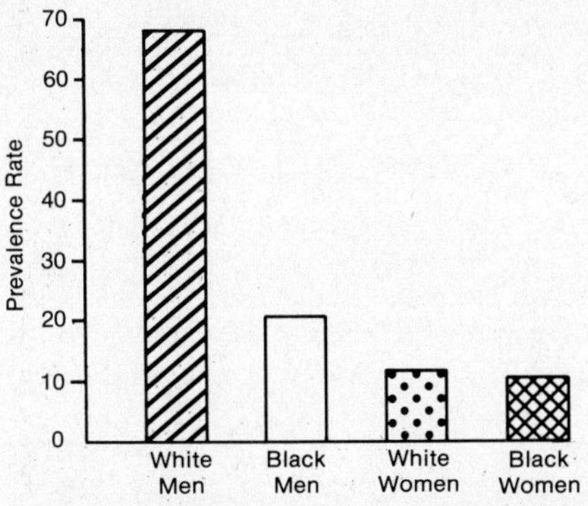

Fig 1.—Age-adjusted prevalence rates per 1,000 population for CHD by sex and ethnic group, Evans County, 1960 through 1962.

possibility exists that this relationship may be changing, and it may vary under different environmental circumstances in the country.

In contrast to the conflicting reports on differences between black and white men, the six difference in CHD rates in whites and the absence of such a sex difference in blacks has consistently been found in all studies on this subject.[11-14] No adequate explanations for this finding seem to be currently available.

In the Evans County, Ga, prevalence study, part of the difference between the black and white men could be explained by an analysis of the rates by social class. For each member of the study population, a social class score was calculated based upon occupation, education, and source of income of the head of the household according to the McGuire and White method.[15] The scores ranged from 16, representing the highest social class, to 84, the lowest. The distribution of scores was divided into deciles. When age-adjusted rates for CHD were compiled for each decile, the analysis revealed a pattern resembling a dichotomy with the rates in the first five deciles similar to each other and considerably higher than those in the remaining five homogeneous deciles.

Accordingly, in subsequent analysis of the 1960 through 1962 prevalence rates, the white men were divided into two social class groups; the upper 50%, which is referred to as high social class, and the lower 50%, which is defined as lower social class. Similar analysis could not be performed for blacks because not only were there too few cases to be divided into two groups, but 95% of the blacks fell into the low social class range of scores. Therefore, in terms of this index, the majority of the black persons would be similar to the low social class whites. Figure 2 shows that when the prevalence data is analyzed in this fashion, most of the white high rates occur in the high social class group and the low social class white men

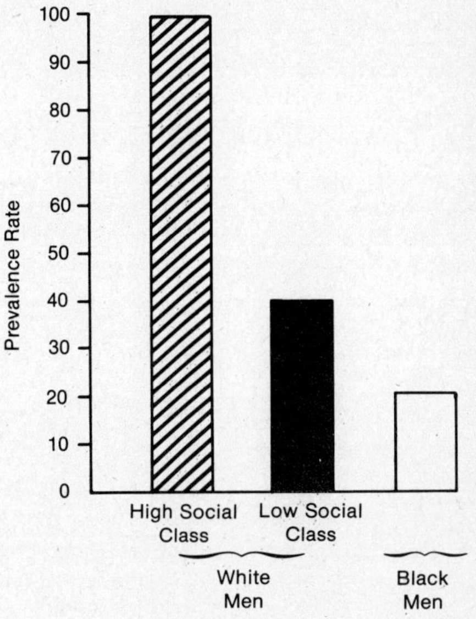

Fig 2.—Age adjusted prevalence rates per 1,000 population for CHD by social class and ethnic group: men only.

Table 1.—Mean Level of Blood Pressure by Ethnic Group, Evans County, 1960 Through 1962 (Men, Aged 45 to 74 Years)[15]*

	Social Class	Total Examined	Mean Age (yr)	Systolic Blood Pressure (mm Hg)	Diastolic Blood Pressure (mm Hg)
White men	High	252	57.2	146.7	91.1
	Low	272	56.0	151.0	92.6
	Total	524	56.6	148.9	91.9
Black men		308	56.5	165.6	101.7

* Individuals with missing data on one or more variables are not included.

Table 2.—Coronary Heart Disease Prevalence in Evans County, 1960 Through 1962 in Men 40 to 74 Years Old by Age Group, Social Class, Race, and Cholesterol Value[15]*

		High Social Class			Low Social Class		
	Age (yr)	Examined	Cases	Rate	Examined	Cases	Rate
White Men							
Cholesterol value less than 240	40-49	148	7	47	212	3	14
	60-74	75	9	120	69	4	60
Cholesterol value more than 240	40-49	60	8	133	50	1	20
	60-74	31	7	226	16	5	313
Black Men							
Cholesterol value less than 240	40-49				227	3	13
	60-74				94	5	53
Cholesterol value more than 240	40-49				49	...	...
	60-74				16	...	...

* Discrepant "case" values from current analysis due to "blind" reevaluation of 1960 through 1962 data based on diagnosis discussed in Cornoni et al paper.[16]

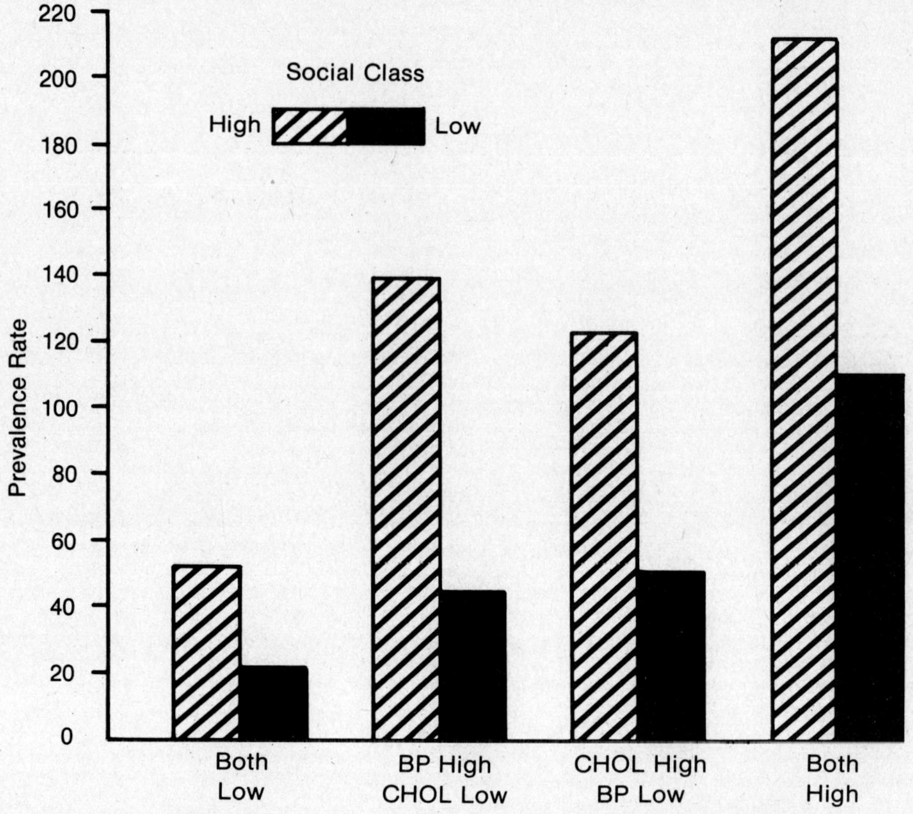

Fig 3.—Age-adjusted prevalence rates per 1,000 population by social class, blood pressure, and cholesterol levels; white men, Evans County, 1960 through 1962. Blood pressure (BP) high = systolic >160 and diastolic <95; cholesterol (Chol) high = >250 mg/100 ml.

have rates not dissimilar to black men. Insofar as the data permitted, attempts were made to explain these ethnic-group and social-class differences on the basis of the variation in several risk factors.

Blood Pressure and Cholesterol Levels.—The first analysis involved the two "standard" risk factors, of blood pressure and serum cholesterol level. Difference in blood pressure seemed unlikely to be an explanation for the differences in these rates for, as Table 1 shows, the mean values of blood pressure (both systolic and diastolic) were, if anything, higher in the low social class than in the high social class white men and considerably higher in black men than in all the whites.

Serum cholesterol levels appeared to be a more likely explanation. The mean level of serum cholesterol in blacks (205.8 mg/100 ml) was slightly lower than in whites (213.3 mg/100 ml), and lower social class whites had values similar to blacks at all ages above 35 years. Accordingly, the rates for CHD were computed for each ethnic and social class group at two levels of serum cholesterol, above and below 240 mg/100 ml, and are shown in Table 2.

From this analysis it can be seen that blacks and low social class whites still have lower rates of CHD than do high social class whites at both low and high levels of cholesterol.

When the joint effects of blood

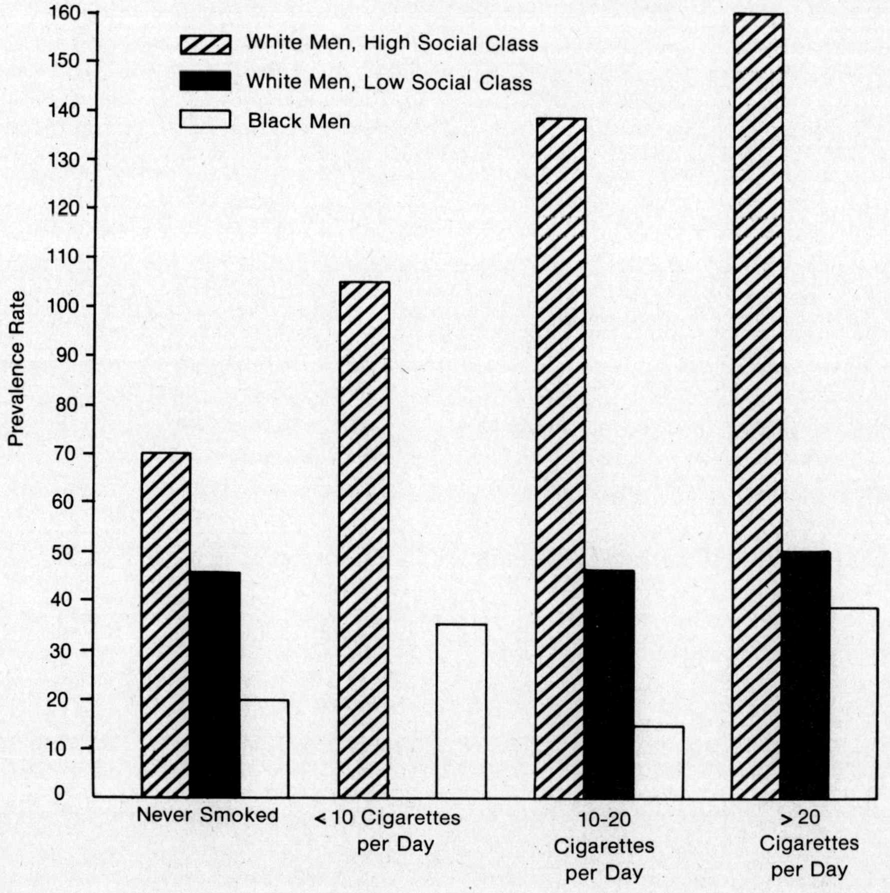

Fig 4.—Age-adjusted prevalence rates per 1,000 population by cigarette smoking history, social class, and ethnic group: men only.

Table 3.—Daily Dietary Intake of Selected Nutrients Among a Random Sample High and Low Social Class White Men and Black Men Aged 40 to 74 Years (Mean and Standard Deviation), Evans County, 1960 through 1962[1]

	White Men		Black Men	Significance (P)		
					Black Men	
	High Social Class (No. = 33)	Low Social Class (N. = 34)	(No. = 23)	High Social Class: Low Social Class	High Social Class	Low Social Class
Carbohydrate (calories as %)	44.8 (5.38)	42.6 (4.70)	47.0 (4.73)	NS*	NS	.001
Protein (calories as %)	12.9 (1.77)	12.4 (2.15)	11.3 (1.85)	NS	.1	.05
Total fat (calories as %)	42.4 (6.8)	45.0 (4.9)	41.5 (4.1)	NS	NS	.01
Animal fat (calories as %)	25.8 (7.7)	30.6 (7.4)	30.1 (6.1)	.02	.05	NS
Saturated fatty acids (gm)	49.1 (17.7)	51.9 (13.4)	50.1 (10.6)	NS	NS	NS
Linoleic acid (gm)	17.2 (7.0)	15.5 (5.8)	13.8 (5.2)	NS	NS	NS
Saturated fatty acids/ linoleic acid	3.37 (1.83)	3.75 (1.40)	3.96 (1.13)	NS	NS	NS
Cholesterol (mg)	608 (220)	650 (214)	527 (190)	NS	NS	NS

* NS = not significant.

pressure and cholesterol level were assessed, there was still an excess in CHD rate in the high social class as is shown in Fig 3.

Thus, differences in blood pressure and cholesterol level could not completely account for the differences in rates observed in these groups.

Cigarette Smoking.—Although there were differences in the cigarette smoking patterns in the different ethnic and social class groups, (15.8% of the high social class white men smoked 20 or more cigarettes a day, for example, as compared to 14.4% of the low social class white men and only 7.6% of the black men), these differences, as shown in Fig 4, did not account for the differences in CHD rates.

Dietary Differences.—Due to limited resources, it was not possible to obtain dietary information on all the subjects. This information was, however, obtained on a 10% random sample of the population. This sample yielded too few cases of CHD to enable case:noncase comparisons to be made, but it was possible to assess the dietary intake of representative samples of the three groups of interest, high and low social class white men and black men.

The results, shown in Table 3, indicated that blacks had higher carbohydrate and lower protein and total fat intake than did whites, but, at the same time, the blacks had slightly higher values for animal fat with no difference by race in saturated fatty acid. Low social class whites did not differ from the high social class except for animal fat intake which, if anything, was slightly higher in the low social class.

From these findings it would appear most unlikely that dietary differences could account for the difference in prevalence rates noted.

Occupation and Physical Activity.—No direct measurement of physical activity was made in the 1960 through 1962 examination, but this could be inferred from the subjects' occupations.

When the occupations were ranked according to the physical activity required on the job, the CHD rates were found to be highest in the most sedentary jobs and lowest in the most active. As is shown in Tables 4 and 5, farm workers had lower rates than nonfarm; within nonfarm occupations there was a gradient from the most sedentary to the most active, and among the farm owners there was a similar gradient according to the amount of physical activity performed.

No subdivision by class or ethnic group was possible as the majority of low social class whites and practically all the blacks were in physically active occupations.

From these findings it was tentatively concluded that differences in habitual physical activity was the most likely explanation for the social class and ethnic differences found in CHD prevalence.

Comment

One of the major problems in drawing inferences from this study, and

Table 4.—Coronary Heart Disease Prevalence Among White Men Aged 40 to 74 Years by Type of Occupation: Evans County, 1960 Through 1962[1]

		Examined	Cases	Cases/1,000 Examined
Nonfarm	Professionals, proprietors, managers	113	10	96
	Clerks, office workers	41	3	77
	Trades, service workers	121	5	48
	Manual laborers	89	3	41
	Unemployed	26	2	55
Farm	Owners	181	17	87
	Sharecroppers, laborers	76	2	31
	Unemployed	17	2	74

one that was recognized at the time of the study, was that it was a cross-sectional prevalence study. Such studies are plagued by two properties which may invalidate any conclusions drawn. First, by definition the study would be restricted to survivors of previous episodes. Accordingly, the low rate among blacks, for example, may not be a reflection of lowered risk of CHD but simply of a higher fatality rate (or migration of susceptibles) prior to the study, leaving fewer remaining cases available for ascertainment. Such a possibility would obviously confound any attempt to assess the effect of the various risk factors on subsequent disease. In the original study an attempt was made to determine whether a differential mortality could account for any of the findings by identifying all deaths which could be attributed to CHD for the four-year period following the initial enumeration of the study population (January 1960 through December 1963). (While it would obviously have been preferable to analyze the death experience *prior* to the initiation of the study, this was not feasible due to the well-known inaccuracies of causes of death derived from death certificate data, especially for blacks, and the difficulties in assigning a social class score to descendants).

While the analysis (Table 6) did not show an excessive death rate in blacks or low social class white men, the possibility still remains that these rates are not an accurate representation of what had occurred previously, nor, of course, do they take into account the problem of selective migration.

The second problem associated with prevalence studies is the difficulty in determining antecedent from consequent. Thus the low CHD rate in manual workers compared to sedentary might represent a change in physical activity following the occurrence of CHD rather than indicating the protective effect of physical activity.

Table 5.—Coronary Heart Disease Prevalence Among White Male Farm Owners Aged 40 to 74 Years by Characteristics of Work: Evans County, 1960 Through 1962[1]

	Examined	Cases	Cases/1,000 Examined*
No supervision, No physical work, (Rent farm land to others)	49 (10)	9 (2)	132
All supervision, No physical work, (All farm work done by others)	40 (1)	5	116
Part supervision, Part physical work, (Some farm work done by others)	34	2	61
No supervision, All physical work, (No farm work done by others)	56 (3)	1	20
Total	179	17	87

* Age-adjusted (indirect method). Characteristics of work were unknown for two examined. Numbers in parentheses represent 14 examined and two cases for whom there is doubt concerning the accuracy of the census classification of farm owner.

Table 6.—Coronary Heart Disease Death Rates* in the Study Population Aged 40 to 74 Years by Sex and Race: Evans County, January 1960 Through December 1963[1]

	Population	CHD Deaths	Rate
High social class white men	337	13	38.0
Low social class white men	370	7	20.2
Total white men	707	20	29.1
Black men	437	3	7.1
White women	743	9	11.2

* Coronary heart disease (CHD) deaths/1,000 population/4 years, age-adjusted (indirect method). No CHD deaths occurred among Negro women

For these reasons it was decided to undertake an incidence study in which the occurrence of CHD in all members of the study population, found in 1960 through 1962 to be free of the disease, could be ascertained. By this means it was hoped to determine whether the initial findings could be confirmed and, if so, whether further insight could be obtained as to the reasons for such differences.

In addition to these reasons, there were a number of other features of the 1960 through 1962 study which required elucidation. In this disease, which is usually regarded as a manifestation of 20th-century urban living, it was rather surprising to find in this very rural county so high a prevalence rate of CHD in one group, the high social class white men. Their rate was as high, if not higher, than the rates found in Framingham, Mass,[17] Albany, NY,[18] Los Angeles,[19] Pittsburgh,[20] and Chicago.[21,22] In part, perhaps this was to be expected as it was known that Evans County is situated in the "high CHD belt" which extends down the Atlantic seaboard,[23] but the surprising feature was that this should affect this one group only.

One possible approach to an explanation was provided by Curtis Hames, MD, who indicated that, based upon his personal knowledge of the majority of this population, the men whom we had labelled high social class, while living in a rural environment, were in fact living a very "urban" way of life. In contrast to their fathers, they were no longer living by the sun but by the clock; they were commuting to work in small industries, their wives were driving car pools, and, even if they were farm owners, they were no longer private entrepeneurs but "employees" of some larger company. Further, there was some evidence that an increasing proportion of the white men in Evans County, even those labeled low social class, were beginning to participate in this 20-century urban "way of life" as the county was rapidly changing from a rural agrarian to a more industrialized economy. If this were so, it would not be unreasonable to expect that these lower social class men would be beginning to develop CHD more frequently and that the social class difference would be diminished. In other words, Evans County might provide a "natural experiment" to identify some of the factors responsible for the spread of this modern epidemic.

References

1. McDonough JR, Hames CG, Stulb SC, et al: Coronary heart disease among Negroes and whites in Evans County, Georgia. *J Chronic Dis* **18**:443-468, 1965.
2. McDonough JR, Garrison GE, Hames CG: Blood pressure and hypertensive disease among Negroes and whites: A study in Evans County, Georgia. *Ann Intern Med* **61**:208-228, 1964.
3. Phillips JH Jr, Burch GE: Cardiovascular diseases in the white and Negro races. *Amer J Med Sci* **238**:97-124, 1959.
4. Blache JO, Handler FP: Coronary artery disease: A comparison of the rates and patterns of development of coronary arteriosclerosis in the Negro and white races with its relation to clinical coronary artery disease. *Arch Path* **50**:189-198, 1950.
5. Weiss MM, Gray WR: Hypertension and myocardial infarction in the Negro. *Amer J Med Sci* **227**:186-187, 1954.
6. Holman RL, McGill AC Jr, Strong JP, et al: The natural history of atherosclerosis. *Amer J Path* **34**:209-236, 1958.
7. Groom D, McKlee E, Webb C, et al: Developmental patterns of coronary and aortic atherosclerosis in Negroes of Haiti and the United States. *Ann Intern Med* **51**:270-289, 1959.
8. Mihaly JP, Whiteman NC: Myocardial infarction in the Negro. Historical survey as it relates to Negroes. *Amer J Cardiol* **2**:464-474, 1958.
9. Stamler J: Cardiovascular diseases in the United States. *Amer J Cardiol* **10**:319-340, 1962.
10. *Vital and Health Statistics*, series 11, publication 6. Heart Disease in Adults, United States 1960-1962: Data from the National Health Survey, National Center for Health Statistics, 1964, p 43.
11. Gager LT, Dunn WL: Heart disease in Washington, D. C.: A study of etiological types and the factors of race, age and sex in 1,200 cases. *Med Ann DC* **2**:112-117, 1933.
12. Holoubek AB: Heart disease in the South. *Amer Heart J* **29**:168-177, 1945.
13. McVay LV Jr, Keil PG: Myocardial infarction with special reference to the Negro. *Arch Intern Med* **96**:762-767, 1955.
14. Stamler J, Kjelsberg M, Hall Y, et al: Epidemiologic studies on cardiovascular-renal diseases. *J Chronic Dis* **12**:440-475, 1960.
15. McGuire C, White GD: *The Measurement of Social Status*, Research Paper in Human Development, No. 3 (revised). Department of Educational Psychology, University of Texas, Austin, 1955.
16. Cornoni JC, Waller LE, Cassel JC, et al: The incidence study–study design and methods. *Arch Intern Med* **128**:896-900, 1971.
17. Dawber TR, Moore FE, Mann GV: Coronary heart disease in the Framingham study. *Amer J Public Health* **47**:4-24, 1957.
18. Doyle JT, Heslin S, Hilliboe HE, et al: Early diagnosis of ischaemic heart disease. *New Eng J Med* **261**:1096-1101, 1959.
19. Chapman JM, Goerke LS, Dixon W, et al: The clinical status of a population group in Los Angeles under observation for two to three years. *Amer J Public Health* **47**:33-42, 1957.
20. Tauber J, Thompson DJ: The prevalence of disease of the heart in an urban center as estimated from medical examination of a probability sample. *J Chronic Dis* **6**:595-605, 1957.
21. Stamler J, Lindberg HA, Berkson DM, et al: Prevalence and incidence of coronary heart diseases in strata of labor force of a Chicago industrial corporation. *J Chronic Dis* **11**:405-420, 1960.
22. Paul O, Lepper MH, Phelan WH, et al: A longitudinal study of coronary heart disease. *Circulation* **28**:20-31, 1963.
23. Sauer HI, Payne GH, Council CR, et al: Cardiovascular disease mortality patterns in Georgia and North Carolina. *Public Health Rep* **81**:455-465, 1966.

The Incidence Study—Study Design and Methods

Joan C. Cornoni, MPH, PhD, Lynn E. Waller, John C. Cassel, MD, MPH, and Herman A. Tyroler, MD, Chapel Hill, NC, and Curtis G. Hames, MD, Claxton, Ga

A biracial sample of 3,102 persons from Evans County, Georgia, was first examined in 1960-1962. Of this original cohort 2,530 persons were reexamined in 1967-1969. From these two observations the incidence rates for the 87-month period of both coronary heart disease and stroke were determined. The recent examination procedure included a complete medical history and physical examination, with a detailed questionnaire for evidence of cerebrovascular disease and symptoms of transient cerebral ischemia, an electrocardiogram, chest x-ray film, laboratory procedures, and sociological and physical activity questionnaires.

Between 1960 and 1962 a study of the prevalence of coronary heart disease was conducted in Evans County, Georgia.[1] For this purpose 100% of the population aged 40 years and older and a 50% random sample of those 15 to 39 years were invited to undergo a complete medical examination. Cooperation was obtained from 3,102 individuals, representing 92% of those eligible for examination.

Received for publication May 13, 1971; accepted Sept 13.

From the Department of Epidemiology, University of North Carolina, Chapel Hill (Drs. Cornoni, Cassel, and Tyroler, and Lynn Waller). Dr. Hames is in private practice in Evans County, Georgia.

Reprint requests to Department of Epidemiology, University of North Carolina, Chapel Hill, NC 27514 (Dr. Cornoni).

Beginning in 1967 a follow-up study was initiated in which all the survivors of this initial cohort were to be reexamined. The results of this reexamination together with an assessment of the causes of all deaths that had occurred between the two time periods would allow a determination of the incidence of new cases occurring since the first examination. The purpose of this paper is to present a description of the methods used in this incidence study.

Identification of the Population at Risk

The first step was to trace all 3,102 persons who had been examined in 1960-1962 in the previous survey. First, by means of a census taken in 1967, the most recent address of those persons still living in Evans County was obtained. Second, the most recent address of those persons who had migrated out of the county was determined. Contacts were made with any relatives, friends, and the US Post Office. Finally, extensive information in regard to any death occurring in this population was gathered. Copies of death certificates, autopsy reports, hospital and physicians records, obituaries from newspapers, and descriptions given by the relatives who were present at the time the death occurred were accumulated.

The flow diagram (Figure) shows that of the 3,102 previously examined population, 2,530 were reexamined in 1967-1969 leaving 572 not reexamined. Of the 572 not reexamined, 264 died within the seven year intervening period and 56 additional deaths occurred during the examination period and before the subjects were contacted for reexamination. Two hundred and twelve of the survivors were not reexamined, 157 of whom had migrated and 55 refused. Tables 1 through 7 give a detailed breakdown of the original sample (3,102); the reexamined population (2,530), the nonreexamined by specific groups; and the rates of reexamination by age, sex, and ethnic groups.

As can be seen from these tables 90.9% of the survivors of the original cohort were reexamined, with black males having the lowest reexamination rate (83.2%) and white females the highest (94.3%). Most of the attrition occurred in the youngest age group (15-24) and thus had a minimal effect on the completeness of the findings of this study, as no case of coronary heart disease occurred under age 40.

Examination Procedures

As explained, the study population in 1967 was 2,530 persons. Each individual underwent an examination averaging from ½ to 2 hours in length. This examination was conducted by two of the study personnel (Alan Bartel, MD, and Siegfried Heyden, MD) and included the following:

A Complete Medical History.—This included a detailed cardiovascular history, including all prior hospitalization, a detailed history of cardiovascular accidents (stroke and transient ischemic attack) and a general history of symptoms and past illnesses. In addition the standardized Rose questionnaire for angina pectoris and myocardial infarction,[2] past and present smoking habits, and a history of changes in body weight and maximum weight attained.[3]

A Complete Physical Examination.—The examination included all systems with special emphasis on heart and neurological signs. Three readings of blood pressure were taken on the left arm with the respondent seated in each case. The first reading was taken at the time of arrival at the clinic, the second was taken 30 to 60 minutes later, and the third, 15 to 20 minutes after the second one.

Electrocardiogram.—A 12 lead ECG was performed in the fasting state in the morning or in the afternoon with no oral intake subsequent to a light breakfast. The ECGs were classified by Alan Bartel, MD with the use of the Minnesota code.[4]

Chest Roentgenogram.—A standard chest X-ray film was taken on each person.

Laboratory Procedures.—The following were determined: (*a*) hemoglobin (oxyhemoglobin method), (*b*) hematocrit (microhematocrit centrifuge method), (*c*) fasting blood glucose (Nelson-Somogyi procedure), (*d*) glucose tolerance load of 100 mg was taken two hours later from approximately 50% of the population and analyzed by the Nelson-Somogyi procedure, (*e*) uric acid (Caraway procedure—modified), (*f*) fasting triglyceride following the modified Carlson method, (*g*) Urine glucose and albumin (Hema-Combistix method), and (*h*) serum cholesterol (Abell-Kendall method).

A Sociological Questionnaire.—This included information on education, occupa-

Table 1.—Status of the 1960-1962 Population at Reexamination in 1967-1969 by Age, Total Population

Total Population Age, yr (1960)	1960-1962 Examined No.	Deaths		Not Reexamined		1967-1969 Reexamined	
		No.	%	No.	%*	No.	%*
15-24	398	5	1.3	88	22.4	305	77.6
25-34	316	5	1.6	30	9.6	281	90.4
35-44	546	16	2.9	47	8.9	483	91.1
45-54	836	57	6.8	55	7.1	724	92.9
55-64	575	86	15.0	20	4.1	469	95.9
65-74	399	131	32.8	11	4.1	257	95.9
75+	32	20	62.5	1	8.3	11	91.7
Total	3,102	320	10.3	252	9.0	2,530	90.9

* Percent of survivors.

Table 2.—Status of the 1960-1962 Population at Reexamination in 1967-1969 by Age, White Males

White Males Age, yr (1960)	1960-1962 Examined No.	Deaths		Not Reexamined		1967-1969 Reexamined	
		No.	%	No.	%*	No.	%*
15-24	118	0	...	16	13.6	102	86.4
25-34	109	2	1.8	11	10.3	96	89.7
35-44	167	5	310	10	6.2	152	93.8
45-54	259	21	8.1	15	6.3	223	93.7
55-64	175	33	18.9	4	2.8	138	97.2
65-74	110	52	47.3	0	...	58	100.0
75+	9	7	77.8	0	...	2	100.0
Total	947	120	12.7	56	6.8	771	93.2

* Percent of survivors.

Table 3.—Status of the 1960-1962 Population at Reexamination in 1967-1969 by Age, Black Males

Black Males Age, yr (1960)	1960-1962 Examined	Deaths		Not Reexamined		1967-1969 Reexamined	
		No.	%	No.	%*	No.	%*
15-24	81	2	2.5	33	41.8	46	58.2
25-34	43	1	2.3	6	14.3	36	83.7
35-44	79	4	5.1	12	16.0	63	84.0
45-54	171	19	11.1	19	12.5	133	87.5
55-64	89	21	23.6	7	10.3	61	89.7
65-74	68	22	32.4	1	2.2	45	97.8
75+	6	4	66.7	0	...	2	100.0
Total	537	73	13.6	78	16.8	386	83.2

* Percent of survivors.

Table 4.—Status of the 1960-1962 Population at Reexamination in 1967-1969 by Age, White Females

White Females Age, yr (1960)	1960-1962 Examined No.	Deaths		Not Reexamined		1967-1969 Reexamined	
		No.	%	No.	%*	No.	%*
15-24	108	1	0.9	12	11.2	95	88.8
25-34	110	1	0.9	8	7.3	101	92.7
35-44	189	3	1.6	11	5.9	175	94.1
45-54	239	8	3.4	10	4.3	221	95.7
55-64	182	15	8.2	6	3.6	161	96.4
65-74	131	31	23.7	4	4.0	96	96.0
75+	13	6	46.2	1	14.3	6	85.7
Total	972	65	6.7	52	5.7	855	94.3

* Percent of survivors.

Table 5.—Status of the 1960-1962 Population at Reexamination in 1967-1969 by Age, Black Females

Black Females Age, yr (1960)	1960-1962 Examined No.	Deaths No.	Deaths %	Not Reexamined No.	Not Reexamined %*	1967-1969 Reexamined No.	1967-1969 Reexamined %*
15-24	91	2	2.2	27	30.3	62	69.7
25-34	54	1	1.8	5	9.4	48	90.6
35-44	111	4	3.6	14	13.1	93	86.9
45-54	167	9	5.4	11	7.0	147	93.0
55-64	129	17	13.2	3	2.7	109	97.3
65-74	90	26	28.9	6	9.4	58	90.6
75+	4	3	75.0	0	...	1	100.0
Total	646	62	9.6	66	11.3	518	88.7

* Percent of survivors.

Table 6.—Status of the 1960-1962 Population of Higher Social Class (HSC) White Males at Reexamination in 1967-1969

White Males (HSC) Age, yr (1960)	1960-1962 Examined No.	Deaths No.	Deaths %	Not Reexamined No.	Not Reexamined %*	1967-1969 Reexamined No.	1967-1969 Reexamined %*
15-24	43	0	...	5	11.6	38	88.4
25-34	48	0	...	5	10.4	43	89.6
35-44	82	1	1.2	4	4.9	77	95.1
45-54	119	9	7.6	6	5.4	104	94.5
55-64	82	14	17.1	4	5.9	64	94.1
65-74	63	27	42.9	0	...	36	100.0
75+	3	3	100.0	0	...	0	...
Total	440	54	12.3	24	6.2	362	93.8

* Percent of survivors.

Table 7.—Status of the 1960-1962 Population of Lower Social Class (LSC) White Males at Reexamination in 1967-1969

White Male (LSC) Age, yr (1960)	1960-1962 Examined No.	Deaths No.	Deaths %	Not Reexamined No.	Not Reexamined %*	1967-1969 Reexamined No.	1967-1969 Reexamined %*
15-24	75	0	0.0	11	14.7	64	85.3
25-34	61	2	3.3	6	10.2	53	89.8
35-44	85	4	4.7	6	7.4	75	92.6
45-54	140	12	8.6	9	7.0	119	93.0
55-64	93	19	20.4	0	...	74	100.0
65-74	47	25	53.2	0	...	22	100.0
75+	6	4	66.7	0	...	2	100.0
Total	507	66	13.0	32	7.2	409	92.7

* Percent of survivors.

Table 8.—Prevalence of Coronary Heart Disease (CHD) and Stroke by Sex and Ethnic Group (1960-1962)

	Total Population Examined 1960	Total Population Examined 1967	CHD Prevalence 1960 No.	CHD Prevalence 1960 Rate*	Stroke Prevalence 1960 No.	Stroke Prevalence 1960 Rate*
White Males	947	771	54	0.0590	20	0.0220
Black Males	537	386	12	.0224	8	.0148
White Females	972	855	18	.0182	11	.0108
Black Females	646	518	9	0.0136	15	0.0236
Total	3,102	2,530	93		54	

* Age adjusted rate by the indirect method using total population as standard.

tion, the religion of the respondent and his family, marital status, family composition, and source of income. It also determined the respondent's perception of worry, his attitude toward goal striving, and his personal affiliations.

Physical Activity.—A short physical activity questionnaire consisting of questions extracted from the physical questionnaire devised by the Health Insurance Plan of New York City was administered. This included an assessment of leisure time as well as on the job activity.[5]

Identification of Cases

Deaths.—As mentioned previously, an attempt to locate every person in the original sample was made and their status as to living or dead was determined. A complete tracing of all death information pertaining to circumstances and cause of death was carried out. After the collection and organization of these data, a panel consisting of three physicians and a cardiologist reviewed all the information gathered for all deaths. Independently a neurologist reviewed all deaths for any evidence of stroke.

Previous to this review, criteria were established in order to identify a death as myocardial infarction, sudden death, or stroke.

Myocardial Infarction.—Death due to coronary heart disease was diagnosed on the basis of a classical history of myocardial infarction or an ECG consistent with myocardial infarction. The World Health Organization criteria were used for defining this history.[6] Criteria used for the evaluation of the ECG were essentially the Class I, Q, and QS patterns of Blackburn et al.[4] Segment depression and T wave inversion was not used. The distinction as to whether a case was definite or probable was based on the assurity of the panel of judges.

Sudden Death.—Sudden death was defined as any unexpected death occurring within 24 hours after the patient was last seen alive if unattended, and within one hour if attended.

Stroke.—A death was attributed to cerebrovascular disease if the death certificate listed stroke as the underlying or contributing cause and if the clinical records indicated that terminal illness began with sudden loss of consciousness without other explanation.

Living Subjects.—At the time of reexamination, the examining physicians made an assessment of the presence or absence of heart disease or stroke. After completion of all examinations, the records of those persons with any suspicion of coronary heart disease were reviewed by two cardiologists and three physicians. (One of the cardiologists, John McDonnough, MD, was one of the examining physicians in the 1960-1962 prevalence study. This helped to insure comparability between the two examinations.) All records were also reviewed by a neurologist for the presence of stroke and transient ischemic attack (TIA).

Without knowledge of the previously determined examining physician's impression, the 1960 record was reviewed. A decision was made on the basis of the original examination data as to whether the subject had been a case in 1960-1962. Then the 1967 record was reviewed and the current diagnosis was made. Cases were designated as definite, probable, possible, or negative angina pectoris, myocardial infarction, chronic heart disease, or stroke.

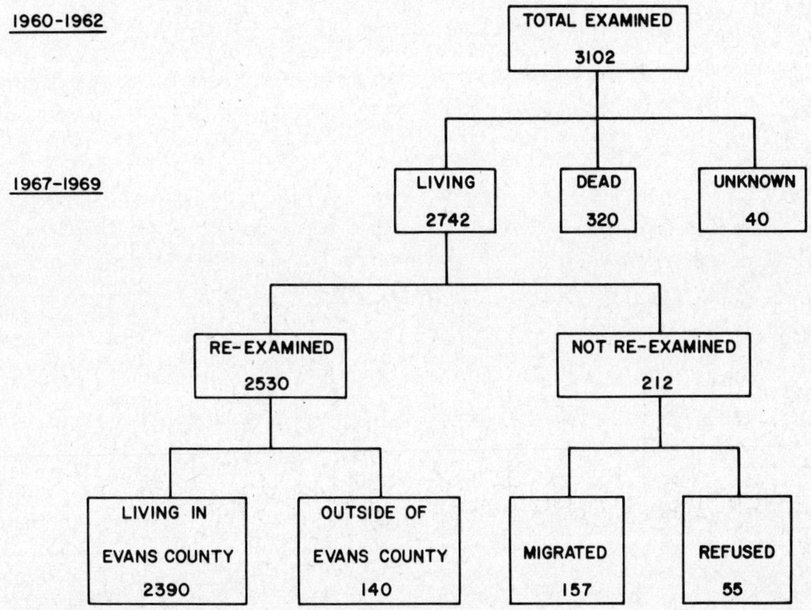

Status of the 1960-1962 population as determined at reexamination in 1967-1969.

Table 9.—Incidence of Coronary Heart Disease (CHD) and Stroke by Sex and Ethnic Group (1960-1962 to 1967-1969)

	CHD Incidence (87 mo)			Stroke Incidence (87 mo)		
	Living	Deaths	Rate*	Living	Deaths	Rate*
White Males	40	32	0.0827	22	13	0.0386
Black Males	6	7	.0238	14	10	.0438
White Females	25	11	.0379	5	7	.0125
Black Females	16	6	0.0343	12	11	0.0365
Total	87	56		53	41	

* Age adjusted rate by the indirect method using sex specific standards.

Coronary Heart Disease.—Angina pectoris was diagnosed according to the criteria of the World Health Organization.[6] Myocardial infarction was diagnosed on the basis of the previously described criteria for death from myocardial infarction. Chronic heart disease was diagnosed using the criteria of the Pooling Project.[7] These criteria were chronic arrythmia or heart failure in the absence of angina pectoris, myocardial infarction, or any other cardiac disorder of known etiology. Cases of congestive heart failure with coexistent hypertension were excluded from this classification. As for assignment of cause of death, the distinction as to whether a case was definite or probable was based on the assurity of the panel of judges.

Stroke and TIA.—Definitions for definite stroke and transient ischemic attack required a clear-cut, classical history of sudden onset of aphasia or unilateral arm and/or weakness in vascular distribution with or without altered consciousness or other focal manifestations. These symptoms had to be associated with residual neurologic findings at the time of examination or a record of laboratory studies (arteriography, spinal fluid) confirming the diagnosis. Probable stroke included a definite history of aphasia or unilateral arm and/or weakness in vascular distribution with or without other neurologic

Table 10.—Prevalence of Coronary Heart Disease and Stroke by Sex and Ethnic Group (1967-1969)*

	CHD Prevalence 1967		Stroke Prevalence 1967	
	No.	Rate†	No.	Rate†
White males	68	0.0950	28	0.0393
Black males	15	.0376	18	.0439
White females	39	.0449	11	.0126
Black females	22	0.0403	18	0.0336
Total	144		75	

* These rates have been age adjusted across ethnic and sex groups for the age attained at time of examination. This, on the average, is 87 months older than that pertaining in the 1960 examination and thus these prevalence rates are not directly comparable to the 1960 prevalence rates.

† Age adjusted rate by the indirect method using six specific standards.

symptoms but with no residual signs found on examination. Possible stroke was diagnosed in the presence of an adequate history of focal neurologic deficit (dysphasia, cerebellar signs, numbness) in vascular distribution (not including arm or leg weakness or aphasia) without residual findings.[8]

The diagnosis of definite transient ischemic attack was considered when a clear-cut history of sudden onset of well-defined transient episode(s) of limb paralysis or monocular amblyopia occurred alone or in combination, or less than 24 hours duration with no residual neurologic manifestations on examination. Probable TIA included a good history of transient focal neurologic deficit(s) in vascular distribution other than limb palsies or amblyopia. The symptoms were reasonably defined and included speech disorder, sensory loss, visual field defect or diplopia with or without syncope, vertigo, or confusion without evidence of anxiety or functional complaints. Finally, possible TIA was defined as a history of transient neurologic episode(s) of nonfocal nature, ie, altered consciousness, dizziness, blurred vision, drop attacks, etc. Focal symptoms if present, were generally vague or poorly defined. Anxiety cannot be totally ruled out as an etiologic factor. Patients with simple syncope, overt labyrinthine disorders, and seizures were excluded from this category.

Tables 8 through 10 give a summary of the cases, both living and dead subjects, and the study population for the different time periods. The prevalence rates for 1960-1962 are based on the number of cases diagnosed as definite or probable in that examination, adjusted for age differences. The prevalence in 1967-1969 include those cases identified in 1960-1962 who had survived the approximate seven year period plus the new cases that occurred during this time. It should be noted that this prevalence rate includes in both the numerator and denominator only those persons in the original cohort who remained in Evans County. This excluded two categories of people: immigrants to Evans County, and those below the age of eligibility in 1960 who had achieved the age by 1967. The incidence rates are restricted to the new cases including both the living and dead occurring during the approximate seven years in individuals judged free of the disease in 1960-1962.

In summary, this study has produced data on a biracial population. It has accumulated prevalence rates of coronary heart disease and stroke at two points in time, 1960-1962 and 1967-1969. In 1960-1962, data was accumulated on medical, nutritional, and laboratory factors related to these diseases. In 1967-1969 the prevalence rates of coronary heart disease and stroke of the survivors of these original cohort was calculated. Also in 1967-1969, in addition to the medical data, information was obtained on sociological and physical activity aspects. As a result of these two measures over time, incidence rates of both coronary heart disease and stroke were determined.

References

1. McDonough JR, Hames CG, Stulb SC, et al: Cardiovascular disease field study in Evans County, Ga. *Pub Health Rep* **78**:1051-1059, 1963.
2. Rose GA, Blackburn H: *Cardiovascular Survey Methods.* Geneva, World Health Organization, 1968.
3. Heyden S, Hames CG, Bartel A: Weight and weight history in relation to cerebrovascular and ischemic heart disease. *Arch Intern Med* **128**:956-960, 1971.
4. Blackburn H, Keys A, Simonson E, et al: The electrocardiogram in population studies: A classification system. *Circulation* **21**:1160-1175, 1960.
5. Frank CW, Weinblatt E, Shapiro S, et al: Myocardial infarction in men: Role of physical activity and smoking in incidence and mortality. *JAMA* **198**:1241-1245, 1966.
6. World Health Organization: Hypertension and coronary heart disease: Classification and criteria for epidemiology studies. *WHO Techn Rep Ser*, No. 168, 1959.
7. Committee on Criteria and Methods, Council on Epidemiology: *Pooling Project*, revised ed. New York, American Heart Association. July 1965.
8. Heyman A, Karp H, Heyden S, et al: Cerebrovascular disease in the biracial population of Evans County, Georgia. *Arch Intern Med* **128**:949-955, 1971.

Incidence of Coronary Heart Disease by Ethnic Group, Social Class, and Sex

John Cassel, MD, MPH, Chapel Hill, NC; Siegfried Heyden, MD, and
Alan G. Bartel, MD, Durham, NC; Berton H. Kaplan, PhD; Herman A. Tyroler, MD;
and Joan C. Cornoni, MPH, PhD, Chapel Hill, NC; and Curtis G. Hames, MD, Claxton, Ga

In a seven-year follow-up of 3,102 Evans County, Georgia, residents examined in the prevalence survey of 1960 through 1962, 143 new cases of coronary heart disease (CHD) occurred, 56 of which resulted in death during the interval. Ethnic differences in CHD among males discovered during 1960 through 1962 were again confirmed. Excess of white males could not be explained by differences in case fatality, diagnostic criteria, missed cases, or by a competing cause of death. In contrast to ethnic differences, differences by social class found in the prevalence survey among white males were not found in the incidence study. Various analyses suggested that the excess prevalence found in the high social class was a reflection of prior high incidence rates in this class. Over time these class differences are disappearing, particularly among younger men.

As indicated previously,[1] the prevalence study in Evans County, Georgia, in 1960 through 1962 had shown marked differences in coronary heart disease (CHD) by ethnic group and social class. White males had an age-adjusted prevalence rate that was almost three times higher than black males (59 per 1,000 compared to 22 per 1,000). Most of this white excess was attributed to the higher social class men who had a rate of 99 compared to 40 for the lower social class. Further, no differences were found by ethnic group for females, the rate for white females being 18 and for black females 14 per 1,000. Thus, within ethnic groups, white males had a five-fold higher rate than white females, while for blacks the ratio was only 2 to 1.

The initial purpose of the incidence study was to determine whether these differences persisted when a population free of CHD was followed over time. Such an analysis would provide an indication of the extent to which the differences in prevalence in the various groups indicated differences in risk of developing CHD as opposed to differences in selective survival or migration, or both. Further, it was hoped that this follow-up study might indicate whether, in the rapidly changing environment of Evans County, a secular trend in these ethnic group-social class patterns was occurring.

The methods by which this study was conducted, including the completeness of ascertainment and examination of the members of the original 1960 through 1962 cohort and the criteria used for diagnosis of the various manifestations of CHD, are described elsewhere.[2]

Results

Differences by Ethnic Group and Sex.—The incidence of all manifestations of definite and probable CHD for the 87-month follow-up period is shown by age, ethnic group, and sex in Table 1 and Fig 1.

As can be seen from these data, the differences in males by ethnic group found in the prevalence study were confirmed, black males having lower rates at all ages than white males, with only minor differences appearing among females. The extraordinarily low rates for black males in comparison to the whites was one of the most intriguing findings of this study and one for which explanations were energetically sought. It is clear from these analyses that black males are definitely protected in some fashion from CHD and that their low rates are not due to selective removal (by a higher case fatality, for example) as was suspected from the prevalence data.

Further analyses (Fig 2 and 3) showed that these black males were at lower risk than whites for all manifestations of CHD (myocardial infarction as well as angina pectoris) and for fatal as well as nonfatal events. In an effort to ensure that these differences were not due to some systematic bias in which black cases were "lost" or were not ascertained to the same degree as whites, some further analyses were performed.

First, the possibility was considered that whites had been "over-

Received for publication May 13, 1971; accepted Aug 3.

From the departments of epidemiology (Drs. Cassel, Tyroler, and Cornoni), University of North Carolina, Chapel Hill; and the departments of cardiology, Duke University Medical Center (Dr. Bartel) and community health sciences, Duke University Medical School (Dr. Heyden), Durham, NC. Dr. Hames is a practicing physician, Evans County, Georgia.

Reprint requests to Department of Epidemiology, University of North Carolina, Chapel Hill, NC 27514 (Dr. Cassel).

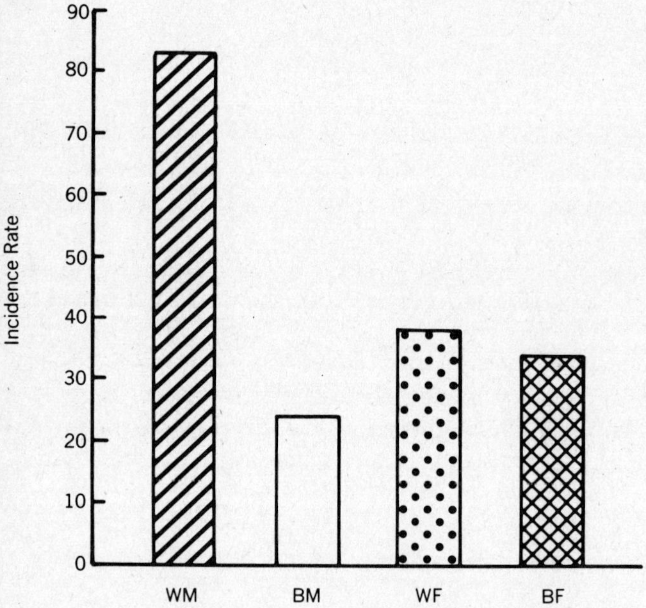

Fig 1.—Age-adjusted incidence rate per 1,000 of coronary heart disease by ethnic group and sex, 1960 through 1962 to 1967 through 1969.

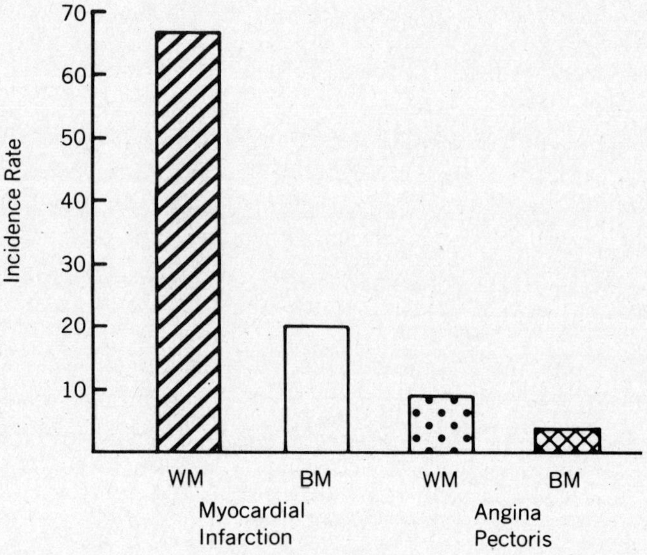

Fig 2.—Age-adjusted incidence rates per 1,000 for myocardial infarction and angina pectoris by ethnic group, 1960 through 1962 to 1967 through 1969 (men only).

diagnosed" (compared to blacks) either due to a failure of the examining physician to elicit a history of myocardial infarction in the living blacks or due to the incompleteness of the record in the case of those blacks who had died. Accordingly, the data were reanalyzed using only electrocardiographically confirmed cases in the living, and deaths ascribed to myocardial infarction in which there was either ECG evidence prior to death or unequivocal autopsy evidence (ie, excluding sudden deaths). Of the 58 cases diagnosed as myocardial infarction in the whites, 30 met these criteria (33.6 cases/1,000 population), while among the black males, six of the 11 cases (11.4 cases/1,000) were diagnosed on the same basis. Thus, using only these criteria which are least likely to have been influenced by the examiners, knowledge of the ethnic group of the subject (ECGs were read blind without knowledge of ethnic group[3]), the white-black gradient in incidence persists.

Second, the problem of the nonexamined living subjects and those deaths for which no cause of death could be ascribed was considered (ie, "missed" black cases). There were 39 black men over the age of 35 years who were not reexamined either due to migration or refusal. Although they were known to be alive and were reported to be in good health by relatives, the possibility could not be excluded that had they been examined a number of new cases of CHD might have been identified. In addition, there were 11 black male deaths for which so little evidence was available that the consultant panel was unwilling to ascribe any cause of death. The computations shown in Tables 2 and 3 were undertaken to determine the number of cases that would have had to be present in these two subsets to have eliminated the difference in the incidence rate between blacks and whites.

In Table 2 it is shown (column 3) that there would have had to have been 24 surviving cases of CHD among the original 401 black men (over the age of 35 years) for the black age-adjusted incidence among the living to be equal to that of the white. Six cases were, in fact, diagnosed (column 4) leaving a deficit of 18 cases which would have had to come from the unexamined 39 men. Thus, the age-adjusted rate in these 39 men would have had to have been 46% or nearly eight times the rate found among white men of the same age.

The same reasoning is applied to the deaths of unknown cause (Table 3). If the black men had had the same CHD mortality rate as the whites, 21 CHD deaths would have been expected (column 3). Seven, in fact, were observed leaving a deficit of 14 CHD deaths which would have had to occur in the 11 cases of death from unknown cause—clearly an impossibility.

It thus appears virtually impossible that sufficient cases could have occurred among those 39 nonexamined and 11 cause unknown deaths to have eliminated the black-white difference in incidence and that the difference is not likely to have been caused by a systematic variation in diagnostic accuracy. Accordingly, it would not seem unrealistic to conclude that this difference is real and thus requires explanation. Subsequent papers in this series[4] attempt explanations in terms of variations in the distributions of a number of risk factors in these populations. Prior to such analyses, however, it was necessary to consider one further category of explanation, namely competing causes of death. Specifically, the known high rate of stroke in blacks has led to the suggestion that many blacks might be dying from stroke in place of CHD.

This argument does not appear to be a likely explanation in Evans County. Between the two examinations ten deaths due to stroke occurred in black males.[5] As can be seen from Table 4, even if, taking the most extreme view, all these cases had lived in subsequently developed CHD, the rates in black males would still have been substantially lower at each age than was the case in white males.

Incidence by Social Class.—As can be seen from Table 5 and Fig 4, the differences by social class found in the 1960 through 1962 prevalence examination were not found in the incidence study, higher social class males having an age-adjusted rate of 84 per 1,000 which is virtually identical to that found in lower social class men (81 per 1,000).

This marked difference in the prevalence by social class and the absence of such a difference in incidence is susceptible to two possible explanations: either the 1960 through 1962 prevalence rates were not a reflection of previous incidence (ie, the low rate in the lower social class was due to a high prior case fatality rate leaving fewer surviving cases in that class to be examined) or there has been a secular change in incidence, with lower social class men beginning to develop the disease at a rate which previously was characteristic of the more favored classes. (A third logical possibility exists, that more higher than lower social class cases were missed due to different rates of nonparticipation in the examination. As there were only 14 out of the 349 eligible high social class men (aged 35 years and older) who were not examined and 15 out of the 471 lower social class men, this possibility seems most unlikely.)

To determine whether the 1960 through 1962 prevalence differences were indeed a reflection of similar differences in incidence, it would be necessary to know whether the death rates prior to 1960 in CHD cases differed in the two social groups. These data, unfortunately, are not available, but the death rates in CHD cases for the follow-up period (that is, subsequent to the 1960 through 1962 examination) can be computed. In the higher social class, 37 cases were

Table 1.—Incidence of Coronary Heart Disease by Age, Ethnic Group, and Sex (87-Month Follow-Up)

Males						
	Whites			Blacks		
Age (yr) at 1960 Through 1962 Examination	No. Examined	New Cases of CHD	Incidence per 1,000	No. Examined	New Cases of CHD	Incidence per 1,000
15-24	118	0	...	81	0	...
25-34	109	0	...	43	0	...
35-44	166	10	60	79	1	13
45-54	249	19	76	166	7	42
55-64	155	20	129	87	1	11
65-74	90	21	233	64	4	63
75+	6	2	333	5	0	...
Total	893	72	81	525	13	25
Age-Adjusted Rate/1,000			83			24

Females						
	Whites			Blacks		
Age (yr) at 1960 Through 1962 Examination	No. Examined	New Cases of CHD	Incidence per 1,000	No. Examined	New Cases of CHD	Incidence per 1,000
15-24	108	0	...	91	1	11
25-34	110	0	...	54	0	...
35-44	189	1	5	111	3	27
45-54	236	7	30	164	6	37
55-64	173	7	40	124	8	65
65-74	126	18	143	89	4	45
75+	12	3	250	4	0	...
Total	954	36	38	637	22	35
Age-Adjusted Rate/1,000			38			34

Table 2.—Incidence of Coronary Heart Disease Necessary in Nonexamined Black Men (Over 35) to Achieve Equal Black-White Incidence Rates

Black Men at Risk (1)	White Living Age-Adjusted Incidence (%) (2)	No. of CHD Cases Expected in Living Blacks (3) = (1) × (2)	No. of CHD Cases Observed in Living Blacks (4)	Black Deficit (5) = (3) − (4)	Black Living Not Re-examined (6)	Age-Adjusted Incidence Rate Required in Non-examined (%) (7)	Relative Risk of B/W in Non-examined (8)
401	6.0	24.01	6	18.01	39	46.18	7.7

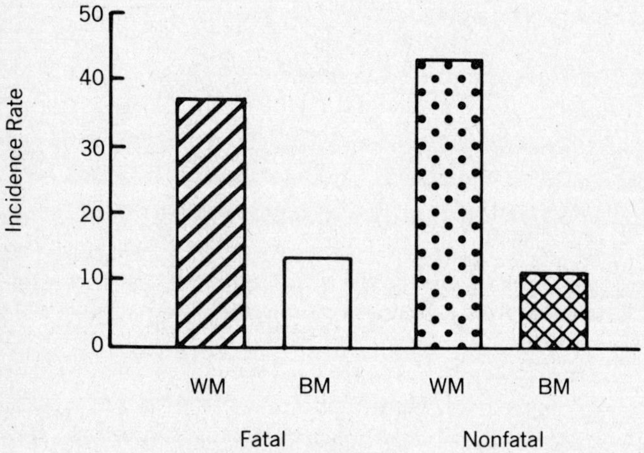

Fig 3.—Age-adjusted incidence rates for fatal and nonfatal events by ethnic group, 1960 through 1962 to 1967 through 1969 (men only). (Fatal events included all deaths ascribed to myocardial infarction and all sudden deaths).

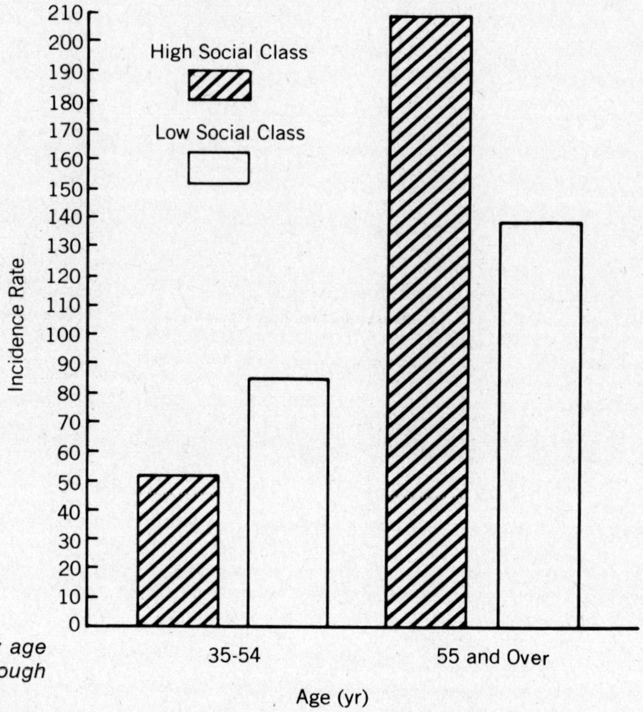

Fig 4.—Incidence of coronary heart disease per 1,000 by age group and social class, 1960 through 1962 and 1967 through 1969 (white men).

diagnosed in the 1960 through 1962 examination and 35 further cases developed between the two examinations. Of these 72 cases, 33 (46%) died from all causes. In the lower social class, 17 cases were initially diagnosed and 37 new cases developed. Of the total 54 cases, 25 (46%) died from all causes. Thus, the death rate among CHD victims in the two social class groups was identical. Unless the case fatality in the lower social class group has dropped dramatically since 1960 through 1962, therefore, it would seem that the lower prevalence rate found at that time in this group was an indication of their lower incidence. Improvements in medical care since 1960 could conceivably have improved the survival rate of the lower social classes to a greater extent than in the higher social classes, but this is most unlikely. The most important change that has occurred in Evans County since that time was the opening of a new hospital in Claxton with a well-equipped coronary care unit. This hospital, however, only started functioning in 1966, while the vast majority of the deaths occurred prior to this time. It would, thus, appear that the alternate explanation, a secular change in incidence, is more likely. This means that either the rates in the lower social class group are increasing or those in the upper social class declining.

Table 3.—Mortality From Coronary Heart Disease Among Black Deaths of Undetermined Cause Required to Achieve Parity With White Rate

Black Men at Risk (1)	Age-Adjusted Mortality Rate for CHD in Whites (2)	No. of CHD Deaths Expected in Blacks (3) = (1) × (2)	No. of Incident Deaths Observed in Blacks (4)	Black Deficit (5) = (3) − (4)	No. of Deaths of Undetermined Cause in Blacks (6)
401	52.5	21.15	7	14.15	11

Table 4.—Incidence of Coronary Heart Disease in Black Men on the Assumption That All Subjects Dying of Strokes Had Lived and Developed Coronary Heart Disease

	Black Men					
Age (yr)	No. Examined	Stroke Deaths	CHD	Total CHD Plus Stroke Deaths	Rate (Total Stroke Deaths and CHD)	White Men Incidence Rate CHD
35-44	79	0	1	1	13	60
45-54	166	4	7	11	67	76
55-64	87	2	1	3	34	129
65+	69	4	4	8	116	240
All ages (over 35)	401	10	13	23	57	108

Comment

The phenomenon of a secular change in the occurrence of CHD by social class is not restricted to Evans County. Although the possibilities that such a change offers for identifying further clues as to the etiology

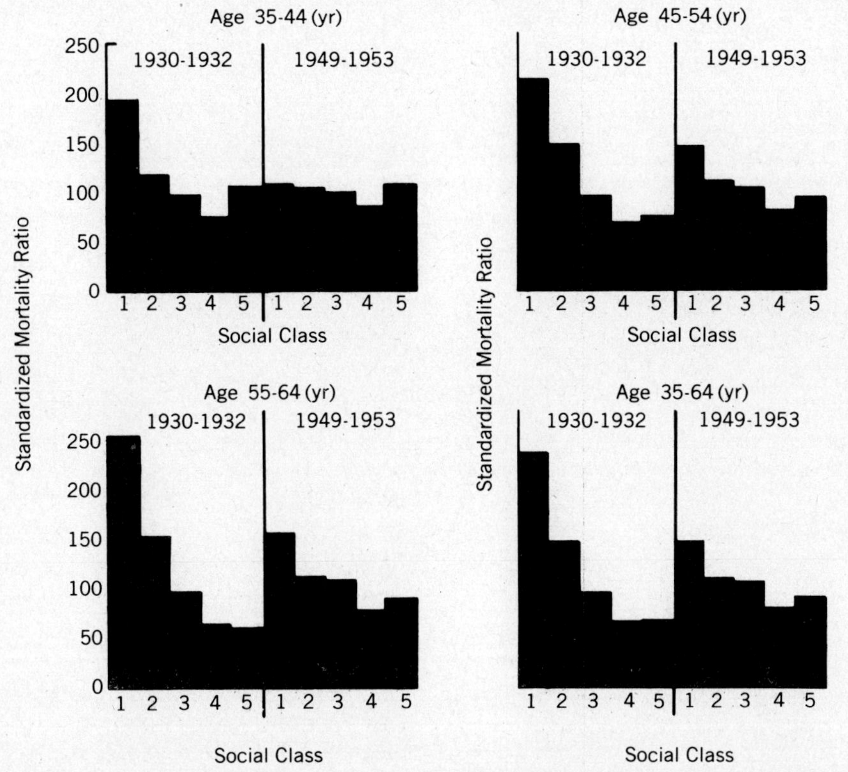

Fig 5.—Standardized mortality ratio for coronary heart disease in men by social class and age, England and Wales, 1930 through 1932 and 1949 through 1953.[6-7] *(Rates for all men for each age based in each period taken as 100).*

Table 6.—Age Specific Death Ratios* From Arteriosclerotic Heart Disease, Including Coronary Disease in Men by Social Class and Age US, Whites 1956 to 1957[8]

	Social Class				
Age (yr)	1	2	3	4	5
25-34	94	99	96	96	139
35-44	93	95	102	97	113
45-54	102	102	103	92	99
55-64	108	99	107	90	90

* Rate for all men in each age group taken as 100.

Table 5.—Incidence of Coronary Heart Disease by Social Class and Age (87-Month Follow-Up) (White Males)

Age (yr) at 1960 Through 1962 Examination	Higher Social Class			Lower Social Class		
	No. Examined	New Cases of CHD	Incidence per 1,000	No. Examined	New Cases of CHD	Incidence per 1,000
15-24	43	0	...	75	0	...
25-34	48	0	...	61	0	...
35-44	81	3	37	85	7	82
45-54	111	7	63	138	12	87
55-64	68	11	162	87	9	103
65-74	51	13	255	39	8	205
75+	1	1	1,000	5	1	200
Total	403	35	87	490	37	76
Age-Adjusted Rate/1,000			84			81

of this disease have not been widely recognized, similar changes over time can be discerned in the mortality data reported both from Britain and the United States.

Figure 5 shows the data from England and Wales for two periods, 1930 through 1932 and 1949 through 1953. For all ages 35 to 64 years, there was a marked gradient in 1930 through 1932 with the highest rates occurring in the highest social class. Twenty years later this gradient had been considerably reduced, with the lower social classes beginning to approach the higher. Further, it can be seen that the greatest change in this gradient has occurred in the youngest age group (35 to 44 years), where the rates in the lowest social class in 1949 through 1953 were equal to those in the highest. By contrast, the original 1930 through 1932 gradient in the older age group (55 to 64 years) still persists in the later period.

It is recognized that any interpretations from these data have to be made with care due to the possibility of noncomparability of diagnoses between the two time periods. The argument here, however, is not whether the overall rates have increased in the 20-year interval but whether at different ages the relationship between social class and this disease has changed. For this change to have been produced by changes in diagnostic custom, it would be necessary to envisage a systematic change in diagnosis which would elevate the rate in 35- to 44-year-old lower social class men (in relation to the higher social class men of the same age) but which would not elevate the rate in 55- to 64-year-old men of the same lower social classes.

The data from the United States are less clear, perhaps in part because the relationship of social class to disease has not been studied as systematically in this country as in Britain and in part because, at any given point in time, this relationship between social class and CHD may differ between the large urban industrialized centers of the country and the more agricultural areas. Nevertheless, by 1950 for the country as a whole mortality rates for CHD showed an age-social class relationship similar to Britain, with no gradient (or perhaps even an inverse gradient) being present in the younger age groups and the gradient steepening as age increases (Table 6).

As the basis of these data, Gordon[8] has suggested a cohort effect, with higher social class men born before about 1900 retaining some of the disadvantageous consequences of their earlier way of life, and that more recently the lower social classes (as represented by the younger men) have begun participating in a similar way of life.

The Evans County data (Table 5 and Fig 4) bear a striking similarity to these British and US data, with lower social class men under the age of 55 years having a higher rate than similar-aged higher social class men and vice versa for the older age groups. The change in Evans County (and perhaps in much of the rural South undergoing industrialization) has, however, occurred later and is taking place more rapidly than was true for Britain or for other parts of this country. The recent changes in the living habits of lower social class white men in Evans County may, thus, hold clues which should advance our knowledge concerning the genesis of this disease.

The differences by ethnic group also suggest important directions for future research. In Evans County the differences found between white and black males in the 1960 through 1962 prevalence study were confirmed in the incidence analysis. This is in contrast to the data for the country as a whole where, in terms of prevalence at least, the US National Survey[8] has found almost identical rates for whites (3.8%) and blacks (3.2%). More detailed studies, however, indicate that this relationship may vary depending upon geographical location. Unfortunately, few biracial prevalence studies and, to our knowledge, no incidence studies with adequate numbers of blacks have been conducted, but the mortality data consistently show a white excess in the more rural areas of the South[9-12] which apparently does not occur in the larger metropolitan areas of the North.[13-14] This suggests that a phenomenon, similar to that occurring among the social groups, may be occurring between the ethnic groups. While changes in the way of life may be occurring more slowly in blacks than in lower social class whites living in rural areas, (so that black rates have not yet changed), such changes do occur when blacks migrate to the urban centers and consequently their rates rise.

What these changes in style of life are is a matter of speculation. Presumably, patterns of living which until recently were characteristic of the more favored segments of white society, which increasingly are being adopted by the less privileged segments of that society but which have not yet involved the majority of blacks, need to be studied. According to current theory, the prime candidates for such changes which are relevant to CHD would be changes in physical activity, diet, psychosocial "stresses," and cigarette smoking. To the extent our data permit, the explanatory power of these factors and their biological correlates, blood pressure, serum cholesterol level, and body weight are explored in subsequent papers. Additional biological risk factors, including blood glucose, uric acid, and catecholamine excretion, unfortunately are only available for the 1967 through 1969 examination. Consequently, their changes in Evans County cannot as yet be assessed, but they, together with some of the factors responsible for clotting, are currently being studied.

References

1. Cassel JC: Review of the 1960 through 1962 cardiovascular disease prevalence study. *Arch Intern Med* **128**:890-895, 1971.
2. Cornoni JC, Waller LE, Cassel JC, et al: The incidence study—study design and methods. *Arch Intern Med* **128**:896-900, 1971.
3. Bartel A, Tyroler HA, Heyden S, et al: Electrocardiographic predictors of coronary heart disease. *Arch Intern Med* **128**:929-937, 1971.
4. Cassel JC: Summary of major findings of the Evans County cardiovascular studies. *Arch Intern Med* **128**:887-889, 1971.
5. Heyman A, Karp H, Heyden S, et al: Cerebrovascular disease in the biracial population of Evans County, Georgia. *Arch Intern Med* **128**:949-955, 1971.
6. Registrar General for England and Wales: *Occupational Mortality*, decennial supplement 1931. London, Her Majesty's Stationery Office, 1938, pt 11a.
7. Registrar General for England and Wales: *Occupational Mortality*, decennial supplement 1951. London, Her Majesty's Stationery Office, 1957, vol 2, pt 2.
8. Gordon T: Heart disease in adults, United States 1960-1962, data from the National Health Survey, in *Vital and Health Statistics*, series 11, No. 6, National Center for Health Statistics, 1964, pp 1-43.
9. Blache JO, Handler FP: Coronary artery disease: A comparison of the rates and patterns of development of coronary arteriosclerosis in the Negro and white races with its relation to clinical coronary artery disease. *Arch Path* **50**:189-198, 1950.
10. Weiss MM, Gray WR: Hypertension and myocardial infarction in the Negro. *Amer J Med Sci* **227**:186-187, 1954.
11. Holman RL, McGill AC Jr, Strong JP, et al: The natural history of atherosclerosis. *Amer J Path* **34**:209-236, 1958.
12. Groom D, McKlee E, Webb C, et al: Developmental patterns of coronary and aortic atherosclerosis in Negroes of Haiti and the United States. *Ann Intern Med* **51**:270-289, 1959.
13. Mihaly JP, Whiteman NC: Myocardial infarction in the Negro: Historical survey as it relates to Negroes. *Amer J Cardiol* **2**:464-474, 1958.
14. Stamler J: Cardiovascular diseases in the United States. *Amer J Cardiol* **10**:319-340, 1962.

Blood Pressure and Cholesterol as Coronary Heart Disease Risk Factors

Herman A. Tyroler, MD, Chapel Hill, NC; Siegfried Heyden, MD; Alan Bartel, MD, Durham, NC;
John Cassel, MD, MPH; Joan C. Cornoni, MPH, PhD, Chapel Hill, NC;
Curtis G. Hames, MD, Claxton, Ga; and David Kleinbaum, PhD, Chapel Hill, NC

Elevations of systolic blood pressure, diastolic blood pressure, and serum cholesterol level were accompanied by an increased risk of developing coronary heart disease (CHD) in Evans County, Georgia. This was true for white men, black men, and white women. Black women did not exhibit an increase in incidence with the rise in risk factor levels. The white male excess in CHD incidence persisted over that of the black male at each categorical level of blood pressure and cholesterol studied. White women appeared to have CHD incidence rates generally similar to those of black women at lower levels of risk factors; at higher levels of risk factors, the white female CHD incidence rate was larger than the black female.

The association of the level of blood pressure and serum cholesterol with coronary heart disease (CHD) has had more epidemiologic investigation and demonstration than any other risk factors identified to date. In this communication we add the Evans County, Georgia, incidence experience to this body of knowledge. The material will be presented from several perspectives. We shall report the relationship of blood pressure and serum cholesterol levels, singly and in combinations, to the incidence of CHD in this rural southern community; and we shall assess the contributions of these risk factors to the higher incidence of CHD in Evans County white men than in black men. It should be noted that the higher white incidence has been reported elsewhere (Cassel et al, p 901).

Received for publication June 13, 1971; accepted Oct 12.

From the departments of epidemiology (Drs. Tyroler, Cassel, Cornoni, and Kleinbaum) and biostatistics (Dr. Kleinbaum), University of North Carolina, Chapel Hill; Department of Community Health Sciences (Dr. Heyden), Duke University Medical School; and Department of Cardiology (Dr. Bartel), Duke University Medical Center, Durham, NC. Dr. Hames is in private practice in Evans County, Georgia.

Reprint requests to Department of Epidemiology, University of North Carolina, Chapel Hill, NC (Dr. Tyroler).

Methods

The first survey examination of this study population (3,102 persons) was carried out between Aug 1, 1960, and June 1, 1962, and consisted of a history of heart disease, stroke, and other illnesses, a physical examination, electrocardiogram, roentgenogram of the chest, urinalysis, and laboratory studies of the blood for cholesterol level and hematocrit reading. The second survey examination of this cohort was made by two of the authors (A. B. and S. H.) between Aug 1, 1967, and Aug 31, 1969, in a clinic established for this purpose. During this seven to nine year follow-up period (average, 87 months), 320 persons had died and 252 had either migrated away from the community or refused to return for the second examination. The examination of the remaining 2,530 persons (90.9% reexamination rate) again consisted of a history, physical examination, and laboratory studies, but also included a detailed questionnaire for evidence of cerebrovascular disease and symptoms of transient cerebral ischemia, a sociological questionnaire, and a physical activities questionnaire. Other laboratory procedures and a complete description of the medical history and physical examination are reported elsewhere (Cornoni et al, p 896).

As in the 1960-1962 study,[1,2] three readings of blood pressure were taken on the left arm with the respondent seated in each case. The second reading was taken 30 to 60 minutes later, and the third, 15 to 20 minutes after the second one. The first recorded casual blood pressure was analyzed for this study. Serum cholesterol level was determined by the Abell-Kendall method after clot retraction occurred in the blood which had been drawn by vacuum syringe (Vacutainer). Intralaboratory and interlaboratory validation and quality control were obtained by participation in the Center for Disease Control Pooling Project.

Results

Age Specific CHD Incidence Rates by Blood Pressure and Serum Cholesterol Levels.—The incidence rates of CHD by levels of systolic blood pressure, diastolic blood pressure, and serum cholesterol for white and black men within ten year age bands, are presented in Fig 1, 2, and 3 (the number of observations upon which these rates are based are presented in Tables 1-6).

Individuals were categorized by their systolic blood pressure levels in 1960-1962 into one of three groupings: pressures equal to or less than 139 called "low"; pressures in the range of 140 to 159, "borderline"; and individuals with systolic blood pressure equal to 160 mm Hg or higher, "high." The incidence of CHD as used in this report refers to the combined manifestations of angina, myocardial infarction, or sudden death.

There is evidence to suggest a continuous effect of blood pressure on incidence of CHD,[3] and we have analyzed the relationship as a continuous one elsewhere (Kleinbaum et al, p 943); the choice of the categorical cutpoints as used here was made to provide comparability with other reported studies[4]; and to place the results within a context more meaningful and relevant to clinical practice.

In Evans County, for white men aged 45 years and older, there is a consistent, sizeable increase in incidence rates of CHD with increasing level of systolic blood pressure (Fig 1). No discernible trends are apparent for the black men. This may be due to the few number of instances of CHD

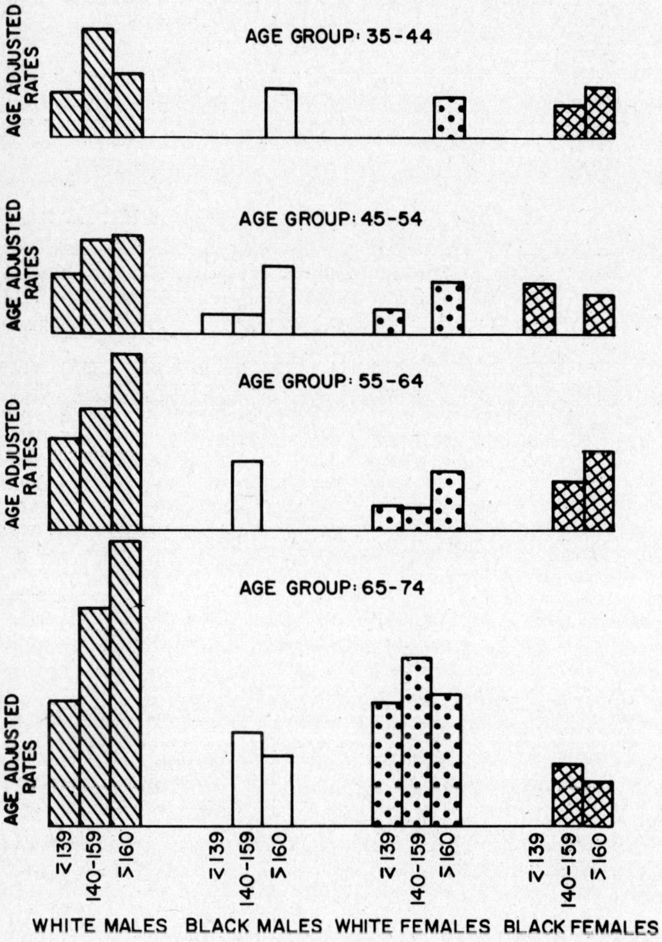

Fig. 1.—Coronary heart disease (CHD) incidence rates by systolic blood pressure levels-race-sex groups by age (rate/1,000). See Tables 1 and 2 for specific values.

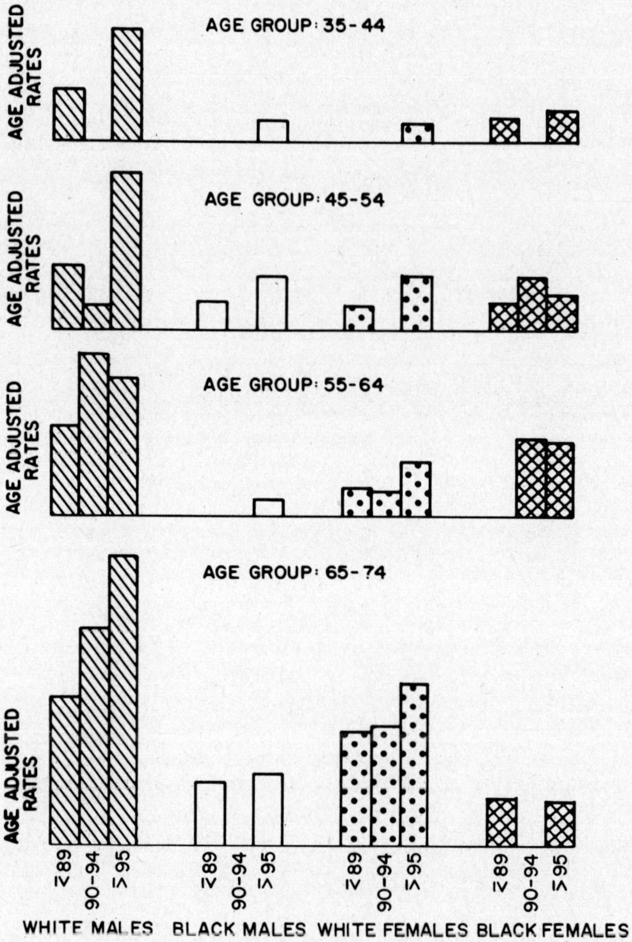

Fig 2.—CHD incidence rates by diastolic blood pressure levels-race-sex groups by age (rate/1,000). See Tables 3 and 4.

in the black man; however, what is apparent is that at each blood pressure level within each age grouping the white male incidence rates are higher than those for the black.

Diastolic blood pressure was categorized into three groupings for reasons similar to those discussed previously for systolic blood pressure. An additional reason for the levels chosen was the existence of clinical trials experience with hypotensive drug therapy.[5,6] Diastolic blood pressure in the 1960-1962 prevalence survey, therefore, was categorized as equal to or less than 89 ("low"), 90 to 94 ("borderline"), or equal to or greater than 95 mm Hg ("high"). The incidence rate was highest for Evans County white men with diastolic pressures equal to or greater than 95 mm Hg, in each age band. The rates at levels of 90 to 94 mm Hg are variable in relationship to individuals with lower and higher diastolic pressure, and, therefore, there is no clear-cut gradient. In no age grouping, for no blood pressure grouping, is the black male incidence rate of CHD equal to the white (Fig 1).

Serum cholesterol levels were categorized by the use of the frequently, but arbitrarily, chosen cutpoints of 220 and 260 mg/100 ml. For white men, at all ages 45 and older, those men with the lowest cholesterol values (ie, equal to or less than 219 mg/100 ml at the time of the 1960 examinations had the lowest incidence rates of CHD during the 1967-1969 follow-up period. There was no regular increment in CHD incidence with increase in cholesterol in the groupings chosen. At each cholesterol level, within each age band, white men in Evans County had higher incidence rates of CHD than did black men (Fig 1).

One reason for presenting the incidence rate data in age specific form was to see if there was any gross difference in the relationship of incidence rates to risk factor levels at different ages. Differences of this

Table 1.—Relationship of Systolic Blood Pressure to all new Coronary Heart Disease by Race and Age, Men

Systolic blood pressure,* mm Hg		≤139		140-159		≥160	
Race		W	B	W	B	W	B
Age, yr							
35-44	PAR†	113	36	36	24	16	19
	Cases	5	0	4	0	1	1
	Rate (%)	44	...	111	...	63	53
45-54	PAR	132	47	64	48	51	71
	Cases	8	1	6	1	5	5
	Rate (%)	61	21	94	21	98	70
55-64	PAR	56	23	49	14	50	49
	Cases	5	0	6	1	9	0
	Rate (%)	89	...	122	71	180	...
65-74	PAR	24	9	18	11	48	44
	Cases	3	0	4	1	14	3
	Rate (%)	125	...	222	91	292	68
75+	PAR	2	1	0	1	4	3
	Cases	1	0	0	0	1	0
	Rate (%)	500	...	...	...	250	...

* Systolic blood pressure unknown: three white men, one black man.
† PAR signifies persons at risk.

Table 2.—Relationship of Systolic Blood Pressure to all new Coronary Heart Disease by Race and Age, Women

Systolic blood pressure,* mm Hg		≤139		140-159		≥160	
Race		W	B	W	B	W	B
Age, yr							
35-44	PAR	130	44	35	29	23	38
	Cases	0	0	0	1	1	2
	Rate (%)	...	...	...	34	43	53
45-54	PAR	112	37	69	30	55	97
	Cases	3	2	0	0	4	4
	Rate (%)	27	54	...	...	73	41
55-64	PAR	43	16	47	20	83	88
	Cases	1	0	1	1	5	7
	Rate (%)	23	...	21	50	60	80
65-74	PAR	16	4	35	16	75	69
	Cases	2	0	6	1	10	3
	Rate (%)	125	...	171	63	133	43
75+	PAR	1	0	2	0	9	4
	Cases	0	0	0	0	3	0
	Rate (%)	...	...	...	...	333	...

* Systolic blood pressure unknown: one white woman.

Table 3.—Relationship of Diastolic Blood Pressure to all new Coronary Heart Disease by Race and Age, Men

Diastolic blood pressure,* mm Hg		≤89		90-94		≥95	
Race		W	B	W	B	W	B
Age, yr							
35-44	PAR	93	20	31	17	41	42
	Cases	5	0	0	0	5	1
	Rate (%)	54	...	...	...	122	24
45-54	PAR	120	36	41	23	86	107
	Cases	8	1	1	0	10	6
	Rate (%)	67	28	24	...	116	56
55-64	PAR	66	22	35	11	54	53
	Cases	6	0	6	0	8	1
	Rate (%)	91	...	171	...	148	19
65-74	PAR	38	15	13	9	39	40
	Cases	6	1	3	0	12	3
	Rate (%)	158	67	231	...	308	75
75+	PAR	1	1	2	1	3	3
	Cases	0	0	1	0	1	0
	Rate (%)	...	...	500	...	333	...

* Diastolic blood pressure unknown: three white men, one black man.

type, for example, have been presented from Framingham[7] with serum cholesterol values more predictive at younger than older ages. Within the limits of the small sample sizes of this study and the risk factor level groupings chosen, there is no evidence in the Evans County data of an age-risk factor: incidence rate interaction. It, therefore, was deemed appropriate to combine the observations within each race-sex group for individuals of all ages; age adjusted incidence rates were calculated for comparisons between the races by the indirect method using ten-year age bands.

Age Adjusted CHD Incidence Rates by Blood Pressure and Serum Cholesterol Levels.—The age adjusted CHD incidence rates for the four race-sex groups by blood pressure and serum cholesterol levels are presented in Fig 4 and Table 7.

Systolic Blood Pressure.—For three of the four race-sex groups (ie, white men, white women, and black men) there is a sizeable and consistent increase in CHD incidence rates with increase in systolic blood pressure levels. For white men the increase is approximately twofold (1.8) from an incidence rate of 59/1,000 at systolic blood pressure levels less than 140 mm Hg to a rate of 108/1,000 at systolic blood pressure levels greater than 160 mm Hg; for white women the rise is 2.5 times from an incidence rate of 22/1,000 to 54/1,000; for the black-man the relative risk is more than fourfold (4.4) with a rise in CHD incidence rates from 7/1,000 at systollic blood pressure levels less than 140 mm Hg to 31/1,000 at systolic blood pressure levels equal to or greater than 160 mm Hg. Thus, for these three groups there is a CHD incidence response with increasing levels of blood pressure. The Evans County black female population is distinctly different from the other three in showing no sizeable nor directionally consistent change in incidence rates with increasing systolic blood pressure levels; for black women the incidence rates are 32/1,000 at systolic blood pressure levels less than 140 mm Hg, 27/1,000 in the range of 140 to 159 mm Hg, and 37/1,000 at a systolic blood pressure equal to or greater than 160 mm Hg.

Diastolic Blood Pressure.—The effect of increasing levels of diastolic blood pressure on CHD incidence rates is generally quite comparable, in relative terms, among the Evans County white male, black male, and white female cohorts: there is an approximately 2:1 relative risk of incidence of CHD, comparing the incidence rate in those with diastolic pressure equal to or greater than 95 mm Hg with those individuals whose 1960 examination diastolic pressure was less than 90 mm Hg (for white men the relative risk is 1.8 on comparing an incidence rate of 115/1,000 with 63/1,000; for black men the relative risk is 2.1 comparing 33/1,000 with 16/1,000; and for white women, 58/1,000 compared with 27/1,000 is also a relative risk of 2.1). The experience of black women is distinctly different: there is only the slightest suggestion of a gradient of CHD incidence rate with increasing levels of diastolic pressure. The incidence

Table 4.—Relationship of Diastolic Blood Pressure to all new Coronary Heart Disease by Race and Age, Women

Diastolic blood pressure,* mm Hg		≤89		90-94		≥95	
Race		W	B	W	B	W	B
Age, yr							
35-44	PAR	113	36	30	18	45	57
	Cases	0	1	0	0	1	2
	Rate (%)	...	28	...	...	22	35
45-54	PAR	124	36	48	18	63	110
	Cases	3	1	1	1	3	4
	Rate (%)	24	28	21	56	48	36
55-64	PAR	67	24	37	12	69	88
	Cases	2	0	1	1	4	7
	Rate (%)	30	...	27	83	58	80
65-74	PAR	58	20	22	7	46	62
	Cases	7	1	3	0	8	3
	Rate (%)	121	50	136	...	174	48
75+	PAR	5	0	1	0	6	4
	Cases	0	0	0	0	3	0
	Rate (%)	...	...	...	...	500	...

* Diastolic blood pressure unknown: two white women.

Table 5.—Relationship of Cholesterol to all new Coronary Heart Disease by Race and Age, Men

Cholesterol level* mg/100 ml		≤219		220-259		≥260	
Race		W	B	W	B	W	B
Age, yr							
35-44	PAR	101	61	42	14	19	3
	Cases	6	1	2	0	2	0
	Rate (%)	59	16	48	...	105	...
45-54	PAR	153	111	62	35	32	16
	Cases	10	5	6	0	3	2
	Rate (%)	65	45	97	...	94	125
55-64	PAR	98	67	35	10	19	9
	Cases	12	1	6	0	2	0
	Rate (%)	122	15	171	...	105	...
65-74	PAR	56	35	25	24	9	4
	Cases	10	1	9	3	2	0
	Rate (%)	179	29	360	125	222	...
75+	PAR	1	2	2	3	2	0
	Cases	0	0	1	0	1	0
	Rate (%)	...	...	500	...	500	...

* Cholesterol level unknown: ten white men, seven black men.

Table 6.—Relationship of Cholesterol to all new Coronary Heart Disease by Race and Age, Women

Cholesterol level* mg/100 ml		≤219		220-259		≥260	
Race		W	B	W	B	W	B
Age, yr							
35-44	PAR	125	70	35	26	26	12
	Cases	0	1	1	1	0	0
	Rate (%)	...	14	29	38	...	...
45-54	PAR	103	101	90	39	41	21
	Cases	3	4	1	0	3	2
	Rate (%)	29	40	11	...	73	95
55-64	PAR	51	55	55	44	65	21
	Cases	2	3	3	4	2	1
	Rate (%)	39	55	55	91	31	48
65-74	PAR	34	35	44	27	46	21
	Cases	2	0	7	2	9	1
	Rate (%)	59	...	159	74	196	48
75+	PAR	2	1	4	2	5	1
	Cases	0	0	2	0	1	0
	Rate (%)	...	...	500	...	200	...

* Cholesterol level unknown: ten white women, sixteen black women (2 cases).

rates for black women were 28/1,000, 33/1,000, and 37/1,000 in the groups with diastolic blood pressure less than 90, 90 to 94, and equal to or greater than 95 mm Hg, respectively.

Serum Cholesterol.—The same three subpopulations (white men and women, black men) which exhibited a systolic and a diastolic blood pressure relationship to CHD incidence also demonstrated increasing incidence with increasing levels of serum cholesterol. White women and black men exhibited relative risks greater than 2:1 contrasting individuals in the highest with those in the lowest cholesterol groupings (for white women the relative risk was 2.4 and there was a stepwise rise in incidence from 21/1,000 to 44/1,000 to 51/1,000; for black men the relative risk was 2.1 and the incidence rates were 22/1,000, 22/1,000 and 47/1,000 in the cholesterol groups less than 219, 220 to 259, and equal to or greater than 260 mg/100 ml, respectively. The change in CHD incidence rates for white men was not a regular rise. The rates were 72/1,000, 109/1,000, and 95/1,000 going from the low to the high cholesterol groups. This is equivalent to a relative risk of CHD incidence of 1.5 in the intermediate contrasted with lowest cholesterol group, and only 1.3 for the highest (ie, equal to or greater than 260 mg/100 ml) contrasted to the lowest cholesterol group (ie, less than 219 mg/100 ml). Black female incidence rates were unrelated, at levels of 29/1,000, 36/1,000, and 34/1,000, respectively, to cholesterol levels.

Ethnic Group Comparisons.—At each level of systolic blood pressure, diastolic blood pressure, and serum cholesterol studied, there is a higher incidence rate of CHD in the white than in the black man. This excess is considerable, and in no instance is the rate less than twofold higher in the white man; the white excess ranges from a white-black male relative risk of 2.2 at serum cholesterol levels equal to or greater than 260 mg/100 ml to 8.5 at systolic blood pressure levels equal to and less than 139 mm Hg; overall, the age adjusted incidence rates are 83/1,000 and 24/1,000 for white and black men, respectively, a relative risk of 3.5 (Table 7).

In contrast to the marked and consistently higher rates for white than for black men, there is little difference between the ethnic groups' CHD incidence rates for women. The overall age adjusted incidence rates are 38/1,000 for white and 34/1,000 for black women. Although the rates are low, there is, however, the suggestion that there is a white female CHD response to increasing levels of risk factors which is not shared by the black woman. This results in the absence of a white/black female excess at low levels of risk factors and the presence of a relative risk of 1.5 at high levels.

In summary, there is evidence from this analysis that the black male incidence rates bear the same general relation to systolic and diastolic blood pressure and serum cholesterol rises as do the white men but at a lower absolute level; and that the white male excess of CHD incidence persists over that of black men when the two groups are studied at comparable levels of these risk factors.

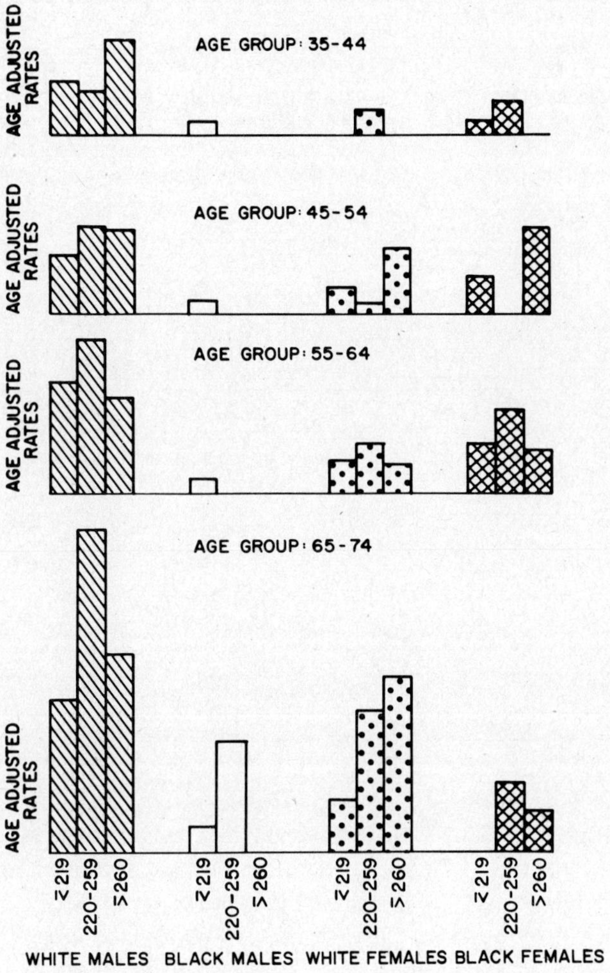

Fig 3.—CHD incidence rates by serum cholesterol levels-race-sex groups by age (rate/1,000). See Tables 5 and 6.

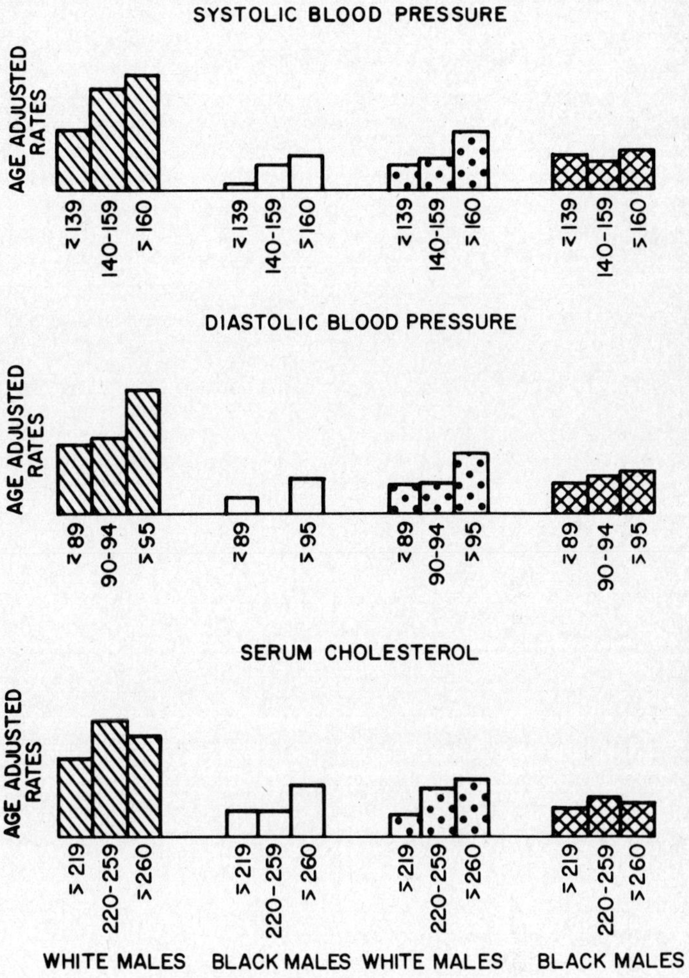

Fig 4.—CHD incidence rates by levels of blood pressure and serum cholesterol in Evans County (rate/1,000). See Table 7.

It should be pointed out that there is not complete comparability of risk factors among the race-sex groups by the method of categorization used. This is a result of the differences in distribution of the risk factors between the races and the use of open-ended groupings. For example, the distribution of blood pressure values in the black is at a considerably higher level than the white[1] and, therefore, values in the black group categorized as systolic pressure equal to or greater than 160 mm Hg are higher than in whites, similarly categorized, and, conversely, the white values categorized as less than 140

Table 7.—Coronary Heart Disease Incidence Rates for 87-Month Follow-Up by Categorical Levels of Blood Pressure and Cholesterol in Evans County

	Age Adjusted Rates/1,000				Relative Risk	
	WM*	BM	WF	BF	WM/BM	WF/BF
Systolic blood pressure, mm Hg						
≤139	59	7	22	32	8.5	0.7
140-159	94	25	28	27	3.8	1.0
≥160	108	31	54	37	3.5	1.5
Diastolic blood pressure, mm Hg						
≤89	63	16	27	28	3.9	1.0
90-94	70	...	29	33	...	0.9
≥95	115	33	58	37	3.5	1.6
Cholesterol						
≤219	72	22	21	29	3.3	0.7
220-259	109	22	44	36	5.0	1.2
≥260	95	47	51	34	2.0	1.5
Totals	83	24	38	34	...	...

* WM signifies white men; BM, black men; WF, white women; and BF, black women.

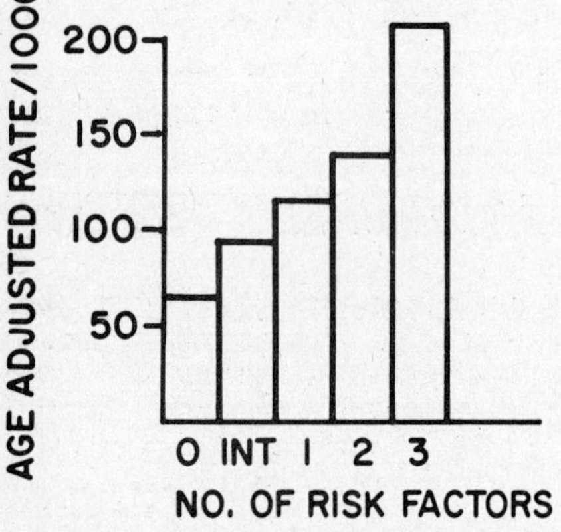

Fig 5.—CHD incidence rates by number of risk factors, white men, age 35+.

Table 8.—Joint Effects of Systolic and Diastolic Blood Pressure on White Male Age Adjusted Incidence Rates of Coronary Heart Disease (Expressed as Incidence Rate/1,000)

Diastolic blood pressure	Systolic Blood Pressure* Low	Medium	High	All SBP Levels
Low	54 (427)†	93 (66)	90 (17)	63
Medium	41 (54)	69 (59)	100 (29)	70
High	148 (31)	111 (78)	113 (127)	115
All DBP Levels	59	94	108	83

* Systolic blood pressure: low = ≤139; medium = 140-159; high = ≥160 mm Hg. Diastolic blood pressure: low = ≤89; medium = 90-94; high = ≥95 mm Hg.
† ( ) = PAR.

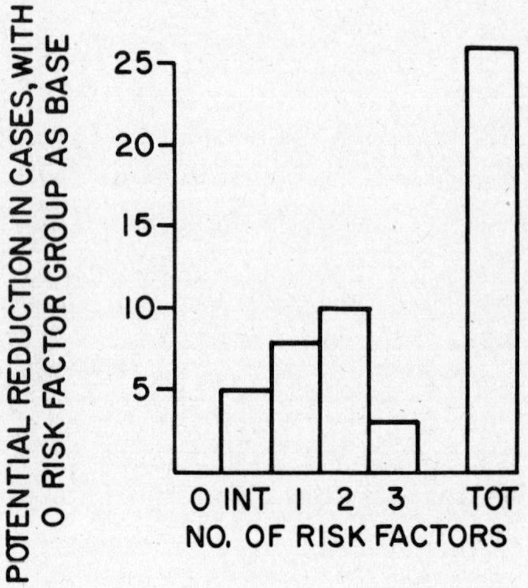

Fig 6.—Potential reduction in number of CHD cases by number of risk factors, white men, age 35+.

mm Hg are lower than are the black. For blood pressure grouping this makes the CHD incidence excess of white men contrasted with black men an underestimate of what it would be at more strictly comparable blood pressure levels. For cholesterol level comparisons the opposite is true, as the distribution of serum cholesterol is considerably lower in the Evans County black than white man.[2]

CHD Incidence Rates by Combinations of Risk Factors.—*The Effects of Concurrent Levels of Systolic and Diastolic Pressure.*—Although there is a high correlation between levels of systolic and diastolic blood pressure, there are pathogenetically different mechanisms for elevations of each, and in population-based studies there are enough individuals with elevations of one but not the other to test their independent effects as risk factors. Data of this type are set out in Table 2 for the CHD incidence in white men in Evans County classified by the joint levels of their systolic and diastolic pressure levels in 1960-1962. The convention for classification of blood pressure is as used previously: for systolic pressure "low" = ≤ 139, "medium" = 140-159, and "high" = ≥ 160 mm Hg; for diastolic pressure "low" = ≤ 89, "medium" = 90-94, and "high" = ≥ 95 mm Hg.

Although the results which follow are based on small subsamples, there is a complex but interesting apparent effect of joint levels of systolic blood pressure (SBP) and diastolic blood pressure (DBP) on the incidence of CHD in white men. At low and medium levels of DBP there is an independent effect as SBP increases with relative risks of approximately 2:1. At low levels of DBP, the incidence increases from 54/1,000 to 93/1,000 as SBP increases from low to medium levels. There is no further increase with increase of SBP to high levels; the incidence rate for those individuals with low DBP and high SBP is 90/1,000.

The independent effect of increasing SBP levels is more striking at medium levels of DBP; in this instance, the incidence rates increase from 41/1,000 to 69/1,000 to 100/1,000 with increasing SBP levels. Similarly, there is an independent effect of increasing DBP levels for individuals with low SBP; in this circumstance the relative risk is almost threefold with rates rising from 54 for individuals with low SBP and low DBP to 148/1,000 for individuals with low SBP and high DBP.

In contrast to the statistically independent effect of each of the blood pressure components when they are low, there is no additional effect of the other component when one is at a high level. Thus, when DBP is high, the CHD incidence rate is 148 in the presence of low SBP, 111 in the presence of medium SBP, and 113 in the presence of high SBP. When SBP is high there is a slight gradient of increasing incidence with increasing DBP from 90/1,000 to 100/1,000 to 113/1,000.

In summary, the major findings are that there is an independent effect of each component when the other is low; there is absence of an independent effect of each blood pressure component when the other one is high, and there is absence of an interactive effect. There is no evidence from this data of a more deleterious consequence of possessing high values of both risk factors (if systolic and diastolic levels are to be considered each as a separate risk factor) contrasted with the consequence of possessing either separately.

The Effect of Concurrent Elevations of Systolic and Diastolic Blood Pressure and Serum Cholesterol Levels.

We now focus our attention on identification of the individuals in Evans County who were at particularly high risk of subsequent development of clinical CHD, although free of detectable CHD at the time of the 1960-1962 examinations. For the reasons previously documented, these are white men, age 35 and over (all the new CHD in white men were of this age) and with evidence of elevations of systolic or diastolic blood pressure or serum cholesterol values. For this analysis an individual was classified by the number of risk factors he possessed. A white man was classified as possessing three risk factors if his systolic blood pressure was equal to or greater than 160 mm Hg, and his diastolic pressure equal to or greater than 95 mm Hg, and his serum cholesterol level equal to or greater than 250 mg/100 ml. He was classified as possessing one or two risk factors if any were in the range specified, in the number indicated. An individual was classified as "free" of risk factors, ie, with a risk factor score of 0, if his systolic pressure was less than 140 and his diastolic less than 90 mm Hg and his serum cholesterol level was less than 250 mg/100 ml. Individuals with one or more risk factors in the range between the cutpoints for definitely "low" and definitely "high" were collectively analyzed an an intermediate group.

Table 9.—Coronary Heart Disease Incidence Rates by No. of Risk Factors, White Men, Age 35+

	No. of Risk Factors					
	0	Intermediate	1	2	3	
PAR age 35+	175	166	166	137	22	666
% Distribution of population by risk factors	26.3	24.9	24.9	20.6	3.3	100%
Observed No. of cases	10	14	20	23	5	72
Observed incidence rate × 10^3	57	84	121	168	227	108
Age adjusted rate × 10^3	66	93	114	140	208	
Relative risk	1.00	1.41	1.72	2.12	3.15	
Attributable risk × 10^3						
With 0 risk group as base		27	48	74	142	
With intermediate group as base			20	47	115	
Potential reduction in cases						
With 0 risk group as base		5	8	10	3	26
With intermediate group as base			3	7	3	12

The results of these observations are set out in Table 9 and Fig 5. The CHD incidence rate was 108/1,000 for all white men age 35 and older. There was a sizeable and consistent increase in the age adjusted incidence rate as the number of risk factors possessed per individual increased. The CHD age adjusted incidence rates for white men with none, one or more intermediate, and one, two, or three high risk factors rose in the respective sequence 66, 93, 114, 140, and 208 per 1,000. Expressed in terms of relative risk, white men with elevations of systolic and diastolic pressure and serum cholesterol level were 3.15 times more likely to develop CHD in the next 87 months than white men with values in the definitely low range.

Comment and Implications

The importance of elevations of serum cholesterol level and blood pressure in predisposing to episodes of coronary heart disease is clear in the Evans County white population. Although there is evidence to suggest that the relationship is continuous and we have analyzed and reported the risk factors in this fashion elsewhere (Kleinbaum et al, p 943), the approach taken here is a categorical one: a given elevation is considered as a risk factor and is either present or not for each individual. This approach facilitates comparisons between populations and also presents the population findings in terms most meaningful for considerations of clinical treatment of individuals and for estimations of the potential impact of community intervention programs.

In contrasting the white and black male incidence rates prior to these analyses, there was the logical possibility of either a different reaction or response to the risk factors in the two groups, or a similar response to a given level of risk factors, but an overall difference in population incidence rates due to differences in prevalence of the risk factors. There is, however, no evidence in our data to suggest that men in the two ethnic groups have basically different responses to increases in the risk factors (although the possibility of a different response in women is strong). There is an increased incidence rate for both white and black men with increase in risk factor levels. These rates, however, consistently show a white excess at each level of risk factors studied. And finally, while overall the lower observed CHD incidence rate in blacks is consistent with the lower serum cholesterol values, the population distribution of blood pressure would lead us to expect higher CHD incidence rates in the black than those observed. The combined effect of blood pressure and cholesterol level is not one which is explanatory of the white-black CHD incidence rate differences; the existence of factors other than blood pressure and serum cholesterol level are manifestly operative in Evans County, either protecting blacks, or predisposing whites to coronary heart disease incidence.

The importance of serum cholesterol level and blood pressure elevations in predisposing to incidence of clinically manifest CHD, and the strength of the association, is apparent from the threefold greater risk of incidence in the presence of elevations of blood pressure and serum cholesterol level contrasted to the incidence in white men with low values. An alternative way, to the relative risk, of studying the importance of risk factors in population studies is that of attributable risk: the relative risk is the ratio of incidence in groups with and without the risk factor; the attributable risk is the difference in the two incidence rates. For example, the age-adjusted rates for white men with all the three risk factors present was 208/1,000; for white men with no risk factor elevations the CHD incidence was 66/1,000 (Table 3 and Fig 5). The relative risk was computed as the ratio of 208:66, ie, 3.15. The attributable risk is the difference between 208 and 66, ie, 142/1,000 and represents the reduction of CHD incidence rate that would obtain if the high risk group were to be influenced in some manner to have the incidence rate of the low risk group. One can postulate that this is the potential for reduction of CHD incidence by eliminating the high risk factors.[7-9] This, of course, is an assumption based only on observational surveys, not experimental clinical trials evidence. It is to be emphasized that there is no data from clinical trials or community intervention reported at the time of this writing to warrant the expectation that reducing elevated serum cholesterol level and blood pressure will bring these groups' experience down to the CHD incidence rate of individuals without elevations. The data are analyzed in the form of attributable risk to present another way of appraising the association of blood pressure and serum cholesterol level with CHD incidence in Evans County, and to estimate the maximally attainable reductions under the (presently unrealistic) assumptions of causality of the risk factors, no misclassifications of examinees, and therapeutic means for totally effective reduction of risk factors with no untoward consequences. The attributable risk among individuals with all three risk factors contrasted with those with none present was 142/1,000 (Table 3 and Fig 6). There were 22 white men age 35 + in Evans County with three risk factors and five of them developed CHD. If they had had the age adjusted CHD incidence experience of the zero risk group, approximately three fewer cases would have occurred. Continuing this argument for each risk group results in a potential reduction of ten, eight, and five cases in the groups with two elevations, one elevation, and intermediate levels and risk factors, respectively. For all groups combined, 26 of the 72 observed cases of new CHD in Evans County white men would not have occurred had the risk groups experienced the CHD incidence rate of the nonrisk group. If one assumes this could have been achieved by lowering of the established risk factors, it indicates a 36% reduction of cases (26:72) by intervening in 74% of the population, ie, 491 of the 666 white men age 35 + were in either the intermediate or one or more risk group categories. Eliminating the intermediate group from consideration, 29% of cases (21:72) theoretically could be prevented by intervention in the men with either elevated blood pressure or cholesterol level; this, however, would still require intervention in 49% of the target population, ie, 325 of the 666 white men age 35 + had elevation of either blood pressure (160/95 mm Hg) or serum cholesterol (260 mg/100 ml).

Obviously a different perspective of the demonstrated association of these risk factors and CHD incidence is obtained when one contrasts the relative and attributable risk arguments. Despite the unquestioned strength of the associations and the importance of blood pressure and serum cholesterol level elevations, the prevalence of these risk factors is so high that interventions would have to include large proportions of the target populations potentially to achieve moderate reductions in incidence. It is clear that much further research in clinical effectiveness and community intervention is required. Similarly, continuing fundamental epidemiologic research into other CHD risk factors in addition to blood pressure and serum cholesterol level is required.

References

1. McDonough JR, Garrison GE, Hames CG: Blood pressure and hypertensive disease among Negroes and whites. *Ann Intern Med* **61**:208-228, 1964.

2. McDonough JR, Hames CG, Stulb SC, et al: Coronary heart disease among Negroes and whites in Evans County, Georgia. *J Chronic Dis* **18**:443-368, 1965.

3. Truett J, Cornfield J, Kannel W: A multivariate analysis of the risk of coronary heart disease in Framingham. *J Chronic Dis* **20**:551-554, 1967.

4. World Health Organization Expert Committee: Arterial hypertension and ischemic heart disease preventive aspects. *WHO Techn Rep Series* 1962, No. 231.

5. Veterans Administration Cooperative Study Group on Antihypertensive Agents: Effects of treatment on morbidity in hypertension. *JAMA* **202**:1028-1034, 1967.

6. Veterans Administration Cooperative Study Group on Antihypertensive Agents: Effects of treatment on morbidity in hypertension: Prescribed results in patients with diastolic blood pressure averaging 90-114 mm Hg. *JAMA* **213**:1143-1152, 1970.

7. Kannel WB, Dawber TR, Kagan A, et al: Factors of risk in the development of coronary heart disease: Six-year follow-up experience. *Ann Intern Med* **55**:33-50, 1961.

8. Cornfield J: Joint dependence of risk of coronary heart disease on serum cholesterol and systolic blood pressure: A discriminant function analysis. *Fed Proc* **21**:58-61, 1962.

9. Tibblin G: High blood pressure in men aged 50. *Acta Med Scand*, suppl 470, pp 5-84, 1967.

Body Weight and Cigarette Smoking As Risk Factors

Siegfried Heyden, MD, Durham, NC; John C. Cassel, MD, MPH, Chapel Hill, NC; Alan Bartel, MD, Durham, NC; Herman A. Tyroler, MD, Chapel Hill, NC; Curtis G. Hames, MD, Claxton, Ga; and Joan C. Cornoni, MPH, PhD, Chapel Hill, NC

In males, the incidence rate of coronary heart disease (CHD) in white noncigarette smokers was 52.7/1,000 and among blacks, 9.8/1,000; among white cigarette smokers the rate was 101/1,000 but in blacks only 32.5/1,000. The incidence rate of CHD in the leanest whites was 95.5/1,000, among the leanest blacks, 24.1/1,000; however, in the most obese whites the rate was 137/1,000 and among the blacks, 53.6/1,000. When comparing white smokers with nonsmokers in the leanest and most obese tertiles, smokers run a substantial risk of developing CHD, increasing with increase in overweight (80, 90, and 150/1,000, respectively). The risk of nonsmokers developing CHD does not increase from the leanest to the moderately overweight and the most obese group, (51, 30, and 64/1,000, respectively). Therefore, obesity in white males seems to enhance the risk of CHD among cigarette smokers but not among nonsmokers.

In the seven-year follow-up study of the Evans County, Georgia, population, it was found that the rate of occurrence of new cases of coronary heart disease (CHD) was higher at each age in white males than in black males. Various analyses of these data have convinced us that these differences are unlikely to be due to variations in diagnostic criteria, to "missing" black cases, or to competing causes of death. Accordingly, attempts are being made to determine the degree to which these differences might be accounted for by differences in the distributions of some of the standard risk factors in whites and blacks. In a separate publication it has been shown that the black rates are lower than the white at comparable levels of blood pressure (both systolic and diastolic) and cholesterol levels. It is the purpose of this paper to present the findings in respect to three other factors which, with varying degrees of certainty, have been suspected to be related to CHD, cigarette smoking, body weight, and hematocrit levels.

Received for publication May 13, 1971; accepted Aug 3.

From the Department of Community Health Sciences, Duke University Medical School (Dr. Heyden) and the Division of Cardiology, Duke University Medical Center (Dr. Bartel), Duke University, Durham, NC, and the Department of Epidemiology, University of North Carolina, Chapel Hill (Drs. Cassel, Tyroler, and Cornoni). Dr. Hames is a practicing physician, Claxton, Ga.

Reprint requests to Department of Community Health Sciences, Duke University Medical School, Durham, NC 27710 (Dr. Heyden).

Methods

Smoking histories were obtained on all subjects examined in the 1960 through 1962 prevalence study. In addition, all subjects had their heights and weights measured with light clothing without shoes and had a hematocrit determination using the microhematocrit centrifuge method. In all individuals judged to be free of CHD in the prevalence examination, the subsequent occurrence of new events was determined by reexamination some 87 months later and a review of all deaths that occurred between the two examinations.

Results

Cigarette Smoking.—For purposes of this analysis the population at risk was classified as either nonsmokers or smokers based upon the 1960 through 1962 smoking history. Smokers included both those who reported at that time that they were currently smoking as well as ex-smokers. Table 1 shows that for both black and white males, smokers had higher rates of CHD than did nonsmokers but that white males had higher rates than blacks whether they were smokers or not. Thus the age-adjusted rate for white nonsmokers was 52.7/1,000, compared to 9.8 for blacks. Similarly, while white smokers had a rate of 101, the rate in black smokers was only 32.5.

Body Weight.—To take into account the joint effect of both height and weight the Quetelet index, $\frac{\text{weight}}{\text{height}^2} \times 100$ was used. Khosla and Lowe[1] determined from a study of 5,000 British males ages 15 to 64 years that this was the best index of obesity. This opinion was also confirmed by Boe et al.[2] The criteria for their choice was that the index be highly correlated with weight but independent of height. To provide convenient categories for analysis, the distribution of the Quetelet index for all males was divided into equal tertiles. This distribution ranged from a value of 2.121, which was the value for the leanest man, to 6.163, for the most obese man. The first tertile included all men with a Quetelet index of less than 3.244. The second tertile included all men whose index ranged between 3.244 and 3.697 and the third tertile was those men with an index of 3.698 or greater.

As shown in Table 2, there was a modest relationship between body size and incidence of CHD in both blacks and whites. While no gradient occurs, whites in the third tertile of the Quetelet index range have an age-adjusted rate 1.43 times as great as those in the first tertile. In blacks the relative risk of being in the third as opposed to the first tertile is 2.22. In each tertile, however, at each age, whites have higher rates than do blacks.

Hematocrit Level.—Considerable controversy exists as to whether blood viscosity, as measured by hematocrit levels, constitutes a risk factor in CHD. Ample physiological evidence exists which would make such a relationship seem plausible. Polycythemia is known to predispose to thrombus formation[3]; reduction in myocardial blood flow occurs when anemic patients are transfused to polycythemic levels[4] and such variations in coronary flow which follow alterations in blood viscosity may be of clinical significance in a setting of atherosclerotic disease.[5]

Studies attempting to document the added risk that high blood viscosity (at least as measured by hematocrit levels) might have for the development of CHD, however, have yielded conflicting results.

Burch and DePasquale found that the hematocrit levels in both male and female patients with myocardial infarction was higher than in controls matched for age-ethnic group and social-class level.[6] These results were confirmed by Mayer in a study of 66 men with coronary disease and 68 controls of the same age and sex.[7] Conley and co-workers did not find any differences between 200 male private patients with acute myocardial infarction and 915 "normal" individuals (including 721 medical students, 136 business executives, and 58 airline pilots).[8] McDonough et al similarly found no difference between cases and controls as far as hematocrit values are concerned.[9]

In part these conflicting results may be accounted for by the difficulties of interpretation that so often accompany any case-control study. These include the effect of the myocardial infarct itself on the hematocrit levels, the adequacy of the controls used, and the problem of selective survival. ("Cases" in such a study are restricted to those who have survived their infarct. Conceivably, individuals with the highest hematocrit values who develop a myocardial infarct may be the ones who die, leaving only those patients with relatively low hematocrit levels available for study.) These problems are to a large extent overcome by prospective or cohort studies, and it is of interest that in the Framingham study, where these phenomena were studied prospectively, both elevated hemoglobin and hematocrit levels were shown to increase the risk of subsequent CHD.[10]

The findings from this study (Table 3) confirm the Framingham findings as far as white males are concerned. The relative risk of a hematocrit level of 50% or greater compared to one of 40% or less was 2.3 (113 cases/1,000 compared to 49 cases/1,000). No such relationship could be observed for blacks, however; also, as in the previous analyses the white rates were higher than the black rates at each level of hematocrit.

It is thus apparent that, as in the case of blood pressure and cholesterol level, black males in Evans County have a lower incidence rate of CHD than do white males at each level of risk factors (cigarette smoking, Quetelet index, and hematocrit value). While the rates in blacks seem

Table 1.—Incidence of CHD by Cigarette Smoking History, Age, and Ethnic Group*

Age (yr)	White Males			Black Males		
	No.	Cases	Rate/1,000	No.	Cases	Rate/1,000
			Nonsmokers			
15-24	62	0	...	16	0	...
25-34	28	0	...	12	0	...
35-44	36	0	...	21	1	48
45-54	68	4	59	40	0	...
55-64	67	4	60	31	0	...
65-74	46	9	196	34	1	29
75+	1	0	...	3	0	...
All ages	308	17	55	157	2	13
Age-adjusted rate			52.7			9.8
			Smokers and Ex-Smokers			
15-24	40	0	...	30	0	...
25-34	67	0	...	24	0	...
35-44	125	10	80	55	0	...
45-54	181	15	83	126	7	56
55-64	88	16	182	56	1	18
65-74	44	12	273	30	3	100
75+	5	2	(400)	1	0	...
All ages	550	55	100	322	11	34
Age-adjusted rate			101			32.5
			Unknown Smoking Status			
15-24	16	0	...	35	0	...
25-34	14	0	...	7	0	...
35-44	5	0	...	3	0	...
45-54	0	0	...	0	0	...
55-64	0	0	...	0	0	...
65-74	0	0	...	0	0	...
75+	0	0	...	1	0	...
All ages	35	0	...	46	0	...

* Eighty-seven-month follow-up period (males only).

to respond to variations in all of these risk factors in a manner similar to whites (with the exception perhaps of hematocrit level), it would appear that some additional factors must be operative which are protective for blacks. As is shown in a subsequent paper, at least one of these additional factors may be sustained and excessive physical activity.

Up to this point the relationship of these risk factors to CHD incidence has been examined one at a time. In view of the potential importance of some of the factors (particularly smoking, body weight, and blood pressure) for intervention purposes, it was decided to determine the combined effects of some of these. While this could not be accomplished for blacks (due to the small number of cases) and, thus, could not contribute any further explanation to the black-white difference, analyzing the relationship in white males only could produce some useful information.

Cigarette Smoking and Body Weight.—In this and subsequent analyses the classification of men into Quetelet index tertiles was recomputed using the distribution of Quetelet index in white males only. As no comparisons were to be made with black males, it was considered that this would provide a more appropriate basis for comparison than the intervals based on the distribution of Quetelet index in all males (black and white) used in the previous analysis. While this reclassification results in a slightly different absolute value for the incidence rates, the relationship between Quetelet index and CHD shown in Table 2 remains unchanged.

One of the reasons for examining the combined effects of body weight and cigarette smoking on incidence was the suspicion we had that the relationship of body weight to CHD could be masked if many of the heavier men had gained weight as a consequence of having given up smoking. Under such circumstances any deleterious effect that overweight might have could conceivably be counterbalanced by cessation of cigarette smoking. Alternatively, the possibility exists that any beneficial effect of giving up smoking might be nullified if there was a subsequent weight gain.

It should be borne in mind that this analysis can at best only provide suggestive answers to these questions as we do not as yet have data showing the incidence of CHD in those individuals whose weight or cigarette smoking patterns have in fact changed. What is available is the subsequent incidence of CHD in those individuals who in 1960 were both over-

Table 2.—Incidence of CHD by Quetelet Index, Age, and Ethnic Group*

Quetelet Index	Age (yr)	White Males No.	White Males Cases	White Males Rate/1,000	Black Males No.	Black Males Cases	Black Males Rate/1,000
First tertile	35-44	50	1	20	24	0	...
	45-54	58	4	69	41	1	24
	55-64	53	5	94	29	0	...
	65-74	32	8	250	22	2	91
	75+	1	1	(1,000)	1	0	...
	All ages	194	19	98	117	3	26
	Age-adjusted rate			95.5			24.1
Second tertile	35-44	53	2	38	30	1	33
	45-54	76	5	66	74	2	29
	55-64	48	7	146	34	0	...
	65-74	28	4	143	20	0	...
	75+	4	1	(250)	3	0	...
	All ages	209	19	91	157	3	19
	Age-adjusted rate			91.3			19.2
Third tertile	35-44	63	7	111	25	0	...
	45-54	115	10	87	55	4	73
	55-64	54	8	148	24	1	42
	65-74	30	9	300	22	2	91
	75+	1	0	...	1	0	...
	All ages	263	34	129	127	7	55
	Age-adjusted rate			137.0			53.6

* Eighty-seven-month follow-up period (males,35 years of age and older).

Table 3.—Incidence of CHD by Hematocrit Level and Ethnic Group*

	Hematocrit Value: 40% No.	Cases	Age-Adjusted Rate/1,000	41% to 49% No.	Cases	Age-Adjusted Rate/1,000	50% No.	Cases	Age-Adjusted Rate/1,000
White	27	2	49	700	51	76	137	14	113
Black	58	2	22	411	11	27	40	0	...

* Eighty-seven-month follow-up period (males only).

Table 4.—Age-Adjusted Incidence Rates of CHD by Quetelet Index and Cigarette Smoking*

Smoking Status at Entry Into Study	Quetelet Index at Entry Into Study: First Tertile No.	Cases	Rate	Second Tertile No.	Cases	Rate	Third Tertile No.	Cases	Rate
Smokers†	183	15	80	161	14	90	127	16	150
Nonsmokers	90	5	51	99	3	30	119	9	64

* Eighty-seven-month follow-up period (white males only).
† Smokers include only those who were smoking cigarettes in 1960. Ex-smokers have been excluded from this table.

weight for their age and height and who smoked cigarettes compared to those with similar weight who did not smoke cigarettes.

Bearing this in mind Table 4 does suggest that part of the effect of increased body weight is indeed being disguised by cessation of cigarette smoking. Lean men (first tertile) who smoke have an age-adjusted incidence rate of CHD of 80. Heavy men who do *not* smoke (third tertile, nonsmokers) only have a rate of 64. By contrast equally heavy men who are smokers have a rate of 150. These latter men obviously have gained weight without giving up smoking. If they had given up smoking their risk of developing CHD presumably would approximate the third tertile nonsmokers (ie, 64) and would, thus, be very different from lean (first tertile) men.

The degree to which the beneficial effect of giving up smoking is mitigated by subsequent weight gain is less clearly demonstrated in Table 4. As mentioned above lean men who smoke (first tertile, smokers) have an incidence rate of 80. If they stop smoking but gain weight, the assumption is that their rate might drop to that of the nonsmoking third tertile men (64). If they stop smoking but do *not* gain weight they might have a slightly greater reduction in risk to 51 (nonsmokers, first tertile).

Table 5.—Age-Adjusted Incidence Rates of CHD by Quetelet Index and Systolic Blood Pressure*

Systolic BP at Entry Into Study	Quetelet Index at Entry Into Study: First Tertile			Second Tertile			Third Tertile		
	No.	Cases	Age-Adjusted Rate/1,000	No.	Cases	Age-Adjusted Rate/1,000	No.	Cases	Age-Adjusted Rate/1,000
≦139	193	6	44	179	9	63	140	7	71
140-154	64	5	78	61	4	70	78	11	138
≦160	45	11	123	54	7	75	74	12	107

* Eighty-seven-month follow-up period (white males only).

The Relationship of Body Weight and Blood Pressure to Coronary Heart Disease

The question of the joint relationship of elevated blood pressure and overweight to CHD is a subject of some controversy. While it is well recognized that a high correlation exists between body weight and blood pressure, no unanimity of opinion exists concerning the possible effect that variations in body weight might have on the prognostic significance of elevated blood pressure.

For over a decade actuarial data have demonstrated the excessive mortality risk in overweight persons with high blood pressures. However, several studies of hypertensive patients in clinical series have shown conflicting results. Bechgaard,[11] Frant and Groen,[12] and Mathisen et al[13] found mortality in obese hypertensive subjects no higher than in nonobese hypertensive persons. Breslin et al[14] in a study of 14 patients with one or more retinal exudates, with or without hemorrhage, but with no papilledema, found that the survival rate was actually better in obese than in nonobese patients. In hypertensive patients without these retinal changes there was no difference in survival between obese and nonobese. The authors concluded at the very least that obesity did not seem to have an adverse effect on the survival in hypertensive patients.

A Japanese study examined the prognostic significance of hypertension in the obese and nonobese by dividing hypertensive patients into five groups according to the percent deviation of their body weight on admission from standard body weight for height. Four-year mortality rates of each group were compared. Average ages and overall severity of hypertension of these five groups were similar. The four-year mortality rates of these five groups were 4.5% in the most obese group (20% or more overweight), 12.5% in the slightly obese group (11% to 19% overweight), 13.0% in the standard weight group, 4.2% in the slightly emaciated group (11% to 19% underweight), and 25% in the most emaciated group (20% or more underweight). The authors could provide no explanation for the better prognosis in the most obese group and the worst prognosis in the most emaciated group.[15]

On the other hand, in two prospective studies[16,17] and in a retrospective study by Levy et al,[18] it was clearly shown that overweight and hypertension are associated with an excess of coronary disease and cerebrovascular disease, especially among men. Severity of hypertensive retinopathy and cardiovascular complications were related to obesity of Tibblins' study of hypertensive disease in men aged 50 years.[19]

This phenomenon was examined in the current study by examining the seven-year incidence of CHD in men classified by their Quetelet index and level of systolic blood pressure in 1960 through 1962.

As can be seen for Table 5, the data tend to support the conclusions of the Japanese study.[15] The relative risk of hypertensives developing CHD in lean men (first tertile) is 2.8 times that of normotensives (incidence of 123 and 44, respectively). In the most overweight third, by contrast, the relative risk of hypertension is only 1.5 (incidence of 107 compared to 71). One possible explanation for these findings may be in the degree of hypertension suffered by the lean as compared to the overweight. In Table 5 the population is stratified into only three blood pressure groups. It is quite possible that the lean men with systolic blood pressures of over 160 mm Hg have considerably higher levels than the overweight men in this category.

Table 5 also produces some suggestive evidence in another aspect of this problem, the effect of weight reduction combined with the reduction of blood pressure compared to the consequences of reduction of blood pressure levels alone. According to these data reduction of systolic blood pressure from over 160 mm Hg to under 140 mm Hg without any change in weight might be expected to reduce the risk of CHD in overweight men from 107 to 71 (these being the relevant incidence rates in men in the third Quetelet index tertile). Reduction of blood pressure levels *and* weight reduction, however, might be expected to lower the risk of CHD from 107 to that of first tertile men with blood pressure under 140 mm Hg, ie, an incidence rate of 44. This of course is but confirmation of a well established clinical impression which makes all the more surprising the lack of attention that weight reduction has received in intervention studies concerned with reducing blood pressures in the hope of preventing cardiovascular complications.

Comment and Conclusions

In this seven-year follow-up study in Evans County, further evidence is produced which shows that black males in this county are at lower risk of developing CHD than are white males, regardless of the level of risk factors. Thus, at comparable levels of body weight and hematocrit level and whether smokers or nonsmokers, black males had age-adjusted incidence rates of CHD which were only one third to one fifth those of white men. In spite of the small number of cases available for analysis in the blacks, their rates did seem to respond to variations in these risk factors in a manner similar to whites (with the possible exception of hematocrit value) but always at a lower level. It would thus appear that, while these risk factors do affect blacks in a manner similar to whites, some additional factors must be operative which either enhance the effect of the risk factors in whites or protect blacks from some of their consequences. As is shown in a subsequent paper, at least one of these additional factors may be sustained and excessive physical activity.

In addition to exploring black-white differences, the joint effects of cigarette smoking and body weight and systolic blood pressure and body weight on the subsequent development of CHD in white males was examined. The data would tend to support the following:

1. The deleterious effect of overweight could be masked if many overweight men in a study had achieved this status as a result of discontinuing smoking.

2. Despite the high correlation known to exist between body weight and hypertension, when systolic hypertension occurs in lean men, it is of graver prognostic significance (as far as subsequent CHD is concerned) than hypertension in overweight men.

3. While reduction of blood pressure levels alone in overweight men can be expected to have a modestly beneficial effect on preventing the occurrence of CHD, the reduction of weight together with lowering of blood pressure in such individuals can be expected to have considerably greater effect.

References

1. Khosla T, Lowe CR: Endices of obesity derived from body weight and height. *Brit J Prev Soc Med* **21**:122-128, 1967.

2. Boe J, Humerfelt S, Wedervang F: The blood pressure in a population. *Acta Med Scand* **321**(suppl):336, 1957.

3. Erf LA: Radioactive phosphorus in the treatment of primary polycythemia (Vera). *Progr Hemat* **1**:153-165, 1956.

4. Regan TJ, Frank MJ, Lehan PH, et al: Influence of red cell mass on myocardial blood flow and oxygen uptake. *Clin Res* **8**:367, 1960.

5. Clifford GO: Determinants of blood viscosity, in James TN, Keyes JW (eds): *The Etiology of Myocardial Infarction*. Boston, Little Brown & Co, 1963, pp 587-597.

6. Burch GE, DePasquale NP: Hematocrit in patients with acute myocardial infarction, abstracted. *Circulation* **26**:694, 1962.

7. Mayer GA: Hematocrit and coronary heart disease. *Canad Med Assoc J* **93**:1151-1153, 1965.

8. Conley CL, Russell RP, Thomas CB, et al: Hematocrit values in coronary artery disease. *Arch Intern Med* **113**:170-176, 1964.

9. McDonough JR, Hames CG, Garrison GE, et al: The relationship of hematocrit to cardiovascular states of health in the Negro and white population of Evans County, Georgia. *J Chron Dis* **18**:243-257, 1965.

10. Dawber TR: Coronary heart disease. *Bibl Cardiol* **13**:9-24, 1962.

11. Bechgaard P: Natural history of benign hypertension, in Ruebi FC, Bock KD, Cattier PT (eds): *Essential Hypertension*. Berlin, Springer-Verlag, pp 198-213, 1960.

12. Frant F, Groen J: Prognosis of vascular hypertension: Nine-year follow-up study of 418 cases, *Arch Intern Med* **85**:727-750, 1950.

13. Mathisen HS, Jensen D, Loken E, et al: Prognosis of essential hypertension. *Amer Heart J* **57**:371-382, 1959.

14. Breslin DJ, Gifford RW Jr, Fairbairn JF III: Essential hypertension: A 20 year follow-up study. *Circulation* **33**:87-97, 1966.

15. Tominaga T, Yoshida M: Prognosis of essential hypertension: Four-year follow-up study of 416 consecutively admitted patients. *Jap Circ J* **31**:55-59, 1967.

16. Stamler J Jr (ed): *Hypertensive Disease—Etiology, Prevalence, Incidence Morbidity, Mortality: Lectures on Preventive Cardiology*. New York, Grune & Stratton Inc, 1967, pp 242-280.

17. Kannel WB, LeBauer EJ, Dawber TR, et al: Relation of body weight to development of coronary heart disease: The Framingham study. *Circulation* **35**:734-744, 1967.

18. Levy RL, White PD, Stroud WD, et al: Overweight: Prognostic significance in relation to hypertension and cardiovascular-renal diseases. *JAMA* **131**:951-953, 1946.

19. Tibblin G: High blood pressure in men aged 50. *Acta Med Scand* **470**(suppl):1-84, 1967.

In a seven-year follow-up study of a total county population, the incidence of coronary heart disease (CHD) was found to be lower in black than in white men in every occupational category except sharecroppers. Among nonfarming occupations the occupational gradient in CHD observed in the 1960 prevalence study was no longer present when incident cases were the basis for comparison. The lower prevalence rate in white farmers compared to nonfarmers, however, was confirmed in the incidence study. The most likely explanation for these findings was that sustained physical activity above a certain critical threshold value was protective against CHD. This explanation received some circumstantial support from the relationship discovered between leisure time and on-the-job physical activity and the prevalence of CHD. Hypotheses concerning the possible pathogenic processes through which physical activity might operate are briefly reviewed.

Occupation and Physical Activity and Coronary Heart Disease

John Cassel, MD, MPH, Chapel Hill, NC; Siegfried Heyden, MD, and Alan G. Bartel, MD, Durham, NC; Berton H. Kaplan, PhD; Herman A. Tyroler, MD; and Joan C. Cornoni, MPH, PhD, Chapel Hill, NC; and Curtis G. Hames, Claxton, Ga

One of the most striking findings of the 1960 through 1962 prevalence study in Evans County, Georgia, was the occurrence of a strong gradient in prevalence of coronary heart disease (CHD) by occupation, with the highest rates occurring in the most sedentary and the lowest in the most active occupations.[1] While no direct measures of physical activity were made at that time, it was inferred from these occupational differences that, in Evans County at least,

1. on-the-job physical activity was probably related to susceptibility to CHD and,
2. variations in on-the-job physical activity were the most likely explanation of the difference in prevalence of CHD between black and white men.

We attempt to determine the degree to which these tentative conclusions can be confirmed using incidence data and some of the 1967-1969 prevalence data.

Method

Two approaches were used as indices of physical activity. One was an individual's occupation; this pertained mainly to the men in the sample. Since no direct measure of activity was obtained in 1960-1962, this variable was used as a substitute. The nonfarm occupations were classified into five groups: (1) professionals, proprietors, managers; (2) clerks, office workers; (3) trades, service workers; (4) manual laborers; and (5) unemployed. Farmers were classified into three groups: (1) farm owners; (2) sharecroppers and farm laborers; and (3) farm workers unemployed. This classificatory scheme, derived from McGuire and White's "The Measurement of Social Status,"[2] can be used both for constructing an index of social status and as a rough index of on-the-job physical activity.

Secondly, in the 1967-1969 follow-up examination, a physical activity questionnaire measuring both on-the-job and leisure time activity was administered. For this purpose the questionnaire used in the HIP study was modified slightly to make the items appropriate for a rural community.[3] The major modifications required were in the leisure time activities categories which were derived from interviews with the first 100 individuals examined. Weights were assigned to each item to approximate as closely as possible those used in the HIP study. Because of the modifications introduced, the absolute value of the scores derived from this questionnaire may not be strictly comparable to the HIP scores, but the rank order of the items within Evans County is probably very similar to that in the New York sample. Thus, while Evans County residents who scored in the most active category, for example, may be more or less active than the New Yorkers with the same score, they would share in common the fact that within each study they were more active than those with a sedentary score.

The items and scores used were as follows:

Physical Activity Questionnaire

	Score Assigned
1. About how much time on the job spent sitting?	
Practically all the time	0
More than ½ the time	1
About ½ the time	2
Less than ½ the time	3
Almost none of the time	4
2. About how much time on the job spent walking?	
Practically all the time	4
More than ½ the time	3
About ½ the time	2
Less than ½ the time	1
Almost none of the time	0
3. About how much walking getting to and from job?	
None	0
Less than ½ mile	2
½ mile or more, but less than 1 mile	4
1 mile or more, but less than 2 miles	5
2 miles or more	6
4. How often do you have to lift heavy weights or carry heavy things on the job?	
Frequently	6
Sometimes	3
Very infrequently (or never)	0

	Frequently	Sometimes	Very Infrequently or Never
Take walks in good weather	2	1	0
Work around house or apartment	2	1	0
Yard work or gardening	2	1	0
Take part in sports			
(i) Active ball game other than golf, bowling, pool or billiards	4	3	0
(ii) Hunting or fishing	4	3	0
(iii) Other sports	3	2	0
In addition to your regular job, do you do any farm work (livestock, feeding hogs, work on farm land, etc.)	4	3	0
Other activities	3	2	0
Any additional types of employment (Specify)________			

Received for publication May 13, 1971; accepted Aug 3.

From the departments of epidemiology (Drs. Cassel, Kaplan, Tyroler, and Cornoni), anthropology, and mental health (Dr. Kaplan), University of North Carolina, Chapel Hill; and departments of community health sciences (Dr. Heyden) and cardiology (Dr. Bartel), Duke University Medical School and Center, Durham, NC. Dr. Hames is in private practice in Claxton, Ga.

Reprint requests to Department of Epidemiology, University of North Carolina, Chapel Hill (Dr. Cassel) NC.

The first survey examination of this study population (3,102 persons) was carried out between Aug 1, 1960, and June 1, 1962, and consisted of a history of heart disease, stroke, and other illnesses; a physical examination; electrocardiogram; roentgenogram of the chest; urinalysis; and laboratory studies of the blood for cholesterol level and hematocrit reading. The second survey examination of this cohort was made by two of us (A. B. and S. H.) between Aug 1, 1967, and Aug 31, 1969, in a clinic established for this purpose. During this seven- to nine-year follow-up period (average, 87 months), 320 persons had died and 252 had either migrated away from the community or refused to return for the second examination. The examination of the remaining 2,530 persons (90.9% reexamination rate) again consisted of a history and physical and laboratory studies, but also included a detailed questionnaire for evidence of cerebrovascular disease and symptoms of transient cerebral ischemia, a sociological questionnaire, and a physical activities questionnaire.

There were 93 cases of coronary heart disease diagnosed in 1960 through 1962, leaving 3,009 persons at risk of developing the disease over the following 87-month period. A detailed description of the response rates and the incidence and prevalence rates by age, ethnic group, and sex are published elsewhere (Cornoni et al, p 896).

For purposes of this study CHD referred to sudden death, myocardial infarction, angina pectoris, and chronic heart disease. Sudden death was defined as any unexpected death occurring within 24 hours after the patient was last seen alive, if unattended, and within 1 hour if attended. In addition, any one of three findings was adequate for a designation of CHD. These included angina pectoris, a history of myocardial infarction, or an ECG consistent with myocardial infarction. The World Health Organization criteria were used for defining angina pectoris and a history of myocardial infarction.[4] Criteria used for the evaluation of the ECG were essentially the class I, Q, and QS patterns of Blackburn et al.[5] ST segment depression and T wave inversion were not used. Chronic heart disease was considered to be probably arteriosclerotic in origin when diagnosed at age 40 or older in the presence of heart failure of chronic arrhythmia and in the absence of angina pectoris, myocardial infarction, or any other cardiac disorder.

This paper is concerned with the incidence of CHD in those men, classified by their 1960 through 1962 occupation, who, at the time of the prevalence examination, were found to be free of any manifestation of CHD. The paper also examines the relationship of the prevalence of CHD found at the second examination (1967 through 1969) to the more direct measure of physical activity, ie, the questionnaire on leisure time and on-the-job activity.

Results

Table 1 shows that there were three occupational groups in which the numbers of blacks were adequate for comparisons to be made (nonfarm laborers, farm owners, and sharecroppers). In the first two groups, the black rates are substantially lower than the white. Among sharecroppers, however, the white rate (31) is as low as the black (39). Significantly, among all the variables explored this is the sole instance in which comparable black and white rates have been discovered. Thus, previous analyses have shown (Tyroler et al, p 907), that at equivalent levels of systolic and diastolic blood pressure, serum cholesterol, and body weight and with similar cigarette smoking histories, the rates in whites were always higher than in blacks.

The most attractive explanation for this finding would be that only as sharecroppers do whites engage in as hard physical labor as do blacks, white farm owners and nonfarm laborers probably being more sedentary than their black counterparts. This tends to support the suggestion that physical activity may be one of the factors accounting for the black-white difference in incidence in Evans County and leads to a more general exploration of the role of physical activity in the genesis of CHD in this country. This explanation will be examined in the white men, as it is only in this group that there are enough cases to permit such an analysis.

As has been mentioned previously, a marked gradient in prevalence by occupation was found in white men in the 1960 through 1962 examination. These data and the relevant findings from the incidence study are reproduced in Fig 1 for ease of comparison. Among the nonfarm occupations the gradient observed in the prevalence data is no longer present when incident cases are the basis for comparison. In fact, except for the surprisingly low rate among professionals, no gradient at all appears in the remaining occupational groups.

The difference between farm owners and sharecroppers found in the prevalence study does, however, persist when these groups are followed over time. Three possible explanations for these data appear likely.

1. The gradient observed in the nonfarm occupations in the prevalence study was not a result of the protective influence of physical activity. Rather, it resulted from men with coronary disease leaving the more physically demanding occupations at periods prior to the first examination (1960 through 1962). Such men might have taken on a more sedentary job (thus swelling the numbers of cases in those occupations) or, more likely, have become unemployed. In either event, the number of cases in the active occupations would have been depleted. Such a possibility is quite reasonable and cannot be refuted from these data.

Even if the original gradient among the nonfarm occupations were due to selective removal rather than the protective influence of physical activity, the difference between farm owners and sharecroppers and between nonfarmers and farmers cannot be explained on this basis. As these differences were observed in the incidence study where the experience of each individual was classified according to his 1960 occupation, the effect of selective removal is obviously eliminated.

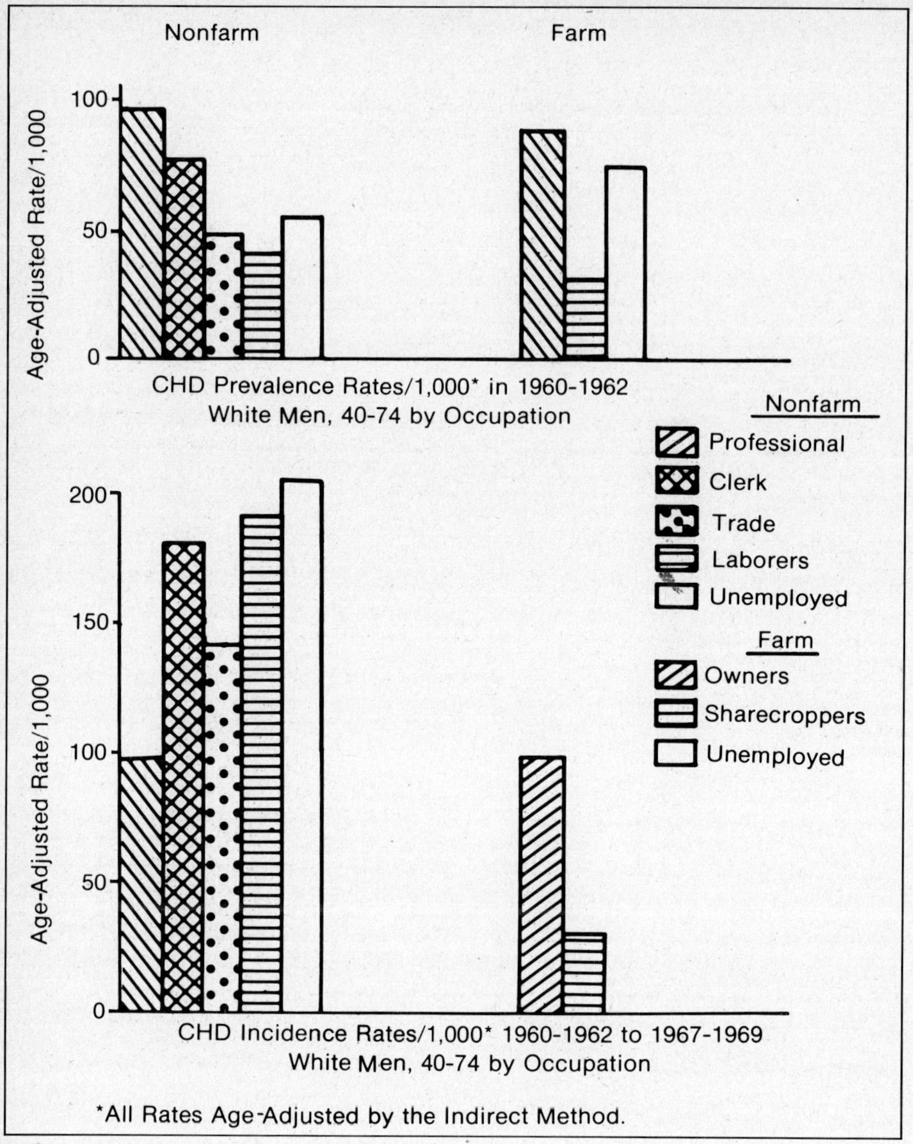

Fig 1.—Coronary heart disease prevalence (1960-1962) and incidence (1960-1962 to 1967-1969) for white men (40-74 years) by occupation.

Fig 2. (Bottom, Left)—Age-adjusted incidence rates per 1,000 (1960-1962 to 1967-1969): coronary heart disease in white men, farmers and nonfarmers (40-74 years), by cigarette smoking status.

Fig 3. (Bottom, Right)—Age-adjusted prevalence rate per 1,000 (1967-1969): coronary heart disease for white men, nonfarmers (40-74 years), by "on-the-job" and "off-the-job" physical activity scores.

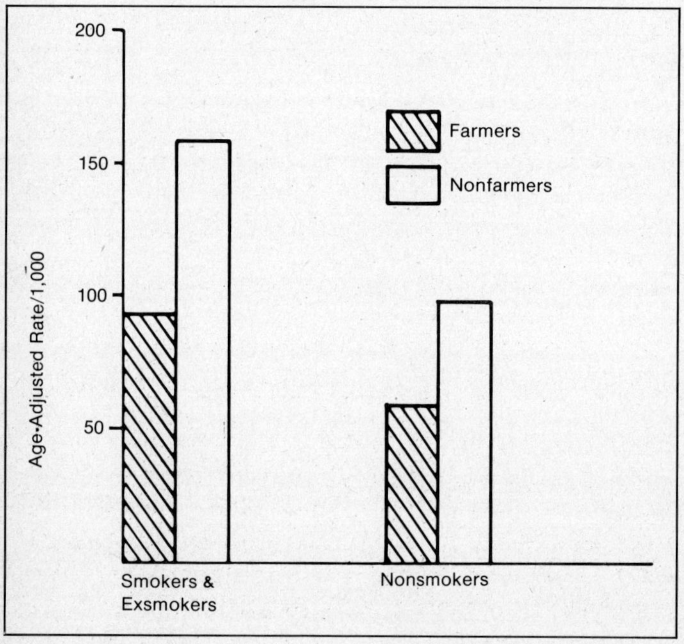

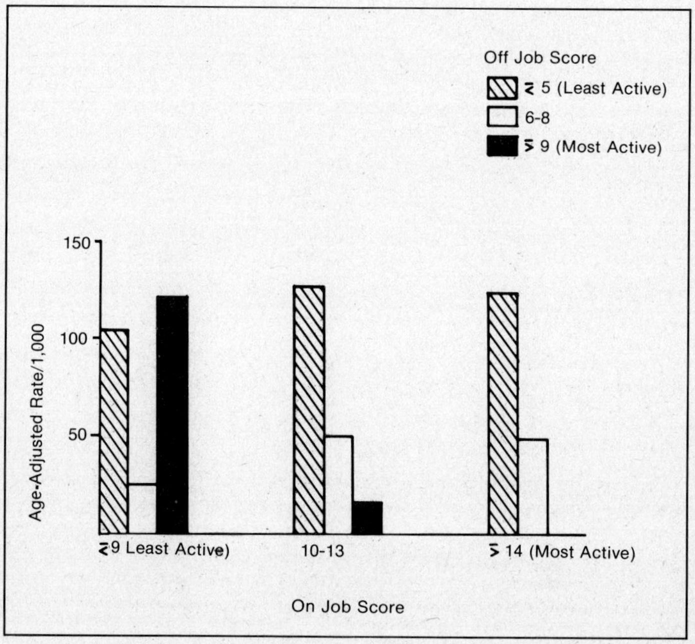

2. The possibility thus exists that physical activity is protective but only above some threshold value, which is exceeded by farmers (particularly sharecroppers) but not by variations in the physical activity required by the nonfarm occupations.

3. A final possibility exists, that at least in part, the gradient observed in 1960 in the nonfarm occupations was a result of variations in physical activity, but that over time, with increasing mechanization, the "active" occupations have become increasingly less physically demanding, or conversely, the men in sedentary occupations have increased their leisure time physical activity, thus accounting for the disappearance in the gradient by 1967.

With the data available it is unfortunately not feasible to determine in any direct fashion the degree to which the first possibility (selective removal) was operative. Some of the existing information can, however, be used to test the likelihood of the second possibility. Implicit in this possibility is the notion that the major difference between farmers and nonfarmers accounting for their different rates is the degree of physical activity, ie, physical activity is protective but only above a threshold value. This notion was tested in two ways. The difference in the other risk factors shown to be related to CHD in this population was examined in farmers and nonfarmers to determine whether these might explain the differences in incidence (Tables 2 and 3). Levels of blood pressure, both systolic and diastolic, were found to be almost identical in the two groups. At each age (except 65-74) farmers did tend to have slightly lower cholesterol levels and, rather surprisingly, to be slightly heavier for their height than nonfarmers. These differences are minimal, however, and are unlikely to account for the marked differences in incidence rates (which were 150/1,000 for nonfarmers as compared to 73/1,000 for farmers).

In contrast to these biological risk factors, there were sizeable differences in the proportion smoking cigarettes, with fewer farmers smoking at each age than nonfarmers (Table 3). Accordingly, before concluding that the difference in incidence between farmers and nonfarmers was

Table 1.—Incidence of CHD* by Occupation, Ethnic Group, and Age (Men, 40 Years and Over)

Age at 1960 Through 1962 Examination	White			Black		
	Examined	Cases	Rate	Examined	Cases	Rate
Nonfarm Occupations						
Professionals, etc						
40-44	21	1	48	1	0	...
45-54	45	1	22	2	0	...
55-64	20	2	100	0	0	...
65-74	13	4	308	0	0	...
75+	1	1	1000	0	0	...
All Ages	100	9	90	3	0	...
Age-adjusted rate			94			...
Trades, etc						
40-44	27	5	185	6	0	...
45-54	51	4	78	9	0	...
55-64	24	4	167	5	0	...
65-74	13	2	154	3	0	...
75+	0	0	...	0	0	...
All Ages	115	15	130	23	0	...
Age-adjusted rate			143			...
Clerks, etc						
40-44	8	1	125	0	0	...
45-54	14	2	143	0	0	...
55-64	9	2	222	0	0	...
65-74	7	2	286	5	0	...
75+	0	0	...	0	0	...
All ages	38	7	184	5	0	...
Age-adjusted rate			180			...
Laborers						
40-44	13	2	154	25	0	...
45-54	45	7	156	46	2	43
55-64	20	4	200	28	1	36
65-74	5	1	200	14	2	143
75+	1	0	...	1	0	...
All ages	84	14	167	114	5	44
Age-adjusted rate			190			46
Farmers						
Farm Owners						
40-44	23	0	...	5	0	...
45-54	58	4	69	16	1	63
55-64	49	6	122	12	0	...
65-74	30	7	233	17	1	59
75+	1	0	...	3	0	...
All ages	161	17	106	53	2	38
Age-adjusted rate			99			30
Sharecroppers and Farm Laborers						
40-44	11	0	...	24	1	42
45-54	33	1	30	86	4	47
55-64	27	0	...	36	0	...
65-74	3	1	333	17	1	59
75+	0	0	...	1	0	...
All ages	74	2	27	164	6	37
Age-adjusted rate			31			39

* Coronary heart disease.

Table 2.—Mean Level of CHD* Risk Factors (1960 Through 1962 Values) in Farmers and Nonfarmers by Age (White Men)

		Nonfarmers			Farmers		
Risk Factor	Age, yr	No.	Mean	SD	No.	Mean	SD
	40-44	72	130.7	16.05	36	136.6	18.32
Systolic blood pressure	45-54	156	142.5	27.17	91	141.6	23.80
	55-64	79	151.0	30.11	76	148.8	25.69
	65-74	47	163.9	33.04	43	156.7	28.22
	75+	4	164.5	43.93	2	195.0	46.67
	All ages	358	145.0	28.82	248	146.1	25.70
	40-44	72	88.1	13.47	36	88.8	12.65
Diastolic blood pressure	45-54	156	91.4	15.16	91	90.8	12.07
	55-64	79	93.1	16.94	76	91.6	12.56
	65-74	47	93.4	15.38	43	91.1	17.50
	75+	4	90.0	7.12	2	114.0	0
	All ages	358	91.3	15.26	248	91.0	13.45
	40-44	71	216.0	39.83	35	202.1	39.34
	45-54	156	216.8	41.91	91	203.9	34.51
Cholesterol	55-64	78	218.4	42.28	74	206.3	35.89
	65-74	72	207.9	39.51	43	209.6	45.51
	75+	4	251.5	26.50	1	...	...
	All ages	356	216.2	41.24	244	205.3	37.59
	40-44	72	358.8	52.6	36	350.0	52.9
Quetelet index	45-54	156	367.4	61.0	91	377.5	59.6
	55-64	78	349.8	53.2	75	364.8	69.5
	65-74	44	343.2	58.9	43	359.7	59.6
	75+	3	339.6	57.0	1	...	...
	All ages	353	358.5	57.8	246	366.3	62.1

* Coronary heart disease.

due to the physical activity involved in farming, the effect of cigarette smoking in farmers and nonfarmers had to be examined.

From Table 4 and Fig 2 it can be seen that, while smoking increased the risk of CHD in both farmers and nonfarmers, farmers had lower rates than nonfarmers whether they smoked or not. The lower rates in farmers must, therefore, be due to some factors other than cigarette smoking.

None of the risk factors shown thus far in this study to be associated with an increased risk of CHD (blood pressure, cholesterol level, body weight, or cigarette smoking) can, therefore, explain the differences found between farmers and nonfarmers, adding weight to the possibility that these differences might in large part be due to variations in physical activity. The possibility exists, of course, that physical activity might be interacting with dietary differences to account for the protection from CHD observed, particularly among sharecroppers (Fig 1). While no dietary data were available in this incidence study, previous reports have indicated that low social class white men (which would include all sharecroppers) were having, if anything, a higher caloric intake with more animal fat and saturated fatty acids than were the higher social class men.[2]

Turning now to the nonfarm occupations, we have suggested that one possible explanation for the lack of any gradient in CHD incidence by occupational group (Fig 1) may be that variations in physical activity in these occupational categories do not exceed a critical threshold value. Data from the HIP study have suggested that if physical activity is in any way protective against coronary disease, its effects are most pronounced in preventing fatal attacks of CHD.[3] Thus, the possibility exists that the variations in physical activity in these different occupation groups may not be sufficient to prevent the occurrence of CHD, but might be adequate to prevent fatality. To test this possibility, the relationship between occupation and CHD mortality was examined (Table 5). To avoid the problem of small numbers, the men in the two most "sedentary" group of occupations (professionals, proprietors, and managers; and clerks and office workers) were grouped and their age specific CHD mortality rate compared with the men in the two most "active" group of occupations (trades and service workers; and manual laborers). In contrast to the lack of any gradient by occupation for the overall incidence of CHD (Fig 1), it can be seen from Table 6 that at each age, except 55 to 64, the CHD mortality was higher in the "sedentary" than the "active" occupations. At ages 55 to 64 the death rates were similar. Given the small numbers in each cell and the lack of any gradient in the overall incidence rate, this consistently higher mortality in the "sedentary" occupations is quite impressive and is difficult to explain except on the grounds of variation in some threshold value of physical activity.

The third possible explanation suggested for the disappearance of the gradient in CHD in the incidence study is that either physical activity of different occupations is changing over time or variations in leisure time activity may be a more important determinant of CHD. As indicated previously, no direct measures of physical activity was made in the 1960 through 1962 study so that any test of this possibility is not feasible. An attempt was made, however, during the 1967 through 1969 examinations to measure the effect of both on-the-job and leisure time physical activity. It was recognized that interpretations drawn from such an analysis would have to be made with care, as they would suffer from the usual limitations of prevalence data, in that any relationships found could equally well be produced by sick people changing their activity as by the effect of physical activity on subsequent disease.

Nevertheless, it was thought that such an analysis might prove useful as, taken together with the previous data, it could provide at least further circumstantial evidence regarding the relative importance of leisure time and on-the-job activity. The analyses were restricted to white men in nonfarm occupations, as the physical activity questionnaire used was least appropriate for full-time farmers.

Tables 6 and 7 show the relationship of CHD prevalence to on-the-job and off-the-job physical activity scores, respectively. In both instances a modest relationship between physical activity and prevalence can be discerned. Table 8 and Fig 3 show the relationship when both on-the-job and off-the-job scores are considered simultaneously. Here, it can be seen that the effect of either score is only manifest when the other score is reasonably high; ie, off-the-job activity is related to prevalence only if the on-the-job activity score is ten or greater. Similarly, on-the-job activity is related to prevalence only in those men who are most physically active off-the-job (with scores of nine or more). In other words, of the three stated possibilities, these data lend support to the notion of a threshold phenomenon as far as physical activity is concerned, and that it is only above a certain level that this becomes protective.

Table 3.—Proportion of Men Smoking Cigarettes (1960 Through 1962) in Farmers and Nonfarmers by Age (White Only)

	Nonfarmers				Farmers			
Age, yr.	No.	% Smokers*	% Nonsmokers	% Unknown	No.	% Smokers*	% Nonsmokers	% Unknown
40-44	72	67	18	15	37	49	32	19
45-54	158	77	22	0.6	91	65	35	0
55-64	79	66	34	0	76	46	52	1.3
65-74	47	70	30	0	43	26	75	0
75+	4	75	25	0	2	100	0	0
All ages	360	72	25	3.3	249	50	47	3.2

* Includes ex-smokers.

Table 4.—Incidence of CHD* (1960-1962 to 1967-1969) in White Men, Farmers and Nonfarmers, by Age and Cigarette Smoking Status

		Farmers (1960 Occupation)			Nonfarmers (1960 Occupation)		
1960 Cigarette Smoking	1960 Age, Yr	No.	Cases	Rate	No.	Cases	Rate
Smokers and exsmokers	40-44	18	0	...	48	5	104
	45-54	59	4	68	122	11	90
	55-64	35	3	86	52	13	250
	65-74	11	4	364	33	8	242
	75+	2	0	...	3	2	667
	All ages	125	11	88	258	39	157
	Age-adjusted rate			93.7			158.2
Non smokers	40-44	12	0	...	13	0	...
	45-54	32	1	31	35	3	86
	55-64	40	3	75	27	1	37
	65-74	32	4	125	14	5	357
	75+	0	0	...	1	0	...
	All ages	116	8	69	90	9	100.0
	Age-adjusted rate			59.6			98.3
Unknown	40-44	7	0	...	11	4	364
	45-54	0	0	...	1	0	...
	55-64	1	0	...	0	0	...
	65-74	0	0	...	0	0	...
	75+	0	0	...	0	0	...
	All ages	8	0	...	12	4	333
	Age-adjusted rate			0			478

* Coronary heart disease.

Comment

The relationship between physical activity and morbidity or mortality from CHD remains a subject of considerable controversy. Despite extensive research on the subject,[6-32] there is no consensus as to whether sustained physical activity is protective against CHD, and if it is, through what pathogenic processes it operates. In population studies a modest inverse relationship between physical activity (inferred from occupational classification or from responses to physical activity questionnaires) and either the incidence prevalence of or mortality from CHD has been found on a number of occasions.[1,13,14,16,23,32] By the same token, a number of other studies have found no such relationship.[27,29,30,33,34] The difficulties encountered in interpreting the results of such studies include the possible lack of validity of the indicators used to measure physical activity (occupational categories or questionnaire methods); the problem of confounding variables, including self-selection into various occupations; and the lack of clarity as to whether any postulated protective effect is a result of prolonged and habitual activity or only recent or current activity (immediate vs delayed effect). In addition, this study would indicate that variations below some threshold value of activity might have no discernible effect and might thus account for the failure to find any relationships in those studies where only modest differences in physical activity occur between the categories. These problems could, therefore, either account for the failure of some studies to find any relationship, even if physical activity were protective, or, alternatively, indicate that where relationships have been found, these are spurious and

Table 5.—Coronary Heart Disease Mortality Rates in "Active" and "Sedentary" Nonfarm Occupations, White Men 1960 Through 1962 to 1967 Through 1969

	"Sedentary" Occupations Professionals, Clerks, etc			"Active" Occupations Trades, Service, and Laborers		
Age	No.	Deaths	Death Rate, %	No.	Deaths	Death Rate, %
40-44	29	0	...	40	0	...
45-54	59	2	33.9	96	2	20.8
55-64	29	2	68.9	44	3	68.2
65-74	20	5	250.0	18	3	166.6
75+	1	1	(1,000)	1	0	...
All ages	138	10	72.5	199	8	40.2

Table 6.—Prevalence of CHD* (1967 Through 1969) by on-the-Job Physical Activity Score White Men, Nonfarmers

	On-The-Job Physical Activity Score ≤9			10-13			≥14		
Age	No.	Cases	Rate	No.	Cases	Rate	No.	Cases	Rate
15-24	21	0	...	30	0	...	18	0	...
25-34	20	0	...	23	0	...	25	0	...
35-44	26	4	154	28	0	...	31	3	97
45-54	40	6	150	47	5	106	33	0	...
55-64	13	1	77	12	3	250	10	3	300
64-74	4	1	250	1	1	(1,000)	0	0	...
75+	0	0	...	0	0	...	0	0	...
All Ages	124	12	97	141	9	64	117	6	51
Age-adjusted rate/1,000			85			68			56

* Coronary heart disease.

Table 7.—Prevalence of CHD* (1967 Through 1969) by off-the-Job Physical Activity Score White Men, Nonfarmers

	Off-The-Job Physical Activity Score ≤5			6-8			≥9		
	No.	Cases	Rate	No.	Cases	Rate	No.	Cases	Rate
15-24	12	0	...	16	0	...	41	0	...
25-34	15	0	...	25	0	...	28	0	...
35-44	25	3	120	27	3	111	33	1	30
45-54	40	5	125	41	2	49	39	4	103
55-64	19	7	368	10	0	...	6	0	...
65-74	2	2	(1,000)	2	0	...	1	0	...
75+	0	0	...	0	0	...	0	0	...
All ages	113	17	150	121	5	41	148	5	34
Age-adjusted Rate/1,000			116			40			45

* Coronary heart disease.

Table 8.—Age Adjusted Prevalence Rates of CHD* (1967 Through 1969) by on-the-Job and off-the-Job Physical Activity Score, White Men, Nonfarmers

Off-the-Job Physical Activity Score		On-the-Job Physical Activity Score ≤9 (Sedentary)	10-13	≥14 Active	Total
(Sedentary)	≤5	105(48)†	127(37)	124(28)	116(117)
	6-8	24(33)	50(43)	47(45)	40(121)
(Active)	≥9	122(43)	22(61)	0(44)	45(148)
	Total	85(124)	68(141)	56(117)	

* Coronary heart disease.
† Numbers in parentheses number of men examined.

have little or nothing to do with physical activity. One finding from this study, however, has been repeatedly and consistenly observed in other studies: the lower rate of CHD in farmers compared to nonfarmers.[9,32] While it is, of course, entirely possible that such differences may be due to factors other than physical activity, no such factor has as yet been identified in this or other studies which would explain these differences. Additionally, the likelihood that such differences are due, at least in part, to differences in physical activity is strengthened by the following observations:

1. There can be little disagreement that farming is a more physically demanding occupation than other occupations (ie, the question of the validity of the index of activity is not in doubt).
2. In this study there is a marked difference in incidence within white farming occupations between the more sedentary farm owners (99/1,000) and the more active sharecroppers (31/1,000 Table 1).
3. Only as sharecroppers do white men have as low an incidence rate (31/1,000) as do blacks (39/1,000, Table 1). This similarity between whites and blacks would tend to reduce the likelihood that genetic factors play a major role in accounting either for the low rates in blacks as a whole compared to whites or for the low rates in white farmers. This is not to say that genetic factors may be unimportant in determining susceptibility to CHD, but only that these factors are unlikely to explain the difference between blacks and whites on the one hand and white sharecroppers and farm owners on the other.

These findings, then, tend to support the proposition that physical activity may be protective against CHD, and taken together with the other findings in this study, suggest that this protection only occurs above some critical threshold value. What such a threshold value might be cannot, unfortunately, be answered from the data available to this study. Conceivably, it might vary in different situations depending upon the dietary intake, the presence or absence of other major risk factors (including some of the personality factors,[35,38] and genetic susceptibility. Under conditions of urban living the Western Electric prospective study[37,38] has shown that there was no important difference in either incidence of or mortality from CHD between active and sedentary men working in the same industry, even though the active men were expending over 50% more calories than the sedentary. These findings would indicate that at least under such circumstances the threshold would have to be greater than 50% above the caloric expenditure of sedentary industrial workers.

Pathogenic Processes.—Even the proponents of the notion that physical activity is protective fail to agree on the pathogenic processes through which this might operate. While a number of hypotheses have been advanced, the one that until recently was most generally subscribed to was that physical activity reduces some of the known coronary risk factors, particularly those predisposing to atherosclerosis. Increasing evidence is making this hypothesis less and less tenable. Thus, Mann et al[39] have concluded from their own studies that

> exercise and fitness are minor elements among risk factors for coronary disease—[and] that physical fitness influences coronary heart disease more directly, that is in ways not measured by the indirect risk factors measured.

These risk factors include hypercholesteremia, a factor long thought to be influenced by physical activity. Neither a vigorous six-month physical education program conducted by Holloszy et al,[40] nor Karvonen et al's[41] Finnish champion cross-country skiers showed any cholesterol lowering effect; Manelis et al[21] demonstrated that the incidence of ischemic heart disease during a 15-year period among over 10,000 40- to 64-year-old men and women in an Israeli kibbutz was two to four times higher in sedentary workers of both sexes compared to active workers; however, no difference in serum lipoproteins or prevalence of obesity or both was found between physical and nonphysical workers. Montoye and Epstein (unpublished data, 1965) compared four different physical activity groups and their physiological measurements; again, no significant differences were observed in the serum cholesterol concentrations in men with different levels of activity. Similar findings are reported by Keys et al[42] for cholesterol and by Roskam et al[44] insofar as β-lipoproteins and total lipid serum concentrations are concerned. Other investigators[34,44-46] have also failed to find any relationship between physical activity, whether measured by occupational category, physical training, or athletic activity and any of the relevant serum lipids. There is, thus, a growing body of experience that would tend to suggest that if physical activity is protective, its effect is not mediated through a reduction in atherosclerosis.

Other hypotheses have included a reduction in predilection to thrombosis, for which there is as yet little evidence either pro or con, and the enhancement of collateral information. This latter notion receives some support from elegant animal experiments by Eckstein[47] who demonstrated collateral growth in dogs following coronary ligation and exercise. Burt and Jackson,[48] however, showed that exercise alone was insufficient to stimulate coronary growth in the absence of coronary narrowing. Rose et al[29] have suggested a further possibility. In their autopsy study they have shown that among active workers the cross-sectional area of the coronary arteries in infarction-free subjects was 75% greater than in the corresponding infarction groups. Among light workers there was little difference. This increased caliber of the coronary vessels might thus make the presence of atherosclerosis less consequential (as far as subsequent ischemic disease is concerned) in the active than in the sedentary. Such a process is at least consistent with the known facts and may indeed provide a plausible biological explanation for the role of physical activity in CHD.

Conclusions

In a seven-year follow-up study of a total county population the incidence of coronary heart disease (CHD) was found to be lower in black than in white men in every occupational category except sharecroppers. Among nonfarming occupations the occupational gradient in CHD observed in the 1960 prevalence study was no longer present when incident cases were the basis for comparison. The lower prevalence rate in white farmers compared to nonfarmers, however, was confirmed in the incidence study. Various explanations for these findings are explored, and it was concluded that, most likely, sustained physical activity above a certain critical threshold value was protective against CHD. This explanation received some circumstantial support from the relationship discovered between leisure time and on-the-job physical activity and the prevalence of CHD in the 1967-1969 examination. Leisure time activity was only related to prevalence when job activity was high. Similarly, on-the-job activity was related to prevalence only in those men who were most physically active off the job.

The various hypotheses concerning the possible pathogenic processes through which physical activity might operate are briefly reviewed, and it was concluded that the suggestion by Rose et al[29] that physical activity leads to an increased caliber of the coronary vessels thus making atherosclerosis less consequential was consistent with the known facts and may provide a plausible biological explanation for the role of physical activity.

References

1. McDonough JR, Hames CG, Stulb SC, et al: Coronary heart disease among Negroes and whites in Evans County, Georgia. *J Chron Dis* **18**:443-468, 1965.

2. McGuire C, White GD: *The Measurement of Social Status: Research Paper in Human Development, No. 3 (revised).* Austin, Tex, Department of Educational Psychology, University of Texas, 1955.

3. Shapiro S, Weinblatt E, Frank CW, et al: The H.I.P. study of incidence and prognosis of coronary heart disease. *J Chron Dis* **18**:527-558, 1965.

4. World Health Organization: Hypertension and coronary heart disease: Classification and criteria for epidemiological studies. *WHO Techn Rep Ser* **168**, 1959.

5. Blackburn H, Keys A, Simonson E, et al: The electrocardiogram in population studies: A classification system. *Circulation* **21**:1160-1175, 1960.

6. Acheson RM: The etiology of coronary heart disease. *Yale J Biol Med* **35**:143-170, 1962.

7. Adelstein AM: Some aspects of cardiovascular mortality in South Africa. *Brit J Prev Soc Med* **17**:29-40, 1963.

8. Bassett DR, Moellering RC Jr, Rosenblatt G, et al: Coronary heart disease in Hawaii: Serum lipids, and cardiovascular anthropometric, and related findings in Japanese and Hawaiian men. *J Chron Dis* **21**:565-583, 1969.

9. Breslow L, Buell P: Mortality from coronary heart disease and physical activity of work in California. *J Chron Dis* **11**:428-444, 1960.

10. Chapman JM, Massey FJ: The inter-relationship of serum cholesterol, hypertension, body weight and risk of coronary disease: Results of the first ten years' follow-up in the Los Angeles heart study. *J Chron Dis* **17**:933-949, 1964.

11. Forssman O, Lindegard B: The post-coronary patient. *J Psychosom Res* **3**:89-169, 1958.

12. Fox SM III: Physical activity and coronary heart disease. *Amer J Cardiol* **23**:298-303, 1969.

13. Frank CW, Weinblatt E, Shapiro S, et al: Myocardial infarction in men: Role of physical activity and smoking in incidence and mortality. *JAMA* **198**:1241-1245, 1966.

14. Frank CW, Weinblatt E, Shapiro S, et al: Physical inactivity as a lethal factor in myocardial infarction among men. *Circulation* **34**:1022-1033, 1966.

15. Heyden S: Physical activity, in Schettler FG, Boyd GS (eds): *Atherosclerosis.* New York, Elsevier Press Inc, 1969, pp 245-269.

16. Higgins ITT, Cochrane AL: Epidemiological studies of coronary disease. *Brit J Prev Soc Med* **17**:153-165, 1963.

17. Kahn HA: The relationship of reported coronary heart disease mortality to physical activity of work. *Amer J Public Health* **53**:1058-1067, 1963.

18. Kannel WB: *The Framingham Heart Study, Habits, and Coronary Heart Disease:* Public Health Service Publication No. 1515. Washington, DC, US Department of Health, Education, and Welfare, 1966.

19. Kasanen A, Kallio V, Forsstrom J: The significance of psychic and socioeconomic stress and other modes of life in the etiology of myocardial infarction. *Ann Med Intern Fenn* **52**(suppl 43):1-dk, 1963.

20. Katz LN: Physical fitness and coronary heart disease: Some basic views. *Circulation* **35**:405-414, 1967.

21. Manelis GE, Altman S, Modan M, et al: Physical activity at work, lipoproteins and the incidence of angina pectoris, myocardial infarction and death due to ischemic heart disease. *Israel J Med Sci* **5**:786-790, 1969.

22. Morris JN, Crawford MD: Coronary heart disease and physical activity at work. *Brit Med J* **2**:1485-1496, 1958.

23. Morris JN, Heady JA, Raffle PAB, et al: Coronary heart disease and physical activity of work. *Lancet* **265**:1053-1057, 1953.

24. Nicolaysen R: Lipids and diet. *Proc Roy Soc London* **156**:365-375, 1962.

25. Paffenbarger RS Jr, Wolf PA, Notkin J: Chronic disease in former college students: I. Early precursors of fatal coronary heart disease. *Amer J Epidem* **83**:314-328, 1966.

26. Paffenbarger RS Jr, Notkin J, Krueger IE, et al: Chronic disease in former college students: II. Methods of study and observations on mortality from coronary heart disease. *Amer J Public Health* **56**:962-971, 1966.

27. Paul O: Physical activity and coronary heart disease. *Amer J Cardiol* **23**:303-306, 1969.

28. Pell S, D'Alonzo CA: Chronic disease morbidity and income level in an employed population. *Amer J Public Health* **60**:116-129, 1970.

29. Rose G, Prineas RJ, Mitchell JRA: Myocardial infarction and the intrinsic calibre of coronary arteries. *Brit Heart J* **29**:548-552, 1967.

30. Stamler J, Lindberg HA, Berkoon DM, et al: Prevalence and incidence of coronary heart disease in strata of the labor force of a Chicago industrial corporation. *J Chron Dis* **11**:405-420, 1960.

31. Taylor HL, Blackburn H, Puchner T, et al: Coronary heart disease in selected occupations of American railroads in relation to physical activity, abstracted. *Circulation* (suppl 3):**39**, **40**:202, 1969.

32. Zukel WJ, Lewis RH, Enterline PE, et al: A short-term community study of the epidemiology of coronary heart disease. *Amer J Public Health* **49**:1630-1639, 1959.

33. Chapman JM, Goerke LS, Dixon W, et al: Measuring the risk of coronary heart disease in adult population group: II. Clinical status of a population in Los Angeles under observation for two or three years. *Amer J Public Health* **47**(April supplement):33-42, 1957.

34. Malhotra SL: Epidemiology of ischaemic heart disease in India with special reference to causation. *Brit Heart J* **29**:895-905, 1967.

35. Rosenman RH, Friedman M, Straus R, et al: Coronary heart disease in the Western Collaborative Group study. *J Chron Dis* **23**:173-190, 1970.

36. Jenkins CD: Psychological and social precursors of coronary disease. *N Eng J Med* **284**:244-255, 307-317, 1971.

37. Paul O, Lepper MH, Phelan WH, Dupertuis GW, et al: A longitudinal study of coronary heart disease. *Circulation* **28**:20-31, 1963.

38. Bliss HA, Graettinger JS: Caloric expenditure at two types of factory work. *Arch Environ Health* **9**:201-208, 1964.

39. Mann GV, Garrett HL, Farhi A, et al: Exercise to prevent coronary heart disease: An experimental study of the effects of training on risk factors for coronary disease in men. *Amer J Med* **46**:12-27, 1969.

40. Holloszy IO, Skinner JS, Toro G, et al: Effects of a six-months program of endurance exercise on the serum lipids of middle-aged men. *Amer J Cardiol* **14**:753-760, 1964.

41. Karvonen MJ, Pekkarinen P, Metsala P, et al: Diet and serum cholesterol of lumberjacks. *Brit J Nutr* **15**:157-dk, 1961.

42. Keys A, Anderson IT, Aresu M, et al: Physical activity and the diet in populations differing in serum cholesterol. *J Clin Invest* **35**:1173-1181, 1956.

43. Roskamm H, Reindell H, König K: Die Bedeutung der körperlichen Aktivität in der Prophylaxe und Therapie von Herz- und Kreislaufkrankheiten. *Allgemeine Therapeutik* **9**:dk, 1964.

44. Taylor HL, Blackburn H, Brozek H, et al: Railroad employers in the United States. *Acta Med Scand* **460**(suppl):55-115, 1967.

45. Cooper RW, Ritota MC, Steinberg M, et al: Hearts and lipids of veteran handball players: A preliminary report. *Angiology* **17**:192-200, 1966.

46. FitzGerald O, Haffernan A, MacFarlane R: Serum lipids and physical activity in normal subjects. *Clin Sci* **28**:83-89, 1965.

47. Eckstein RW: Effect of exercise and coronary artery narrowing on coronary collateral circulation. *Circulation Res* **5**:230-235, 1967.

48. Burt JJ, Jackson R: The effects of physical exercise on the coronary collateral circulation of dogs. *J Sports Med* **5**:203-206, 1965.

Electrocardiographic Predictors of Coronary Heart Disease

Alan Bartel, MD; Siegfried Heyden, MD, Durham, NC;
Herman A. Tyroler, MD, Chapel Hill, NC; Enayatollah Tabesh, MD, Dayton, Ohio;
John C. Cassel, MD, MPH, Chapel Hill, NC; and Curtis G. Hames, MD, Claxton, Ga

Ischemic heart disease (IHD) differs in Evans County, Georgia, white and black males in terms of its lower occurrence in black males, less definite age relationship, and less dependence on the usual coronary risk factors. The common electrocardiographic manifestations or precursors of IHD differ markedly in frequency and prognostic import in the two groups. The ECG patterns of Evans County black males are much more similar to those of Jamaican and South African black males than to those of Evans County white males or white males in other studies performed in the United States or elsewhere.

The Evans County Study of 1960-1962 indicated that overt ischemic heart disease (IHD) manifested by a history of angina pectoris or myocardial infarction or electrocardiographic evidence of myocardial infarction was distinctly less common in blacks than whites and less frequent in females than males.[1] Lower incidence of IHD in blacks has also been reported in Jamaica,[2] Africa,[3,4] and Baltimore.[5] It has also been described in reports by Phillips and Burch,[6] Chapman et al[7] and others.[8-15]

Received for publication July 25, 1971; accepted Sept 7.

From the Department of Cardiology, Duke University Medical Center (Dr. Bartel); Department of Community Health Sciences, Duke University Medical School (Dr. Heyden), Durham, NC; Department of Epidemiology, University of North Carolina, Chapel Hill (Drs. Tyroler and Cassel); Department of Medicine, Department of Cardiology, Veterans Administration Hospital, Dayton, Ohio (Dr. Tabesh). Dr. Hames is in private practice in Evans County, Georgia.

Reprint requests to Department of Cardiology, Duke University Medical Center, Durham, NC 27710 (Dr. Bartel).

Since hypertension is one of the most important risk factors in the development of IHD, and blacks in Evans County, Georgia, had higher mean blood pressure levels (systolic and diastolic, at all age levels),[16] one would predict higher rates of IHD among black males than white males. However, Tyroler et al (p 907) reported in a previous paper of this issue that the observed of coronary heart disease (CHD) incidence is lower in blacks than whites at similar blood pressure levels. Regarding other risk factors, there was a lower observed incidence rate in blacks at comparable levels of serum cholesterol (Tyroler et al, p 907), body weight, and cigarette smoking (Heyden et al, p 915).

The present study is an attempt to test another well-known risk factor, ECG abnormalities, as a predictor of the development of IHD and to compare its predictive ability in whites and blacks. For this purpose, the distribution of selected ECG abnormalities in each race-sex group was determined and the incidence of new coronary events was measured for each of a number of selected abnormalities. Comparisons between Evans County and other populations in terms of the selected ECG abnormalities may provide useful data regarding the high occurrence of CHD in

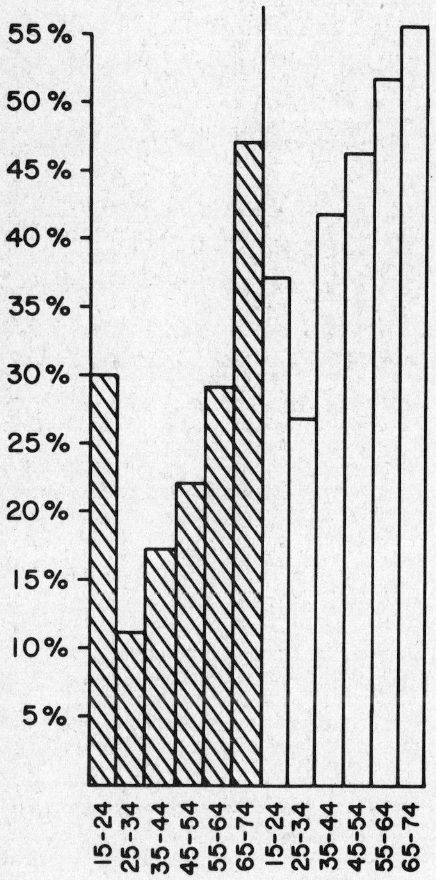

Fig 1.—Age specific prevalence of any specified electrocardiogram abnormality. Evans County study, white and black males, 1960-1962 (rate/100).

Evans County white males and the low rates in Evans County black males.

The ECGs were performed in the fasting state in the morning, or in the afternoon with no oral intake subsequent to a light breakfast. All ECGs were reviewed by the principal author without knowledge of the subject's race, sex, age, name, clinical history, or previous ECG diagnosis. The ECGs were classified according to the Minnesota code.[17]

The demographic description of the Evans County Study has been given in this issue by Cornoni et al (p 896).

Table 1.—Age Adjusted Prevalence Rate (1960-1962) of Electrocardiogram Abnormalities per 100 Examinees*

	Males		Females	
	Black	White	Black	White
No. of examinees	516	889	626	951
Any specified abnormality	44.5	25.5	54.5	22.1
Increased QRS (3-1)†	27.2	10.4	19.1	4.9
Major T (5-1, 5-2)	11.6	3.3	20.0	4.3
Minor T (5-3)	7.2	3.5	14.9	6.5
Sinus tachycardia (8-7)			11.2	6.3
ST changes (4-1, 4-2)			7.7	3.3
Prolonged P-R (6-3)	3.6	1.8	1.6	0.6
Sinus tachycardia (8-7)	4.9	5.1		
LAD (2-1)	4.9	5.4	4.3	2.3
ST changes (4-1, 4-2)	3.4	2.3		
Left and right bundle branch block (7-1, 7-2)	0.6	1.6	0.4	0.6

* Examinees are all subjects with ECG and free of evidence of past and present coronary heart disease (CHD) at time of examination.

† ( ) signifies Minnesota code.

Fig 2.—Age specific prevalence of ECG abnormalities. Evans County study, white and black males, 1960-1962 (rates/100).

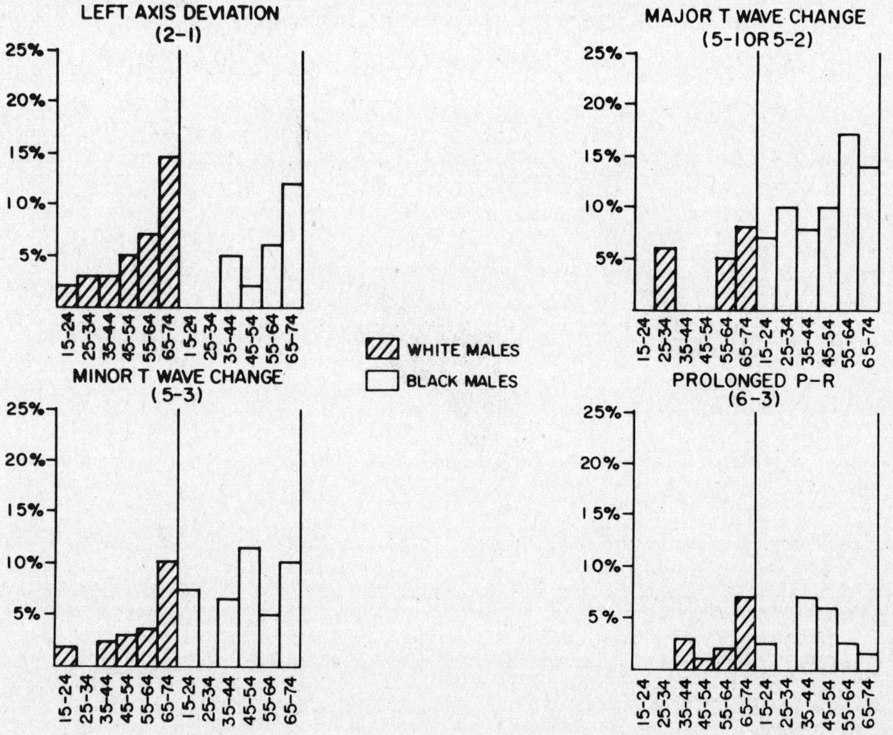

Table 2.—Age Adjusted CHD Incidence by Specified ECG Abnormality, Evans County 1960-1962 to 1967-1969 (Average, 87 mo) Rates per 1,000*

	White Males	Black Males	White Females	Black Females
No specified abnormality				
Cases	41	6	19	10
Par	661	277	724	273
Rate	68.7	23.3	29.0	43.0
Any specified abnormality				
Cases	29	7	14	10
Par	217	221	198	306
Rate	109.3	27.2	50.8	29.6
Left axis deviation (2-1)				
Cases	7	2	3	2
Par	46	20	22	18
Rate	159.7	90.2	124.7	125.5
Increased QRS voltage (3-1)				
Cases	6	3	5	4
Par	88	133	41	98
Rate	63.9	23.6	91.6	47.4
ST changes (4-1 or 4-2)				
Cases	6	1	4	1
Par	19	12	26	38
Rate	307.6	87.0	136.1	28.9
Major T wave change (5-1 or 5-2)				
Cases	5	2	3	3
Par	27	55	37	107
Rate	209.9	34.4	65.7	30.5
Minor T wave changes (5-3)				
Cases	7	3	5	4
Par	28	39	59	87
Rate	235.1	80.6	79.0	48.3
Prolonged P-R (6-3)				
Cases	5	0	0	0
Par	16	19	6	9
Rate	238.4	. . .	. . .	. . .
Left or right bundle branch block (7-1 or 7-2)				
Cases	3	0	0	0
Par	14	3	6	2
Rate	283.6	. . .	. . .	. . .

* See Table 1, footnote.

Methods

The first survey examination of this study population (3,102 persons) was carried out between Aug 1, 1960, and June 1, 1962, and consisted of a history of heart disease, stroke, and other illnesses; a physical examination; ECG; roentgenogram of the chest; urinalysis; and laboratory studies of the blood for cholesterol and hematocrit. The second survey examination of this cohort was made by two of the authors (A. B. and S. H.) between Aug 1, 1967, and Aug 31, 1969, in a clinic established for this purpose. During this seven to nine year follow-up period (average, 87 months), 320 persons had died and 252 had either migrated away from the community or refused to return for the second examination. The examination of the remaining 2,530 persons (90.0% reexamination rate) again consisted of a history, physical examination, and laboratory studies, but also included a detailed questionnaire for evidence of cerebrovascular disease and symptoms of transient cerebral ischemia, a sociological questionnaire, and a physical activities questionnaire.

In 1960-1962 93 cases of CHD were diagnosed, leaving 3,009 persons at risk of developing the disease over the following 87 month period. A detailed description of the response rates and incidence and prevalence rates by age, ethnic group, and sex are published elsewhere (Cornoni et al, p 896).

For purposes of this study CHD referred to sudden death, myocardial infarction, angina pectoris, and chronic heart disease. Sudden death was defined as any unexpected death occurring within 24 hours after the patient was last seen alive, if unattended, and within one hour if attended. In addition, any one of three findings was adequate for a designation of CHD. These included angina pectoris, a history of myocardial infarction or an ECG consistent with myocardial infarction. The World Health Organization criteria were used for defining angina pectoris and a history of myocardial infarction.[18] Criteria used for the evaluation of the ECG were essentially the class I, Q, and QS patterns of Blackburn et al.[18] ST segment depression and T wave inversion were not used. Chronic heart disease was considered to be probably arteriosclerotic in origin when diagnosed at age 40 or older in the presence of

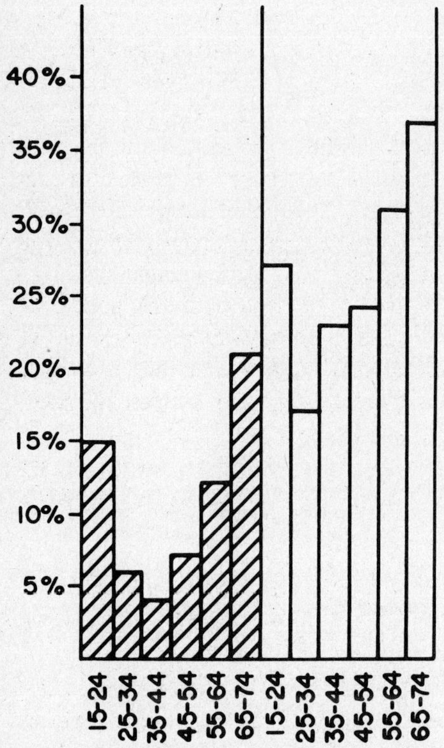

Fig 3.—Age specific prevalence of ECG abnormalities. Evans County study, white and black males, 1960-1962 (rates/100), increased QRS voltage (3-1).

Table 3.—Age Specific Prevalence* of ECG Abnormalities: Evans County, White Males, 1960-1962

		Age, yr						
		15-24	25-34	35-44	45-54	55-64	65-74	75+
Total population at risk†		117	109	164	245	148	89	6
No specified abnormality	No.	82	97	136	191	105	47	3
	Rate	70.1	89.0	82.9	78.0	70.9	52.8	50.0
Any specified abnormality	No.	35	12	28	54	43	42	3
	Rate	29.9	11.0	17.1	22.0	29.1	47.2	50.0
Left axis deviation (2-1)	No.	2	3	5	12	10	13	1
	Rate	1.7	2.8	3.0	4.9	6.8	14.6	16.7
Increased QRS voltage (3-1)	No.	18	7	7	18	18	17	3
	Rate	15.4	6.4	4.3	7.3	12.2	19.1	50.0
ST changes (4-1 or 4-2)	No.	0	1	0	3	10	4	1
	Rate	...	0.9	...	1.2	6.8	4.5	16.7
Major T wave changes (5-1 or 5-2)	No.	7	0	0	5	8	7	0
	Rate	6.0	...	...	2.0	5.4	7.9	...
Minor T wave changes (5-3)	No.	2	0	4	7	5	9	1
	Rate	1.7	...	2.4	2.9	3.4	10.1	16.7
Prolonged P-R (6-3)	No.	0	0	5	2	3	6	0
	Rate	...	...	3.0	0.8	2.0	6.7	...
Left or right bundle branch block (7-1 or 7-2)	No.	0	0	2	7	2	3	0
	Rate	...	...	1.2	2.9	1.4	3.4	...
Sinus tachycardia (8-7)	No.	11	3	7	15	5	4	0
	Rate	9.4	2.8	4.3	6.1	3.4	4.5	...
Increased QRS voltage without ST changes (3-1 w/o 4-1 or 4-2)	No.	18	6	7	17	15	17	2
	Rate	15.4	5.5	4.3	6.9	10.1	19.1	33.3
Increased QRS voltage with ST changes (3-1 w/4-1 or 4-2)	No.	0	1	0	1	3	0	1
	Rate	...	0.9	...	0.4	2.0	...	16.7
ECG's not complete	No.	...	...	1	...	3	...	...

* Rates per 100.
† All with heart disease excluded.

heart failure or chronic arrhythmia and in the absence of angina pectoris, myocardial infarction, hypertension, or any other cardiac disorder.

Results

The age-adjusted prevalence rate for each selected ECG abnormality at intake examination (1960-1962) is presented in Table 1 by sex and ethnic group. The abnormalities are ordered by their relative frequency. A twofold excess of one group over the other was selected as a cutoff arbitrarily. The age-adjusted prevalence rate of "any specified ECG abnormality" was markedly higher for blacks than whites: 45% of black males had abnormalities, contrasted with only 25% white males; 54% of black females, contrasted with only 22% of white females. The major contributors to this black excess in males were the findings of increased QRS voltage, T abnormalities (both major and minor), and prolonged PR intervals. The same abnormalities were more frequently present in black than white females; in addition, black females had higher rates than white females for ST changes and sinus tachycardia. There were no marked differences in prevalence of abnormalities between blacks and whites for the less frequently present left axis deviation (LAD) in both males and females, nor for sinus tachycardia and ST segment changes in males. There was only one instance of the recorded abnormalities, bundle branch block, wherein the whites had a twofold excess over the blacks. However, the overall prevalence is low and differences are based upon small numbers of cases. The analyses were repeated excluding all individuals with either the clinical roentgenographic or ECG diagnosis of hypertensive heart disease and no major

Table 4.—Age Specific Prevalence* of ECG Abnormalities: Evans County, Black Males, 1960-1962

		Age, yr						
		15-24	25-34	35-44	45-54	55-64	65-74	75+
Total population at risk†		81	41	74	158	81	59	4
No specified abnormality	No.	51	30	43	86	39	26	2
	Rate	63.0	73.2	58.1	54.4	48.1	44.1	50.0
Any specified abnormality	No.	30	11	31	72	42	33	2
	Rate	37.0	26.8	41.9	45.6	51.9	55.9	50.0
Left axis deviation (2-1)	No.	0	0	4	3	5	7	1
	Rate	...	...	5.4	1.9	6.2	11.9	25.0
Increased QRS voltage (3-1)	No.	22	7	17	38	25	22	2
	Rate	27.2	17.1	23.0	24.1	30.9	37.3	50.0
ST changes (4-1 or 4-2)	No.	0	1	1	4	2	3	1
	Rate	...	2.4	1.4	2.5	2.5	5.1	25.0
Major T wave changes (5-1 or 5-2)	No.	6	4	5	16	14	8	2
	Rate	7.4	9.8	6.8	10.1	17.3	13.6	50.0
Minor T wave changes (5-3)	No.	6	0	5	18	4	6	0
	Rate	7.4	...	6.8	11.4	4.9	10.2	...
Prolonged P-R (6-3)	No.	2	0	5	9	2	1	0
	Rate	2.5	...	6.8	5.7	2.5	1.7	...
Left or right bundle branch block (7-1 or 7-2)	No.	0	0	0	0	1	2	0
	Rate	...	...	...	...	1.2	3.4	...
Sinus tachycardia (8-7)	No.	0	1	2	13	7	3	0
	Rate	...	2.4	2.7	8.2	3.6	5.1	...
Increased QRS voltage without ST changes (3-1 w/o 4-1 or 4-2)	No.	22	7	17	36	23	21	1
	Rate	27.2	17.1	23.0	22.8	28.4	35.6	25.0
Increased QRS voltage with ST changes (3-1 w/4-1 or 4-2)	No.	0	0	0	2	2	1	1
	Rate	...	...	...	1.3	2.5	1.7	25.0
ECG's not complete	No.	...	1	3	3	1	1	...

* Rates per 100.
† All with heart disease excluded.

changes in the relationships, as presented, were found.

The relationship of the prevalence of ECG abnormalities to age is presented in Fig 1-3. For the prevalence of any "specified abnormality" there is a sizeable and marked increase with increasing age with the exception of the youngest age groups in this sample (ie, ages 15 to 24). Inspection of the figures for each of the specified abnormalities discloses that the excess among the young is attributable primarily to increased QRS voltage, a finding which is expected and may be considered normal for adolescence. From age 25 on there is an increase in prevalence of ECG abnormalities with advancing age, the most marked increase occurring in the 65+ age group. These age relationships are present for black as well as white males with the exception of prolonged PR interval abnormalities, the prevalence of which declines in blacks after age 35.

The age-adjusted prevalence rate of the different ECG abnormalities varied considerably between the sexes within ethnic groups. For example, for any specified abnormality the prevalence was quite similar for white: 26% of white males and 22% of white females exhibiting any abnormality; there was, however, an excess in the black female contrasted with the black males: 55% of black females and 45% of black males exhibiting any specified abnormality. Increased QRS voltage was more common in both black and white males than females. The T wave changes, both major and minor, however, were more prevalent in the female than the male for both blacks and whites. ST segment changes were markedly more prevalent in the black female than the black male (7.7% contrasted with 3%).

The Incidence of Coronary Disease by Presence or Absence of Selected ECG Abnormalities

In computing incidence rates, individuals with diagnosed hypertensive heart disease in 1960-1962 were excluded; the rationale for this was that there might well have been coexistent coronary disease not clinically detectable in such individuals. The age-adjusted incidence rates of CHD were, therefore, calculated for those initially free of coronary and hypertensive heart disease for the follow-up period (average of 87 months). The incidence rates are presented in Table 2 and the tabular data upon which they are based are presented in Tables 3 to 6.

In contrast to the marked excess of ECG abnormalities in the blacks noted in the prevalence examinations, white males had a markedly higher incidence than did black males of new coronary events in the presence of each ECG abnormality (the statement was true for males; the ratios were not as clear-cut for females). The relative risks ranged from a low of 1.8 for excess of CHD incidence in white contrasted with black males with left axis deviation to a high of 6.1 in the presence of major T wave changes (Table 7).

Thus, among white males, increased QRS voltage with ST changes, prolonged PR intervals, bundle branch block, and sinus tachycardia were associated with increased new coronary events. In contrast, no black males with these abnormalities developed ischemic heart disease in the follow-up period. To phrase this differently, each of the specified ECG abnormalities carried an increased risk of coronary disease for white males but not for black males. The nonpredictability of the ECG abnormalities for the black male is highlighted by the fact that black males with "any of the specified abnormalities" had no increased CHD incidence compared to black males with none of the specified abnormalities. White females had higher rates of CHD with ECG findings of left axis deviation, increased QRS voltage, ST changes, and major and minor T wave changes. Black females, however, had increased CHD incidence rates only with left axis deviation.

Table 5.—Age Specific Prevalence* of ECG Abnormalities: Evans County, White Females, 1960-1962

		Age, yr						
		15-24	25-34	35-44	45-54	55-64	65-74	75+
Total population at risk†		107	110	185	227	165	116	12
No specified abnormality	No.	92	91	155	191	116	72	7
	Rate	86.0	82.7	83.8	84.1	70.3	62.1	58.3
Any specified abnormality	No.	15	19	30	36	49	44	5
	Rate	14.0	17.3	16.2	15.9	29.7	37.9	41.7
Left axis deviation (2-1)	No.	0	0	1	2	5	13	1
	Rate	...	...	0.5	0.9	0.3	11.2	8.3
Increased QRS voltage (3-1)	No.	2	2	4	5	13	13	2
	Rate	1.9	1.8	2.2	2.2	7.9	11.2	16.7
ST changes (4-1 or 4-2)	No.	0	1	0	5	7	13	0
	Rate	...	0.9	...	2.2	4.2	11.2	...
Major T wave changes (5-1 or 5-2)	No.	2	3	3	9	6	13	1
	Rate	1.9	2.7	1.6	4.0	3.6	11.2	8.3
Minor T wave changes (5-3)	No.	6	5	6	8	20	12	2
	Rate	5.6	4.5	3.2	3.5	12.1	10.3	16.7
Prolonged P-R (6-3)	No.	1	0	1	1	0	3	0
	Rate	0.9	...	0.5	0.4	...	2.6	...
Left or right bundle branch block (7-1 or 7-2)	No.	0	1	0	1	1	3	0
	Rate	...	0.9	...	0.4	0.6	2.6	...
Sinus tachycardia (8-7)	No.	7	9	17	13	7	4	0
	Rate	6.5	8.2	9.2	5.7	4.2	3.4	...
Increased QRS voltage without ST changes (3-1 w/o 4-1 or 4-2)	No.	2	2	4	4	13	12	2
	Rate	1.9	1.8	2.2	1.8	7.9	10.3	16.7
Increased QRS voltage with ST changes (3-1 w/ 4-1 or 4-2)	No.	0	0	0	1	0	1	0
	Rate	...	...	...	0.4	...	0.9	...
ECGs not completed	No.	...	...	...	1	...	2	1

* Rates per 100.
† All with heart disease excluded.

Comparisons With Other Population Studies

Realizing the inherent difficulties in comparing populations, the rates of the specified ECG abnormalities (Minnesota code) in Evans County white males and black males are compared with the population studies in Lawrence Tavern, Jamaica,[2] Tecumseh, Mich,[19] Framingham, Mass,[20] five European countries,[21] Greece,[22] Italy,[22] and US railroad workers,[22] and Rhondda Fach, South Wales,[20] (Table 8).

As far as the rates of P-R prolongation and ST and T wave changes are concerned, Evans County white males are surprisingly similar to white males in Tecumseh, Mich, Framingham, Mass, and Europe. The higher rates of increased QRS voltage and P-R prolongation for black males in Evans County were also found in Jamaican black males. However, the black males of Evans County have higher rates of both major and minor T wave changes than the Jamaican black males or any other comparison group. These may be explained by a combination of persistent "juvenile T waves," "nonspecific," nonischemic T waves, and hypertensive changes. The abnormal T wave changes appear to have a different prognostic significance for CHD in the blacks than in the whites. The prevalence and incidence rates of hypertension among the Evans County black population is higher than in other black populations within this country and in Jamaica.[2] Electrocardiogram abnormalities are not as predictive for the development of CHD among the blacks as the whites and may, in part, be explained by hypertension. It should be noted here that only the data for CHD has been analyzed for this paper. Data for incidence of hy-

Table 6.—Age Specific Prevalence* of ECG Abnormalities: Evans County, Black Females, 1960-1962

		Age, yr						
		15-24	25-34	35-44	45-54	55-64	65-74	75+
Total population at risk†		86	51	106	152	112	68	4
No specified abnormality	No.	45	22	59	80	42	25	0
	Rate	52.3	43.1	55.7	52.6	37.5	36.8	...
Any specified abnormality	No.	41	29	47	72	70	43	4
	Rate	47.7	56.9	44.3	47.4	62.5	63.2	100.0
Left axis deviation (2-1)	No.	0	0	1	3	9	4	1
	Rate	...	...	0.9	2.0	8.0	5.9	25.0
Increased QRS voltage (3-1)	No.	4	6	12	21	31	23	1
	Rate	4.7	11.8	11.3	13.8	27.7	33.8	25.0
ST changes (4-1 or 4-2)	No.	0	2	3	7	12	12	2
	Rate	...	3.9	2.8	4.6	10.7	17.6	50.0
Major T wave changes (5-1 or 5-2)	No.	18	13	16	18	28	12	2
	Rate	20.9	25.5	15.1	11.8	25.0	17.6	50.0
Minor T wave changes (5-3)	No.	15	7	10	26	15	12	2
	Rate	17.4	13.7	9.4	17.1	13.4	17.6	50.0
Prolonged P-R (6-3)	No.	0	0	2	5	0	2	0
	Rate	...	...	1.9	3.3	...	2.9	...
Left or right bundle branch block (7-1 or 7-2)	No.	0	0	1	0	0	1	0
	Rate	...	...	0.9	...	...	1.5	...
Sinus tachycardia (8-7)	No.	9	9	15	17	10	4	1
	Rate	10.5	17.6	14.2	11.2	8.9	5.9	25.0
Increased QRS voltage without ST changes (3-1 w/o 4-1 or 4-2)	No.	4	5	11	18	26	17	0
	Rate	4.7	9.8	10.4	11.8	23.2	25.0	...
Increased QRS voltage with ST changes (3-1 w/ 4-1 or 4-2)	No.	0	1	1	3	5	6	1
	Rate	...	2.0	0.9	2.0	4.5	8.8	25.0
ECGs not completed	No.	4	...	1	4	...	2	...

* Rates per 100.
† All with heart disease excluded.

pertensive heart disease will be reported later.

Comment

For many years, the ECG has been used as a clinical tool in the diagnosis and management of IHD. The limitations of the standard ECG and also the protean manifestations of IHD become more evident in studying patients by means of refined techniques such as vector cardiography, exercise cardiography, and coronary angiography. Although the standard ECG is a very frequently performed test, there is surprisingly little "hard data" relative to the distribution of various ECG abnormalities in the unselected population, the association of these abnormalities with IHD and the electrocardiographic precursors of overt IHD. Racial differences in IHD have received little attention in the literature. The data obtained from the previously described analysis confirms the association of certain ECG abnormalities with IHD, the age dependence of these variables, and their relative importance in terms of the risk of developing overt IHD, particularly in white males.

The use of a standardized electrocardiographic coding system in which the defined abnormalities are based upon easily measured indices, has the disadvantage of lack of agreement regarding the interpretation of those indices, especially relative to clinical applicability. In spite of this, the use of such a system (ie, the Minnesota code)[17] has the great advantage of comparability of data in serial examinations, long-term follow-up studies and data comparisons among populations.

The distribution of ECG abnormalities among Evans County white males is similar to those of large population studies performed in the United States and in several foreign countries. The distribution of certain ECG abnormalities in black males is strikingly different from Evans County white males and appears to differ in significance. The occurrence of major T wave changes, for example, is 3.6 times more frequent in black males. Among those black males with T wave inversion, however, the incidence of overt IHD is one sixth that of Evans County white males and only slightly higher than black males with no ECG abnormality. T wave inversion, therefore, is a risk factor for CHD in white males but not for black males. Table 1 and Fig 1 to 3 show the differences between white and black males and the prognostic implications of all the ECG abnormalities specified. The most marked differences occurred with ST abnormalities, major and minor T wave changes, increased QRS voltage with ST-T changes, prolonged P-R interval, bundle branch block, and sinus tachycardia.

Most comparison of the progression and severity of anatomical evidence of coronary and aortic atherosclerosis between races have demonstrated decreased occurrence in black vs white.[2-4,6,9] The frequency of myocardial infarction and angina pectoris in the presence of higher blood pressures has been much lower in black than white males in Evans County,[1] as well as almost all reported studies.[3,6-15] Sudden death is also less frequent in black males.[5]

The high rates of ST and T wave abnormalities in Evans County black males are consistent with many other ECG studies.[2,4,6,23,24] These studies also emphasize the benign nature of this ECG change. In white males of Evans County as well as many other studies,[20,25-28] even minor T wave changes increase the risk of developing IHD, although these changes may be transient and unstable.[19]

Studies performed in Jamaican males,[2] a population of rural blacks of African descent, in whom symptomatic IHD and atheromatous lesions of the coronary arteries and aorta are rare but hypertension and diabetes common, provide an interesting population for ECG comparisons. The frequencies of the specified ECG abnormalities in Jamaican black males and Evans County black males are strikingly similar (Table 7); the only

Table 7.—Black-White Relative Risk* of CHD Incidence by Specified Abnormality

	Males	Females
No specified abnormality	68.7/23.3 = 2.948	29.0/43.0 = .674
Any specified abnormality	109.3/27.2 = 4.018	50.8/29.6 = 1.716
Left axis deviation (2-1)	159.7/90.2 = 1.770	124.7/125.5 = .994
Increased QRS voltage (3-1)	63.9/23.6 = 2.708	91.6/47.4 = 1.932
ST changes (4-1 or 4-2)	307.6/87.0 = 3.536	136.1/28.9 = 4.709
Major T wave changes (5-1 or 5-2)	209.9/34.4 = 6.102	65.7/30.5 = 2.154
Minor T wave changes (5-3)	235.1/80.6 = 2.917	79.0/48.3 = 1.636
Prolonged PR (6-3)	...	...
Left or right bundle branch (7-1 or 7-2)	...	...
Sinus tachycardia (8-7)	...	19.2/43.0 = .446

* Relative risk: white race/black race.

Table 8.—Comparison Between Evans County and Other Populations of the Prevalence of ECG Abnormalities (Rates per 100)

	Evans County		Jamaica	5 European Countries	Tecumseh	Framingham	Greece	Italy	US Railroad Workers	Rhondda Fach
Race	White	Black	Black	White	White	White	White	White	White	White
Sex	M	M	M	M	M	M	M	M	M	M
Age range	15-74	15-74	35-64	40-59	16-80+	30-62		40-59	40-59	36-64
No.	878	498	526	4,317	2,449	2,336	683	993	1,682	537
ECG abnormality										
Left axis deviation (2-1)	5.3	4.0	3.8		6.0		4.5	4.1	2.9	
Increased QRS voltage (3-1)	10.0	26.7	29.3	4.6	6.0	7.8	5.1	5.5	2.5	4.7
ST changes (4-1 or 4-2)	2.2	2.4	2.3	2.1	2.0	1.7				4.6
Major T wave change (5-1 or 5-2)	3.1	11.1	3.6	1.8	2.7	2.2	0.59	1.7	0.89	4.1
Minor T wave change (5-3)	3.2	7.8	5.3	2.9	8.9	7.5				2.6
Prolonged P-R (6-3)	1.8	3.8	4.7		1.9	0.7†				3.2†
Left or right bundle branch block (7-1 or 7-2)	1.6	0.6	1.3	0.42*	0.73	2.9‡	0.73‡	1.5‡	1.4‡	5.4‡
Sinus tachycardia (8-7)	5.1	5.2	4.2							

* Left bundle branch block only (7-1).
† 6-1 through 6-4.
‡ 7-1 through 7-4 all IVCD.

discrepant category was a greater prevalence of major T wave abnormalities in Evans County black males. The authors suggested that the ECG abnormalities in Jamaican black males may be derived from causes other than IHD. Valvular heart disease was uncommon in both Jamaica and Evans County, as were parasitic infections involving the heart. Cardiomyopathy and "small artery disease" as well as hypertension and IHD were suggested as contributors to heart disease in Jamaica.

Comparisons of South African Bantu and white populations[4] reveal a much higher prevalence in the Bantu of inverted T waves, ST changes, and increased QRS voltage. Coronary heart disease is rare among Bantu and the authors have been unable to associate definite pathological lesions with those ECG changes or demonstrate any adverse prognostic significance.

Lower incidence rates of overt IHD in black males and marked differences in the significance of risk factors and electrocardiographic manifestations in the present follow-up study confirm the prevalence findings reported earlier.[1] Evans County white males appear much more similar to other in the United States and elsewhere populations in IHD manifestations than do Evans County black males. Evans County black males appear more to resemble Jamaican black males and South African blacks than US or European white males; hence, it appears that black males in some way are "protected" from developing IHD even in the presence of the "usual" coronary risk factors such as hypertension and electrocardiographic abnormalities. It is possible that genetic determinants may play a role in this regard.

References

1. McDonough JR, Hames CG, Stulb SC, et al: Coronary heart disease among Negroes and whites in Evans County, Georgia. *J Chronic Dis* **18**:443-468, 1968.
2. Miall WE, Del Campo E, Fodor J, et al: A longitudinal study of heart disease in a Jamaican rural population. *Bull WHO*, to be published, 1971.
3. Pepler WJ, Meyer BJ: Interarterial coronary anastomoses and coronary arterial pattern: A comparative study of South African Bantu and European hearts. *Circulation* **22**:14-24, 1960.
4. Walker ARP, Walker BF: The bearing of race, sex, age, and nutritional state on the precordial electrocardiograms of young South African Bantu and Caucasian subjects. *Amer Heart J* **77**:441-459, 1969.
5. Kuller L: Sudden death in arteriosclerotic heart disease. *Amer J Cardiol* **24**:617-628, 1969.
6. Phillips JH, Burch GE: A review of cardiovascular diseases in the white and Negro races. *Medicine* **39**:241-288, 1960.
7. Chapman JM, Coulson AH, Clark V: Negro-white differences in risk factors and disease incidence in an epidemiologic study of ischemic heart disease. *Circulation* **42**(suppl III):143, 1970.
8. Lilienfeld AM: Variation in mortality from heart disease: Race, sex, and socioeconomic status. *Public Health Rep* **71**:545-552, 1956.
9. Blacke JO, Handler FP: Coronary artery disease: A comparison of the rates and patterns of development of coronary arteriosclerosis in the Negro and white races and its relation to clinical coronary artery disease. *Arch Path* **50**:189-198, 1950.
10. McVay LF, Keil PG: Myocardial infarction with special reference to the Negro. *Arch Intern Med* **96**:762-767, 1955.
11. Thomas WA, Blanche JO, Lee KI: Race and the incidence of acute myocardial infarction. *Arch Intern Med* **100**:423-429, 1957.
12. Roberts DW, Meck PG, Grueger DE: Prevalence of heart disease in the population of Baltimore. *Circulation* **14**:988-989, 1956.
13. Moriyama I, Woolsey TD, Stamler J: Observations on possible causative factors responsible for the sex and race trends in cardiovascular-renal disease mortality in the United States. *J Chronic Dis* **7**:401-412, 1958.
14. Moriyama IM, Woolsey TD: Statistical studies of heart disease: IX. Race and diseases. *Public Health Rep* **66**:355-368, 1951.
15. Pennel MY, Lehman JL: Statistical studies of heart disease: VIII. Mortality from heart disease among Negroes as compared with white persons. *Public Health Rep* **66**:57-80, 1951.
16. McDonough JR, Garrison GE, Hames CG: Blood pressure and hypertensive disease among Negroes and whites in Evans County, Georgia. *Ann Intern Med* **61**:208-228, 1964.
17. Blackburn H, Keys A, Simonson E, et al: The electrocardiogram in population studies: A classification system. *Circulation* **21**:1160-1175, 1960.
18. World Health Organization: Hypertension and coronary heart disease: Classification and criteria for epidemiological studies. *WHO Techn Rep Ser* 1959, No. 168.
19. Ostrander LD: Serial electrocardiographic findings in a prospective epidemiological study. *Circulation* **34**:1069-1080, 1966.
20. Higgins IT, Kannel WB, Dawber TR: The electrocardiogram in epidemiological studies. *Brit J Prev Soc Med* **19**:53-68, 1965.
21. Rose GA, Ahmetelli M, Checcacci L, et al: Ischaemic heart disease in middle-aged men: Prevalence comparisons in Europe. *Bull WHO* **38**:885-895, 1968.
22. Blackburn H, Vasquez CL, Keys A: The aging electrocardiogram. *Amer J Cardiol* **20**:618-627, 1967.
23. Gottschalk CW, Craig E: A comparison of the precordial S-T and T waves in the electrocardiograms of 600 healthy young Negro and white adults. *Southern Med J* **49**:453-457, 1956.
24. Lamb LE, Averill KH: *First International Symposium on Cardiology in Aviation.* Brooks Air Force Base, Tex, US Air Force, 1959.
25. Ostrander LD: The relation of "silent" T Wave inversion to cardiovascular disease in an epidemiologic study. *Amer J Cardiol* **25**:325-328, 1970.
26. Ungerleider HE: The prognostic implications of the electrocardiogram. *Amer J Cardiol* **6**:35-44, 1965.
27. Blackburn H: The electrocardiogram in cardiovascular epidemiology. *Ann NY Acad Sci* **126**:882-905, 1965.
28. Blackburn H, Parlin RW: Antecedents of disease: Insurance mortality experience. *Ann NY Acad Sci* **134**:965-1017, 1966.

Occupational Mobility and Coronary Heart Disease

Berton H. Kaplan, PhD; John C. Cassel, MD, MPH; Herman A. Tyroler, MD; Joan C. Cornoni, MPH, PhD; David G. Kleinbaum, PhD, Chapel Hill, NC; and Curtis G. Hames, Claxton, Ga

Using prevalence data of white men in Evans County, Ga, this paper studies the relationship between coronary heart disease (CHD) and social mobility. Two basic findings are (1) that in both types of mobility, intragenerational and intergenerational, persons in the two lower social classes are more at risk if upwardly mobile than the stable populations; and (2) that upwardly mobile persons among the upper social classes show lower rates than the stable, a reversal of the other finding.

One of the striking findings of the cardiovascular incidence study conducted in Evans County, Georgia, between 1960-1962 and 1967-1969 was the changing relationship between coronary heart disease (CHD) and social class that had occurred during this time period (Cassel et al, p 901). Social class was assessed by the McGuire-White scale[1] (a rural version of the Warner scale), which uses occupation, education, and source of income to derive a social class index score. Social class analysis was restricted to white men. In 1960 those in the upper half of the range of social class scores were found to have age adjusted rates of CHD that were more than twice as high as those with scores in the lower half of the range. By 1967, however, this social class difference had disappeared with the "lower" social class men having the same rates as the "higher." Various analyses have convinced us that these changing relationships represent a change in incidence by social class rather than being the effects of selective survival or migration (Cassel et al, p 901). Furthermore, it would appear that the equality in rates in the two social class groups has been achieved by an increase in the rates for the "lower" social class men (particularly younger men), rather than a decrease in the "higher" social class.

This increase in the rates of CHD in the lower social class is occurring at a time when Evans County is undergoing a fairly rapid transition from a rural agrarian to a more "modern" industrialized economy. Until comparatively recently the only people participating in this change of "style of life" to any large extent were the "higher" social class men. It was the clinical impression of one of us (Hames, p 883), based upon a lifetime of experience in this county, that in recent years "lower" social class men were beginning to participate in these changes to an ever increasing extent. Thus, in microcosm Evans County may be recapitulating the changes in style of life and accompanying CHD rates that have characterized the urban developed countries over the past half century. What those particular styles of life are, particularly those which may be relevant to the risk of developing CHD, is a matter of speculation. There is no evidence that major changes in diet have occurred. Changes in cigarette smoking and physical activity surely have occurred, but as shown elsewhere (Cassel, p 890), these are unlikely to have accounted for all of these social class findings. An additional possibility that requires exploration is that some of the psychosocial factors that accompany such social change may be implicated; we present a preliminary attempt at examining some of these factors.

Theoretical Orientation

A broad spectrum, ranging from total disbelief to complete conviction, exists today as to whether psychosocial factors can influence the risk of developing CHD, and if so, which factors and by what mechanisms.[2] Paradoxically, some of the more convincing evidence comes from animal experiments, where a number of investigators have shown quite convincingly that variations in the social milieu with all aspects of the physical environment and genetic stock held constant can produce marked alterations in health status, including the development of hyperten-

Received for publication July 25, 1971; accepted Oct 13.

From the departments of epidemiology (Drs. Kaplan, Cassel, Tyroler, Cornoni, and Kleinbaum) and biostatistics (Dr. Kleinbaum), University of North Carolina, Chapel Hill, NC. Dr. Hames is in private practice in Evans County, Georgia.

Reprint requests to Department of Epidemiology, University of North Carolina, Chapel Hill, NC 27514 (Dr. Kaplan).

Table 1.—Intergenerational Mobility, Evans County, White Men

Type of Mobility	No.	%
Upward	271	42.4
Downward	209	31.2
Stable	158	26.4
Totals	638	100.0

sion and arteriosclerosis.[3-12] Furthermore, many of the neuroendocrine changes which might account for such changing health status have been elucidated, providing a rational biological explanation for these phenomena.[13,14] Convincing as this evidence is, however, the relevance to human health remains unproved, and no consensus exists as to the appropriate analogues in the human social system. The changes in the social milieu in the animal experiments have to a large extent been produced by varying the size of the group in which the animals interact and by situations which lead to confusion over territorial control. Attempts to demonstrate that these same situations (particularly crowding and increased population density) in humans lead to poorer health have been unconvincing and have led to confusing and often conflicting results.[15] Cassel has suggested elsewhere[16] that, as a more likely possibility, the social process linking high population density to enhanced susceptibility to disease in animals is not the crowding per se but the disordered relationships that inevitably accompany such animal crowding. These, while being manifest by many unusual behaviors, often have in common a failure of the behavior on the part of one animal to elicit appropriate responses on the part of the others. This failure of the behavioral patterns to modify the relationships between animals frequently leads to repetition of these behaviors with concomitant alterations in autonomic nervous system arousal and endocrine activity.

It is thus possible that in human populations the absence of adequate evidence (feedback) that actions were leading to predictable consequences, particularly if these consequences were of considerable importance to the individual, would increase susceptibility to disease. Furthermore, our theory (reported by Cassel[17]) would suggest that the health consequences of such lack of adequate feedback would be most extreme in those individuals deprived of meaningful social support.

Sociologists have long maintained that social mobility is accompanied by both these phenomena. Various authors have shown that such mobility is associated with powerlessness, role and value conflicts,[18] reduction in family ties,[19] alienation,[20] social isolation,[21] anomie,[22] and status inconsistency.[23-25] Furthermore, the effects of such mobility should be greatest in the lower social class groups, as these are the least socially prepared, ie, the least skilled or competent to adapt to the strains of upward social mobility. As Kohn's[26] recent review indicates, lower class life contains more "vulnerability," and mobility in higher social classes less discontinuity. These notions were put to a test in the Evans County data.

Methodology

The sample consists of all white men in the original cohort. Since this sociological data was not included in the first phase, our data is in the character of prevalence, not incidence, with all the restrictions imposed, therefore, on prevalence data. The major limitation that such a prevalence study poses for this analysis is the fact that, by definition, we are dealing with survivors only, and there may have been selective survival.

We used the Hollingshead[27] occupational classification to measure occupational levels which were classified 1 (high status) through 7 (low status). Intergenerational mobility was defined by the difference between the occupational rank of the respondent and the occupational rank of the respondent's father or head of household, on these Hollingshead rankings. Consequently, using this method of classification, the respondents were ranked as either up, if the respondent had a higher occupation than his father; stable, if the respondent was the same rank as his father; and downward, if the respondent was lower than his father. Small numbers precluded any measure of the extent of mobility. (Due to small numbers, we will only analyze for main effects. Duncan's cautions, reported by Simpson, are well recognized.[21] Small numbers precluded accounting for effects due to class of origin or class of destination.) Intragenerational mobility was measured in terms of changes in occupational rank of the respondents within their own lifetime. For this purpose respondents were classified as upwardly mobile, downwardly mobile, or stable on the basis of the ranking of their first and last

Table 2.—Intragenerational Mobility, Evans County, White Men

Type of Mobility	No.	%
Upward	401	63.4
Downward	53	8.4
Stable	178	29.2
Totals	632	101.0

job. It should be emphasized that occupational mobility is measured by the status rankings of occupations. Social class was measured by the McGuire-White scale, which, as previously indicated, uses occupation of respondent (current), education, and source of income to derive a social class index score.[1] Thus, for example, an upper social class person could still be upwardly mobile on both the intergenerational and intragenerational measures if his current job was higher ranking than his father's and higher than his own first job.

The accurate assessment of occupational status is one of the most difficult problems in sociological field work.[28] We tried to overcome this problem by the following methods: (1) very careful training of our coders; and (2) securing very detailed information on the type of work, work skill of job, income, and specific job title. Throughout the data processing, the information on occupation was coded independently by two coders. The two coders had an agreement of approximately 90% on the coding of the first 100 cases. All these differences were reconciled by securing additional data, if data was missing, and by a third coder who coded independently of the other two. After the first 100 cases, there was virtual agreement by the two coders, with about 1% adjudicated for the differences in coding.

The first survey examination of this study population (3,102 persons) was carried out between Aug 1, 1960, and June 1, 1962, and consisted of a history of heart disease, stroke, and other illnesses, a physical examination, electrocardiogram, roentgenogram of the chest, urinalysis, and laboratory studies of the blood for cholesterol level and hematocrit reading. The second survey examination of this cohort was made by two examiners between Aug 1, 1967, and Aug 31, 1969, in a clinic established for this purpose. During this seven to nine year follow-up period (average, 87 months), 320 persons had died and 252 had either migrated away from the community or refused to return for the second exam-

Table 3.—Coronary Heart Disease Prevalence Rates by Intergenerational Mobility Status—White Men

Mobility Status	PAR	Cases	Crude Rate	Age Adjusted Rate
Upward	271	27	99.6	117.3
Downward	209	15	100.5	89.9
Stable	158	15	94.9	86.2

Table 4.—Coronary Heart Disease Prevalence by Intergenerational Mobility and Social Class—White Men

	Social Class							
	I, II, III (higher)				IV, V (lower)			
Mobility Status	PAR*	Cases	Crude Rate/ 1,000	Age Adjusted Rate/1,000†	PAR	Cases	Crude Rate/ 1,000	Age Adjusted Rate/1,000†
Upward	156	13	83.3	98.3	115	14	121.7	142.8
Downward	73	5	68.5	73.8	136	16	117.6	96.4
Stable	78	9	115.4	114.9	80	6	75.0	62.7

* Persons at risk.
† Age adjustment by the indirect method.

ination. The examination of the remaining 2,530 persons (90.9% reexamination rate) again consisted of a medical history, physical examination, and laboratory studies, but also included a detailed questionnaire for evidence of cerebrovascular disease and symptoms of transient cerebral ischemia, a sociological questionnaire, and a physical activities questionnaire.

For purposes of this study CHD referred to sudden death, myocardial infarction, angina pectoris, and chronic heart disease. Sudden death was defined as any unexpected death occurring within 24 hours after the patient was last seen alive, if unattended, and within one hour if attended. In addition, any one of three findings was adequate for a designation of CHD. These included angina pectoris, a history of myocardial infarction, or an ECG consistent with myocardial infarction. The World Health Organization criteria were used for defining angina pectoris and a history of myocardial infarction.[29] Criteria used for the evaluation of the ECG were essentially the class I, Q, and QS patterns of Blackburn and Keys[30]; segment depression and T wave inversion were not used. Chronic heart disease was considered to be probably arteriosclerotic in origin when diagnosed at age 40 or older in the presence of heart failure or chronic arrhythmia and in the absence of angina pectoris, myocardial infarction, or any other cardiac disorder. In the presnet group of white men, 63 cases were so diagnosed.

Results

We were first interested in the extent of occupational mobility as an index of social change, namely, industrialization. Table 1 documents the large involvement in the new division of labor. Specifically, 73.6% are involved in either upward or downward intergenerational mobility: 42.4% are upwardly mobile, indicating the higher skill level of greater industrialization; yet, almost one third, 31.2%, are downwardly mobile. Only 26.4% were stable.

In terms of intragenerational mobility, ie, changes in occupational rank of the respondents within their own lifetime, Table 2 indicates the extensive sifting and sorting in a context of a changing division of labor—brought on by industrialization, the shift from agricultural economic base to industrial occupations. Sixty-three and four-tenths percent are upwardly mobile between their first full-time job and their current or most recent occupation. In a single lifetime, then, there has been a very considerable change. Eight and four-tenths percent were downwardly mobile by intragenerational mobility and 29.2% were stable. Thus, 71.8% were either upward or downward in mobility—over two thirds of the population caught up in both types of mobility. Tables 1 and 2 thus document the very extensive changes in the division of labor, both intergenerationally and intragenerationally, that have occurred in Evans County (a social context in which mobility is expected, if not institutionalized).

Table 3 deals with the relationship of intergenerational mobility to CHD. It appears that there is a modest excess in the age adjusted rates in upwardly mobile white men, ie, 117.3/1,000 when compared to the downwardly mobile, 89.9/1,000, and to the stable 86.2/1,000.

In examining our hypothesis, it is necessary to determine how these mobility classified rates vary by current social class. For this purpose the population was divided into two, those in the upper half of the social class range (equivalent to social classes I, II, and III) and those in the lower half of the range (equivalent to social classes IV and V), thus replicating the method originally used in the analysis of the 1960 prevalence study (Cassel et al, p 890). This analysis is presented in Table 4, which emphasizes the current social context in which mobility is experienced.

There is clearly an excess rate in the upwardly mobile in the two lower social classes (Table 4). The upwardly mobile within those two lower social classes have an age adjusted rate of 142.8, compared to 96.4 in the downwardly mobile, and 62.7 in the stable population. (This entire exercise is, of course, limited by the problem of small numbers. However, trends can be suggested.) In the upper three social classes, no excess risk in the upwardly mobile is apparent, the relevant rates being 98.3 for the upwardly mobile, 73.8 for the downward, and 114.9 for the stable.

To further emphasize the point that upward mobility may have a more deleterious effect as social class decreases, Table 5 shows the class gradient on a four point interval. Table 5 includes the rates for the upwardly mobile *only* and by a fourfold social class breakdown. The risk of CHD increases among the upwardly mobile with decreasing social class status. For example, classes I and II have an age adjusted rate of 63.9/1,000; class III, 111.7/1,000; class IV, 139.0/1,000; and class V, 158.6/1,000. Under the restriction of small numbers introduced by an expanded table, it would appear that the least socially prepared, those in the last two social classes, are the least skilled or competent to adapt to the strains of upward social mobility; this is in keeping with our hypothesis.

It is important to contrast the difference between the effects of intergenerational and intragenerational mobility. Table 6 shows the rates of CHD prevalence by intragenerational mobility.

In both measures of mobility, the two lower social classes are more at risk, if upwardly mobile, than is the stable population. In the case of intergenerational mobility (Table 4), the two lower social classes, if upwardly mobile, have an age adjusted rate of 142.8 compared to 62.7 in the stable. In the case of intragenerational mobility (Table 6) in the lower two social classes, the upward mobility rate is 104.3 compared to the stable rate of 83.0. Insofar as one can extrapolate from prevalence data, both measurements of mobility suggest the same phenomena, as predicted by our hypothesis, that upward mobility in the lower social classes increases the risk of CHD. In relative risk terms, in the lower social classes the intergenerational upwardly mobile have a relative risk of 2.3 compared to the stable individuals, while the intragenerational upwardly mobile have a relative risk of 1.2 compared to the stable, a negligible difference. It would appear, therefore, that the intergenerational process is a more sensitive indicator of increased risk to CHD.

Somewhat surprisingly, we find a reversal of these findings amid the upper social classes in which upward mobility appears, if anything, to be protective. Among the intergenerational upwardly mobile, we find a rate of 98.3, compared to a slightly higher rate of 114.9 for the stable. Among the intragenerational upwardly mobile, we find a rate of 83.1, compared to a stable rate of 155.9, a relative risk for stable individuals of 1.9.

There are too few cases in the downwardly mobile in Table 6 to even speculate about class comparisons.

Comment and Conclusions

A review of the pertinent literature presents a contrasting picture. Syme and Reader[31] and Syme et al,[32] Bruhn et al,[33,34] Shekelle et al,[35] Caffrey,[36] and Bakker and Levinson[37] all found that social mobility was associated with the risk of CHD. Williams[38] and Lehman et al[39] and Hinkle et al[40] found no such association. Hence, we have conflicting evidence. Since Hinkle et al and Williams studied industrial populations, selection may be at work. And it must be pointed out that these studies used different measures of mobility, and usually did not distinguish mobility types—up and down—or rate variations by class contexts. These studies have been carefully reviewed by Smith,[41] Marks,[42] and, most recently, by Jenkins.[2]

Table 5.—Coronary Heart Disease Prevalence by Upward Intergenerational Occupational Mobility and Social Class Groups—White Men

Social Class	PAR*	Cases	Crude Rate	Age Adjusted Rate†
I, II	47	3	63.8	63.9
III	109	10	91.7	117.3
IV	95	11	115.8	139.0
V*	20	3	150.0	158.6

* Persons at risk.

† It is possible to be mobile yet still in social class V since current social class is defined by summing the index based on source of income, education, and occupation, while mobility is the difference between the respondent's occupational level and the occupational level of the respondent's father.

Table 6.—Coronary Heart Disease Prevalence by Intragenerational Occupation Mobility and Social Class—White Men

	Social Class							
	I, II, III (higher)				IV, V (lower)			
Mobility Status	PAR*	Cases	Crude Rate/ 1,000	Age Adjusted Rate/ 1,000	PAR	Cases	Crude Rate/ 1,000	Age Adjusted Rate/ 1,000
Upward	229	18	78.6	83.1	172	19	110.5	104.3
Downward	13	1	76.9	113.4	40	6	150.0	147.3
Stable	61	8	131.1	155.9	117	11	94.0	83.0

* Persons at risk.

It is not surprising that the lower social classes, IV and V, experience mobility as more deleterious. Work in competence theory,[43] anomie,[44] and social disintegration-integration[45] all point to the lack of appropriate preparation, social support, and interferences in lower class life that would make upward mobility in these groups more difficult.

But why does upward mobility in the upper three social classes, especially intragenerational mobility, appear to be protective? This was unexpected and we have no ready explanation from our data. Elder,[43] however, found that the upwardly mobile middle class men (compared to working class) experienced more work satisfaction, communal ties, and more personal competence. If these factors are at work in Evans County, the reversal of findings makes sense. Blau's[46,47] review of mobility studies has pointed out that upward mobility, per se, need not be deleterious at all, provided comfortable acculturation takes place, ie, the successful acquisition of new life styles. Our case may be in keeping with Blau's observation.

It should be emphasized that these data do not necessarily confirm either that the psychosocial processes are important in the genesis of CHD, or that if they are, they necessarily explain the recent increase in rates in the lower social class men. At least, they are consistent with such notions and certainly do not refute them.

Glen Elder, PhD; Jay Turner, PhD; and Robert J. Klein, PhD, assisted in our application of the mobility theory.

References

1. McGuire C; White GD: *The Measurement of Social Status, Research Paper in Human Development No. 3.* Austin, Tex, University of Texas, 1955.

2. Jenkins CD: Psychological and social precursors of coronary disease. *New Eng J Med* **284**:244-255, 307-317, 1971.

3. Calhoun JB: Population density and social pathology. *Sci Amer* **206**:139, 1962.

4. Ratcliffe HL; Cronin MTI: Changing frequency of arteriosclerosis in mammals and birds at the Philadelphia zoological garden. *Circulation* **18**:41-52, 1958.

5. Swinyard EA; Clark LD; Miyahara JT; et al: Studies on the mechanism of amphetamine toxicity in aggregated mice. *J Pharmacol Exp Ther* **132**:97-102, 1961.

6. Davis DE; Read CP: Effect of behavior on development of resistance in trichinosis. *Proc Soc Exp Biol Med* **99**:269-272, 1958.

7. Ader R; Hahn EW: Effects of social environment on mortality to whole body: X-irradiation in the rat. *Psychol Rep* **13**:214-215, 1963.

8. Ader R; Kreutner A; Jacobs HL: Social environment, emotionality and alloxan diabetes in the rat. *Psychosom Med* **25**:60-68, 1963.

9. King J; Lee YCP; Visacher MB: Single versus multiple cage occupancy and convulsion frequency in CH mice. *Proc Soc Exp Biol Med* **88**:661-663, 1955.

10. Andervont HB: Influence of environment on mammary cancer in mice. *J Nat Cancer Inst* **4**:579-581, 1944.

11. Christian JJ; Williamson HO: Effect of crowding on experimental granuloma formation in mice. *Proc Soc Exp Biol Med* **99**:385-387, 1958.

12. Henry JP; Meehan JP; Stephens PM: The use of psychosocial stimuli to induce prolonged hypertension in mice. *Psychosom Med* **29**:408-432, 1967.

13. Mason JW: Psychological influences on the pituitary-adrenal-cortical system, in Pincus G (ed): *Recent Progress in Hormone Research.* New York, Academic Press Inc, 1959, pp 345-389.

14. Mason JW, Brady JV: The sensitivity of the psycho-endocrine systems to social and physical environment, in Leiderman PH, Shapiro D (eds): *Psychobiological Approaches to Social Behavior.* Stanford, Calif, Stanford University Press, 1964.

15. Cassel JC: The relation of the urban environment to health: Towards a conceptual frame of research strategy, to be published.

16. Cassel JC: Health consequences of population density and crowding, in *Consequences of Population Change and Implications for National and International Policies.* Washington, DC National Academy of Sciences, to be published.

17. Cassel JC: An epidemiological perspective of psychosocial factors in disease etiology. Read before American Public Health Association, Houston, 1970.

18. Simpson ME: Social mobility, normlessness and powerlessness in two cultural contexts. *Amer Sociol Rev* **35**:1002-1013, 1970.

19. Stuckert RP: Occupational mobility and family relationships. *Social Forces* **41**:301-307, 1963.

20. Seeman M: On the meaning of alienation. *Amer Sociol Rev* **24**:783-791, 1959.

21. Warner W, Abegglen JC: *Big Business Leaders in America.* New York, Harper Brothers, 1955.

22. Meier D, Bell W: Anomia and differential access to the achievement of life goals. *Amer Sociol Rev* **24**:189-207, 1959.

23. Blalock HM Jr: Status and consistency, social mobility and structural effects. *Amer Sociol Rev* **21**:750-801, 1967.

24. Lenski G: Comment. *Publ Opin Quart* **28**:326-330, 1964.

25. Bloombaum M: Mobility dimension and status consistency. *Soc Soc Res* **58**:340-347, 1964.

26. Kohn M: Class, family and schizophrenia: A reformulation. *Social Forces* to be published, 1971.

27. Hollingshead AB: *Two Factor Index of Social Position.* New Haven, Conn, Yale University Press, 1957.

28. Turner RJ: Social mobility and schizophrenia. *J Health Hum Behav* **9**:194-201, 1968.

29. World Health Organization: Hypertension and coronary heart disease: Classification and criteria for epidemiological studies. *WHO Techn Rep Ser* 1959; No. 168, pp 1-28.

30. Blackburn H; Keys A: Simonson E; et al: The electrocardiogram in population studies: A classification system. *Circulation* **21**:1160-1175, 1960.

31. Syme SL; Reader LG: Social stress and cardiovascular disease. *Milbank Mem Fund Quart* **45** (suppl):175-180, 1967.

32. Syme SL; Hymen MM; Enterline TE: Some social and cultural factors associated with the occurrence of coronary heart disease. *J Chronic Dis* **17**:277-289, 1964.

33. Bruhn JG; Wolfe S; Lynn TN; et al: Social aspects of coronary heart disease in a Pennsylvania German community. *Soc Sci Med* **2**:201-212, 1968.

34. Bruhn JG; Chandler B; Miller MC; et al: Social aspects of coronary heart disease in two adjacent ethnically different communities. *Amer J Public Health* **56**:1493-1506, 1966.

35. Shekelle RS; Ostfeld AM; Paul O: Social status in the incidence of coronary heart disease. *J Chronic Dis* **22**:381-394, 1969.

36. Caffrey B: Behavior patterns and personality characteristics related to prevalence rates of coronary heart disease in American monks. *J Chronic Dis* **22**:93-103, 1969.

37. Bakker CB; Levinson RM: Determinants of angina pectoris. *Psychosom Med* **29**:621-633, 1967.

38. Williams CA: *The Relationship of Occupational Change to Blood Pressure, Serum Cholesterol and Specific Overt Behavior Patterns,* PhD dissertation. University of North Carolina, Chapel Hill, 1968.

39. Lehman EW; Shulman J; Hinkle L: Coronary deaths in organizational mobility: The 30 year experience of 1,160 men. *Arch Environ Health* **15**:455-461, 1967.

40. Hinkle LE Jr; Whitney LH; Lehman EW; et al: Occupation, education and coronary heart disease. *Science* **161**:238-246, 1968.

41. Smith T: Factors involving sociocultural incongruity and change: A review of empirical findings. *Milbank Mem Fund Quart* **45**:23-37, 1967.

42. Marks RU: Factors involving social and demographic characteristics: A review of empirical findings. *Milbank Mem Fund Quart* **45**:51-108, 1967.

43. Elder GH: Occupational mobility, life patterns, and personality. *J Health Soc Behav* **10**:321-322, 1969.

44. Cloward MB (ed): *Anomie and Deviant Behavior.* Glencoe Ill, Free Press, 1964.

45. Kaplan BH: Social disorganization and poverty, in *Encyclopedia of Social Work.* New York, American Council on Social Work, 1971.

46. Blau P: Social mobility and interpersonal relations. *Amer Sociol Rev* **21**:290-295, 1956.

47. Blau P: Structural effects. *Amer Sociol Rev* **24**:178-193, 1960.

Multivariate Analysis of Risk of Coronary Heart Disease in Evans County, Georgia

David G. Kleinbaum, PhD; Lawrence L. Kupper, PhD; John C. Cassel, MD, MPH; and Herman A. Tyroler, MD, Chapel Hill, NC

To determine how various risk factors help to explain the incidence deficit of coronary heart disease (CHD) in black males as compared with white males in Evans County, Georgia, multivariate analyses involving use of multiple logistic functions were employed. Four variables found to be the best predictors of CHD for white males were smoking, electrocardiogram, and the interactive relationships between blood pressure and age and cholesterol and age. When risks for the black population were computed by applying the best white male model adjusted for black incidence to the black male data, it was concluded that blacks respond to the four risk factors similarly to whites but always at a lower level of CHD (due to unmeasured factors).

Cornfield[1] and Truett et al[2] have demonstrated the utility of discriminant analysis techniques in longitudinal studies designed to investigate the joint effects of several risk factors on the risk of developing coronary heart disease (CHD). In fact, the use of such methodology becomes almost mandatory when the number of risk factors or variables under consideration is large enough to make multiple cross-classification techniques impractical. In addition, there is something to be said for avoiding the problem of how to categorize the data since, in many cases, the choice of groupings is both coarse and arbitrary and can lead to loss of information.

In all that follows, we will assume that the probability (or risk) of a person with variable values $X_1, X_2, \ldots, X_k$ developing CHD is given by the *multiple logistic function*

$$P(X_1, X_2, \ldots, X_k) = \left(1+\exp\left[-\beta_0 - \sum_{i=1}^{k} \beta_i X_i\right]\right)^{-1}, \quad (1)$$

Received for publication May 13, 1971; accepted Aug 16.

From the departments of biostatistics (Drs. Kleinbaum and Kupper) and epidemiology (Drs. Cassel and Tyroler), University of North Carolina, Chapel Hill.

Reprint requests to Department of Biostatistics, University of North Carolina, Chapel Hill, NC 27514 (Dr. Kleinbaum).

where $\beta_0, \beta_1, \beta_2, ..., \beta_k$ are indexes to be estimated.

When the joint distribution of $X_1, X_2, ..., X_k$ in both the well (NCHD) and diseased (CHD) populations is multivariate normal with respective mean vectors $\underset{\sim}{\mu}_0 = (\mu_{01}, \mu_{02}, ..., \mu_{0k})$ and $\underset{\sim}{\mu}_1 = (\mu_{11}, \mu_{12}, ..., \mu_{1k})$ and with a *common* covariance matrix Σ, then the $\{\beta_i\}$ are simply the coefficients in Fisher's linear discriminant function.[3] In particular, if the element in the i-th row and j-th column of Σ^{-1} is σ^{ij}, then

$$\beta_i = \sum_{j=1}^{k} \sigma^{ij} (\mu_{1j} - \mu_{0j}), \quad i = 1, 2, \ldots, k, \qquad (2)$$

and

$$\beta_0 = -\tfrac{1}{2} \sum_{j=1}^{k} \beta_j (\mu_{0j} + \mu_{1j}) - \log_e \frac{(1-p)}{p} \frac{c_{10}}{c_{01}}, \qquad (3)$$

where p is the a priori or unconditional probability of developing CHD, and where $c_{01}(c_{10})$ is the cost of misclassifying a member of the CHD(NCHD) population as a member of the NCHD(CHD) population. The corresponding index estimates are obtained directly from (2) and (3) by using for σ^{ij} the i, j-th element $\hat{\sigma}^{ij}$ in the inverse of the pooled sample covariance matrix, for μ_{0j} and μ_{1j} the corresponding sample means $\bar{X}_{0j}$ and $\bar{X}_{1j}$, and for p the ratio $N_1/(N_0+N_1)$, where N_0 and N_1 are the numbers of individuals in the NCHD and CHD groups, respectively. The choice of the cost ratio c_{10}/c_{01} is at the discretion of the investigator but is not without consequence, as we shall see later. Cornfield[1] and Truett et al[2] took this ratio to be unity.

It is not necessary that the expression in the exponent of (1) be linear in the Xs. As a matter of fact, even if the multivariate normality assumption holds (which, in practice, will hardly ever be the case), a violation of the common covariance matrix assumption means that terms of the second order in the Xs (eg, X_1^2, X_2X_3, etc) should also be included in the model.

However, as long as the expression in the exponent of (1), namely the "discriminant function," is linear in its coefficients, the described estimation procedure can be used no matter how the Xs are defined. For example, X_1 could represent the product term (age) × (cholesterol), X_2 could be (systolic blood pressure)$^{1/2}$. The analogy to multiple regression should be apparent.

Such an interpretation affords us a very general approach with regard to the problem of determining the "best" form of the multiple logistic function to be used in a given situation. (The concept of what constitutes a "best" model will be discussed in the next section.) This approach has the desired flexibility of allowing various functions of risk factors to be included in the model if they are important predictors of risk.

As an illustration of the value of such a general approach, Truett et al[2] noted that a significant interaction between age and cholesterol was evident in the Framingham data, which indicates that a multiple logistic function containing this interaction term would almost certainly discriminate better than the one actually used (which was linear in the Xs). Significant interactions between various risk factors were also expected to appear to the Evans County, Georgia, data.

In the following section, the general statistical methodology associated with the problem of determining how various risk factors can account for the difference in incidence of CHD in black and white males in Evans County is discussed.

Methodology and Related Results

One of the primary objectives of this study was to compare white and black males in Evans County with respect to the effects of blood pressure, cholesterol (CHOL) level, age, smoking history (SMK), electrocardiogram abnormality, and Quetelet index (QI) (a measure of "size" defined as weight/[height]^2) on the risk of developing CHD. In this regard, it was desired to show that there was evidence in support of the following statement, henceforth referred to as (†):

(†) Differences in the distributions of the above risk factors in the white and black male data sets are *not* sufficient to account completely for the higher observed incidence of CHD in white males; it therefore follows that this difference in incidence must, in addition, be due to the fact that the above risk factors and/or possibly other factors are related to the risk of developing CHD in different ways in white males and black males in Evans County, Georgia.

Now, since we are assuming that (1) expresses the general form of the relationship between risk and risk factors, it follows, in particular, that (†) is not true when the multiple logistic function defining the exact relationship between risk of CHD and various risk factors for white males is identical to the one for black males. By this is meant that the two functions not only involve exactly the same risk factors but also that the values of corresponding coefficients agree. If this was indeed the case, then coefficients calculated using the white male data would estimate the same indexes as coefficients calculated from the black male data, regardless of differences in the distributions of the risk factors in blacks and whites.

From these remarks, it is clear that two fairly direct approaches for determining whether (†) is true or not suggest themselves. Generally speaking, the first would be to compare the "best" form of (1) determined from white male data with the "best" form of (1) obtained from black male data. If these functions turn out to be significantly different in structure, this would be evidence in support of (†). The second approach would also involve finding the "best" white male model from available data. The next step would then require using the black male data itself to estimate the coefficients of the risk factors appearing in the "best" white male model.

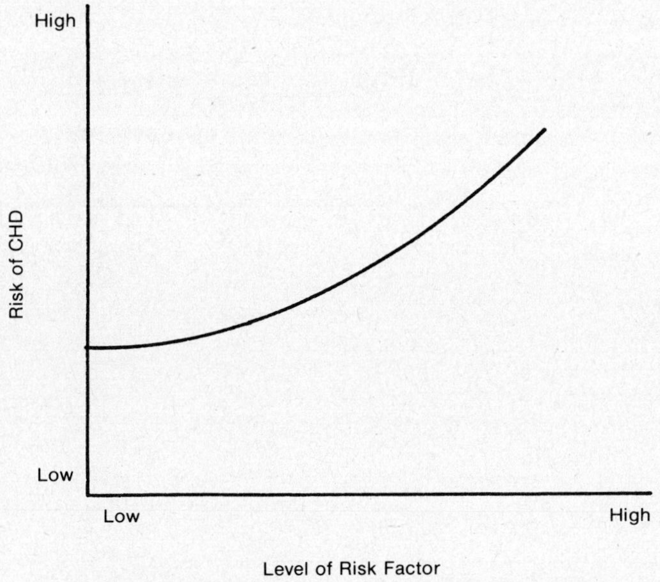

Fig 1.—General relationship to risk of cardiovascular heart disease of any risk factor in the best white male model for fixed levels of the other three factors.

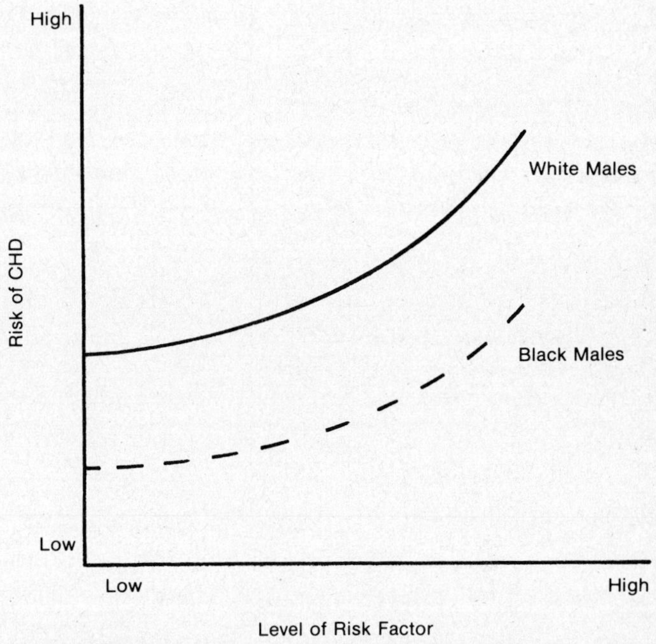

Fig 2.—General relationship between white male and black male logistic functions.

Evidence for (†) would be found if at least one of these estimated coefficients was significantly different from the corresponding one in the "best" white male model. Standard statistical techniques are available for making the comparisons required in this second approach.

The major problem in implementing these approaches was to find some optimal way of choosing these so-called best models. In this respect, the following methodology was used. Based primarily on present medical knowledge of CHD, twenty variable combinations were selected for consideration as possible important predictors of risk. They were AGE, CHOL level, diastolic blood pressure (DBP), systolic blood pressure (SBP), SMK, ECG, and QI, as well as the second-order combinations QI×AGE, QI×CHOL, QI×DBP, QI×SBP, SBP×CHOL, DBP×CHOL, AGE×DBP, AGE×SBP, AGE×CHOL, $(AGE)^2$, $(CHOL)^2$, $(DBP)^2$ and $(SBP)^2$. A stepwise discriminant analysis procedure was used to determine the important predictors of risk from this basic set of variables. In such a procedure, one variable is included in the discriminant function at each step, this variable being the one that results in the largest F value when testing for equality of means in the NCHD and CHD groups. (This F is actually a "partial F" since it is adjusted for the variables already included in the model.) This step-by-step procedure continues until no further "significant" gain in discrimination can be achieved by the addition of more variables to the discriminant function. The level of this "significance" can be controlled in the sense that a variable will not be included unless its partial F exceeds a number, called the "F to enter," which is to be specified beforehand by the researcher (for significance level α, this number is the α percentage point of the F distribution alluded to above). Of course, different choices of α can possibly lead to different models, so that care must be exercised in interpreting the results.

Previous studies of CHD risk which utilized the multiple logistic function adopted the policy of specifying beforehand which variables to include in (1). This is an especially arbitrary and inexact procedure when a large number of risk factors or combinations of these factors or both, are worthy of consideration. The improvement on such a technique which can be expected by using a stepwise discriminant analysis approach is that of being able to examine at every stage of the analysis the importance both of variables which have been included and which are candidates for inclusion in the discriminant function. (In addition to the "F to enter" criterion described, a variable already included may be removed from the model at a given step if its partial F fails to exceed an "F to remove," a number also specified beforehand by the researcher.) For example, a variable which may have appeared to be fairly important at an early stage may, at a later stage, be superfluous because of the relationships between it and other variables already included in the model. Such redundancy among variables would go unnoticed when these variables are "forced" into the discriminant function and could, in fact, lead to a loss in discriminatory power.

An application of stepwise discriminant analysis ($\alpha=0.10$) to the white male data ($N_0=761$, $N_1=71$) resulted in the following estimated multiple logistic function:

$$\hat{P}_w(X_1, X_2, X_3, X_4) = (1+\exp[5.7901 - 0.0289X_1 - 0.677X_2 - 0.770X_3 - 0.0122X_4])^{-1}, \quad (4)$$

where $X_1=(\text{DBP}\times\text{AGE})/100$, $X_2=\text{SMK}$(1 if there is a history of smoking and 0 if not), $X_3=\text{EKG}$(1 if abnormal and 0 if not), and $X_4=(\text{CHOL}\times\text{AGE})/100$. The variables are numbered in the order in which they

Table 1.—Expected and Observed Cases of Coronary Heart Disease for White Males Using the Best Fitting White Male Model (4)

Decile No.	Observed Cases	Expected Cases
1	23	23.517
2	14	12.983
3	12	9.255
4	11	7.110
5	3	5.537
6	3	4.168
7	4	3.231
8	1	2.352
9	0	1.518
10	0	0.737
Total	71	70.408

Table 2.—Expected and Observed Cases of Coronary Heart Disease for Black Males Using the Best Fitting White Male Model (4)

Decile No.	Observed Cases	Expected Cases
1	2	16.550
2	4	10.057
3	3	7.239
4	0	5.722
5	1	4.649
6	2	3.627
7	0	2.652
8	1	1.920
9	0	1.167
10	0	0.567
Total	13	54.150

Table 3.—Expected and Observed Cases of Coronary Heart Disease for Black Males Using the Best Fitting White Male Model (4) With an Adjusted Constant

Decile No.	Observed Cases	Expected Cases
1	2	5.478
2	4	2.812
3	3	1.918
4	0	1.472
5	1	1.172
6	3	0.898
7	0	0.645
8	1	0.461
9	0	0.276
10	0	0.133
Total	13	15.265

entered into the model. Very generally speaking, then, in terms of power to discriminate between the white male NCHD and CHD groups, X_1 is the "most powerful" variable; X_2, the second most powerful. The standard errors of the estimated coefficients were significantly different 0.0135, 0.2596, 0.3002, and 0.0055, respectively, indicating that all the estimated coefficients were significantly different from zero. The above model is somewhat unusual in the sense that the risk factors blood pressure, CHOL, and AGE enter into the model only as interactions.

In Table 1 a comparison of deciles of risk is given between observed numbers of cases of CHD for white males and expected numbers calculated using (4). It is easy to see that (4) "fits" the data fairly well, although this should not by any means be the main criterion for choosing the "best" model. In fact, a model which provides excellent discrimination between the NCHD and CHD groups might be preferred over one which, to paraphrase Truett et al[2] gives good agreement between observation and expectation but does not lead to as sharp a gradient of risk. The use of a stepwise discriminant analysis procedure was actually motivated by this primary consideration of finding a model which was best in terms of discriminatory power.

Perhaps this is also a good time to point out that the magnitudes of the expected numbers of cases in each decile of Table 1 can be drastically altered by simply varying the cost ratio c_{10}/c_{01}. For example, if the costs were chosen to be inversely proportional to the prior probabilities in the sense that $c_{10}/c_{01} = p/(1-p)$, then the expected numbers of cases would be much larger than those in Table 1, reflecting the fact that an error in classifying a person with CHD as a member of the NCHD group is now considered to be much more costly than a mistake in the opposite direction. As mentioned earlier, in all previous studies these costs have been taken to be equal; this was also done here. In terms of "goodness of fit" of the model, anyway, this assumption of equal costs seems to be a realistic one.

Since the use of a stepwise discriminant analysis approach is not claimed to be a panacea, it was important to be able to base the decision as to the choice of a best model on at least one other criterion as well. This was done by comparing models on the basis of tables constructed as Table 1. From such a table, two meaningful numerical measures can be calculated. The first is like a Pearson χ^2 type of statistic and is a reflection of the "closeness of fit" of the proposed model to the data. It is of the form

$$C^2 = \Sigma_{i=1}^{k} (O_i - E_i)^2/E_i,$$

where O_i and E_i are, respectively, the numbers of observed and expected cases of CHD in the i-th category, the number of categories k possibly being less than ten (deciles) since we agree to pool all deciles with expected numbers less than one (unless the sum of all these numbers is still less than one, in which case the next decile is included in the pool.) The second measure, $G = \Sigma_{i=1}^{10} i^2 O_i$, is inversely related to the sharpness of the "gradient of risk." To compare two models, A and B say, we compute

$$Q = (C_A/C_B)^{\gamma} (G_A/G_B)^{\delta}$$

and argue for model A if $Q<1$ and for model B if $Q>1$; here, C_A^2 and G_A are the values of C^2 and G for the table constructed using model A, C_B^2 and G_B are the values for the table associated with model B, and γ and δ are nonnegative numbers specified by the researcher (ideally, before seeing the tables) according to how much importance or weight he wants to give to the closeness-of-fit criterion C relative to the "gradient of risk" criterion G. In general, if $\gamma/\delta<1$, then discriminatory power is given more weight than goodness of fit; if $\gamma/\delta>1$, the converse is true. In the Evans County study, we chose to place more emphasis on the G criterion by setting $\gamma=1$ and $\delta=2$. It is important to emphasize, however, that there are no specific guidelines for choosing the values of γ and δ in a given situation, and any such choice must necessarily involve a certain amount of subjectivity. Thus, in the situation, for example, when several values of a particular choice of Q are fairly close to one, any decision about what model is best should also involve a careful comparison of the structures, interpretations, and other factors of the models involved.

Several different models involving subsets of the 20 basic variable combinations listed earlier (among these one containing all 20 basic combinations and one a function only of the seven linear effects) were individually compared to (4) using the Q criterion with $\gamma=1$ and $\delta=2$. (It was not necessary to consider all possible combinations since some were obviously inferior.) In every case, the model found by stepwise discriminant analysis was observed to be the better one. Hence, (4) was our choice as the best white male model.

We are now in a position to try to utilize the approaches mentioned earlier in an effort to show that (†) is true. In this regard, two models were fit to the black male data ($N_0=439$, $N_1=13$). The first, obtained by using the exact same methodology which resulted in (4), took the form

$$\hat{P}_B(X_2,X_5) = [1+\exp(5.2276-2.263X_2-0.0105X_5)]^{-1}, \quad (5)$$

where X_2 is SMK (as before) and X_5 is (QI×AGE)/100; the coefficient of X_2 in $\hat{P}_B(X_2,X_5)$ was significantly different from zero since its standard error was 0.6035. The second model,

$$\hat{P}_B(X_1,X_2,X_3,X_4) = (1+\exp[6.0245-0.0124X_1-0.150X_2-1.073X_3-0.0097X_4)]^{-1}, \quad (6)$$

was obtained by using the black male data to fit a model with exactly the same variables as in (4). In this case, the four variables entered in the order X_4,X_2,X_1,X_3, and none of the estimated coefficients were significantly different from zero, the standard errors being 0.0248, 0.6016, 0.5823, and 0.0118 for the coefficients of X_1, X_2, X_3, and X_4, respectively.

Now, if the five estimated coefficients in (6) are compared with the corresponding ones in (4), no significant differences are found. Thus, from earlier arguments, (5) appears to support (†) but (6) does not. However, such an interpretation should not be accepted at face value since the models (5) and (6) are estimated from data on only 13 black males with CHD, quite a small number from which to expect reliable results. In contrast, the minimum number of people with CHD for any of the models fit by Truett et al[2] was 39. In fact, one reason that no significant differences were found between corresponding coefficients in (4) and (6) was because the standard errors of the estimated coefficients in (6) were quite large due to the small sample size in the black male CHD group.

To combat this small sample size problem, a procedure to find evidence in support of (†) was developed which was based essentially on an examination of how well the best white male model (4) predicted CHD incidence in black males.

First of all, a computation using (4) of observed and expected cases of CHD by deciles of risk for the black male data is presented in Table 2. It is clear by inspection that (4) significantly overpredicts incidence of CHD in black males. Before discussing a possible reason for this overprediction, let us point out now that it is not simply due to the fact that we are guilty of a mistake often made in the course of a regression analysis, namely that of using the fitted model to predict outside the region of experimentation. Such is definitely not the case here because the variables AGE, CHOL, and DBP have quite comparable ranges for black and white males in both the NCHD and CHD groups.

Now, the obvious discrepancies between expected and observed cases of CHD in Table 2 are, in themselves, significant evidence in support of (†), since they indicate, from remarks made at the beginning of this section, that the multiple logistic function which (4) is estimating is not the same as the one giving the relationship between risk of CHD and related risk factors for black males in Evans County.

Let us pursue this a step further. From (3), it can be seen that the value of the constant term in (4) was calculated (assuming equal costs) as

$$\tfrac{1}{2}(0.0289[\bar{X}_{01}+\bar{X}_{11}]+0.677[\bar{X}_{02}+\bar{X}_{12}]+0.770[\bar{X}_{03}+\bar{X}_{13}]+0.0122[\bar{X}_{04}+\bar{X}_{14}])+\log_e\frac{761}{71}, \quad (7)$$

where $\bar{X}_{0j}$ and $\bar{X}_{1j}$ are the mean values of the j-th variable in (4), j=1,2,3,4, for the white male NCHD and CHD groups, respectively. If we now replace these mean values by the corresponding ones for black males and we use instead of 761/71 the ratio of sample sizes for the black male groups (namely, 439/13), then (7) changes to 7.2509, a value which is dependent on the white male data set only insofar as its computation involved the estimated risk factor coefficients appearing in (4). If this adjusted constant is used in (4) in place of 5.7901, the effect will be to lower the value of the estimated risk for any individual. Table 3 illustrates this phenomenon for the black male data. The second columns in Tables 2 and 3 are identical since a change in the constant in (4) does not affect the relative standings of individuals with regard to estimated risk. As a general rule, changing the constant will only alter the fit of the multiple logistic function and not the gradient of risk.

If one decides that Table 3 is indicative of a fairly good fit between expected and observed (which, despite the lack of an absolute criterion of fit, is certainly not an unreasonable decision) then an appropriate conclusion to be drawn, based on previous remarks, is that the true multiple logistic functions for black and white males in Evans County both are functions of the same risk factors which appear in (4) and that they differ only in the value of the constant term, this value being larger in the case of the black male model. Such an interpretation would imply that a black male in Evans County would have less of a chance of developing CHD than a white male with the same values of the risk factors in (4). In other words, black males appear to have factors other than the ones already discussed which protect them against CHD. On the other hand, a bad fit would indicate that either a different model is needed to describe the relationship between risk of CHD and related risk factors for black males or that a model of the form (4) with different values for one or more of the five coefficients is appropriate. In any case, the significant overprediction of black males incidence using (4) is evidence that the relationship between risk of CHD and associated risk factors is not the same for white males and black males in Evans County over and above differences in the distributions of the risk factors.

Conclusions

In an attempt to determine whether or not the deficit in incidence of CHD in black males as compared to white males in Evans County could be completely accounted for by differences in the distributions of the measured risk factors in the two ethnic groups, a multivariate analysis involving the use of multiple logistic functions was employed.

First, the best fitting multiple logistic function for white males was determined. Of the 20 variables measured in 1960 to be considered for the model, four were found to be the best predictors of CHD occurring in the next seven to nine years. These four variables were, in order of importance, DBP×AGE product (a measure of interaction), ECG, SMK, and CHOL×AGE product. Two of these variables involve the three basic risk factors, AGE, CHOL, and blood pressure; but, whereas previous studies assumed that these factors made independent, linear contributions to the risk of CHD, our results show that the interactive relationships between these variables provide much of the predictive power of the model.

The general relationship between any one of the risk factors in (4) and the risk of developing CHD (for fixed values of the other three factors in the model) are graphically illustrated in Fig 1.

The most direct approach for determining whether the lower incidence of CHD in blacks was due entirely to differences in their distributions of risk factors as compared to those for whites would be to find the best black male model from the black male data and then to determine whether this model was different from the best model for whites. However, there were unfortunately not enough black cases to give a "reliable" black male model.

Accordingly, as an alternative approach, the white model was applied to the black data; ie, risks for the black population were computed using the white male model. If the predicted number of black cases was approximately equal to the number of black cases actually observed, this would be evidence that the best white male model was also applicable to the blacks. Consequently, the black deficit in incidence would be explained completely by the fact that the distributions of risk factors for blacks were different from those for whites. If, however, the white model did not predict the number of black cases accurately, it would suggest differences in the two models over and above differences in the distributions of the risk factors. In other words, either the regression coefficients associated with the risk factors (ie, $\beta_1, \beta_2, \ldots, \beta_k$) are different in blacks and whites, or the constant term β_0 (which is related to the effects of unmeasured variables) is different in the two ethnic groups, or both.

The result of applying the white male model to the black male data was that 54 black cases were predicted when, in fact, only 13 were observed. Clearly, then, this is evidence that the white male model is not applicable to the black male data.

To determine whether this discrepancy was due only to differences in the unmeasured factors (the β_0 value) was not to differences in the regression coefficients, a further analysis was performed, this time using a β_0 value based on the black incidence rate. The expected number of black cases using this adjusted model was 15 (compared to the observed 13), which is clearly a much better fit than the first model.

From these two analyses, then, it can be inferred that blacks are responding to the risk factors in a manner similar to the whites but always at a lower level of CHD. This relationship is schematically represented in Fig 2.

As indicated in a separate publication,[4] while there may be many potential factors, as yet unmeasured, which account for this possible difference in the β_0 value for blacks and whites, one strong possibility is habitual physical activity.

Jo Maready assisted with data management and processing. Rudi Meir performed the laboratory analyses, and Bobbie Daniels assisted with the sociological questionnaire. Luretha Tillman served as interviewer and Lynn Waller assisted as bibliographic and editorial assistant. Anna Nevius served as statistical assistant by performing statistical calculations and running statistical computer programs.

References

1. Cornfield J: Joint dependence of risk of coronary heart disease on serum cholesterol and systolic blood pressure: A discriminant function analysis. *Fed Proc* **21**:58-61, 1962.

2. Truett J, Cornfield J, Kannel W: A multivariate analysis of the risk of coronary heart disease in Framingham. *J Chronic Dis* **20**:511-524, 1967.

3. Fisher RA: The use of multiple measurements in taxonomic problems. *Ann Eugenics* **7**:179-188, 1936.

4. Cassel JC, Heyden S, Bartel A, et al: Occupation and physical activity and coronary heart disease. **128**:920-928, 1971.

Cerebrovascular Disease in the Biracial Population of Evans County, Georgia

Albert Heyman, MD, Durham, NC; Herbert R. Karp, MD, Atlanta; Siegfried Heyden, MD; and Alan Bartel, MD, Durham, NC; John C. Cassel, MD, MPH; and Herman A. Tyroler, MD, Chapel Hill, NC; and Curtis G. Hames, MD, Claxton, Ga

An epidemiologic study was made of cerebrovascular disease in a biracial semirural community in Georgia. During an 87-month period, 94 of the 3,000 persons studied developed their first cerebrovascular event. The incidence of stroke among white men (4.7/1,000/year) was almost four times that in white women and more than twice that reported for white men in other sections of the country. The incidence rates of stroke in black men and women were equal (5.8/1000/yr). The risk factors predisposing to stroke in white men appeared to be severe hypertension, obesity, high hematocrit levels, and electrocardiographic abnormalities. The high incidence of cerebrovascular disease in this study supports previous reports of increased mortality for stroke in this region and represents an unusual situation with an undetermined cause.

Mortality studies in the United States indicate that death rates from cerebrovascular disease are greater among blacks than whites and higher in both races in the southeastern section of the country. Recent studies designed to authenticate these death rates have shown that the high mortality for cerebrovascular disease which appears on death certificates is probably an accurate indication of an increased incidence of stroke in the southeastern United States.[1,2] There is a need, therefore, for further studies to determine the clinical and environmental factors which may be responsible for this unique racial and geographical problem. This report presents our findings on the prevalence and incidence of cerebrovascular disease in Evans County, Georgia, a small rural community with a 60% white and 40% black population. This report also describes the relationship between cerebrovascular disease and the presence of conditions thought to favor its development, such as hypertension, hypercholesterolemia, and obesity. Previous epidemiologic studies of this community have described the sampling techniques and the socioeconomic and population characteristics of the study area.[3] The prevalence of ischemic heart disease and hypertension as related to race, social class, and occupational groups in this community have also been reported.[4,5]

Received for publication May 13, 1971; accepted July 21.

From the Center for Cerebrovascular Research, Duke University Medical Center, Durham, NC; the Division of Neurology, Emory School of Medicine, Atlanta; Department of Epidemiology, University of North Carolina, Chapel Hill; and the Department of Public Health, Evans County, Georgia.

Reprint requests to Center for Cerebrovascular Research, Box 3203, Duke University Medical Center, Durham, NC 27710 (Dr. Heyman).

Methods

The first survey examination of this study population (3,102 persons) was carried out between Aug 1, 1960, and June 1, 1962, and consisted of a history of heart disease, stroke, and other illnesses; a physical examination; electrocardiogram; roentgenogram of the chest; urinalysis; and laboratory studies of the blood for cholesterol and hematocrit values. The second survey examination of this cohort was made by two of us (A. B. and S.H.) between Aug 1, 1967, and Aug 31, 1969, in a clinic established for this purpose. During this seven- to nine-year follow-up period (average, 87 months), 320 persons had died and 252 had either migrated away from the community or refused to return for the second examination (Table 1). The examination of the remaining 2,530 persons (90.9% reexamination rate) again consisted of a history, physical, and laboratory studies but also included a detailed questionnaire for evidence of cerebrovascular disease and symptoms of transient cerebral ischemia, a sociological questionnaire, and a physical activities questionnaire. All persons with a history of physical findings of any type of neurologic disorder and particularly those whose response to the questionnaire suggested transient cerebral ischemia or stroke were referred to the neurologists (A. H., and H. R. K.) and for further evaluation. In addition, the records containing the questionnaire responses of all 2,530 persons were reviewed by one of us (A. H.) and all persons having neurologic symptoms suggesting even a remote possibility of cerebrovascular disease were called back for neurologic evaluation. Examinations were conducted in the home of the subjects who were unable to visit the clinic because of disability due to stroke or other illnesses. Members of the subject's family were also interviewed if an adequate history could not be obtained because of aphasia, confusion, or memory loss due to brain damage.

A review was made by the neurologists of the clinical records to confirm the cause of death in each of the subjects whose death certificate listed stroke as a causative factor. Although autopsies were made in approximately 30% of the 320 deaths during this interval, the brain was usually not included in the postmortem examination. Spinal fluid and neuroradiologic diagnostic studies were rarely part of the clinical examination during the subject's terminal illness. For these reasons, differentiation of cerebral hemorrhage from cerebral infarction was generally not possible and no such distinction has been made in the individual subjects.

Criteria for the diagnosis of cerebrovascular disease were established for those examined by the neurologists and for the cases listed as having a stroke on death certificates. In both groups the subject was considered to have a *definite* stroke if there was a history of sudden onset of aphasia or hemiparesis and the appropriate neurologic or physical abnormalities were noted during the neurologists' examination or during the subject's terminal illness. Arteriographic, spinal fluid, or autopsy findings of cerebral thrombosis or hemorrhage were also considered to be evidence of definite cerebrovascular disease. Subjects were classified as having a *probable* stroke if, at the time of his examination, the neurologist obtained a definite history of sudden onset of aphasia or unilateral arm or leg weakness in vascular distribution, but no residual signs could be found on his examination. A diagnosis was made of death probably caused by cerebrovascular disease if the death certificate listed stroke as the underlying or contributing cause and if the clinical records indicated that the terminal illness began with sudden loss of consciousness without other explanation even though there was no mention in the clinical records of hemiplegia or focal neurologic deficits. Patients with transient cerebral ischemia only, ie, neurological deficit less than 24-hours duration, were not included in the present study.

The prevalence rate of stroke is the frequency and distribution of the disease found in the 2,530 persons reexamined in 1967 through 1969. The incidence rate of cerebrovascular disease is based on the number of persons developing a fatal or nonfatal stroke in the seven to nine year follow-up period among the 3,048 subjects who were judged free of the illness at the initial examination in 1960 through 1962.

Table 1.—Distribution of Sample Population by Age and Sex in the Two Survey Examinations

	White Men	White Women	Black Men	Black Women	Total
Cases in first examination (1960 to 1962)	947	972	537	646	3,102
Died 1960 to 1967	120	65	73	62	320
Migrated, refused, etc	56	52	78	66	252
Cases in second examination (1967 to 1969)	771	855	386	518	2,530
Percentage of eligible cases in second examination (1967 to 1969)	93.2%	94.3%	83.2%	88%	90.9%

Results

Prevalence of Cerebrovascular Disease.—During the second examination in 1967 through 1969, 75 persons were diagnosed as having a definite or probable stroke (57 and 18 cases, respectively). Of these, 53 had developed a stroke during the interval between the two survey examinations, and 22 had a history of cerebrovascular disease prior to the first examination in 1960 through 1962. The age-adjusted rates were higher in men than in women and were higher in blacks than in whites (Table 2). Black women had almost three times the rates of white women. Although the prevalence of stroke generally increased with age, this tendency was not as marked among black men who had moderately high rates in middle age (45 to 65 years). The diagnosis in almost every case was thought to be cerebral thrombosis since those with cerebral hemorrhage were not likely to have survived to be included in this reexamination. One subject, however, a black man, gave a good history of subarachnoid hemorrhage, and two other subjects (both white men) had a diagnosis of cerebral embolism.

These prevalence rates are not likely to be in error due to the inaccessability of persons who refused reexamination or migrated out of the community. This group consisted largely of young individuals, under the age of 35 years, in whom the likelihood of cerebrovascular disease is quite small.[6]

Incidence of Cerebrovascular Disease.—During the interval between the two examinations (an average of 87 months) cerebrovascular disease developed in 94 persons, in whom the diagnosis was definite in 65 cases and probable in 29 others (Table 3). Fifty-three of the 94 persons were alive at the time of the second examination. The remaining 41 died shortly after onset of their stroke. Twenty-three other subjects may also have had a stroke in the 1960 through 1967 interval but were excluded from this incidence table because of insufficient clinical information. They consisted of nine subjects who were said to have had a stroke, but died of other

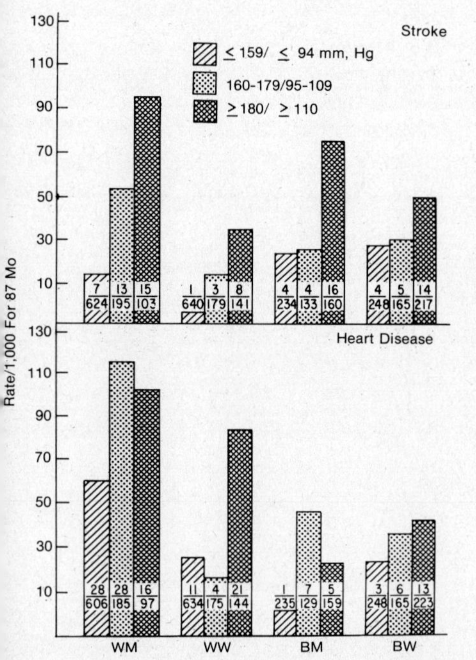

Fig 1.—Risk of stroke or ischemic heart dis-se according to blood pressure on entry—age-djusted. In this figure and in the subsequent es, the numbers within each bar indicate the pulation at risk in the denominator and the bjects developing either stroke or ischemic art disease in the numerator.

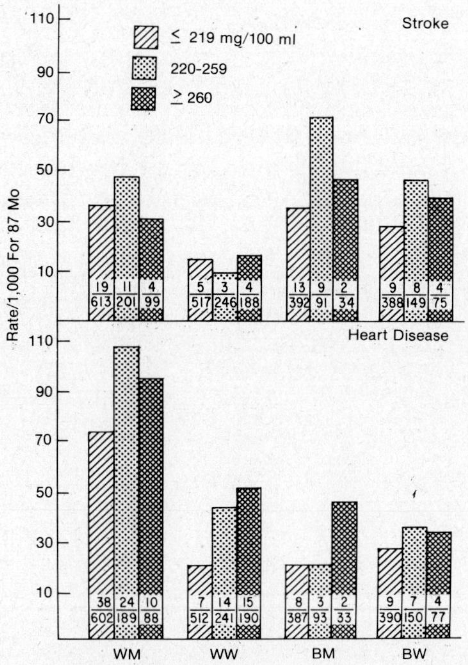

Fig 2.—Risk of stroke or ischemic heart disease according to level of serum cholesterol on entry—age-adjusted.

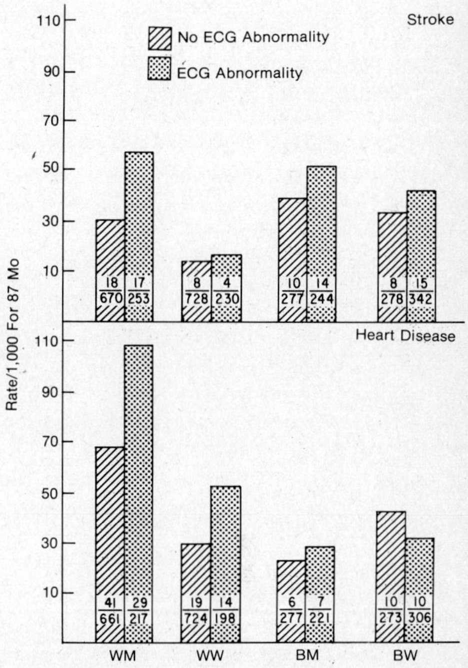

Fig 3.—Risk of stroke or ischemic heart disease according to ECG abnormalities on entry—age-adjusted.

causes. These cases were excluded because the clinical evidence for the diagnosis of stroke prior to death was poorly documented, particularly among the blacks. In 14 additional subjects stroke was listed on the death certificates as the underlying or contributory cause, but the information which was available in their medical records was not sufficient to confirm this diagnosis.

The age-adjusted incidence rates for cerebrovascular disease were highest among the black men (6.0/1,000/yr). The rates for white men,

Table 2.—Age-Specific Prevalence Rates of Stroke (per 1,000) Found in Examination, 1967 Through 1969

Age At Time of First Examination, yr	White Men			White Women			Black Men			Black Women		
	Population Examined	No. of Cases	Rate	Population Examined	No. of Cases	Rate	Population Examined	No. of Cases	Rate	Population Examined	No. of Cases	Rate
≦34	198	...	...	196	1	5.1	82	...	...	110	...	...
35-44	152	3	19.7	175	...	...	63	2	31.7	93	2	21.5
45-54	223	9	40.4	221	2	9.0	133	9	67.6	147	7	47.6
55-64	138	7	50.7	161	5	31.0	61	5	82.0	109	2	18.3
≧65*	60	9	150.0	102	3	29.4	47	2	42.6	59	7	118.6
Total												
≦35 yr	573	28		659	10		304	18		408	18	
All ages	771	28		855	11		386	18		518	18	
Age-adjusted rate												
≦35			53.2			15.0			58.6			43.4
All ages			40.9			12.7			45.0			33.4

* Only 11 persons were greater than 75 years of age, two of whom had cerebrovascular disease.

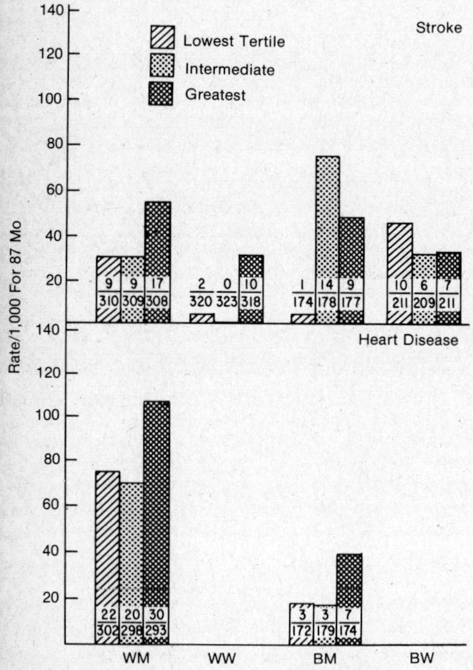

Fig 4.—Risk of stroke or ischemic heart disease according to degree of obesity (by tertiles)—age-adjusted.

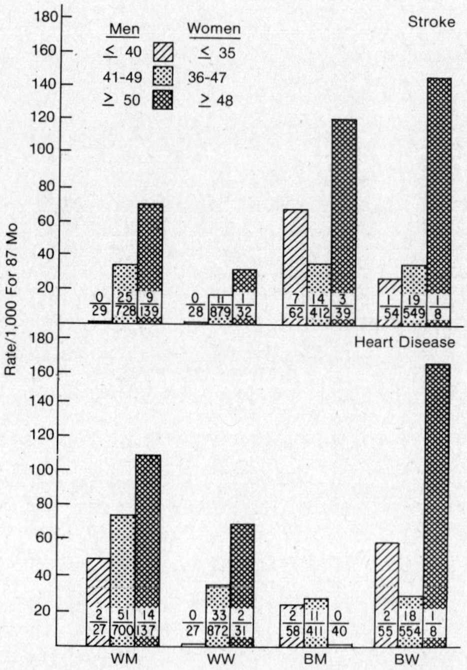

Fig 5.—Risk of stroke or ischemic disease according to level of hematocrit—age-adjusted.

however, were only slightly lower (5.3/1,000/yr). It should be noted that these age-adjusted rates underestimate the black-white differences. The white male population has a higher proportion of men aged 65 years and over than the black population. At all other ages the blacks have a higher incidence rate than the whites and particularly at the 55- to 64-year age group the blacks have a twofold excess. The rates for white and black women were 1.7 and 5.0/1,000/yr, respectively. After adjusting the county's age distribution to that of the 1950 United States populations, the estimated rate for white men was 4.7; for white women, 1.2; and for black men and black women, 5.8 each.

As shown in Table 3, the age-specific rates increased generally with advancing age. The white and black men, however, tended to have relatively high rates in their middle ages as well as in older age groups. The slight decreases in the incidence of stroke in white men aged 55 to 64 years and in black men 65 years or older probably represent artefacts resulting from inadequate documentation of the terminal illness of several men in these age-race groups. Although their clinical records suggested the possibility of stroke, the rigid criteria established in this study for the diagnosis of cerebrovascular disease did not permit their inclusion in the stroke category.

Comparison With Other Studies.—The annual age-specific incidence rates found in our white study population are compared in Table 4 with those found in other small population

Table 3.—Age-Specific Incidence Rates of New Cases of Stroke, 1960 Through 1969 (Cases/1,000/yr)

	White Men			White Women			Black Men			Black Women		
Age at Time of Initial Examination, yr	No. at Risk	No. of Cases	Rate	No. at Risk	No. of Cases	Rate	No. at Risk	No. of Cases	Rate	No. at Risk	No. of Cases	Rate
≦34	227	...	...	218	1	0.6	124	...	...	145	2 (2)	1.9
35-44	166	3 (1)*	2.5	189	...	...	79	2 (0)	3.5	111	2 (0)	2.5
45-54	257	12 (5)	6.4	237	2 (2)	1.2	167	9 (4)	7.4	165	6 (2)	5.0
55-64	168	7 (1)	5.8	179	4 (1)	3.1	86	8 (2)	12.8	125	5 (3)	5.5
≧65†	109	13 (6)	16.5	138	5 (4)	5.0	73	5 (4)	9.4	85	8 (4)	13.0
Total	927	35 (13)		961	12 (7)		529	24 (10)		631	23 (11)	
Age-adjusted rate (all ages)			5.3			1.7			6.0			5.0
Adjusted to US 1950 Population			4.7			1.2			5.8			5.8

* Figures in parentheses indicate number of subjects in whom the stroke was fatal.
† Only 24 persons were over 75 years of age, five of whom had developed cerebrovascular disease.

Table 4.—Age-Specific Annual Incidence Rates (per 1,000) for Stroke in Five US Population Studies*

Age (yr)	Evans County, Georgia	Middlesex County, Conn	Rochester, Minn	Framingham, Mass	Mid-Missouri
		White Men			
≦34	0	0	0.03	0.8	0
35-44	2.5	0	0.5	0.3	0
45-54	6.4	1.2	1.8	1.9	0.3
55-64	5.8	4.6	3.9	3.7	3.9
65-74	14.9	11.9	12.6	5.8	7.4
75-84	35.0	24.3	22.5	...	23.5
Age-adjusted rate—all ages	4.7†	1.9†	2.0†	2.1	2.2
		White Women			
≦34	0.6	0	0.02	0	0.3
35-44	0	0.2	0.2	0.4	0
45-54	1.2	1.0	1.4	1.2	0
55-64	3.1	3.5	3.5	2.7	2.6
65-74	5.4	7.2	9.5	8.9	4.6
75-84	0	20.0	22.2	...	22.5
Age-adjusted rate—all ages	1.2†	1.5†	1.8†	1.8	1.8

* Data from references 7 through 10.
† Adjusted to age distribution, US population, 1950.

studies.[7-10] It is apparent that the incidence of stroke in white men for all ages in Evans County is more than twice that found in other sections of the country. In contrast, the incidence figures for white women in our sample population are compatible with those found in the other studies. The only published report of the incidence of stroke in black men and women is the Mid-Missouri Stroke Survey[10] which is based on small numbers of cases. Nevertheless, the annual age-adjusted incidence rate obtained in three rural counties in Mid-Missouri was 5.9 (per 1,000 for all ages) for black men and 3.5 for black women, figures similar to those found in the Evans County black population.

Risk Factors.—The incidence rates for the initial episodes of either stroke or ischemic heart disease during the 87-month study period was determined in the sample population stratified according to the presence or absence of certain "risk" factors observed on entry into the study. An analysis was made of the following clinical and laboratory characteristics: arterial blood pressure, serum cholesterol and hematocrit levels, electrocardiographic findings, and body weight. The criteria for the diagnosis of ischemic coronary heart disease have been described elsewhere,[6] and include patients with acute myocardial infarction, angina pectoris, and other clinical evidence or arteriosclerotic heart disease.

Risk of Stroke or Ischemic Heart Disease According to Blood Pressure.—The age-adjusted incidence of cerebrovascular or ischemic heart disease according to the level of blood pressure on entry into the study is shown in Fig 1. The study population was classified into three blood pressure categories: those with normal or borderline pressures (equal to or less than 159/94 mm Hg), those with moderate hypertension (160 to 179/95 to 109 mm Hg), and those with severe hypertension (180/110 mm Hg or greater). While the gradient between level of blood pressure and disease was clearer in the case of stroke than in ischemic heart disease, hypertension clearly increased the risk of both diseases in all four race-sex groups.

Risk of Stroke or Ischemic Heart Disease According to Serum Cholesterol Levels.—The incidence of cerebrovascular disease in our subjects according to their level of serum cholesterol on entry into the study is shown in Fig 2. For the entire age range, the percentage of men or women (black or white) developing stroke was not significantly different in the subjects with low or intermediate cholesterol levels as compared with those with high cholesterol levels (260 mg/100 ml or greater). An analysis of the cholesterol levels among the stroke cases in the younger age groups (less than 55 years) likewise failed to show any significant relationships. In contrast, there is a modest relationship between ischemic heart disease and elevated serum cholesterol levels for whites, both men and women, and for black men though not for black women.

Risk of Stroke or Ischemic Heart Disease According to Electrocardiographic Abnormalities.—In white men, the presence of antecedent electrocardiographic abnormalities, (such as Q-waves, first-degree block, and ST-T abnormalities) was associated with a definite increase in susceptibility to stroke as well as ischemic heart disease (Fig 3). A slightly increased risk of developing cerebrovascular disease was also observed in black men and women with prior electrocardiographic changes. The association of electrocardiographic abnormalities with subsequent ischemic heart disease was also noted in white women, but not in black men or women.

Risk of Stroke or Ischemic Heart Disease According to Body Weight.—The degree of overweight in our subjects was determined by the Quetelet index (weight in pounds divided by the square of the height in inches) and the results were stratified into those with lowest, intermediate, and highest weight by height indices.[11] The risk of developing stroke or ischemic heart disease was increased in severely overweight white men and to some extent in black men as well (Fig 4). White women with the highest indices also seemed to be more susceptible to stroke, but surprisingly this relationship was not evident in black women. An analysis of the possible association of Quetelet index to ischemic heart disease in white and black women was not computed because of insufficient information.

Risk of Stroke or Ischemic Heart Disease According to Hematocrit.—As shown in Fig 5, white men and women with very high hematocrit levels had an increased risk of developing stroke or ischemic heart disease. Although a similar trend was present among black women with very high hematocrit levels, the number of cases of heart disease or stroke in this group was very small and the findings are not considered significant. It is apparent from these analyses that the clinical and laboratory characteristics favoring the development of stroke are not always the same as those associated with the development of ischemic heart disease.

Comment

The results of this study indicate that the incidence of cerebrovascular disease in this rural population of Southeastern Georgia is considerably higher than that in other sections of the country. Similar high stroke morbidity rates have been reported by Kuller and his associates in the white population of the nearby urban community of Savannah.[1] These workers also noted a high ratio of the incidence of stroke in men to that in women in this area of Georgia as well as in North Carolina. The reason for the increased incidence of stroke in the southeastern portion of the United States is not known, but there is evidence to suggest that the high prevalence of hypertension in this area of the country is one of the most important etiologic factors.[2]

The significance of hypertension and other risk factors in the development of stroke has been described in other prospective epidemiologic studies of cerebrovascular disease. Elevation of arterial blood pressure, particularly, is known to be a major predisposing factor in cerebral hemorrhage. In the study of Japanese men and women in Hiroshima, hypertension was associated with a definitely increased risk of developing cerebrovascular disease.[12] As in the present study, the degree of hypertension was found to be a more useful indicator of stroke than of ischemic heart disease. In the Framingham, Mass, population, hypertension increased the probability of developing cerebral thrombosis about fivefold over that of normotensive individuals.[13] In the Los Angeles study of male city employees reported by Chapman et al, there were 2% strokes among the normotensive population as compared to 9% among those with hypertension, the increased risk being more apparent in cerebral hemorrhage than in cerebral thrombosis.[14]

Our observations on the association of hypercholesterolemia with vascular disease have also been confirmed in other studies. Although high serum cholesterol levels are recognized as a risk factor in coronary artery disease, particularly in the younger age groups, its relationship to the development of cerebrovascular disease is less well established. Chapman et al reported little or no increase in the risk of stroke associated with high serum cholesterol levels except in those without hypertension.[14] In the Framingham population there was an increase in the incidence of stroke associated with elevated serum cholesterol levels only in subjects under the age of 50 years.[13] In older age groups, elevated lipid levels are not reliable indicators of susceptibility to either stroke or heart disease. Although the Hiroshima population generally had low cholesterol levels, hypercholesterolemia (values exceeding 220 mg/100 ml) was found to be associated with added risk of stroke in both men and women, particularly the latter.[12]

Our observations on the relationship of stroke to antecedent electrocardiographic abnormalities were also noted in the Framingham study. The presence of left ventricular hypertrophy, intraventricular block, and nonspecific electrocardiographic abnormalities were associated with a very high risk of cerebral infarction in the Framingham population.[13] Similarly, in Japanese men and women, electrocardiographic evidence of left ventricular hypertrophy (as well as cardiac enlargement by radiographic examination) increased the risk of stroke almost three to five times.[12]

Extreme obesity was found to be associated with an increase in the risk of stroke in men and in white women in the Evans County population. Similar findings were obtained in both the Framingham and Japanese populations.[12,13] The results of the Los Angeles study also suggested an increased risk of cerebral thrombosis with increasing weight.[14]

Only a very few studies have been reported on the relationship of high hematocrit levels to subsequent development of stroke. It is noteworthy that Japanese women with elevated hemoglobin or hematocrit levels seemed to have an increased risk of developing a stroke, but no significant association was found in Japanese men.[12] In the present study, there was some evidence to indicate that high hematocrit levels were associated with increased susceptibility of stroke in white and black men. The incidence of ischemic heart disease may also be higher in the white men and women with elevated hematocrit levels on entry into the study.

Many of the factors which were found in this study to increase the susceptibility to stroke have also been reported in other studies of cerebrovascular disease. Our observations on the incidence of stroke, however, differ from those noted in other areas of the country. In the northeastern and mid-western sections of the United States, for example, the incidence of stroke in white men is similar to (or perhaps only slightly higher than) that in women, whereas the rates for ischemic heart disease in men are usually several times that found in white women.[7,10] In our sample population, the incidence of stroke in white men was almost four times that of white women, a ratio even greater than that noted for ischemic heart disease in this community. Despite this similarity in the incidence of stroke and heart disease, the risk factors predisposing to stroke were not necessarily applicable to heart disease. It is noteworthy in this regard that relatively few of our subjects with ischemic heart disease developed cerebrovascular disease, a phenomena emphasized particularly in the Framingham study and frequently observed in clinical practice. The type of stroke most commonly associated with ischemic heart disease is that caused by atherosclerotic occlusive disease of the extracranial portion of the carotid or vertebral arteries or by cerebral embolism associated with cardiac arrhythmias, valvular disease, or mural thrombus due to recent myocardial infarction. It is our clinical impression that most of the subjects found to have stroke on neurologic examination had intracranial vascular disease. The usual manifestations of extracranial carotid disease such as a history of transient cerebral ischemia and the presence of carotid bruits were noted in only very few cases. The possibility that a specific type of stroke accounts for the race, sex, and area differences within the United States has been offered by Kuller and his associates.[1] They suggested that populations characterized by a high prevalence of hypertension and low lipid levels should have a higher ratio of intracranial to extracranial vascular disease. This particular combination of risk factors was a common pattern in our stroke cases and tends to support the hypothesis suggested by these workers.

This investigation was supported in part by Public Health research grants NS-HE-06233 and HE-03341.

William Stuart, MD, performed neurologic evaluations. Joan Cornoni, MPH, PhD, was responsible for data analysis. Linda Davis assisted with data analysis.

References

1. Kuller L, Bolker A, Saslaw MS, et al: Nationwide cerebrovascular disease morbidity study. *Stroke* **1**:86-99, 1970.
2. McDonough JR, Hames CG, Stulb SC, et al: Cardiovascular disease field study in Evans County, Ga. *Public Health Rep* **78**:1051-1059, 1963.
3. McDonough JR, Hanes CG, Stulb SC, et al: Coronary heart disease among negroes and whites in Evans County, Georgia. *J Chron Dis* **18**:443-468, 1964.
4. McDonough JR, Garrison GE, Hames CG: Blood pressure and hypertensive disease among Negroes and whites. *Ann Intern Med* **61**:208-228, 1964.
5. Cornoni JC, Waller LE, Cassel JC, et al: The incidence study—study design and methods. *Arch Intern Med* **128**:896-900, 1971.
6. Eisenberg H, Morrison JT, Sullivan P, et al: Cerebrovascular accidents: Incidence and survival rates in a defined population, Middlesex County, Connecticut. *JAMA* **189**:883-888, 1964.
7. Whisnant JP, Fitzgibbons JP, Kurland LT, et al: Natural history of stroke in Rochester, Minnesota, 1945 through 1954. *Stroke* **2**:11-21, 1971.
8. *Framingham Study: An Epidemiological Investigation of Cardiovascular Disease.* US Government Printing Office, 1968.
9. Eckstrom PT, Brand FR, Edlavitch SA, et al: Epidemiology of stroke in a rural area. *Public Health Rep* **84**:878-882, 1969.
10. Khosla T, Lowe CR: Indices of obesity derived from body weight and height. *Brit J Prev Soc Med* **21**:122-218, 1967.
11. Johnson KG, Yamo K, Kato H: Cerebral vascular disease in Hiroshima, Japan. *J Chron Dis* **20**:545-559, 1967.
12. Kannel WB, Dawber TR, McNamara PM, et al: Vascular disease of the brain—Epidemiologic aspects: The Framingham study. *Amer J Public Health* **55**:1355-1365, 1965.
13. Chapman JM, Reeder LG, Borun ER, et al: Epidemiology of vascular lesions affecting the central nervous system: The occurrence of strokes in a sample population under observation for cardiovascular disease. *Amer J Public Health* **56**:191-201, 1966.
14. Chapman JM, Clark VA, Coulson AH, et al: Risk factors and the development of stroke in the Los Angeles study area, abstracted. Read before the Council on Epidemiology, American Heart Association Meeting, New Orleans, 1970.

Weight and Weight History in Relation to Cerebrovascular and Ischemic Heart Disease

Siegfried Heyden, MD, Durham, NC; Curtis G. Hames, MD, Claxton, Ga; Alan Bartel, MD, Durham, NC; and John C. Cassel, MD, MPH; Herman A. Tyroler, MD; and Joan C. Cornoni, MPH, PhD, Chapel Hill, NC

The main findings from this study, as well as several others, tend to favor the concept of a definite risk factor of overweight *and* excessive weight gain after age 20 for the development of cerebrovascular disease. However, overweight and excessive weight gain after age 20 seem to be of no major importance in the etiology of myocardial infarction.

The relationship of weight to the development of stroke or of ischemic heart disease (IHD) is uncertain. Several studies have shown that overweight as measured in a variety of ways is a factor favoring the development of stroke and IHD. Other reports indicate only a slight or no relationship.

Relationship of Overweight to Stroke.—In the Los Angeles Epidemiologic Study of Vascular Disease the differences in stroke incidence according to relative body weight (based upon the index by Sheldon) were far less striking than the differences in the risk according to blood pressure. No association was found between weight and cerebral hemorrhage or nondifferentiated cerebrovascular disease. However, there appeared to be a gradient for *cerebral thrombosis* with rates of 5.6 in the lowest weight group, 13.7 in the intermediate, to 30.8 in the highest weight group.[1]

In a prospective study of cerebrovascular disease in Hiroshima, a significant correlation was noted between relative body weight and the risk of cerebrovascular disease, especially in women.[2]

In the Framingham Study[3] Kannel, on the basis of 16 years of experience, stated:

> The role of excess weight in atherosclerotic disease is rather uncertain. No significant nor impressive contribution of excess weight to the risk of any manifestation of atherosclerosis could be demonstrated . . . Obesity may be hazardous in brain infarction, particularly in subjects predisposed to stroke with hypertension and electrocardiographic abnormalities.

A positive relationship between obesity and stroke was noted by Paffenbarger and Wing[4] in a long-term follow-up study of college students: "Ponderal index differentiated subsequent cases of fatal stroke from controls at time of college case-tak-

Received for publication Sept 7, 1971; accepted Sept 16.

From the departments of community health sciences (Dr. Heyden) and cardiology (Dr. Bartel), Duke University Medical School, Durham, NC; and the Department of Epidemiology, University of North Carolina, Chapel Hill (Drs. Cassel, Tyroler, and Cornoni). Dr. Hames is in private practice in Evans County, Georgia.

Reprint requests to Department of Community Health Sciences, Duke University Medical School, Durham, NC 27710 (Dr. Heyden).

ing." They found a 50% increased risk of death from stroke for individuals with excesses of body weight.[4] In a longitudinal study of fatal coronary heart disease (CHD) and stroke in longshoremen, Paffenbarger et al[5] reported that

> an excess of CHD death rate of 35% attended men with body weight above mean levels as compared with the rate of those less heavy. Independent correlations between characteristics of high risk and coronary mortality suggested a rank order by decreasing strength of heavier cigarette smoking, higher blood pressure level, increased weight for height and physical activity of work.

Of the four risk factors, only systolic blood pressure correlated significantly with the risk of fatal stroke.[5]

Relationship Between Overweight and Ischemic Heart Disease.—Data from the Tecumseh Study suggest that an overweight condition increases the risk for the development of IHD independent of blood pressure (in men) and independent of its association with hyperglycemia and with serum cholesterol concentrations. Epstein et al concluded "that overweight is a definite risk factor in its own right and not merely a consequence of an association between overweight and high blood pressure."[6] However, Epstein admitted in his review article that the unexpected discrepancy among prospective epidemiological studies in regard to overweight and IHD is a paradox:

> At this time there is little doubt that obesity per se is a less potent risk factor than either serum cholesterol or blood pressure level so that control of obesity alone is not likely to make a major dent in the frequency of coronary disease.[7]

In a retrospective interracial comparison study of Japanese and Hawaiian men with myocardial infarction, "overweight, carbohydrate intolerance and hypertension were the factors . . . relate[d] most clearly to the very high coronary heart disease rate observed in Hawaiian men."[8]

Yes	No	
______	______	"Between the ages of 20 and (up to 35) did you gain weight?"
		If "YES",
	______	more than 10 lb?
	______	less than 10 lb?
		If "NO",
	______	did you lose weight?
	______	was your weight stable?
		"What was your approximate weight at ages"
______		20 yr
______		30 yr
______		40 yr
______		50 yr
______		60 yr
______		70 yr
		(Write xxx against nonapplicable age)
______		"What was your maximum weight?"
______		"What age were you?"

Questions used to obtain weight history and maximum weight gain.

There was no relationship between overweight and myocardial infarction in the findings of the International Cardiovascular Epidemiologic Study by Keys.[9] The Framingham Study reported that antecedent relative weight and gain in weight after age 25 were strongly related to the risk of angina pectoris and sudden death but not associated with myocardial infarction.[10]

The prevalence study by Spain et al[11] revealed that overweight per se is not an important contributory factor to the development of CHD. In fact, after exclusion of diabetics and hypertensive patients, overweight was not associated with a higher prevalence rate of CHD than normal or average weight. The authors concluded that the "relative muscle mass rather than an increase in adipose tissue probably has a more direct association with the prevalence of coronary atherosclerotic heart disease."[11]

Gofman and Young[12] spoke of the imperfect association of overweight and atherosclerosis and suggested as a reasonable implication of these findings "that overweight per se must be relatively or totally unimportant in acceleration of the process of atherosclerosis." Apart from the association of overweight with diastolic blood pressure level and with serum lipoprotein level, "no residual independent contribution of overweight per se to risk of coronary heart disease can be discerned."[12]

Gertler et al[13] are very outspoken on obesity and its relation to the "Coronary Profile":

> It is noteworthy that weight is absolutely useless as a classifier, and it is further emphasized that obesity was a very popular predictor at one time, but has now fallen into disuse in spite of the fact that this was pointed out by this group more than 15 years ago.[13]

Paul et al[14] found no statistically significant differences in mean height and weight between the noncoronary population and the coronary group in a prospective epidemiologic study of over four years' duration. The findings from this study suggested that endomorphic dominance may be important in the development of coronary disease since there was an excess of coronary cases in the group characterized by endomorphic dominance.[14]

The same group reporting on cere-

Table 1.—The Distribution of the Number of Cases of Cerebrovascular Disease and Ischemic Heart Disease for Men 40 Years of Age or Older in Each of the Defined Subgroups

Illness	Subgroups 1	2	3	4	Total
Cases of cerebrovascular disease	6	3	12	6	27
Cases of ischemic heart disease total	12	5	16	4	37
Cases of myocardial infarction only	8	1	11	3	23
Cases of angina pectoris only	2	1	4	1	8
Total No. of persons at risk	150	59	204	69	482

Table 2.—Age Adjusted Incidence of Stroke (Survivors Only) in White Men by Weight at Age 20 and Degree of Weight Gain

	Weight at Age 20	
	≤68.0 kg (150 lb)	>150 lb
Max weight, ≤30	38	52
Gain >30	59	90

Table 3.—Age Adjusted Incidence of Ischemic Heart Disease (Survivors Only) in White Men by Weight at Age 20 and Degree of Weight Gain

	Weight at Age 20	
	≤150 lb	>150 lb
Max weight ≤30	76	97
Gain >30	84	66

Table 4.—Age Adjusted Incidence of Myocardial Infarction (Survivors Only) in White Men by Weight at Age 20 and Degree of Weight Gain

	Weight at Age 20	
	≤150 lb	>150 lb
Max weight ≤30	51	(19)*
Gain >30	57	49

*Rate is based on one case only.

brovascular disease incidence in Hiroshima stated that, in contrast to cerebrovascular disease, overweight is of no predictive value in CHD.[15]

One of the possible reasons for those conflicting findings is that in all the studies reviewed, with the exception of the paper by Kannel et al,[10] the only relationship examined was between obesity or overweight in middle-age and incidence of either stroke or IHD. The possibility exists that weight in young adulthood may be more importantly related to subsequent cerebrovascular or cardiovascular disease than weight in middle-age, or alternatively, the degree of weight gain—after growth has been completed—may be the biologically more important process.

This paper, then, is an attempt to explore the relationship between weight at age 20 and subsequent weight gain to the incidence of stroke and IHD.

Method

The first survey examination of this study population (3,102 persons) was carried out between Aug 1, 1960, and June 1, 1962, and consisted of a history of heart disease, stroke, and other illnesses, a physical examination, electrocardiogram, roentgenogram of the chest, urinalysis, and laboratory studies of the blood for cholesterol level and hematocrit reading. The second survey examination of this cohort was made by two of the authors (A. B. and S. H.) between Aug 1, 1967, and Aug 31, 1969, in a clinic established for this purpose. During this seven to nine year follow-up period (average, 87 months), 320 persons had died and 252 had either migrated away from the community or refused to return for the second examination. The examination of the remaining 2,530 persons (90.9% reexamination rate) again consisted of a history, physical examination, and laboratory studies, but also included a detailed questionnaire for evidence of cerebrovascular disease and symptoms of transient cerebral ischemia, a sociological questionnaire, and a physical activities questionnaire.

In 1960-1962, 93 cases of IHD were diagnosed, leaving 3,009 persons at risk of developing the disease over the following 87 month period. A detailed description of the response rates and the incidence and prevalence rates by age, ethnic group, and sex is given in the paper by Cassel et al (p 901).

For purposes of this study IHD referred to sudden death, myocardial infarction, angina pectoris, and chronic heart disease. Sudden death was defined as any unexpected death occurring within 24 hours after the patient was last seen alive, if unattended, and within one hour if attended. In addition, any one of three findings was adequate for a designation of IHD. These included angina pectoris, a history of myocardial infarction, or an ECG consistent with myocardial infarction. The World Health Organization criteria were used for defining angina pectoris and a history of myocardial infarction.[16] Criteria used for the evaluation of the ECG were essentially the class I, Q, and QS patterns of Blackburn and Keys.[17] ST segment depression and T wave inversion were not used. Chronic heart disease was considered to be probably arteriosclerotic in origin when diagnosed at age 40 or older in the presence of heart failure or chronic arrhythmia and in the absence of angina pectoris, myocardial infarction, or any other cardiac disorder, including hypertension.

During the 1967-1969 examination of the Evans County, Georgia, population each individual was asked in detail about his weight at age 20 and the subsequent maximum weight gain. The specific questions used to obtain this information are given in the Figure. The analysis in this paper is limited to white men over 40 years of age, since there was only a small number of cases surviving stroke or IHD in the other three sex and ethnic groups.

It might be argued that we are relying on poorly reproducible data when asking a person to recall his weight at age 20. However, the white persons in our sample did appear to be certain of their weight at age 20 and their maximum weight gain. Weight at age 20 in white men generally coincided with army induction or college attendance.

Results

The weight history (ie, the weight at age 20 and subsequent maximum weight gain) could only be obtained in survivors who lived to be examined in 1967-1969. As a result, any conclusions may be biased by selective survival with the possibility existing that those who were heaviest at age 20 or who showed maximal weight gain may already have died. Any relationships found in this investigation, therefore, might well underrepresent the true relationship.

The following groups were defined to study the possible relationships. White men were categorized at age 20 as being above or below 150 lb (68 kg) and maximal weight gain in subsequent years classified into 30 lb (13.6 kg) or less and 31 lb (14.1 kg) or more.

Subgroup 1.—Weight at age 20 less than 150 lb, maximum weight gain 30 lb or less.

Subgroup 2.—Weight at age 20, 150 lb or greater, maximum weight gain 30 lb or less.

Subgroup 3.—Weight at age 20 less than 150 lb, maximum weight gain over 30 lb.

Subgroup 4.—Weight at age 20, 150 lb or greater, maximum weight gain over 30 lb.

The number of white men in each of these subgroups is given in Table 1.

Table 5.—Correlation Coefficients of Weight and Blood Pressure

	P	
	Weight Gain	Weight at Age 20
Systolic blood pressure	.118	.011
Diastolic blood pressure	.285	.028

Table 2 shows the relationship of weight at age 20 and subsequent weight gain to the incidence of stroke and definite transient ischemic attacks among the survivors of the 1960 cohort. In each case we were able to determine the age at maximum weight, and in none of the stroke patients did this maximum weight gain occur after the clinical event. The lowest incidence rates of cerebrovascular disease were found in individuals who at age 20 weighed less than 150 lb and had gained less than 30 lb, and the highest incidence rates were found in individuals who weighed over 150 lb at age 20 and gained more than 30 lb.

Further, it can be seen that both weight at age 20 and degree of weight gain exert an independent effect on subsequent cerebrovascular disease incidence. Among those individuals who gained less than 30 lb, for example, the incidence rate of stroke was 38 if they weighed 150 lb or less at age 20, but 52 if they weighed more than 150 at that age. A similar effect of weight at age 20 is manifest in those who gained more than 30 lb, where the relevant cerebrovascular disease rates are 59 for the "lean" at age 20 and 90 for the "heavy" men. On the other hand weight gain itself is shown to have an effect on subsequent incidence, regardless of whether the subjects were below or above 150 lb at age 20, the rates increasing from 38 to 59 in the former and from 52 to 90 in the latter.

In contrast, as seen in Table 3, weight at age 20 and subsequent weight changes did not correlate with IHD. Reanalyzing this, the data for those individuals who had myocardial infarction (ie, excluding the cases of angina pectoris without myocardial infarction and the so-called chronic heart disease cases) were separated out and there was again no correlation demonstrated between weight history and myocardial infarction (Table 4). This confirms the report from the Framingham Study.[10]

With only eight cases of angina pectoris among survivors (white men) in our incidence study, it is impossible to state any association with either weight gain or weight at age 20. The Framingham Study reported that antecedent relative weight and gain in weight after 25 years of age was strongly related to the risk of angina pectoris and sudden death but not associated with myocardial infarction.[10]

Reported weight at age 20 and degree of weight gain since age 20 thus seems to be related to the risk of developing cerebrovascular disease but not to IHD. One possible explanation for these findings may be in the relationship between body weight history and level of blood pressure. While elevated blood pressure increases the risk of both stroke and IHD, hypertension is more strongly related to cerebrovascular than cardiovascular complications.

To explore this possibility, a stepwise regression analysis was calculated to examine the relationship between reported weight at age 20 and reported amount of weight gained to systolic and diastolic blood pressure. A statistically significant relationship between weight change and both systolic and diastolic blood pressure was found, while the relationship between weight at age 20 and blood pressure levels was not significant. The beta value for weight change was significant at the .01 level. The beta value for weight at age 20 was not significant. (The correlation coefficients are shown in Table 5.) From this analysis it would appear likely that the effect of weight gain on the subsequent occurrence of stroke is mediated through the rise in blood pressure that accompanies such an increase. Weight in young adulthood, however, is related to subsequent stroke through some mechanism other than a rise in blood pressure.

Comment

With decreasing physical activity, usually occurring in white men around age 20 (after completion of military service, marriage, in many instances related to regular meal pattern, taking up predominantly sedentary occupations, etc), *any* weight increase beyond age 20 can be regarded as pure accumulation of adipose fat tissue. It is noteworthy that about 80% of the world's population maintain their weight at (and without appreciably rising after) age 25, whereas European and North American standards "allow" for increases in weight from one decade to the next.[18]

At age 20 musculoskeletal growth is usually completed and the rapid and often excessive weight gain at this point in life in our sedentary society therefore represents no further muscular development but rather an excess of fat tissue. The concomitant development of hypercholesterolemia, hypertriglyceridemia, hyperuricemia, hyperglycemia, and hypertension have all been well documented.[19] But the discrepancy in the consequences of these hemodynamic and metabolic changes in regard to the development of myocardial infarction and thrombotic brain infarction is not understood. An explanation of this paradox is impossible at this time. The fact that obesity is so common in the United States that a differentiating effect is lost has been mentioned frequently. It is rather unlikely that this is true since there is a very strong relationship between overweight and stroke on the one hand, and a very low or absent relationship between overweight and myocardial infarction on the other hand.

An additional unexpected puzzle is the observation from the Framingham Study that the development of angina pectoris and sudden death are strongly related to obesity and weight gain, whereas myocardial infarction is not related to obesity or weight gain. (However, in the Evans County Study, overweight is not related to sudden death!) Since changes in body weight are known to affect blood pressure and cholesterol levels it is possible that the contribution of excess weight to the increased risk of angina pectoris and sudden death is due to the association with the level of blood pressure and cholesterol. However, this would again not explain the absent association between overweight and myocardial infarction. It was, therefore, interesting that Kannel et al reported that "even among those men who had neither an elevated blood pressure nor cholesterol level the obese appeared to develop an excess of angina pectoris or sudden death. Conversely, independent effects of blood pressure and cholesterol level, quite distinct from the effects of adiposity, are also operative."[10] Our conclusion from the presently available data is that this problem of the relationship between overweight and *different manifestations of ischemic heart disease* may only be resolved through future long-term observations. It may well turn out that the obvious statistical discrepancies without a valid biologic explanation could be artifacts on the basis of small numbers of actual cases.

References

1. Chapman JM, Reeder LG, Borum ER, et al: Epidemiology of vascular lesions affecting the central nervous system: The occurrence of strokes in a sample population under observation for cardiovascular disease. *Amer J Public Health* **56**:191-201, 1966.
2. Johnson KG, Yano K, Kato H: Cerebral vascular disease in Hiroshima, Japan. *J Chronic Dis* **20**:545-559, 1967.
3. Kannel WB: Epidemiology of cerebrovascular disease: An epidemiologic study of cerebrovascular disease, in Millikan CH, Siekert RG, Whisnant JP, (eds): *Cerebrovascular Disease.* New York, Grune & Stratton Inc, 1966.
4. Paffenbarger RS Jr, Wing AL: Characteristics in youth predisposing to fatal stroke in later years. *Lancet* **1**:753-754, 1967.
5. Paffenbarger RS Jr, Laughlin ME, Gima AS, et al: Work activity of longshoremen as related to death from coronary heart disease and stroke. *N Eng J Med* **282**:1109-1114, 1970.
6. Epstein FH, Ostrander LD Jr, Johnson BC, et al: Epidemiologic studies of cardiovascular disease in a total community–Tecumseh, Michigan. *Ann Intern Med* **62**:1170-1187, 1965.
7. Epstein FH: The epidemiology of coronary heart disease: A review. *J Chronic Dis* **18**:735-774, 1965.
8. Basset DR, Moellering RC Jr, Rosenblatt G, et al: III. Coronary heart disease in Hawaii: Serum lipids, and cardiovascular, anthropometric, and related findings in Japanese and Hawaiian men. *J Chronic Dis* **21**:565-583, 1969.
9. Keys A: *Coronary Heart Disease in Seven Countries*, American Heart Association monograph 29. New York, American Heart Association, 1970.
10. Kannel WB, LeBauer EJ, Dawber TR, et al: Relation of body weight to development of coronary heart disease: The Framingham study. *Circulation* **35**:734-744, 1967.
11. Spain DM, Nathan DJ, Gellis M: Weight, body type and the prevalence of coronary atherosclerotic heart disease in males. *Amer J Med Sci* **245**:63-69, 1963.
12. Gofman JW, Young W: The filtration concept of atherosclerosis and serum lipids in the diagnosis of atherosclerosis, in Sandler M, Bourne GH, (eds): *Atherosclerosis and Its Origin.* New York, Academic Press Inc, 1963, pp 197-230.
13. Gertler MM, White PD, Cady LD, et al: Coronary heart disease. *Amer J Med Sci* **248**:377-398, 1964.
14. Paul O, Lepper MH, Phelan WH, et al: A longitudinal study of coronary heart disease. *Circulation* **28**:20-31, 1963.
15. Johnson KG, Yano K, Kato H: Coronary heart disease in Hiroshima, Japan: A report of a six-year period of surveillance, 1958-1964. *Amer J Public Health* **58**:1355-1367, 1968.
16. World Health Organization: Hypertension and coronary heart disease: Classification and criteria for epidemiological studies. *WHO Techn Rep Ser* No. 168, 1959.
17. Blackburn H, Keys A, Simonson E, et al: The electrocardiogram in population studies: A classification system. *Circulation* **21**:1160-1175, 1960.
18. McGanity WJ: Obesity. *JAMA* **186**:39-40, 1963.
19. Heyden S: Weight gain after reaching adulthood versus obesity, in Schettler FG, Boyd GS, (eds): *Atherosclerosis.* Amsterdam, Elsevier Press Inc, 1969, pp 234-244.

Angina Pectoris and the Rose Questionnaire

Siegfried Heyden, MD, and Alan G. Bartel, MD, Durham, NC;
Enayatollah Tabesh, MD, Dayton, Ohio; John C. Cassel, MD, MPH; Herman A. Tyroler, MD;
and Joan C. Cornoni, MPH, PhD, Chapel Hill, NC; and Curtis G. Hames, MD, Claxton, Ga

White men who responded positively to the Rose questionnaire but who were judged on clinical grounds to be free of angina pectoris resembled true cases of angina pectoris insofar as their blood pressure and cholesterol level was concerned. This was true for results obtained at the time of the current examination, as well as those taken seven years prior to this examination. Variability in response to the questionnaire at an interval of one year was assessed. "True" cases of angina showed as much variation (changing from positive to negative responses) as did the "false positives." This would suggest that, in large part, this variation is a reflection of the natural history of the disease rather than unreliability of the questionnaire. The Rose questionnaire was found to have a sensitivity of 81% and a specificity of 97% when compared to clinical judgment.

After 4½ years of a prospective epidemiologic study, Paul and co-workers reported findings on the association of a history of chest pain among 2,080 men at intake examination to subsequent coronary heart disease.[1] Of particular interest was the follow-up of men who, at the time of the first examination, gave a history of some type of chest discomfort which was not considered adequate for a diagnosis of angina pectoris. Among those who eventually developed coronary heart disease, 31% gave a positive history of "noncardiac" chest discomfort, whereas only 16% of those who did not develop clinical coronary disease gave such a history.[1]

Many clinicians are aware of the vagaries of an atypical history of angina pectoris. There is usually a ready agreement between cardiologists when a patient gives a history of exertional chest pain, lasting less than five minutes and relieved by rest and nitroglycerin, but so-called noncardiac chest discomfort without any obvious muscle or bone pathologic findings in the chest can be a serious challenge to the responsibility of the cardiologist.

The Rose questionnaire[2,3] was designed to help discriminate between cardiac and noncardiac chest pain. It was introduced to elicit angina pectoris not in the physician's office but in the general community and has been used in many countries around the world on an experimental basis. In the Evans County study this questionnaire was administered (in addition to a complete medical examination) to 2,500 adults, black and white, men and women. Results will be presented only on the case findings among the white men.

The purpose of this paper is twofold: (1) to discuss the validity of the Rose questionnaire for detecting angina pectoris when compared with the clinical diagnosis by the physician, and (2) to describe certain characteristics associated with a positive response to the questionnaire. We are particularly interested in comparing the characteristics of persons with a positive response to the Rose ques-

Received for publication May 13, 1971; accepted July 26.

From the Department of Community Health Sciences, Duke University (Dr. Heyden) and the Department of Cardiology, Duke University Medical Center (Dr. Bartel), Durham, NC; departments of cardiology and medicine, Veterans Administration Hospital, Dayton, Ohio (Dr. Tabesh); and the Department of Epidemiology, University of North Carolina, Chapel Hill (Drs. Cassel, Tyroler, and Cornoni). Dr. Hames is with the Evans County Health Department, Claxton, Ga.

Reprint requests to Department of Community Health Sciences, Duke University, Durham, NC (Dr. Heyden).

Table 1.—Distribution of Cases by Clinical Evaluation and Rose Questionnaire Response

Rose Questionnaire Response	Clinical Evaluation of Angina Pectoris: Positive	Negative	Totals
Positive	Group 1 n = 25	Group 2 n = 22	47
Negative	Group 3 n = 6	Group 4 n = 712	718
Total	31	734	765

tionnaire whose cases were diagnosed by the physician as angina pectoris with those who responded positively to the Rose questionnaire but whose cases were not diagnosed as angina pectoris. The latter group may harbor undetected ischemic heart disease with "noncardiac" chest discomfort, and, therefore, we wish to identify these persons by differences in selected characteristics.

Methods

In the Evans County population we recorded a positive response for those who answered positively to the following questions (section A of the Rose questionnaire)[2]:

1. Have you ever had any pain or discomfort in your chest? (yes)
2. Do you get it when you walk uphill or hurry? (yes)
3. Do you get it when you walk at an ordinary pace on the level? (yes or no)
4. What do you do if you get it while you are walking? (stop or slow down)
5. If you stand still, what happens to it? (relieved)
6. How soon? (ten minutes or less)
7. Will you show me where it was? (indicate where pain was)
8. Do you feel it anywhere else? (yes or no)
9. Did you see a doctor because of this pain (or discomfort)? (yes or no; if yes, what did he say it was)

Table 2.—Age Adjusted Means of Diastolic Blood Pressure by Response and Evaluation Groups (1967-1969 Data)

Rose Questionnaire Response	Clinical Evaluation of Angina Pectoris: Positive	Negative
Positive	Group 1 84.4 n = 25	Group 2 93.8 n = 22
Negative	Group 3 95.8 n = 6	Group 4 87.2 n = 712

Table 3.—Age Adjusted Means of Systolic Blood Pressure by Response and Evaluation Groups (1967-1969 Data)

Rose Questionnaire Response	Clinical Evaluation of Angina Pectoris: Positive	Negative
Positive	Group 1 140.2 n = 25	Group 2 152.3 n = 22
Negative	Group 3 153.0 n = 6	Group 4 141.7 n = 712

The questionnaire was administered to 768 white men, age 22 to 78 in 1967, who were the survivors of all the Evans County white males aged 40 to 70 in 1960 and a 50% random sample of those aged 15 to 39 in 1960. Data on the clinical status of three of these men was incomplete at the time of this analysis, and the report is thus restricted to 765 subjects.

After completion of the questionnaire, a regular interview was conducted by the examining physician in which the medical history and history of possible chest pain was elicited in the usual fashion. At the end of the examination, the physicians reached their conclusion as to the presence or absence of ischemic heart disease and assigned a diagnosis of definite, probable, possible or negative ischemic heart disease to each case. All cases with a diagnosis of possible, probable, or definite angina pectoris were presented to a cardiologist who reached his conclusion after taking his own history and doing a thorough clinical examination.

At the end of the study in 1969 a panel of two cardiologists, the two examining physicians, and two epidemiologists conducted a chart review of every case initially diagnosed as possible, probable, or definite coronary heart disease. At this session the 1960 chart, including electrocardiogram; the 1967 chart, including ECG; and the additional notes from the cardiologist were reviewed. The two cardiologists made their decision as to the possible, probable, or definite status of angina pectoris independently of results of the Rose questionnaire. The Rose questionnaire was considered an experimental tool for the diagnosis of chest pain in the general population and, therefore, never influenced the clinical diagnosis of angina pectoris by the two cardiologists.

Results

Since a standard is necessary for measuring validation, the final clinical diagnosis by the two cardiologists was accepted as the criterion for comparison. Table 1 gives the number responding positively or negatively to the Rose questionnaire in relation to the clinical diagnosis. In a total of 712 men, the response to the Rose questionnaire was essentially negative, and the clinical evaluation based on the examination and interview was that these men did not suffer from angina pectoris. The men in this group, therefore, can be termed to be true negatives and comprise group 4 in our analysis.

There were six cases of clinically diagnosed angina pectoris, with negative response to the Rose questionnaire. These "false negatives" comprise group 3 in Table 1.

Because of our interest in the delineation of risk factors associated with

Table 4.—Age Adjusted Means of Cholesterol Level by Response and Evaluation Groups (1967-1969 Data)

Rose Questionnaire Response	Clinical Evaluation of Angina Pectoris	
	Positive	Negative
Positive	Group 1 221.4 n = 25	Group 2 223.0 n = 22
Negative	Group 3 230.1 n = 6	Group 4 212.0 n = 712

Table 5.—Age Adjusted Means of Diastolic Blood Pressure by Response and Evaluation Groups (1960-1962 Data)

Rose Questionnaire Response	Clinical Evaluation of Angina Pectoris	
	Positive	Negative
Positive	Group 1 90.1 n = 25	Group 2 92.5 n = 22
Negative	Group 3 93.1 n = 6	Group 4 86.1 n = 712

a positive response to the Rose questionnaire, our analysis centered around the two remaining groups. In group 1, the "true positives" (n = 25), the cardiologists came to the conclusion that angina pectoris was present (probable or definite), and in group 2, the "false positives" (n = 22), with a similarly positive response to the Rose questionnaire, the cardiologists came to the conclusion that angina pectoris was not present.

Table 1 shows the distribution of the cases in relation to both the clinical diagnosis and the response to the Rose questionnaire. Validation was assessed in terms of sensitivity, the percent of clinically judged positive identified as positive by the test; and specificity, the percent of clinically judged negatives identified by the test as negative. The validity of the Rose questionnaire was tested in an earlier study by Rose,[4] and he concluded that the questionnaire diagnosis of angina showed reasonable (about 83%) sensitivity and high specificity as compared with diagnosis by physicians. In another study Rose tests the validity of the questionnaire by comparison with ECG findings.[3] By calculating these measures in our study, the sensitivity of the Rose questionnaire is 81% and the specificity, 97%.

For the purpose of this paper, two risk factors—serum cholesterol level and blood pressure—will be considered in association with the results from the Rose questionnaire. These risk factors were first considered in terms of the average values reported for each of the defined groups at the time of the 1967-1969 examinations when the Rose questionnaire was administered. Second, the mean values of these two risk factors measured in 1960-1962 for these same groups were examined as an estimate of their predictive power. Since there was a slight difference in the mean age among the four groups, with those in group 1 being oldest, all the means of the two risk factors were adjusted for this variable.

For the 1967-1969 results, the highest means for diastolic and systolic blood pressure and cholesterol level were found in group 3, those with clinically diagnosed angina pectoris but a negative Rose questionnaire. However, little can be inferred from this group since it represents only six men. It is interesting to find that among all those who were judged on clinical grounds to be free of angina pectoris, those with a positive Rose questionnaire (group 2) had a higher mean diastolic and systolic blood pressure and mean cholesterol level than the group who were true negatives. While the only difference that achieved statistical significance (at the 5% level) was diastolic blood pressure, the consistency of this pattern given the small number of subjects involved is quite impressive (Tables 2-4).

Table 6.—Age Adjusted Means of Systolic Blood Pressure by Response and Evaluation Groups (1960-1962 Data)

Rose Questionnaire Response	Clinical Evaluation of Angina Pectoris	
	Positive	Negative
Positive	Group 1 145.1 n = 25	Group 2 143.5 n = 22
Negative	Group 3 137.0 n = 6	Group 4 137.3 n = 712

Table 7.—Age Adjusted Means of Cholesterol Level by Response and Evaluation Groups (1960-1962 Data)

Rose Questionnaire Response	Clinical Evaluation of Angina Pectoris	
	Positive	Negative
Positive	Group 1 216.6 n = 25	Group 2 213.7 n = 22
Negative	Group 3 183.7 n = 6	Group 4 201.2 n = 705

The 1960-1962 examination data showed similar results (Tables 5-7). The means of diastolic and systolic blood pressure and cholesterol were higher in group 2 than in those men also judged to be free of angina pectoris but who responded negatively to the Rose questionnaire (group 4). In this analysis, also, the difference in the mean diastolic pressure achieved significance at the 5% level.

Thus, on two separate occasions—at the time of this examination and seven years prior to this—white men complaining of atypical chest pain were shown to have somewhat higher risk factors than men without this complaint. Should these results be confirmed by replication, it would not be unrealistic to suggest that men with atypical "noncardiac" chest pain, ie, those responding positively to the Rose questionnaire but judged clinically free of angina pectoris, are at increased risk of ischemic heart disease and should be followed-up by means of exercise ECG and, if feasible, by coronary angiography.

Repeatability of the Rose Questionnaire Over Time

All subjects in groups 1 and 2 were reinterviewed one year following their examination, and the Rose questionnaire was readministered. Of the 25 subjects in group 1, 2 died of myocardial infarction, 13 gave the same answers to the Rose questionnaire as they had previously, and 10 patients changed their answers from "yes" to "no." Of the 22 persons in group 2, 11 gave negative and 11, positive responses to the questionnaire.

These results are not very dissimilar from those obtained by Rose.[4] On reinterviewing 995 of 1,136 men who had originally answered the Rose questionnaire, he found that one year later 14 of the 33 initially positive were still positive. From the data available to him, however, he could not determine to what extent this variability in response was a function of variations in anginal symptoms over time and to what extent it represented unreliability of the questionnaire. If the men in group 1 in the Evans County study are regarded as true cases of angina (both on the grounds of the clinical diagnosis and the subsequent high coronary heart disease mortality in this group), a large proportion of the variability in response is a function of the natural history of this disease.

Implications for Identification of Early Coronary Disease

Currently, there is general consensus that one of the more accurate methods for identification of early coronary artery involvement is coronary angiography. Even this procedure, however, does not provide a foolproof method for the diagnosis of ischemic heart disease.

From a recent study conducted by Dwyer et al,[5] it would appear that even patients with normal coronary arteriograms can have angina pectoris. Detailed analyses of the clinical and hemodynamic features in 10 patients with angina pectoris but normal coronary arteriograms, and 11 patients with angina and abnormal coronary arteriograms demonstrated many of the high risk features and physical findings expected in atherosclerotic heart disease (eg, abnormal lipid and carbohydrate metabolism, family history of diabetes or coronary artery disease, abnormal ECG after exercise, heavy smoking history) occurred with the same frequency in both groups. In addition, James[6] had drawn attention to the possibility that an unknown number of patients with angina without coronary disease on angiography have occlusive disease of the small coronary arteries (0.1 to 1.0 mm in diameter), in the terminal distribution of all the coronary arteries. In most coronary arteriograms it is impossible to make any interpretation at all concerning small coronary arteries, but James feels that "it is improbable that the majority of patients with angina and allegedly normal coronary arteriograms have abnormal small coronary arteries."[6] He points out that errors in interpretation of arteriograms can easily occur, and that the incidence of such errors is inversely related to the experience of the coronary angiographer. The conclusion seems to be justified that selected coronary angiography is not the sole answer in the detection of ischemic heart disease but will be a valuable help in evaluating the extent of coronary atherosclerosis in most patients with chest pain. On the other hand, it is obviously not the generally available diagnostic method in the community. Until other methods have been invented, it seems advisable to consider a positive response to the Rose questionnaire in association with elevated blood pressure and cholesterol levels as indirect indicator of underlying ischemic heart disease. This suggestion receives additional support from a study by Lim et al[7] who found that eight (30%) of 24 patients with atypical chest pain had destructive changes in the coronary arteries when examined by coronary angiography. Follow-up observations over the next three to five years of the group in Evans County with positive responses to the Rose questionnaire but judged clinically negative for angina pectoris will provide more definitive answers to this possibility.

References

1. Paul O, Lepper MH, Phelan WH, et al: A longitudinal study of coronary heart disease. *Circulation* **28**:20-31, 1963.
2. Rose GA, Blackburn H: *Cardiovascular Survey Methods.* Geneva, World Health Organization, 1968, annex 6, p 172.
3. Rose GA: Chest pain questionnaire. *Milbank Mem Fund* **43**:32-39, 1965.
4. Rose GA: The diagnosis of ischemic heart pain and intermittent claudication in field surveys. *Bull WHO* **27**:645-658, 1962.
5. Dwyer EM, Wiener L, Cox JW: Angina pectoris in patients with normal and abnormal coronary arteriograms. *Amer J Cardiol* **23**:639-646, 1969.
6. James TN: Angina without coronary disease (sic). *Circulation* **42**:189-191, 1970.
7. Lim HF, Dreifus LS, Kasparian H, et al: Chest pain, coronary artery disease and coronary cine-arteriography. *Chest* **57**:41-46, 1970.

The major findings of family aggregation of blood pressure in the Evans County Prevalence Survey are that (1) similarities for first degree genetic relatives, as measured by correlation coefficients, are of the same order of magnitude in blacks and whites and of the same order of magnitude as reported in other populations; (2) categorical, mating-type analysis applied to the data indicates the dependence of offspring prevalence of both systolic and diastolic high blood pressure upon parental type, and this is greater in the white than the black; (3) evidence from both categorical and correlational analyses indicates spouse similarity in the white pairs, not in the black pairs; and (4) for white spouse pairs aggregation is a function of wife's age and is maximal at approximately the age of 50 years.

Family Aggregation of Blood Pressure in Evans County, Georgia

Carl G. Hayes, MPH, PhD; Herman A. Tyroler, MD; and John C. Cassel, MD, Chapel Hill, NC

The study of family aggregation in cardiovascular epidemiology is of importance for both theoretic and substantive reasons. Interest focused on aggregation of risk factors, in addition to aggregation of the diseases themselves, promises insights into the processes responsible for population distributions. A priori, it would be anticipated that most health-relevant characteristics would be determined by family factors; the joint effect of genetic and cultural transmission mechanisms, plus shared physical and social environments, could be predicted to maximize similarities of individuals within families. Each variable studied in this manner, however, must be subjected to the empiric test. There are, for example, differences reported from population studies in the magnitude of within-family similarities of serum cholesterol levels and blood pressures[1,2] and conflicting reports of similarities of blood pressure in genetically unrelated household members.[3,4]

This paper is a report of the study of family aggregation of blood pressures in the biracial community of Evans County, Georgia, at the time of the cardiovascular prevalence survey performed in 1960 through 1962.[5-7]

The analyses were undertaken with two primary objectives in mind, to attempt to throw further light on the question of aggregation among spouses and to determine whether, in view of their higher prevalence of elevated blood pressure, black families displayed a different pattern of aggregation from whites. Answers to the latter question might well provide clues as to whether the search for determinants of elevated pressure should focus on different factors in ethnic groups.

Materials and Methods

The Sample.—The eligible study population consisted of all individuals residing in Evans County in 1960, ages 40 through 74 years and a 50% random sample of those ages 15 through 39. In addition, residents of specified contiguous militia districts in Bullock County were enumerated, and all blacks ages 40 through 74 years were included to increase the number of blacks in the study. The details of the original sampling procedure are presented elsewhere.[5]

The participation rate was 92% of those identified as eligible by private census. As the original survey was oriented toward identifying and examining individuals, family relationships were not determined, except for members residing in the same household and for twins residing in the county.[8] Subsequently, in 1964 one of us (C.H.) organized a family linkage study. An attempt was made to ascertain, identify, and link all examined residents of Evans and Bullock Counties in sibship, parent-child, and spouse-pair relationships, whether living in the same household, or physically separate, one from another. The information linkage was accomplished by lifetime residents of

Received for publication May 13, 1971; accepted July 13.

From the Department of Epidemiology, School of Public Health, University of North Carolina, Chapel Hill. Dr. Hayes is now with the Environmental Protection Agency, Research Triangle Park, NC.

Portions of this work were reported in the unpublished doctoral dissertation, Hayes CG: *Familial Aggregation of Blood Pressure in a Biracial Community*. University of North Carolina, Chapel Hill, 1969.

Reprint requests to Environmental Protection Agency, Research Triangle Park, NC 27711 (Dr. Hayes).

Evans County, some of whom had previously worked as census-takers, and by interviews with selected respondents of the original survey sample. No attempt was made to construct extended geneologies nor to describe the complete membership of nuclear families, if some individuals had died or migrated. The linkage was restricted to spouses and the first degree genetic relatives resident in Evans County and examined in 1960 through 1962. Although efforts were made to determine genetic relatives, this was not validated and in some instance the definitions of relatedness are social in nature.

Analysis of Blood Pressure.—The blood pressure of each subject was measured and recorded by one of two examining physicians at the time of the original survey. This was performed after completion of a standardized history and at the beginning of the physical examination with the use of mercury sphygmomanometers with cuff widths of 14 cm. First and fifth phase (disappearance) of Korotkoff sounds were employed to designate systolic and diastolic pressures. Efforts to maximize interobserver comparability, and to adjust for noted instrument differences, are described elsewhere.[6]

The literature on the analysis of population distributions of blood pressure is extensive, varied in the approaches used, and at present contains nonstandardized, controversial approaches: Hamilton et al,[9] Miall and Oldham,[10] Ostfeld and Paul,[11] Platt,[12] Morrison and Morris,[13] McDonough et al,[6] Gearing et al,[14] Gordon and Waterhouse,[15] Johnson et al,[2] Murphy,[16] Winkelstein,[17] Priore,[18] Acheson,[19] and Borhani.[20] These varied approaches have been stimulated by two major problems, one primarily theoretic, the other methodologic. The theoretic problem issues from the controversy regarding the nature of hypertension, that is, whether or not there is a unique entity, identifiable by blood pressure level and permitting classification of individuals as either normal or abnormal. The conviction or belief referrable to this question influences the choice of statistical analysis. If there is an entity, essential hypertension, classifiable by blood pressure readings, a categorical disease orientation, and nonparametric statistical analysis is indicated; if high blood pressure is one end of a continuous distribution of values, either ordinal or parametric measures of association at all points of the continuum are more appropriate. Since there are no critical tests of either of these hypotheses available to us and since we wish to compare our data with other surveys, we have analyzed the data in both manners.

The second general problem is more methodologic: as blood pressure is so highly influenced by age and sex, techniques of standardization are mandatory in most aggregation studies, where sample size is inadequate to tabulate multiple, age-sex-specific comparisons. Hamilton et al,[9] compute age-sex-standardized scores with an attempt to adjust for increased variance with age; Johnson et al[2] regard the age-variance adjustment unnecessary; Priore[18] uses an ordac, distribution-free method for age-sex scoring; and Winkelstein[3] a modified ordinal classification scheme designed to reduce misclassification.

We have replicated, with slight modification, the methods of Johnson et al[2] and of Winkelstein et al,[3] treating blood pressure as a continuous variable. When the categorical approach was used, independence of the blood pressures of relatives was tested by χ^2. Diastolic blood pressure was classified as abnormal if equal to or greater than 95 mm Hg; for systolic blood pressure analyses, we were unable to use the more commonly adopted cut-point of 160 mm Hg due to inadequate numbers and arbitrarily chose a value of 150 mm Hg sacrificing specificity, race-specific, age-sex standardized prevalence ratios were computed.

Results

Of the 3,092 examinees, 1,954 (63%) had a spouse, 767 (19%) had one or both parents, and 554 (18%) had one or more siblings included in the surveyed population. The proportion of individuals with ascertained relatives is influenced markedly by the nature of the relationship and the age, sex, and race of the propositus. These relationships are set out in Table 1 and presented graphically in Fig 1. The proportion of examined individuals with spouse included in the survey was higher for males than females and higher for whites than blacks. The age relationship is different in the two sexes; for males the percent with spouse present is generally the same at all ages past 30 years, with values in the range of 80% for whites and 65% for blacks; for females the percent with spouse present drops sharply past the ages of 30 through 39 years, from 93% at the ages of 30 through 39 years to 42% at the ages of 60 through 74 years for whites, and from 66% at the ages of 40 through 49 years to only 30% at the ages of 60 through 74 years for blacks.

Some of the difference in ascertainment of black and white relatives is due to the original sampling procedure. The number of blacks examined in the coronary heart disease prevalence survey was increased by examining all blacks ages 40 through 74 years in portions of Bullock County adjacent to Evans County. This leads to ascertainment of proportionately fewer black relationships with one or both of the relatives less than 40 years of age. The effect is greatest for the parent-offspring relationship and least for spouse and sibship relationships.

The differences in percent of examinees with spouse present reflect the combined effects of widowhood, separation, and divorce, as well as the relatively small proportion of individuals never married. Although the data presented are cross-sectional in nature, and although specific, detailed marital history information was not collected at the time of the original survey, it is safe to postulate that most of the sex differences are due to differential mortality, with excess male mortality in middle and older ages resulting in progressively small proportions of examined females with spouse present. The lower proportions of blacks than whites with spouses ascertained is similarly a result of higher mortality, although how much is also due to greater social fragility of the marital state in the Black was not determined in this survey.

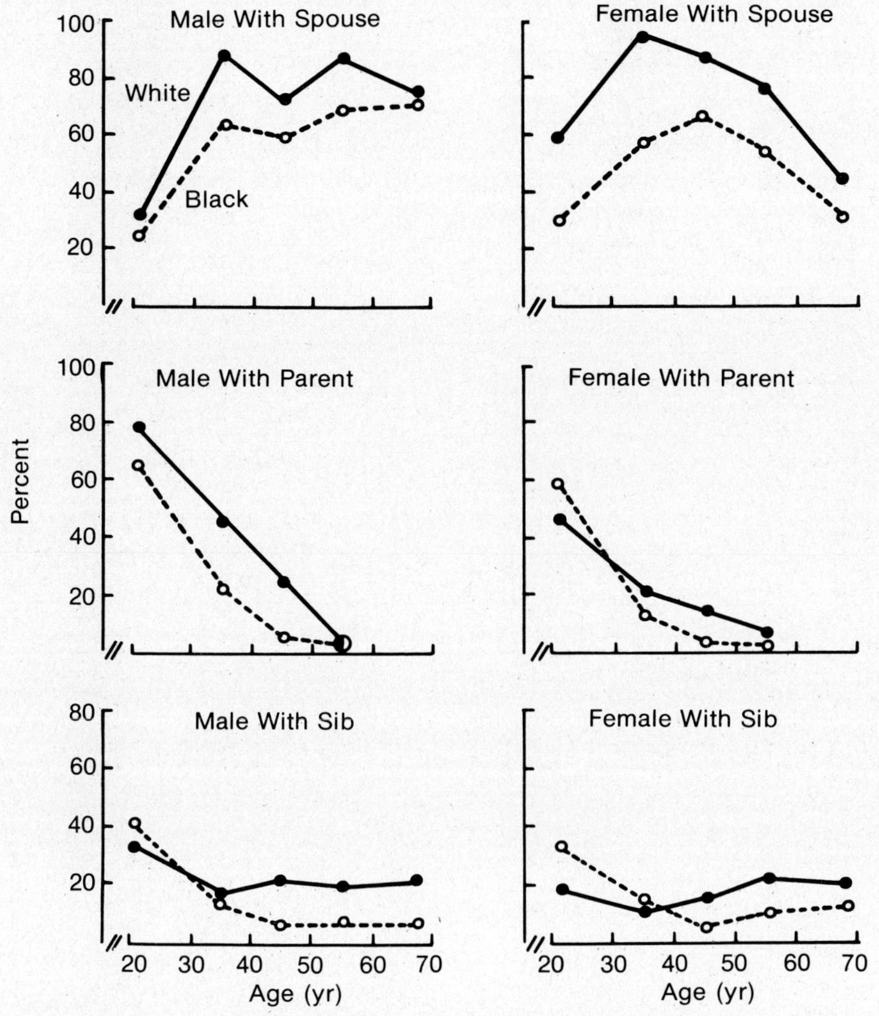

Fig 1.—Percent of examined individuals with ascertained relative(s) by type of relationship in age-race-sex groups.

The proportion of examinees with one or more parents present drops precipitously from 60% to 80% at the ages of 15 to 29 years, to 2% to 7% at the ages of 50 to 59. (Not surprisingly, there were no examinees aged 60 years and older in the survey with living parents, as the upper limit of age. eligibility in the survey sample was 74 years). The marked decrease in ascertained parent-child relationships with age is due to the combined effects of sampling method mortality and migration. The relatively small numbers of intergenerational pairs in this community survey highlight the difficulties in using prevalence data in familial studies of a disease expressed in middle age.

This evidence of strong selective forces in the ascertainment of relationships raises questions regarding the comparability of blood pressure in ascertained relationships with that in relationships not ascertained due to these selected forces. Unfortunately, no data are available upon which estimates of this comparability could be based. Similarly, comparisons of blood pressures in those individuals removed from the scope of the survey through this selection are not available.

Preliminary clues regarding the effect of the selective forces are sought in the comparison of blood pressures in those persons with and those without ascertained relationships at the time of the prevalence survey in 1960 through 1962. The prevalence of elevated diastolic blood pressure (> 95 mm Hg) was compared in those with and without ascertained relatives for each of the four race-sex groups. Due to the strong age effect as previously discussed, the prevalence figures were age-adjusted, by the indirect method, using the age groups 15 through 29, 30 through 39, 40 through 49, 50 through 59, and 60+ years for each race-sex group. For example, for all examined white males the observed prevalence of elevated diastolic blood pressure was 27.3%; for those with ascertained spouses the prevalence was 30.3%, contrasted with 19.9% for examined white males without spouse. The age distribution, however, was as expected quite dissimilar; males without spouse were much younger than males with ascertained spouse. After age adjustment, the prevalence rate was 27.7% for white men with spouse, 25.9% for white men without spouse. Referring both values to the overall prevalence of 27.3% for all white results in age-standardized prevalence ratios of 102 and 95. In white females, where the proportions with and without spouse are possibly even more highly influenced by selection, there was little difference in the prevalence of elevated blood pressure between those with and without spouse, the standardized prevalence ratio of elevated diastolic blood pressure for women with a spouse being 101 and 98 for those without a spouse. As can be seen then from Tables 2 and 3, none of the four race-sex groups

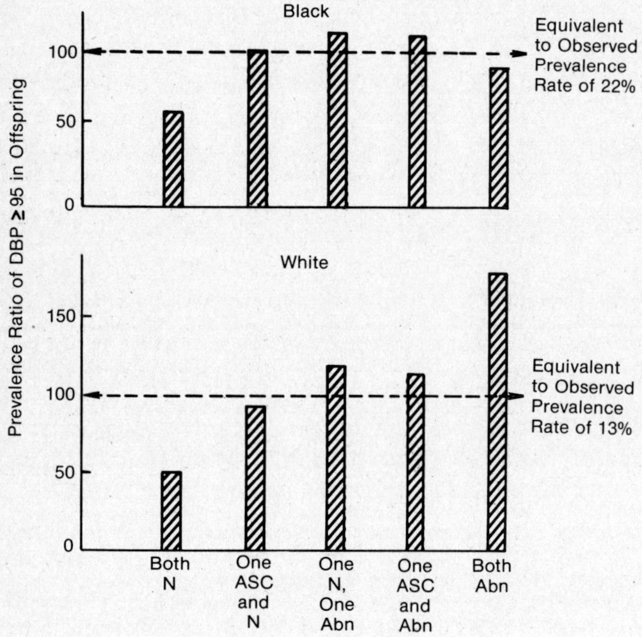

Fig 2.—Standardized prevalence ratios of diastolic blood pressure, 95 mm Hg, in offspring by parental type. Prevalence ratios are race-specific, age-sex standardized. N = normal, ASC = ascertained, and Abn = abnormal.

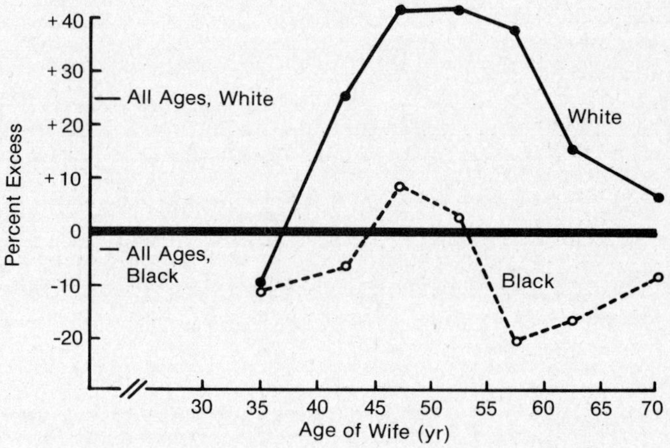

Fig 3.—Aggregation of diastolic blood, 95 mm Hg, in spouse pairs: Evans County Prevalence Survey. Percent of excess = $\frac{O-E}{E} \times 100$ *where O = observed number of pairs, both members with diastolic blood pressure ≧ 95; E = expected number of pairs, given independence of blood pressure between members of spouse pair, and computed using the age-race-sex specific prevalence rates for Evans County married individuals.*

showed strong differences in elevated systolic or diastolic blood pressure prevalence when individuals were classified by the presence or absence of spouse.

Similarly, there are only the slight differences in the age-standardized prevalence ratios of elevated diastolic blood pressure for those with and without ascertained parents, but prevalence of elevated systolic blood pressure appears somewhat higher in both white males and white females with parents than those without.

The only other sizable differences in these tables appear in the comparison of blood pressures in those with and without sibs. For white females and black males, the prevalence of elevated diastolic pressure is lower in those with sibs in the community, and for all except white males the prevalence of elevated systolic pressure is lower among those with sibs.

Similar results to these are obtained when comparisons are made of means and variances of both diastolic and systolic blood pressure treated as continuous variables.

These data suggest that despite strong selection on the attributes of age, race, and sex, the blood pressures do not differ in any systematic fashion in those propositi with ascertained relatives from those without such relatives. Attention was next directed toward analysis of the similarities between pairs of ascertained relatives. Pearson product moment correlation coefficients were computed based on standard scores. Means and standard deviations were computed for each of the race-sex categories in ten-year age groupings. The standard score was derived as the algebraic difference between the observed value and the mean for that age-race-sex group, divided by the standard deviation for the same grouping. As displayed in Table 4, the correlation coefficients, based on standard scores, for first-degree genetic relatives for systolic and diastolic blood pressure range from 0.13 to 0.26. These values are all statistically significantly different from zero, are quite comparable to values reported from other populations,[2] and with the exception of parent-offspring correlations of 0.26 for systolic blood pressure for blacks contrasted with 0.13 for whites, show no sizeable difference between the races. Correlation coefficients for height are included here primarily as "bench mark" comparisons, although these values are also of anthropometic interest and height often is cited as the human characteristic most illustrative of polygenic inheritance.[21] The correlation coefficients for height, ranging from 0.34 to 0.44 for first-degree genetic relatives residing in Evans County, are consistent with studies of other populations[2] and lend added

Table 1.—Number and Percent of Examined Individuals With Ascertained Relatives by Age, Race, and Sex; Evans County Prevalence Survey, 1960 Through 1962*

Age (yr)	15-29	30-39	40-49	50-59	60-74	All ages
No. examined in original survey						
White male	170	113	249	218	191	941
Black male	105	36	150	132	112	535
White female	161	127	238	207	239	972
Black female	114	59	181	144	146	644
% with ascertained spouse						
White male	33.5	88.5	74.1	86.2	74.9	71.0
Black male	24.8	63.9	59.3	68.9	70.5	57.6
White female	59.0	92.9	84.9	74.4	42.3	68.8
Black female	29.8	57.6	66.3	53.5	29.5	47.8
% with ascertained parent(s)						
White male	78.8	45.1	24.1	3.7	0	26.9
Black male	64.8	22.2	4.7	2.3	0	16.1
White female	46.6	21.3	14.3	6.8	0	15.4
Black female	59.6	13.6	4.4	2.1	0	13.5
% with ascertained sibling(s)						
White male	32.9	16.8	21.7	20.2	21.5	22.7
Black male	41.0	13.9	6.7	6.8	6.3	13.8
White female	18.0	10.2	15.1	22.2	20.9	17.9
Black female	32.5	15.3	5.5	11.1	13.7	14.3

* There were six white males, two black males, and two black females, the status of whose relatives was not determined.

Table 2.—Prevalence of Diastolic Blood Pressure ≧ 95 mm Hg in Individuals With and Without Ascertained Relatives by Race-Sex Classes

Total Survey Sample	No.	Observed Prevalence (% of DPB* ≧ 95 mm Hg)	Age-Standardized Prevalence Ratio
White male	941	27.3	100
Black male	535	52.0	100
White female	972	25.0	100
Black female	644	54.8	100

Age-Standardized Prevalence Ratio of Individuals	With Spouse	Without Spouse	With Parent(s)	Without Parent(s)	With Sib(s)	Without Sib(s)
White male	102	95	104	99	105	98
Black male	98	104	97	100	77	102
White female	101	98	98	100	88	103
Black female	101	99	94	100	103	99

* DBP = diastolic blood pressure.

confidence to the techniques of ascertainment of family relationship, which were used here.

In contrast to the consistency between the findings in Evans County and other population studies of similarities of blood pressure levels between genetic relatives, the finding of significant similarity between blood pressures of white spouse pairs (the correlation coefficient is 0.08 for diastolic and 0.13 for systolic blood pressure) has not been generally reported[1] and in this study was not true for the black couples.

The concordance of pairs of relatives were studied, treating high blood pressure as a categorical variable with cut points of 95 mm Hg for diastolic and 150 mm Hg for systolic blood pressure, adjusting the age-race-sex prevalences. As set out in Table 5, there is an observed/expected ratio of 120 (20% excess) of concordant white sib pairs, and an observed/expected ratio of 122 (22% excess) of concordant black sibling pairs, both oldest members of sibships presenting high diastolic blood pressures. The comparable figures for systolic blood pressure (Table 6) are 8% excess for white and 31% excess for black sibships. The model used is one of expectations under the independence hypothesis tested by χ^2 with the sample size reduced from 416 to 194 for white pairs and reduced for 308 to 83 in the blacks by the restriction of analyses to the two oldest members of the sibship; with the dichotomous treatment of the variable, none of the categorical analyses of sib concordance reach statistical significance. Based on other studies,[22-24] however, there is little doubt of the meaning of the relationship for sib pairs and the significant correlational analyses of the Evans County Survey. The values, however, do not indicate gross differences in comparisons of blacks and whites.

Categorizing individuals as either having or not having elevated blood pressure permits an analysis of the dependence of offspring types on those of both parents, analogous to the genetical mating test. In this approach the prevalence of the abnormality (high blood pressure) in offspring is determined for each parental mating type: those with both, one, or neither parent abnormal. In the Evans County Prevalence Survey data there are two additional categories, (ignoring the sex of each parent), in which one parent was not ascertained and the other was, respectively, normal or abnormal. The observed number with high blood pressure (for each set of offspring) was adjusted to the age-sex composition of that race group by the indirect method and divided by the observed prevalence for all ascertained offspring in that race group to obtain a race specific, age-sex standardized prevalence ratio. The values for diastolic blood pressure are presented in Table 7 and Fig 2. For white children the standardized prevalence ratio rises from 51 when both parents are normal to 178 when both parents were ascertained and abnormal. The intermediate increments in prevalence were not stepwise: with one parent normal and one abnormal, 118, and with only one parent ascertained and abnormal, 114. In contrast to the threefold gradient for whites, the black children presented only a 1.5 to 1 gradient, with standardized prevalence ratios of 90 when both parents were ascertained and abnormal and 60 when both were normal. Similar gradients but more clearly stepwise, and of greater magnitude, were observed for systolic blood pressure. For whites there was a six fold gradient: the standardized prevalence ratio rising from 22 in children of parents both normal to 129 in children, both parents abnormal. For blacks the gradient was less marked rising from 85 to 142. Thus, for both systolic and diastolic blood pressure, there was a positive mating test: the prevalence of elevated values is sensitive to the joint effect of father and mother's blood pressure type. The effect was more pronounced in the white than the black.

In analyzing spouse concordance of high blood pressure, the model of independence-tested χ^2 was used; expected instances of concordant pairs were calculated under the independence hypothesis as the product of the observed age-race-sex prevalence of high blood pressure levels. As set out in Table 8, there was a 25% excess of white spouse pairs concordant for diastolic blood pressure equal to or greater than 95 mm Hg; this excess was statistically significant ($P < .05$). For blacks, the number of observed concordantly high spouse pairs was slightly less than those expected under the independence hypothesis, the ratio of observed to expected being 0.95. Similar results were obtained analyzing for concordance of systolic blood pressure equal to or greater than 150 (Table 9). For whites there was an observed to expected ratio of 1.13 for pairs concordant on high systolic blood pressure (a 13% excess, not reaching statistical significance) and for blacks an observed prevalence of concordance extremely close to that expected under independence. These tables also document the same types of analysis in the instances where each member of a spouse pair was examined by a different physician. The possibility of systematic observer differences creating spurious

Table 3.—Prevalence of Systolic Blood Pressure ≧ 150 mm Hg in Individuals With and Without Ascertained Relatives by Race Sex Classes

	Total Survey Sample: No.	Total Survey Sample: Observed Prevalence (% of SBP* ≧ 150 mm Hg)	Age-Standardized Prevalence Ratio
White male	941	28.8	100
Black male	535	46.4	100
White female	972	35.0	100
Black female	644	56.5	100

	Age-Standardized Prevalence Ratio of Individuals: With Spouse	Without Spouse	With Parent(s)	Without Parent(s)	With Sib(s)	Without Sib(s)
White male	98	107	112	98	101	100
Black male	99	101	91	101	86	102
White female	100	100	115	98	98	101
Black female	105	95	100	100	93	101

* SBP = systolic blood pressure

Table 4.—Similarities Between Ascertained Relatives

	No. of Pairs	Correlation Coefficients*: Diastolic Blood Pressure	Systolic Blood Pressure	Height
Spouse Pairs				
White	669	.08†	.13‡	.13‡
Black	308	−.05	−.03	.11
Sib Pairs				
White	545	.17‡	.20‡	.41‡
Black	191	.19‡	.14†	.34‡
Parent-Offspring Pairs				
White	635	.14‡	.13‡	.44‡
Black	263	.17†	.26‡	.40‡

* Product moment correlation coefficients were computed based on standard scores, computed in ten-year age groupings, race-sex specific.
† $P < .05$.
‡ $P < .01$.

Table 5.—Concordance of Diastolic Blood Pressure ≧ 95 mm Hg in Sib Pairs

	Total No. of Pairs	Observed No. of Pairs, Both Members With DBP* ≧ 95 mm Hg	Expected No. of Pairs, Both Members With DBP ≧ 95 mm Hg†	Observed × 100 Expected
Two oldest members:				
White sibships	194	17	14.19	120
Black sibships	83	21	17.21	122

* DBP = diastolic blood pressure.
† Expected number of pairs: computed under the assumption of independence between the members of the pair, given age-sex-race-specific prevalences of elevated diastolic blood pressure.

Table 6.—Concordance of Systolic Blood Pressure ≧ 150 mm Hg in Sib Pairs

	Total No.	Observed No. of Pairs, Both Members With SBP* ≧ 150 mm Hg	Expected No. of Pairs, Both Members With SBP ≧ 150 mm Hg†	Observed × 100 Expected
Two oldest members:				
White sibships	194	36	33.24	108
Black sibships	83	19	15.54	131

* SBP = systolic blood pressure.
† Expected number of pairs: computed under the assumption of independence between the members of the pair, given age-sex-race-specific prevalence of elevated systolic blood pressure.

Table 7.—Prevalence of Diastolic Blood Pressure ≧ 95 mm Hg in Offspring by Parental Type

Parental Type	No. of Offspring	Observed No. With HBP*	Age-Sex-Adjusted No. Prevalence of HBP	Standardized Prevalence Ratio
	White			
Both normal	117	5	6.9	51
One ascertained and normal	93	16	12.4	91
Two ascertained, one normal, one abnormal	90	9	16.0	118
One ascertained and abnormal	64	17	15.5	114
Both abnormal	39	8	24.2	178
All parental types with one or more child age 15-59	403	55	13.6	100
	Black			
Both normal	16	2	13.2	60
One ascertained and normal	43	11	22.0	100
Two ascertained, one normal, one abnormal	36	6	24.9	113
One ascertained and abnormal	41	14	24.2	110
Both abnormal	37	5	19.8	90
All parental types with one or more child age 15-59	173	38	22.0	100

* HBP = high blood pressure.

correlations was ruled out by this means; there were 416 white spouse pairs in which each member was examined by a different physician and under those examining circumstances the excess concordance of elevated diastolic pressure was 24% ($P < .05$) and for systolic pressure, 13% ($P < .05$).

Winkelstein[3] has reported spouse concordance of elevated blood pressure in Buffalo, NY, as a function of length of marriage. The method he uses for coding blood pressure is designed to minimize misclassifications, ie, intraindividual variation in blood pressure coding is supposedly reduced. In addition, dividing the blood pressure range in five intervals (116, 116 to 134, 136 to 154, 156 to 174, 176+) exploits the continuous nature of blood pressure and also offers more ordinal possibilities of classification than does the simple classification of "high blood pressure" contrasted with "normal blood pressure." Using this method and computing expected members of concordant spouse pairs, based on age-sex-specific prevalence rates and the assumption of statistical independence, we observed 122 concordant spouse pairs under circumstances where 114 would be expected on the basis of chance alone. This results in an observed to expected ratio of 1.07. Interestingly, although this method corroborates Winkelstein's findings, the results are not statistically significant, in contrast to the categorical analysis already described, the results of which do reach statistical significance. Regardless of the potential theoretic desirability of using Winkelstein's method, it would appear that its power in detecting spouse concordance is somewhat less than that of either the correlational or dichotomous categorical approach. This follows from the multilevel classification system used and the fact that no weight is given to similar values unless they fall into the same class interval.

The data from Tecumseh, Mich,[2] indicate the possibility of associations in those marital pairs where female age is 50 years, although the investigators, in a subsequent publication, question its importance. We did not have data on duration of marriage and, therefore, repeated our analyses stratifying spouse pairs by age of wife. As set out in Table 10 and depicted in Fig 3, it can be seen that for the white pairs, the aggregation or concordance of diastolic blood pressure is an interesting function of wife's age; there is no evidence of concordance in the spouse pairs in which the wife's age is less than 40 years. The excess of concordant pairs above those expected by chance then increases to reach a maximum at wife's age of 50 and declines virtually to zero in the older age group. For systolic blood pressure the slight excess of concordant pairs is present only when the wife's age is 50 years or older.

Table 8.—Concordance of Diastolic Blood Pressure ≧ 95 mm Hg in Spouse Pairs

	Total No. of Pairs	Observed No. of Pairs, Both Members With DBP* ≧ 95 mm Hg	Expected No. of Pairs, Both Members With DBP ≧ 95 mm Hg†	Observed × 100 Expected
All-white pairs	669	73	58.24	125
White pairs with husband and wife examined by different observers	416	45	36.23	124
All-black pairs	308	102	107.31	95

* DBP = diastolic blood pressure.
† Expected number of pairs: computed under the assumption of independence between the members of the pair, given age-sex-race-specific prevalances of elevated diastolic blood pressure.

Table 9.—Concordance of Systolic Blood Pressure ≧ 150 mm Hg in Spouse Pairs

	Total No. of Pairs	Observed No. of Pairs, Both Members With SBP* ≧ 150 mm Hg	Expected No. of Pairs, Both Members With SBP ≧ 150 mm Hg†	Observed × 100 Expected
All-white pairs	670	101	90.23	...
White pairs with husband and wife examined by different observers	416	67	59.39	113
All-black pairs	180	65	64.30	101

* SBP = systolic blood pressure.
† Expected number of pairs: computed under the assumption of independence between the members of the pair, given age-sex-race-specific prevalances of elevated systolic blood pressure.

Table 10.—Number of Spouse Pairs Concordant for Elevated Blood Pressure by Age of Wife

	White: No. of Concordant Pairs					
	Diastolic BP 95 mm Hg			Systolic BP 150 mm Hg		
Wife's Age (yr)	Observed	Expected*	O/E × 100	Observed	Expected*	O/E × 100
15-29	0	0.19	...	0	0.04	...
30-39	2	2.33	86	3	1.95	154
40-49	26	18.98	137	15	14.92	101
50-59	27	19.28	140	37	32.97	112
60+	18	17.46	103	45	40.35	112
All ages	73	58.24	125	101	90.23	111

* Expected number of pairs—computed under the assumption of independence between the pair, given age-sex-race-specific prevalence of elevated blood pressure.

Comment

The family study of blood pressure levels in Evans County, Ga, has generally confirmed the results of other population-based studies. The similarity between putatively genetical first degree relatives is of the same magnitude here and, interestingly, is of approximately the same magnitude for blacks and whites, despite the much higher prevalence of elevated blood pressure in the black. No attempt has been made in this study to separate secondary from primary hypertension, and there was no attempt to standardize for time of examination nor antecedent activity; the similarity coefficients are based on casual blood pressure readings. One must be impressed with these levels of similarity in the presence of the known marked intraindividual variation of blood pressure and differential response to nonstandardized psychologic, physiologic, and physical environmental stimuli. No light is shed on the black-white differences in population levels of blood pressure; the similarity of blood pressure concordance for white and black genetic relatives residing in Evans County is suggestive that there are factors influencing aggregation with the same force and acting on population values whose means are, in effect, set at different levels. It is, of course, possible that totally different factors are responsible for the production of similar levels of blood pressure concordance in blacks and whites. Nothing in the observational data, for example, rules out the possibility that ethnically idiosyncratic, environmental factors result in higher population mean levels and also family aggregation of blood pressure in the black and

Table 11.—Deaths in White Spouse Pairs in 87 Months' Follow-up by Presence of Diastolic Hypertension in 1960

Blood Pressure of Both as Associated With Age of Wife (yr)		No. of Pairs in 1960	No. of Pairs Removed Due to Death				Death Removal Rate %		
		(1)	(2)	(3)	(4)	(5)	6 = (5)*/(1)	7 = (2) + (4)†/(1)	8 = (3) + (4)‡/(1)
						Total Pair Removal	Pairs	Individuals	
Men	Women		Men	Women	Both			Men	Women
35-44		166	7	2	1	10	6.0	4.8	1.8
N§	N	87	4	1	0	5	5.7	4.6	1.1
N	H‖	24	0	0	0	0	0	0	0
¶						2	3.1		
H	N	41	2	0	0	2	4.9	4.9	0
H	H	14	1	1	1	3	21.4	14.3	14.3
45-54		196	25	6	0	31	15.8	12.8	3.1
N	N	104	11	3	0	14	13.5	10.6	2.9
N	H	27	3	1	0	4	14.8	11.1	3.7
¶						9	14.3		
H	N	36	5	0	0	5	13.9	13.9	0
H	H	29	6	2	0	8	27.6	20.7	6.9
55-64		108	23	5	3	31	28.7	24.1	7.4
N	N	42	5	2	1	8	19.0	14.3	7.1
N	H	25	3	3	1	7	28.0	16.0	16.0
¶						15	33.3		
H	N	20	8	0	0	8	40.0	40.0	0
H	H	21	7	0	0	8	38.1	38.1	5.0
65-74		48	17	7	8	32	66.7	52.1	31.3
N	N	18	3	4	2	9	50.0	27.8	33.3
N	H	10	2	2	3	7	70.0	50.0	50.0
¶						17	73.9		
H	N	13	9	1	0	10	76.9	69.2	7.7
H	H	7	3	0	3	6	85.7	85.7	42.9

* The values in the sixth column are equal to the respective values in the fifth column divided by the respective values in the first column, times 100.

† The values in the seventh column are equal to the respective values in the second column plus the respective values in the second column, divided by the respective values in the first column, times 100.

‡ The values in the eighth column are equal to the respective values in the third column plus the respective values in the fourth column, divided by the respective values in the first column, times 100.

§ N = normotensive.

‖ H = hypertensive.

¶ Vertical braces indicate the combined category of spouse pairs with one hypertensive and one normotensive member, irrespective of sex.

contrariwise, shared genes result in family aggregation of blood pressure in the white. Numerous other logical possibilities exist which cannot be ruled out from this set of observational data. At this stage of our knowledge, however, it seems more potentially productive and parsimonious to accept the levels of family aggregation as indicative of the common effect of shared factors, of a similar nature, in the black and white.

Whether these shared family factors are genetical, environmental, or an interactive effect of both genetical and environmental factors, cannot be determined from these data. The mating test, for example (Tables 7 and 8), is highly suggestive of the operation of genetic influences. Lillienfeld,[25] however, has presented clear instances of positive mating tests for characteristics which are social in determination. Clearly, community-based family studies, of the type reported here, cannot prove the operation and relative importance of genetic determinants. General consensus from studies more genetically oriented in design, including twin studies, leaves little doubt of the importance of genetic factors in the etiology of hypertension. What remains uncertain is the genetic mechanism operative.

Although community-based family studies may not contribute to knowledge of genetic mechanisms, they do provide empiric information of the levels of similarities between genetic relatives, and they clearly can add to our knowledge of the importance of shared environmental factors. Winklestein[3] has pointed out the paucity and importance of such inquiries. Our data for the white population of Evans County is confirmatory of his results in disclosing both significant similarity of spouse levels of blood pressure and an age effect, ie, spouse similarity of blood pressure is maximal at wife's age of 50 years.

The explanation offered by Winkelstein is that shared spouse experiences for several years are necessary before expression of similarities is manifested. Johnson et al,[2] noting a similar age effect, speak of the possibility of a spurious solitary, significant correlation but also offer the possibility of endocrine changes coincident with the menopause, which permit a greater relative role to be played by environmental influences at this age. However, as noted earlier, Deutscher et al,[1] interpreting the same data, deny the existence of spouse aggregation. The replication of this finding in Evans County white spouse pairs, after its demonstration in the Buffalo, NY, and Tecumseh, Mich, studies, makes the random occurrence explanation unlikely.

The interpretation of this finding presumably lies in the sharing of life experiences of the marital partners.

Either social-psychological (eg, family interaction) or biologic (eg, diet, water) experiences could reasonably be postulated as accounting for such similarity. Alternate explanations for these findings include the possibility of (1) bias in the ascertainment of data; (2) secondary associations due to assortative mating for characteristics related to blood pressure level, and (3) the more remote possibility of a cohort effect, ie, the observed age effect on the degree of association is a reflection of a change over time in the nature of the marital bond and not duration of marriage.

The first of these categories of alternate explanations arises as a result of the examination of both members of spouse pairs by the same physician and with the same manometer. It was found, however, that (*a*) there was a tendency for the members of spouse pairs to be examined by different physicians and (*b*) a similar association is seen when only those pairs whose members were examined by different physicians were tested. In addition, there was a tendency for both members to appear for examinations simultaneously, which raises the possibility of bias due to known circadian or seasonal variations in blood pressure. These effects would be expected to apply to all ages, however, and do not seem consistent with the observed age association.

The secondary association of blood pressure with other physical characteristics for which there is known assortative mating (eg, height and weight) would similarly be an unlikely explanation for blood pressure associations only at the age of 50 years.

While shared spouse experience, thus, appears a reasonable explanation for the occurrence of spouse aggregation in middle but not at younger ages, the disappearance of such aggregation at older ages is at first sight rather surprising. In reviewing the nature of the known selective processes, however, a not unlikely explanation becomes apparent. If it is borne in mind that removal of any one member of a spouse pair leads (in the absence of remarriage) to removal of the total pair from further consideration, then the question resolves into a consideration of the factors that might lead to faster removal of individuals from middle-aged concordantly high blood pressure couples than from discordant (high-low) couples. The major selective force operating on hypertensive individuals in this population will be death, and death rates from this disease are known to be higher in males than females. Furthermore, by definition 100% of the concordantly high pairs will contain a male, while in the discordant pairs there will by definition be fewer males as there is a female preponderance of hypertension. Consequently, the concordantly high couples in middle age will contain a higher proportion of the more vulnerable sex (males with high blood pressure) than will the discordant couples. By the age of 65 or 70 years, therefore, it can be expected there will have been a greater number of withdrawals (due to death) from the concordant than from the discordant couples, which leads to a reduction in the proportion of concordant couples.

To test this assumption we determined the mortality in spouse pair members in the follow-up period after the 1960 examinations. The data set out in Table 11 show cohorts of spouse pairs classified by their joint diastolic blood pressure levels within ten-year age bands. As anticipated, male death rates are higher than female mortality at all ages and blood pressure levels, and individuals with elevated diastolic pressure have a higher mortality for both sexes at all ages (Table 11, columns 7 and 8). Also as anticipated, the removal rates of spouse pairs (due to death of either member) are higher when both members have elevated diastolic pressure than when only one member does (Table 11, column 6); the removal rate of pairs due to deaths is 21.4% when both individuals have elevated diastolic pressure. This rate contrasts with 3.1% when only one member has elevated pressure at the age of 35 to 44 years, 27.6% with 14.3% at the age of 45 to 54, 38.1% with 33.3% at the age of 55 to 64, and 85.7% with 73.9% at the age of 55 to 64. Thus, one component of the inferred dynamics producing the age relationship of concordantly elevated diastolic pressure has been observationally confirmed; selective removal of spouse pairs, concordant on elevated pressure, due to mortality. The additional assumption that concordance increases with age due to shared experiences has not at this time been tested by us and will require standardization of the blood pressure measurements performed on cohorts at two points in time.

One unanticipated finding which emerged in the preparation of the data for analysis of mortality in relation to blood pressure concordance is the suggestion that mortality rates for men with diastolic hypertension are higher when their wives also have elevated diastolic pressure. For the spouse pairs with wives age 35 to 44 years, men with diastolic elevations have a mortality of 14.3% (2/14) if their wives also have elevated pressure and 4.9% (2/41) when their wives are normotensive; at the age group of 45 to 54 years, the mortality rates are 20.7% (6/29) contrasted with 13.9 (5/36), and at the ages of 65 to 74 years, the men in concordantly elevated diastolic pressure spouse pairs have a mortality rate of 85.7% (6/7) contrasted with 69.2% (10/13) for those living with normotensive wives; only in one of the four wives' age bands analyzed, the age band 55 to 64 years, was there no difference: here the mortality rates were 38.1% (8/21) and 40.0% (8/20) (Table 11, column 6). These findings have not been analyzed in detail; the number of observations is small and could well have arisen by chance variation. The age of men living with hypertensive wives may be systematically higher and their expected mortality consistently higher; further, any interpretation offered is post hoc. However, it is intriguing to speculate that we have further indirect evidence of shared environmental factors related to blood pressure, in this instance the possibility of higher case fatality rates in the more susceptible man when the inferred environmental factor is qualitatively or quantitatively different enough to produce elevated pressure in both husband and wife. This, of course, is highly speculative and is offered as a challenge for further empirical investigation.

It is perhaps this age effect on spouse similarity (a resultant of the combined effects of shared experience and subsequent selective removal) that explains the contradictory results that have been obtained in other studies concerned with spouse aggregation. According to our explanation the degree of such aggregation will be highly influenced by the age of the sample and should in all cases be examined by specific age groups.

The failure to demonstrate this relationship in black spouse pairs in Evans County is the one striking difference between the races found in this study. One possible explanation is that of different environmental mechanisms operative, both in producing high blood pressure and in producing its family aggregation in the black and the white. An alternate explanation is that higher mortality forces in the black combined with higher divorce and separation rates produce shorter average durations of shared experience and selective withdrawal of spouse pairs, thus, reducing instances of concordance. There will be the opportunity to test some of these hypotheses with follow-up studies of the examined cohort of 1960 through 1962.

References

1. Deutscher S, Epstein FH, Kjelsberg MO: familial aggregation of factors associated with coronary heart disease. *Circulation* **33**:911-924, 1966.
2. Johnson BC, Epstein FH, Kjelsborg MO: Distribution and familial studies of blood pressure and serum cholesterol levels in a total community—Tecumseh, Michigan. *J Chron Dis* **18**:147-160, 1965.
3. Winkelstein W, Kantor S, Ibrahim M, et al: Familial aggregation of blood pressure: Preliminary report. *JAMA* **195**:848-850, 1966.
4. Gearing FR, Leonard MA, Schweitzer MD: Hypertension among the relatives of hypertensives. Read before the Conference on Cardiovascular Disease Epidemiology, Chicago, 1965.
5. McDonough JR, Hames CG, Stulb SC, et al: Cardiovascular disease field study in Evans County, Georgia: Characteristics of the study population. *Public Health Rep* **78**:1051-1059, 1963.
6. McDonough JR, Garrison GE, Hames CG: Blood pressure and hypertensive disease among Negroes and whites: A study in Evans County, Georgia. *Ann Intern Med* **61**:208-228, 1964.
7. McDonough JR, Hames CG, Stulb SC, et al: Coronary heart disease among Negros and whites in Evans County, Georgia. *J Chron Dis* **18**:443-468, 1965.
8. McDonough JR, Hames CG, Greenberg BG, et al: Observations on serum cholesterol levels in the twin population of Evans County, Georgia. *Circulation* **25**:962-969, 1962.
9. Hamilton J, Pickering GW, Roberts JAF, et al: The etiology of essential hypertension. *Clin Sci* **13**:37-49, 1954.
10. Miall WE, Oldham PH: The hereditary factor in arterial blood pressure. *Brit Med J* **5323**:75-79, 1963.
11. Ostfeld AM, Paul O: The inheritance of hypertension. *Lancet* **1**:575-579, 1963.
12. Platt R: Essential hypertension: Incidence, cause and heredity. *Ann Intern Med* **55**:1-11, 1961.
13. Morrison SL, Morris JN: Epidemiological observations on high blood pressure without evident cause. *Lancet* **2**:864-870, 1959.
14. Gearing FR, Clark EG, Perera GA, et al: Hypertensions among relatives of hypertensives: Progress report of a family study. *Amer J Public Health* **52**:2058-2065, 1962.
15. Gordon T, Waterhouse AM: Hypertension and hypertensive heart disease. *J Chron Dis* **19**:1089-1100, 1966.
16. Murphy EA: One cause? Many causes? The argument from the bimodal distribution. *J Chron Dis* **17**:301-324, 1964.
17. Winkelstein W: Study of blood pressure in Buffalo, N.Y. *Ann NY Acad Sci* **107**:570-575, 1963.
18. Priore RL: The Ordac method of making age adjustments in data. *J Chron Dis* **17**:241-263, 1964.
19. Acheson R: On the inheritance of stature and blood pressure. *J Chron Dis* **20**:731-745, 1967.
20. Borhani NO, Slansky D, Gaffey W, et al: Family aggregation of blood pressure. *Amer J Epidem* **89**:537-546, 1969.
21. Roberts JAF: Multifactorial inheritance and disease, in Steinberg AG, Bearn AG (eds): *Progress in Medical Genetics.* New York, Grune & Stratton Inc, 1964, vol 3, pp 178-216.
22. Thomas CB, Cohen BH: The familial occurrence of hypertension and coronary artery disease, with observations concerning obesity and diabetes. *Ann Intern Med* **42**:90-127, 1955.
23. Soybe P: Heredity in essential hypertension and nephro-sclerosis, in *Genetic-Clinical Study of 200 Propositi Suffering From Nephrosclerosis.* Copenhagen, A Busek, Nyt Nordisk, 1948.
24. Speransky II, Beljaeva N: The influence of hereditary and environmental factors on the course of hypertensive disease: (On the basis of long-term observation of patients). *Amer Heart J* **60**:855-862, 1960.
25. Lillienfeld AM: Sampling techniques and significance tests, in Burdette WJ (ed): *Methodology in Human Genetics.* San Francisco, Holden-Day Inc, 1962, pp 3-16.

The Relation of Migration to Coronary Heart Disease Risk Factors

Helen Wetherbee, MPH, Jackson, Miss; and Herman A. Tyroler, MD, Chapel Hill, NC

Migration out of Evans County, Georgia, was sizeable and, in an 87 month follow-up period, amounted to 14% of the cohort originally examined for the cardiovascular survey of 1960-1962. Migration was selective of young individuals and differentially selective of blacks for long-distance moves out of Georgia, and selective of whites for short-distance migration. There was no evidence of significant migration selection on the coronary heart disease risk factors of blood pressure and cholesterol adjusting for the age, race, and sex of migrants.

Migration is one of the major demographic forces influencing population structure and, thereby, the distribution of health and diseases in populations. It is particularly important in the context of the Evans County Study as Evans County, Georgia, is located in the rural South, which has been the origin of large scale outmigration during the past two or three decades. Outmigration could have biased the incidence findings of this survey if there were systematic differences in the coronary heart disease (CHD) risk factors of individuals who did and did not migrate, and if the two groups were not equally ascertained for the measurement of CHD incidence. Although ascertainment rates were generally high (Cornoni et al, p 896) and although differential ascertainment was found to be an unlikely explanation of any of the major differences observed in Evans County CHD incidence rates in subpopulations (Cassel et al, p 901), this study of the CHD risk factors in migrants is necessary to complete the analysis of possible selective bias. Migration information is also of intrinsic interest and importance for reasons additional to its bearing on the interpretation of the Evans County survey incidence data. Migration is of large proportions and increasing; it is known to be selective of individuals with certain psychological and social characteristics[1,2] and there is the possibility that there is also selection, direct or indirect, on biologic characteristics such as height,[3] some of which may be related to CHD. We report on analysis of this question of the relationship of CHD risk factors and migration from Evans County.

Received for publication June 13, 1971; accepted Sept 7.

From the Department of Planning and Evaluation, Tufts-Delta Health Center, Mound Bayou, Miss (Miss Wetherbee); and Department of Epidemiology, University of North Carolina, Chapel Hill (Dr. Tyroler). Miss Wetherbee is now with the Department of Obstetrics and Gynecology, University of Mississippi Medical Center, Jackson.

Reprint requests to Department of Obstetrics and Gynecology, University of Mississippi Medical Center, 2500 N State St, Jackson, Miss (Miss Wetherbee).

Method

The first survey examination of this study population (3,102 persons) was carried out between Aug 1, 1960, and June 1, 1962, and consisted of a history of heart disease, stroke, and other illnesses, a physical examination, electrocardiogram, roentgenogram of the chest, urinalysis, and laboratory studies of the blood for cholesterol level and hematocrit reading. The second survey examination of this cohort was made by two of the authors (A. B. and S. H.) between Aug 1, 1967, and Aug 31, 1969, in a clinic established for this purpose. During this seven to nine year follow-up period (average, 87 months), 320 persons had died and 252 had either migrated away from the community or refused to return for the second examination. The examination of the remaining 2,530 persons (90.9% reexamination rate) again consisted of a history, physical examination, and laboratory studies, but also included a detailed questionnaire for evidence of cerebrovascular disease and symptoms of transient cerebral ischemia, a sociological questionnaire, and a physical activities questionnaire.

There were 93 cases of CHD diagnosed in 1960-1962, leaving 3,009 persons at risk of developing the disease over the following 87 month period. A detailed description of the response rates and the incidence and prevalence rates by age, ethnic group and sex are published elsewhere (Cornoni et al, p 896).

For purposes of this study CHD referred to sudden death, myocardial infarction, angina pectoris, and chronic heart disease. Sudden death was defined as any unexpected death occurring within 24 hours after the patient was last seen alive, if unattended, and within one hour if attended. In addition, any one of three findings was adequate for a designation of CHD. These included angina pectoris, a history of myocardial infarction, or an ECG consistent with myocardial infarction. The World Health Organization criteria were used for defining angina pectoris and a history of myocardial infarction.[4] Criteria used for the evaluation of the ECG were essentially the class I, Q, and QS patterns of Blackburn et al.[5] ST segment depression and T wave inversion were not used. Chronic heart disease was considered to be probably arteriosclerotic in origin when diagnosed at age 40 or older in the presence of heart failure of chronic arrhythmia and in the absence of angina pectoris, myocardial infarction, or any other cardiac disorder.

Unlike the prior analyses, for the purposes of this study individuals were classified as migrants if their place of residence in 1967 was in a county different from that at the time of their 1960-1962 prevalence examination. This information was ascertained from local informants, county records, changed mail addresses, interviews with relatives and friends, and in some instances direct follow-up and inter-

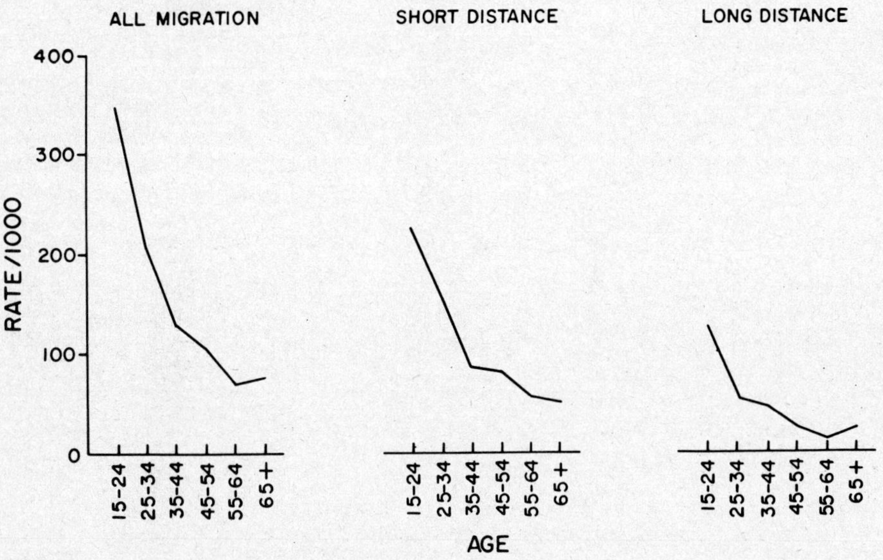

Fig 1.—Migration rates per 1,000 of Evans County, Georgia; all race-sex groups combined by age and by distance of migration.

Table 1.—CHD* Risk Factors in 1960-1962 Examinees by Subsequent Migratory Status—Means Values of Risk Factors

	SBP† (mm Hg)	DBP† (mm Hg)	Serum Cholesterol (mg/100 ml)	Height (in)	Weight (lb)	Age (yr)	Population Size
All migrants	141.2	87.5	195.1	64.9	148.3	37.5	434
Nonmigrants	149.4	92.0	211.2	64.5	152.7	48.0	2668
All Evans County examinees	148.7	91.4	208.9	64.6	152.1	46.5	3102

* Coronary heart disease.
† Systolic blood pressure; diastolic blood pressure.

Table 2.—CHD* Risk Factors in 1960-1962 Examinees by Subsequent Migratory Status—Race-Sex % Distributor

	WM†	BM	WF	BF	
All migrants	27.4	18.9	29.7	24.0	100%
Nonmigrants	31.0	17.1	31.6	20.3	100%
All Evans County examinees	30.5	17.3	31.3	20.8	99.9%

* Coronary heart disease.
† White male, black male, white female ,and black female.

view. Those known to have entered the military were so coded, and the remainder classified as migrants. Migratory status was further subclassified by distance: individuals were classified as short-distance migrants if they had moved out of Evans County (or, if they were black, Bulloch County) but still resided within the state of Georgia; long-distance migrants were defined as individuals with their new place of residence outside of the state. Thus, for the purposes of this analysis, classification as a migrant is restricted to individuals definitely known to have changed their county place of residence and to have remained in a residence in 1967 different from that in 1960 (eg, mobile individuals who would not be classified as migrants are those who migrated out of Evans County and returned prior to 1967, or who changed residence within Evans County). Decedents presented a particular problem. It was not feasible to obtain detailed, next-of-kin interviews to determine residential histories, and death certificate information was not regarded as adequate for our purposes. For example, migrants could possibly have returned to Georgia with terminal illnesses and, living with relatives at time of death, had Evans County entered as residence on the death certificate, leading to false classification as nonmigrants; alternatively, nonmigrants dying out of state could have the place of death erroneously listed as place of residence leading us falsely to classify them as migrants. For these reasons, no decedents were classified by us as migrants. In the analyses, the CHD risk factors in migrants were compared with the group classified as nonmigrants in two ways: with decedents included and with the decedents excluded from the nonmigrant group.

Results

The original cohort examined in 1960-1962 numbered 3,102 individuals; of these, 434 were ascertained and classified as migrants in 1967-1969; the remaining 2,668 individuals not classified as migrants included 320 decedents. The major CHD risk factors of blood pressure, serum cholesterol, age, race, and sex are contrasted in migrants and nonmigrants in Tables 1 and 2.

The mean values for individuals subsequently migrating (Table 1, row 1) compared with nonmigrants (Table 1, row 2) are systolic blood pressure of 141.2 compared with 149.4 mm.Hg; diastolic blood pressure, 87.5 compared with 92.0 mm Hg; serum cholesterol level, 195.1 compared with 211.2 mg/100 ml; height of 64.9 compared with 64.5 inches; weight of 148.3 lb (67.2 kg) compared with 152.7 lb (69.2 kg); and age of 37.5 compared with 48.0 years for the mean values of migrants and nonmigrants, respectively. Thus, there is a clear statistical picture of individuals who subsequently migrate: in Evans County in 1960-1962, future migrants had lower levels of blood pressure and serum cholesterol, were taller, leaner, and younger. The race-sex distribution of individuals who subsequently migrated was generally similar to that for nonmigrants, although proportionately there were slightly more black males among migrants than nonmigrants (18.9% vs 17.1%), slightly more black females (24.0% vs 20.3%) and, conversely, proportionately slightly fewer white males and females among migrants than nonmigrants.

Thus, from an overall population perspective, migrants are statistically dissimilar to nonmigrants in their mean values of CHD risk factors. What is not answered from the data of Tables 1 and 2 is how much of the blood pressure and serum cholesterol level differences between migrants and nonmigrants is explainable by the age differences between these groups. A more detailed, prospectively oriented, analysis of migration rates by age is required to answer this question. The outmigration rates for Evans County ten-year age cohorts, for the years 1960-1967, in 1960 are set out by age in Table 3 and Fig 1.

Table 3 and Fig 1 indicate that the probability of migration is highly age dependent. Although the overall migration rate was 140/1,000, the rate varied fivefold from a high of 349/1,000 in individuals aged 15 to 24 years, to a low of 70/1,000 in individuals aged 55 to 64 years. There was a decrease in migration rate with each ten-year increment of age to age 65; the observed rates for all migration were 349, 206, 129, 105, and 70 per 1,000 respectively. These data, and their graphic representation in Fig 1, indicate that the relation of migration rate to age is that of a decreasing exponential function to age 50, and that there are no sizeable nor consistent changes past age 50.

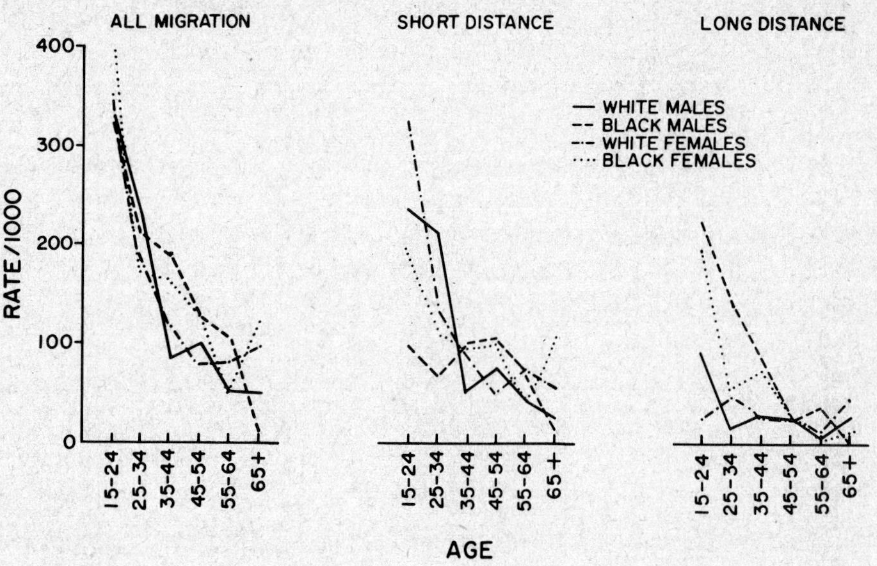

Fig 2.—Migration rates per 1,000 out of Evans County, by age, race, sex, and distance of migration.

Table 3.—Migration Rates out of Evans County, 1960-1967, by Age

Age, yr	Total No.	Short Distance Migration No.	Short Distance Migration Rate/1,000	Long Distance Migration No.	Long Distance Migration Rate/1,000	All Migration No.	All Migration Rate/1,000
15-24	398	89	224	50	125	139	349
25-34	316	48	152	16	53	64	206
35-44	549	46	84	25	46	71	129
45-54	838	67	80	21	25	88	105
55-64	569	33	58	7	12	40	70
65+	432	22	51	10	23	32	74
Total	3102	305	98	129	42	434	140

Table 4.—Migration Rates per 1,000 out of Evans County by Age, Race, Sex, and Distance of Migration

Race, Sex	15-24	25-34	35-44	45-54	55-64	65+	All Ages
			Long-Distance Migration				
WM*	93	18	30	23	6	25	30
BM	222	140	88	23	35	0	71
WF	28	45	26	25	11	44	28
BF	198	57	71	29	8	11	56
All White							29
All Black							63
			Short-Distance Migration				
WM	237	211	54	77	45	25	96
BM	99	70	100	104	71	13	82
WF	324	144	95	51	71	55	105
BF	198	113	97	100	48	105	105
All White							101
All Black							95
			All Migration				
WM	330	229	84	100	51	50	126
BM	321	210	188	127	106	13	153
WF	352	189	121	76	82	99	133
BF	396	170	168	129	56	116	161
All White							129
All Black							157

* White male, black male, white female, and black female.

Each of the four race-sex groups shows a similar relation of migration rates to age (Table 4, part 3 and Fig 1). Although there are slight differences in total migration rates among the race-sex groups in each age band, no clear-cut, or consistent, differences are apparent. For all ages combined, the total migration rate is higher for blacks: the black's migration rate was 157/1,000, the white's 129/1,000. The rates were slightly higher for females than males. The migration rates for the four race-sex groups across all ages were 161/1,000 and 153/1,000 for black females and males, respectively, and 133/1,000 and 126/1,000 for white females and males, respectively.

These generally similar total rates of migration among the four race-sex groups obscure major differences in the probability of migration, which are related to the distance of migration. Major differences, of potential CHD incidence importance, are apparent when migration rates within and out of the state of Georgia are analyzed separately (Table 4). The long-distance migration rates are more than two times higher for blacks than whites across all ages (63/1,000 for blacks, 29/1,000 for whites), and in the younger age groups some of the black rates are seven times higher than those of whites (eg, at ages 15 to 24, the long distance migration rate for black females was 198/1,000, for white females only 28/1,000; at ages 25 to 34 the long-distance migration rate for black males was 140/1,000, for white males only 18/1,000). Conversely, at younger ages, where the migration rates are highest, whites have short-distance migration rates 1½ to 3 times higher than do blacks (eg, at age 15 to 24 the short-distance migration rate was 324/1,000 for white females, 198/1,000 for blacks; at ages 25 to 34 the short-distance migration rate was 211/1,000 for white males, 70/1,000 for blacks).

There also are differences in migration rates between the sexes when analyses are performed by distance of migration. The long-distance migration rates are higher for males than females, particularly at younger ages, and the converse is true for short distance migration, for which females have higher rates than males.

Thus, the overall similarity of total migration rates in the race-sex groups is the resultant effect of a much higher rate for short-distance migration among the young white individuals and a much higher rate for long-distance migration among the young blacks; the sum of these two different rates balance out one another and result in generally similar rates for total migration in the two ethnic groups.

Returning to the question of the comparison of risk factors in migrants and nonmigrants, analyses were performed by age in 1960 for individuals classified by distance of subsequent migration. Detailed tabulation of mean values within the four race-sex groups were computed and are available upon request. No major, consistent, clear-cut differences are apparent. To summarize this data and to take into account the large effect of age, standardized scores were computed within each group. These scores are presented in Table 5. Each CHD risk factor measurement was converted to an age standardized score (within ten year age groups) by subtracting the observed value from the average for all individuals of the same race-sex group and then dividing by the standard deviation. The mean value of the score for all individuals in each race-sex group across all age groups is zero and the standard deviation one. The mean value for each migratory status group, if different from zero, represents the departure, either positive or negative, from the average for like race and sex individuals of the same age, expressed in standard deviation units. Thus, white male long-distance migrants had a mean systolic blood pressure age-standardized score of −0.25 (Table 5). The blood pressure equivalent of this value is different at different ages, as the mean systolic blood pressure and its standard deviation vary with age. For example, the mean systolic blood pressure of all white males age 15 to 24 was 126.7 mm Hg and the standard deviation 13. Therefore, the standardized score of −0.25 is equivalent to a systolic blood pressure 3.25 mm Hg (−0.25 × 13) lower than 126.7, ie, 123.45 mm Hg. At age 45 to 54, the Evans County white male population had a mean systolic pressure of 142.4 mm Hg with a standard deviation of 26; the age standardized score of −0.25 in long distance migrants is equivalent to an average systolic blood pressure of 135.9 mm Hg [142.4 − (0.25 × 26)] among 45 to 54 year olds.

In the Evans County cohort, white males who subsequently migrated long distances had lower, age-adjusted systolic blood pressure scores than surviving nonmigrants (the standard score of the latter was close to zero, the average for all of that age). Similarly, the diastolic blood pressure and serum cholesterol level age standardized scores of white male long-distance migrants were lower and their height scores higher (the score values were −0.32 and +0.41, respectively). Although the analysis discloses these differences, the differences are small in magnitude, without consistent pattern by distance of migration, show no relationships across race-sex groups, and none of the risk factors analyzed are statisti-

Table 5.—Mean Age Standardized Scores of CHD* Risk Factors by Migration Status

	White Male				White Female				Black Male			
	Migrants		Nonmigrants		Migrants		Nonmigrants		Migrants		Nonmigrants	
	Long-Distance	Short-Distance	Living	Dead	Long-Distance	Short-Distance	Living	Dead	Long-Distance	Short-Distance	Living	Dead
No.	27	91	709	120	27	102	778	65	38	44	382	73
SBP†	−0.25	−0.02	−0.07	+0.44	+0.27	+0.01	−0.06	+0.59	−0.04	−0.01	−0.06	+0.31
DBP†	−0.32	+0.08	−0.07	+0.42	−0.25	+0.04	−0.04	+0.52	−0.06	+0.12	−0.04	+0.23
Cholesterol	−0.20	−0.14	+0.02	+0.13	+0.33	−0.08	−0.01	+0.16	+0.05	+0.04	+0.01	−0.02
Height	+0.41	−0.01	0.00	−0.01	−0.10	+0.05	+0.01	−0.06	−0.13	−0.03	+0.04	−0.14
Weight	+0.13	−0.03	0.00	−0.07	+0.12	−0.03	0.00	−0.02	−0.10	−0.03	+0.02	−0.03

* Coronary heart disease.
† Systolic blood pressure; diastolic blood pressure.

cally different in migrants than in nonmigrants.

In contrast to the absence of consistent or sizeable differences in CHD risk factors in migrants, there were statistically significant higher blood pressure values in individuals examined in 1960 who died in the period 1960-1967. The detailed study of the antecedents of mortality is not the purpose of this presentation; the data is discussed in this context to illustrate and document the power of the method used. For individuals who subsequently died of all causes, elevated age-standardized scores ranging from +0.23 to +0.59 were present for systolic and diastolic blood pressure (Table 5) in each of the four race-sex groups. It is to be emphasized that these higher age-standardized blood pressure scores were demonstrated in white and black, male and female cohorts who subsequently died of many causes in addition to those of the cardiovascular-renal system, for which elevated blood pressure is a known risk factor. The analyses were not refined to be specific. Rather, it is apparent that the method used is capable of detecting age-standardized differences in risk factors for nonspecific disease mortality in sample sizes approximately the same size for subsequent decedents as for migrants. Clearly, if there is any migration selection out of Evans County on blood pressure, it is not of the same statistical dimension as blood pressure selection out of the population by death.

Comment

Residential mobility is extremely high in the United States[6-8] and, even as restricted by the operational definitions of outmigration as used in this study, amounted to 14% of the original Evans County cohort. It is important to recognize that the analyses as performed by us were motivated by interest in the relation of selective forces to CHD incidence and were not primarily addressed to residential mobility nor the migration process itself. The fundamental unit of study for CHD incidence is a population of individuals, each of whom either does or does not newly manifest CHD. Migration is a socially conditioned process, and family members may passively accompany others who actively migrate. For example, the 14% migration rate we report does not distinguish between the active migration rates of single, self-determining adults and the passive migration of dependent children, physically dependent older individuals, nor wives who accompany their husbands in residential moves for new jobs. Thus, the overall migration rate and the relationships of individual characteristics such as age, race, and sex to migration, are valid measures of the flow of subpopulations out of Evans County in the years 1960-1969; however, they do not necessarily reflect the importance of these characteristics in studies of self-selection factors in migration.

Migration selection on youthful individuals results in an older residual population in Evans County. Although a repeat private census of the entire county was not performed by us in 1969 and although inmigration was not measured, it can be confidently predicted that there was net outmigration of younger individuals from Evans County. The remaining older population is at higher risk of CHD, and the burden of this disease in Evans County is higher in absolute terms than it would have been in the absence of migration. There is no evidence from our data, however, that those who remained would be expected to have significantly higher age specific CHD incidence rates. Long-distance migrants had slightly lower systolic and diastolic blood pressure and slightly lower serum cholesterol values if they were white males; differences were small and inconsistent for other groups. This finding is interesting in light of the high CHD death rate geographic band ex-

Black Female			
Migrants		Nonmigrants	
Long-Distance	Short-Distance	Living	Dead
36	68	480	62
+0.21	−0.01	−0.08	+0.51
+0.14	−0.09	−0.05	+0.42
+0.16	−0.01	+0.01	−0.20
+0.13	−0.10	+0.01	−0.08
+0.28	−0.04	−0.05	+0.20

tending through the southeastern seaboard, which includes Evans County.[9] Outmigration selection, from Evans County, of low CHD risk white males, leaving high risk individuals residing in Evans County was considered as a possible determinant of the geographic findings; it is possible the number of white males in the Evans County cohort who migrated long distances may have been too small (only 27) statistically to demonstrate such selective effect; however, it appears unlikely that migration selection on risk factors of this magnitude could account for the marked CHD death rate excess observed in the coastal plains of the eastern United States.

Height, weight, and derived measures of physique have often been studied as CHD risk factors, and indices of them have been demonstrated to be risk factors in Evans County (Heyden et al, p 915). For that reason, and because other investigations have disclosed migration selection on these characteristics,[3] we included analyses of these characteristics in our study. Although white male long-distance migrants were taller than nonmigrants, these findings were not statistically significant, and height differences were not consistently demonstrated across the Evans County race-sex groups.

A comparison study of migration and health is provided by the follow-up study of the Commission on Chronic Diseases which reported residential mobility of a biracial cohort of residents of Baltimore. In both the Evans County and Baltimore studies, migration was maximal in youth and decreased with age; intercounty and interstate outmigration was higher for blacks than whites from Baltimore; from Evans County the black rate was higher for interstate migration. These differences clearly are related to the rural South as the origin, and the urban North as the destination, for black migration. Of interest in relation to health is Bright's finding in the Baltimore study[10-12] that "outmigration among whites tends to be selective of those with lower mortality." However, this was primarily manifest among short-distance, ie, intercounty migrants, from the city of Baltimore and may reflect selection of high socioeconomic status (SES) individuals out of the city to the suburbs, characteristics possibly associated with lower mortality in the urban North but probably unrelated to forces of outmigration operative on the Evans County rural population. Of more probable relationship to the Evans County findings are the Baltimore findings[10-12] that "age for age, health status as reported on interview has little to do with whether individuals will change residence and, for those who move, with the destination of the move." These findings are not directly comparable to, but are consistent with, our observations of little relationship between prevalence of CHD risk factors and subsequent migration.

Gordon Goode, MD, coordinated the collection of migration status information.

References

1. Murphy HBM: Migration and the major mental disorders: A reappraisal, in Kantor MB (ed): *Mobility and Mental Health.* Springfield, Ill, Charles C Thomas Publisher, 1965, pp 5-29.
2. Bogue DJ: Internal migration, in Hauser PM, Duncan OD (eds): *The Study of Population.* Chicago, University of Chicago Press, 1959, pp 486-510.
3. Schreider E: Possible selective mechanism of social differentiation in biological traits. *Hum Biol* **39**:14-21, 1967.
4. World Health Organization: Hypertension and coronary heart disease: Classification and criteria for epidemiological studies. *WHO Techn Rep Ser* 1959, No. 168.
5. Blackburn H, Keys A, Simonson E, et al: The electrocardiogram in population studies: A classification system. *Circulation* **21**:1160-1175, 1960.
6. Hamilton CH: Continuity and change in southern migration, in McKinney JC, Thompson ET (eds): *The South in Continuity and Change.* Durham, NC, Duke University Press, 1965.
7. Hamilton CH: Educational selectivity of migration from farm to urban and to other non-farm communities, in Kantor MB (ed): *Mobility and Mental Health.* Springfield, Ill, Charles C Thomas Publisher, 1965.
8. Hamilton CH: The Negro leaves the south. *Demography* **1**:273-279, 1964.
9. Sauer HI, Payne GH, Council CR, et al: Cardiovascular disease mortality patterns in Georgia and North Carolina. *Public Health Rep* **81**:445-463, 1966.
10. Bright MB: A follow-up study of the commission on chronic illness morbidity survey in Baltimore: I. Tracing a large population sample over time. *J Chronic Dis* **20**:707-716, 1967.
11. Bright MB: A follow-up study of the commission on chronic illness morbidity survey in Baltimore: II. Race and sex differences in mortality. *J Chronic Dis* **20**:717-729, 1967.
12. Bright MB: A follow-up study of the commission on chronic illness morbidity survey in Baltimore: III. Residential mobility and prospective studies. *J Chronic Dis* **21**:749-759, 1969.

Decrease of Serum Cholesterol Level and Blood Pressure in the Community

Seven to Nine Years of Observation in the Evans County Study

Siegfried Heyden, MD, Durham, NC; Leo Walker, MD, Chapel Hill, NC; Curtis G. Hames, MD, Claxton, Ga; and Herman A. Tyroler, MD, Chapel Hill, NC

There is a tendency to replace long-term epidemiologic studies of vascular diseases with intervention studies in the hope to prevent them. Two main factors singled out for intervention on a community level are hypertension and hypercholesterolemia. It was learned from clinical studies in the past, usually involving small numbers of subjects, that for lack of health education, money, and transportation and because of poor motivation or the development of side effects, or both, drug therapy of asymptomatic chronic conditions other than diabetes is being frequently interrupted or stopped. Before embarking on an intervention study, we were interested in finding out to what extent the present medical management has influenced hypertension and hypercholesterolemia in the community over an 87-month period. Significant decreases of blood pressure had occurred in 6.5% of whites and 4.6% of blacks, significant decreases in cholesterol in 7.4% of whites and 5.6% of blacks.

Many epidemiologic studies have been concerned with the relationship of hypercholesterolemia and hypertension to the development of ischemic heart disease (IHD) based on the level of hypercholesterolemia or hypertension, or both, at the intake examination. Relatively little attention has been directed towards epidemiologic study of those individuals in the community who either had elevated baseline serum cholesterol concentrations or hypertension and who subsequently have decreased to normal values.

The purpose of the study was twofold. The first was to define the percentage of people in the total population examined twice (1960 through 1962 and 1967 through 1969) who significantly decreased their cholesterol level or blood pressure. The second goal was to investigate the possible relationship between decreases of cholesterol level or blood pressure and changes in dietary habits or continued use of medication, or both, in persons remaining free of vascular disease.

1. Cholesterol levels were determined during both examinations in a total of 2,272 persons. Of these 1,507 were white, 711 white males (WM) and 796 white females (WF). The black sample consisted of a total of 765 persons: 321 black males (BM) and 444 black females (BF). This sample white to black ratio represents the racial distribution of the total community very closely.

Hypercholesterolemia was arbitrarily defined as a level of 240 mg/100 ml or above. Changes in cholesterol levels were compared from the intake examinations (1960 through 1962) to the second round of examinations (1967 through 1969). Significant decreases were defined as those occurring in persons who had a baseline serum cholesterol concentration of 240 mg/100 ml or higher which in 1967 had decreased at least 40 mg/100 ml. Persons with decreases of serum cholesterol concentrations were matched for race, sex, and age ($\pm$ 3 yr) with control individuals who either remained at their baseline level or had increased levels.

2. Persons with systolic blood pressure (SBP) $\geq$ 160 mm Hg or diastolic blood pressure (DBP) $\geq$ 95 mm Hg at their baseline examination (casual single reading, sitting position, right arm) were classified as hypertensive. We searched for all hypertensive persons who had achieved a decrease of their SBP of 20 mm Hg or more *and* a decrease of their DBP of 10 mm Hg or more into the nonhypertensive range. At the time of the second examination, all persons in this group had an SBP < 160 mm Hg *and* a DBP < 95 mm Hg.

Received for publication July 25, 1971; accepted Sept 23.

From the Department of Community Health Sciences, Duke University Medical School, Durham, NC (Dr. Heyden), and the Department of Epidemiology, University of North Carolina, Chapel Hill (Drs. Walker and Tyroler). Dr. Hames is a practicing physician, Evans County, Georgia.

Reprint requests to Department of Community Health Sciences, Duke University Medical School, Durham, NC 27710 (Dr. Heyden).

3. Our intention was to interview each healthy person with significant decreases who had remained free of heart disease and stroke and one control person in order to evaluate reasons for decreases. There were only two refusals. A small number of people had migrated but were known to be alive and healthy. Interviews were conducted in the homes and S.H. interviewed all black persons, L.W. all white persons. Prior to and during the interviews, techniques were standardized in order to assure greatest possible comparability between the two interviewers. The questionnaire comprised 26 items, covering major changes in the person's diet between the first and second examination (1960 through 1962 and 1967 through 1969). Medication as a factor in lowering cholesterol levels could be dismissed but played some role in hypertension control. We were mainly interested in dietary habits and particularly changes in the consumption of visible fat and types of meat.

As will be seen, only a few persons actually decreased either cholesterol level or blood pressure to a significant degree and remained free of vascular diseases.

Table 1.—Distribution of Cholesterol ≥240 mg/100 ml by Age in Race-Sex Groups, 1960 Through 1962 Cohort

Age yr	White Men		White Females		Black Males		Black Females	
	Par	Cases	Par	Cases	Par	Cases	Par	Cases
15-24	118	2	108	2	81	0	91	3
25-34	109	15	110	11	43	3	54	2
35-44	167	35	189	43	79	11	111	18
45-54	259	61	239	79	171	33	167	45
55-64	175	42	182	93	89	13	129	44
65-74	110	25	131	71	68	10	90	32
75+	9	3	13	6	6	2	4	2
Total	947	183	972	305	537	72	646	146

Percent With Cholesterol ≥240 mg/100 ml	WM	WF	BM	BF
15-24	1.7	1.9	0	3.3
25-34	13.8	10.0	7.0	3.7
35-44	21.0	22.8	13.9	16.2
45-54	23.6	33.1	19.3	26.9
55-64	24.0	51.1	14.6	34.1
65-74	22.7	54.2	14.7	35.6
75+	33.3	46.2	33.3	50.0
Total	19.3	31.4	13.4	22.6

Results

1. Hypercholesterolemia (≥ 240 mg/100 ml) at the baseline examination was found almost twice as frequently in females as in males of both races, ie, 19% in WM but 31% in WF and 13% in BM but 23% in BF (Table 1).

For WM there is a steady increase in percentage of hypercholesterolemic individuals up to the age of 55 to 64 years followed by a slight decrease in the age group 65 to 74. For WF there is a sharp increase in the prevalence of hypercholesterolemia at age of menopause (at the ages of 45 to 54 years, the prevalence is higher than in males of the same age) and a further increase of hypercholesterolemia subjects after menopause (twice as many females as males of the same age group). For BM except at the age of 45 to 54 years, there is no sizeable increase in percentage of hypercholesterolemic subjects at each age. There is a higher prevalence of hypercholesterolemia in the white than the black with increasing age. The age relationship for black females is similar to that for whites.

In view of the known relationship of IHD incidence and hypercholesterolemia in general[1] and in Evans County, Georgia, the lowering of cholesterol levels might be considered of potential benefit. Fifty-seven whites with hypercholesterolemia in 1960 died prior to reexamination. Of 458 WM and WF survivors with hypercholesterolemia (as defined at the baseline examination) and reexamined in 1967 through 1969, only 34 showed a decrease of cholesterol levels ≥ 40 mg/100 ml and were found free of vascular disease. An additional 23 persons (5% of 458 WM and WF) also had a decrease of cholesterol levels but were diagnosed with vascular disease. It is interesting to note, therefore, that of the total white population with hypercholesterolemia only 7.4% had significant reductions in serum cholesterol concentrations and were healthy after an average 87-month period.

Table 2.—All Persons With Hypercholesterolemia (≥240 mg/100 ml) at Intake Examination Who Survived to the Second Examination and Whose Cholesterol Values Decreased ≥ 40 mg/100 ml

Status, August 1970	57 Whites	18 Blacks
Vascular disease	23	9
Migration, L & W*	6	1
Interviewed, L & W	27	7
Not interviewed, L & W	1	1

* L & W = live and well.

Among the blacks, 24 individuals with hypercholesterolemia died prior

Table 3.—Dietary Changes—Comparison of Persons With Decreases in Cholesterol Levels and Controls With Increases in Serum Cholesterol Concentrations

Hypercholesterolemia	27 White Males and Females		27	Controls	7 Black Males and Females		7	Controls
Dietary								
Changes	25	(93%)	17	(63%)*	6		2	
Average No. of changes		3		2		2		1
Diabetes mellitus	4		5		0		1	
With dietary changes		4		4		...		1
Without dietary changes		...		1		...		...
Medication (thyroid hormones)	4		1		0		1	
Gastrectomy	1		0					

* Probability significant at the 5% level.

Table 4.—Number of Individuals Who Changed Dietary Habits

Food Items Eliminated	"Cholesterol Decreasers"	"Cholesterol Increasers"
Fried Foods	16/27	4/27
Eggs	11/27	4/27
Hard Fat	10/27	5/27
Desserts	10/27	5/27
Pork	12/27	8/27

to reexamination. Of the 196 BM and BF survivors with hypercholesterolemia, only nine persons (5.6%) had a decrease in cholesterol levels ≥ 40 mg/100 ml during the same observation time. In 1967 through 1969 an additional nine black persons (5.6%) also had a decrease of cholesterol levels but were diagnosed as having vascular disease. Table 2 shows the status of the subjects in August of 1970 when an attempt was made to locate all persons with decreases of serum cholesterol level for interviews.

In an attempt to elicit reasons for lowering of cholesterol levels in the general community where no drug intervention campaign or any other effort had been directed toward this specific problem, we examined the dietary habits among this group (Table 3).

To make the dietary interview meaningful, control persons with high cholesterol levels who either had remained hypercholesterolemic or increased further were asked the same questions. Quite marked differences in changes of dietary habits appeared between the "decreasers" (93%) and controls (63%) among whites, whereas numbers among blacks were too small to permit any conclusion. Specific dietary changes are enumerated in Table 4.

The table indicates that more than twice as many persons with decreases of cholesterol levels eliminated certain food items from their diets than persons whose cholesterol levels remained at the same level or increased. These changes are particularly interesting in view of the drastic cholesterol reductions among the 27 white persons interviewed. The mean level in 1960 through 1962 was 293 mg/100 ml and in 1967 through 1969, 220 mg/100 ml; the 27 control individuals started at a mean level of 260 mg/100 ml with a subsequent increase in 1967 through 1969 to 289 mg/100 ml (+ 29 mg/100 ml).

As expected, dietary changes were encountered mainly in diabetics with hypercholesterolemia regardless of whether they belonged to the "decreasers" or to the controls: out of ten diabetics nine reported several alterations in dietary customs.

2. Hypertension is a very frequent finding in this community. During the 1960 through 1962 examination, 33% of WM in all age groups were hypertensive, 34% of all WF, 56% of all BM, and 61% of all BF. When taking only those 45 years and older, the percentage of hypertensives among the Evans County population increased to 45% of WM, 48% of WF, 70% of BM, and 78% of BF, which demonstrates an excessive increase of hypertension particularly in the blacks after the age of 45 years.

The great majority of these hypertensives remained at the baseline blood pressure or increased further over the ensuing seven to nine years. Of 488 whites (224 WM and 264 WF) with hypertension found in 1960 through 1962, a total of 76 had a decrease of blood pressures (SBP ≥ 20 mm Hg *and* DBP ≥ 10 mm Hg). However, only 37 previously hypertensive patients became nonhypertensives, ie, were found below 160 mm Hg systolic *and* below 95 mm Hg diastolic. Five of these 37 were diagnosed with vascular disease which most likely had caused the drop in blood pressure; therefore, *only 32 were healthy with significant decreases into nonhypertensive blood pressures representing 6.5% of the total hypertensive white population.*

Of 513 blacks (202 BM and 311 BF) with hypertension found in 1960 through 1962, a total of 106 showed decreases of blood pressures (SBP ≥ 20 mm Hg *and* DBP ≥ 10 mm Hg). However, only 37 previously hypertensive patients had a sufficient reduction to become nonhypertensive (below 160 mm Hg systolic *and* below 95 mm Hg diastolic). Thirteen of

Table 5.—Decreases in Hypertensive Blood Pressure Levels ($\geq$160 mm Hg or $\geq$95 mm Hg or Both) Over a Seven to Nine-Year Period (1960 Through 1962 and 1967 Through 1969) Into Normotension or Borderline Normotension

Status, August 1970	37 Whites	37 Blacks
Vascular disease	5	13
Migration, L & W*	6	3
Interviewed, L & W	21	20
Not interviewed, L & W	5	1

* L & W = live and well.

Table 6.—Dietary Changes, Continued Use of Medication, and Changes in Salt Intake—Comparison of Persons With Decreases in Blood Pressure and Controls With Increases in Blood Pressure

	21 White Males and Females		21	Controls	20 Black Males and Females		20	Controls
Dietary changes	18	(89%)	15	(71%)	5	(25%)	7	(35%)
Average No. (excluding salt)		2		2		1		2
Diabetes mellitus	5		2		1		4	
With dietary changes		5		2		1		1
Without dietary changes		...		...		...		3
No dietary changes	3		6		15		13	
Less salt intake	6		2		3		4	
Medication	5		3		6		7	

these 37 were diagnosed with vascular disease; therefore, *only 24 were healthy with significant decreases in their blood pressure levels, representing 4.6% of the total hypertensive black population.*

After exclusion of migrating hypertensives and those who were not interviewed for other reasons, we finally interviewed 21 white hypertensives with significant decreases and 20 black hypertensives with significant decreases of their blood pressure levels (Table 5).

As can be seen from Table 6 the majority of the 21 WM and WF previously hypertensive subjects had made on the average two dietary changes. In contrast among the 20 BM and BF previously hypertensive subjects, only a small minority had made dietary changes. In both whites and blacks, a small number reported less salt intake over the seven to nine years.

Those hypertensives who at the same time had diabetes mellitus reported dietary changes in each case.

Medication was reported as a probable reason for lowering blood pressures in five of 21 white individuals and six of 20 black individuals—a number which is not surprising in view of general estimates[2] that only 50% of all hypertensives are diagnosed as such and of these 50% only half receive adequate medication.

Comment

McDonough et al[3] reported from the prevalence examination in Evans County that blacks "have significantly more calories in the diet" than whites, but that black males weighed less. "Significant differences were noted in animal fat intake," providing more saturated fatty acids and less linoleic acid in the average diet of blacks compared to the diet of whites. In spite of these differences, the cholesterol levels in 1960 through 1962 were significantly higher in whites. The reexamination in 1967 through 1969 revealed essentially the same differences in dietary intake and again fewer black persons with high cholesterol levels than white persons, though not at a significant level.

The conclusion seems unavoidable that cholesterol levels are less influenced by the life-long fat intake among blacks and that—once serum cholesterol concentrations are in the high range—they do not carry the same high risk as in whites.

The causes of hypercholesterolemia are still shrouded with uncertainties as to which are more important in an individual case, genetic or environmental (ie, dietary) factors. However the influence of diet on hypercholesterolemia, eg, dietary manipulation by less dietary cholesterol intake and increase of polyunsaturated fatty acids is well documented in human experiments, such as secondary and primary prevention in dietary trials of groups with and without heart disease and under metabolic ward conditions.[4] One purpose of this study was to find the possible effects of dietary influences on hypercholesterolemic individuals in the community. The number of individuals free of vascular disease displaying a significant decrease of cholesterol levels was distressingly small, leaving only 27 white and 7 black individuals for analysis. It is felt that this small percentage of the hypercholesterolemic segment of the total community becoming normocholesterolemic (7.4% whites, 5.6% blacks) in itself is interesting data for the planning of future intervention studies.

As far as one can judge from the small numbers involved, changes in dietary customs among the white hypercholesterolemic subjects who were interviewed might indeed have contributed to the significant reduction of the serum cholesterol level from an initial mean value of 293 mg/100 ml to a desirable mean value of 220 mg/100 ml. We were able to rule out seasonal variations with the well known cholesterol lowering effect occurring during the spring and summer months. In only four cases was the time of the first blood drawing during winter and the time of the second blood drawing during summer. In all other cases, the time of blood drawing was identical as far as season is concerned and, therefore, reductions beyond 40 mg/100 ml as cutoff point in this study could not be explained by either seasonal variations nor by intraindividual changes which in reliable laboratories are reported to amount to between ± 5 and ± 30 mg/100 ml.

Another factor influencing cholesterol levels in the community is age. Generally speaking, after a steep increase of cholesterol levels from the age of 20 to 50 years, the serum cholesterol concentrations level off without further increase. This was shown in the prevalence study by McDonough et al.[3] However, no decrease after the age of 50 to account for almost 70 mg/100 ml in our 27 white persons who were interviewed has been reported in any population study. In addition it should be noted that these 27 men and women were spread over the entire age range of the population.

The results of our study may lead one to ask whether it would be desirable or even necessary to change the dietary habits of the black community. If neither the incidence of cerebrovascular disease nor the incidence of ischemic heart disease—as demonstrated in other publications from this study—is markedly influenced by the cholesterol concentration in the serum of blacks, one might well concentrate on other dietary aspects in blacks. Undoubtedly, the salt content of the diet among black men and women would be a more important target for intervention as a contributing factor in the control of hypertension. Likewise, among blacks the considerably higher carbohydrate and total caloric intake would require dietary advice among the large number of black women with decreased glucose tolerance.

Finally, the overall picture in decreases of hypertensive blood pressure levels reflects the present system of medical management of hypertension in the community. The urgency for changes in this management is particularly brought out in the summary of our interviews on hypertensive control persons (Table 6). They were those hypertensives who were already classified as such during the baseline examination in 1960 through 1962 and were found again hypertensive in 1967 through 1969 or had even higher blood pressure levels. Only three of 21 white hypertensive controls were presently under drug therapy. Two of 21 white hypertensive controls reported less salt intake and four of 20 black hypertensive controls reported less salt intake over the past seven to nine years. No dietary changes were reported in six of 21 white hypertensive controls and 13 out of 20 black hypertensive controls. The observation that 71% of the white hypertensive controls changed their diet but only 35% of 20 black hypertensive controls made changes in their customary diets is a reflection of overall changes in nutrition in Evans County with the preferential use of vegetable oil and margarine among the white community, whereas the black community still adheres to the traditional way of eating and heavy use of animal fat, in particular the salt-rich bacon drippings and lard. The extremely small number of hypertensive individuals with significant decreases in blood pressure levels (6.5% whites, 4.6% blacks) over a relatively long period of time in the total adult community is another urgent reminder of the need for public health action on a community wide basis, coinciding with efforts by the National Institute of Heart and Lung Disease to initiate intervention studies for the control of hypertension in the community.

References

1. Kannel WB, Castelli WP, Gordon T, et al: Serum cholesterol, lipoproteins, and the risk of coronary heart disease: The Framingham study. *Ann Intern Med* **74**:1-12, 1971.
2. Wilber JA, Barrow JG: Reducing elevated blood pressure: Experience found in a community. *Minn Med* **52**:1303-1305, 1969.
3. McDonough JR, Hames CG, Stulb SC, et al: Coronary heart disease among Negroes and whites in Evans County, Georgia. *J Chron Dis* **18**:443-486, 1965.
4. Heyden S: Epidemiology, in Schettler FG, Boyd GS (eds): *Atherosclerosis*. New York, Elsevier Pub Co, 1969.

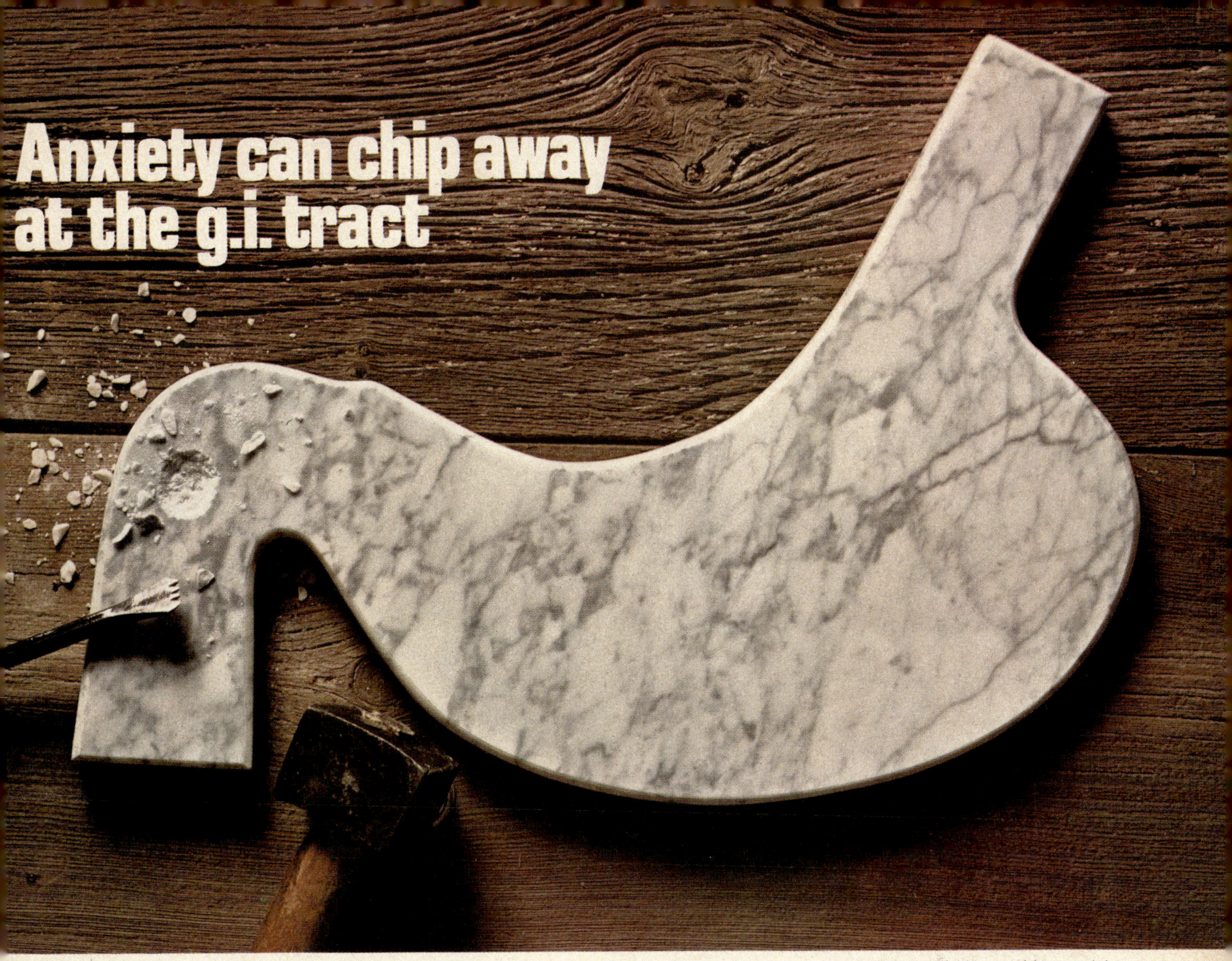

Probably no bodily system is as vulnerable to the relentless pounding of excess anxiety as the g.i. tract. Patients unable to cope with emotional pressures often show such stress physically, as ulcer or other g.i. disorders. 'Combid' can help control the patient's anxiety as well as spasm and excess secretion—round-the-clock with just b.i.d. dosage.

Combid®

Trademark

Each capsule contains: Compazine® (brand of prochlorperazine) 10 mg., as the maleate; Darbid® (brand of isopropamide) 5 mg., as the iodide.

Spansule®

brand of sustained release capsules

Before prescribing, see complete prescribing information, including symptoms and treatment of overdosage, in SK&F literature or *PDR.*

Indications: For adjunctive therapy in peptic ulcer.

Contraindications: Patients with known hypersensitivity to prochlorperazine or isopropamide, existing drug-induced C.N.S. depression, glaucoma, pyloric obstruction, prostatic hypertrophy, bladder neck obstruction, obstructive intestinal lesions and/or ileus, jaundice, hepatic disease, blood dyscrasias, or bone marrow depression. Nausea and vomiting associated with intestinal obstruction or brain tumor. Children under 12 years of age.

Warnings: Use with caution in patients with a past history of jaundice, hepatic abnormality, or blood dyscrasia. Caution patients about concomitant use of alcohol and other C.N.S. depressants because of possible additive effects. Also caution against activities requiring mental alertness (driving, operating machinery). Use in pregnancy, nursing mothers, and in women of childbearing age only when necessary. An inhibiting effect on lactation may occur.

Precautions: Patients sensitive to other drugs may be more liable to have a reaction to prochlorperazine. Use with caution in elderly patients. Discontinue one week prior to I^{131} uptake and PBI tests, as the iodine in isopropamide iodide may alter results.

Adverse Reactions: Drowsiness, dry mouth, blurred vision, urinary retention, dilated pupils, photophobia, constipation and tachycardia. Less frequently, palpitation, nausea, dysphagia, fever, and nasal congestion. Rarely, hypotension, agranulocytosis, cholestatic jaundice, leukopenia, extrapyramidal symptoms (parkinsonism-like symptoms, spasticity, painful constriction of skeletal muscles, or dystonias, chiefly of head, neck and shoulders, oculogyric crises, carpopedal spasms) have occurred with prochlorperazine.

Other Adverse Effects reported with one or more phenothiazines: Some adverse effects are dose-related, others involve patient sensitivity, some occur more frequently in patients with special medical problems, for example, mitral insufficiency or pheochromocytoma. Opisthotonos, hyperreflexia, akathisia, dyskinesia, sometimes lasting months or years; *grand mal* convulsions; altered cerebrospinal fluid proteins; cerebral edema, potentiation of C.N.S. depressants (opiates, analgesics, antihistamines, barbiturates, alcohol) and atropine, heat and phosphorus insecticides; headache, adynamic ileus, inhibition of ejaculation; reactivation of psychotic processes, catatonic-like states; hypotension (sometimes fatal; cardiac arrest); pancytopenia, thrombocytopenic purpura, eosinophilia; lactation, galactorrhea, gynecomastia, menstrual irregularities, false positive pregnancy tests; photosensitivity, itching, erythema, urticaria, eczema, exfoliative dermatitis; asthma, laryngeal edema, angioneurotic edema, anaphylactoid reactions; peripheral edema; reversed epinephrine effect; hyperpyrexia; pigmentary retinopathy; with prolonged administration of substantial doses, skin pigmentation, epithelial keratopathy, and lenticular and corneal deposits. EKG changes—particularly nonspecific, usually reversible Q and T wave distortions—have been reported, but relationship to myocardial damage is not confirmed. Sudden discontinuance in long-term patients may cause temporary nausea, vomiting, dizziness, tremulousness.

NOTE: Sudden death has been reported, though a relationship to phenothiazine administration has not been determined. In some cases the cause appeared to be asphyxia due to failure of the cough reflex; in others, no cause could be determined.

Supplied: Bottles of 50 capsules.

SK&F Smith Kline & French Laboratories

Initiation of Ventricular Tachycardia

Douglas P. Zipes, MD, and Charles Fisch, MD, Indianapolis

The importance of a premature ventricular complex (PVC) initiating ventricular tachycardia (VT) or ventricular fibrillation (VF) when the PVC occurs during the vulnerable period of the antecedent T wave has been stressed in the literature.[1] The vulnerable period represents an interval of 20 to 40 msec located near the apex of the T wave during which the heart, when stimulated, is more prone to developing VT or VF. The stimulus may be from an intrinsic source such as PVC (Fig 1) or from an extrinsic source such as a pacemaker (Fig 2).[2] During the interval of the vulnerable period, maximal electrical nonuniformity in the ventricular muscle is present; that is, ventricular muscle fibers are at varying stages of recovery of excitability. Some fibers have completely repolarized, others only partially repolarized and still others may be completely refractory. Therefore, stimulation during this stage establishes nonuniform conduction with some areas of slowed conduction or actual block and sets the stage for repetitive reentrant excitation.

In Fig 3, a continuously discharging pacemaker fortuitously outlines the vulnerable period. Up to an interval of 0.24 second after the onset of the QRS complex, the ventricles are completely refractory to the pacemaker stimulus. From 0.25 second to 0.27 second the pacemaker elicits a paced beat followed by a QRS complex with similar morphological features that is not preceded by a pacing artifact of a P wave. This extra beat represents a repetitive ventricular response produced by pacemaker discharge occurring during the vulnerable period of the sinus-initiated QRS complex which precedes the paced beat. When the pacemaker discharges 0.28 second or later after the onset of the sinus-initiated QRS complex, a single ventricular systole results, and is not followed by a repetitive beat. Thus, pacing stimuli outline the effective refractory period (up to 0.24 second after the onset of electrical systole) and the vulnerable period (0.25 second to 0.27 second after the onset of electrical systole) for this patient.

Myocardial ischemia enhances electrical nonuniformity which occurs normally during the vulnerable period; this fact explains the ominous importance of PVCs in patients with acute myocardial infarction. Slow heart rates also seem to create a greater disparity in the normal recovery process and may predispose to ectopic beating. At times, simply increasing the heart rate may eliminate PVCs or recurrent VT which occurs in the setting of sinus bradycardia.[3]

Patients who have congenitally prolonged Q-T intervals appear to

Received for publication July 29, 1971; accepted Sept 17.

From the Department of Medicine, Indiana University School of Medicine, and the Krannert Institute of Cardiology, Marion County General Hospital, Indianapolis.

Reprint requests to 1100 W Michigan St, Indianapolis 46202 (Dr. Zipes).

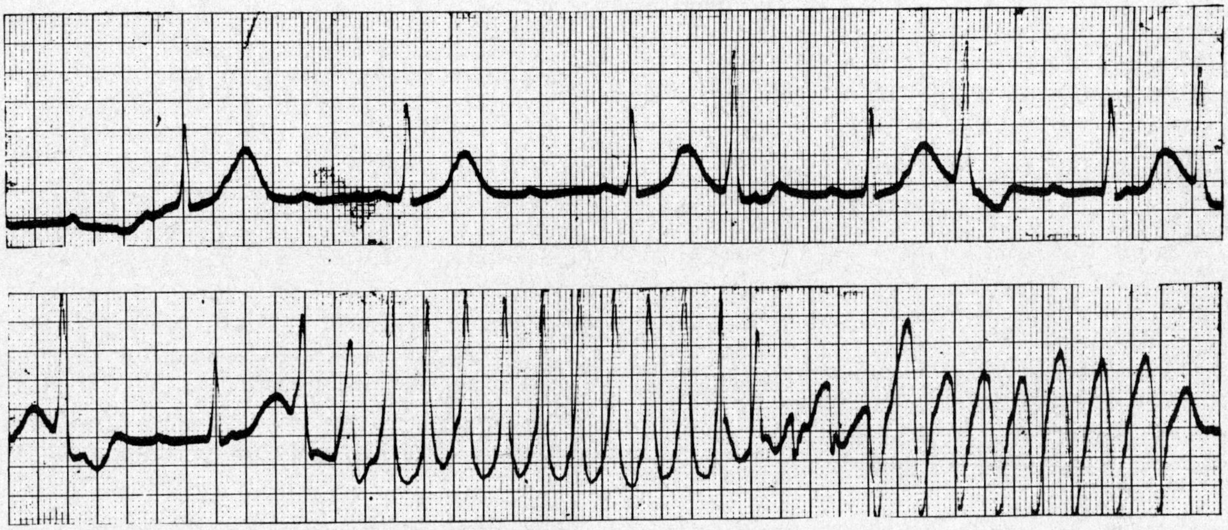

Fig 1.—Initiation of ventricular tachycardia. In the top tracing premature ventricular complexes occur at a coupling interval of 620 to 680 msec (0.62 to 0.68 second), well outside the vulnerable period. Lower tracing documents that when the premature ventricular complex arrives earlier (560 msec), it strikes during vulnerable period of antecedent T wave and initiates ventricular tachycardia. Underlying rhythm is basically 3:1 conduction.

Fig 2.—Initiation of ventricular tachycardia. A continuously discharging ventricular pacemaker competes with sinus rhythm and precipitates ventricular tachycardia on three separate occasions when pacing stimulus discharges during vulnerable period.

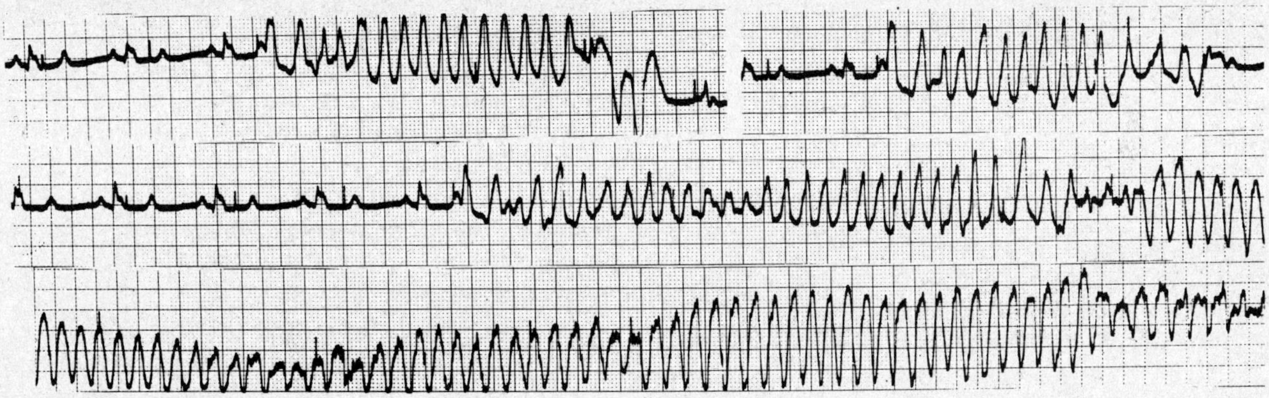

represent a group with a greater than normal risk of developing VT or VF. In such patients, the normal safety feature of slowed conduction through the A-V node may not delay sufficiently a premature *supraventricular* beat from reaching the ventricles during the vulnerable period of the antecedent T wave. Thus, under these circumstances, a premature atrial systole may initiate VT or VF.[4] Similarly, it has been demonstrated experimentally in some young mammals that when A-V conduction is quite rapid, a premature atrial impulse may discharge the ventricles during the vulnerable period and precipitate VT or VF.[5]

The VT or VF may begin in other ways as well. It may start suddenly "out of the blue," without preexisting or precipitating PVCs[6] (Fig 4). Also, if electrical disorganization occurs during periods of asystole, the beat which terminates a lengthy pause may initiate VT. Speeding the heart rate may be useful in this latter situation. Very rapid ventricular rates, such as that which may occur as a response to atrial fibrillation during

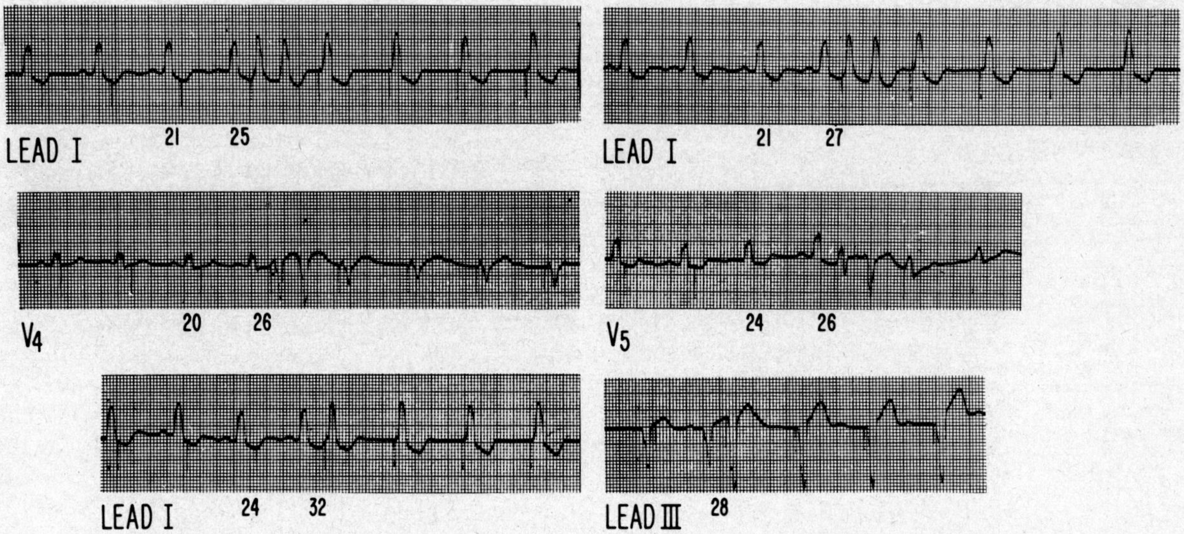

Fig 3.—Continuously discharging ventricular pacemaker competing with normal sinus rhythm. Left bundle branch block is present. Numbers indicate time interval in hundredths of a second between onset of QRS complex and the following pacemaker artifact. Repetitive ventricular activity occurs when pacemaker artifact discharges 0.25 to 0.27 second after the onset of sinus-initiated QRS complex.

Fig 4.—Ventricular tachycardia. Monitor lead. VT begins without preexisting or precipitating PVCs in a patient with an acute myocardial infarction.

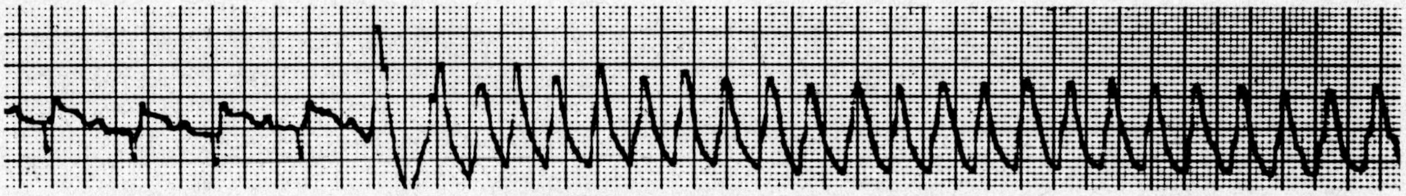

the preexcitation (Wolff-Parkinson-White) syndrome, may also result in ventricular tachycardia or fibrillation.[7]

Other interesting or unusual manifestations of ventricular tachycardia such as retrograde Wenckebach conduction, exit block, and parasystolic beating will be discussed in future articles after concepts and mechanisms underlying these basic disorders have been introduced.

References

1. Smirk FH, Palmer DG: A myocardial syndrome: With particular reference to the occurrence of sudden death and of premature systoles interrupting antecedent T waves. *Amer J Cardiol* **6**:620-629, 1960.

2. Tavel ME, Fisch C: Repetitive ventricular arrhythmia resulting from artificial internal pacemaker stimulation. *Circulation* **30**:493-500, 1964.

3. Zipes DP: The clinical significance of bradycardic rhythms in acute myocardial infarction. *Amer J Cardiol* **24**:814-825, 1969.

4. James TN: Congenital deafness and cardiac arrhythmias. *Amer J Cardiol* **19**:627-643, 1967.

5. Preston JB, McFadden S, Mow GK: Atrioventricular transmission in young mammals. *Amer J Physiol* **197**:236-240, 1959.

6. Dhurandhar RW, MacMillan RL, Brown KWG: Primary ventricular fibrillation complicating acute myocardial infarction. *Amer J Cardiol* **27**:347-351, 1971.

7. Boineau JP, Moore EN: Evidence for propagation of activation across an accessory artioventricular connection in types A and B preexcitation. *Circulation* **41**:375-397, 1970.

Editorial

The History and Clinical Usefulness of Pi

The clinician setting out to dilate a stricture needs to know what size instrument will pass through it. The trial-and-error method for catheters, endoscopes, and bougies will work, but there is an easier way. One need only measure the diameter in millimeters of the narrowed segment on the roentgenogram and multiply by pi to get the circumference. This gives the French number of the bougie that should pass snugly.

With an esophageal stricture, for example, the film should show the narrowed segment fully distended with barium sulfate, as in the Figure. The diameter (arrows) must be corrected for magnification by multiplying by 0.83 using films taken with an overhead tube and a target-to-film distance of at least 36 inches.[1] In order to find the proper bougie, one employs the following formula:

$$C = \pi D$$

where C is the circumference to be found, π is 3.14, and D the diameter as measured on the films and corrected for magnification. Therefore, if the stricture measures 7 mm, the actual width of the stricture is 5.8 mm, and the bougie that should fit snugly is 3.14 × 5.8 or 18.2 mm or 18 F. Spot films produce a greater magnification and ought not to be relied on for measurements.[1]

A simpler procedure uses the following formula:

$$C = 2.6\ D'$$

where D′ is the diameter measured on the film, and 2.6 is the product of the correction factor, 0.83, and π, 3.14. The result gives the same value as in the example above, C = 2.6 × 7 = 18.2 mm or an 18 F bougie. Note that a fiberesophagoscope (Olympus EF) measures 13 mm in diameter at the tip, equivalent to a 40.8 mm circumference, and this would not be expected to pass through this stricture unless it were very pliable.

The French scale for bougies and catheters was introduced about 1850 by the Parisian instrument maker Joseph François Bernard Charrière (1803-1876).[2] The circumference of each tube in millimeters is its French number.[3] Although two other scales also found general use, Charrière's gradually came to be preferred in Europe and the United States. Some definitions of "French scale" use the less accurate relationship of ⅓ mm for each increment in French number.[2]

The idea of a constant, useful value for C/D of a circle of any size began early in recorded history. The Babylonians of 2,000 BC recognized that

From the Tufts University School of Medicine and the Gastroenterology Service, Department of Medicine, New England Medical Center Hospitals, Boston.

Reprint requests to New England Medical Center Hospitals, 171 Harrison Ave, Boston 02111 (Dr. Norton).

C/D was approximately 3.[4(p40)] In the same era, the Egyptian Ahmes gave directions for finding the area of a circular field as $(D - \frac{1}{9} D)^2$ where D is the diameter; this assumes π to be 3.1604, an inaccuracy of only 0.6%.[4(p7)]

Barium-filled esophagus with a stricture. Arrows show the point of greatest narrowing.

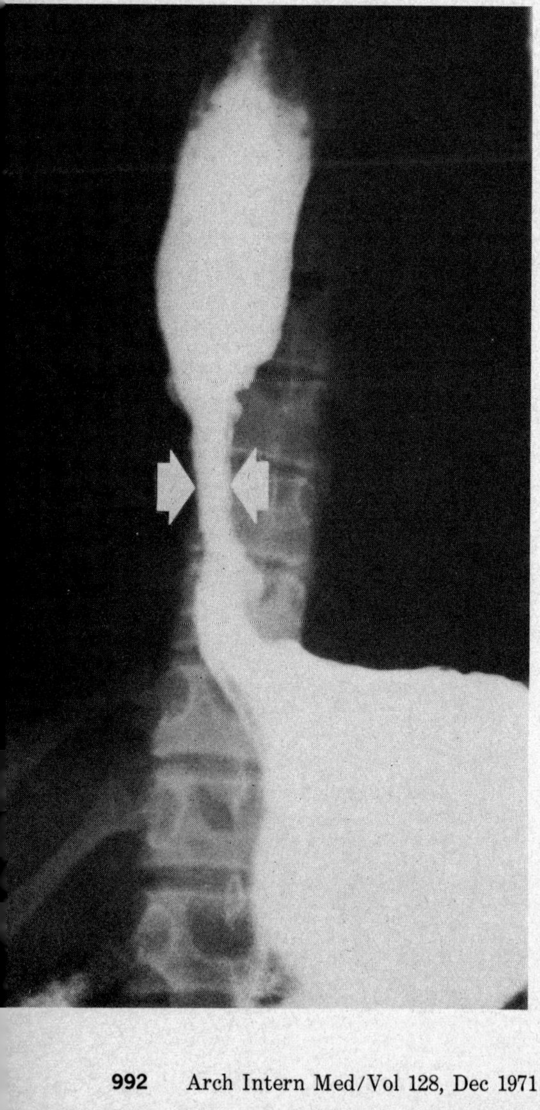

The ancient Hebrews assumed C/D to be 3.0, an error of 4.5%.[5] Archimedes (287-212 BC) proved that π was less than $3\frac{1}{7}$ and greater than $3\frac{10}{71}$; he did this by inscribing and circumscribing 96-sided regular polygons.[4(p67)] Ptolemy of Alexandria (died 168 AD) gave $3\frac{17}{120}$ as the approximate value of π, the equivalent of 3.1416.[7] Brahmagupta in India in the early seventh century AD took $\sqrt{10}$ or 3.16227 as the value of π, an inaccuracy of 0.66%.[4(p150)]

In 1610, L. van Ceulen obtained the value of C/D to 35 decimal places after a lifetime of study.[4(p236)] In 1706, W. Jones was the first to use the single symbol π to represent the ratio of C/D. Mathematicians since the ancient Greeks had previously referred to the periphery of a circle by this symbol.[6] Leonhard Euler (1707-1783) popularized the newer use of π in his *Introductio in Analysin Infinitorum*, published in 1748.

In 1874, William Shanks computed π to 707 decimal places, a task which required bits of leisure time during 15 years.[7] The digital computer has now extended further this process of calculation. Genuys used a computer in 1958 to find 10,000 decimal places, and in 1962 Daniel Shanks and John Wrench used a more advanced computer to produce 100,000 decimal places.[8]

In the meantime, however, the whole matter had been laid to rest by Lindemann in 1882 when he proved that π is transcendent, that it satisfies no algebraic equation with integers as coefficients.[6] Thus, from the viewpoint of ordinary algebra, the circle cannot be squared.[6]

From the beginning of civilization Man has needed accurate measurements and an understanding of π. Today these tools assist the clinician as he plans his attack on the narrowed viscus.

RICHARD A. NORTON, MD
Boston

References

1. Norton RA, Sultan M: Esophageal contractility and diameter in achalasia. *Lahey Clin Found Bull* **17**:117-119, 1968.
2. *World Who's Who in Science: From Antiquity to the Present.* Chicago, Marquis-Who's Who Inc, 1968, p 323.
3. Winter CC: *Practical Urology.* St. Louis, CV Mosby, 1969, p 5.
4. Ball WWR: *A Short Account of the History of Mathematics.* New York, Dover, 1960.
5. I Kings 7:23. Also II Chronicles 4:2. *The New English Bible.* London, Oxford University Press, 1970, pp 382, 480.
6. Kramer EE: *The Main Stream of Mathematics.* Greenwich, Conn, Fawcett Publications Inc, 1951, p 51.
7. Leonhardy A: Introductory College Mathematics. New York, John Wiley & Sons Inc, 1952, p 73.
8. Pathria RK: A statistical study of randomness among the first 10,000 digits of π. *Mathemat Computation* **16**:188-197, 1962.

Cold Pressor Test and Arteriosclerosis

To the Editor.—I read with interest the article entitled "Mortality and Coronary Heart Disease Among Men Studied for 23 Years," by Ancel Keys et al in August 1971 issue of the *Archives of Internal Medicine.*[1]

Unfortunately, the authors failed to cite prior and original published research from this laboratory.[2-7] Keys et al assert that "the most significant single variable for coronary disease predilection proved to be the rise of diastolic blood pressure in the cold-pressor test." Keys continues "one of the major surprises in the present analysis was the discovery of the value of information from the cold-pressor test." Since the cold-pressor test was dismissed ". . . as being unreliable in predicting hypertension . . . interest in the test evaporated, but no one looked at the question of what other signifiance the cold-pressor test might have." This is a misstatement.

In my studies based upon over 1,000 cold-pressor tests in normotensives, pure arteriosclerotics, pure hypertensives, and hypertensives with superimposed arteriosclerosis,[2-8] I have shown that vascular sclerosis is associated with exaggerated systolic and pulse pressure cold-pressor response; and that the cold-pressor test may be used as a screening test for the detection of already existing arteriosclerosis.

One of my papers published in the January 1970 issue of the newly established *Journal of Surgical Oncology* was abstracted in the Oct 5, 1970, issue of *Modern Medicine.* Keys et al submitted their work for publication in the *Archives of Internal Medicine* on Dec 7, 1970—two months after the appearance of the abstract of my paper in *Modern Medicine.* In February 1971, the manuscript from my laboratory appeared in *Angiology.* This same original paper was presented at the 16th annual meeting of the American College of Angiology in June 1970 and was also abstracted in the April 12, 1971, issue of *JAMA.* I reported a highly significant correlation between retinal arteriosclerosis and exaggerated cold-pressor response. Additionally, there was an excellent correlation between the cold-pressor response and calcification of the aorta and/or its branches. Arteriosclerotic heart disease was much more prevalent among the hyperreactors.

A final caution regarding my own experience with the cold-pressor test seems indicated in that the physician, per se, is a hypertensive stimulus. Blood pressure may rise considerably in the presence of the physician even after 30 minutes' rest. Valid basal blood pressures taken prior to cold-pressor test could only be obtained by a medical assistant in a dark room with the patient lying in a comfortable hospital bed. Only under such a setting are basal blood pressures, cold-pressor response, and reproducibility of the cold-pressor test valid.[7,9-11]

Ignatios J. Voudoukis, MD
Detroit

References

1. Keys A, Taylor HL, Blackburn H, et al: Mortality and coronary heart disease among men studied for 23 years. *Arch Intern Med* **128**:201-214, 1971.

2. Voudoukis IJ: Exaggerated cold-pressor response: An aid in the detection of systemic arteriosclerosis, abstracted. *Clin Res* **14**:264, 1966.

3. Voudoukis IJ: Exaggerated cold-pressor response in patients with systemic arteriosclerosis, abstracted. *Clin Res* **15**:95, 1967.

4. Voudoukis IJ, Caldwell JR: Correlation of coronary heart disease, retinal arteriosclerosis, vascular calcification, and cold-pressor response in hypertensive patients, abstracted. *Circulation* **36**(suppl 2):42, 1967.

5. Voudoukis IJ: Exaggerated cold-pressor response in hypertensive patients with superimposed atherosclerotic vascular disease, abstracted. *Circulation* **38**(suppl 6):25, 1968.

6. Voudoukis IJ: Exaggerated cold-pressor response in hypertensive patients with superimposed arteriosclerosis. *J Surg Oncol* **2**:83-87, 1970, abstracted, *Mod Med* **38**:125, 1970.

7. Voudoukis IJ: Exaggerated cold-pressor response in patients with atherosclerotic vascular disease. *Angiology* **22**:57-62, 1971, abstracted, *JAMA* **216**:369, 1971.

8. Voudoukis IJ: Exaggerated cold-pressor response in arteriosclerosis, abstracted. *Circulation*, to be published.

9. Caldwell JR, Hollinger FW: The importance of basal blood pressure. *Henry Ford Hosp Med Bull* **3**:175, 1955.

10. Smirk FH: *High Arterial Pressure.* Oxford, England, Blackwell Scientific Publications, 1957.

11. Laing VO, Voudoukis IJ: Reproducibility of the standard cold-pressor test, abstracted. *Clin Res* **15**:211, 1967.

Books

Interpretation of Diagnostic Tests. By Jacques Wallach, MD. Price, $6.95. Pp 441, with 5 illustrations. Little Brown & Co, 34 Beacon St, Boston 02106, 1970.

This is truly a handy book (pun intended!). It is a pocket book, but will probably also find its way into the doctor's bag or the glove compartment of his car.

Its obvious advantages are as follows:

1. the index—45 pages (10% of the book!);

2. 60 tables—ranging from one showing the normal leukocyte differential count at 12 different points in the first year of life (as well as 11 other points to the age of 21) to seven tables on antibiotics and infections (usual antibiotic susceptibility, microorganisms *uniformly* sensitive, antibiotic combinations, etc);

3. its organization—in addition to the usual sections on "Normal Values" and "Specific Laboratory Examinations," there is a 275-page section on "Diseases of Organ Systems." This last section is comprehensive: from listing the times of abnormalities of phase reactants in a disease to "Myocardial Disease Associated with Marked Eosinophilia."

There are a few errors, eg, showing the *normal* specific gravity of serous fluids as ranging from 1.010 to 1.026, but these are explained in later sections.

Frankly, I like the book and recommend it to students, house officers, and practitioners (even faculty!).

NICHOLAS J. COTSONAS, Jr, MD
Peoria, Ill

Communications to this Department may be sent directly to Robert H. Moser, MD, the Maui Medical Group, Maui Professional Center, Wailuku, Maui, Hawaii 96793, or to the Chief Editor for transmittal to him.

Parenthood: Its Psychology and Psychopathology. Edited by E James Anthony, MD, DPM; Therese Benedek, MD. Price, $15. Pp 644, with illustrations. Little Brown. & Co, 34 Beacon St, Boston 02106, 1970.

This monumental volume, the product of no less than two editors and 29 authors, aims in the words of the Preface "to present parenthood as a function of biology and . . . a tool of civilisation." Broadly, it succeeds in both aims, and is a useful consensus of current Freudian views on the problems of parenthood.

Curiously, 28 of the 29 authors deal only with parental reactions to the first child and make no mention of those aroused by the second and third, presumably because they feel that such problems would be essentially similar—though, here, Adler would not have agreed with them. Not that this would have worried most of these authors, who seem to be, with two or three exceptions, sublimely indifferent to—even unconscious of—any views outside the charmed circle of Freudian thought.

The book is divided into six parts, the sixth being a brief summing-up. The opening chapter of part 1 is a fascinating ethological study by Charles Kaufman on the biology of parenthood. It is drawn mainly from research on the parent-child behavior of two contrasting species of monkey—"pig-tailed" and "bonnet" macaques. The chapter abounds in what seem to be valuable simian hints on such matters as weaning and the infantile drive towards independence, but in the end we are warned, disappointingly, that "such a study could never tell us how to bring up a child." (In spite of this warning I must stoutly declare my conviction that any child of mine should be brought up on bonnet rather than pigtail lines.)

This first part of the book, and parts 3, 4, and 5 are based solidly on research and clinical observation, not on opinion. Part 2, on the other hand, written exclusively by one of the coeditors, Therese Benedek, presents the theoretic approach to parenthood from the strictly Freudian standpoint. It is a brilliant but curiously limited performance, comparable to that of an enthusiastic teacher of physics who had never heard of the Quantum theory. There is a missing dimension. Benedek writes of love like the queen of an ant colony. She does confess (p 112) to feeling "almost embarrassed" at her attempt "to abstract from love . . . its interpersonal dynamics." Well she may.

In parts 3, 4, and 5 the clinical approach is resumed, and we are back for the most part in a real world of human values. A number of excellent chapters ensue, including two brilliant essays (chapters 12 and 14) by the other co-editor, James Anthony, on "Parental Reactions"—to the so-called Oedipal child, and to "Adolescents." It is well to remind us, as Anthony does, that "the child of today is growing into a world so different from his parents (that) . . . the discrepancy in life-styles may be as large as that between immigrant parents and their children"; and it may reassure nervous university professors to remember, amid campus alarms, that "adolescents have always been regarded as dangerous by adults, from primitive times till now." In the Middle Ages, for instance, "the candidate was required to take an oath that he would not take vengeance on the examiner." Nowadays we no longer prescribe controlling rituals, but nevertheless "the adolescent is surrounded by a mysterious apprehensiveness; his milieu has all the tensity of a roomful of people who expect the latest arrival to throw a bomb." This kind of writing is of real value today. It is cathartic to the most dangerous collective emotions of our time.

The latter two thirds of this comprehensive study of parenthood contains so much first-class clinical material that it would be invidious to single out particular chapters. Any such selection can therefore be regarded as no more than a personal choice. Two chapters which impressed me were Donald Winnicott's essay (chapter 10) on the "Mother-Infant Experience of Mutuality," and the contribution (chapter 16) by Norman Paul on "Parental Empathy." In both, a whole man speaks in direct and compassionate terms of the value of reaching, at least occasionally and momentarily, an empathic rapport with another human being. Admittedly, it is difficult, and can even be dangerous. As Harold Pinter is quoted as saying, "to enter into someone else's life is too frightening." But the therapeutic result may be the saving of that life.

Chapter 22, which should surely be required reading for every hospital intern, is a discussion by Brandt Steele on that sickening aberration of parental care which results in "The Battered Baby," and offers guidance on the constructive approach to this appalling calamity.

In the final chapter Anthony presents a provocative study of the bizarre phenomenon known as "Folie a Deux," in which the child is, so to speak, infected with the mother's psychosis. This, as Anthony points out, "deals a blow to the classic psychoanalytic theory of a gradual evolution of neurosis or psychosis out of infantile traumas"; and he makes a gallant effort to rescue the theory by a reconciling hypothesis of his own. He might have been wiser to let the theory drop—basic though it is to Freudian thinking. It is strange to find him supporting his hypothesis with the sadly out-of-date views of Ferenzi (as expressed in a book published 55 years ago) on the supposedly malign influence of fairy tales and legends on the mental development of children. It is difficult to believe that Freudians in America are still clinging to this out-worn creed. Do they still think that their own restricted "sense of reality" is the final truth to which man must adapt, or perish?

If so, someone should bring to their notice that the very different "sense of reality" experienced by children and primitives is now in process of being revalued and in some particulars even shared by contemporary physicists and mathematicians. When distinguished scientists begin to make responsible statements to the effect that the "quantum" must be large enough to cover a 100-inch mirror, and small enough to enter an atom, and certain substances can be given such a degree of fluidity that they pass easily through a hole *which does not exist*—we are not far from the realm of legend and fairy-tale, from the mighty dwarf of the Finnish *Kalevala* who was, like the quantum, "smaller than small yet bigger than big," or of genies of incalculable power escaping from bottles (biochemists' bottles?) and being imprisoned in them again.

The world which contemporary science is beginning to reveal is essentially this kind of world, a magical, self-contradictory place in which the impossible is always happening: nearer by far to the realm of legend, myth, and fairy-tale and to the naive imagination of a child, than to the claustrophobic "adult" world which the 19th century realism of the Freudian approach is still setting up as our goal.

In spite of the constricted mental atmosphere of much of this book, however, a great deal of solid research has gone into it. The amount of genuine clinical information it provides is impressive, and on this score alone, the book is to be recommended.

ALAN MCGLASHAN, MRGS, LRCP, DPM
London

S. Weir Mitchell, M.D.—Neurologist: A Medical Biography. By Richard D Walter. Price, $9.75. Pp 232. Charles C Thomas Publisher, 301-327 E Lawrence Ave, Springfield, Ill 62703, 1970.

"The bias of this biography is medical" according to the author. Medical biography of an individual is most difficult, especially if the man is subordinated to his field. This is particularly true if the subject is a man of such diverse and unrelated fields of interest as Weir Mitchell. Indeed, while this book is a review of Mitchell's medical experiences, it consists mainly of lengthy portions from his notes and writings; an underlying coherence is not apparent.

A critical review of the man's contributions to modern neurology is lacking. Unfortunately, this book does not fill the need.

J. PARK BIEHL, MD
Cincinnati

Recent Results in Cancer Research: Advances in the Treatment of Acute (Blastic) Leukemias. Edited by Georges Mathe. Price, $10.50. Pp 177, with 84 figures. Springer-Verlag New York Inc, 175 Fifth Ave, New York 10010, 1970.

This is the 30th volume in the series of recent results in cancer research. It deals with advances in the treatment of acute (blastic) leukemia as presented at the plenary session of the European Organization for Research on Treatment of Cancer (EORTC) in 1969. This group, comprised of a number of European medical centers, is actively engaged in basic cancer research, drug development, and collaborative clinical research. Several American investigators have also contributed to this two-day meeting and have reported results of cooperative study groups in the United States.

The first chapter contains an impressive amount of information on several drugs that have recently come to clinical trial, such as daunomycin (Daunorubicin) and asparaginase. Some interesting animal studies and clinical trial with immunotherapy are described.

In the second chapter different therapeutic approaches to acute myeloblastic leukemia are discussed. Most progress has been made in acute lymphoblastic leukemia (ALL) of childhood with multiple drug regimens; however, also in adult acute myeloblastic leukemia (AML), multiple drug regimens have increased the response rate from a meager 10% with mercaptopurine alone to 50% with cytarabine (Cytosar), cyclophosphamide, vincristine sulfate (Oncovin), and prednisone (COAP). Most important, there is a clear increase in survival of responders compared to the nonresponders.

Cytarabine is the first drug to show

evidence of prolongation of remissions in AML.

In ALL, consolidation treatment of patients who have been brought to remission, followed by maintenance treatment, has greatly prolonged the remission duration and ultimately the survival. In both AML and ALL complete remissions last longer than partial remissions.

In the third chapter, treatment for blastic crisis of chronic leukemias and polycythemia vera are discussed, but the newer regimens which have been so effective in AML and ALL, have had very little influence on the terminal course of the chronic leukemias.

In the concluding chapter, long-term survivors of the different treatment regimens are discussed. Life table analysis indicates that the percentage of five-year survivors is increasing. Burchenal found in his survey of long-term survivors that the chance of relapse of five-year survivors is only about 50%. The first attack on the disease should, therefore, be vigorous with different drug combinations and with supportive measures such as antibiotics and blood components transfusions. This is best administered in specialized centers. Further care during the subsequent maintenance phase can then be carried out by patient's local physician in cooperation with the center.

This monograph can be highly recommended to all physicians who are involved in the care of patients with acute leukemias.

JOHANNES BLOM, MD
Washington, DC

Indications and Alternatives in X-Ray Diagnosis. By Melvyn H Schreiber, MD. Price, \$4.50. Pp 117. Charles C Thomas Publisher, 301-327 E Lawrence Ave, Springfield, Ill 62703, 1970.

The purpose of this book (which might be subtitled "What Every Radiologist Knows") is to survey the usefulness and limitations of the roentgenographic examinations available for study of different organ systems, and to recommend those believed to be appropriate or their alternatives, if there is a choice. The book is written for doctors' helpers, medical students, general physicians, and nonradiologic specialists. The first three might profit from reading this survey.

Perhaps the nonradiologic specialist also could find something of interest in this slim, relatively inexpensive paperback, provided that he was uncertain of what the indications and alternatives were, or he wished to update his knowledge.

MARCUS J. SMITH, MD
Santa Fe, NM

The Cerebellum: In Health and Disease. Edited by William S Fields, MD; William D Willis, Jr, MD, PhD. Price, \$27.50. Pp 557. Warren H Green Inc, 10 S Brentwood Blvd, St. Louis 63105, 1970.

This book is a record of the recent Dallas Neurological Symposium on the cerebellum. The volume offers the reader a wide and varied review of the many aspects of cerebellar research and unsolved clinical problems. The symposium is divided into three parts: (*a*) historical and anatomical aspects; (*b*) physiologic aspects; and (*c*) clinical and pathologic aspects.

The "Historical Review of Cerebellar Investigation" by Robert S. Dow is helpful but sobering when one realizes the limitations of our knowledge in this field. A sample of the titles of three papers in the anatomic and physiologic sections will illustrate the ground that is covered. A paper on "Light and Electron Microscopic Studies of Two Cerebellar Relay Nuclei" by Fred Walberg is offered. J. C. Eccles' paper is on "The Topography of the Mossy and Climbing Fiber Inputs to the Anterior Lobe of the Cerebellum." The "Cerebellar Influences on Units in Sensory Areas of Cerebellar Cortex" by R. S. Snyder and J. Mitre are discussed. In all, 13 papers are offered in the anatomic and physiologic sections. Their appeal is mainly to individuals interested in or actively engaged in research in this area.

There are seven papers on the clinical and pathological aspects of cerebellar disease. Topics such as viral disease and the developing cerebellum, diphenylhydantoin sodium (Dilantin) intoxication and the cerebellum, the nutritional and metabolic diseases of the cerebellum, and the management of cerebellar and other posterior fossa tumors are discussed. The paper on the "Spinocerebellar Degenerations" by Robert P. Segwick is written with a sense of balance, style, and wit.

The papers on the clinical and pathologic aspects of cerebellar disease would be of interest to the neurologist and neurosurgeon. The internist would find the paper on the "Nutritional and Metabolic Diseases of the Cerebellum" by Victor and Ferrendelli especially useful.

This volume brings together a cogent review and summary of our present knowledge of cerebellar anatomy, physiology, and clinical correlations. The participants are leaders in the field. For the most part, this is a highly specialized volume of interest to research workers in the field, neurologists, and neurosurgeons. Its appeal to a practicing internist is limited.

DAVID GREEN, MB, BS
Albany, NY

Medical Pharmacology, Principles and Concepts, ed 5. By Andres Goth, MD. Price, \$16.50. Pp 665, with 108 illustrations. CV Mosby Co, 3207 Washington Blvd, St. Louis 63103, 1970.

This is a well-written, well-organized introductory textbook. It places commendable emphasis on the pharmacological principles and concepts relevant to medicine. Despite its modest size, all of the more significant drugs appear to be included; it is well illustrated and referenced extensively. It provides the student with a means for conducting a quick, no frills review of the basic facts prior to a pharmacology test or a National Board exam.

This edition contains a useful appendix on drug interactions and an excellent chapter on contemporary drug abuse written by Gregory G. Dimijian. A few areas appear to require updating: for example, antibiotics, and there is no mention of proinsulin. The format is of high quality, and the book seems larger than it actually is because of its heavy glossy paper. It is not intended to be a reference work, but it is rather expensive compared to the widely used pharmacology reference tests. A rough calculation shows that the reference texts provide about 61,000 words per dollar, while Goth provides only about 16,000 words per dollar. In summary, this is an excellent text for students who want a clear presentation of the basic facts (and only the basic facts).

JAMES F. LENNEY, PhD
Honolulu

Endocrine Function Tests. By Arturo Atria, MD. Price, $9. Pp 126. Charles C Thomas Publisher, 301-327 E Lawrence Ave, Springfield, Ill 62703, 1970.

The information contained in this book is readily available from other sources. Even though it was published in 1970, it contains many outdated theories and techniques and has many factual errors. Acquisition of this book by physicians, medical students, paramedical personnel, and libraries cannot be advised. I doubt that it would be helpful to cite specific examples of its inadequacy. However, it might be worth asking is it possible to publish a useful book on a subject now advancing at such a rapid rate?

A book on endocrine function tests might achieve satisfactory timeliness by having its sections prepared by well informed subspecialists; each section could be updated just before publication. With the time required for production and distribution of books these days, this technique will still result in a delay of months to years. Even if the book were satisfactory when purchased, it would need revision in six months or a year.

One alternative might be to model a book on the old looseleaf treatises of medicine still displayed in some medical libraries. A reader who wants to gather data on endocrine function testing might buy a loose-leaf book with current information together with an n year subscription service which updates the book with inserts distributed every four months or so.

Another alternative is a telephone-contactable updated data bank on endocrine function tests. This might be done on a fee for service or subscription basis. Good advice on planning a well informed laboratory investigation of patients with endocrine disease would often result in substantial savings. The fee for consultation on planning a patient's work-up could be passed on to the patient or to the financially responsible third party. One of the large clinical laboratories might offer this as a service to its customers.

C. A. NUGENT, MD
Tucson, Ariz

Research on the Cerebral Circulation. Edited by John Stirling Meyer, MD; Martin Reivich, MD; Helmut Lechner, MD; Otto Eichhorn, MD. Price, $22.25. Pp 297. Charles C Thomas Publisher, 301-327 E Lawrence Ave, Springfield, Ill 62703, 1970.

This volume is another in a series of "instant books" containing the papers presented at a specific meeting. The date of the fourth Salzburg conference is not given. Thirty-five papers by the more than 60 participants were presented in six major headings. The attempt to organize the data is in general successful, but this volume has the many defects of all such "compilations." In many ways this book is better than average. Most of the chapters are short and contain essential elements without rehashing previously published data. Some repetitions occur, but they do not appear excessive.

The chapters concerning changes in small vessels of the brain in cerebral vascular disease, and particularly the chapter on the blood supply and angioarchitecture, are quite good, as are those on the intracerebral steal syndromes. Three chapters are devoted to methods for measuring cerebral blood flow, but the chapter "Sources of Error in External Measurements of Isotopes in Human Brain" is perhaps the most useful.

The fourth section deals with clinical, experimental, and morphologic studies of cerebral vascular disease and includes an excellent chapter on regional changes in autoregulation following cerebral trauma.

Section five deals with cerebral blood flow, metabolism, and electroencephalography in cerebral disorders and is highlighted by an excellent section on cerebral blood flow in organic dementias by Ingvar. He points out that intellectual impairment parallels a reduction in the relative weight and blood flow in the cerebral gray matter. In senile dementias abnormalities in blood flow in the white matters are rare, but they are more common in the presenile dementias. This perhaps suggests a different pathogenosis in senile and presenile dementias. Also, abnormalities in the frontotemporal region are most pronounced in the senile dementia but there may be a patchy or focal type of impairment in blood flow in the presenile types.

The final section, in my judgment, should not have been published. It contains four chapters, one of which is virtually identical to one presented earlier in the book, and one of which consists of two paragraphs.

In summary, this is a potpourri of topics relating to cerebral circulation; some are excellent and others do not merit comment. There is little here for the practicing physicians and only slightly more for those who have a specific interest in current research on cerebral circulation.

ARNOLD A. BANK, MD
Philadelphia

Emotional Issues in the Lives of Physicians. By John C Duffy, MD. Price, not given. Pp 92. Charles C Thomas Publisher, 301-327 E Lawrence Ave, Springfield, Ill 62703, 1970.

Duffy has favored himself, and every member of his medical profession, with a very great service indeed, in working-up and publishing this excellent little book. I report whole, the concise and comprehensive first paragraph of his Preface:

> Every man in his personal journey through life must chart a course marked

by uncertainty and danger from within and without. The bond of human nature determines that many of the demands and stresses of living are common to all. Fear, poverty, disease, prejudice, and numerous other ancient adversaries have tested the mettle of man's health and emotional maturity. Since antiquity there have been groups of men who, by their choice of profession, must cope with special issues inherent in their life work which pose unique problems and emotional risks. The medical profession represents a group of men, who by their oath and their practice are indeed special. Their role as physician is a point of glory at best, a punishing test of emotional health at worst.

There is no greater, or more fatal, delusion than the belief that health is a kind of natural outcome of life which requires no careful and continuous cultivation. No one can be any more healthy than he requires himself to become. Human living is emotional living. Whatever exists in men, exists emotionally. Whether or not I am able to be aware of my emotionality does not affect its existence. It is greatly to my advantage to be able to be aware that I am an emotional person, however. For instance, entirely unsuspected as such, my facial pallor may be an expression of my habit of mind of living in despair, or constant fear; or my flush, an unrealized sign of my habit of mind of feeling constantly ashamed, or outraged; and so on and on.

In *Science*, June 1970, Carroll E. Izard of Vanderbilt University insightfully pointed out the value of being able to experience unpleasant feelings as being biologically adequate *conscious signals* of the way a person is conducting his living:

"We have been taught that the emotions, especially what we call negative emotions, are dangerous and bad. But each of the emotions, like any other significant part of the human being, has an inherently adaptive function."

Duffy's volume consists of a fine preface and nine excellent chapters, each of which excites and sustains my personal, including professional, interest: "Changing Image of the Physician"; "The Young Physician"; "The Physician's Family"; "Professional Relationships"; "The Woman Physician"; "The Incompetent Physician"; "The Medical Man's Menopause"; "The Physically Handicapped Physician"; and "Suicide." His important and timely study concludes with a statement every physician will take to heart:

"All human life has value beyond measure, but when a great portion of that life has been devoted to education and training in medicine for the service of mankind, the loss of that life to society is indeed great."

I highly and heartily recommend this practical and propitious monograph, *Emotional Issues in the Lives of Physicians*, to everyone working in the field of health.

JOHN M. DORSEY, MD
Detroit

Standardization in Hematology. Edited by G Astaldi, C Sirtori, G Vanzetti. Price, 7,000 lire. Pp 352, with 209 figures and tables. Franco Angeli Editore, Viale Monza 106, 20127 Milano, Italy, 1970.

This book is a summary of the proceedings of the conference sponsored by the International Committee for Standardization in Hematology which was held in New York in 1968 and of the International Symposium on Standardization of Hematological Methods held in Milan in 1968. It is a pleasure to find discussions of the work of international experts on quality control and standardization in hematology compiled in one book.

The first conference concentrated on the standardization of the determination of hemoglobin because worldwide experiences are now documented and essential basic approaches and requirements have become well delineated.

The second conference presented the progress made in other areas of hematology, such as cell counts, coagulation, and enzyme assays. The well thought-out organization of the symposia led to logical presentation of material, problems, and criticisms. Discussion on a given subject is easily located.

During the first conference, different international groups critically examined the preparation, distribution, and use of the international cyanmethemoglobin reference solution. It is good to see the responsibilities of both producer and user emphasized. The producer must closely adhere to an acceptable mode of preparation and use the designated procedures for reliable characterization of physical and chemical properties. The producer's effectiveness in applying criteria for characterization depends on his controlling the many potential sources of cumulative error. For instance, the setting of the wave length scale, selection of slit width, and fluctuation of voltage can affect adversely the calibration of reference solutions with the spectrophotometer.

Human differences in technique, questionable statistical practices, and nonrecognition of trends in conditions in the laboratory also may contribute to total error in calibration of the reference solution. The producer should maintain a quality control system that covers all factors of performance, with particular emphasis on factors that validate the criteria based on spectrophotometric measurements. An extended trial apparently is still needed to determine the efficacy of the suggestion that carbon yellow or Chance glass be the practical means of calibrating the photometric scale.

Yet, probably the most interesting, and in the long run the most highly beneficial concept is the need for the user to assume more responsibility in employing the reference solution product. He should institute and follow proper directions and exercise precautions by continually being alert to changes in the reference materials.

It is useful to have reports on studies of (1) possible modes of preparing reagents, (2) potential reference methods, (3) limitations of measuring turbidity, (4) availability of standard glasses and emission sources for calibration of wave length and optical density, and (5) measurement of an accurate absorption coefficient. The discussions suggest that concensus is needed to determine what choices of wave length and what upper limits of acceptable absorption are best for measuring turbidity. The difficulties experienced by six surveys revealed the standardization problems usually encountered in determining the "normal" range of the individual or of groups and in delineating different nutritional or disease states.

Several reports critically evaluated sample measurements, reagent addition, and turbidity estimations. The papers by Lewis should be disturbing to the careless worker. The discussions rightfully suggest that it is much more desirable to prevent turbidity or to demand its absence in the reference solution than to measure it. Nomographic and numerical corrections for turbidity should be considered only as necessary evils, and turbidity should be eliminated as soon as possible. There is no substitute for a nonturbid, stable reference solution.

The last half of the book contains an examination of most of the known sources of errors involved in the standardization of clinical hematological tests. The problems in the use of cell suspensions, stability of substances to be measured, errors in sampling and dilution, misuses of spectrophotometry, inherent difficulties in automation, and errors made in calculating results give an investigator an insight into the difficulties and limitations of standardizing hematological tests. Directions for using reference standard solutions for hematological tests must emphasize problems of aliquot measurement, lack of contamination and preservation, and control of pH and interfering substances. The different reference cell suspensions or constituent solutions should be tested for applicability to different instrument and automation systems. Investigators were challenged not only to measure the magnitude of statistical errors, but also to indicate the sources of error. Several papers restated the need to define clearly the highly variable term "precision."

This book is remarkable in maintaining easy readability even when technical and statistical details are presented. The concise report of the conference and the symposium makes available a comprehensive review of the problems and proposed solutions in the field of hematological standardization. Obviously, points of view from industrial, clinical, and academic groups were presented and communicated. The book emphasizes a heartening trend: recognized experts in the field of hematology are accepting the challenge to create acceptable international standards.

My criticisms of the book are few. The printing of some of the charts and graphs is of poor quality. A few papers reveal poor experimental design and inadequate presentation of data.

The book covers the many standardization problems common to hematology laboratories. I recommend it to anyone interested in quality control, proficiency testing, and standardization.

GERALD R. COOPER, MD, PhD
Atlanta

Principles and Techniques of Cardiac Pacing. By Seymour Furman, MD, Doris JW Escher, MD. Price, $12.50. Pp 269, with 284 Illustrations. Harper & Row Publishers Inc, 49 E 33rd St, New York 10016, 1970.

The distinguished authors of this book are to be congratulated on achieving what might be subtitled *The Compleat Pacer.* No conceivable aspect of electric stimulation of the heart has been neglected. Every theoretic and practical consideration is covered, bracketed by a concise review of the history of pacing and by commercial aspects of currently available equipment. A great number of helpful illustrations are carefully keyed to the text.

The authors and publisher may take particular pride in the production of this book which is of especial help to the reader (who, in this case, is also a user). Section and subsection headings are produced in large, bold, contrasting type faces distributed over well-indented, clearly printed text, so that categorical information is quickly and easily located. One could, in fact, reconstruct the authors' outline quite easily. The illustrations, taken by themselves, are a veritable atlas of pacing. Anyone interested in teaching, learning, or practicing pacing will regard Furman and Escher as a masterpiece. At $12.50, this book is a steal.

DAVID H. SPODICK, MD
Boston

Nephrology: Proceedings of the 4th International Congress of Stockholm 1969. By N Alwall; F Berglund; B Josephson. Price, $30. Pp 880, with 396 figures and 143 tables. Albert J Phiebig Inc, PO Box 352, White Plains, NY 10602, 1970.

The International Congress of Nephrology is a happy event that takes place every three years. The first Congress was held in 1960 in Evian, and occurred thereafter in Prague, Washington, and most recently in Stockholm. Three slender volumes contain the proceedings of the Fourth International Congress of Nephrology and are divided into volume 1 (Embryology, Ultrastructure, Physiology), volume 2 (Endocrinology, Metabolic Aspects), and volume 3 (Clinical Nephrology, Immunology). Within these volumes are state of the art lectures and free communications grouped by subject. The latter obviously range over the entire face of modern nephrology in its physiologic, anatomic, and clinical aspects. A mere catalogue of the subject matter would require all of the space available for this review. For the nephrologists, the proceedings are an invaluable compendium of current opinion, experimental data, and clinical results of various therapies.

The index provides a valuable survey of those topics under the most active investigation and debate. For example, volume 1 includes a section on renal medullary function, and another on the excretion of macromolecules. In volume 2, one finds an emphasis on renin, angiotensin, aldosterone, natruretic hormone, and the ever elusive uremic toxins. Volume 3 heavily stresses the immunologic aspects of glomerulonephritis including immunosuppressive treatments. Sections on dialysis and transplant are present. It is a pleasure to note that pyelonephritis has ceased to be a nephrological obsession.

Those with a casual interest in nephrology are unlikely to be entranced by these proceedings. The nephrologist, and particularly one who has attended the congresses, will find himself nostalgic for Stockholm and resolve to be in Mexico City in 1972.

LEONARD B. BERMAN, MD
Cleveland

Liver Pathophysiology: Its Relevance to Human Disease. By Charles S Davidson, MD. Price, $10. Pp 279, with 68 illustrations. Little, Brown & Co, 34 Beacon St, Boston 02106, 1970.

Revered principles in health care and medical education are being attacked and considered shibboleths of the past. The charisma of basic sciences and even that of its recently most glamorous branch, molecular biology, is fading. Their relevance is being challenged, and organ-directed specialization is frowned upon. Several new deities have appeared in medical education, such as integration, core curriculum, and erasing of the borders between basic sciences. Thus, as discipline-oriented textbooks lose their popularity in medical school teaching, the syllabus has appeared as the best device to serve the new deities. While I favor them as an excellent challenge for the teacher and an essential device for coordination of the course, they are not necessarily the ideal solution. They consist usually of drab mimeographed sheets with drawing exercises of questionable esthetic value. They vary in quality and organization even in the same institution, particularly if the responsible author, the teacher, is not convinced of the usefulness of the syllabus. During this quarrelsome battle about value and style of syllabi going on in many medical schools, a handsome, not expensive book (possibly cheaper than the cost of the production of a syllabus) suddenly appears which combines the good things of the old revered principles and of the new deities, even bowing to one of the new cliches, "pathophysiology."

It is a paperback—easy to read and pleasant to look at—though I am not quite sure which riddle is to be solved by looking at the cover. In concise, lucid, and elegant fashion, liver disease is discussed for the medical student and for those physicians who want to refresh their knowledge in this field and learn about specific problems. Basic science is made relevant by interweaving it with pertinent clinical information. Moreover, illustrative case histories are inserted in a casual fashion to whet the appetite of the reader. They provide valuable cross references to pertinent facts in different diseases.

The greatest feat is to leave material out and, here, Davidson exhibits the discipline of the "pro." He covers the common diseases of the liver without letting the student even know whether he is dealing with clinical science, or the sciences basic to medicine, or whether he wants to impress him with sound therapeutic principles. The patient orientation disguises the large amount of hard information presented. The nomenclature, troublesome in liver disease, is simple and clear. This is a book written by a clinician, a scientist, and a scholar, and, although its main purpose is to intrigue the neophyte, even the seasoned hepatologist may pick up a few refreshing pearls. He may not agree with every detail, which reveals the subjectivity of the seasoned clinician.

Up to now, I have offered only praise, but I want to prove my objectivity by protesting the quality of many of the photomicrographs, including the electron micrographs. I have been carried away by genuine enthusiasm in the description of this book and apologize for dispensing with the abbreviated table of contents expected in a book review. Davidson has given us a standard for the modern student textbook. It will be hard to match. It took courage to write it at this time. My hat is off to him for a smashing success.

HANS POPPER, MD
New York

BOOKS RECEIVED

Anesthesia for Outpatient Surgery. By David D Cohen, MD; John B Dillon, MD. Price, $5.75. Pp 67. Charles C Thomas Publisher, 301-327 E Lawrence Ave, Springfield, Ill 62703, 1970.

The Hormones: Endocrine Physiology. By Clark T Sawin, MD. Price, $9.75. Pp 308, with few illustrations. Little Brown & Co, 34 Beacon St, Boston 02106, 1969.

Spectrophotometry of Haemoglobin Derivatives. By OW Van Assendelft, MD. Price, $15.75. Pp 152. Charles C Thomas Publisher, 301-327 E Lawrence Ave, Springfield, Ill 1971.

Rheumatology: The Immunochemistry and Bio Connective Tissue and Its Disease States. Price, $16.20. Pp 227. Albert J Phiebig Inc, PO Box 352, White Plains, NY 10602, 1970.

Anatomical Studies on the Motion of the Heart and Blood. By William Harvey, MD. Price, $4.50. Pp 151. Charles C Thomas Publisher, 301-327 E Lawrence Ave, Springfield, Ill, 1970.

Overcoming the Fear of Death. By David Cole Gordon. Price, $3.95. Pp 115. Macmillan Co, 866 Third Ave, New York 10022, 1970.

Drugs With Possible Ocular Side-Effects. By Hugh Green, and John Spencer. Price, $20. Pp 213. St. Martin's Press, 175 Fifth Ave, New York 10010, 1970.

Psychologic Cues in Forecasting Physical Illness. By Samuel Silverman, MD. Price, $12. Pp 403. Appleton-Century-Crofts Inc, Educational Division, Meredith Corporation, 440 Park Ave S, New York 10016, 1970.

Tumours of the Testicle. By John P Blandy, DM, MCH, FRCS; HF Hope-Stone, MB, BS, DMRT, FFR; Anthony D Dayan, BSC, MD, MRC (PATH). Price, $7. Pp 199. Grune & Stratton Inc, 757 Third Ave, New York 10017; 23 Bedford Sq, London, WC1, 1970.

Anaesthesiology and Resuscitation: Anaesthesiologie und Wiederbelebung: Anesthésiologie et Réanimation. Intensivtherapie Beim Akuten Nierenversagen. By E Buchborn, and O Heidenreich. Price, $6.80. Pp 78, with 31 illustrations. Springer-Verlag, New York, 1970.

ERRATUM

In the book review entitled "Ulcerative Colitis" by Robert S. Nelson, MD, which appeared in the October issue (*Arch Intern Med* **128**:644-645, 1971), an error appeared on page 644. The second sentence should read "Its etiology is **not** known. . . ."

AUTHOR INDEX TO VOLUME 128

In this Index in alphabetical order are listed the names of authors of all articles. Full citation is given under first author only; reference is made from joint authors.

A

Abram HS: The psychology of physical illness as portrayed in Thomas Mann's *The Magic Mountain*, 446 (Se)

Abrams HL see Dobrzinsky SJ

Acacio I see Goldberg MF

Adams WS see Williams RA

Alexander SJ see Swezey RL

Allison AC: Lysosmes and the toxicity of particulate pollutants, 131 (Jy)

Alpert SM, Schwartz BB, Lee SD and Lewis TR: Alveolar protein accumulation, 69 (Jy)

Anderson JT see Keys A

Armstrong D see Wolfe MS

Assaykeen TA, Castellino RA, Love TA and Stamey TA: Peripheral and renal vein renin activity, 378 (Se)

Aviram A see Viskoper RJ

B

Balint JA see Fromm H

Barry KG see Scurry MT

Bartel AG, Heyden S, Tyroler HA, Tabesh E, Cassel JC and Hames CG: Electrocardiographic predictors of coronary heart disease, 929 (De)

See also Cassel JC; Heyden S; Heyman A; Tyroler HA

Berger HM, Goldman R, Gonick HC and Waisman J: Epidermoid carcinoma of the lip after renal transplantation, 609 (Oc)

Berman LB: The Goldblatt kidney, 306 (Au)

Bethune JE see Speckart PF

Bhoopalam N, Lee BM, Yakulis VJ and Heller P: IgM heavy chain fragments in Waldenstrom's macroglobulinemia, 437 (Se)

Bierman CW see Jordan MC

Biggar WD, Meuwissen HJ and Good RA: Successful defense against *Histoplasma capsulatum* in hypogammaglobulinemia, 585 (Oc)

Blackburn H see Keys A

Blevins A see Wolfe MS

Blomfield J, Dixon SR and McCredie DA: Potential hepatotoxicity of copper in recurrent hemodialysis, 555 (Oc)

Bloodworth JMB Jr see Shelp WD

Blumenschein GR see Grant JA

Boak R see Warren SL

Bobroff LM see Robboy SJ

Bogdonoff MD: The challenge and the opportunities of the Weed system, 832 (No)
Consumerism in medicine, 469 (Se)
The funding of graduate education, 144 (Jy)
Societal health and medical services, 636 (Oc)

Borowsky SA see Goldberg MF

Brazil S see Rocha H

Bross IDJ, Shimaoka K and Tidings J: Some epidemiological clues in thyroid cancer, 755 (No)

Brozek J see Keys A

Bruton J see Scurry MT

Buckley CE see Grant JA

Bunn SM Jr see Rogers PW

Burch GE, Tsui C-Y, Harb JM and Colcolough HL: Pathologic findings in the pancreas of mice infected with coxsackievirus B4, 40 (Jy)

C

Carr DT see Lillington GA

Carrasco H see Lang TW

Cassel JC: Review of 1960 through 1962 cardiovascular disease prevalence study, 890 (De)
Summary of major findings of the Evans County Cardiovascular Studies, 887 (De)
Heyden S, Bartel AG, Kaplan BH, Tyroler HA, Cornoni JC and Hames CG: Incidence of coronary heart disease by ethnic group, social class and sex, 910 (De)
Heyden S, Bartel AG, Kaplan BH, Tyroler HA, Cornoni JC, and Hames CG: Occupation and physical activity and coronary heart disease, 920 (De)
See also Bartel AG; Cornoni JC; Hayes CG; Heyden S; Heyman A; Kaplan BH; Kleinbaum DG; Tyroler HA

Castellino RA see Assaykeen TA

Chaco J see Viskoper RJ

Charache S see Goldberg MF

Chazan JA and Garella S: Glutethimide intoxication, 215 (Au)

Cherubin CE: Infectious disease problems of narcotic addicts, 309 (Au)

Christlieb AR see Dobrzinsky SJ

Chuquimia R see Rahimtoola SH

Clapp JR see Robinson RR

Coffin DL see Huber GL

Cohen RJ see Erickson CC

Colcolough HL see Burch GE

Colman RW see Robboy SJ

Coltman CA Jr: Pagophagia (corres.), 472 (Se)

Corday E see Lang TW

Cornoni JC, Waller LE, Cassel JC, Tyroler HA and Hames CG: The incidence study—study design and methods, 896 (De)
See also Cassel JC; Heyden S; Kaplan BH; Tyroler HA

Cotlier E see Goldberg MF

Council on the Kidney in Cardiovascular Disease of the American Heart Association: Criteria for the evaluation of the severity of established renal disease, 304 (Au)

Counts GW, Nitzkin JL, Hennekens CH Jr, and Ehrenkranz NJ: Shiga bacillus dysentery acquired in Nicaragua, 582 (Oc)

Creger WP see Poth JL

Crocker TT see Wang IY

Crowder JG, Gilkey and White AC: *Serratia marcescens* bacteremia, 247 (Au)

D

Degenshein G see Kozinn PJ

Denison EK, Peters RL and Reynolds TB: Portal hypertension in a patient with osteopetrosis, 279 (Au)

Dexter M see Koch-Weser J

Di Chiro G: see Sherman BM

DiGilio MM see Rahimtoola SH

Dixon SR see Blomfield J

Dobrzinsky SJ, Voegeli E, Grant HA, Christlieb AR, Abrams HL and Hickler RB: Spontaneous reestablishment of renal function after complete occlusion of a renal artery, 266 (Au)

Dorff GJ, Geimer NF, Rosenthal DR and Rytel MW: *Pseudomonas* septicemia, 591 (Oc)

Dowell AR, Kilburn KH and Pratt PC: Short-term exposure to nitrogen dioxide [Dowell], 74 (Jy)

E

Ehrenkranz NJ see Counts GW

Eichhorn RD see Jenkins DE

Enat R see Goldberg MF

Ensinck JW see Williams RH

Erickson CC, Lagios MD, Schoenfeld P and Cohen RJ: Effect of bilateral nephrectomy in postpartum nephrosclerosis, 448 (Se)

Evans MJ, Stephens RJ and Freeman G: Effects of nitrogen dioxide on cell renewal in the rat lung, 57 (Jy)

F

Fass RJ and Saslaw S: Earth day histoplasmosis, 588 (Oc)

Feinstein AR and Niebyl JR: Changes in the diagnostic process during 40 years of clinicopathologic conferences, 774 (No)

Figueroa-Casas JC see Jenkins DE

Finer DC see Koch-Weser J

Fisch C see Zipes DP

Fishenscher LG see Goldberg MF

Frame B, Guiang HL, Frost HM, Reynolds WA: Osteomalacia induced by laxative (phenolphthalein) ingestion, 794 (No)

Franciosa JA and Lawrinson W: Coronary artery occlusion due to neoplasm, 797 (No)

Freeman G see Evans MJ

Fritzhand M see Hueter FG

Fromm H, Wilson FA, Rodgers JB Jr and Balint JA: Granulomatous bowel (Crohn's) disease, 739 (No)

Frost HM see Frame B

G

Gardner DE see Huber GL

Garella S see Chazan JA

Gause EM see Rowlands JR

Geimer NF see Dorff GJ

George RP Jr see Poth JL

Gilkey GH see Crowder JG

Gold H see Lang TW

Goldberg MF, Charache S and Acacio I: Ophthalmologic manifestations of sickle cell thalassemia, 33 (Jy)
Cotlier E, Fichenscher LG, Kenyon K, Enat R and Borowsky SA: Macular cherry-red spot, corneal clouding, and β-galactosidase deficiency, 387 (Se)

Goldfine ID see Lawrence AM

Goldman R see Berger HM

Goldman RH see Yamashiro KM

Gonick HC see Berger HM

Good RA see Biggar WD

Gorden P see Sherman BM

Gorman CA see Ivy HK

Gould VE and Smuckler EA: Alveolar injury in acute carbon tetrachloride intoxication, 109 (Jy)

Grant HA see Dobrzinsky SJ

Grant JA, Blumenschein GR and Buckley CE III: Familial paraproteinemia, 427 (Se)

Grob PJ see Morandi LP

Guiang HL see Frame B

Gunnar RM see Rahimtoola SH

Gurwith MJ, Stinson EB, Remington JS: *Aspergillus* infection complicating cardiac transplantation, 541 (Oc)

H

Hadley JG see Roehm JN

Haff RC see Marr JJ

Hames CG: Evans County Cardiovascular and Cerebrovascular Study; introduction, 883 (De)
See also Bartel A; Cassell JC; Cornoni JC; Heyden S; Heyman A; Kaplan BH; Tyroler HA

Hampers CL see Kominami N

Harb JM see Burch GE

Harris D see Yamashiro KM

Hart RJ Jr and McCurdy PR: Psychosis in vitamin B_{12} deficiency, 596 (Oc)

Hayes CG, Tyroler HA and Cassel JC: Family aggregation of blood pressure in Evans County, Georgia, 965 (De)

Hearey CD Jr see Rocha H

Heller P see Bhoopalam N

Hennekens CH Jr see Nitzkin GW

Heyden S, Walker L, Hames CG and Tyroler HA: Decrease of serum cholesterol level and blood pressure in the community, 982 (De)
Cassel JC, Bartel A, Tyroler HA, Hames CG and Cornoni JC: Body weight and cigarette smoking as risk factors, 915 (De)
Hames CG, Bartel A, Cassel JC, Tyroler HA and Cornoni JC: Weight and weight history in relation to cerebrovascular and ischemic heart disease, 956 (De)
Bartel AG, Tabesh E, Cassel JC, Tyroler HA, Cornoni JC and Hames CG: Angina pectoris and the Rose questionnaire, 961 (De)
See also Bartel AG; Cassel JC; Heyman A; Tyroler HA

Heyman A, Karp HR, Heyden S, Bartel A, Cassel JC, Tyroler HA and Hames CG: Cerebrovascular disease in the biracial population of Evans County, Georgia, 949 (De)

Hicler RB see Dobrzinsky SJ

Howard RP and Keaty EC: Evaluation of equilin 3-monosulfate and other estrogens, 229 (Au); correction, 654 (Oc)

Huber GL, Mason RJ, LaForce M, Spencer NJ, Gardner DE and Coffin DL: Alterations in the lung following the administration of ozone, 81 (Jy)

Hueter FG and Fritzhand M: Oxidants and lung biochemistry, 48 (Jy)

Hurst JW: The art and science of presenting a patient's problems (as an extension of the Weed system), 463 (Se)
How to implement the Weed system (in order to improve patient care, education, and research by improving medical records), 456 (Se)
The problem-oriented record and the measurement of excellence, 819 (No)

I

Ivy HK, Wahner HW and Gorman CA: "Triiodothyronine (T_3) toxicosis," 529 (Oc)

J

Jacobson BM see Robboy SJ

Jenkins DE, Malik SK, Figueroa-Casas JC and Eichhorn RD: Sequential observations on pulmonary functional derangements in bagassosis, 535 (Oc)

Jordan MC and Kirby WMM: Pyogenic vertebral osteomyelitis, 405 (Se)
Bierman CW and VanArsdel PP Jr: Allergic bronchopulmonary aspergillosis, 576 (Oc)

Jordan PH Jr see Twomey JJ

K

Kanarek P see Koch-Weser J

Kanovitz BS see Leb DE

Kao YS see Twomey JJ

Kaplan BH, Cassel JC, Tyroler HA, Cornoni JC, Kleinbaum DG and Hames CG: Occupational mobility and coronary heart disease, 938 (De)
See also Cassel JC

Karp HR see Heyman A

Keaty EC see Howard RP

Kem DC, Weinberger MH, Mayes DM and Nugent CA: Saline suppression of plasma aldosterone in hypertension, 380 (Se)

Kenyon K see Goldberg MF

Keys A, Taylor HL, Blackburn H, Brozek J, Anderson JT and Simonson E: Mortality and coronary heart disease among men studied for 23 years, 201 (Au)

Khero BA and Mullins CB: Cardiac syncope due to glossopharyngeal neuralgia, 806 (No)

Kleinbaum DG, Kupper LL, Cassel JC, and Tyroler HA: Multivariate analysis of risk of coronary heart disease in Evans County, Georgia, 943 (De)
See also Kaplan BH; Tyroler HA

Kilburn KH see Kowell AR

Kirby WMM see Jordan MC

Kirk JW see Rocha H

Koch-Weser J, Sidel VW, Dexter M, Parish C, Finer DC and Kanarek P: Adverse reactions to sulfisoxazole, sulfamethoxazole, and nitrofurantoin, 399 (Se)

Kominami N, Tyler HR, Hampers CL and Merrill JP: Variations in motor nerve conduction velocity in normal and uremic patients, 235 (Au)

Kozinn PJ and Degenshein G: Treatment of *Candida* infection (corres.), 639 (Oc)

Kupper LL see Kleinbaum DG

Kurtzman NA see Rogers PW

L

LaForce M see Huber GL

Lagios MD see Erickson CC

Lang T-W, Corday E, Meerbaum S, Lozano JR, Carrasco H and Gold H: Ascending aorta synchronized pulsation, 258 (Au)

Langford HG see Summers WE

Laughter AH see Twomey JJ

Lawrence AM, Pinsky SM and Goldfine ID: Conventional radiation therapy in acromegaly, 369 (Se)

Lawrinson W see Franciosa JA

Leb DE, Weisskopf B and Kanovitz BS: Chromosome aberrations in the child of a kidney transplant recipient, 441 (Se)

Lebovitz HE see Shultz KT

Lee BM see Bhoopalam N

Lee SD see Alpert SM

Levy M see Zlotnick A

Lewis TR see Alpert SM

Lidsky MD see Twomey JJ

Liebes DM see Warren SL

Lillington GA, Carr DT and Mayne JG: Rheumatoid pleurisy and effusion, 764 (No)

Loeb HS see Rahimtoola SH

Lorian V: The mode of action of antibiotics on gram-negative bacilli, 623 (Oc)

Louria DB see Wolfe MS

Love TA see Assaykeen TA

Lozano JR see Lang TW

Lyon LW, McCormick WF and Schochet SS Jr: Progressive multifocal leukoencephalopathy, 420 (Se)

M

McCormick WF see Lyon LW

McCredie DA see Blomfield J

McCurdy PR see Hart RJ Jr

Maher JF see Nolph KD; Tamm HS

Malik SK see Jenkins DE

Marmor L see Warren SL

Marr JJ and Haff RC: Superinfection of an amoebic abscess by *Salmonella enteritidis,* 291 (Au)

Marver HS see Wang IY

Mason RJ see Huber GL

Mayes DM see Kem DC

Mayne JG see Lillington GA

Medalle R, Webb R and Waterhouse C: Lactic acidosis and associated hypoglycemia, 273 (Au)

Meerbaum S see Lang TW

Mendeloff AI see Nair PP

Menzel DB see Roehm JN

Merrill JP see Kominami N

Meuwissen HJ see Biggar WD

Mezey E see Nair PP

Morandi LP and Grob PJ: Retroperitoneal fibrosis, 295 (Au)

Mullins CB see Khero BA

Murty HS see Nair PP

N

Nair PP, Mezey E, Murty HS, Quartner J and Mendeloff AI: Vitamin E and porphyrin metabolism in man, 411 (Se)

Neal RA: Enzymic mechanism of metabolism of the phosphorothionate insecticides, 118 (Jy)

Neelon JA see Shultz KT

Nicoloff JT see Speckart PF

Niebyl JR see Feinstein AR

Nilsen LB see Shultz KT

Nitzkin JL see Counts GW

Nolph KD, Stoltz M and Maher JF: Calcium free peritoneal dialysis, 809 (No)
See also Tamm HS

Norton RA: The history and clinical usefulness of *Pi,* 991 (De)

Noyes R Jr: The care and management of the dying, 299 (Au)

Nugent CA see Kem DC

O

Orgain ES see Spencer WH III

P

Parish C see Koch-Weser J

Peter RH see Spencer WH III

Peters RL see Denison EK

Pinsky SM see Lawrence AM

Pollock AA: Combination therapy (corres.), 473 (Se)

Poth JL, George RP Jr, Creger WP, and Schrier SL: Acute myelogenous leukemia following localized radiotherapy, 802 (No)

Pratt PC see Dowell AR

Q

Quartner J see Nair PP

R

Ragsdale B see Robby SJ

Rahimtoola SH, DiGilio MM, Sinno MZ, Loeb HS, Rosen KM and Gunnar RM: Cardiac performance three to eight weeks after acute myocardial infarction, 220 (Au)
Sinno MZ, Loeb HS, Chuquimia R, Rosen KM and Gunnar RM: Lidocaine infusion in acute myocardial infarction, 416 (Se)

Rasmussen RE see Wang IY

Remington JS see Gurwith MJ

Reynolds TB see Denison EK

Reynolds WA see Frame B

Rhoades RA see Williams RA

Richters V see Sherwin RP

Rieselbach RE see Shelp WD

Robboy SJ, Salisbury K, Ragsdale B, Bobroff LM, Jacobson BM and Colman RW: Mechanism of *Aspergillus*-induced microangiopathic hemolytic anemia, 790 (No)

Robinson RR and Clapp JR: AMA drug evaluations; a praiseworthy venture, 147 (Jy)

Rocha H, Brazil S, Kirk JW and Hearey CD Jr: Prolonged *Salmonella* bacteremia in patients with *Schistosoma mansoni* infection, 254 (Au)

Rodgers JB Jr see Fromm H

Roehm JN, Hadley JG and Menzel DB: Antioxidants vs lung disease, 88 (Jy)

Rogers PW, Bunn SM Jr, Kurtzman NA and White MG: Schönlein-Henoch syndrome associated with exposure to cold, 782 (No)

Rosen KM see Rahimtoola SH

Rosenthal DR see Dorff GJ

Rowlands JR and Gause EM: Reaction of nitrogen dioxide with blood and lung components, 94 (Jy)

Rutsky EA: Bradycardic rhythms during peritoneal dialysis, 445 (Se)

Rytel MW see Dorff GJ

S

Salisbury K see Robboy SJ

Saslaw S see Fass RJ

Schochet SS Jr see Lyon LW

Schoenfeld P see Erickson CC

Schrier SL see Poth JL

Schwartz BB see Alpert SM

Scurry MT, Burton J, and Barry KG: The effect of chorionic gonadotropin on steroid excretion, 561 (Oc)

Seymour JL: Easing the pain (corres.), 149 (Jy)

Shelp WD, Bloodworth JMB Jr, and Rieselbach RE: Effect of azathioprine on renal histology and function in lupus nephritis, 566 (Oc)

Shepherd GR: Diabetes mellitus of juvenile onset with 40 years' survival and no gross damage, 284 (Au)

Sherman BM, Gorden P and Di Chiro G: Postmeningitic selective hypopituitarism with suprasellar calcification, 600 (Oc)

Sherwin RP and Richters V: Lung capillary permeability, 61 (Jy)

Sherwood WC: Palmar varices and gastrointestinal bleeding, 598 (Oc)

Shimaoka K see Bross IDJ

Shultz KT, Neelon JA, Nilsen LB and Lebovitz HE: Mechanism of postgastrectomy hypoglycemia, 240 (Au)

Sidel VW see Koch-Weser J

Simonson E see Keys A

Sinno MZ see Rahimtoola SH

Smuckler EA see Gould VE

Speckart PF, Nicoloff JT and Bethune JE: Screening for adrenocortical insufficiency with cosyntropin (synthetic ACTH), 761 (No)

Spencer NJ see Huber GL

Spencer WH III, Peter RH and Orgain ES: Detection of a left atrial myxoma by echocardiography, 787, (No)

Stamey TA see Assaykeen TA

Stephens RJ see Evans MF

Stinson EB see Gurwith MJ

Stoltz M see Nolph KD

Summers WE, Watson RL, Wooldridge WH and Langford HG: Hypertension, obesity, and fibromyomata uteri, as a syndrome, 750 (No)

Swezey RL and Alexander SJ: Erosive osteoarthritis and the main en lorgnette deformity, 269 (Au); correction, 840 (No)

T

Tabesh E see Bartel AG; Heyden S

Tamm HS, Nolph KD and Maher JF: Factors affecting plasma calcium concentration during hemodialysis, 769 (No)

Tashima CK: Autonomic hyperreflexia in spinal cord injury (corres.), 472 (Se)

Taylor HL see Keys A

Tidings J see Bross IDJ

Tsui C-Y see Burch GE

Twomey JJ, Laughter AH, Villanueva ND, Kao YS, Lidsky MD and Jordan PH Jr: Gastric secretory and serologic studies on patients with neoplastic and immunologic disorders, 746 (No)

Tyler HR see Kominami N

Tyroler HA, Heyden S, Bartel AG, Cassel JC, Cornoni JC, Hames CG and Kleinbaum D: Blood pressure and cholesterol as coronary heart disease risk factors, 907 (De)
See also Bartel AG; Cassel JC; Cornoni JC; Hayes CG; Heyden S; Heyman A; Kaplan BH; Kleinbaum DG; Wetherbee H

U

Uyeda CT see Yamashiro KM

V

VanArsdel PP Jr see Jordan MC

Villanueva ND see Twomey JJ

Viskoper RJ, Chaco J and Aviram A: Nerve conduction velocity in the assessment of hypertension, 574 (Oc)

Voegeli E see Dobrzinsky SJ

Voudoukis IJ: Cold pressor test and arteriosclerosis (corres.), 993 (De)

W

Wahner HW see Ivy HK

Waisman J see Berger HM

Walker L see Heyden S

Waller LE see Cornoni JC

Wang IY, Marver HS, Rasmussen RE and Crocker TT: Enzymatic conversion of benzo[α]pyrene, 125 (Jy)

Warren SL, Marmor L and Liebes DM: Chronic lesions of the vertebral column and joints in older mice, 614 (Oc)
Marmor L, Boak R and Liebes DM: Transmission of an active agent from rheumatoid arthritis synovial tissue to chicks, 619 (Oc)

Waterhouse C see Webb R

Watson RL see Summers WE

Webb R see Medalle R

Weibel ER: Oxygen effect on lung cells, 54 (Jy)

Weinberger MH see Kem DC

Weisskopf B see Leb DE

Wetherbee H and Tyroler HA: The relation of migration to coronary heart disease risk factors, 976 (De)

White AC see Crowder JG

White MG see Rogers PW

Williams RA, Rhoades RA and Adams WS: The response of lung tissue and surfactant to nitrogen dioxide exposure, 101 (Jy)

Williams RH and Ensinck JW: Current studies regarding diabetes, 820 (No)

Wilson FA see Fromm H

Wolfe MS, Armstrong D, Louria DB and Blevins A: Salmonellosis in patients with neoplastic diseases, 546 (Oc)

Wooldridge WH see Summers WE

Y

Yakulis VJ see Bhoopalam N

Yamashiro KM, Goldman RH, Harris D and Uyeda CT: Pasteurella pseudotuberculosis, 605 (Oc)

Z

Zipes DP and Fisch C: Initiation of ventricular tachycardia; ECG analysis no. 5, 988 (De)
Premature A-V junctional contractions; ECG analysis no. 3, 633 (Oc)
Premature atrial contraction; ECG analysis no. 2, 453 (Se)
Premature ventricular beats; ECG analysis no. 1, 140 (Jy)
Ventricular tachycardia; ECG analysis no. 4, 815 (No)

Zlotnick A and Levy M: A heavy chain disease, 432 (Se)

SUBJECT INDEX TO VOLUME 128

The following Index is an alphabetical list of significant subjects presented in this volume. Books are listed alphabetically by first author under the heading "BOOK REVIEW."

A

Abdominal Neoplasms
α heavy chain disease; variant of Mediterranean lymphoma [Zlotnick], 432 (Se)

Acetylcholinesterase
enzymic mechanism of metabolism of phosphorothionate insecticides [Neal], 118 (Jy)

Acidosis
lactic, and associated hypoglycemia [Medalle], 273 (Au)

Acne
epidemiological clues in thyroid cancer [Bross], 755 (No)

Acromegaly
conventional radiation therapy [Lawrence], 369 (Se)
effect of chorionic gonadotropin on steroid excretion [Scurry], 561 (Oc)

ACTH see Cosyntropin

Adrenal Gland Hypofunction
screening for adrenocortical insufficiency with cosyntropin (synthetic ACTH) [Speckart], 761 (No)

Adrenocorticotropic Hormone see Cosyntropin

Agammaglobulinemia
successful defense against *Histoplasma capsulatum* in hypogammaglobulinemia [Biggar], 585 (Oc)

Age Factors
blood pressure and cholesterol as coronary disease risk factors [Tyroler], 907 (De)
cerebrovascular disease in biracial population of Evans County, Georgia [Heyman], 949 (De)
chronic lesions of vertebral column and joints in older mice; induction by active agent from rheumatoid synovial tissue [Warren], 614 (Oc)
epidemiological clues in thyroid cancer [Bross], 755 (No)

Air Pollution
oxidants and lung biochemistry [Hueter], 48 (Jy)

Aldosterone, Secretion
saline suppression of plasma aldosterone in hypertension [Kem], 380 (Se)

Allergy see Hypersensitivity

Amebiasis, Hepatic see Liver Abscess, Amebic

Amenorrhea
evaluation of equilin 3-monosulfate and other estrogens [Howard], 229 (Au); correction, 654 (Oc)

American Medical Association
drug evaluations; praiseworthy venture [Robinson], 147 (Jy)

Anaphylaxis
Schönlein-Henoch syndrome associated with exposure to cold [Rogers], 782 (No)

Androgens, Urine
effect of chorionic gonadotropin on steroid excretion [Scurry], 561 (Oc)

Anemia, Hemolytic
effect of bilateral nephrectomy in postpartum nephrosclerosis [Erickson], 448 (Se)
mechanism of *Aspergillus*-induced microangiopathic hemolytic anemia [Robboy], 790 (No)

Anemia, Hypochromic
pagophagia (corres.) [Coltman], 472 (Se)

Anemia, Pernicious
psychosis in vitamin B 12 deficiency [Hart], 596 (Oc)

Anemia, Sickle Cell
ophthalmologic manifestations of sickle cell thalassemia [Goldberg], 33 (Jy)

Angina Pectoris
and the Rose questionnaire [Heyden], 961 (De)

Angioid Streaks
ophthalmologic manifestations of sickle cell thalassemia [Goldberg], 33 (Jy)

Angiotensin
the Goldblatt kidney [Berman], 306 (Au)

Antecubital Veins
renin activity [Assaykeen], 378 (Se)

Antibiotics, Pharmacodynamics
mode of action of antibiotics on gram-negative bacilli [Lorian], 623 (Oc)

Antioxidants see Guaiacol; Vitamin E

Aorta, Thoracic
ascending aorta synchronized pulsation [Lasng], 258 (Au)

Appetite, Abnormal
pagophagia (corres.) [Coltman], 472 (Se)

Arrhythmia see also Bradycardia
premature atrial contraction; ECG analysis no. 2, [Zipes], 453 (Se)
premature A-V junctional contractions; ECG analysis no. 3 [Zipes], 633 (Oc)
premature ventricular beats; ECG analysis no. 1, [Zipes], 140 (Jy)

Arrhythmia, Drug Therapy
lidocaine infusion in acute myocardial infarction [Rahimtoola], 416 (Se)

Arteriosclerosis, Diagnosis
cold pressor test and arteriosclerosis (corres.) [Voudoukis], 993 (De)

Arthritis, Rheumatoid
chronic lesions of vertebral column and joints in older mice; induction by active agent from rheumatoid synovial tissue [Warren], 614 (Oc)
gastric secretory and serologic studies [Twomey], 746 (No)
rheumatoid pleurisy with effusion [Lillington], 764 (No)
transmission of active agent from rheumatoid arthritis synovial tissue to chicks [Warren], 619 (Oc)

Asbestosis
lysosomes and toxicity of particulate pollutants [Allison], 131 (Jy)

Aspergillosis
allergic bronchopulmonary aspergillosis [Jordan], 576 (Oc)
Aspergillus infection complicating cardiac transplantation [Gurwith], 541 (Oc)
mechanism of *Aspergillus*-induced microangiopathic hemolytic anemia [Robboy], 790 (No)

Azathioprine, Adverse Effects
chromosome aberrations in child of kidney transplant recipient [Leb], 441 (Se)

Azathioprine, Therapeutic Use
effect on renal histology and function in lupus nephritis [Shelp], 566 (Oc)

B

Bacteremia see Septicemia

Bacterial Proteins, Biosynthesis
mode of action of antibiotics on gram-negative bacilli [Lorian], 623 (Oc)

Bagassosis see Pneumoconiosis

Bed Rest see Rest

Benzopyrenes
enzymatic conversion of benzo[*a*]pyrene [Wang], 125 (Jy)

Blood Pressure
decrease of serum cholesterol level and blood pressure in the community [Heyden], 982 (De)
family aggregation of blood pressure in Evans County, Georgia [Hayes], 965 (De)
mortality and coronary heart disease among men studied for 23 years [Keys], 201 (Au)

Blood Protein Disorders, Familial and Genetic
familial paraproteinemia [Grant], 427 (Se)

Blood Proteins
alveolar protein accumulation [Alpert], 69 (Jy)
lung capillary permeability; nitrogen dioxide exposure and leakage of tritiated serum [Sherwin], 61 (Jy)

Blood Vessels, Revascularization
spontaneous reestablishment of renal function after complete occlusion of renal artery [Dobrzinsky], 266 (Au)

Body Weight
and cigarette smoking as coronary risk factors [Heyden], 915 (De)
weight and weight history in relation to cerebrovascular and ischemic heart disease [Heyden], 956 (De)

Bougie
history and clinical usefulness of pi (π) [Norton], 991 (De)

Bradycardia
bradycardic rhythms during peritoneal dialysis [Rutsky], 445 (Se)
cardiac syncope due to glossopharyngeal neuralgia [Khero], 806 (No)

Bronchial Diseases
allergic bronchopulmonary aspergillosis [Jordan], 576 (Oc)

BOOK REVIEWS
Aaron B and Osmond H, eds. Psychedelics, 652 (Oc)
Abramoff P and La Via MF. Biology of the immune response, 643 (Oc)
Alwall N and others. Nephrology: proceedings of the International Congress of Nephrology, 999 (De)
AMA Council on Drugs. AMA drug evaluations 1971, 474 (Se)
Anthony EJ and Benedek T, eds. Parenthood: its psychology and psychopathology, 994 (De)
Ashizawa S and Kidokoro T. Endoscopic color atlas of gastric diseases, 835 (No)
Astaldi G and others, eds. Standardization in hematology, 998 (De)
Atria A. Endocrine function tests, 997 (De)
Barzel US, ed. Osteoporosis, 482 (Se)
Benjamin B and Benjamin AF. In case of emergency: what to do until the doctor arrives, 840 (No)

BOOK REVIEWS, cont.
Braverman IM. Skin signs of systemic disease, 481 (Se)
Brooks FP. Control of gastrointestinal function, 646 (Oc)
Brown H. Hepatic failure, 837 (No)
Caldwell AE. Origins of psychopharmacology: from CPZ to LSD, 476 (Se)
Cantor MO. Abdominal trauma, 652 (Oc)
Cawley LP. Electrophoresis and immunoelectrophoresis, 650 (Oc)
Cerasi R and Luft CR. Pathogenesis of diabetes mellitus, 314 (Au)
Christian GD and Feldman FJ. Atomic absorption spectroscopy: applications in agriculture, biology, and medicine, 649 (Oc)
Cooper IS. Involuntary movement disorders, 648 (Oc)
Crue BL Jr, ed. Pain and suffering, 479 (Se)
Cummack DH. Gastrointestinal x-ray diagnosis, 647 (Oc)
Davidson CS. Liver pathophysiology: its relevance to human disease, 1000 (De)
Dekornfeld TJ. Inhalation therapy procedure manual, 477 (Se)
Dewhurst K, ed. Oxford medicine, 654 (Oc)
Dubin D. Rapid interpretation of EKG's, 653 (Oc)
Duffy JC. Emotional issues in the lives of physicians, 997 (De)
Educational Aids from the Tampa Tracings, 483 (Se)
Eichler O and others, eds. Handbook of experimental pharmacology, 838 (No)
Elliott HW and others, eds. Annual review of pharmacology, 152 (Jy)
Fields WS and Willis WD Jr, eds. The cerebellum: in health and disease, 996 (De)
Fox CL Jr and Nahas G, eds. Body fluid replacement in the surgical patient, 479 (Se)
Furman S and Escher DJW. Principles and techniques of cardiac pacing, 999 (De)
Goligher JC and others. Ulcerative colitis, 644 (Oc); correction, 1000 (De)
Goth A. Medical pharmacology, principles and concepts, ed. 5, 996 (De)
Grace WJ and Keyloun V. The coronary care unit, 152 (Jy)
Hamburger JI. Diagnosis and management of common thyroid problems, 477 (Se)
Harders HH, ed. Advances in microcirculation, 652 (Oc)
Harris JE and Sinkovics JG. The immunology of malignant disease, 838 (No)
Harvey AM and Bordley J III. Differential diagnosis: the interpretation of clinical evidence, 643 (Oc)
Haymaker W and Schiller F eds. The founders of neurology, 835 (No)
Hicks RE and others, eds. Psychedelic drugs, 652 (Oc)

BOOK REVIEWS, cont.
Hill DW. Electronic measurement techniques in anaesthesia and surgery, 647 (Oc)
Hobby GL, ed. Antimicrobial agents and ehemotherapy - 1969, 150 (Jy)
Hurst JW and Logue RB, eds. The heart, arteries, and veins, 314 (Au)
Jakab I. Art interpretation and art therapy, 649 (Oc)
Johnson JE III, ed. Rational therapy and control of tuberculosis, 480 (Se)
Keefer CS and Wilkins RW, eds. Medicine: essentials of clinical practice, 640 (Oc)
Leevy CM and Britton RC, eds. The hepatic circulation and portal hypertension, 481 (Se)
Luisada AA. Pulmonary edema in man and animals, 839 (No)
Mac-Bryde CM and Blacklow RS. Signs and symptoms, 640 (Oc)
McGraw-Hill Book Co. McGraw-Hill encyclopedia of science and technology, 644 (Oc)
McLetchie NCB. Coronary atheroma: a diary of discovery, 642 (Oc)
Maddin S, ed. Current dermatologic management, 150 (Jy)
Masserman JH, ed. Current psychiatric therapies, vol 10, 479 (Se)
Mathe G. Recent results in cancer research: advances in the treatment of acute (blastic) leukemias, 995 (De)
Meyer JS and others, eds. Research on the cerebral circulation, 997 (De)
Moritz AR. Handbook of legal medicine, 153 (Jy)
Nelson RS. Recent results in cancer research: endoscopy in gastric cancer, 477 (Se)
New York Heart Association. Interferon, 475 (Se)
Paulson M, ed. Gastroenterologic medicine, 474 (Se)
Philipp EE, and others, eds. Scientific foundation of obstetrics and gynecology, 317 (Au)
Pridgen JE and others, eds. Penetrating wounds of the abdomen, 482 (Se)
Raab W. Preventive myocardiology: fundamentals and targets, 478 (Se)
Regamey RH and others, eds. Progress in immunobiological standardization, 839 (No)
Schneeberg NG. Essentials of clinical endocrinology, 838 (No)
Schreiber MH. Indications and alternatives in x-ray diagnosis, 996 (De)
Selye H. Experimental cardiovascular diseases, part 1, 475 (Se)
Sikuv MR and Mahlum DD, eds. Radiation biology of the fetal and juvenile mammal, 645 (Oc)
Smith H, ed. Antibiotics in clinical practice, 315 (Au)
Speer F, ed. Allergy of the nervous system, 317 (Au)

BOOK REVIEWS, cont.
Stead WA. Fundamentals of tuberculosis today, 653 (Oc)
Stefanini M. Progress in clinical pathology, 645 (Oc)
Stewart WD and others. Synopsis of dermatology, 476 (Se)
Stuart AE. The reticuloendothelial system, 153 (Jy)
Sunderman FW and Sunderman FW Jr, eds. Laboratory diagnosis of diseases caused by toxic agents, 480 (Se)
Swanson DW and others. The paranoid, 480 (Se)
Talbott JH. Biographical history of medicine, 653 (Oc)
Teltscher HO. Handwriting revelation of self: a source book of psychographology, 641 (Oc)
Thompson RB. A short textbook of haematology, 316 (Au)
Utz JP and Gordan GS. Modern treatment. Vol 7, no. 3. Treatment of the systemic mycosis: treatment of calcium disorders, 654 (Oc)
Viers ER. So you have glaucoma, 651 (Oc)
Wallach J. Interpretation of diagnostic tests, 994 (De)
Walter RD. S. Weir Mitchell, MD. - neurologist: a medical biography, 995 (De)
Wang Y and Paoletti P, eds. Radionuclide applications in neurology and neurosurgery, 651 (Oc)
Wiener AS ed. Advances in blood grouping III, 837 (No)
Williams R, ed. Fifth symposium on advanced medicine, 646 (Oc)
Wintrobe MM and others. Principles of internal medicine, 836 (No)
Wittig HJ and others. A primer on immunologic disorders, 317 (Au)
Zugibe FT. Diagnostic histochemistry, 478 (Se)
Zuppinger A and Ruckensteiner E, eds. Encyclopedia of medical radiology. Vol 17. Radiation therapy of benign diseases, 648 (Oc)

C

Calcinosis
postmeningitic selective hypopituitarism with suprasellar calcification [Sherman], 600 (Oc)

Calcium
calcium free peritoneal dialysis [Nolph], 809 (No)

Calcium, Blood
factors affecting plasma calcium concentration during hemodialysis [Tamm], 769 (No)

Capillary Permeability
lung capillary permeability [Sherwin], 61 (Jy)

Carbon Tetrachloride
alveolar injury in acute carbon tetrachloride intoxication [Gould], 109 (Jy)

Carcinoma
gastric secretory and serologic studies [Twomey], 746 (No)

Carcinoma, Epidermoid
acute myelogenous leukemia following localized radiotherapy [Poth], 802 (No)
coronary occlusion due to neoplasm [Franciosa], 797 (no)
of lip after renal transplantation [Berger], 609 (Oc)

Carcinoma, Squamous Cell see Carcinoma, Epidermoid

Cardiography
detection of a left atrial myxoma by echocardiography [Spencer], 787 (No)

Cathartics see Phenolphthaleins

Catheterization
history and clinical usefulness of pi (π) [Norton], 991 (De)

Cell Division
effects of nitrogen dioxide on cell renewal in rat lung [Evans], 57 (Jy)

Cell Membrane
mode of action of antibiotics on gram-negative bacilli [Lorian], 623 (Oc)

Cell Wall
mode of action of antibiotics on gram-negative bacilli [Lorian], 623 (Oc)

Central America
Shiga bacillus dysentery acquired in Nicaragua [Counts], 582 (Oc)

Cerebrovascular Disorders, Occurrence
Evans County Cardiovascular and Cerebrovascular Study; papers, 833-986 (De)
in biracial population of Evans County, Georgia [Heyman], 949 (De)
incidence study—study design and methods [Cornoni], 896 (De)
weight and weight history in relation to cerebrovascular disease [Heyden], 956 (De)

Cholesterol, Blood
decrease of serum cholesterol level and blood pressure in the community [Heyden], 982 (De)

Cholinesterase Inhibitors see Parathion

Chromosome Aberrations
in child of kidney transplant recipient [Leb], 441 (Se)

Clinicopathologic Conferences
changes in the diagnostic process during 40 years [Feinstein], 774 (No)

Cold
Schönlein-Henoch syndrome associated with exposure to cold [Rogers], 782 (No)

Cold Pressor Test
and arteriosclerosis (corres.) [Voudoukis], 993 (De)

Collateral Circulation see Blood Vessels, Revascularization

Communicable Diseases
infectious disease problems of narcotic addicts [Cherubin], 309 (Au)

Consanguinity
macular cherry-red spot, corneal clouding, and β-galactosidase deficiency [Goldberg], 387 (Se)

Consumer Satisfaction
consumerism in medicine [Bogdonoff], 469 (Se)

Copper, Poisoning
potential hepatotoxicity of copper in recurrent hemodialysis [Blomfield], 555 (Oc)

Corneal Opacity
macular cherry-red spot, corneal clouding, and β-galactosidase deficiency [Goldberg], 387 (Se)

Coronary Disease, Diagnosis
angina pectoris and the Rose questionnaire [Heyden], 961 (De)

Coronary Disease, Occurrence
blood pressure and cholesterol as risk factors [Tyroler], 907 (De)
body weight and cigarette smoking as risk factors [Heyden], 915 (De)
electrocardiographic predictors of coronary disease [Bartel], 929 (De)
Evans County Cardiovascular and Cerebrovascular Study; papers, 883-986 (De)
incidence by ethnic group, social class, and sex [Cassel], 901 (De)
incidence study—study design and methods [Cornoni], 896 (De)
mortality and coronary heart disease among men studied for 23 years [Keys], 201 (Au)
multivariate analysis of risk of coronary disease in Evans County, Georgia [Kleinbaum], 943 (De)
occupation and physical activity [Cassel], 920 (De)
occupational mobility and coronary disease [Kaplan], 938 (De)
relation of migration to coronary disease risk factors [Wetherbee], 976 (De)
review of 1960 through 1962 cardiovascular disease prevalence study [Cassel], 890 (De)
summary of major findings of Evans County cardiovascular studies [Cassel], 887 (De)
weight and weight historyin relation to ischemic heart disease [Heyden], 956 (De)

Coronary Vessels
occlusion due to neoplasm; rare cause of myocardial infarction [Franciosa], 797 (No)

Corticotropin see Cosyntropin

Cortisol see Hydrocortisone

Cosyntropin
screening for adrenocortical insufficiency with cosyntropin (synthetic ACTH) [Speckart], 761 (No)

Counterpulsation (Arterial)
ascending aorta synchronized pulsation [Lang], 258 (Au)

Coxsackie Virus Infections
pathologic findings in pancreas of mice infected with coxsackievirus B4 [Burch], 40 (Jy)

Crohn's Disease see Enteritis Regional

D

Death
care and management of the dying [Noyes Jr], 299 (Au)

Dexamethasone, Therapeutic Use
retroperitoneal fibrosis; response to corticosteroid therapy [Moranki], 295 (Au)

Diabetes Insipidus
postmeningitic selective hypopituitarism with suprasellar calcification [Sherman], 600 (Oc)

Diabetes Mellitus
current studies; review [Williams], 820 (No)

Diabetes Mellitus, Complications
calcium free peritoneal dialysis; treatment of vitamin D intoxication [Nolph], 809 (No)
Pasteurella pseudotuberculosis; acute sepsis with survival [Yamashiro], 605 (Oc)

Diabetes Mellitus, Etiology
pathologic findings in pancreas of mice infected with coxsackievirus B4 [Burch], 40 (Jy)

Diabetes Mellitus, Juvenile
diabetes mellitus of juvenile onset with 40 years' survival and no gross damage [Shepherd], 284 (Au)

Diagnosis
changes in diagnostic process during 40 years of clinicopathologic conferences [Feinstein], 774 (No)

DNA
enzymatic conversion of benzo[*a*]pyrene [Wang], 125 (Jy)

DNA, Bacterial
mode of action of antibiotics on gram-negative bacilli [Lorian], 623 (Oc)

Drug Addiction, Complications
infectious disease problems of narcotic addicts [Cherubin], 309 (Au)

Drugs
AMA drug evaluations; praiseworthy venture [Robinson], 147 (Jy)

Dysentery, Bacillary
Shiga bacillus dysentery acquired in Nicaragua [Counts], 582 (Oc)

E

Echocardiography see Ultrasonics, Diagnostic Use

Ecthyma
Pseudomonas septicemia; illustrated evolution of its skin lesion [Dorff], 591 (Oc)

Education, Medical
art and science of presenting a patient's problems; (as extension of the Weed system) [Hurst], 463 (Se)

Education, Medical, Graduate
funding [Bogdonoff], 144 (Jy)

Electrocardiography
initiation of ventricular tachycardia; ECG analysis no. 5 [Zipes], 988 (De)
predictors of coronary disease [Bartel], 929 (De)
premature atrial contraction; ECG analysis no. 2 [Zipes], 453 (Se)
premature A-V junctional contractions; ECG analysis no. 3 [Zipes], 633 (Oc)
premature ventricular beats; ECG analysis no. 1 [Zipes], 140 (Jy)
ventricular tachycardia; ECG analysis no. 4 [Zipes], 815 (No)

Electron Spin Resonance
reaction of nitrogen dioxide with blood and lung components [Rowlands], 94 (Jy)

Endocarditis, Bacterial
infectious disease problems of narcotic addicts [Cherubin], 309 (Au)

Enteritis, Regional
granulomatous bowel (Crohn's) disease; retrospective study of course and treatment [Fromm], 739 (No)

Equilin see Estrogens, Pharmacodynamics

Ergocalciferol
calcium free peritoneal dialysis; treatment of vitamin D intoxication [Nolph], 809 (No)

ERRATA
154 (Jy); 654 (Oc); 840 (No); 1000 (De)

Erythrocyte Aggregation, Intravascular
mechanism of *Aspergillus*-induced microangiopathic hemolytic anemia [Robboy], 790 (No)

Esophageal Stenosis
history and clinical usefulness of pi (π) [Norton], 991 (De)

Estrogens, Pharmacodynamics
evaluation of equilin 3-monosulfate and other estrogens [Howard], 229 (Au); correction, 654 (Oc)

Ethnic Groups see Jews

Evans County (Georgia) Cardiovascular and Cerebrovascular Study
introduction [Hames], 883 (De)
papers, 883-986 (De)
summary of major findings [Cassel], 887 (De)

Exertion
occupation and physical activity and coronary disease [Cassel], 920 (De)

Ex-Lax see Phenophthaleins

Extracorporeal Circulation see Counterpulsation (Arterial)

Eye Manifestations see also Corneal Opacity
ophthalmologic manifestations of sickle cell thalassemia [Goldberg], 33 (Jy)

F

Fibroid, Uterine see Leiomyoma

Fibromyoma see Leiomyoma

Fibrosis see Asbestosis; Silicosis

G

Galactosidase, Metabolism
macular cherry-red spot, corneal clouding, and β-galactosidase deficiency [Goldberg], 387 (Se)

Gamma Globulins
IgM heavy chain fragments in Waldenstrom's macroglobulinemia [Bhoopalam], 437 (Se)
prophylactic, for prevention of endemic hepatitis [Cooperative Study], 723 (No)

Gantanol see Sulfamethoxazole, Adverse Effects

Gastric Juice, Secretion
gastric secretory and serologic studies on patients with neoplastic and immunologic disorders [Twomey], 746 (No)

Glomerulonephritis
effect of azathioprine on renal histology and function in lupus nephritis [Shelp], 566 (Oc)
Schönlein-Henoch syndrome associated with exposure to cold [Rogers], 782 (No)

Glossopharyngeal Nerve
cardiac syncope due to glossopharyngeal neuralgia [Khero], 806 (No)

Glucose
rheumatoid pleurisy with effusion [Lillington], 764 (No)

Glutethimide, Poisoning
prospective study of 70 patients treated conservatively without hemodialysis [Chazan], 215 (Au)

Goiter, Exophthalmic
"triiodothyronine (T_3) toxicosis;" its role in Graves' disease [Ivy], 259 (Oc)

Gonadotropins, Chorionic
effect on steroid excretion [Scurry], 561 (Oc)

Gonadotropins, Urine
evaluation of equilin 3-monosulfate and other estrogens [Howard], 229 (Au); correction 654 (Oc)

Granulomatous Bowel see Enteritis, Regional

Graves' Disease see Goiter, Exophthalmic

Guaiacol
antioxidants vs lung diseases [Roehm], 88 (Jy)

H

Hand, Blood Supply
palmar varices and gastointestinal bleeding [Sherwood], 598 (Oc)

Hand Deformities, Acquired
erosive osteoarthritis and the main en lorgnette deformity [Swezey], 269 (Au); correction, 840 (No)

Heart, Transplantation
Aspergillus infection complicating cardiac transplantation [Gurwith], 541 (Oc)

Heart Atrium
detection of left atrial myxoma by echocardiography [Spencer], 787 (No)
premature atrial contraction; ECG analysis, no. 2 [Zipes], 453 (Se)

Heart Conduction System
premature A-V junctional contractions; ECG analysis no. 3 [Zipes], 633 (Oc)

Heart Neoplasms
coronary artery occlusion due to neoplasm; rare cause of acute myocardial infarction [Franciosa], 797 (No)
detection of left atrial myxoma by echocardiography [Spencer], 787 (No)

Heart Ventricle
cardiac performance three to eight weeks after acute myocardial infarction [Rahimtoola], 220 (Au)
lidocaine infusion in acute myocardial infarction [Rahimtoola], 416 (Se)

Heavy Chain Disease
α variant of Mediterranean lymphoma [Zlotnick], 432 (Se)

Hemochromatosis
Pasteurella pseudotuberculosis; acute sepsis with survival [Yamashiro], 605 (Oc)

Hemodialysis
factors affecting plasma calcium concentration during hemodialysis [Tamm], 769 (No)
potential hepatotoxicity of copper in recurrent hemodialysis [Blomfield], 555 (Oc)

Hemoglobin
reaction of nitrogen dioxide with blood and lung components [Rowlands], 94 (Jy)

Hemolysis, Chemically Induced
potential hepatotoxicity of copper in recurrent hemodialysis [Blomfield], 555 (Oc)

Hemorrhage, Gastrointestinal
palmar varices and gastrointestinal bleeding [Sherwood], 598 (Oc)

Hepatitis, Chemically Induced
potential hepatotoxicity of copper in recurrent hemodialysis [Blomfield], 555 (Oc)

Hepatitis, Infectious
infectious disease problems of narcotic addicts [Cherubin], 309 (Au)
prophylactic gamma globulin for prevention of endemic hepatitis [Cooperative Study], 723 (No)

Histoplasmosis
Earth Day histoplasmosis; new type of urban pollution [Fass], 588 (Oc)
successful defense against *Histoplasma capsulatum* in hypogammaglobulinemia [Biggar], 585 (Oc)

Hormones see Gonadotropins, Chorionic

Hydrochloric Acid, Gastric see Gastric Juice

Hydrocortisone, Blood
screening for adrenocortical insufficiency with cosyntropin (synthetic ACTH) [Speckart], 761 (No)

17-Hydroxycorticosteroids, Urine
effect of chorionic gonadotropin on steroid excretion [Scurry], 561 (Oc)

Hydroxylation
enzymatic conversion of benzo[*a*]pyrene [Wang], 125 (Jy)

Hypercalcemia
calcium free peritoneal dialysis; treatment of vitamin D intoxication [Nolph], 809 (No)

Hypercholesteremia
and blood pressure as coronary disease risk factors [Tyroler], 907 (De)
decrease of serum cholesterol level in the community [Heyden], 982 (De)
mortality and coronary heart disease among men studied for 23 years [Keys], 201 (Au)

Hypersensitivity
allergic bronchopulmonary aspergillosis; report of two cases and evaluation of tests for hypersensitivity [Jordan], 576 (Oc)
epidemiological clues in thyroid cancer [Bross], 755 (No)

Hypertension
and cholesterol as coronary heart disease risk factors [Tyroler], 907 (De)
autonomic hyperreflexia in spinal cord injury (corres.) [Tashima], 472 (Se)
cold pressor test and arteriosclerosis (corres.) [Voudoukis], 993 (De)
decrease of serum cholesterol level and blood pressure in the community [Heyden], 982 (De)
family aggregation of blood pressure in Evans County, Georgia [Hayes], 965 (De)
hypertension, obesity, and fibromyomata uteri, as a syndrome [Summers], 750 (No)
nerve conduction velocity in assessment [Viskoper], 574 (Oc)
saline suppression of plasma aldosterone [Kem], 380 (Se)

Hypertension, Portal
in patient with osteopetrosis [Denison], 279 (Au)

Hypertension, Renal
effect of bilateral nephrectomy in postpartum nephrosclerosis [Erickson], 448 (Se)
the Goldblatt kidney [Berman], 306 (Au)
spontaneous reestablishment of renal function after complete occlusion of a renal artery [Dobrzinsky], 266 (Au)

Hyperthyroidism
"triiodothyronine (T_3) toxicosis;" its role in Graves' disease [Ivy], 529 (Oc)

Hypertonic Solutions
easing the pain (corres.) [Seymour], 149 (Jy)

Hypoglycemia
and lactic acidosis [Medalle], 273 (Au)
mechanism of postgastrectomy hypoglycemia [Shultz], 240 (Au)

Hypogonadism
effect of chorionic gonadotropin on steroid excretion [Scurry], 561 (Oc)
postmeningitic selective hypopituitarism with suprasellar calcification [Sherman], 600 (Oc)

Hypopituitarism
effect of chorionic gonadotropin on steroid excretion [Scurry], 561 (Oc)
postmeningitic selective hypopituitarism with suprasellar, calcification [Sherman], 600 (Oc)

Hypothalamo-Hypophyseal System
postmeningitic selective hypopituitarism with suprasellar calcification [Sherman], 600 (Oc)

I

Immunity
successful defense against *Histoplasma capsulatum* in hypogammaglobulinemia [Biggar], 585 (Oc)

Immunoglobulin see Gamma Globulin

Income
funding of graduate education [Bogdonoff], 144 (Jy)

Infectious Diseases see Communicable Diseases

Injections, Intrathecal
easing the pain (corres.) [Seymour], 149 (Jy)

Insecticides see Parathion

INTERNAL MEDICINE AT LARGE
5 (Jy); 185 (Au); 333 (Se), 513 (Oc); 691 (No); (De)

Internship and Residency
funding of graduate education [Bogdonoff], 144 (Jy)

Intrinsic Factor, Secretion
gastric secretory and serologic studies on patients with neoplastic and immunologic disorders [Twomey], 746 (No)

Islands of Langerhans
pathologic findings in pancreas of mice infected with coxsackievirus B4 [Burch], 40 (Jy)

Isotonic Solutions
saline suppression of plasma aldosterone in hypertension [Ken], 380 (Se)

J

Jews
epidemiological clues in thyroid cancer [Bross], 755 (No)

Joint Diseases
chronic lesions of vertebral column and joints in older mice; induction by active agent from rheumatoid synovial tissue [Warren], 614 (Oc)

K

17-Ketosteroids, Urine
effect of chorionic gonadotropin on steroid excretion [Scurry], 561 (Oc)

Kidney, Artificial see Hemodialysis; Peritoneal Dialysis

Kidney, Blood Supply
spontaneous reestablishment of renal function after complete occlusion of a renal artery [Dobrzinsky], 266 (Au)

Kidney, Transplantation
chromosome aberrations in child of kidney transplant recipient [Leb], 441 (Se)
epidermoid carcinoma of lip after renal transplantation [Berger], 609 (Oc)

Kidney Failure, Acute see Nephrosclerosis, Malignant

Kidney Failure, Chronic
criteria for evaluation of severity of established renal disease [Council on the Kidney in Cardiovascular Disease of the American Heart Association], 304 (Au)

Klinefelter's Syndrome
effect of chorionic gonadotropin on steroid excretion [Scurry], 561 (Oc)

Kyphosis
chronic lesions of vertebral column and joints in older mice; induction by active agent from rheumatoid synovial tissue [Warren], 614 (Oc)

L

Lactates, Blood
lactic acidosis and associated hypoglycemia [Hedalle], 273 (Au)

Latin American see Central America

Laxatives see Phenolphthaleins

Leiomyoma
hypertension, obesity, and fibromyomata uteri, as a syndrome [Summers], 750 (No)

Leukemia, Complications
salmonellosis [Wolfe], 546 (Oc)

Leukemia, Lymphocytic
IgM heavy chain fragments in Waldenstrom's macroglobulinemia [Bhoopalam], 437 (Se)

Leukemia, Myeloblastic
acute myelogenous leukemia following localized radiotherapy [Poth], 802 (No)

Leukoencephalopathy, Progressive Multifocal
associated with macroglobulinemia, case [Lyon], 420 (Se)

Lidocaine
infusion, in acute myocardial infarction [Rahimtoola], 416 (Se)

Lip Neoplasms
epidermoid carcinoma, after renal transplantation [Berger], 609 (Oc)

Lipids
reaction of nitrogen dioxide with blood and lung components [Rowlands], 94 (Jy)

Liver Abscess, Amebic
superinfection by *Salmonella enteritidis* [Marr], 291 (Au)

Lung
enzymatic conversion of benzo-[*a*]pyrene [Wang], 125 (Jy)

Lung Abscess
combination therapy (corres.) [Pollock], 473 (Se)

Lung Compliance
short-term exposure to nitrogen dioxide [Dowell], 74 (Jy)

Lung Diseases, Fungal
allergic bronchopulmonary aspergillosis [Jordan], 576 (Oc)
Aspergillus infection complicating cardiac transplantation [Gurwith], 541 (Oc)
Earth Day histoplasmosis; new type of urban pollution [Fass], 588 (Oc)

Lung Neoplasms
coronary occlusion due to neoplasm [Franciosa], 797 (No)

Lungs, Cytology
effects of nitrogen dioxide on cell renewal in rat lung [Evans], 57 (Jy)
oxygen effect on lung cells [Weibel], 54 (Jy)

Lungs, Metabolism
oxidants and lung biochemistry [Hueter], 48 (Jy)

Lungs, Physiopathology
sequential observations on pulmonary functional derangements in bagassosis [Jenkins], 535 (Oc)

Lupus Erythematosis, Systemic
effect of azathioprine on renal histology and function in lupus nephritis [Shelp], 566 (Oc)

Lymphatic Diseases
gastric secretory and serologic studies [Twomey], 746 (No)

Lymphoma
α heavy chain disease; a variant of Mediterranean lymphoma [Zlotnick], 432 (Se)

Lymphoma, Complications
salmonellosis [Wolfe], 546 (Oc)

Lymphosarcoma, Radiotherapy
acute myelogenous leukemia following localized radiotherapy [Poth], 802 (No)

Lysosomes
and toxicity of particulate pollutants [Allison], 131 (Jy)

M

Macroglobulinemia
and progressive multifocal leukoencephalopathy, case [Lyon], 420 (Se)
IgM heavy chain fragments in Waldenstrom's macroglobulinemia [Bhoopalam], 437 (Se)

Macrophages
alterations in lung following administration of ozone [Huber], 81 (Jy)
lysosomes and toxicity of particulate pollutants [Allison], 131 (Jy)

Macula Lutea
macular cherry-red spot, corneal clouding, and β-galactosidase deficiency [Goldberg], 387 (Se)

Main en Lorgnette Deformity see Hand Deformities, Acquired

Massachusetts General Hospital
changes in the diagnostic process during 40 years of clinicopathologic conferences [Feinstein], 774 (No)

Median Nerve, Physiopathology
nerve conduction velocity in assessment of hypertension [Viskoper], 574 (Oc)

Medical Records
art and science of presenting a patient's problems; (as an extension of the Weed system) [Hurst], 463 (Se)
challenge and opportunities of the Weed system [Bogdonoff], 832 (No)
how to implement the Weed system; (in order to improve patient care, education, and research by improving medical records) [Hurst], 456 (Se)
problem-oriented record and measurement of excellence [Hurst], 818 (No)

Medicine, Social Aspects
consumerism in medicine [Bogdonoff], 469 (Se)

Medicine, U.S.
societal health and medical services [Bogdonoff], 636 (Oc)

Medicine in Literature
psychology of physical illness as portrayed in Thomas Mann's *The Magic Mountain* [Abram], 466 (Se)

Meningitis, Tuberculous see Tuberculosis, Meningeal

Metabolism, Inborn Errors, Enzymology see Galactosidase, Metabolism

Methylprednisolone
alveolar protein accumulation [Alpert], 69 (Jy)

Microscopy, Electron
alveolar injury in acute carbon tetrachloride intoxication [Gould], 109 (Jy)

Microsomes, Liver
enzymatic conversion of benzo[*a*] pyrene [Wang], 125 (Jy)
enzymic mechanism of metabolism of phosphorothionate insecticides [Neal], 118 (Jy)

Migration
relation to coronary disease risk factors [Wetherbee], 976 (De)

Military Medicine
effects of US gamma globulin upon incidence of viral hepatitis and other infectious diseases in US soldiers abroad [Cooperative Study], 723 (No)

Moniliasis
treatment of *Candida* infection (corres.) [Kozinn], 639 (Oc)

Motor Nerve see Ulnar Nerve

Motor Neurons
nerve conduction velocity in assessment of hypertension [Viskoper], 574 (Oc)

Multiple Myeloma
familial paraproteinemia [Grant], 427 (Se)
gastric secretory and serologic studies [Twomey], 746 (No)

Multivariate Analysis
of risk of coronary disease in Evans County, Georgia [Kleinbaum], 943 (De)

Myeloma, Plasma Cell see Multiple Myeloma

Myocardial Infarct
cardiac performance three to eight weeks after acute infarction [Rahimtoola], 220 (Au)
lidocaine infusion in acute infarction [Rahimtoola], 416 (Se)
rare cause; coronary artery occlusion due to neoplasm [Franciosa], 797 (No)

Myxoma
detection of left atrial myxoma by echocardiography [Spencer], 787 (No)

N

Neoplasms, Complications
coronary artery occlusion due to neoplasm [Franciosa], 797 (No)
salmonellosis [Wolfe], 546 (Oc)

Nephrectomy
effect of bilateral nephrectomy in postpartum nephrosclerosis [Erickson], 448 (Se)

Nephritis, Lupus see Glomerulonephritis

Nephrosclerosis, Malignant
effect of bilateral nephrectomy in postpartum nephrosclerosis [Erickson], 448 (Se)

Neural Conduction
nerve conduction velocity in assessment of hypertension [Viskoper], 574 (Oc)
variations in motor nerve conduction velocity in normal and uremic patients [Kominami], 235 (Au)

Neuroses
psychology of physical illness as portrayed in Thomas Mann's *The Magic Mountain* [Abram], 466 (Se)

Nicaragua see Central America

Nitrofurantoin, Adverse Effects
manifestations and specific reaction rates during 2,118 courses of therapy [Koch-Weser], 399 (Se)

Negroes, Diseases
blood pressure and cholesterol as coronary disease risk factors [Tyroler], 907 (De)
body weight and cigarette smoking as coronary risk factors [Heyden], 915 (De)
cerebrovascular disease in the biracial population of Evans County, Georgia [Heyman], 949 (De)
electrocardiographic predictors of coronary disease [Bartel], 929 (De)
Evans County Cardiovascular and Cerebrovascular Study; papers, 883-986 (De)
family aggregation of blood pressure in Evans County, Georgia [Hayes], 965 (De)
incidence of coronary heart disease by ethnic group, social class and sex [Cassel], 901 (De)
incidence study—study design and methods [Cornoni], 896 (De)
multivariate analysis of risk of coronary disease in Evans County, Georgia [Kleinbaum], 943 (De)
occupation and physical activity and coronary disease [Cassel], 920 (De)
relation of migration to coronary disease risk factors [Wetherbee], 976 (De)
review of 1960 through 1962 cardiovascular disease prevalence study [Cassel], 890 (De)
summary of major findings of Evans County cardiovascular studies [Cassel], 887 (De)

Nitrogen Dioxide
antioxidants vs lung diseases [Roehm], 88 (Jy)
effects on cell renewal in rat lung [Evans], 57 (Jy)
reaction with blood and lung components [Rowlands], 94 (Jy)
response of lung tissue and surfactant to nitrogen dioxide exposure [Williams], 101 (Jy)
short-term exposure to nitrogen dioxide [Dowell], 74 (Jy)

Nitrogen Dioxide, Adverse Effects
lung capillary permeability [Sherwin], 61 (Jy)
oxidants and lung biochemistry [Hueter], 48 (Jy)

O

Obesity
hypertension, obesity, and fibromyomata uteri, as a syndrome [Summers], 750 (No)

Occupation
and physical activity and coronary disease [Cassel], 920 (De)
occupational mobility and coronary disease [Kaplan], 938 (De)

Occupational Diseases see Pneumoconiosis

Opera-Glass Hand see Hand Deformities, Acquired

Organic Dust Diseases see Pneumoconiosis

Organophosphates see Parathion

Osteoarthritis
erosive, and the main en lorgnette deformity [Swezey], 269 (Au); correction, 840 (No)

Osteomalacia
induced by laxative (phenolphthalein) ingestion [Frame], 794 (No)

Osteomyelitis, Therapy
pyogenic vertebral osteomyelitis; treatment with antimicrobial agents and bed rest [Jordan], 405 (Se)

Osteopetrosis
portal hypertension in patient with oteopetrosis [Denison], 279 (Au)

Oxygen, Adverse Effects
oxygen effect on lung cells [Weibel], 54 (Jy)

Ozone
alterations in lung following administration of ozone [Huber], 81 (Jy)
alveolar protein accumulation [Alpert], 69 (Jy)
antioxidants vs lung diseases [Roehm], 88 (Jy)
oxidants and lung biochemistry [Hueter], 48 (Jy)

P

Pacemaker, Artificial
cardiac syncope due to glossopharyngeal neuralgia; treatment with transvenous pacemaker [Khero], 806 (No)

Pagophagia see Appetite Disorders

Pain, Therapy
easing the pain (corres.) [Seymour], 149 (Jy)

Pancreas, Pathology
pathologic findings in pancreas of mice infected with coxsackievirus B4 [Burch], 40 (Jy)

Parathion
enzymic mechanism of metabolism of phosphorothionate insecticides [Neal], 118 (Jy)

Pasteurella Infections
Pasteurella pseudotuberculosis; acute sepsis with survival [Yamashiro], 605 (Oc)

Palm see Hand

Paraproteinemia, Familial see Blood Protein Disorders, Familial and Genetic

Penicillin, Therapeutic Use
combination therapy of lung abscess (corres.) [Pollock], 473 (Se)

Peritoneal Dialysis
bradycardic rhythms during peritoneal dialysis [Rutsky], 445 (Se)
calcium free; treatment of vitamin D intoxication [Nolph], 809 (No)

Phenolphthaleins
osteomalacia induced by laxative (phenolphthalein) ingestion [Frame], 794 (No)

Phosphorothionates see Parathion

Photochemistry
oxidants and lung biochemistry [Hueter], 48 (Jy)

Physical Activity see Exertion

Pituitary Gland, Radiotherapy
conventional radiation therapy in acromegaly [Lawrence], 369 (Se)

Pleural Effusion, Analysis
rheumatoid pleurisy with effusion [Lillington], 764 (No)

Pneumoconiosis, Physiopathology
sequential observations on pulmonary functional derangements in bagassosis [Jenkins], 535 (Oc)

Pneumonia
infectious disease problems of narcotic addicts [Cherubin], 309 (Au)

Porphyrin, Metabolism
vitamin E and porphyrin metabolism in man [Nair], 411 (Se)

Postgastrectomy Syndromes
mechanism of postgastrectomy hypoglycemia [Shultz], 240 (Au)

Postoperative Complications
salmonellosis in patients with neoplastic diseases [Wolfe], 546 (Oc)

Posture
peripheral and renal vein renin activity [Assaykeen], 378 (Se)

Precipitin Tests
Serratia marcescens bacteremia [Crowder], 247 (Au)

Prednisone, Therapeutic Use
retroperitoneal fibrosis; response to corticosteroid therapy [Moranki], 295 (Au)

Pregnancy Complications
effect of bilateral nephrectomy in postpartum nephrosclerosis [Erickson], 448 (Se)

Pseudomonas Infections
septicemia; illustrated evolution of its skin lesion [Dorff], 591 (Oc)

Psychoses, Etiology
psychosis in vitamin B 12 deficiency [Hart], 596 (Oc)

Pulmonary Alveoli
alterations in lung following administration of ozone [Huber], 81 (Jy)
alveolar injury in acute carbon tetrachloride intoxication [Gould], 109 (Jy)
alveolar protein accumulation [Alpert], 69 (Jy)
effects of nitrogen dioxide on cell renewal in rat lung [Evans], 57 (Jy)
response of lung tissue and surfactant to nitrogen dioxide exposure [Williams], 101 (Jy)

Pulmonary Edema
short-term exposure to nitrogen dioxide [Dowell], 74 (Jy)

Purpura
Schönlein-Henoch syndrome associated with exposure to cold [Rogers], 782 (No)

Q

Questionnaires
angina pectoris and the Rose questionnaire [Heyden], 961 (De)

R

Radiotherapy, Adverse Effects
acute myelogenous leukemia following localized radiotherapy [Poth], 802 (No)

Reflex, Abnormal
autonomic hyperreflexia in spinal cord injury (corres.) [Tashima], 472 (Se)

Regression
psychology of physical illness as portrayed in Thomas Mann's *The Magic Mountain* [Abram], 466 (Se)

Renal Artery Obstruction
the Goldblatt kidney [Berman], 306 (Au)
spontaneous reestablishment of renal function after complete occlusion of renal artery [Dobrzinsky], 266 (Au)

Renal Veins
renin activity [Assaykeen], 378 (Se)

Renin
the Goldblatt kidney [Berman], 306 (Au)
peripheral and renal vein renin activity [Assaykeen], 378 (Se)

Respiratory Function Tests
sequential observations on pulmonary functional derangements in bagassosis [Jenkins], 535 (Oc)

Rest
pyogenic vertebral osteomyelitis; treatment with antimicrobial agents and bed rest [Jordan], 405 (Se)

Retina, Pathology
ophthalmologic manifestations of sickle cell thalassemia [Goldberg], 33 (Jy)

Retroperitoneal Fibrosis
response to corticosteroid therapy [Morandi], 295 (Au)

RNA, Bacterial
mode of action of antibiotics on gram-negative bacilli [Lorian], 623 (Oc)

Rose Questionnaire see Questionnaires

S

Salmonella Infections
in patients with neoplastic disease [Wolfe], 546 (Oc)
prolonged *Salmonella* bacteremia in patients with *Schistosoma mansoni* infection [Rocha], 254 (Au)
superinfection of amoebic abscess by *Salmonella enteritidis* [Marr], 291 (Au)

Schistosomiasis
prolonged *Salmonella* bacteremia in patients with *Schistosoma mansoni* infection [Rocha], 254 (Au)

Schönlein-Henoch Purpura see Purpura

Semantics
how to implement the Weed system; (in order to improve patient care, education, and research by improving medical records) [Hurst], 456 (Se)

Septicemia
Pasteurella pseudotuberculosis; acute sepsis with survival [Yamashiro], 605 (Oc)
prolonged *Salmonella* bacteremia in patients with *Schistosoma mansoni* infection [Rocha], 254 (Au)
Pseudomonas septicemia; illustrated evolution of its skin lesion [Dorff], 591 (Oc)
Serratia Marcescens bacteremia [Crowder], 247 (Au)

Serrati Marcescens see Septicemia

Sex Factors
blood pressure and cholesterol as coronary heart disease risk factors [Tyroler], 907 (De)
electrocardiographic predictors of coronary disease [Bartel], 929 (De)
epidemiological clues in thyroid cancer [Bross], 755 (No)
incidence of coronary heart disease [Cassel], 901 (De)
relation of migration to coronary disease risk factors [Wetherbee], 976 (De)

Sex Hormones see Androgens

Shiga Bacillus see Dysentery, Bacillary

Shock, Cardiogenic
ascending aorta synchronized pulsation; new form of circulatory assist [Lang], 258 (Au)

Silicosis
lysosomes and toxicity of particulate pollutants [Allison], 131 (Jy)

Skin Manifestations
Pseudomonas septicemia; illustrated evolution of its skin lesion [Dorff], 591 (Oc)

Smoking
and body weight as coronary risk factors [Heyden], 915 (De)

Social Class
incidence of coronary heart disease [Cassell], 901 (De)
occupational mobility and coronary disease [Kaplan], 938 (De)

Social Mobility
occupational mobility and coronary disease [Kaplan], 938 (De)

Social Problems
societal health and medical services [Bogdonoff], 636 (Oc)

Socioeconomic Factors
societal health and medical services [Bogdonoff], 636 (Oc)

Sodium Chloride
saline suppression of plasma aldosterone in hypertension [Kem], 380 (Se)

Solvents see Carbon Tetrachloride

Sprinal Cord Injuries
autonomic hyperreflexia in (corres.) [Tashima], 472 (Se)

Spinal Diseases
chronic lesions of vertebral column and joints in older mice; induction by active agent from rheumatoid synovial tissue [Warren], 614 (Oc)
pyogenic vertebral osteomyelitis; treatment with antimicrobial agents and bed rest [Jordan], 405 (Se)

Steroids see 17-Ketosteroids

Stomach, Secretion
gastric secretory and serologic studies on patients with neoplastic and immunologic disorders [Twomey], 746 (No)

Sulfamethoxazole, Adverse Effects
manifestations and specific reaction rates during 2,118 courses of therapy [Koch-Weser], 399 (Se)

Sulfisoxazole, Adverse Effects
manifestations and specific reaction rates during 2,118 courses of therapy [Koch-Weser], 399 (Se)

Surface Tension
response of lung tissue and surfactant to nitrogen dioxide exposure [Williams], 101 (Jy)

Surface-Active Agents
response of lung tissue and surfactant to nitrogen dioxide exposure [Williams], 101 (Jy)

Symposium on Pollution and Lung Biochemistry
papers, 48-139, (Jy)

Syncope
cardiac syncope due to glossopharyngeal neuralgia [Khero], 806 (No)

T

Tachycardia
initiation of ventricular tachycardia; ECG analysis no. 5 [Zipes], 988 (De)
ventricular; ECG analysis no. 4 [Zipes], 815 (No)

Tetanus
infectious disease problems of narcotic addicts [Cherubin], 309 (Au)

Tetracycline
combination therapy of lung abscess (corres.) [Pollock], 473 (Se)

Thyroid Neoplasms
epidemiological clues; tonsillectomy, acne, allergy, ethnicity [Bross], 755 (No)

Tonsillectomy
epidemiological clues in thyroid cancer [Bross], 755 (No)

Triiodothyronine, Blood
"triiodothyronine (T_3) toxicosis;" its role in Graves' disease [Ivy], 529 (Oc)

Tritium
lung capillary permeability; nitrogen dioxide exposure and leakage of tritiated serum [Sherwin], 61 (Jy)

Tuberculosis, Meningeal
postmeningitic selective hypopituitarism with suprasellar calcification [Sherman], 600 (Oc)

Tuberculosis, Pulmonary
psychology of physical illness as portrayed in Thomas Mann's *The Magic Mountain* [Abram], 466 (Se)

U

Ulnar Nerve, Physiopathology
nerve conduction velocity in assessment of hypertension [Viskoper], 574 (Oc)
variations in motor nerve conduction velocity in normal and uremic patients [Kominami], 235 (Au)

Ultrasonics, Diagnostic Use
detection of a left atrial myxoma by echocardiography [Spencer], 787 (No)

Uremia
variations in motor nerve conduction velocity in normal and uremic patients [Kominami], 235 (Au)

Uterine Neoplasms
hypertension, obesity, and fibromyomata uteri, as a syndrome [Summers], 750 (No)

V

Vagotonia see Vagus Nerve

Vagus Nerve
bradycardic rhythms during peritoneal dialysis [Rutsky], 445 (Se)

Varicose Veins
palmar varices and gastrointestinal bleeding [Sherwood], 598 (Oc)

Ventricular Fibrillation
initiation of ventricular tachycardia; ECG analysis no. 5 [Zipes], 988 (De)

Vitamin B 12 Deficiency
psychosis in [Hart], 596 (Oc)

Vitamin D 2 see Ergocalciferol

Vitamin E
and porphyrin metabolism in man [Nair], 411 (Se)
antioxidants vs lung diseases [Roehm], 88 (Jy)

W

Weed (Lawrence) System see Medical Records